Atkinson's Principles of Clinical Pharmacology

Atkinson's Principles of Clinical Pharmacology

Fourth Edition

Edited by

Shiew-Mei Huang
Deputy Director, Office of Clinical Pharmacology (OCP), Center for Drug Evaluation Research (CDER), Food and Drug Administration (FDA), Silver Spring, MD, United States

Juan J.L. Lertora
Adjunct Professor, Division of Clinical Research, Pennington Biomedical Research Center, Louisiana State University, Baton Rouge, LA, United States
Adjunct Professor, Department of Medicine, Duke University School of Medicine, Durham, NC, United States

Paolo Vicini
Chief Development Officer, Confo Therapeutics NV, Ghent, Belgium

Arthur J. Atkinson, Jr.
Department of Pharmacology, Feinberg School of Medicine, Northwestern University, Chicago, IL, United States

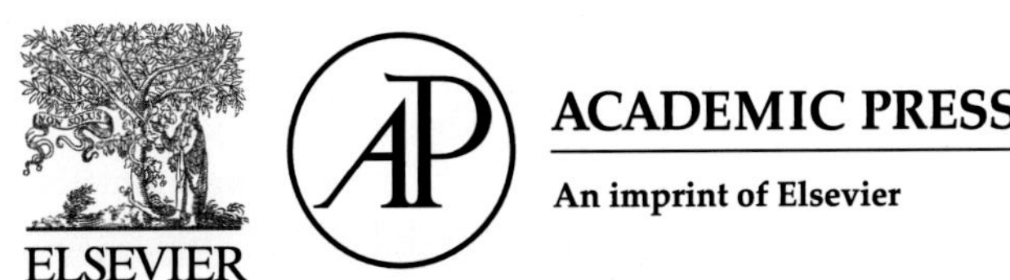

Academic Press is an imprint of Elsevier
125 London Wall, London EC2Y 5AS, United Kingdom
525 B Street, Suite 1650, San Diego, CA 92101, United States
50 Hampshire Street, 5th Floor, Cambridge, MA 02139, United States
The Boulevard, Langford Lane, Kidlington, Oxford OX5 1GB, United Kingdom

Library of Congress Cataloging-in-Publication Data
A catalog record for this book is available from the Library of Congress

British Library Cataloguing-in-Publication Data
A catalogue record for this book is available from the British Library

ISBN 978-0-12-819869-8

For information on all Academic Press publications
visit our website at https://www.elsevier.com/books-and-journals

Publisher: Andre Gerhard Wolff
Acquisitions Editor: Erin Hill-Parks
Editorial Project Manager: Samantha Allard
Production Project Manager: Selvaraj Raviraj
Cover Designer: Christian J. Bilbow

Typeset by STRAIVE, India

Contents

15. Biochemical mechanisms of drug toxicity

Jack Uetrecht, Denis M. Grant, and Peter G. Wells

16. Pharmacogenomic mechanisms of drug toxicity

Shiew-Mei Huang, Ligong Chen, and Kathleen M. Giacomini

17. Biomarkers in drug development

Robert N. Schuck, Jana G. Delfino, Christopher Leptak, and John A. Wagner

Contributors

Numbers in parenthesis indicate the pages on which the authors' contributions begin.

Darrell R. Abernethy (479), Office of Clinical Pharmacology, Food and Drug Administration, Silver Spring, MD, United States

Balaji Agoram (573), Arcus Biosciences, Hayward, CA, United States

John M. Allen (73), Department of Pharmacotherapy and Translational Research, College of Pharmacy, University of Florida; Department of Internal Medicine, College of Medicine, University of Central Florida, Orlando, FL, United States

Mark E. Arnold (169), Labcorp Drug Development, Westampton, NJ, United States

Arthur J. Atkinson, Jr. (1, 11, 27, 43, 61, 73), Department of Pharmacology, Feinberg School of Medicine, Northwestern University, Chicago, IL, United States

Thomas J. Bateman (563), Merck & Co. Inc., Kenilworth, NJ, United States

Kimberly Bergman (691), Office of Clinical Pharmacology, Office of Translational Sciences, Center for Drug Evaluation and Research, U.S. Food and Drug Administration, Silver Spring, MD, United States

Brian Booth (169), Office of Clinical Pharmacology, Office of Translational Sciences, Center for Drug Evaluation and Research, US Food and Drug Administration, Silver Spring, MD, United States

David W. Boulton (653), Astra Zeneca Global Clinical Pharmacology and Quantitative Pharmacology, Gaithersburg, MD, United States; Astra Zeneca Global Clinical Pharmacology and Quantitative Pharmacology, Gothenburg, Sweden; Astra Zeneca Global Clinical Pharmacology and Quantitative Pharmacology, Cambridge, United Kingdom

Robert A. Branch (91), Orenda Health, Pittsburgh, PA, United States

Gilbert J. Burckart (455), Office of Clinical Pharmacology, U.S. Food and Drug Administration, Silver Spring, MD, United States

Mary Buschmann (691), Department of Pediatrics, University of California San Diego School of Medicine; Scripps Institution of Oceanography, UCSD, La Jolla, CA, United States

Owen Carmichael (343), Pennington Biomedical Research Center, Baton Rouge, LA, United States

Christine Chamberlain (499), Food and Drug Administration Office of Surveillance and Epidemiology, Division of Pharmacovigilance, Silver Spring, MD, United States

Ligong Chen (303), Department of Bioengineering and Therapeutic Sciences, University of California, San Francisco, CA, United States

Charles E. Daniels (519), Skaggs School of Pharmacy and Pharmaceutical Sciences, University of California, San Diego, CA, United States

Promi Das (691), Department of Pediatrics, University of California San Diego School of Medicine; Scripps Institution of Oceanography, UCSD, La Jolla, CA, United States

Jana G. Delfino (323), Office of New Drugs, Center for Drug Evaluation and Research, U.S. Food and Drug Administration, Silver Spring, MD, United States

John N. Van Den Anker (455), Division of Pediatric Clinical Pharmacology and Medical Toxicology, Children's National Hospital, Washington, DC, United States

Albert W. Dreisbach (61), Department of Internal Medicine, Division of Nephrology, University of Mississippi Medical Center, Jackson, MS, United States

Michael Dyszel (537), Global Portfolio & Program Management, Mallinckrodt Pharmaceuticals, Bedminster, NJ, United States

Justin C. Earp (359), Office of Clinical Pharmacology, Office of Translational Sciences, Center for Drug Evaluation and Research, US Food and Drug Administration, Silver Spring, MD, United States

M. Khair ElZarrad (691), Office of Medical Policy, Center for Drug Evaluation and Research, U.S.

Food and Drug Administration, Silver Spring, MD, United States

Osatohanmwen J. Enogieru (213), Department of Bioengineering and Therapeutic Sciences, University of California, San Francisco, CA, United States

Elimika Pfuma Fletcher (681), Office of Clinical Pharmacology, Office of Translational Sciences, Center for Drug Evaluation and Research, U.S. Food and Drug Administration, Silver Spring, MD, United States

David M. Foster (113), Department of Bioengineering, University of Washington, Seattle, WA, United States

Marilynn C. Frederiksen (425), Department of Obstetrics and Gynecology, Northwestern University Feinberg School of Medicine, Chicago, IL, United States

Aleksandra Galetin (241), Centre for Applied Pharmacokinetic Research, School of Health Sciences, The University of Manchester, Manchester, United Kingdom

Pamela D. Garzone (611), Anixa Biosciences, San Jose, CA, United States

Kathleen M. Giacomini (213, 303), Department of Bioengineering and Therapeutic Sciences, University of California, San Francisco, CA, United States

Megan A. Gibbs (653), Astra Zeneca Global Clinical Pharmacology and Quantitative Pharmacology, Gaithersburg, MD, United States; Astra Zeneca Global Clinical Pharmacology and Quantitative Pharmacology, Gothenburg, Sweden; Astra Zeneca Global Clinical Pharmacology and Quantitative Pharmacology, Cambridge, United Kingdom

Jack A Gilbert (691), Department of Pediatrics, University of California San Diego School of Medicine; Scripps Institution of Oceanography, UCSD, La Jolla, CA, United States

Danijela Gnjidic (479), School of Pharmacy, Faculty of Medicine and Health, and Charles Perkins Centre, The University of Sydney, Sydney, NSW, Australia

Charles T. Gombar (537), HIV Drugs, Bill & Melinda Gates Foundation, Seattle, WA, United States

Denis M. Grant (267), Department of Pharmacology and Toxicology, University of Toronto, Toronto, ON, Canada

Charles Grudzinskas (537), NDA Partners LLC, Rochelle, VA, United States

Bengt Hamren (653), Astra Zeneca Global Clinical Pharmacology and Quantitative Pharmacology, Gaithersburg, MD, United States; Astra Zeneca Global Clinical Pharmacology and Quantitative Pharmacology, Gothenburg, Sweden; Astra Zeneca Global Clinical Pharmacology and Quantitative Pharmacology, Cambridge, United Kingdom

Nicholas H.G. Holford (377, 389), Department of Pharmacology and Clinical Pharmacology, University of Auckland, Auckland, New Zealand

Shiew-Mei Huang (213, 241, 303, 681, 691), Office of Clinical Pharmacology, Office of Translational Sciences, Center for Drug Evaluation and Research, U.S. Food and Drug Administration, Silver Spring, MD, United States

Renee Iacona (653), Astra Zeneca Oncology Biometrics, Gaithersburg, MD, United States

Nina Isoherranen (151), Department of Pharmaceutics, School of Pharmacy, University of Washington, Seattle, WA, United States

Denise Jin (573), Gilead Sciences, Menlo Park, CA, United States

Bridgette L. Jones (455), Department of Pediatrics, University of Missouri-Kansas City School of Medicine, Children's Mercy, Kansas City, MO, United States

Gregory L. Kearns (455), Department of Medical Education and Pediatrics, Texas Christian University and UNTHSC School of Medicine, Fort Worth, TX, United States

Cindy Kortepeter (499), Food and Drug Administration Office of Surveillance and Epidemiology, Division of Pharmacovigilance, Silver Spring, MD, United States

Elizabeth Kunkoski (691), Office of Medical Policy, Center for Drug Evaluation and Research, U.S. Food and Drug Administration, Silver Spring, MD, United States

S.W. Johnny Lau (479), Office of Clinical Pharmacology, Food and Drug Administration, Silver Spring, MD, United States

Christopher Leptak (323), Office of New Drugs, Center for Drug Evaluation and Research, U.S. Food and Drug Administration, Silver Spring, MD, United States

Juan J.L. Lertora (61, 91, 359), Adjunct Professor, Division of Clinical Research, Pennington Biomedical Research Center, Louisiana State University, Baton Rouge, LA; Adjunct Professor, Department of Medicine, Duke University School of Medicine, Durham, NC, United States

Lawrence J. Lesko (681), Center for Pharmacometrics and Systems Pharmacology, College of Pharmacy, University of Florida, Lake Nona in Orlando, FL, United States

Jiang Liu (359), Office of Clinical Pharmacology, Office of Translational Sciences, Center for Drug Evaluation and Research, US Food and Drug Administration, Silver Spring, MD, United States

Qi Liu (691), Office of Clinical Pharmacology, Office of Translational Sciences, Center for Drug Evaluation and Research, U.S. Food and Drug Administration, Silver Spring, MD, United States

Rajanikanth Madabushi (681), Office of Clinical Pharmacology, Office of Translational Sciences, Center for Drug Evaluation and Research, U.S. Food and Drug Administration, Silver Spring, MD, United States

Raymond Miller (137), Advanced Pharmacometrics, Quantitative Clinical Pharmacology, Daiichi Sankyo Inc, Basking Ridge, NJ, United States

Diane R. Mould (389), Projections Research Inc, Phoenixville, PA, United States

Monica Muñoz (499), Food and Drug Administration Office of Surveillance and Epidemiology, Division of Pharmacovigilance, Silver Spring, MD, United States

Thomas D. Nolin (61, 73), Department of Pharmacy and Therapeutics, and Department of Medicine, Renal-Electrolyte Division, University of Pittsburgh Schools of Pharmacy and Medicine, Pittsburgh, PA, United States

Robert Joseph Noveck (603), Noveck Consultancy, Durham, NC, United States

R. Scott Obach (151), ADME Sciences Group, Medicinal Sciences, Pfizer Inc., Groton, CT, United States

Michael Pacanowski (189), Office of Clinical Pharmacology, Office of Translational Sciences, Center for Drug Evaluation and Research, US Food and Drug Administration, Silver Spring, MD, United States

Mary F. Paine (405), Department of Pharmaceutical Sciences, College of Pharmacy and Pharmaceutical Sciences, Washington State University, Spokane, WA, United States

Carl C. Peck (389), Department of Bioengineering and Therapeutic Sciences, University of California at San Francisco, San Francisco, CA, United States

Anuradha Ramamoorthy (189), Office of Clinical Pharmacology, Office of Translational Sciences, Center for Drug Evaluation and Research, US Food and Drug Administration, Silver Spring, MD, United States

A. David Rodrigues (241), ADME Sciences, Medicine Design, Worldwide Research & Development, Pfizer Inc., Groton, CT, United States

Malcolm Rowland (589), Centre for Applied Pharmacokinetic Research, Manchester School of Pharmacy, University of Manchester, Manchester, United Kingdom; Department of Bioengineering and Therapeutic Sciences, Schools of Pharmacy and Medicine, University of California San Francisco, CA, United States

Chandrahas G. Sahajwalla (681), Office of Clinical Pharmacology, Office of Translational Sciences, Center for Drug Evaluation and Research, U.S. Food and Drug Administration, Silver Spring, MD, United States

Martina Dagmar Sahre (603), Office of Clinical Pharmacology, Food and Drug Administration, Silver Spring, MD, United States

Robert N. Schuck (323), Office of Clinical Pharmacology, Center for Drug Evaluation and Research, U.S. Food and Drug Administration, Silver Spring, MD, United States

Khushboo Sharma (537), Office of New Drugs, CDER, US FDA, Silver Spring, MD, United States

Tristan Sissung (189), Clinical Pharmacology Program, National Cancer Institute, National Institutes of Health, Bethesda, MD, United States

Catherine S. Stika (425), Department of Obstetrics and Gynecology, Northwestern University Feinberg School of Medicine, Chicago, IL, United States

Chris H. Takimoto (573), Gilead Sciences, Menlo Park, CA, United States

Helen Tomkinson (653), Astra Zeneca Global Clinical Pharmacology and Quantitative Pharmacology, Gaithersburg, MD, United States; Astra Zeneca Global Clinical Pharmacology and Quantitative Pharmacology, Gothenburg, Sweden; Astra Zeneca Global Clinical Pharmacology and Quantitative Pharmacology, Cambridge, United Kingdom

Jack Uetrecht (267), Faculty of Pharmaceutical Sciences, University of Toronto, Toronto, ON, Canada

Paolo Vicini (113), Confo Therapeutics NV, Ghent, Belgium

Karen D. Vo (405), Department of Pharmaceutical Sciences, College of Pharmacy and Pharmaceutical Sciences, Washington State University, Spokane, WA, United States

John A. Wagner (323), Cygnal Therapeutics, Cambridge, MA, United States

Yaning Wang (359), Office of Clinical Pharmacology, Office of Translational Sciences, Center for Drug Evaluation and Research, US Food and Drug Administration, Silver Spring, MD, United States

Yow-Ming C. Wang (611), Office of Clinical Pharmacology, Office of Translational Sciences, Center for

Drug Evaluation and Research, Food and Drug Administration, Silver Spring, MD, United States

Peter G. Wells (267), Faculty of Pharmaceutical Sciences, University of Toronto, Toronto, ON, Canada

Michael J. Wick (573), Preclinical Research, XenoSTART, San Antonio, TX, United States

Sook Wah Yee (213), Department of Bioengineering and Therapeutic Sciences, University of California, San Francisco, CA, United States

Ophelia Yin (137), Advanced Pharmacometrics, Quantitative Clinical Pharmacology, Daiichi Sankyo Inc, Basking Ridge, NJ, United States

Nathalie K. Zgheib (91), Department of Pharmacology and Toxicology, American University of Beirut Faculty of Medicine, Beirut, Lebanon

Lei Zhang (213. 241), Office of Research and Standards, Office of Generic Drugs, Center for Drug Evaluation and Research, U.S. Food and Drug Administration, Silver Spring, MD, United States

Hao Zhu (691), Office of Clinical Pharmacology, Office of Translational Sciences, Center for Drug Evaluation and Research, U.S. Food and Drug Administration, Silver Spring, MD, United States

Preface to the first edition

The rate of introduction of new pharmaceutical products has increased rapidly over the past decade, and details learned about a particular drug become obsolete as it is replaced by newer agents. For this reason, we have chosen to focus this book on the principles that underlie the clinical use and contemporary development of pharmaceuticals. It is assumed that the reader will have had an introductory course in pharmacology and also some understanding of calculus, physiology, and clinical medicine.

This book is the outgrowth of an evening course that has been taught for the past 3 years at the NIH Clinical Center. Wherever possible, individuals who have lectured in the course have contributed chapters corresponding to their lectures. The organizers of this course are the editors of this book and we also have recruited additional experts to assist in the review of specific chapters. We also acknowledge the help of William A. Mapes in preparing much of the artwork. Special thanks are due to Donna Shields, Coordinator for the ClinPRAT training program at NIH, whose attention to myriad details has made possible both the successful conduct of our evening course and the production of this book. Finally, we were encouraged and patiently aided in this undertaking by Robert M. Harington and Aaron Johnson at Academic Press.

Preface to the fourth edition

In the two decades since the first edition of *Principles of Clinical Pharmacology* was published, major advances have been made in our understanding of many areas of this discipline, including pharmacogenetics/pharmacogenomics, drug transporters, the mechanism of adverse drug reactions, and biomarkers. The primary physical base of clinical pharmacology has also migrated from academia to the pharmaceutical industry and the U.S. Food and Drug Administration (FDA), where the discipline plays an increasingly prominent role in the development and regulation of new pharmaceuticals. Evidence for this transition is provided by the proliferation of FDA Guidance Documents that are cited in many chapters of the current edition of our text. However, as in previous editions, some linkage remains with the online lecture series that continues to be offered by the Clinical Center at the National Institutes of Health.[a]

We are indebted to the authors from previous editions who returned to update their chapters. However, the recent advances in clinical pharmacology have been paralleled by a change in the demographics of the discipline. This is reflected in our text by the addition of many new scientists to our roster of chapter authors. Our editorial leadership has also evolved in order to maintain its relevance and vitality. In launching this new edition of the textbook, the editorial team and the publisher wish to acknowledge the pioneering work of Dr. Arthur J. Atkinson, Jr., who conceived the first edition as an introductory textbook emphasizing fundamental principles to guide drug discovery, drug development, drug regulation, and drug utilization in clinical medicine. His outstanding leadership and dedication to this educational endeavor is thus recognized by the present edition being published as *Atkinson's Principles of Clinical Pharmacology*.

Many of the illustrations in the text appeared originally in *Clinical Pharmacology and Therapeutics*, and we thank the American Society for Clinical Pharmacology and Therapeutics for allowing us to reproduce these free of charge. Finally, special thanks are due the Elsevier Production Staff who together provided the ongoing support that has been invaluable for the successful production of this book.

---

[a] https://ocr.od.nih.gov/courses/principles-clinical-pharmacology.html.

Chapter 1

Introduction to clinical pharmacology

Arthur J. Atkinson, Jr.
Department of Pharmacology, Feinberg School of Medicine, Northwestern University, Chicago, IL, United States

Fortunately a surgeon who uses the wrong side of the scalpel cuts his own fingers and not the patient; if the same applied to drugs they would have been investigated very carefully a long time ago.

Rudolph Buchheim, Beitrage zur Arzneimittellehre, 1849 [1]

Background

Clinical pharmacology can be defined as the study of drugs in humans. Clinical pharmacology often is contrasted with basic pharmacology. Yet *applied* is a more appropriate antonym for *basic* [2]. In fact, many basic problems in pharmacology can only be studied in humans. This text will focus on the basic principles of clinical pharmacology. Selected applications will be used to illustrate these principles, but no attempt will be made to provide an exhaustive coverage of applied therapeutics. Other useful supplementary sources of information are listed at the end of this chapter.

Leake [3] has pointed out that pharmacology is a subject of ancient interest but is a relatively new science. Reidenberg [4] subsequently restated Leake's listing of the fundamental problems with which the science of pharmacology is concerned:

1. The relationship between dose and biological effect.
2. The localization of the site of action of a drug.
3. The mechanism(s) of action of a drug.
4. The absorption, distribution, metabolism, and excretion of a drug.
5. The relationship between chemical structure and biological activity.

These authors agree that pharmacology could not evolve as a scientific discipline until modern chemistry provided the chemically pure pharmaceutical products that are needed to establish a quantitative relationship between drug dosage and biological effect.

Clinical pharmacology has been termed a bridging discipline because it combines elements of classical pharmacology with clinical medicine. The special competencies of individuals trained in clinical pharmacology have equipped them for productive careers in academia, the pharmaceutical industry, and governmental agencies, such as the National Institutes of Health (NIH) and the Food and Drug Administration (FDA). Reidenberg [4] has pointed out that clinical pharmacologists are concerned both with the optimal use of existing medications and with the scientific study of drugs in humans. The latter area includes both evaluation of the safety and efficacy of currently available drugs and development of new and improved pharmacotherapy.

Optimizing use of existing medicines

As the opening quote indicates, the concern of pharmacologists for the safe and effective use of medicine can be traced back at least to Rudolph Buchheim (1820–79), who has been credited with establishing pharmacology as a laboratory-based discipline [1]. In the United States, Harry Gold and Walter Modell began in the 1930s to provide the foundation for the modern discipline of clinical pharmacology [5]. Their accomplishments include the invention of the double-blind design for clinical trials [6], the use of effect kinetics to measure the absolute bioavailability of digoxin and characterize the time course of its chronotropic effects [7], and the founding of *Clinical Pharmacology and Therapeutics.*

Atkinson's Principles of Clinical Pharmacology. https://doi.org/10.1016/B978-0-12-819869-8.00012-4

Few drugs have focused as much public attention on the problem of adverse drug reactions as thalidomide, which was first linked in 1961 to catastrophic outbreaks of phocomelia by Lenz in Germany and McBride in Australia [8]. Although thalidomide had not been approved at that time for use in the United States, this tragedy prompted passage in 1962 of the Harris-Kefauver Amendments to the Food, Drug, and Cosmetic Act. This act greatly expanded the scope of the FDA's mandate to protect the public health. The thalidomide tragedy also provided the major impetus for developing a number of NIH-funded academic centers of excellence that have shaped contemporary clinical pharmacology in this country. These US centers were founded by a generation of vigorous leaders, including Ken Melmon, Jan Koch-Weser, Lou Lasagna, John Oates, Leon Goldberg, Dan Azarnoff, Tom Gaffney, and Leigh Thompson. Colin Dollery and Folke Sjöqvist established similar programs in Europe. In response to the public mandate generated by the thalidomide catastrophe, these leaders quickly reached consensus on a number of theoretically preventable causes that contribute to the high incidence of adverse drug reactions [5]. These include:

1. Inappropriate polypharmacy.
2. Failure of prescribing physicians to establish and adhere to clear therapeutic goals.
3. Failure of medical personnel to attribute new symptoms or changes in laboratory test results to drug therapy.
4. Lack of priority given to the scientific study of adverse drug reaction mechanisms.
5. General ignorance of basic and applied pharmacology and therapeutic principles.

The important observations also were made that, unlike the teratogenic reactions caused by thalidomide, most adverse reactions encountered in clinical practice occurred with drugs that had been in clinical use for a substantial period of time, rather than newly introduced, drugs, and were dose related, rather than idiosyncratic [5, 9, 10].

Recognition of the considerable variation in response of different patients treated with standard drug doses has provided the impetus for the development of what has been called "personalized medicine" [11] or, more recently, "precision medicine" [12]. Despite the recent introduction of these terms, they actually describe a continuing story that can be divided into three chapters in which different complementary technologies were developed and are being applied to improve patient therapy by coping with this variability [13]. In the earliest chapter, laboratory methods were developed to measure drug concentrations in patient blood samples and to guide therapy, an approach now termed "therapeutic drug monitoring" [10]. The routine availability of these measurements then made it possible to apply pharmacokinetic principles in routine patient care to achieve and maintain these drug concentrations within a prespecified therapeutic range. Despite these advances, *serious adverse drug reactions* (defined as those adverse drug reactions that require or prolong hospitalization, are permanently disabling, or result in death) continue to pose a severe problem and have been estimated to occur in 6.7% of hospitalized patients [14]. Although this figure has been disputed, the incidence of adverse drug reactions probably is still higher than is generally recognized [15]. In the third chapter that is still being written, genetic approaches are being developed and applied to meet both this challenge and to improve the efficacy and safety of drug therapy [16]. Thus pharmacogenetics is being used to identify slow drug-metabolizing patients who might be at increased risk for drug toxicity and rapid metabolizers who might not respond when standard drug doses are prescribed. In a parallel development, pharmacogenomic methods are increasingly used to identify subsets of patients who will either respond satisfactorily or be at increased risk of an adverse reaction to a particular drug.

The fact that most adverse drug reactions occur with commonly used drugs focuses attention on the last of the preventable causes of these reactions: the inadequate training that prescribing physicians receive in pharmacology and therapeutics. Buchheim's comparison of surgery and medicine is particularly apt in this regard [5]. Most US medical schools provide their students with only a single course in pharmacology that traditionally is part of the second-year curriculum, when students lack the clinical background that is needed to support detailed instruction in therapeutics. In addition, Sjöqvist [17] has observed that most academic pharmacology departments have lost contact with drug development and pharmacotherapy. As a result, students and residents acquire most of their information about drug therapy in a haphazard manner from colleagues, supervisory house staff and attending physicians, pharmaceutical sales representatives, and whatever independent reading they happen to do on the subject. This unstructured process of learning pharmacotherapeutic technique stands in marked contrast to the rigorously supervised training that is an accepted part of surgical training, in which instantaneous feedback is provided whenever a retractor, let alone a scalpel, is held improperly.

Evaluation and development of medicines

Clinical pharmacologists have made noteworthy contributions to the evaluation of existing medicines and development of new drugs. In 1932 Paul Martini published a monograph entitled *Methodology of Therapeutic Investigation* that summarized his experience in scientific drug evaluation and probably entitles him to be considered the "first clinical pharmacologist" [18]. Martini described the use of placebos, control groups, stratification, rating scales, and the "n of 1" trial design, and emphasized the need to estimate the adequacy of sample size and to establish baseline conditions before beginning a trial. He also introduced the term "clinical pharmacology." Gold [6] and other academic clinical pharmacologists also have made important contributions to the design of clinical trials. More recently, Sheiner [19] outlined a number of improvements that continue to be needed in the use of statistical methods for drug evaluation, and asserted that clinicians must regain control over clinical trials in order to ensure that the important questions are being addressed.

Contemporary drug development is a complex process that is conventionally divided into preclinical research and development and a number of clinical development phases, as shown in Fig. 1.1 for small molecule drugs licensed by the US FDA [20]. After a drug candidate is identified and put through in vitro screens and animal testing, an Investigational New Drug application (IND) is submitted to the FDA. When the IND is approved, Phase 1 clinical development begins with a limited number of studies in healthy volunteers or patients. The goal of these studies is to establish a range of tolerated doses and to characterize the drug candidate's pharmacokinetic properties and initial toxicity profile. If these results warrant further development of the compound, short-term Phase 2 studies are conducted in a selected group of patients to obtain evidence of therapeutic efficacy and to explore patient therapeutic and toxic responses to several dose regimens. These dose-response relationships are used to design longer Phase 3 trials to confirm therapeutic efficacy and document safety in a larger patient population. The material obtained during preclinical and clinical development is then incorporated in a New Drug Application (NDA) that is submitted to the FDA for review. The FDA may request clarification of study results or further studies before the NDA is approved and the drug can be marketed. Adverse drug reaction monitoring and reporting is mandated after NDA approval. Phase 4 studies, conducted after NDA approval, may include studies to support FDA licensing for additional therapeutic indications or "over-the-counter" (OTC) sales directly to consumers. The development pathway of biologic products is similar and leads to submission of a Biologics License Application (BLA).

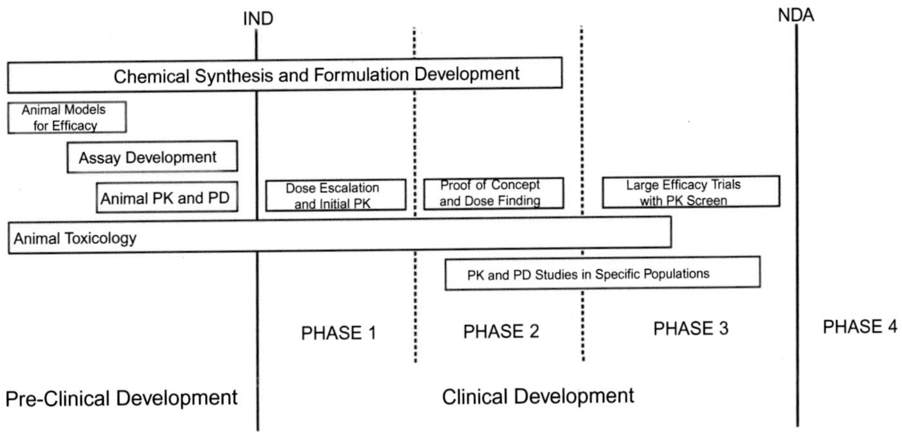

FIG. 1.1 The process of new drug development in the United States. (PK indicates pharmacokinetic studies; PD indicates studies of drug effect or pharmacodynamics.) Further explanation is provided in the text. *(Modified from Peck CC, Barr WH, Benet LZ, Collins J, Desjardins RE, Furst DE, et al. Opportunities for integration of pharmacokinetics, pharmacodynamics, and toxicokinetics in rational drug development. Clin Pharmacol Ther 1992;51:465–473.)*

Although the expertise and resources needed to develop new drugs are primarily concentrated in the pharmaceutical industry, clinical investigators based in academia have played an important catalytic role in championing the development of a number of drugs [21]. For example, dopamine was first synthesized in 1910 but the therapeutic potential of this compound was not recognized until 1963 when Leon Goldberg and his colleagues provided convincing evidence that dopamine mediated vasodilation by binding to a previously undescribed receptor [22]. These investigators subsequently demonstrated the clinical utility of intravenous dopamine infusions in treating patients with hypotension or shock unresponsive to plasma volume expansion. This provided the basis for a small pharmaceutical firm to bring dopamine to market in the early 1970s.

Academically based clinical pharmacologists have a long tradition of interest in drug metabolism. Drug metabolism generally constitutes an important mechanism by which drugs are converted to inactive compounds that usually are more rapidly excreted than the parent drug. However, some drug metabolites have important pharmacologic activity. This was first demonstrated in 1935 when the antibacterial activity of prontosil was found to reside solely in its metabolite, sulfanilamide (Fig. 1.2) [23]. Advances in analytical chemistry over the last 30 years have made it possible to measure on a routine basis plasma concentrations of drug metabolites as well as parent drugs. Further study of these metabolites has demonstrated that several of them have important pharmacologic activity that must be considered for proper clinical interpretation of plasma concentration measurements [24].

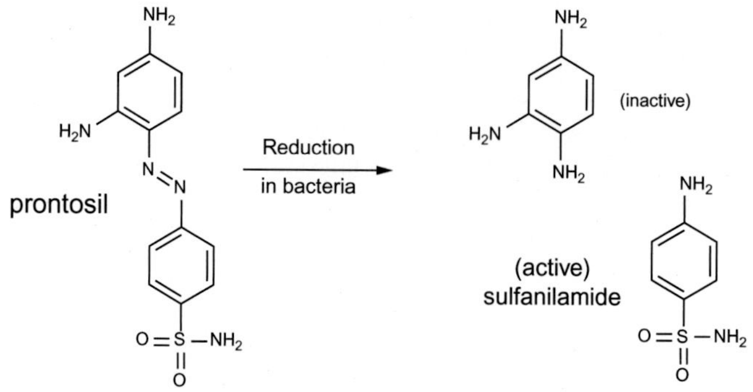

FIG. 1.2 Azo-reduction of prontosil to form sulfanilamide and 1,2,4-triaminobenzene.

In some cases, clinical pharmacologists have demonstrated that drug metabolites have pharmacologic properties that make them preferable to marketed drugs. For example, when terfenadine (Seldane), the prototype of nonsedating antihistamine drugs, was reported to cause *torsades de pointes* and fatality in patients with no previous history of cardiac arrhythmia, Woosley and his colleagues [25] proceeded to investigate the electrophysiologic effects of both terfenadine and its carboxylate metabolite (Fig. 1.3). These investigators found that terfenadine like quinidine, an antiarrhythmic drug with known propensity to cause *torsades de pointes* in susceptible individuals, blocked the delayed rectifier potassium current. However, terfenadine carboxylate, which actually accounts for most of the observed antihistaminic effects when patients take terfenadine, was found to be devoid of this proarrhythmic property. These findings provided the impetus for commercial development of the carboxylate metabolite as a safer alternative to terfenadine. This metabolite is now marketed as fexofenadine (Allegra).

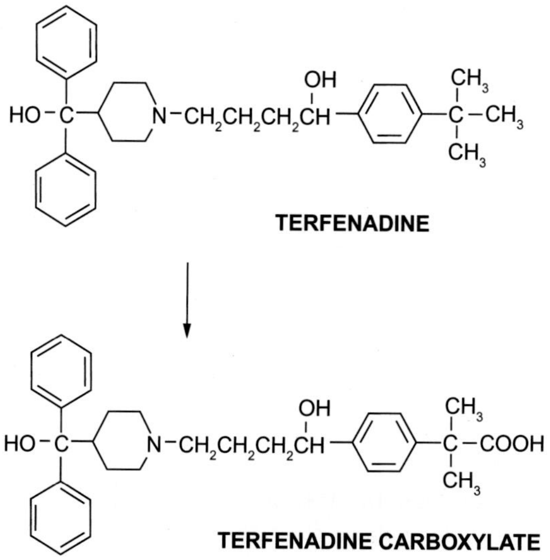

FIG. 1.3 Chemical structures of terfenadine and its carboxylate metabolite. The acid metabolite is formed by oxidation of the *t*-butyl side chain of the parent drug.

The potential impact of pharmacogenetics on drug prescribing and development is illustrated by the example of tamoxifen, a selective estrogen receptor modifier that has been used as therapy and recurrence prevention in patients with breast cancer. As shown in Fig. 1.4, tamoxifen is converted by cytochrome P450 (CYP) enzymes to several metabolites that have more potent antiestrogenic activity than the parent compound. Although 4-hydroxy-tamoxifen had been thought to be the primary pharmacologically active tamoxifen metabolite, Flockhart and colleagues [26] demonstrated that endoxifen plasma concentrations averaged more than 10 times those of 4-hydroxy-tamoxifen in women treated with tamoxifen and that both compounds had equal in vitro potency in suppressing breast cancer cell proliferation. Unfortunately, there is still no agreement on the clinical utility of using genotype biomarkers to assess the extent of endoxifen formation to guide breast cancer therapy with tamoxifen, so therapeutic monitoring of endoxifen plasma concentrations is being evaluated for this purpose [27, 28]. These findings also have provided the rationale for current efforts to develop endoxifen as a replacement for tamoxifen that would not be subject to pharmacogenetic variation or drug interactions affecting CYP2D6 activity [29, 30].

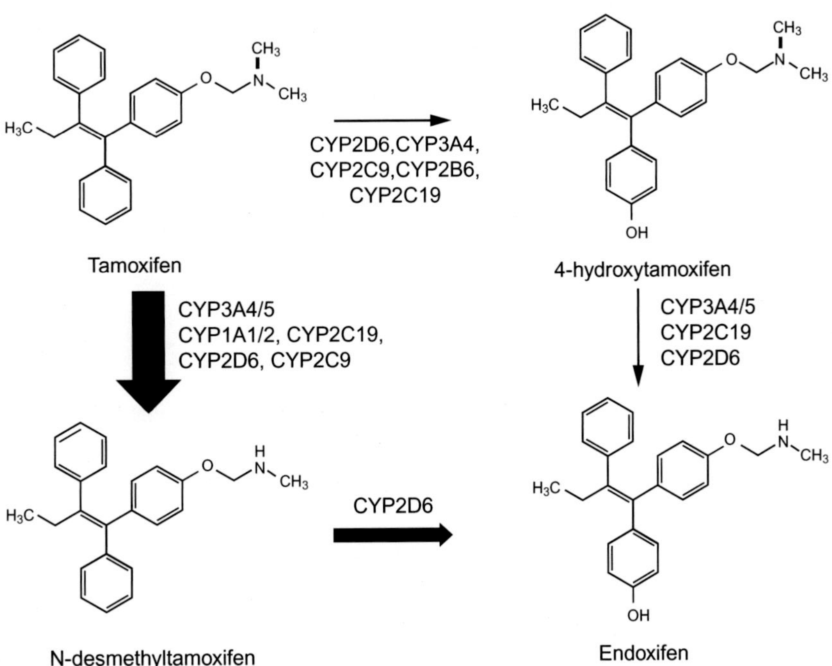

FIG. 1.4 Partial metabolic pathway of tamoxifen showing metabolite structures and the CYP enzymes involved. The relative contribution of each metabolic step is indicated by the thickness of the *arrows*.

Pharmacokinetics

Pharmacokinetics is defined as the quantitative analysis of the processes of drug absorption, distribution, and elimination that determine the time course of drug action in response to an administered drug dose. *Pharmacodynamics* deals with the mechanism of drug action. Hence, pharmacokinetics and pharmacodynamics constitute two major subdivisions of pharmacology.

Since as many as 70%–80% of adverse drug reactions are dose related [9], our success in preventing these reactions is contingent on our grasp of the principles of pharmacokinetics that provide the scientific basis for dose selection. This becomes critically important when we prescribe drugs that have a narrow therapeutic index. Pharmacokinetics is inescapably mathematical. Although 95% of pharmacokinetic calculations required for clinical application are simple algebra, some understanding of calculus is required to fully grasp the principles of pharmacokinetics.

The concept of clearance

Because pharmacokinetics comprises the first few chapters of this book and figures prominently in subsequent chapters, we will pause here to introduce the clinically most important concept in pharmacokinetics: the concept of *clearance*. In 1928 Möller et al. [31] observed that, above a urine flow rate of 2 mL/min, the rate of urea excretion by the kidneys is proportional to the amount of urea in a constant volume of blood. They introduced the term "clearance" to describe this proportionality and defined urea clearance as the volume of blood which one minute's excretion serves to clear of urea. Since then, creatinine clearance (CL_{CR}) has become most commonly used in clinical practice when renal functional status is directly measured and is calculated from the following equation:

$$CL_{CR} = UV/P$$

where U is the concentration of creatinine excreted over a certain period of time in a measured volume of urine (V) and P is the serum concentration of creatinine. This is really a first-order differential equation since UV is simply the rate at which creatinine is being excreted in urine (dE/dt). Hence,

$$dE/dt = CL_{CR} \cdot P$$

If, instead of looking at the rate of creatinine excretion in urine, we consider the rate of change of creatinine in the body (dX/dt), we can write the following equation:

$$dX/dt = I - CL_{CR} \cdot P \tag{1.1}$$

Here I is the rate of *synthesis* of creatinine in the body and $CL_{CR} \cdot P$ is the rate of creatinine *elimination*. At steady state, these rates are equal and there is no change in the total body content of creatinine ($dX/dt = 0$), so:

$$P = I/CL_{CR} \tag{1.2}$$

This equation explains why it is hazardous to estimate the status of renal function solely from serum creatinine results in patients who have a reduced muscle mass and a concomitant decline in creatinine synthesis rate. For example, creatinine synthesis rate may be substantially reduced in elderly patients, so it is not unusual for serum creatinine concentrations in these patients to remain within normal limits, even though renal function is markedly impaired.

Clinical estimation of renal function

In routine clinical practice, it is not practical to collect the urine samples that are needed to measure creatinine clearance directly. However, creatinine clearance in adult patients can be estimated either from a standard nomogram or from equations such as that proposed by Cockcroft and Gault [32]. For men, creatinine clearance can be estimated from this equation as follows:

$$CL_{CR}(\text{mL/min}) = \frac{(140 - \text{age})(\text{weight in kg})}{72(\text{serum creatinine in mg/dL})} \tag{1.3}$$

For women, this estimate should be reduced by 15%. By comparing Eq. (1.2) with Eq. (1.3), we see that the terms *(140 − age)(weight in kg)/72* simply provide an estimate of the creatinine formation rate in an individual patient.

Since the Cockcroft-Gault equation was introduced, there has been substantial improvement in reducing the variability and analytical bias in automated methods for measuring creatinine concentrations and these measurements are now calibrated to values obtained by isotope dilution mass spectrometry [33]. In addition, the Cockcroft-Gault equation overestimates true glomerular filtration rate (GFR) as measured by inulin clearance because creatinine is secreted by the renal tubule in addition to being filtered at the glomerulus [34]. For these reasons, data from the Modification of Diet in Renal Disease (MDRD) Study have been used by Levey and colleagues [35] to develop a series of equations that more accurately estimate GFR from standardized serum creatinine measurements and other patient characteristics. This group of investigators [36] has used measured renal clearance of iothalamate as a reference to compare GFR estimates and drug dosing recommendations based on the Cockcroft-Gault equation with those obtained using the following 4-variable version of the MDRD Study equation:

$$\text{GFR} = 175 \times \text{SCR}^{-1.154} \times \text{age}^{-0.203} \times 1.212\,(\text{if African American}) \times 0.742\,(\text{if female})$$

Standardized serum creatinine (SCR) measurements were used in both equations without correcting the Cockcroft-Gault equation for this change in analytical precision. Nonetheless, the concordance rates of dosing recommendations for a panel of 15 medications were 88% for the MDRD Study equation and 85% for the Cockcroft-Gault equation when compared with measured GFR. Consequently, the authors recommended basing drug dosing adjustments in patients with impaired renal function on more recent GFR estimating equations rather than on the Cockcroft-Gault equation. Subsequent estimating equations have been developed to extend the prediction range from patients with chronic kidney disease and GFR less than $60\,\text{mL/min}/1.73\,\text{m}^2$ to individuals with higher GFR (CKD-EPI) [37] and to incorporate serum concentration of cystatin C, another endogenous GFR marker [38].

Neither the Cockcroft-Gault equation nor the previously described GFR estimating equations can be used to estimate creatinine clearance in pediatric patients because muscle mass has not reached the adult proportion of body weight. Therefore, Schwartz and colleagues [39, 40] developed the following equation to predict creatinine clearance in these patients:

$$CL_{CR}(\text{mL/min}/1.73\text{m}^2) = \frac{k \cdot L(\text{in cm})}{\text{plasma creatinine in mg/dL}}$$

where L is the body length and k varies by age and sex. For children 1–13 years of age, the value of k had been 0.55 but Schwartz et al. [41] have revised this to 0.413, to reflect the introduction of SCR measurements. The original Schwartz formula also recommended discrete values of k for neonates and children under 1 year of age (0.45), and for females (0.57) and males (0.70) between the ages of 13 and 20. Pottel et al. [42] subsequently proposed the following modification of the Schwartz formula in which k for children between 1 and 14 years of age is expressed as the following age-dependent continuous variable:

$$k = 0.0414 \times \ln(\text{age}) + 0.3018$$

In all these equations body length is used as a surrogate for muscle mass in order to estimate creatinine generation rate.

The assessment of renal function in the elderly also has been problematic and this dilemma prompted the Berlin Initiative Study (BIS) to develop two separate equations for patients aged 70 years or older that were modeled on iohexol clearance as a GFR reference [43]. The first equation (BIS1) is creatinine based and includes age and sex as additional variables:

$$GFR = 3736 \times SCR^{-0.87} \times age^{-0.95} \times 0.82\,(\text{if female})$$

A second equation was developed that included measurement of cystatin C but was not deemed as suitable for routine clinical use because of the high cost of cystatin C analysis. A subsequent attempt also has been made to develop an SCR-based equation for estimating GFR as a continuous function across all age groups [44]. However, these latter methods have not been independently validated nor used to guide drug dosage and a recent review of four different methods found that each had limited accuracy [45].

The 2012 clinical guidelines issued by the Kidney Disease: Improving Global Outcomes (KDIGO) group [46] recommend that clinical laboratories report GFR using the 2009 CKD-EPI equations and that an estimating equation incorporating cystatin C be used if confirmation is needed in patients without "markers of kidney damage." Fortunately, CKD-EPI equation results can be automatically calculated by clinical laboratories but are normalized to a body surface area of 1.73 m^2, requiring further calculation to obtain a result that is more consistent with an individual patient's muscle mass. Given this complexity, the simpler Cockcroft and Gault equation still finds widespread use among clinicians involved in patient care. Unfortunately, estimating equations based on serum creatinine measurements are inaccurate in patients whose renal function is changing rapidly, for example in acute renal failure, [47], and frequently underestimate GFR in trauma and burn patients or in those requiring intensive care in whom augmented renal clearance is common, so measured creatinine clearance must be relied on [48]. On the other hand, creatinine clearance is likely to overestimate renal function in patients with low creatinine production due to cirrhosis, cachexia, or age-related skeletal muscle atrophy [47].

Dose-related toxicity often occurs when impaired renal function is unrecognized

Failure to appreciate that a patient has impaired renal function is a frequent cause of dose-related adverse drug reactions with digoxin and other drugs that normally rely primarily on the kidneys for elimination. As presented in Table 1.1, an audit of patients with high plasma concentrations of digoxin (≥3.0 ng/mL) demonstrated that 19 of 44, or 43% of 44 patients with digoxin toxicity had serum creatinine concentrations within the range of normal values, yet had estimated creatinine clearances less than 50 mL/min [49]. Hence, assessment of renal function is essential if digoxin and many other drugs are to be used safely and effectively, and is an important prerequisite for the application of clinical pharmacologic principles to patient care.

TABLE 1.1 Status of renal function in 44 patients with digoxin toxicity.

	CL_{CR} (mL/min)		
Serum creatinine (mg/dL)	≥50	<50	%
≤1.7	4	19	52%
>1.7	0	21	48%

Data from Piergies AA, Worwag EM, Atkinson AJ Jr. A concurrent audit of high digoxin plasma levels. Clin Pharmacol Ther 1994;55:353–358.

Decreases in renal function are particularly likely to be unrecognized in older patients whose creatinine clearance declines as a consequence of aging rather than overt kidney disease. It is for this reason that the Joint Commission on Accreditation of Healthcare Organization has placed the estimation or measurement of creatinine clearance in patients of 65 years of age or older at the top of its list of indicators for monitoring the quality of medication use [50]. Fortunately, computerized laboratory reporting systems have been programmed to automatically report MDRD or CKD-EPI estimates of GFR, a task that was relatively easy to accomplish because these calculations can be performed without access to patient weight. This undoubtedly is an important advance in that it should increase prescriber awareness of a patient's renal functional status.

Although the developers of the MDRD equation advocated its further use in calculating drug dosage [36], there is a substantial existing body of published dosing guidelines that are based on the Cockcroft-Gault equation. In the final analysis, it may not matter in most cases which equation is used as the basis for adjusting oral doses of many drugs as the accuracy of either equation in estimating renal function generally exceeds the level of adjustment permitted by available oral formulations, or even the accuracy with which tablets can be split.

References

[1] Holmstedt B, Liljestrand G. Readings in pharmacology. Oxford: Pergamon; 1963.

[2] Reidenberg MM. Attitudes about clinical research. Lancet 1996;347:1188.

[3] Leake CD. The scientific status of pharmacology. Science 1961;134:2069–2079.

[4] Reidenberg MM. Clinical pharmacology: the scientific basis of therapeutics. Clin Pharmacol Ther 1999;66:2–8.

[5] Atkinson AJ Jr, Nordstrom K. The challenge of in-hospital medication use: an opportunity for clinical pharmacology. Clin Pharmacol Ther 1996;60:363–367.

[6] Gold H, Kwit NT, Otto H. The xanthines (theobromine and aminophylline) in the treatment of cardiac pain. JAMA 1937;108:2173–2179.

[7] Gold H, Catell MK, Greiner T, Hanlon LW, Kwit NT, Modell W, et al. Clinical pharmacology of digoxin. J Pharmacol Exp Ther 1953;109:45–57.

[8] Taussig HB. A study of the German outbreak of phocomelia: the thalidomide syndrome. JAMA 1962;180:1106–1114.

[9] Melmon KL. Preventable drug reactions – causes and cures. N Engl J Med 1971;284:1361–1368.

[10] Koch-Weser J. Serum drug concentrations as therapeutic guides. N Engl J Med 1972;287:227–231.

[11] Piquette-Miller M, Grant DM. The art and science of personalized medicine. Clin Pharmacol Ther 2007;81:311–315.

[12] Collins FS, Varmus H. A new initiative on precision medicine. N Engl J Med 2015;372:793–795.

[13] Atkinson AJ Jr. Individualization of drug therapy: an historical perspective. Transl Clin Pharmacol 2014;22:52–54.

[14] Lazarou J, Pomeranz BH, Corey PN. Incidence of adverse drug reactions in hospitalized patients: a meta-analysis of prospective studies. JAMA 1998;279:1200–1205.

[15] Bates DW. Drugs and adverse drug reactions. How worried should we be? JAMA 1998;279:1216–1217.

[16] Zhang G, Nebert DW. Personalized medicine: genetic risk prediction of drug response. Pharmacol Ther 2017;175:75–90.

[17] Sjöqvist F. The past, present and future of clinical pharmacology. Eur J Clin Pharmacol 1999;55:553–557.

[18] Shelley JH, Baur MP. Paul Martini: the first clinical pharmacologist? Lancet 1999;353:1870–1873.

[19] Sheiner LB. The intellectual health of clinical drug evaluation. Clin Pharmacol Ther 1991;50:4–9.

[20] Peck CC, Barr WH, Benet LZ, Collins J, Desjardins RE, Furst DE, et al. Opportunities for integration of pharmacokinetics, pharmacodynamics, and toxicokinetics in rational drug development. Clin Pharmacol Ther 1992;51:465–473.

[21] Flowers CR, Melmon KL. Clinical investigators as critical determinants in pharmaceutical innovation. Nat Med 1997;3:136–143.

[22] Goldberg LI. Cardiovascular and renal actions of dopamine: potential clinical applications. Pharmacol Rev 1972;24:1–29.

[23] Tréfouël J, Tréfouël Mme J, Nitti F, Bouvet D. Activité du *p*-aminophénylsulfamide sur les infections streptococciques expérimentales de la souris et du lapin. C R Soc Biol (Paris) 1935;120:756–758.

[24] Atkinson AJ Jr, Strong JM. Effect of active drug metabolites on plasma level-response correlations. J Pharmacokinet Biopharm 1977;5:95–109.

[25] Woosley RL, Chen Y, Freiman JP, Gillis RA. Mechanism of the cardiotoxic actions of terfenadine. JAMA 1993;269:1532–1536.

[26] Stearns V, Johnson MD, Rae JM, Morocho A, Novielli A, Bhargava P, et al. Active tamoxifen metabolite plasma concentrations after coadministration of tamoxifen and the selective serotonin reuptake inhibitor paroxetine. J Natl Cancer Inst 2003;95:1758–1764.

[27] Binkhorst L, Mathijssen RHJ, Jager A, van Gelder T. Individualization of tamoxifen therapy: much more than just *CYP2D6* genotyping. Cancer Treat Rep 2015;41:289–299.

[28] de Vries Schultink AHM, Huitema ADR, Beijnen JH. Therapeutic drug monitoring of endoxifen as an alternative for *CYP2D6* genotyping in individualizing tamoxifen therapy. Breast 2018;42:38–40.

[29] Ahmad A, Shahabuddin S, Sheikh S, Kale P, Manjunath K, Rane RC, et al. Endoxifen a new cornerstone for breast cancer therapy: demonstration of safety, tolerability, and systemic bioavailability in healthy human subjects. Clin Pharmacol Ther 2010;88:814–817.

[30] Goetz MP, Suman VJ, Reid JM, Northfelt D, Mahr MA, Ralya AT, et al. First-in-human phase I study of the tamoxifen metabolite Z-endoxifen in women with endocrine-refractory metastatic breast cancer. J Clin Oncol 2017;35:3391–3430.

[31] Möller E, McIntosh JF, Van Slyke DD. Studies of urea excretion. II. Relationship between urine volume and the rate of urea excretion in normal adults. J Clin Invest 1928;6:427–465.

[32] Cockcroft DW, Gault MH. Prediction of creatinine clearance from serum creatinine. Nephron 1976;16:31–41.

[33] Myers GL, Miller WG, Coresh J, Fleming J, Greenberg N, Greene T, et al. Recommendations for improving serum creatinine measurement: a report from the National Kidney Disease Education Program. Clin Chem 2006;52:5–18.

[34] Bauer JH, Brooks CS, Burch RN. Clinical appraisal of creatinine clearance as a measurement of glomerular filtration rate. Am J Kidney Dis 1982;2:337–346.

[35] Levey AS, Coresh J, Greene T, Stevens LA, Zhang L, Hendriksen S, et al. Using standardized serum creatinine values in the Modification of Diet in Renal Disease Study equation for estimating glomerular filtration rate. Ann Intern Med 2006;145:247–254.

[36] Stevens LA, Nolin TD, Richardson MM, Feldman HI, Lewis JB, Rodby R, et al. Comparison of drug dosing recommendations based on measured GFR and kidney function estimating equations. Am J Kidney Dis 2009;54:33–42.

[37] Levey AS, Stevens LA, Schmid CH, Zhang Y, Castro III AF, Feldman HI, et al. A new equation to estimate glomerular filtration rate. Ann Intern Med 2009;150:604–612.

[38] Inker LA, Schmid CH, Tighiouart H, Eckfeldt JH, Feldman HI, Greene T, et al. Estimating glomerular filtration rate from serum creatinine and cystatin C. N Engl J Med 2012;367:20–29.

[39] Schwartz GJ, Feld LG, Langford DJ. A simple estimate of glomerular filtration rate in full-term infants during the first year of life. J Pediatr 1984;104:849–854.

[40] Schwartz GJ, Gauthier B. A simple estimate of glomerular filtration rate in adolescent boys. J Pediatr 1985;106:522–526.

[41] Schwartz GJ, Muñoz A, Schneider MF, Mak RH, Kaskel F, Warady BA, et al. New equations to estimate GFR in children with CKD. J Am Soc Nephrol 2009;20:629–637.

[42] Pottel H, Mottaghy FM, Zaman Z, Martens F. On the relationship between glomerular filtration rate and serum creatinine in children. Pediatr Nephrol 2010;25:927–934.

[43] Schaeffner ES, Ebert N, Delanaye P, Frei U, Caedeke J, Jakob O, et al. Two novel equations to estimate kidney function in persons aged 70 years or older. Ann Intern Med 2012;157:471–481.

[44] Pottel H, Hoste L, Dubourg L, Ebert N, Schaeffner E, Eriksen BO, et al. An estimated glomerular filtration rate equation for the full age spectrum. Nephrol Dial Transplant 2016;31:798–806.

[45] da Silva Selistre L, Rech DL, de Souza V, Iwaz J, Lemoine S, Dubourg L. Diagnostic performance of creatinine-based equations in estimating glomerular filtration rate in adults 65 years and older. JAMA Intern Med 2019;179:796–804.

[46] KDIGO Group. KDIGO 2012 clinical practice guideline for the evaluation and management of chronic kidney disease. Kidney Int Suppl 2013;3:1–150.

[47] Perrone RD, Madias NE, Levey AS. Serum creatinine as an index of renal function: new insights into old concepts. Clin Chem 1992;38:1933–1953.

[48] Atkinson AJ Jr. Augmented renal clearance. Transl Clin Pharmacol 2018;26:176–181.

[49] Piergies AA, Worwag EM, Atkinson AJ Jr. A concurrent audit of high digoxin plasma levels. Clin Pharmacol Ther 1994;55:353–358.

[50] Nadzam DM. A systems approach to medication use. In: Cousins DM, editor. Medication use. Oakbrook Terrace, IL: Joint Commission on Accreditation of Healthcare Organizations; 1998. p. 5–17.

Additional sources of information

General

Bruton LL, Hilal-Dandan R, Knollman B, editors. Goodman & Gilman's The pharmacological basis of therapeutics. 13th ed. New York: McGraw-Hill; 2018.

This is the standard reference textbook of pharmacology. It contains good introductory presentations of the general principles of pharmacokinetics, pharmacodynamics and therapeutics. Appendix II contains a useful tabulation of the pharmacokinetic properties of many commonly-used drugs.

Carruthers SG, Hoffman BB, Melmon KL, Nierenberg DW, editors. Melmon and Morrelli's Clinical pharmacology. 4th ed. New York: McGraw-Hill; 2000.

This is the classic textbook of clinical pharmacology with introductory chapters devoted to general principles and subsequent chapters covering different therapeutic areas. A final section is devoted to core topics in clinical pharmacology.

Waldman SA, Terzic A, editors. Pharmacology and therapeutics: principles to practice. Philadelphia: Saunders-Elsevier; 2009.

This is an introductory textbook that is divided into initial chapters that present pharmacologic principles and later chapter that are devoted to therapeutic applications in a wide number of clinical areas.

Pharmacokinetics

Gibaldi M, Perrier D. Pharmacokinetics. 2nd ed. New York: Marcel Dekker; 1982.

This is a standard reference in pharmacokinetics and is the one most often cited in the "methods section" of papers that are published in journals covering this area.

Rowland M, Tozer TN. Clinical pharmacokinetics and pharmacodynamics: concepts and applications. 4th ed. Philadelphia: Lippincott Williams & Wilkins; 2010.

This is a well-written book that is very popular as an introductory text.

Drug metabolism

Pratt WB, Taylor P, editors. Principles of drug action: the basis of pharmacology. 3rd ed. New York: Churchill Livingstone; 1990.

This book is devoted to basic principles of pharmacology and has good chapters on drug metabolism and pharmacogenetics.

Drug therapy in special populations

Evans WE, Schentag JJ, Jusko WJ, editors. Applied pharmacokinetics: principles of therapeutic drug monitoring. 3rd ed. Vancouver, WA: Applied Therapeutics; 1992.

This book contains detailed information that is useful for individualizing dose regimens of a number of commonly-used drugs.

Drug development

Gallin J, Ognibene F, Johnson LL. Principles and practice of clinical research. 4th ed. San Diego: Academic Press/Elsevier; 2018.

This book is based on a long-standing and successful course taught at the Clinical Center of the National Institutes of Health and provides a practical introduction to the conduct of clinical research.

Spilker B. Guide to clinical trials. Philadelphia: Lippincott-Raven; 1996.

This book contains detailed discussions of many practical topics that are relevant to the process of drug development.

Yacobi A, Skelly JP, Shah VP, Benet LZ, editors. Integration of pharmacokinetics, pharmacodynamics, and toxicokinetics in rational drug development. New York: Plenum; 1993.

This book describes how the basic principles of clinical pharmacology currently are being applied in the process of drug development.

Journals

British Journal of Clinical Pharmacology.

Clinical Pharmacology and Therapeutics.

Journal of Pharmaceutical Sciences.

Journal of Pharmacokinetics and Biopharmaceutics.

Websites

American Society for Clinical Pharmacology and Therapeutics (ASCPT). http://www.ascpt.org/.

The American Board of Clinical Pharmacology (ABCP). http://www.abcp.net/.

Chapter 2

Clinical pharmacokinetics

Arthur J. Atkinson, Jr.
Department of Pharmacology, Feinberg School of Medicine, Northwestern University, Chicago, IL, United States

Pharmacokinetics is a valuable adjunct for prescribing and evaluating patient therapy with many drugs, particularly those that have a *narrow therapeutic index*, the ratio of toxic/therapeutic drug concentrations. In addition, pharmacokinetics plays an important role in the conduct of both basic and applied pharmacological research, and is an essential component of the drug development process. For most clinical and many other applications, pharmacokinetic analyses can be simplified by representing drug distribution within the body by a *single compartment* in which drug concentrations are uniform [1]. Clinical application of pharmacokinetics usually entails relatively simple calculations, carried out in the context of what has been termed *the target concentration strategy*. We shall begin by discussing this strategy.

The target concentration strategy

The rationale for measuring concentrations of drugs in plasma, serum, or blood is that *concentration-response* relationships are often less variable than are *dose-response* relationships [2]. This is true because individual variation in the processes of drug absorption, distribution, and elimination affects dose-response relationships, but not the relationship between free (nonprotein-bound) drug concentration in plasma water and intensity of effect (Fig. 2.1). The rationale of therapeutic drug monitoring was first elucidated over 90 years ago when Otto Wuth recommended monitoring bromide levels in patients treated with this drug [3]. However, its more widespread clinical application has been possible only

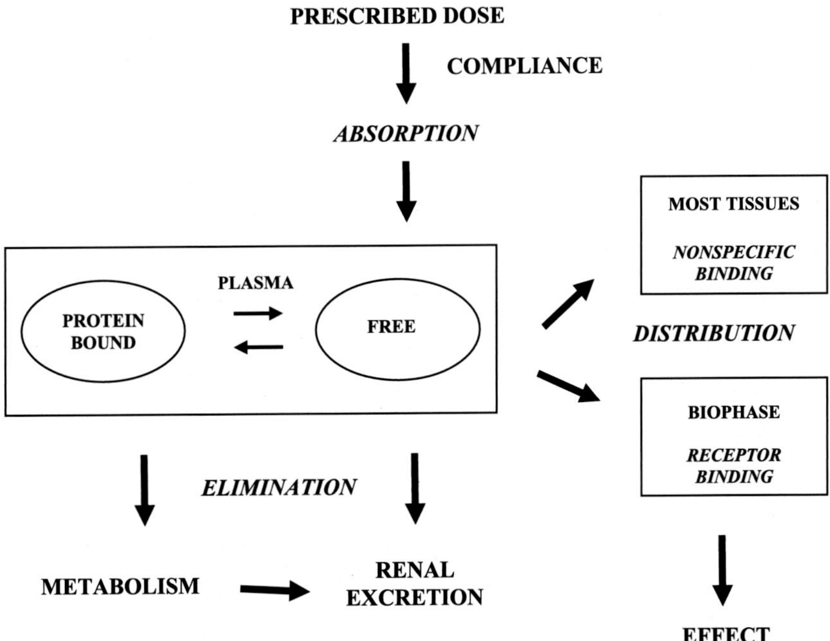

FIG. 2.1 Diagram of factors that account for variability in observed effects when standard drug doses are prescribed. Some of this variability can be compensated for by using plasma concentration measurements to guide dose adjustments.

Atkinson's Principles of Clinical Pharmacology. https://doi.org/10.1016/B978-0-12-819869-8.00021-5

because major advances have been made over the past 50 years in developing analytical methods capable of routinely measuring drug concentrations in patient serum, plasma, or blood samples, and because of increased understanding of basic pharmacokinetic principles [4, 5]

Because most adverse drug reactions are dose related, therapeutic drug monitoring has been advocated as a means of improving therapeutic efficacy and reducing drug toxicity [6]. Drug concentration monitoring is most useful when combined with pharmacokinetic/pharmacogenetic-based dose selection in an integrated management plan as outlined in Fig. 2.2. This approach to drug dosing is termed the *target concentration strategy*. Pharmacokinetics has been most useful in estimating initial drug doses, particularly for loading doses and for maintenance doses of drugs that are primarily eliminated by renal excretion, and in making subsequent dose adjustments based on plasma concentration measurements. Recent advances in pharmacogenetics and pharmacogenomics are finding increasing clinical utility in guiding drug selection and in providing dose estimates for drugs that are primarily eliminated by certain metabolic pathways.

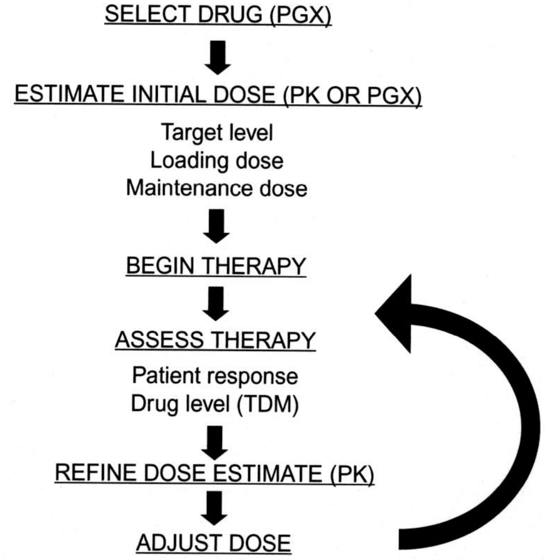

FIG. 2.2 Target concentration strategy in which pharmacogenetics (PGX), pharmacokinetics (PK), and drug concentration measurements (TDM) are integral parts of a therapeutic approach that extends from initial drug selection and dose estimation to subsequent patient monitoring and dose adjustment. *(Reproduced with permission from Atkinson AJ Jr. Individualization of drug therapy: an historical perspective. Transl Clin Pharmacol 2014;22:52–54.)*

Monitoring serum concentrations of digoxin as an example

Given the advanced state of modern chemical and immunochemical analytical methods, the greatest current challenge is the establishment of the range of drug concentrations in blood, plasma, or serum that correlate reliably with therapeutic efficacy or toxicity. This challenge is exemplified by the results shown in Fig. 2.3 that are taken from the attempt by Smith and Haber

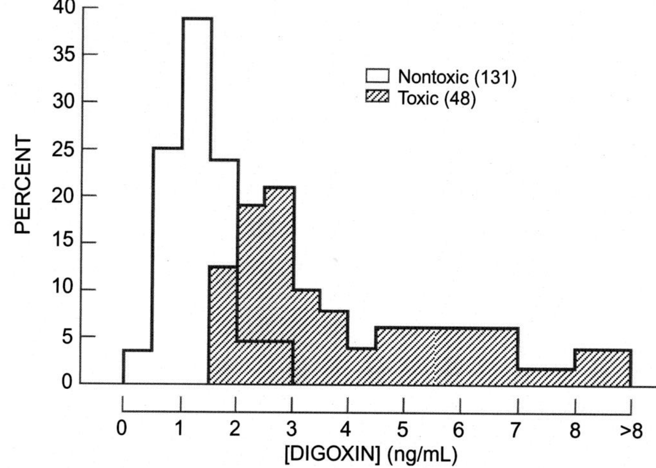

FIG. 2.3 Superimposed frequency histograms in which serum digoxin concentrations are shown for 131 patients without digoxin toxicity and 48 patients with electrocardiographic evidence of digoxin toxicity. *(Reproduced with permission from Smith TW, Haber E. Digoxin intoxication: the relationship of clinical presentation to serum digoxin concentration. J Clin Invest 1970;49:2377–2386.)*

[7] to correlate serum digoxin levels with clinical manifestations of toxicity. It can be seen that no patient in this study with digoxin levels below 1.6 ng/mL was toxic and that all patients with digoxin levels above 3.0 ng/mL had evidence of digoxin intoxication. However, there was a large intermediate range between 1.6 and 3.0 ng/mL in which patients could be either nontoxic or toxic. Accordingly, laboratory reports of digoxin concentration have traditionally been accompanied by the following guidelines:

Usual therapeutic range	0.8–1.6 ng/mL
Possibly toxic levels	1.6–3.0 ng/mL
Probably toxic levels	>3.0 ng/mL

Additional clinical information is often necessary to interpret drug concentration measurements that are otherwise equivocal. Thus Smith and Haber found that all toxic patients with serum digoxin levels less than 2.0 ng/mL had coexisting coronary heart disease, a condition known to predispose the myocardium to the toxic effects of this drug. Conversely, 4 of the 10 nontoxic patients with levels above 2.0 ng/mL were being treated with antiarrhythmic drugs that might have suppressed electrocardiographic evidence of digoxin toxicity.

Although traditional digoxin serum level recommendations were based largely on studies in which digoxin toxicity or intermediate inotropic endpoints were measured, more recent studies have focused on correlating digoxin serum levels with the long-term clinical outcome of patients treated with this drug. The Digitalis Investigation Group trial, in which nearly 1000 patients were enrolled, has forced a major revaluation of digoxin dosing guidelines [8]. The investigators concluded that, compared to placebo, digoxin therapy decreased the need for hospitalization and reduced the incidence of death from congestive heart failure, but not overall mortality. Post hoc analysis of this data indicated that all-cause mortality was only lessened in men whose serum digoxin concentrations ranged from 0.5 to 0.9 ng/mL [9]. Higher levels were associated with progressively greater mortality and did not confer other clinical benefit. Based on the pharmacokinetic properties of digoxin, one would expect levels in this range to be obtained with a daily dose of 0.125 mg. However, most patients with serum digoxin levels in this range were presumed to be taking a 0.25-mg daily digoxin dose, a dose that in patients with normal renal function generally provides a steady-state plasma level of 1.4 ng/mL. In addition, the serum digoxin levels were only measured in a subset of the patients at a single time point, whereas outcomes were followed for a duration of 28–58 months [10].

As a result of subsequent observational studies and meta-analyses, a revised therapeutic range of 0.5–0.9 ng/mL has been recommended with a 56% increase in mortality risk being observed with levels ≥1.2 ng/mL [11, 12]. The strongest support for using digoxin is to control rapid heart rate in patients with atrial fibrillation whose blood pressure is only marginally adequate [12]. Digoxin is also recommended for patients with congestive heart failure and reduced cardiac ejection fraction as it has been shown to reduce mortality, morbidity, and hospitalization frequency. However, it has been estimated that only 20% of patients hospitalized for congestive heart failure in recent years were receiving digoxin therapy, whereas in the 1990s more than two-thirds of heart failure patients entering clinical trials were being treated with this drug [13]. In part, this decrease reflects the advent of more effective diuretics and other drugs that unload the left ventricle [12]. However, this may also reflect the fact that appropriate monitoring of digoxin plasma levels and knowledge of pharmacokinetics required to use digoxin safely and effectively is regarded as too much of an inconvenience by most clinicians. So some cardiologists have advocated creating a cadre of dedicated medical heart failure specialists who would have the requisite expertise in these areas [13].

General indications for drug concentration monitoring

Unfortunately, controlled studies documenting the clinical benefit of drug concentration monitoring are limited. In addition, one could not justify concentration monitoring for all prescribed drugs even if this technical challenge could be met. Thus drug concentration monitoring is most helpful for drugs that have a narrow therapeutic index and that have no clinically observable effects that can be easily monitored to guide dose adjustment. Generally accepted indications for measuring drug concentrations are as follows:

1. To evaluate concentration-related toxicity
   - Unexpectedly slow drug elimination
   - Accidental or purposeful overdose
   - Surreptitious drug taking
   - Dispensing errors

2. To evaluate lack of therapeutic efficacy
   - Patient noncompliance with prescribed therapy
   - Poor drug absorption
   - Unexpectedly rapid drug elimination
3. To ensure that the dose regimen is likely to provide effective prophylaxis.
4. To use pharmacokinetic principles to guide dose adjustment.

Unfortunately, dose-related adverse reactions still occur frequently with digoxin, phenytoin, and many other drugs for which drug concentration measurements are routinely available. The persistence in contemporary practice of these adverse reactions most likely reflects inadequate understanding of basic pharmacokinetic principles. This is illustrated by the following case history [4]:

> *A 39-year-old man with mitral stenosis was hospitalized for mitral valve replacement. He had a history of chronic renal failure resulting from interstitial nephritis and was maintained on hemodialysis. His mitral valve was replaced with a prosthesis and digoxin therapy was initiated postoperatively in a dose of 0.25 mg/day. Two weeks later, he was noted to be unusually restless in the evening. The following day, he died shortly after he received his morning digoxin dose. Blood was obtained during an unsuccessful resuscitation attempt, and the measured plasma digoxin concentration was 6.9 ng/mL.*

Later in this chapter we will demonstrate that the ostensibly surprising delayed onset of this fatal adverse event was pharmacokinetically consistent with this initial therapeutic decision.

Concepts underlying clinical pharmacokinetics

Pharmacokinetics provides a scientific basis for dose selection, and the process of dose regimen design can be used to illustrate with a single-compartment model the basic concepts of *apparent distribution volume* (V_d), *elimination half-life* ($t_{1/2}$), and *elimination clearance* (CL_E). A schematic diagram of this model is shown in Fig. 2.4 along with the two primary pharmacokinetic parameters of distribution volume and elimination clearance that characterize it.

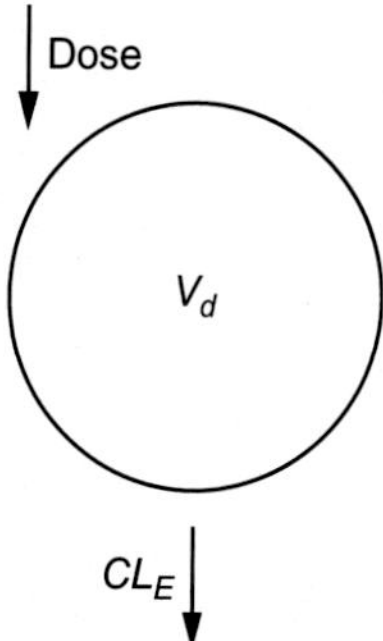

FIG. 2.4 Diagram of a single-compartment model in which the primary kinetic parameters are the apparent distribution volume of the compartment (V_d) and the elimination clearance (CL_E).

Initiation of drug therapy (concept of apparent distribution volume)

Sometimes drug treatment is begun with a loading dose to produce a rapid therapeutic response. Thus a patient with atrial fibrillation might be given a 0.375 mg intravenous loading dose of digoxin as initial therapy to control ventricular rate. The expected plasma concentrations of digoxin are shown in Fig. 2.5. Inspection of this figure indicates that the log plasma-concentration-vs.-time curve eventually becomes a straight line. This part of the curve is termed the *elimination phase*. By extrapolating this elimination-phase line back to time zero, we can estimate the plasma concentration (C_0) that would have occurred if the loading dose were instantaneously distributed throughout the body. Measured plasma digoxin concentrations lie above the back-extrapolated line for several hours because distribution equilibrium actually is reached only slowly after a digoxin dose is administered. This part of the plasma-level-vs.-time curve is termed the *distribution phase*. This phase reflects the underlying *multicompartmental* nature of digoxin distribution from the intravascular space to peripheral tissues.

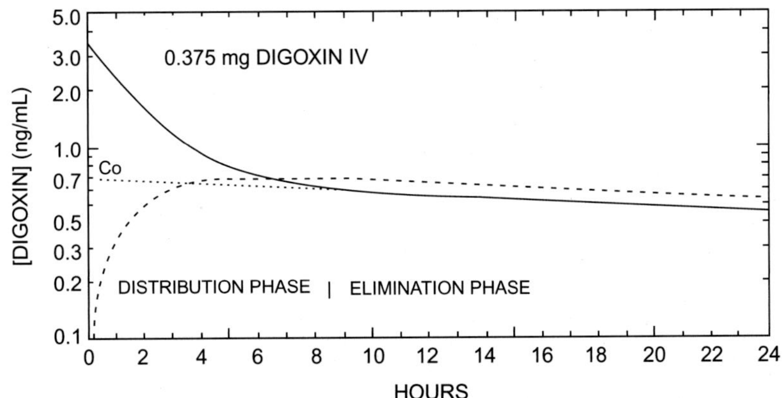

FIG. 2.5 Simulation of plasma (*solid line*) and tissue (*heavy dashed line*) digoxin concentrations after intravenous administration of a 0.375-mg loading dose to a 70-kg patient with normal renal function. A value of 0.7 ng/mL for C_0 is estimated by back-extrapolating (*dotted line*) the elimination-phase plasma concentrations. A value of 536 L for V_d is calculated by dividing the administered drug dose by this estimate of C_0, as shown in the text. Tissue concentrations are referenced to the apparent distribution volume of a peripheral compartment that represents tissue distribution. *(Simulation based on pharmacokinetic model of Reuning RH, et al. Role of pharmacokinetics in drug dosage adjustment. I. Pharmacologic effect kinetics and apparent volume of distribution of digoxin. J Clin Pharmacol New Drugs 1973;13:127–141.)*

As shown in Fig. 2.5, the back-extrapolated estimate of 0.7 ng/mL for C_0 can be used to calculate the apparent volume ($V_{d(extrap)}$) of a hypothetical single compartment into which digoxin distribution occurs:

$$V_{d(extrap)} = \text{Loading dose}/C_0 \tag{2.1}$$

In this case,

$$V_{d(extrap)} = 0.375\,\text{mg}/0.7\,\text{ng/mL}$$
$$V_{d(extrap)} = 536\,\text{L}$$

This distribution volume is much larger than anatomically possible. However, this discrepancy occurs because digoxin has a much higher binding affinity for tissues than for plasma, and the *apparent* distribution volume is the volume of *plasma* that would be required to provide the observed dilution of the loading dose. Despite this anomaly, the concept of distribution volume is clinically useful because it defines the relationship between plasma concentration and the total amount of drug in the body. Further complexity arises from the fact that $V_{d(extrap)}$ is only one of three different distribution volume estimates that we will encounter. Because the distribution process is neglected in calculating this volume, it represents an overestimate of the sum of the volumes of the individual compartments involved in drug distribution.

The time course of the myocardial effects of digoxin parallels its concentration profile in peripheral tissues (Fig. 2.5), so there is a delay between the attainment of peak plasma digoxin concentrations and the observation of maximum inotropic and chronotropic effects. The range of therapeutic and toxic digoxin concentrations has been estimated from observations made during the elimination phase, so blood should not be sampled for digoxin assay until distribution equilibrium is nearly complete. In clinical practice, this means waiting for at least 6 h after a digoxin dose has been administered. In an audit of patients with measured digoxin levels of 3.0 ng/mL or more, it was found that nearly one-third of these levels were not associated with toxicity but reflected procedural error, in that blood was sampled less than 6 h after digoxin administration [14].

For other drugs, such as thiopental [15] or lidocaine [16], the locus of pharmacologic action (termed the *biophase* in classical pharmacology) is in rapid kinetic equilibrium with the intravascular space. The distribution phase of these drugs represents their somewhat slower distribution from intravascular space to pharmacologically inert tissues, such as skeletal muscle. In this way, the pharmacological effects of single doses of these drugs may be rapidly terminated by the process of distribution even though only a small fraction of the dose has been eliminated from the body. Plasma levels of these drugs reflect therapeutic and toxic effects throughout the dosing interval and blood can be obtained for drug assay without waiting for the elimination phase to be reached.

Continuation of drug therapy (concepts of elimination half-life and clearance)

After starting therapy with a loading dose, maintenance of a sustained therapeutic effect usually necessitates administering additional drug doses to replace the amount of drug that has been excreted or metabolized. Fortunately, the elimination of most drugs is a *first-order* process in that the rate of drug elimination is directly proportional to the drug concentration in plasma.

Elimination half-life

It is convenient to characterize the elimination of drugs with first-order elimination rates by their *elimination half-life*, the time required for half an administered drug dose to be eliminated. If drug elimination half-life can be estimated for a patient, it is often practical to continue therapy by administering half the loading dose at an interval of one elimination half-life. In this way, drug elimination can be balanced by drug administration and a steady state maintained from the onset of therapy. Because digoxin has an elimination half-life of 1.6 days in patients with normal renal function, it is inconvenient to administer digoxin at this interval. When renal function is normal, it is customary to maintain digoxin therapy by administering daily doses equal to one-third of the required loading dose.

Another consequence of first-order elimination kinetics is that a constant fraction of total body drug stores will be eliminated in a given time interval. Thus if there is no urgency in establishing a therapeutic effect, the loading dose of digoxin can be omitted and 90% of the eventual steady-state drug concentration will be reached after administering daily doses for a period of time equal to 3.3 elimination half-lives. This is referred to as the *Plateau Principle*. The classical derivation of this principle is provided later in this chapter, but for now brute force will suffice to illustrate this important concept. Suppose that we elect to omit the 0.375 mg digoxin loading dose shown in Fig. 2.5 and simply begin therapy with a 0.125 mg/day maintenance dose. If the patient has normal renal function, we can anticipate that one-third of the total amount of digoxin present in the body will be eliminated each day and that two-thirds will remain when the next daily dose is administered. As shown in Scheme 2.1, the patient will have digoxin body stores of 0.326 mg just after the fifth daily dose (3.3×1.6 day half-life = 5.3 days), and this is 87% of the total body stores that would have been provided by a 0.375 mg loading dose.

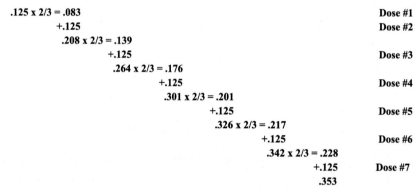

.125 x 2/3 = .083	**Dose #1**
+.125	**Dose #2**
.208 x 2/3 = .139	
+.125	**Dose #3**
.264 x 2/3 = .176	
+.125	**Dose #4**
.301 x 2/3 = .201	
+.125	**Dose #5**
.326 x 2/3 = .217	
+.125	**Dose #6**
.342 x 2/3 = .228	
+.125	**Dose #7**
.353	

SCHEME 2.1 "Brute force" demonstration of drug cumulation when maintenance doses are administered repeatedly.

The solid line in Fig. 2.6 shows ideal matching of digoxin loading and maintenance doses. When the digoxin loading dose (called *digitalizing dose* in clinical practice) is omitted, or when the loading dose and maintenance dose are not matched appropriately, steady-state levels are reached only asymptotically. However, the most important concept that this figure

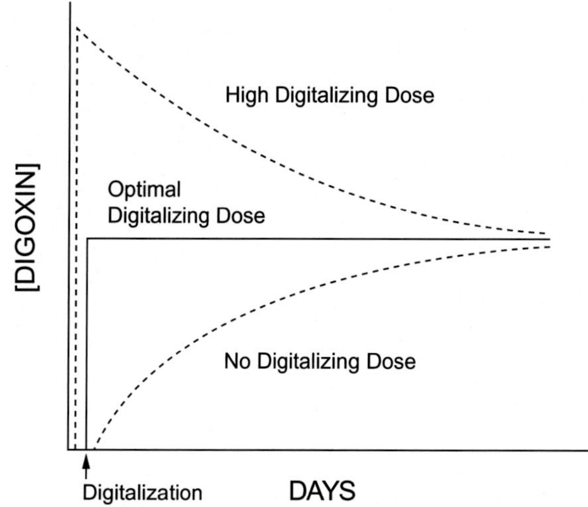

FIG. 2.6 Expected digoxin plasma concentrations after administering perfectly matched loading and maintenance doses (*solid line*), no initial loading dose (*bottom dashed line*), or a high loading dose that is large in relation to the subsequent maintenance dose (*upper dashed line*).

demonstrates is that *the eventual steady state level is determined only by the maintenance dose*, regardless of the size of the loading dose. Selection of an inappropriately high digitalizing dose only exposes patients to an interval of added risk without achieving a permanent increase in the extent of digitalization. Conversely, when a high digitalizing dose is required to help control ventricular rate in patients with atrial fibrillation or flutter, a higher than usual maintenance dose also will be required.

Elimination clearance

Just as creatinine clearance is used to quantitate the renal excretion of creatinine, the removal of drugs eliminated by first-order kinetics can be defined by an *elimination clearance* (CL_E). In fact, elimination clearance is the primary pharmacokinetic parameter that characterizes the removal of drugs that are eliminated by first-order kinetics. When drug administration is by intravenous infusion, the eventual steady-state concentration of drug in the body (C_{ss}) can be calculated from the following equation (note the similarity to Eq. 1.2), where the drug infusion rate is given by I:

$$C_{ss} = I/CL_E \tag{2.2}$$

When intermittent oral or parenteral doses are administered at a dosing interval, τ, the corresponding equation is:

$$\overline{C}_{ss} = \frac{Dose/\tau}{CL_E} \tag{2.3}$$

where $\overline{C}_{ss}$ is the mean concentration during the dosing interval. Under conditions of intermittent administration, there is a continuing periodicity in maximum ("peak") and minimum ('trough") drug levels so that only a quasi-steady state is reached. However, unless particular attention is directed to these peak and trough levels, no distinction generally is made in clinical pharmacokinetics between the true steady state that is reached when an intravenous infusion is administered continuously and the quasi-steady state that results from intermittent administration.

Because there is a directly proportionate relationship between administered drug dose and steady-state plasma level, Eqs. (2.2), (2.3) provide a straightforward guide to dose adjustment for drugs that are eliminated by first-order kinetics. Thus, to double the plasma level, the dose simply should be doubled. Conversely, to halve the plasma level, the dose should be halved. It is for this reason that Eqs. (2.2), (2.3) are the most clinically important pharmacokinetic equations. Note that, as is apparent from Fig. 2.6, these equations also stipulate that the steady-state level is determined only by the maintenance dose and elimination clearance. The loading dose does not appear in the equations and does not influence the eventual steady-state level.

In contrast to elimination clearance, elimination half-life ($t_{1/2}$) is not a primary pharmacokinetic parameter because it is determined by distribution volume as well as by elimination clearance:

$$t_{1/2} = \frac{0.693\, V_{d(area)}}{CL_E} \tag{2.4}$$

The value of V_d in this equation is not $V_{d(extrap)}$ but represents a second estimate of distribution volume, referred to as $V_{d(area)}$ or $V_{d(\beta)}$ that generally is estimated from measured elimination half-life and clearance. The similarity of these two estimates of distribution volume reflects the extent to which drug distribution is accurately described by a single-compartment model, and obviously varies from drug to drug [17].

Fig. 2.7 illustrates how differences in distribution volume affect elimination half-life and peak and trough plasma concentrations when the same drug dose is given to two patients with the same elimination clearance. If these two hypothetical patients were given the same nightly dose of a sedative-hypnotic drug for insomnia, $\overline{C}_{ss}$ would be the same for both. However, the patient with the larger distribution volume might not obtain sufficiently high plasma levels to fall asleep in the evening, and might have a plasma level that was high enough to cause drowsiness in the morning.

Drugs not eliminated by first-order kinetics

Unfortunately, the elimination of some drugs does not follow first-order kinetics. For example, the primary pathway of phenytoin elimination entails initial metabolism to form 5-(parahydroxyphenyl)-5-phenylhydantoin (*p*-HPPH), followed by glucuronide conjugation (Fig. 2.8). The metabolism of this drug is not first order but follows *Michaelis-Menten* kinetics because the microsomal enzyme system that forms *p*-HPPH is partially saturated at phenytoin concentrations of 10–20 μg/mL that are therapeutically effective. The result is that phenytoin plasma concentrations rise hyperbolically as dosage is increased (Fig. 2.9).

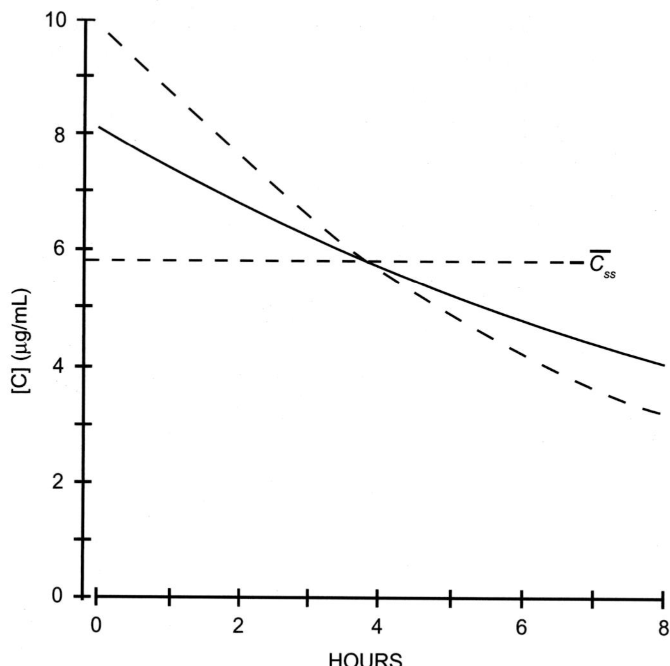

FIG. 2.7 Plasma concentrations after repeated administration of the same drug dose to two hypothetical patients whose elimination clearance is the same but whose distribution volumes differ. The patients have the same $\overline{C}_{ss}$ but the larger distribution volume results in lower peak and higher trough plasma levels (*solid line*) than when the distribution volume is smaller (*dashed line*).

PHENYTOIN → *p* - HPPH → *p* - HPPH GLUCURONIDE

FIG. 2.8 Metabolism of phenytoin to form *p*-HPPH and *p*-HPPH glucuronide. The first step in this enzymatic reaction sequence is rate limiting and follows Michaelis-Menten kinetics, showing progressive saturation as plasma concentrations rise within the range that is required for anticonvulsant therapy to be effective.

For drugs eliminated by first-order kinetics, the relationship between dosing rate and steady-state plasma concentration is given by rearranging Eq. (2.3) as follows:

$$Dose/\tau = CL_E \cdot \overline{C}_{ss} \tag{2.5}$$

The corresponding equation for phenytoin is:

$$Dose/\tau = \frac{V_{\max}}{K_m + \overline{C}_{ss}} \cdot \overline{C}_{ss} \tag{2.6}$$

where $V_{\max}$ is the maximum rate of drug metabolism and K_m is the apparent Michaelis-Menten constant for the enzymatic metabolism of phenytoin.

Although phenytoin plasma concentrations show substantial interindividual variation when standard doses are administered, they average 10 µg/mL when adults are treated with a 300-mg total daily dose, but rise to an average of 20 µg/mL when the dose is increased to 400 mg [18]. This nonproportional relationship between phenytoin dose and plasma concentration complicates patient management and undoubtedly contributes to the many adverse reactions that are seen in patients treated with this drug. Although several pharmacokinetic approaches have been developed for estimating dose adjustments, it is safest to change phenytoin doses in small increments and to rely on careful monitoring of clinical response and phenytoin plasma levels. The pharmacokinetics of phenytoin were studied in both patients shown in Fig. 2.9 after they became toxic when treated with the 300 mg/day dose that is routinely prescribed as initial therapy for adults [19]. The figure demonstrates that the entire therapeutic range is traversed in these patients by a dose increment of less than 100 mg/day. This presents an obvious therapeutic challenge because the phenytoin oral formulation that is most commonly prescribed for adults is a 100 mg capsule.

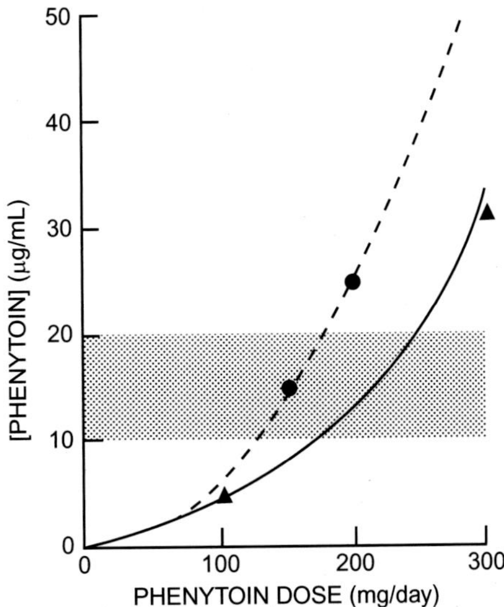

FIG. 2.9 The *lines* show the relationship between dose and steady-state plasma phenytoin concentrations predicted for two patients who became toxic after initial treatment with 300mg/day. Measured steady-state plasma concentrations are shown by the *solid circles* and *triangles*. The *shaded area* shows the usual range of therapeutically effective phenytoin plasma concentrations. *(Reproduced with permission from Atkinson AJ Jr. Individualization of anticonvulsant therapy. Med Clin North Am 1974;58:1037–1049.)*

Even though many drugs in common clinical use are eliminated by drug-metabolizing enzymes, relatively few of them have Michaelis-Menten elimination kinetics (e.g., aspirin and ethyl alcohol). The reason for this is that K_m for most drugs is much greater than $\overline{C}_{ss}$. Hence for most drugs, $\overline{C}_{ss}$ can be ignored in the denominator of Eq. (2.6) and this equation reduces to:

$$Dose/\tau = \frac{V_{max}}{K_m} \cdot \overline{C}_{ss}$$

where the ratio V_{max}/K_m is equivalent to CL_E in Eq. (2.5). Thus, even for most metabolized drugs, a change in dose will change steady-state plasma concentrations proportionately, a property that is termed *dose proportionality*.

Mathematical basis of clinical pharmacokinetics

In the following sections we will review the mathematical basis of some of the important relationships that are used when pharmacokinetic principles are applied to the care of patients. The reader also is referred to other literature sources that may be helpful [1, 17, 20].

First-order elimination kinetics

For most drugs, the amount of drug eliminated from the body during any time interval is proportional to the total amount of drug present in the body. In pharmacokinetic terms, this is called *first-order* elimination and is described by the equation:

$$dX/dt = -kX \tag{2.7}$$

where X is the total amount of drug present in the body at any time (t) and k is the elimination rate constant for the drug. This equation can be solved by separating variables and direct integration to calculate the amount of drug remaining in the body at any time after an initial dose:

Separating variables:

$$dX/X = -kdt$$

Integrating from zero time to time $= t$:

$$\int_{X_0}^{X} dX/X = -k\int_0^t dt$$

$$\ln X\Big|_{X_0}^{X} = -kt\Big|_0^t$$

$$\ln\frac{X}{X_0} = -kt \tag{2.8}$$

$$X = X_0 e^{-kt} \tag{2.9}$$

Although these equations deal with total amounts of drug in the body, the equation $C = X/V_d$ provides a general relationship between X and drug concentration (C) at any time after the drug dose is administered. Therefore C can be substituted for X in Eqs. (2.7), (2.8) as follows:

$$\ln\frac{C}{C_0} = -kt \tag{2.10}$$

$$C = C_0 e^{-kt} \tag{2.11}$$

Eq. (2.10) is particularly useful because it can be rearranged in the form of the equation for a straight line ($y = mx + b$) to give:

$$\ln C = -kt + \ln C_0 \tag{2.12}$$

Now when data are obtained after administration of a single drug dose and C is plotted on base 10 semilogarithmic graph paper, a straight line is obtained with 0.434 times the slope equal to k ($\log x/\ln x = 0.434$) and an intercept on the ordinate of C_0. In practice C_0 is never measured directly because some time is needed for the injected drug to distribute throughout body fluids. However, C_0 can be estimated by back-extrapolating the straight line given by Eq. (2.12) (Fig. 2.5).

Concept of elimination half-life

If the rate of drug distribution is rapid compared with the rate of drug elimination, the terminal exponential phase of a semilogarithmic plot of drug concentrations vs. time can be used to estimate the elimination half-life of a drug, as shown in Fig. 2.10. Because Eq. (2.10) can be used to estimate k from any two concentrations that are separated by an interval t, it can be seen from this equation that when $C_2 = ½\, C_1$:

$$\ln 1/2 = -kt_{1/2}$$

$$\ln 2 = kt_{1/2}$$

So:

$$t_{1/2} = \frac{0.693}{k}, \text{ and } k = \frac{0.693}{t_{1/2}} \tag{2.13}$$

For digoxin, $t_{1/2}$ is usually 1.6 days for patients with normal renal function and $k = 0.43\ \text{day}^{-1}$ ($0.693/1.6 = 0.43$). As a practical point, it is easier to estimate $t_{1/2}$ from a graph such as Fig. 2.10 and to then calculate k from Eq. (2.13), than to estimate k directly from the slope of the elimination-phase line.

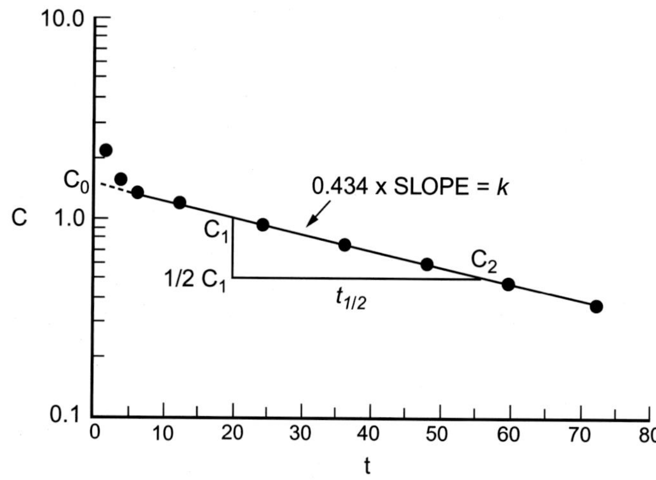

FIG. 2.10 Plot of drug concentrations vs. time on semilogarithmic coordinates. Back extrapolation (*dashed line*) of the elimination phase slope (*solid line*) provides an estimate of C_0. The elimination half-life ($t_{1/2}$) can be estimated from the time required for concentrations to fall from some point on the elimination-phase line (C_1) to $C_2 = ½C_1$, as shown by the *dotted lines*.

Relationship of k to elimination clearance

In Chapter 1, we pointed out that the creatinine clearance equation:

$$CL_{CR} = \frac{UV}{P}$$

could be rewritten in the form of the following first-order differential equation:

$$dX/dt = -CL_{CR} \cdot P$$

If this equation is generalized by substituting CL_E for CL_{CR}, it can be seen from Eq. (2.7) that, since $P = X/V_d$:

$$k = \frac{CL_E}{V_d} \tag{2.14}$$

Eq. (2.4), that was previously cited, is derived by substituting Cl_E/V_d for k in Eq. (2.13). Although V_d and Cl_E are the two primary parameters of the single-compartment model, confusion arises because k is initially calculated from experimental data. However, k is influenced by changes in distribution volume as well as clearance and does not reflect just changes in drug elimination.

Cumulation factor

In the steady-state condition, the rate of drug administration is exactly balanced by the rate of drug elimination. Gaddum [21] first demonstrated that the maximum and minimum drug levels that are expected at steady state (quasi-steady state) can be calculated for drugs that are eliminated by first-order kinetics. Assume that just maintenance doses of a drug are administered without a loading dose (Fig. 2.6, lowest curve). Starting with Eq. (2.9):

$$X = X_0 e^{-kt}$$

where X_0 is the maintenance dose and X is the amount of drug remaining in the body at time t. If τ is the dosing interval, let:

$$p = e^{-k\tau}$$

Therefore, just before the second dose:

$$X_{1(\min)} = X_0 p$$

Just after the second dose:

$$X_{2(\max)} = X_0 + X_0 p = X_0(1+p)$$

Similarly, after the third dose

$$X_{3(\max)} = X_0 + X_0 p + X_0 p^2 = X_0\left(1+p+p^2\right)$$

and after the nth dose:

$$X_{n(\max)} = X_0\left(1+p+\ldots\ldots p^{n-1}\right)$$

or,

$$X_{n(\max)} = X_0 \frac{(1-p^n)}{(1-p)}$$

Since $p < 1$, as $n \to \infty$, $p^n \to 0$. Therefore

$$X_{\infty(\max)} = X_0/(1-p)$$

or, substituting for p

$$X_{\infty(\max)} = \frac{X_0}{(1-e^{-k\tau})}$$

The value of X_∞ is the maximum *total body content* of the drug that is reached during a dosing interval at steady state. The maximum *concentration* is determined by dividing this value by V_d. The *minimum* value is given by multiplying either of these maximum values by $e^{-k\tau}$.

Note that the respective maximum and minimum drug concentrations after the first dose are:

$$\text{Maximum}: \ C_0$$

$$\text{Minimum}: \ C_0 e^{-k\tau}$$

The expected steady-state counterparts of these initial concentration values can be estimated by multiplying them by the *cumulation factor* (CF):

$$CF = \frac{1}{1 - e^{-kt}} \tag{2.15}$$

The plateau principle

Although the time required to reach steady state cannot be calculated explicitly, the time required to reach *any specified fraction (f) of the eventual steady state* can be estimated. In clinical practice, $f = 0.90$ is usually a reasonable approximation of the eventual steady state. For dosing regimens in which drugs are administered as a constant infusion, the pharmacokinetic counterpart of Eq. (1.1) in which both creatinine synthesis and elimination are considered is:

$$dX/dt = I - kX$$

Separation of variables and integration of this equation yields:

$$X = \frac{I}{k}\left(1 - e^{-kt}\right)$$

Because infinite time is required for X to reach its steady state, $X_{ss} = I/k$ and

$$f_{.90} = \frac{X_{.90}}{X_{ss}} = \left(1 - e^{-kt_{.90}}\right)$$

By definition $X_{.90}/Xss = 0.90$, also $k = \ln 2/t_{1/2}$ (Eq. 2.13), so:

$$t_{.90} = 3.3t_{1/2} \tag{2.16}$$

For dosing regimens in which drugs are administered at a constant dosing interval, Gaddum [21] showed that the number of drug doses (n) required to reach any fraction of the eventual steady-state amount of drug in the body can be calculated as follows:

$$f = \frac{X_n}{X_\infty} = \frac{X_0(1 - p^n)^0}{(1 - p)} \cdot \frac{(1 - p)}{X_0} = 1 - p^n \tag{2.17}$$

Once again, taking $f = 0.90$ as a reasonable approximation of eventual steady state, substituting this value into Eq. (2.17), and solving for n:

$$0.90 = 1 - e^{-nk\tau}$$

$$e^{-nk\tau} = 0.1$$

$$n = -\frac{\ln 0.1}{k\tau}$$

$$n = \frac{2.3}{k\tau}$$

Again from Eq. (2.13), $k = \ln 2/t_{1/2}$, so the number of doses needed to reach 90% of steady state is:

$$n = 3.3\,t_{1/2}/\tau \tag{2.18}$$

and the corresponding time is:

$$n\tau = 3.3\,t_{1/2} \tag{2.19}$$

Not only are drug accumulation greater and steady-state drug levels higher in patients with a prolonged elimination half-life, but an important consequence of Eq. (2.18) is that it also takes these patients longer to reach steady state. For example, the elimination half-life of digoxin in patients with normal renal function is 1.6 days, so that 90% of the expected steady state is reached in 5 days when daily doses of this drug are administered. However, the elimination half-life of digoxin is approximately 4.3 days in functionally anephric patients, such as the one described in the illustrative case history, and 14 days would be required to reach 90% of the expected steady state. This explains why this patient's adverse reaction occurred 2 weeks after starting digoxin therapy.

Application of Laplace transforms to pharmacokinetics

The Laplace transformation method of solving differential equations falls into the area of *operational calculus* that we will use in deriving several pharmacokinetic equations. Operational calculus was invented by an English engineer, Sir Oliver Heaviside (1850–1925), who had an intuitive grasp of mathematics [22]. Although Laplace provided the theoretical basis for the method, some of Sir Oliver's intuitive contributions remain (e.g., the Heaviside Expansion Theorem utilized in Chapter 3). The idea of operational mathematics and Laplace transforms perhaps is best understood by comparison with the use of logarithms to perform arithmetic operations. This comparison is diagrammed in the flow charts shown in Scheme 2.2.

Just as there are tables of logarithms, there are tables to aid the mathematical process of obtaining Laplace transforms ($\mathcal{L}$) and inverse Laplace transforms ($\mathcal{L}^{-1}$). Laplace transforms can also be calculated directly from the integral:

$$\mathcal{L}[F(t)] = f(s) = \int_0^{\infty} F(t)e^{-st}dt$$

We can illustrate the application of Laplace transforms by using them to solve the simple differential equation that we have used to describe the single-compartment model (Eq. 2.7) Starting with this equation:

$$dX/dt = -kX$$

we can use a table of Laplace transform operations (Appendix I) to take Laplace transforms of each side of this equation to create the *subsidiary equation*:

For X on the right side of the equation:

$$\mathcal{L}F(t) = f(s)$$

For dX/dt on the left side of the equation:

$$\mathcal{L}F'(t) = sf(s) - F(0)$$

Since $F(0)$ represents the *initial condition*, in this case the amount of drug in the model compartment at time zero, X_0, the subsidiary equation can be written:

$$sf(s) - X_0 = -kf(s)$$

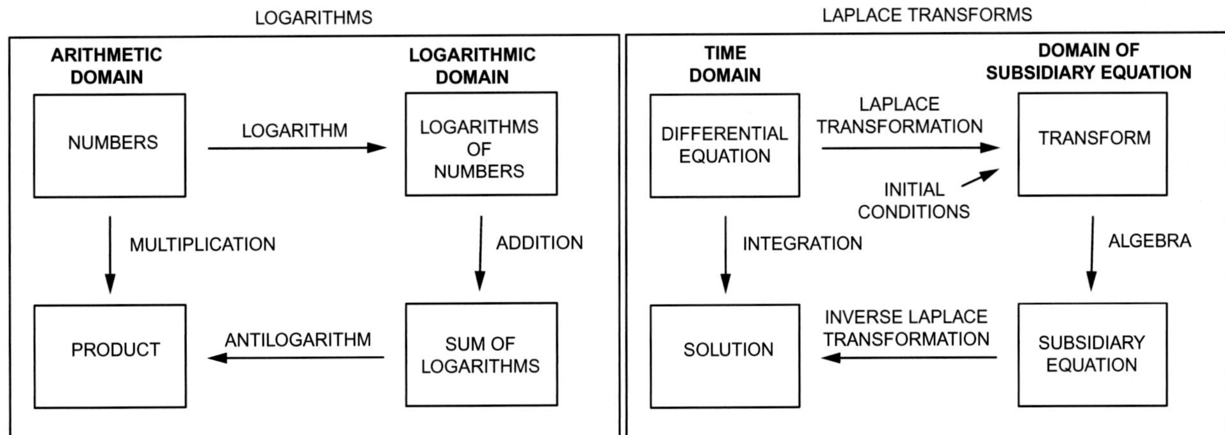

SCHEME 2.2 Analogy between use of logarithms and Laplace transforms.

This can be rearranged to give:

$$(s+k)f(s) = X_0$$

Or,

$$f(s) = \frac{X_0}{s+k}$$

A table of *inverse Laplace transforms* indicates:

$$\mathcal{L}^{-1}\frac{1}{s-a} = e^{at}$$

Therefore the solution to the differential equation is:

$$X = X_0 e^{-kt}$$

and this is the same result that we obtained as Eq. (2.9).

In other words, the Laplace operation transforms the differential equation from the time domain to another functional domain represented by the subsidiary equation. After algebraic simplification of this subsidiary equation, the inverse transformation is used to return the solved equation to the time domain. We have selected a simple example to illustrate the use of Laplace transform methods. A more advanced application is given in the next chapter in which equations are derived for a two-compartment model. It will be shown subsequently that Laplace transform methods also are helpful in pharmacokinetics when convolution/deconvolution methods are used to characterize drug absorption processes.

References

[1] Atkinson AJ Jr, Kushner W. Clinical pharmacokinetics. Annu Rev Pharmacol Toxicol 1979;19:105–127.

[2] Atkinson AJ Jr, Reidenberg MM, Thompson WL. Clinical pharmacology. In: Greenberger N, editor. MKSAP VI syllabus. Philadelphia: American College of Physicians; 1982. p. 85–96.

[3] Wuth O. Rational bromide treatment: new methods for its control. JAMA 1927;88:2013–2017.

[4] Atkinson AJ Jr, Ambre JJ. Kalman and Clark's Drug assay: the strategy of therapeutic drug monitoring. 2nd ed. New York: Masson; 1984.

[5] Atkinson AJ Jr. Individualization of drug therapy: an historical perspective. Transl Clin Pharmacol 2014;22:52–54.

[6] Koch-Weser J. Serum drug concentrations as therapeutic guides. N Engl J Med 1972;287:227–231.

[7] Smith TW, Haber E. Digoxin intoxication: the relationship of clinical presentation to serum digoxin concentration. J Clin Invest 1970;49:2377–2386.

[8] The Digitalis Investigation Group. The effect of digoxin on mortality and morbidity in patients with heart failure. N Engl J Med 1997;336:525–533.

[9] Rathore SS, Curtis JP, Wang Y, Bristow MR, Krumholz HM. Association of serum digoxin concentration and outcomes in patients with heart failure. JAMA 2003;289:871–878.

[10] Ambrosy AP, Gheorghiade M. Targeting digoxin dosing to serum concentration: is the Bullseye too small? Eur J Heart Fail 2016;18:1082–1084.

[11] Adams KF Jr, Ghali JK, Patterson H, Stough WG, Butler J, Bauman JL, et al. A perspective on re-evaluating digoxin's role in the current management of patients with chronic systolic heart failure: targeting serum concentration to reduce hospitalization and improve safety profile. Eur J Heart Fail 2014;16:483–493.

[12] Whayne TF. Clinical use of digitalis: a state of the art review. Am J Cardiovasc Drugs 2018;18:427–440.

[13] Packer M. Why is the use of digitalis withering? Another reason that we need medical heart failure specialists. Eur J Heart Fail 2018;20:851–852.

[14] Piergies AA, Worwag EW, Atkinson AJ Jr. A concurrent audit of high digoxin plasma levels. Clin Pharmacol Ther 1994;55:353–358.

[15] Goldstein A, Aronow L. The durations of action of thiopental and pentobarbital. J Pharmacol Exp Ther 1960;128:1–6.

[16] Benowitz N, Forsyth RP, Melmon KL, Rowland M. Lidocaine disposition kinetics in monkey and man. I. Prediction by a perfusion model. Clin Pharmacol Ther 1974;16:87–98.

[17] Gibaldi M. Biopharmaceutics and clinical pharmacokinetics. 4th ed. Philadelphia: Lea & Febiger; 1991.

[18] Kutt H, McDowell F. Management of epilepsy with diphenyhydantoin sodium. JAMA 1968;203:969–972.

[19] Atkinson AJ Jr. Individualization of anticonvulsant therapy. Med Clin North Am 1974;58:1037–1049.

[20] Rowland M, Tozer TN. Clinical pharmacokinetics and pharmacodynamics: concepts and applications. 4th ed. Philadelphia: Lippincott Williams & Wilkins; 2010.

[21] Gaddum JH. Repeated doses of drugs. Nature 1944;153:494.

[22] Van Valkenberg ME. The Laplace transformation. In: Network analysis. Englewood Cliffs, NJ: Prentice-Hall; 1964. p. 159–181.

Study problems

Select the *one* lettered answer or statement completion that is BEST. It may be helpful to carry out dimensional analysis by including units in your calculations. Answers are provided in Appendix II.

1. A 35-year-old woman is being treated with gentamicin for a urinary tract infection. The gentamicin plasma level is 4 µg/mL shortly after initial intravenous administration of an 80 mg dose of this drug. The distribution volume of gentamicin is:
   A. 5 L
   B. 8 L
   C. 10 L
   D. 16 L
   E. 20 L
2. A 58-year-old man is hospitalized in a cardiac intensive care unit following an acute myocardial infarction. He has had recurrent episodes of ventricular tachycardia that have not responded to lidocaine and an intravenous infusion of procainamide will now be administered. The patient weighs 80 kg and expected values for his procainamide distribution volume and elimination half-life are 2.0 L/kg and 3 h, respectively.
   What infusion rate will provide a steady-state plasma procainamide level of 4.0 µg/mL?
   A. 2.5 mg/min
   B. 5.0 mg/min
   C. 7.5 mg/min
   D. 10.0 mg/min
   E. 12.5 mg/min
3. A patient with peritonitis is treated with gentamicin 80 mg every 8 h. Plasma gentamicin levels are measured during the first dosing interval. The gentamicin plasma level is 10 µg/mL at its peak after initial intravenous administration of this drug, and is 5 µg/mL when measured 5 h later.
   The cumulation factor can be used to predict an expected steady-state peak level of:
   A. 10 µg/mL
   B. 12 µg/mL
   C. 15 µg/mL
   D. 18 µg/mL
   E. 20 µg/mL
4. A 20-year-old man is hospitalized after an asthmatic attack precipitated by an upper respiratory infection but fails to respond in the emergency room to two subcutaneously injected doses of epinephrine. The patient has not been taking theophylline-containing medications for the past 6 weeks. He weighs 60 kg and you estimate that his apparent volume of theophylline distribution is 0.45 L/kg. Bronchodilator therapy includes a 5.6 mg/kg loading dose of aminophylline, infused intravenously over 20 min, followed by a maintenance infusion of 0.63 mg/kg per hour (0.50 mg/kg per hour of theophylline). Forty-eight hours later, the patient's respiratory status has improved. However, he has nausea and tachycardia, and his plasma theophylline level is 24 µg/mL.
   For how long do you expect to suspend theophylline administration in order to reach a level of 12 µg/mL before restarting the aminophylline infusion at a rate of 0.31 mg/kg per hour?
   A. 5 h
   B. 10 h
   C. 15 h
   D. 20 h
   E. 25 h
5. Digitoxin has an elimination half-life of approximately 7 days and its elimination is relatively unaffected by decreased renal function. For this latter reason, the decision is made to use this drug to control ventricular rate in a 60-year-old man with atrial fibrillation and a creatinine clearance of 25 mL/min.
   If no loading dose is administered and a maintenance dose of 0.1 mg/day is prescribed, how many days would be required for digitoxin levels to reach 90% of their expected steady-state value?
   A. 17 days
   B. 19 days
   C. 21 days
   D. 23 days
   E. 24 days
6. A 75-year-old man comes to your office with anorexia and nausea. Five years ago he was found to have congestive heart failure that initially responded to treatment with a loop diuretic, a β-blocker, and an angiotensin-converting enzyme inhibitor. Three years ago his exercise tolerance was found to have deteriorated and digoxin was added to

the regimen in a dose of 0.25 mg/day. This morning he omitted his digoxin dose because of these symptoms and your office electrocardiogram showed frequent bigeminal extrasystoles. On hospitalization, the patient's serum creatinine and digoxin plasma digoxin levels were 1.4 mg/dL and 2.4 ng/mL, respectively. Twenty-four hours later, the digoxin level is 1.9 ng/mL. At that time you decide that it would be advisable to let the digoxin level fall to 0.6 ng/mL, within the current therapeutic range of 0.5–0.9 ng/mL, before restarting a daily digoxin dose of 0.0625 mg.
For how many *more* days do you anticipate having to withhold digoxin before your target level of 0.6 ng/mL is reached?
A. 2 days
B. 3 days
C. 4 days
D. 5 days
E. 6 days

7. A 50-year-old man is being treated empirically with gentamicin and a cephalosporin for pneumonia. The therapeutic goal is to provide a maximum gentamicin level of *more than* 8 µg/mL 1 h after intravenous infusion and a minimum concentration, just before dose administration, of *less than* 1 µg/mL. His estimated plasma gentamicin clearance and elimination half-life are 100 mL/min and 2 h, respectively. Which of the following dosing regimens is appropriate?
A. 35 mg every 2 h
B. 70 mg every 4 h
C. 90 mg every 5 h
D. 110 mg every 6 h
E. 140 mg every 8 h

8. You start a 19-year-old man on phenytoin in a dose of 300 mg/day to control generalized (grand mal) seizures. Ten days later, he is brought to an emergency room following a seizure. His phenytoin level is found to be 5 µg/mL and the phenytoin dose is increased to 600 mg/day. Two weeks later, he returns to your office complaining of drowsiness and ataxia. At that time his phenytoin level is 30 µg/mL.
Assuming patient compliance with previous therapy, which of the following dose regimens should provide a phenytoin plasma level of 15 µg/mL (therapeutic range: 10–20 µg/mL)?
A. 350 mg/day
B. 400 mg/day
C. 450 mg/day
D. 500 mg/day
E. 550 mg/day

Chapter 3

Compartmental analysis of drug distribution

Arthur J. Atkinson, Jr.
Department of Pharmacology, Feinberg School of Medicine, Northwestern University, Chicago, IL, United States

All models are wrong but some are useful.

George E.P. Box, 1979 [1]

Drug distribution can be defined as the postabsorptive transfer of drug from one location in the body to another. Absorption after various routes of drug administration is not considered part of the distribution process and is dealt with separately. In most cases, the process of drug distribution is symmetrically reversible and requires no input of energy. However, there is increasing awareness that receptor-mediated endocytosis and carrier-mediated active transport also play important roles in either increasing or limiting the extent of drug distribution. The role of these processes in drug distribution will be considered in Chapter 13.

Fit-for-purpose modeling of drug distribution

In the previous chapter we neglected distribution-phase data and considered drug distribution within the body to be represented by a single homogeneous compartment. Although both anatomically and physiologically wrong, this model nonetheless is useful for most clinical applications. In fact, most routine pharmacokinetic studies are performed using *noncompartmental* methods which provide useful estimates of drug elimination clearance and total distribution volume. This approach will be described in greater detail in Chapter 8.

A multicompartmental system was first used to model the kinetics of drug distribution in 1937 by Teorell [2]. The two body distribution compartments of this model consisted of a central compartment corresponding to intravascular space and a peripheral compartment representing nonmetabolizing body tissues. Drug elimination was modeled as proceeding from the central compartment. Since then, more complex physiologically based multicompartmental models have been developed using a *bottom-up* approach in which different anatomical organs or groups of organs are represented by separate compartments that are linked by blood flows in a model that incorporates *drug physical chemical* characteristics. Price [3] pioneered this approach in 1960 by analyzing thiopental distribution after intravenous dosing with a four-compartment model that combined previously published values for organ weight and blood flow with values for thiopental's tissue/blood partition ratio. Distribution was considered to be instantaneous in the intravascular space and then proceeded at different rates to visceral organ, lean tissue, and fat compartments. The brain, heart, splanchnic organs, and kidneys were lumped together into a single visceral compartment because their distribution characteristics were similar. Price used this model to compare measured thiopental concentrations in blood and fat with model-predicted values and to demonstrate that the termination of this drug's central nervous system pharmacologic effect was primarily due to redistribution from the brain to skeletal muscle and other lean tissues rather than to fat, as had previously been believed. Thiopental elimination from the body was considered to be relatively insignificant during the study period, so was not included in the model. This a priori approach was further extended by Bischoff and Dedrick [4] whose expanded model included parameters for drug metabolism, protein binding, and lipid solubility, while using a similar compartmental model structure. They compared their pharmacokinetic predictions with previously published human blood concentration results and with measured blood, visceral, lean tissue, and adipose concentrations in dogs.

This type of *physiologically based pharmacokinetics* has become increasingly popular in recent years and typical models now include 14 different tissues linked by arterial and venous blood compartments. They have been further

Atkinson's Principles of Clinical Pharmacology. https://doi.org/10.1016/B978-0-12-819869-8.00026-4

modified to incorporate increasingly detailed information regarding drug physicochemical properties and drug interactions, and drug absorption, distribution, and eliminating organ function in specific patient populations [5, 6]. These models can now be implemented using commercially available software and, as described in Chapter 31, are playing an increasingly important role in drug development and regulatory review [7, 8].

Because physiologically based pharmacokinetic models contain more parameters than can be identified from the analysis of experimental data, compartmental analysis of this data is usually made with systems that model drug distribution with only one, two, or three compartments [9]. Therefore this chapter will focus on the two- and three-compartment models that are most commonly used for this purpose. In most applications, these models retain Price's assumption that distribution within the intravascular space occurs instantaneously after intravenous administration. However, the onset of pharmacologic action of intravenously administered anesthetic agents occurs within seconds of administration and this necessitates consideration of the kinetics of intravascular mixing [10]. So, the appropriate selection of a given modeling approach and model type is very much dependent on the intended purpose of the analysis—what might be termed "fit-for-purpose pharmacokinetics."

Despite their varying complexity, all pharmacokinetic models represent parsimonious simplifications of real-world systems and, in the sense of the opening quote, are "wrong." However, after reaching that conclusion, Box [1] explained that parsimony is desirable because (i) when essential aspects of the system are simple, simplicity illuminates and complication obscures; (ii) parsimony typically results in increasingly precise model parameter estimates; and (iii) indiscriminate model elaboration is not practical because "the road is endless." Similarly, Cobelli et al. [11] pointed out that the validity of a model depends on its adequacy for a well-defined and limited set of objectives, rather than on whether it is a true representation of all facets of an underlying system. Berman [12] made the further distinction between mathematical models in which functions or differential equations are used without regard to the mechanistic aspects of a system, and physical models, which have features that have physiological, biochemical, or physical significance. Dollery [13] has referred to the former as "abstractions derived from curve fitting" that provide minimal mechanistic insight. So this chapter will focus on identifying mechanistic elements of the compartmental models most commonly used for pharmacokinetic data analysis that can be linked to underlying features of human physiology and drug physical chemistry. This can be conceptualized as a *top-down* approach to linking pharmacokinetics to physiology.

Physiological significance of drug distribution volumes

The physiological concept of body compartments evolved slowly from desiccation of cadavers to measure total body water to exsanguination to measure intravascular space [14]. However, in the 20th century the dilution principle was introduced and various indicator compounds were used to measure physiologic spaces. This empirical approach also is taken when experimental data are used to analyze the pharmacokinetics of drug distribution. Unfortunately, digoxin is typical of most drugs in that its distribution volume, averaging 536 L in 70-kg subjects with normal renal function, is not readily interpreted by reference to physiologically defined fluid spaces. However, some drugs and other compounds appear to have distribution volumes that are physiologically identifiable. Thus the total distribution volumes of inulin, quaternary neuromuscular blocking drugs, and the initial distribution volumes of aminoglycoside antibiotics approximate expected values for extracellular fluid space (ECF). The distribution volumes of urea, antipyrine, ethyl alcohol, and caffeine also can be used to estimate total body water (TBW) [9].

Binding to plasma proteins affects drug distribution volume estimates. Initial attempts to explain the effects of protein binding on drug distribution were based on the assumption that the distribution of these proteins was confined to the intravascular space. However, "plasma" proteins distribute throughout ECF, so the distribution volume of even highly protein bound drugs exceeds plasma volume and approximates ECF in many cases [9]. For example, thyroxine is 99.97% protein bound and its distribution volume of 0.15 L/kg [15] approximates ECF estimates of 0.16 ± 0.01 L/kg made with inulin [16]. Distribution volumes are usually larger than ECF for uncharged drugs that are less tightly protein bound to plasma proteins. Theophylline is a methylxanthine, similar to caffeine, and its nonprotein bound, or free fraction is like caffeine in that it distributes throughout TBW. The fact that theophylline is normally 40% bound to plasma proteins accounts for the finding that its 0.5 L/kg apparent volume of distribution is intermediate between expected values for ECF and TBW (Fig. 3.1). The impact on distribution volume (V_d) of changes in the extent of theophylline binding to plasma proteins can be estimated from the following equation:

$$V_d = \mathrm{ECF} + f_U\,(\mathrm{TBW} - \mathrm{ECF}) \tag{3.1}$$

where f_U is the unbound fraction of theophylline that can be measured in plasma samples [17]. An additional correction has been proposed to account for the fact that interstitial fluid protein concentrations are less than those in plasma [18].

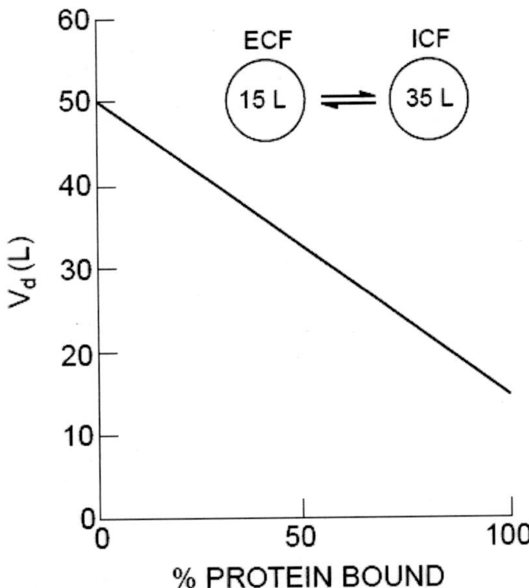

FIG. 3.1 Analysis of theophylline V_d in terms of protein binding, ECF, and intracellular fluid (ICF) components of TBW in a hypothetical 70-kg subject. Theophylline is normally 40% bound, so its V_d approximates 35 L or 0.5 L/kg. *(Reproduced with permission from Atkinson AJ Jr, Ruo TI, Frederiksen MC. Physiological basis of multicompartmental models of drug distribution. Trends Pharmacol Sci 1991;12:96–101.)*

However, this correction does not account for the heterogeneous nature of interstitial fluid composition and entails additional complexity that may not be warranted [9].

Many drugs have distribution volumes that exceed expected values for TBW or are considerably larger than ECF despite extensive binding to plasma proteins. The extensive tissue binding of these drugs increases the apparent distribution volume that is calculated by reference to drug concentrations measured in plasma water. By modifying Eq. (3.1) as follows:

$$V_d = \text{ECF} + \Phi f_U\,(\text{TBW} - \text{ECF}) \tag{3.2}$$

published kinetic data can be used to estimate the tissue-binding affinity (Φ) of these drugs.

For many drugs, the extent of tissue binding is related to their lipophilicity. Although the octanol/water partition coefficient (P_{oct}) measured at pH 7.4 is the in vitro parameter traditionally used to characterize lipophilicity and is appropriate for neutral compounds, this coefficient fails to take into account the fact that many acidic and basic drugs are ionized at physiological pH. Because only unionized drug generally partitions into tissues, a distribution coefficient (D_{oct}) is thought to provide a better correlation with the extent to which a drug distributes into tissues [19]. Thus for drugs that are monoprotic bases:

$$\log D_{oct} = \log P_{oct} + \left[1/\left(1 + 10^{\text{pK}_a - \text{pH}}\right)\right]$$

where pK_a is the dissociation constant of the drug. For monoprotic acids, the exponent in this equation becomes pH − pK_a. In Fig. 3.2, published experimentally determined values for $\log D_{oct}$ are compared with estimates of $\log \Phi$. Eq. (3.2) was rearranged to calculate Φ from literature values for f_u and distribution volume [20, 21], and estimates of ECF (0.16 L/kg) and TBW (0.65 L/kg) were obtained from a study of inulin and urea distribution kinetics [16].

Since the parameters f_u and D_{oct} can be obtained by in vitro measurements, Lombardo et al. [21] have used the reverse of this approach to predict drug distribution volume in humans in order to facilitate compound optimization and selection during the early stages of drug development. Although this type of approach would not be expected to provide an accurate prediction of the distribution volume of drugs that bind to specific subcellular components, this is not necessarily the case. For example, digoxin incorporates a steroid molecule (aglycone) but is relatively polar because three glycoside (sugar) groups are attached to it. It is a neutral compound and has an octanol/water partition coefficient of 18 (log = 1.25), but also binds very tightly to the enzyme Na/K-ATPase that is present in most body tissues. Since digoxin is only 25% bound to plasma proteins ($f_U = 0.75$), Eq. (3.2) can be used to estimate that a 536-L distribution volume of this drug corresponds to a Φ value of 20.4 (log = 1.31), consistent with the relationship between lipophilicity and tissue partitioning shown in Fig. 3.2. However, an important consequence of its binding to Na/K-ATPase is that digoxin can be displaced from its binding sites on this enzyme by concurrent administration of quinidine, causing a decrease in digoxin distribution volume [22]. As discussed in Chapter 5, Sheiner et al. [23] showed that elevations in serum creatinine concentration, resulting from impaired renal function, also are associated with

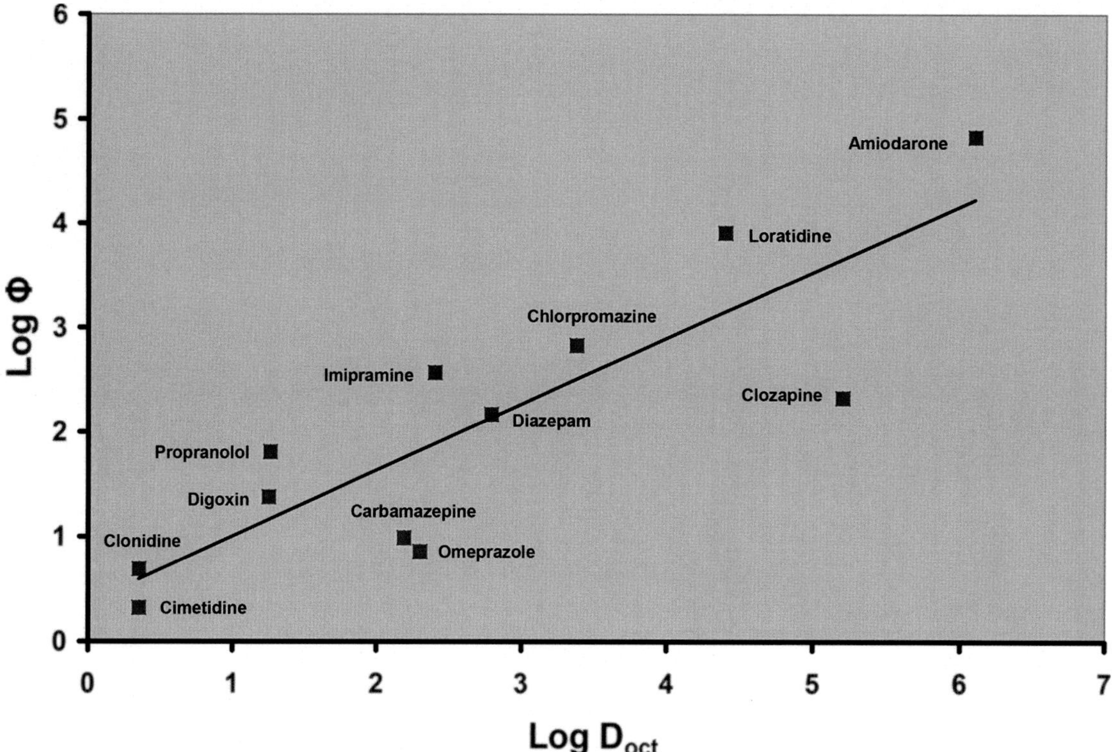

FIG. 3.2 Relationship between lipophilicity, estimated from D_{oct}, and tissue/plasma partition ratio (Φ) for several commonly used drugs.

decreases in digoxin distribution volume. This presumably parallels the impairment in Na/K-ATPase activity that makes these patients more susceptible to toxicity when digoxin levels are ≥3.0 ng/mL [24].

Physiological basis of multicompartmental models of drug distribution

Formulation of multicompartmental models

The construction of multicompartmental models for data analysis entails consideration of the *identifiability*, the structural *uniqueness*, and, for physiologically relevant models, the biological *plausibility* of the model. Identifiability of model parameters is problematic when there is a mismatch between the limited data provided by a pharmacokinetic study and the complexity of the proposed model structure [11]. However, a plot of plasma concentration data vs. time from a pharmacokinetic experiment can be resolved in many cases into a number of discrete exponential phases and characterized by a *sum of exponentials* data equation, such as described later in this chapter. This provides a guide to allowable model complexity in that the minimal number of exponential terms in the data equation corresponds to the number of compartments that can be specified in the model [12]. In addition, the total number of independently identifiable model parameters can not exceed the number of parameters in the data equation. Because of this restriction, drug elimination is usually modeled as proceeding only from the central compartment rather than from several model compartments. Drug transfer between model compartments is best characterized by *intercompartmental clearance*, a term coined by Sapirstein et al. [25] to describe the volume-independent parameter that quantifies the rate of analyte transfer between the compartments of a kinetic model. Thus elimination clearance and intercompartmental clearance are primary pharmacokinetic parameters because they share the property of volume independence and are not affected by changes in compartment volume. However, a number of compartment and parameter configurations are compatible with the data equation in most cases and additional information about the underlying system may be required to arrive at a unique model structure.

Basis of multicompartmental structure

In contrast to Teorell's model, the central compartment of most two-compartment models often exceeds expected values for intravascular space, and three-compartment models are required to model the kinetics of many other drugs. The situation has been further complicated by the fact that some drugs have been analyzed with two-compartment models on some occasions and with three-compartment models on others. To some extent, these discrepancies reflect differences in experimental design. Particularly for rapidly distributing drugs, a tri-exponential plasma-level-vs.-time curve is likely to be observed only when the drug is administered by rapid intravenous injection and blood samples are obtained frequently in the immediate postinjection period.

The central compartment of a pharmacokinetic model usually is the only one that is directly accessible to sampling. When attempting to identify this compartment as intravascular space, the erythrocyte/plasma partition ratio must be incorporated in comparisons of central compartment volume with expected blood volume if plasma levels, rather than whole blood levels, are used for pharmacokinetic analysis. Models in which the central compartment corresponds to intravascular space are of particular physiological interest because the process of distribution from the central compartment then can be identified as transcapillary exchange (Fig. 3.3). In three-compartment models of this type, it might be tempting to conclude that the two peripheral compartments are connected in series (*catenary* model) and represent interstitial fluid space and intracellular water. Urea is a marker of TBW and the kinetics of its distribution could be analyzed with a three-compartment catenary model of this type. On the other hand, a three-compartment model is also required to model distribution of inulin from a central compartment that corresponds to plasma volume. Since inulin distributes only within ECF, this implies that interstitial fluid is kinetically heterogeneous and suggests that the *mammillary* system shown in Fig. 3.3 is the proper unique configuration for models of both inulin and urea distribution kinetics [9, 16].

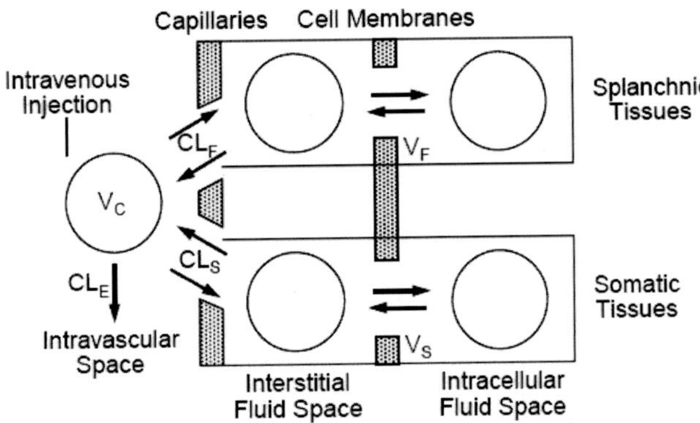

FIG. 3.3 Multicompartmental model of the kinetics of inulin and urea distribution and elimination. After injection into a central compartment corresponding to intravascular space (V_C), both compounds distribute to rapidly (V_F) and slowly (V_S) equilibrating peripheral compartments (*rectangles*), at rates of transcapillary exchange that are characterized by intercompartmental clearances CL_F and CL_S. These peripheral compartments contain both interstitial and intracellular fluid components but transfer of urea between them is too rapid to be distinguished kinetically. Inulin is limited in its distribution to the interstitial fluid components of the peripheral compartments. *(Reproduced with permission from Odeh YK, Wang Z, Ruo TI, Wang T, Frederiksen MC, Pospisil PA, Atkinson AJ Jr. Simultaneous analysis of inulin and* $^{15}N_2$*-urea kinetics in humans. Clin Pharmacol Ther 1993:53:419–425.)*

The proposed physiological basis for this model is that transfer of relatively small polar compounds, like urea and inulin, occurs rapidly across fenestrated and discontinuous capillaries that are located primarily in the splanchnic vascular bed, but proceeds more slowly through the interendothelial cell junctions of less porous capillaries that have a continuous basement membrane and are located primarily in skeletal muscle and other somatic tissues. Direct evidence to support this proposal has been provided by kinetic studies in which the volume of the rapidly equilibrating compartment was found to be reduced in animals whose spleen and lower intestine had been removed [26]. Indirect evidence also has been provided by a study of the distribution and pharmacologic effects of *insulin*, a compound with molecular weight and extracellular distribution characteristics similar to *inulin*. As shown in Fig. 3.4, insulin distribution kinetics were analyzed together with the rate of glucose utilization needed to stabilize plasma glucose concentrations (glucose clamp) [27]. Since changes in the rate of glucose infusion paralleled the rise and fall of insulin concentrations in the slowly equilibrating peripheral compartment, it was inferred that this compartment is largely composed of skeletal muscle. This *pharmacokinetic-pharmacodynamic* (PK-PD) study is also of interest because it illustrates one of the few examples in which a distribution compartment can be plausibly identified as the site of drug action or *biophase*.

Mechanisms of transcapillary exchange

At this time, the physiological basis for the transfer of drugs and other compounds between compartments can only be inferred for mammillary systems in which the central compartment represents intravascular space and intercompartmental

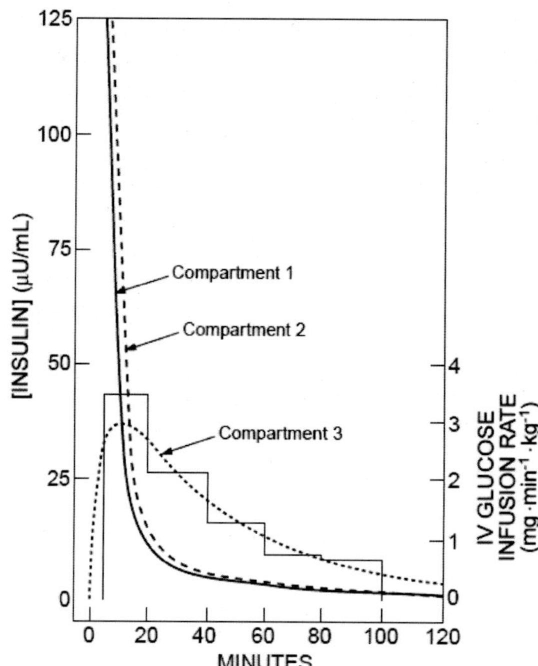

FIG. 3.4 Measured plasma concentrations of insulin in compartment 1 (intravascular space) after intravenous injection of a 25-mU/kg dose and computer-derived estimates of insulin concentration in presumed splanchnic (compartment 2) and somatic (compartment 3) components of interstitial fluid space. The bar graph indicates the glucose infusion rate needed to maintain blood glucose concentrations at the basal level. *(Reproduced with permission from Sherwin RS, Kramer KJ, Tobin JD, Insel PA, Liljenquist JE, Berman M, Andres R. A model of the kinetics of insulin in man. J Clin Invest 1974;53:1481–1492.)*

clearance can be equated with transcapillary exchange. In the case of inulin and urea, intercompartmental clearance (CL_I) can be analyzed in terms of the rate of blood flow (Q) through exchanging capillary beds and the permeability coefficient-surface area product ($P\bullet S$) characterizing diffusion through capillary fenestrae (primarily in splanchnic capillary beds) or small pores (primarily in somatic capillary beds). The following permeability-flow equation has a long developmental history [28] but was first used by Renkin [29] for analyzing transcapillary exchange of nongaseous solutes in an isolated perfused hind limb preparation before being incorporated in multicompartmental pharmacokinetic models [30],

$$CL_I = Q\left(1 - e^{-P\cdot S/Q}\right) \quad (3.3)$$

In order to estimate both Q and $P\bullet S$ from measured values of CL_I it was necessary to study both inulin and urea kinetics simultaneously. The additional assumption needed to be made that the ratio of urea/inulin $P\bullet S$ values for each compartment was the same as the ratio of their free water diffusion coefficients. Calculations based on this assumption yielded estimates of the sum of blood flows to the peripheral compartments that were in close agreement with independently measured cardiac output when studies were conducted in both dogs [31] and humans [16]. We will see in Chapter 6 that this modeling approach has been particularly useful in characterizing the physiological basis of the pharmacokinetic changes that occur during hemodialysis.

Although there have been few studies designed to interpret actual drug distribution results in physiological terms, one approach has been to administer the drug under investigation along with reference compounds such as inulin and urea. In one study, it was found that the molecular charge of gallamine retards its transcapillary exchange to the ECF [32]. In a second study, it was found that the intercompartmental clearances of theophylline to its two peripheral compartments corresponded to the compartmental blood flow components of urea and inulin transcapillary exchange [33]. Given that the free water diffusion coefficient of theophylline is less (slower) than that of urea, yet its intercompartmental clearances were more rapid than the corresponding urea clearances, its transcapillary exchange presumably occurs by carrier-mediated facilitated diffusion. Very lipid soluble compounds also appear to pass directly though capillary walls at rates limited only by blood flow (i.e., $P\bullet S \gg Q$ in Eq. 3.3). On the other hand, large molecular size retards transcapillary exchange and molecules considerably larger than inulin are probably transported through small-pore capillaries by convection rather than diffusion (Fig. 3.5) [34]. These observations lead to the classification of transcapillary exchange mechanisms presented in Table 3.1.

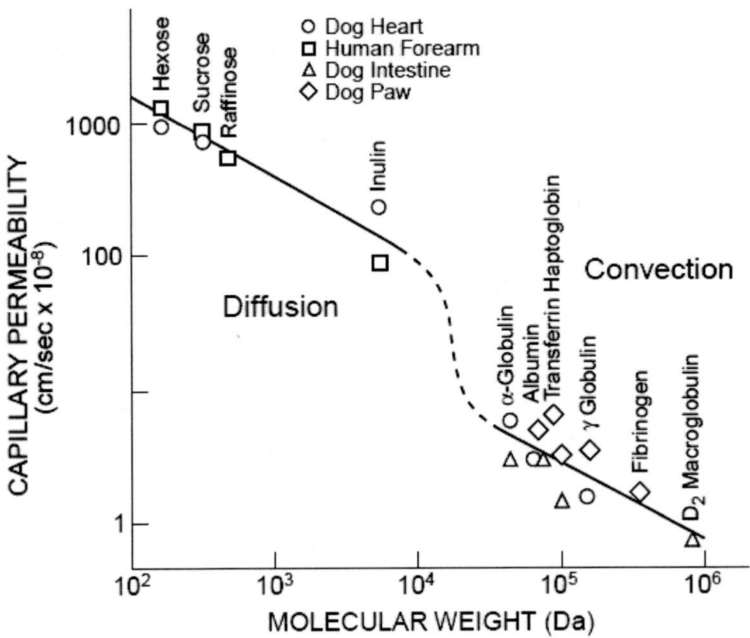

FIG. 3.5 Plot of capillary permeability vs. molecular weight. *(Reproduced with permission from Dedrick RL, Flessner MF. Pharmacokinetic considerations on monoclonal antibodies. Prog Clin Biol Res 1989;288:429–438.)*

TABLE 3.1 Classification of transcapillary exchange mechanisms.

1. Diffusive transfer of small molecules (<6000 Da)
   - Transferred at rates proportional to their free water diffusion coefficients
     – Polar, uncharged compounds (e.g., urea, inulin)
   - Transferred more slowly than predicted from free water diffusion coefficients
     – Highly charged compounds (e.g., quaternary skeletal muscle relaxants)
     – Compounds with intermediate polarity that interact with capillary walls (e.g., procainamide)
   - Transferred more rapidly than predicted from free water diffusion coefficients
     – Highly lipid soluble compounds that freely penetrate endothelial cells (e.g., anesthetic gases)
     – Compounds transferred by carrier-mediated facilitated diffusion (e.g., theophylline)
2. Convective transfer of large molecules (>50,000 Da)

Clinical consequences of different drug distribution patterns

The process of drug distribution can account for both the slow onset of pharmacologic effect of some drugs (e.g., digoxin) and the termination of pharmacologic effect after bolus intravenous injection of others (e.g., thiopental and lidocaine). Because conventional pharmacokinetic studies do not have the resolving power to identify distribution to smaller but pharmacologically important regions such as the brain or heart, the clinical consequences of different drug distribution patterns are generally inferred from observations of drug effect. For example, theophylline was often administered by rapid intravenous injection to asthmatic patients when it was introduced in the 1930s. It was only after several fatalities were reported that the current practice was adopted of initiating therapy in emergency situations with a slow intravenous infusion. Nonetheless, excessively rapid intravenous administration of theophylline still contributes to the frequency of serious adverse reactions to this drug [35]. The rapidity of carrier-mediated theophylline distribution to the brain and heart probably contributes to the infusion rate dependency of these serious adverse reactions.

The impact of physiological changes on drug distribution kinetics has not been studied extensively. As described in Chapter 6, changes in intercompartmental clearance occur during hemodialysis and have important effects on the extent of drug removal during this procedure. In addition, physiological changes in body fluid compartment volumes and protein binding both affect drug distribution in pregnant subjects. As discussed in Chapter 23, Eq. (3.1) has been used to correlate pregnancy-associated changes in theophylline distribution with this altered physiology [17].

Drugs with faster elimination than distribution

For most drugs whose plasma-level-vs.-time curve demonstrates more than one exponential phase, the terminal phase primarily, but not entirely, reflects the process of drug elimination, and the initial phase or phases primarily reflect the process of drug distribution. However, the sequence of *distribution* and *elimination phases* is reversed for some drugs, and these drugs are said to exhibit "*flip-flop*" kinetics. For example, Schentag and colleagues [36] have shown that the elimination phase precedes the distribution phase of gentamicin, an aminoglycoside antibiotic, and accounts for the long terminal half-life that is seen after a course of therapy (Fig. 3.6). In this case, the reported central compartment of drug distribution probably corresponds to ECF because aminoglycosides are highly charged and do not passively diffuse across mammalian cell membranes. However, they are taken up by proximal renal tubular cells by a saturable receptor-mediated endocytic mechanism in which megalin serves as the endocytic receptor [37]. Accordingly, in one of the few studies in which drug concentrations actually were measured in human tissues, Schentag et al. [38] demonstrated that the kidneys account for the largest fraction of drug in the peripheral compartment.

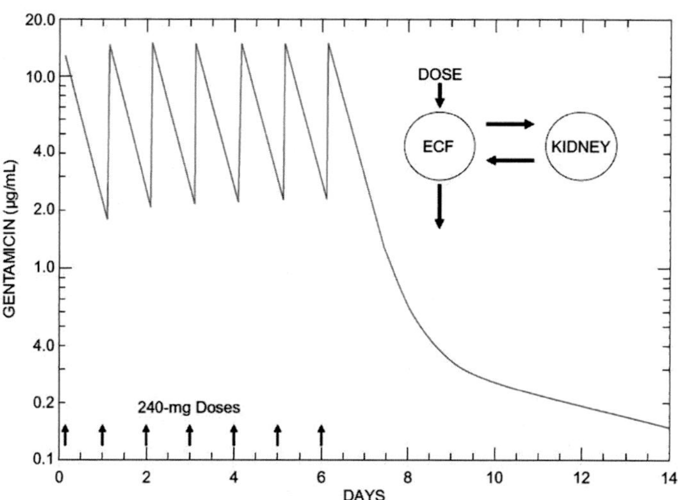

FIG. 3.6 Simulated serum gentamicin concentrations in a patient during and after a typical 1-week course of therapy (240 mg infused intravenously every 24 h). The half-life of serum levels observed during repeated dosing is primarily reflective of renal elimination. The terminal half-life seen after therapy was stopped is the actual distribution phase. *(Data were simulated with the two-compartment model shown in the figure using pharmacokinetic parameters reported by Colburn WA, Schentag JJ, Jusko WJ, Gibaldi M. A model for the prospective identification of the prenephrotoxic state during gentamicin therapy. J Pharmacokinet Biopharm 1978;6:179–186.)*

Not surprisingly, nephrotoxicity is a major concern in treating patients with aminoglycosides. However, the nephrotoxic effects of aminoglycosides exhibit *dose regimen dependency* in that daily administration of high aminoglycoside doses has been shown to be associated with a lower probability of nephrotoxicity than when the same total amount is administered more frequently [39, 40]. The physiological basis for these observations is that megalin transport is saturable at high aminoglycoside concentrations, so that renal tubular uptake is limited and toxicity is minimized with daily dosing. But even with similar dose regimens, the extent of gentamicin distribution into tissues was found to be much greater in patients who exhibited nephrotoxicity than in those whose renal function was preserved (Fig. 3.7) [41].

In technical terms, we can say that the approximation of a single-compartment model represents *misspecification* of what is really a two-compartment system for gentamicin. However, the distribution phase for this drug is not even apparent until therapy is stopped. As a result, most clinical pharmacokinetic calculations are made with the initial assumption that gentamicin distributes in a single compartment that roughly corresponds to ECF. If the dose and dose interval are kept constant, steady-state peak and trough levels can be predicted for this assumed single-compartment model simply by multiplying initial peak and trough levels by the *cumulation factor* (CF). As derived in Chapter 2,

$$CF = 1/\left(1 - e^{-k\tau}\right) \tag{3.4}$$

where k is $\ln 2/t_{1/2}$ and τ is the dosing interval. However, it can be expected that peak and trough levels will initially rise more rapidly than predicted from Eq. (3.4), reflecting the fact that some drug is accumulating in the "tissue" compartment rather than being eliminated by renal excretion. Of course, deterioration in renal function can also cause gentamicin peak and trough levels to increase, but usually this occurs only after five or more days of therapy.

An important point about drugs that exhibit flip-flop kinetics is that the terminal exponential phase usually is reached only when plasma drug levels are subtherapeutic. For this reason, the half-life corresponding to this terminal exponential phase (greater than 4 days in the example shown in Fig. 3.7) cannot be used in selecting an appropriate dosing interval. If the

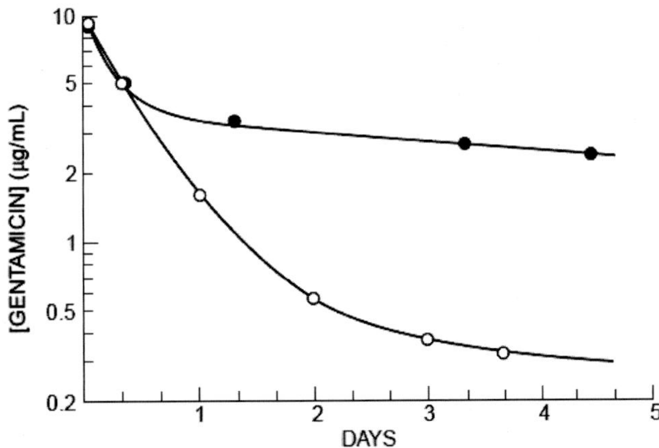

FIG. 3.7 Decline in serum gentamicin concentrations after therapy was stopped in a patient with nephrotoxicity (●) and a patient who did not have this adverse reaction (○). Both patients had been treated with gentamicin at an 8-h dosing interval and had nearly identical elimination-phase half-lives and peak and trough levels. *(Reproduced with permission from Colburn WA, Schentag JJ, Jusko WJ, Gibaldi M. A model for the prospective identification of the prenephrotoxic state during gentamicin therapy. J Pharmacokinet Biopharm 1978;6:179–186.)*

actual extent of drug accumulation is known from the ratio of steady-state/initial plasma levels, the observed cumulation factor (CF_{obs}) during repetitive dosing can be used to estimate an effective elimination rate constant (k_{eff}) by rearranging Eq. (3.4) to the form:

$$k_{eff} = \frac{1}{\tau} \ln\left(\frac{CF_{obs}}{CF_{obs} - 1}\right)$$

and the effective half-life ($t_{1/2\ eff}$) can be calculated as:

$$t_{1/2eff} = \ln 2 / k_{eff}$$

The effective half-life can then be used to design dose regimens for drugs that have a terminal exponential phase representing the disposition of only a small fraction of the total drug dose [42].

Estimating model parameters from experimental data

Derivation of equations for a two-compartment model

After rapid intravenous drug injection, sequentially measured plasma concentrations may follow a pattern similar to that shown by the solid circles in Fig. 3.8. For most drugs, the elimination phase is reached when the data points fall on the line marked "β." The distribution phase occurs prior to that time. In this case, the curve contains two exponential phases and can be described by the following sum of exponentials *data equation*:

$$C = A' e^{-\alpha t} + B' e^{-\beta t} \tag{3.5}$$

where A' and B' are the back-extrapolated intercepts, and α and β are the slopes shown in the figure. The drug concentration in the central compartment at time zero (C_0) equals the sum of $A' + B'$. For convenience in the derivation that follows, we normalize the values of these intercepts:

$$A = A' V_1 / C_0 V_1 = A' / C_0$$

$$B = B' V_1 / C_0 V_1 = B' / C_0$$

Since $A + B = 1$, the administered dose also has a normalized value of 1.

There are two exponential terms in the data equation, so the data are consistent with a two-compartment model and, because the data equation only has a total of four coefficients and exponents, the model can have only four independently identifiable parameters. In addition, the assumption usually is made that both intravenous administration and subsequent drug elimination proceed via the central compartment. Accordingly, the model is drawn as shown in Fig. 3.9. We are

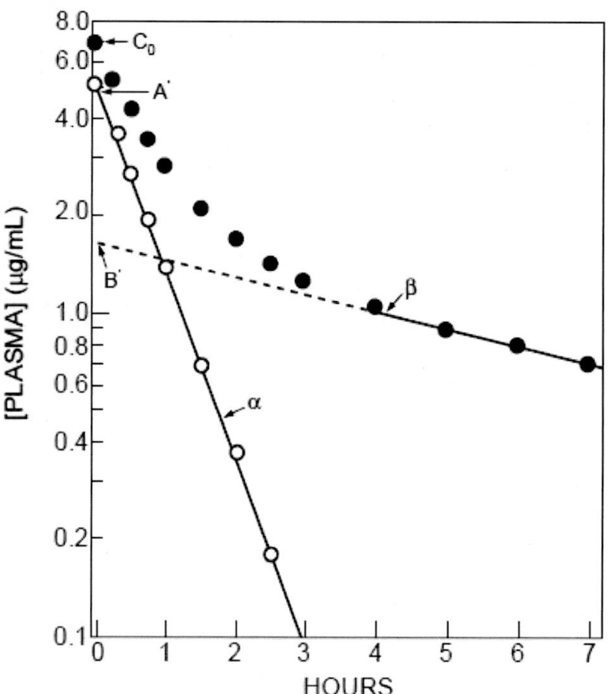

FIG. 3.8 "Curve-peeling" technique used to estimate the coefficients and exponents of Eq. (3.5). Data points (●) are plotted on semilogarithmic coordinates and the points for the α-curve (○) are obtained by subtracting back-extrapolated β-curve values from the experimental data.

FIG. 3.9 Schematic drawing of a two-compartment model with central and peripheral (Periph.) compartments. The number of primary model parameters (V_1, V_2, CL_E, and CL_I) that can be identified from the data cannot exceed the total number of coefficients and exponents in the data equation.

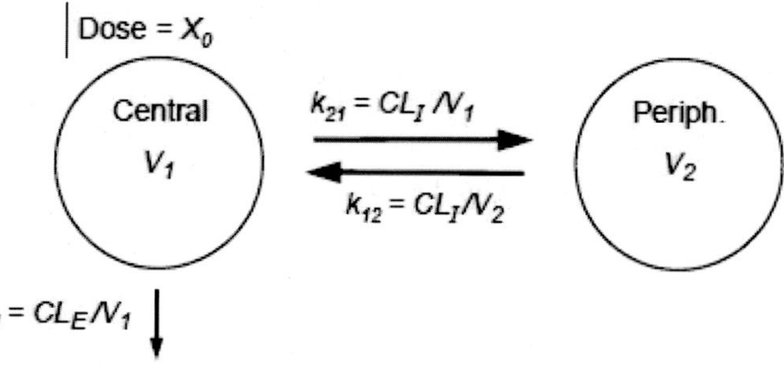

interested in obtaining values for the parameters of this model in terms of the parameters of the data equation (Eq. 3.5). Whereas the data equation is written in the concentration units of the data, the equations for the model shown in Fig. 3.9 usually are developed in terms of the amounts of drug in each compartment (X_1 and X_2), the micro-rate constants describing drug transfer between or out of compartments (k's), and a single drug dose (X_0). The model itself can be described in terms of two first-order linear differential equations (*model equations*):

$$dX_1/dt = -k_{01}X_1 - k_{21}X_1 + k_{12}X_2$$
$$dX_2/dt = k_{21}X_1 - k_{12}X_2$$

Combining terms:

$$dX_1/dt = -(k_{01} + k_{21})X_1 + k_{12}X_2$$
$$dX_2/dt = k_{21}X_1 - k_{12}X_2$$

Laplace transforms can be used to transform this system of linear differential equations in the time domain into a system of linear equations in the Laplace domain. From the table of Laplace operations (Appendix I) we obtain:

$$sX_1 - X_1(0) = -(k_{01} + k_{21})X_1 + k_{12}X_2$$
$$sX_2 - X_2(0) = k_{21}X_1 - k_{12}X_2$$

If a single drug dose is injected intravenously, the entire administered dose is initially in compartment 1 and, because of normalization, $X_1(0)$ equals 1. The amount of drug in compartment 2 at zero time [$X_2(0)$] is 0. We can now write the following nonhomogenous linear equations:

$$(s + k_{01} + k_{21})X_1 - k_{12}X_2 = 1$$
$$-k_{21}X_1 + (s + k_{12})X_2 = 0$$

The method of determinants (Cramer's Rule) can be used to solve the equations for each model compartment. However, we will focus only on the solution for the central compartment, which is the one usually sampled for concentration measurements.

$$X_1 = \frac{\begin{vmatrix} 1 & -k_{12} \\ 0 & s + k_{12} \end{vmatrix}}{\begin{vmatrix} s + k_{01} + k_{21} & -k_{12} \\ -k_{21} & s + k_{12} \end{vmatrix}}$$

$$X_1 = \frac{s + k_{12}}{s^2 + (k_{01} + k_{21} + k_{12})s + k_{01}k_{12}} \quad (3.6)$$

This solution is in the form of a quotient of two polynomials, $P(s)/Q(s)$. $Q(s)$ can be expressed in terms of its factors as follows:

$$X_1 = \frac{s + k_{12}}{(s + \alpha)(s + \beta)}$$

where the roots of the polynomial $Q(s)$ are $R_1 = -\alpha$ and $R_2 = -\beta$. The Heaviside Expansion Theorem states:

$$X_i = \sum_{i=1}^{n} \frac{P(R_i)}{Q'(R_i)} e^{R_i t}$$

Since:

$$Q(s) = s^2 + (\alpha + \beta)s + \alpha\beta \quad (3.7)$$
$$Q'(s) = 2s + \alpha + \beta$$

Therefore,

$$X_1 = \frac{k_{12} - \alpha}{-2\alpha + \alpha + \beta} e^{-\alpha t} + \frac{k_{12} - \beta}{-2\beta + \alpha + \beta} e^{-\beta t}$$

$$X_1 = \frac{k_{12} - \alpha}{\beta - \alpha} e^{-\alpha t} + \frac{k_{12} - \beta}{\alpha - \beta} e^{-\beta t} \quad (3.8)$$

In order to estimate the model parameters from the data equation, we also need to specify the rate of drug elimination from the central compartment (V_1). The rate of elimination from this compartment, dE/dt is given by the equation:

$$dE/dt = k_{01}X_1$$

So total elimination is:

$$E = k_{01} \int_0^{\infty} X_1 \, dt$$

Since E equals the administered dose, which has been normalized to 1,

$$k_{01} = \frac{1}{\int_0^{\infty} X_1 \, dt} \quad (3.9)$$

If X_1 is written in the form of the data equation (Eq. 3.5):

$$X_1 = Ae^{-\alpha t} + Be^{-\beta t} \tag{3.10}$$

We obtain,

$$\int_0^\infty X_1\,dt = -(A/\alpha)\,e^{-\alpha t} - (B/\beta)\,e^{-\beta t}\Big|_0^\infty$$

$$= A/\alpha + B/\beta$$

Substituting this result into Eq. (3.9):

$$\boxed{k_{01} = \frac{1}{A/\alpha + B/\beta}} \tag{3.11}$$

By comparing Eqs. (3.6), (3.7), it is apparent that:

$$Q(s) = s^2 + (k_{01} + k_{21} + k_{12})\,s + k_{01}k_{12}$$

So from Eq. 3.7:

$$\alpha + \beta = k_{01} + k_{21} + k_{12} \tag{3.12}$$

$$\alpha\beta = k_{01}k_{12} \tag{3.13}$$

Rearranging Eq. (3.13):

$$k_{12} = \frac{\alpha\beta}{k_{01}}$$

Substituting for k_{01} as defined by Eq. (3.11):

$$\boxed{k_{12} = \beta A + \alpha B} \tag{3.14}$$

Eq. (3.12) can be rearranged to give:

$$k_{21} = \alpha + \beta - k_{01} - k_{12}$$

$$= \alpha + \beta - \frac{\alpha\beta}{k_{12}} - k_{12}$$

$$= -\frac{k_{12}^2 - (\alpha + \beta)\,k_{12} + \alpha\beta}{k_{12}}$$

$$= -\frac{(k_{12} - \alpha)(k_{12} - \beta)}{k_{12}} \tag{3.15}$$

by comparing Eqs. (3.8), (3.10):

$$A = \frac{k_{12} - \alpha}{\beta - \alpha} \quad \text{so,} \quad k_{12} - \alpha = -A(\alpha - \beta)$$

and:

$$B = \frac{k_{12} - \beta}{\alpha - \beta} \quad \text{so,} \quad k_{12} - \beta = B(\alpha - \beta)$$

Therefore, substitution of these results into Eq. (3.15) yields a solution for k_{21}.

$$\boxed{k_{21} = \frac{AB(\alpha - \beta)^2}{k_{12}}} \tag{3.16}$$

These techniques also can be applied to develop equations for three-compartment and other commonly used pharmacokinetic models.

Calculation of rate constants and compartment volumes from data

Values for the data equation parameters can be obtained by the technique of "curve peeling" that is illustrated in Fig. 3.8. After plotting the data, the first step is to identify the terminal exponential phase of the curve, in this case termed the *β-phase*, and then back-extrapolate this line to obtain the ordinate intercept (B'). It is easiest to calculate the value of β by first calculating the half-life of this phase. The value for β then can be estimated from the relationship: $\beta = \ln 2/t_{½\beta}$. The next step is to subtract the corresponding value on the back-extrapolated β-phase line from each of the data point values obtained during the previous exponential phase. This generates the α-line from which the α-slope and A' intercept can be estimated.

After calculating the normalized intercept values A and B, the rate constants for the model can be obtained from Eqs. (3.11), (3.14), (3.16). The volume of the central compartment is calculated from the ratio of the administered dose to the back-extrapolated value for C_0 (which equals $A'+B'$) as follows:

$$V_1 = \frac{Dose}{C_0}$$

Since $k_{21} = CL_I/V_1$, and $k_{12} = CL_I/V_2$,

$$k_{21} V_1 = k_{12} V_2$$

and

$$V_2 = V_1 (k_{21}/k_{12})$$

The sum of V_1 and V_2 is termed the apparent volume of distribution at steady state ($V_{d(ss)}$) and is the third distribution volume that we have described. Note also that $CL_I = k_{21}V_1 = k_{12}V_2$.

Even though computer programs now are used routinely for pharmacokinetic analysis, most require initial estimates of the model parameters. As a result of the least-squares fitting procedures employed, these computer programs generally yield the most satisfactory results when the technique of curve peeling is used to make reasonably accurate initial estimates of parameter values.

Different estimates of apparent volume of distribution

The three estimates of distribution volume that we have encountered have slightly different properties [43]. Of the three, $V_{d(ss)}$ has the strongest physiologic rationale for multicompartment systems of drug distribution. It is independent of the rate of both drug distribution and elimination and is the volume that is referred to in Eqs. (3.1), (3.2). On the other hand, estimates of $V_{d(area)}$ are most useful in clinical pharmacokinetics, since it is this volume that links elimination clearance to elimination half-life in the equation:

$$t_{1/2} = \frac{0.693\, V_{d\,(area)}}{CL_E}$$

Because the single-compartment model implied by this equation makes no provision for the contribution of intercompartmental clearance to elimination half-life, estimates of $V_{d(area)}$ are larger than $V_{d(ss)}$.

Estimates of $V_{d(extrap)}$ are also based on a single-compartment model in which drug distribution is assumed to be infinitely fast. However, slowing of intercompartmental clearance reduces estimates of B', the back-extrapolated β-curve intercept in Fig. 3.8, to a greater extent than it prolongs elimination half-life. As a result, $V_{d(extrap)}$ calculated from the equation:

$$V_{d\,(extrap)} = Initial\ Dose / B'$$

is even larger than $V_{d(area)}$. Thus when the plasma-level-vs.-time curve includes more than a single exponential component, the relationship of the three distribution volume estimates to each other is:

$$V_{d\,(extrap)} > V_{d\,(area)} > V_{d\,(ss)}$$

References

[1] Box GEP. Robustness in the strategy of scientific model building. In: Launer RL, Wilkinson GN, editors. Robustness in statistics. New York: Academic Press; 1979. p. 231–6.

[2] Teorell T. Kinetics of distribution of substances administered to the body: I. The extravascular modes of administration. Arch Int Pharmacodyn Ther 1937;57:205–25.

[3] Price HL, Kovnat PJ, Safer JN, Conner EH, Price ML. The uptake of thiopental by body tissues and its relation to the duration of narcosis. Clin Pharmacol Ther 1960;1:16–22.

[4] Bischoff KB, Dedrick RL. Thiopental kinetics. J Pharm Sci 1968;57:1346–51.

[5] Sager JE, Yu J, Ragueneau-Majlessi I, Isoherranen N. Physiologically based pharmacokinetic (PBPK) modeling and simulation approaches: a systematic review of published models, applications and model verification. Drug Metab Dispos 2015;43:1823–37.

[6] Kuepfer L, Niederalt, Wendl T, SchlenderJ-F, Willmann S, Lippert J, et al. Applied concepts in PBPK modeling: how to build a PBPK/PD model. CPT Pharmacometrics Syst Pharmacol 2016;5:516–31.

[7] Rowland M, Peck C, Tucker G. Physiologically-based pharmacokinetics in drug development and regulatory science. Annu Rev Pharmacol Toxicol 2011;51:45–75.

[8] Huang S-M, Abernethy DR, Wang Y, Zhao P, Zineh I. The utility of modeling and simulation in drug development and regulatory review. J Pharm Sci 2013;102:2812–23.

[9] Atkinson AJ Jr, Ruo TI, Frederiksen MC. Physiological basis of multicompartmental models of drug distribution. Trends Pharmacol Sci 1991;12: 96–101.

[10] Henthorn TK, Krejcie TC, Avram MJ. Early drug distribution: a generally neglected aspect of pharmacokinetics of particular relevance to intravenously administered anesthetic agents. Clin Pharmacol Ther 2008;84:18–22.

[11] Cobelli C, Carson ER, Finkelstein L, Leaning MS. Validation of simple and complex models in physiology and medicine. Am J Physiol 1984;246: R259–66.

[12] Berman M. The formulation and testing of models. Ann N Y Acad Sci 1963;108:182–94.

[13] Dollery CT. The challenge of complexity. Clin Pharmacol Ther 2010;88:13–5.

[14] Atkinson AJ Jr. Physiological spaces and multicompartmental pharmacokinetic models. Transl Clin Pharmacol 2015;23:38–41.

[15] Larsen PR, Atkinson AJ Jr, Wellman HN, Goldsmith RE. The effect of diphenylhydantoin on thyroxine metabolism in man. J Clin Invest 1970;49:1266–79.

[16] Odeh YK, Wang Z, Ruo TI, Wang T, Frederiksen MC, Pospisil PA, Atkinson AJ Jr. Simultaneous analysis of inulin and $^{15}N_2$-urea kinetics in humans. Clin Pharmacol Ther 1993;53:419–25.

[17] Frederiksen MC, Ruo TI, Chow MJ, Atkinson AJ Jr. Theophylline pharmacokinetics in pregnancy. Clin Pharmacol Ther 1986;40:321–8.

[18] Øie S, Tozer TN. Effect of altered plasma protein binding on apparent volume of distribution. J Pharm Sci 1979;68:1203–5.

[19] Lombardo F, Shalaeva MY, Tupper KA, Gao F. ElogD$_{oct}$: a tool for lipophilicity determination in drug discovery. 2. Basic and neutral compounds. J Med Chem 2001;44:2490–7.

[20] Thummel KE, Shen DD, Isoherranen N, Smith HE. Design and optimization of dosage regimens: pharmacokinetic data. In: Bruton LL, Lazo JS, Parker KL, editors. Goodman & Gilman's the pharmacological basis of therapeutics. 11th ed. New York: McGraw-Hill; 2006. p. 1787–888.

[21] Lombardo F, Obach RS, Shalaeva MY, Gao F. Prediction of human volume of distribution values for neutral and basic drugs. 2. Extended data set and leave-class-out statistics. J Med Chem 2004;47:1242–50.

[22] Hager WD, Fenster P, Mayersohn M, Perrier D, Graves P, Marcus FI, Goldman S. Digoxin-quinidine interaction: pharmacokinetic evaluation. N Engl J Med 1979;300:1238–41.

[23] Sheiner LB, Rosenberg B, Marathe VV. Estimation of population characteristics of pharmacokinetic parameters from routine clinical data. J Pharmacokinet Biopharm 1977;5:445–79.

[24] Piergies AA, Worwag EW, Atkinson AJ Jr. A concurrent audit of high digoxin plasma levels. Clin Pharmacol Ther 1994;55:353–8.

[25] Sapirstein LA, Vidt DG, Mandel MJ, Hanusek G. Volumes of distribution and clearances of intravenously injected creatinine in the dog. Am J Physiol 1955;181:330–6.

[26] Sedek GS, Ruo TI, Frederiksen MC, Frederiksen JW, Shih S-R, Atkinson AJ Jr. Splanchnic tissues are a major part of the rapid distribution spaces of inulin, urea and theophylline. J Pharmacol Exp Ther 1989;251:963–9.

[27] Sherwin RS, Kramer KJ, Tobin JD, Insel PA, Liljenquist JE, Berman M, Andres R. A model of the kinetics of insulin in man. J Clin Invest 1974;53:1481–92.

[28] Yim D-S. "Physiological spaces and multicompartmental pharmacokinetic models": fundamentals that pharmacokinetics textbooks do not tell you. Transl Clin Pharmacol 2015;23:35–7.

[29] Renkin EM. Effects of blood flow on diffusion kinetics in isolated perfused hindlegs of cats: a double circulation hypothesis. Am J Physiol 1953;183:125–36.

[30] Stec GP, Atkinson AJ Jr. Analysis of the contributions of permeability and flow to intercompartmental clearance. J Pharmacokinet Biopharm 1981;9:167–80.

[31] Bowsher DJ, Avram MJ, Frederiksen MC, Asada A, Atkinson AJ Jr. Urea distribution kinetics analyzed by the simultaneous injection of urea and inulin: demonstration that transcapillary exchange is rate limiting. J Pharmacol Exp Ther 1984;230:269–74.

[32] Henthorn TK, Avram MJ, Frederiksen MC, Atkinson AJ Jr. Heterogeneity of interstitial fluid space demonstrated by simultaneous kinetic analysis of the distribution and elimination of inulin and gallamine. J Pharmacol Exp Ther 1982;222:389–94.
[33] Belknap SM, Nelson JE, Ruo TI, Frederiksen MC, Worwag EM, Shin S-G, Atkinson AJ Jr. Theophylline distribution kinetics analyzed by reference to simultaneously injected urea and inulin. J Pharmacol Exp Ther 1987;243:963–9.
[34] Dedrick RL, Flessner MF. Pharmacokinetic considerations on monoclonal antibodies. Prog Clin Biol Res 1989;288:429–38.
[35] Camarata SJ, Weil MH, Hanashiro PK, Shubin H. Cardiac arrest in the critically ill. I. A study of predisposing causes in 132 patients. Circulation 1971;44:688–95.
[36] Schentag JJ, Jusko WJ, Plaut ME, Cumbo TJ, Vance JW, Abrutyn E. Tissue persistence of gentamicin in man. JAMA 1977;238:327–9.
[37] Nagai J, Takano M. Molecular aspects of renal handling of aminoglycosides and strategies for preventing the nephrotoxicity. Drug Metab Pharmacokinet 2004;19:159–79.
[38] Schentag JJ, Jusko WJ, Vance JW, Cumbo TJ, Abrutyn E, DeLattre M, Gerbracht LM. Gentamicin disposition and tissue accumulation on multiple dosing. J Pharmacokinet Biopharm 1977;5:559–77.
[39] Verpooten GA, Giuliano RA, Verbist L, Eestermans G, De Broe ME. Once-daily dosing decreases renal accumulation of gentamicin and netilmicin. Clin Pharmacol Ther 1989;45:22–7.
[40] Murry KR, McKinnon PS, Mitrzyk B, Rybak MJ. Pharmacodynamic characterization of nephrotoxicity associated with once-daily aminoglycoside. Pharmacotherapy 1999;19:1252–60.
[41] Colburn WA, Schentag JJ, Jusko WJ, Gibaldi M. A model for the prospective identification of the prenephrotoxic state during gentamicin therapy. J Pharmacokinet Biopharm 1978;6:179–86.
[42] Boxenbaum H, Battle M. Effective half-life in clinical pharmacology. J Clin Pharmacol 1995;35:763–6.
[43] Gibaldi M, Perrier D. Pharmacokinetics. 2nd ed. New York: Marcel Dekker; 1982. p. 199–219.

Study problems

1. Single dose and steady-state multiple dose plasma concentration-vs.-time profiles of tolrestat, an aldose reductase inhibitor, were compared. The terminal exponential-phase half-life was 31.6h at the conclusion of multiple dose therapy administered at a 12-h dosing interval. However, there was little apparent increase in plasma concentrations with repetitive dosing and the cumulation factor, based on measurements of the area under the plasma-level-vs.-time curve (*AUC*), was only 1.29. Calculate the effective half-life for this drug (Boxenbaum H, Battle M. Effective half-life in clinical pharmacology. J Clin Pharmacol 1995;35:763–766).
2. The following data were obtained in a Phase 1 dose-escalation tolerance study after administering a 100-mg bolus of a new drug to a healthy volunteer:

Plasma concentration data

Time (h)	[Plasma] (μg/mL)
0.10	6.3
0.25	5.4
0.50	4.3
0.75	3.5
1.0	2.9
1.5	2.1
2.0	1.7
2.5	1.4
3.0	1.3
4.0	1.1
5.0	0.9
6.0	0.8
7.0	0.7

a. Use two-cycle, semilogarithmic graph paper to estimate α, β, A, and B by the technique of curve peeling.

b. Draw a two-compartment model with elimination proceeding from the central compartment (V_1). Use Eqs (3.11), (3.14), (3.16) to calculate the rate constants for this model.
c. Calculate the central compartment volume and the elimination and intercompartmental clearances for this model.
d. Calculate the volume for the peripheral compartment for the model. Sum the central and peripheral compartment volumes to obtain $V_{d(ss)}$ and compare your result with the volume estimates, $V_{d(extrap)}$ and $V_{d(area)}$, *that are based on the assumption that the* β-slope represents elimination from a one-compartment model. Comment on your comparison.

Chapter 4

Drug absorption and bioavailability

Arthur J. Atkinson, Jr.
Department of Pharmacology, Feinberg School of Medicine, Northwestern University, Chicago, IL, United States

Drug absorption

The study of drug absorption is of critical importance in developing new drugs and in establishing the therapeutic equivalence of new formulations or generic versions of existing drugs. A large number of factors can affect the rate and extent of absorption of an oral drug dose. These are summarized in Fig. 4.1.

Biopharmaceutic factors include drug solubility and formulation characteristics that impact the rate of drug disintegration and dissolution. From the physiologic standpoint, passive nonionic diffusion is the mechanism by which most drugs are absorbed once they are in solution. Absorption by passive diffusion is largely governed by the molecular size and shape, degree of ionization, and lipid solubility of a drug.

Classical explanations of the rate and extent of drug absorption have been based on the pH-partition hypothesis. According to this hypothesis, weakly acidic drugs are largely unionized and lipid soluble in acid medium, and hence should be absorbed best by the stomach. Conversely, weakly basic drugs should be absorbed primarily from the more alkaline contents of the small intestine. Absorption would not be predicted for drugs that are permanently ionized, such as quaternary ammonium compounds. In reality, the stomach does not appear to be a major site for the absorption of even acidic drugs. The surface area of the intestinal mucosa is so much greater than that of the stomach that this more than compensates for the decrease in absorption rate per unit area. Table 4.1 presents results that were obtained when the stomach and small

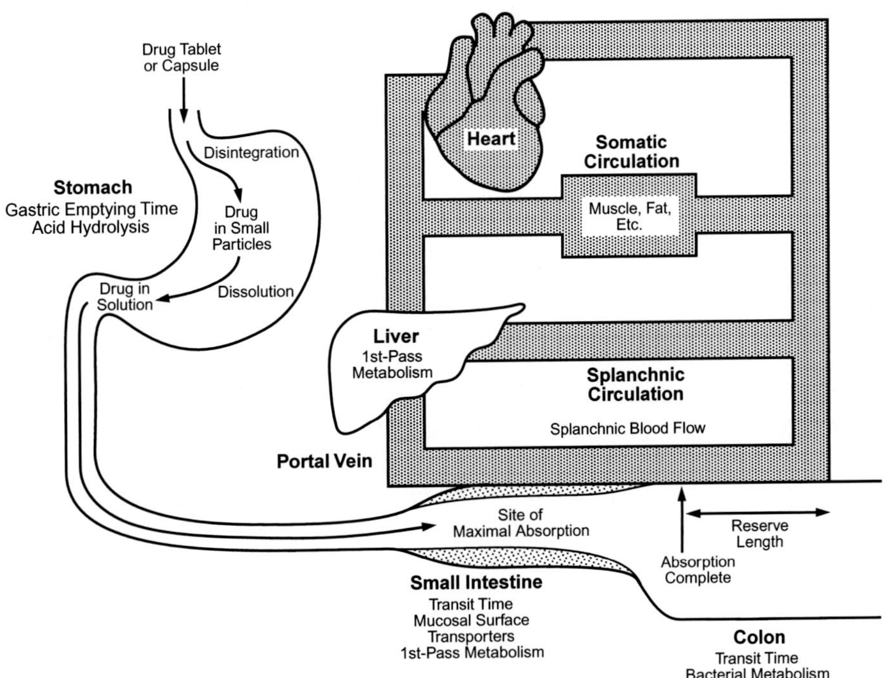

FIG. 4.1 Summary of biopharmaceutic and physiologic processes that affect the rate and extent of absorption of an orally administered drug dose. Further explanation is provided in the text.

Atkinson's Principles of Clinical Pharmacology. https://doi.org/10.1016/B978-0-12-819869-8.00027-6

TABLE 4.1 Aspirin (ASA) absorption from simultaneously perfused stomach and small intestine.

	ASA absorption (μmol/100 mg protein/h)		
pH	Stomach	Small intestine	ASA serum level (mg/100 mL)
3.5	346	469	20.6
6.5	0	424	19.7

Data from Hollander D, Dadugalza VD, Fairchild PA. Intestinal absorption of aspirin: Influence of pH, taurocholate, ascorbate, and ethanol. J Lab Clin Med 1981;98:591–598.

intestine of rats were perfused with solutions of aspirin at two different pH values [1]. Even at a pH of 3.5, gastric absorption of aspirin makes only a small contribution to the observed serum level, and the rate of gastric absorption of aspirin is less than the rate of intestinal absorption even when normalized to organ protein content. Furthermore, it is a common misconception that the pH of resting gastric contents is always 1–2 [2]. Values exceeding pH 7 may occur after meals, and achlorhydria is common in the elderly.

In addition to passive diffusion, specialized small intestine transport systems play an important role in both enhancing and reducing the intestinal absorption of some drugs [3]. Both influx and efflux transporters are located on the apical and basal membranes of enterocytes. The influx transporters belong to the solute carrier transporter superfamily. A member of this superfamily, peptide transporter protein-1 (PEPT-1), facilitates the absorption of penicillin, cephalosporin, and angiotensin-converting enzyme inhibitors. The efflux transporters belong to the adenosine triphosphate binding cassette (ABC) superfamily and are instrumental in limiting the absorption of a large number of drugs, including digoxin, verapamil, cyclosporine, and methotrexate. P-glycoprotein (P-gp) is the efflux transporter that has been studied most extensively, but multidrug resistance-associated protein 2 (MRP2) and breast cancer related protein (BCRP) are other ATP-dependent efflux transporters that limit the extent to which some drugs are absorbed [4]. In the case of sulfasalazine, this lipophilic prodrug would be expected to rapidly cross the small intestinal mucosa but it reaches its intended site of action in the colon without significant prior absorption because it is a substrate for both the MRP2 and BCRP efflux transport in the small intestine [5].

Since absorption from the stomach is poor, the rate of gastric emptying becomes a prime determinant of the rate of drug absorption. Two patterns of gastric motor activity have been identified that reflect whether the subject is fed or fasting [6]. Fasting motor activity has a cyclical pattern. Each cycle lasts 90–120 min and consists of the following three phases:

Phase 1: A period of quiescence lasting approximately 60 min.
Phase 2: A 40-min period of persistent but irregular contractions that increase in intensity as the phase progresses.
Phase 3: A short burst of intense contractions that are propagated distally from the stomach to the terminal ileum. These have been termed migrating motor complexes (MMC) or "housekeeper waves."

After feeding, the MMCs are inhibited and there is uncoupling of proximal and distal gastric motility such that the resting tone of the antrum is decreased. However, solid food stimulates intense and sustained antral contractions that reduce the particle size of gastric contents. The pylorus is partially constricted and, although liquids and particles less than 2 mm in diameter can pass through to the small bowel, larger particles are retained in the stomach. Studies employing γ-scintigraphy have confirmed that, as a result of these patterns of motor activity, a tablet taken in the fasting state will generally leave the stomach in less than 2 h but may be retained in the stomach for more than 10 h if taken following a heavy meal [7].

Slow gastric emptying may not only retard drug absorption but, in some cases, may lead to less complete drug absorption as well. Thus penicillin is degraded under acid conditions and levodopa is decarboxylated by enzymes in the gastric mucosa. Accordingly, patients should be advised to take these medications before meals. On the other hand, the prolonged gastric residence time that follows feeding may be needed to optimize the absorption of saquinavir and other drugs that are either poorly soluble or are prepared in formulations that have a slow rate of disintegration [8]. Concurrent administration of drugs that modify gastric motility may also affect drug absorption. Hence, metoclopramide stimulates gastric emptying and has been shown to increase the rate of acetaminophen absorption, whereas propantheline delays gastric emptying and retards acetaminophen absorption [9].

Transit through the small intestine is more rapid than generally has been appreciated. Small intestinal transit time averages 3 ± 1 h (±SE), is similar for large and small particles, and is not appreciably affected by fasting or fed state [10]. Rapid transit through the small intestine may reduce the absorption of compounds that either are relatively insoluble

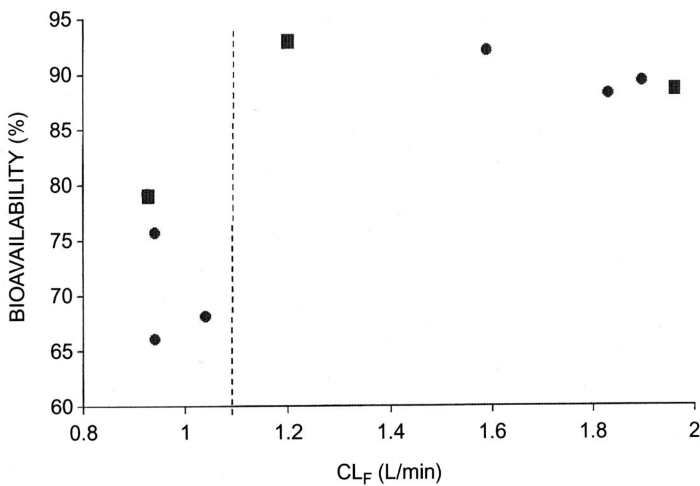

FIG. 4.2 Relationship between extent of absorption and intercompartmental clearance between the intravascular space and rapidly equilibrating splanchnic tissues (CL_F) as an indirect indicator of splanchnic blood flow. Absorption of NAPA was reduced in both healthy subjects (▪) and heart disease patients (●) when CL_F was less than 1.1 L/min (P = .0286, Fisher's exact test). *(Reproduced with permission from Atkinson AJ Jr. The stable isotope method for determining absolute bioavailability. Transl Clin Pharmacol 2017;25:53–58.)*

or are administered as extended-release formulations that have an absorption window with little reserve length. *Reserve length* is defined as the anatomical length over which absorption of a particular drug can occur, less the length at which absorption is complete (Fig. 4.1) [11]. Digoxin is an important example of a compound that has marginal reserve length. Consequently, the extent of absorption of one formulation of this drug is influenced by small bowel motility, being decreased when coadministered with metoclopramide and increased when an atropinic was given shortly before the digoxin dose [12]. Mucosal integrity of the small intestine also may affect the absorption of drugs that have little reserve length. Thus the extent of digoxin absorption was found to be less than one-third of normal in patients with D-xylose malabsorption due to sprue, surgical resection of the small intestine, or intestinal hypermotility [13].

Splanchnic blood flow may also influence the rate and extent of drug absorption but most studies of this effect have only been conducted in animals [14]. As described in Chapter 3, drug transfer between the intravascular space and splanchnic tissues can be characterized by an intercompartmental clearance (CL_F) that is partly determined by splanchnic blood flow. When the extent of *N*-acetylprocainamide (NAPA) oral absorption was studied in a small number of healthy subjects and patients with congestive heart failure, it was found, as shown in Fig. 4.2, that absorption reached a plateau of between 89% and 93% when splanchnic CL_F exceeded 1.1 L/min but fell to as low as 66% when it was lower [15]. This variation in absorption most likely reflects differences in splanchnic blood flow and the pattern is typical of the relation between absorption and flow rate reported in previous animal studies in which the extent of absorption ascends to a plateau as intestinal blood flow rates increase [16].

Metabolism by intestinal bacteria

Administered drug may be lost in transit through the intestine due to metabolism by intestinal bacteria. Most enteric bacteria reside in the large intestine, so this is seldom a problem for drugs that are rapidly and completely absorbed in the small bowel. However, at least 30 drugs have been identified as substrates for intestinal bacteria, and this is most likely to have important consequences for drugs that have minimal reserve length [17]. A variety of chemical reactions are catalyzed by bacterial enzymes but the most important are hydrolysis and reduction [18]. In Chapter 1, the conversion of the classic prodrug prontosil to its active metabolite sulfanilamide was described. It subsequently was shown that the extent of sulfanilamide formation was markedly reduced in rats which received antibiotics prior to prontosil oral administration and that little sulfanilamide was formed when prontosil was administered intravenously [19]. On this basis, it was concluded that cecal bacteria were the major site for this azoreduction reaction. Subsequently, digoxin was found to be metabolized to inactive dihydro compounds by *Eggerthella lenta* (formerly known as *Eubacterium lentum*), a constituent of normal bacterial flora in some individuals [20]. Not all individuals who had *E. lentum* colonies in their intestines inactivated digoxin, just those in whom the cardiac glycosidase reductase operon had been upregulated [21]. In contrast to the microbial specificity of cardiac glycosidase reductase, azoreductases and β-glucuronidases are more widely distributed throughout intestinal bacteria.

Drug metabolism by intestinal bacteria has been shown to also underlie some toxic drug reactions. Irinotecan is metabolized in the liver by carboxylesterases to form its active metabolite, SN-38, which is inactivated by glucuronidation before being excreted in bile. However, β-glucuronidases produced by gut bacteria hydrolyze this metabolite back to SN-38, resulting in therapy-limiting severe diarrhea [18]. Intestinal metabolism of sorivudine, an oral antiviral drug introduced in Japan to treat patients with herpes zoster, had particularly serious consequences that resulted in the death of 18 patients who were treated concurrently with the anticancer drug 5-fluorouracil (5-FU). Okuda et al. [22] found that sorivudine undergoes intestinal metabolism by *Bacteroides* species to (*E*)-5-(2-bromovinyl)-uracil (BVU), which when absorbed and further converted in the liver to dihydro-BVU, then binds covalently to and inactivates dihydropyrimidine dehydrogenase (*suicide inhibition*). Because this enzyme is primarily responsible for metabolizing 5-FU, plasma 5-FU concentrations reached toxic levels in the patients who died while being treated with these two drugs. This adverse reaction led to the withdrawal of sorivudine from the market.

On the other hand, intestinal metabolism has been beneficially exploited to target topical therapy for patients with inflammatory bowel disease. This was demonstrated first with sulfasalazine, a prodrug in which 5-aminosalicylic acid (5-ASA) is linked by an azo bond to sulfapyridine [23]. As described before, this drug is not absorbed in the small bowel but reaches the colon where azoreductase in enteric bacteria liberates 5-ASA, thus maximizing delivery of its topical antiinflammatory effects to the affected mucosa and accounting for its particular efficacy in treating patients with ulcerative colitis. However, the sulfopyridine moiety limits the tolerability of sulfasalazine, so delayed-release formulations of 5-ASA, now referred to as mesalamine, currently are used to target colonic delivery of this compound.

Presystemic elimination

Orally administered drugs also can be eliminated before reaching the systemic circulation, either through metabolism or efflux transport in their first pass through intestinal mucosal cells or after delivery by the portal circulation to the liver. Cytochrome P450 (CYP) 3A (CYP3A4+CYP3A5) accounts for 80% of the intestinal P450 content and is strategically placed at the apex of intestinal villi [24]. CYP3A4 is the predominant CYP3A cytochrome, so it plays the major role in the intestinal metabolism of drugs and other xenobiotics [25]. Studies in anhepatic patients have demonstrated that intestinal CYP3A4 may account for as much as half of the first-pass metabolism of cyclosporine that normally is observed [26]. P-gp shares considerable substrate specificity with CYP3A4 and may act in concert with intestinal CYP3A to synergistically reduce the net absorption of a variety of lipophilic drugs [3]. However, some drugs (e.g., digoxin) are substrates for P-gp but not CYP3A4 and others (e.g., midazolam) are substrates for CYP3A4 but not P-gp [4].

Marzolini et al. [27] compiled a list of drugs that are P-gp substrates, and some of these are listed in Table 4.2 along with the extent to which they are absorbed after oral administration [28]. The underlined names indicate drugs that also are known to be CYP3A4 substrates. As expected, many drugs that are combined P-gp and CYP3A4 substrates are poorly absorbed. But it is surprising that the absorption of some P-gp substrate drugs exceeds 70%. In part, this can be explained by the fact that some highly water-soluble drugs that rapidly penetrate the intestinal mucosa, and so are classified as having high membrane permeability, may saturate the P-gp transport mechanism [29], as has been shown to occur with indinavir [30]. Other drugs have also been shown to saturate CYP3A or both P-gp and CYP3A [31]. This is particularly likely to occur with drugs that are administered in greater than 100-mg doses. In addition, P-gp transport is nondestructive, so some less permeable non-CYP3A4 substrate drugs that are extruded by P-gp in the proximal small intestine may continue to be reabsorbed along the length of the intestinal tract, as shown in Fig. 4.3. This is probably the case for digoxin and would account for the fact that this drug has a limited reserve length and absorption that is affected by changes in intestinal motility. On the other hand, P-gp substrate drugs that also are CYP3A4 substrates would repeatedly be exposed to metabolism in the intestinal mucosa acting synergistically with P-gp to further reduce their absorption [3].

After intestinal absorption, some highly lipophilic drugs (e.g., cyclosporine) associate intracellularly with colloidal lipoproteins, thus enabling them to enter intestinal lymphatics and be directly transported to the systemic circulation [32]. However, the rate of portal blood flow is approximately 500-fold higher than that of intestinal lymph, so most drugs absorbed by the intestine are transported by the portal vein to the liver which represents a final barrier that they must traverse before reaching the systemic circulation. Here they enter hepatocytes, either by diffusion or carrier-mediated transport, where they may undergo further metabolism [33]. The P450 enzymes again play a major role in this stage of first-pass metabolism but the relative abundance of P450 isoforms differs from that in the intestine. For example, CYP3A accounts for only 40% of hepatic P450 content [24]. This partly accounts for the fact that intestinal metabolism is primarily responsible for the first-pass elimination of some drugs, whereas hepatic metabolism predominates for others [34]. The

TABLE 4.2 Extent of absorption (*F*) of some P-glycoprotein substrates.[a]

>70% Absorption		30%–70% Absorption		<30% Absorption	
Drug	***F*** **%**	**Drug**	***F*** **%**	**Drug**	***F*** **%**
Phenobarbital	100	Digoxin	70	Cyclosporine	28
Levofloxacin	99	Indinavir	65	Tacrolimus	25
Methadone	92	Ondansetron	62	Morphine	24
Phenytoin	90	Cimetidine	60	Verapamil	22
Methylprednisolone	82	Clarithromycin	55	Nicardipine	18
Tetracycline	77	Itraconazole	55	Sirolimus	15
		Etoposide	52	Saquinavir	13
		Amitriptyline	48	Atorvastatin	12
		Amiodarone	46	Paclitaxel	10
		Diltiazem	38	Doxorubicin	5
		Losartan	36		
		Erythromycin	35		
		Chlorpromazine	32		

[a]*Underlined drugs are also substrates for CYP3A4 (data from references [27, 28]).*

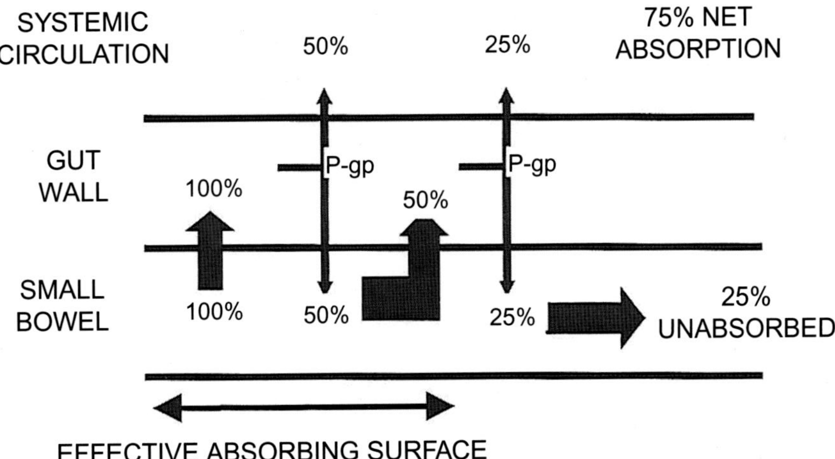

FIG. 4.3 Possible explanation for >70% absorption of some P-glycoprotein (P-gp) substrates that have a reserve length that permits repeated absorption opportunities.

products of hepatic drug metabolism and some of the unmetabolized drug are then to some extent secreted by P-gp and other transporters into the bile. In this way, some intestinally absorbed drug returns to the intestine via the biliary system, in what is termed *enterohepatic circulation* [33].

Morphine, organic nitrates, propranolol, lidocaine, and cyclosporine are some commonly used drugs that have extensive presystemic elimination. As a result, effective oral doses of these drugs are substantially higher than intravenously administered doses. Despite the therapeutic challenge that this poses for some drugs, first-pass metabolism provides important protection from some potentially noxious dietary xenobiotics. Thus hepatocytes contain monoamine oxidase that inactivates tyramine present in Chianti wine, and in cheddar and other aged cheeses. Patients treated with monoamine oxidase inhibitors lack this protective barrier. So tyramine in foods and beverages can reach the systemic circulation of these patients, causing norepinephrine release from sympathetic ganglia and potentially fatal hypertensive crises [35]. On the other hand, first-pass sulfation of swallowed isoproterenol minimizes the systemic side effects experienced by patients using isoproterenol nebulizers.

Drug-drug and food-drug interactions

In addition to their effects on gastrointestinal motility, drug-drug [36] and food-drug [37] interactions can have other effects on drug absorption. Clinically significant drug-drug interactions may affect drug absorption either by altering CYP3A or P-gp-mediated presystemic elimination [38]. Other mechanisms of drug-drug interactions may include a direct chemical interaction between drugs, for example antacids that chelate with tetracycline or complex with fluoroquinolones [39], or alterations in intestinal pH or other aspects of gastrointestinal physiology. These interactions are discussed in further detail in Chapter 14. Grapefruit juice is probably the most widely studied food that interacts with drug absorption and can inhibit CYP 3A enzymes to increase drug absorption, or with organic anion-transporting polypeptides (OATPs) to decrease drug absorption [40]. The former effect may persist for 3 days after grapefruit juice ingestion, whereas OATP inhibition is shorter lived. Obviously, the clinical consequences of this CYP3A inhibition are only of clinical relevance for drugs, such as hydroxy-3-methylglutaryl coenzyme A inhibitors (statins), that are only poorly absorbed in the absence of grapefruit juice. Fexofenadine is an example of a drug whose absorption is reduced by grapefruit juice inhibition of OATP.

Bioavailability

Bioavailability is the term most often used to characterize drug absorption. This term has been defined as the relative amount of a drug administered in a pharmaceutical product that enters the systemic circulation in an unchanged form, and the rate at which this occurs [41]. When bioavailability is reported as a percent, it only relates to the extent of absorption. Implicit in the concept of bioavailability is that a comparison is being made. If the comparison is made between an oral and an intravenous formulation of a drug, which by definition has 100% bioavailability, the *absolute bioavailability* of the drug is estimated. If the comparison is made between two different oral formulations, then the *relative bioavailability* of these formulations is determined. As shown in Fig. 4.4, three indices of a drug's oral bioavailability usually are estimated: the maximum drug concentration in plasma (C_{max}), the time needed to reach this maximum (t_{max}), and the **a**rea **u**nder the plasma or serum-concentration-vs.-time **c**urve (*AUC*). Generally, there is also an initial lag period (t_{lag}) that occurs before drug concentrations are measurable in plasma.

The *AUC* resulting from administration of a drug dose is related to the extent of drug absorption in the following way. Generalizing from the analysis of creatinine clearance that we presented in Chapter 1, the first-order differential equation describing rate of drug elimination from a single-compartment model is:

$$dE/dt = CL \cdot C$$

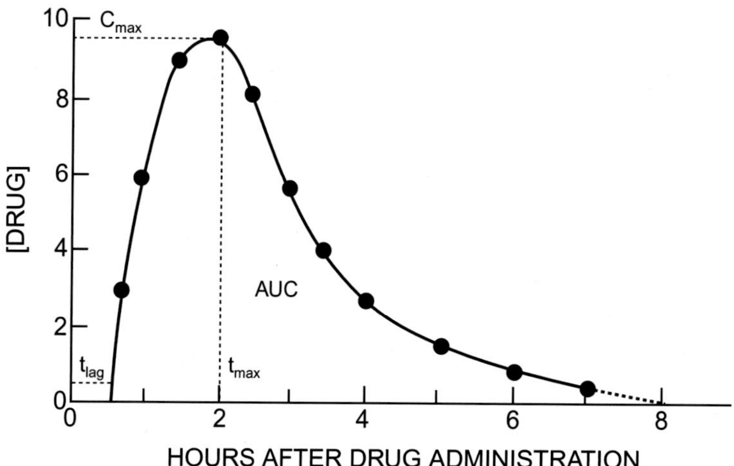

FIG. 4.4 Hypothetical plasma concentration-vs.-time curve after a single oral drug dose. Calculation of the area under the plasma level-vs.-time curve (*AUC*) requires extrapolation of the elimination phase curve beyond the last measurable plasma concentration, as shown by the *dotted line*.

where dE/dt is the rate of drug elimination, CL is the elimination clearance, and C is the concentration of drug in the compartment. Separating variables and integrating yields the result:

$$E = CL \int_0^{\infty} C\,dt \tag{4.1}$$

where E is the total amount of drug eliminated in infinite time. By mass balance, E must equal the amount of the drug dose that is absorbed. The integral is simply the AUC. Thus for an oral drug dose (D_{oral}):

$$D_{oral} \cdot F = CL \cdot AUC_{oral} \tag{4.2}$$

where F is the fraction of the dose that is absorbed and AUC_{oral} is the AUC resulting from the administered oral dose.

Absolute bioavailability

In practice, absolute bioavailability most often is estimated by sequentially administering single intravenous and oral doses (D_{IV} and D_{oral}) of a drug and comparing their respective $AUCs$. Extent of absorption of the oral dose can be calculated by modifying Eq. (4.2) as follows:

$$\%\,\text{Bioavailability} = \frac{CL \cdot D_{IV} \cdot AUC_{oral}}{CL \cdot D_{oral} \cdot AUC_{IV}} \times 100$$

$$= \frac{D_{IV} \cdot AUC_{oral}}{D_{oral} \cdot AUC_{IV}} \times 100$$

In the conventional assessment of bioavailability, a two-formulation, two-period, two-sequence crossover design is used to control for administration sequence effects. $AUCs$ frequently are estimated using the linear trapezoidal method, the log trapezoidal method, or a combination of the two [42]. Alternatively, bioavailability can be assessed by comparing the amounts of unmetabolized drug recovered in the urine after giving the drug by the intravenous and oral routes. This follows directly from Eq. (4.1), since urinary excretion accounts for a constant fraction of total drug elimination when drugs are eliminated by first-order kinetics.

In either case, the assumption usually is made that the elimination clearance of a drug remains the same in the interval between drug doses. This problem can be circumvented by administering an intravenous dose of the stable isotope-labeled drug intravenously at the same time that the test formulation of unlabeled drug is given orally. Although the feasibility of this technique was first demonstrated in normal subjects [43], the method entails only a single study and set of blood samples and is ideally suited for the efficient evaluation of drug absorption in patients, as shown for a patient with heart disease in Fig. 4.5 [44], or in specific population groups. An example of the latter was the use of the stable isotope method to assess the absolute bioavailability of a controlled-release formulation of terbutaline in eight children with asthma [45].

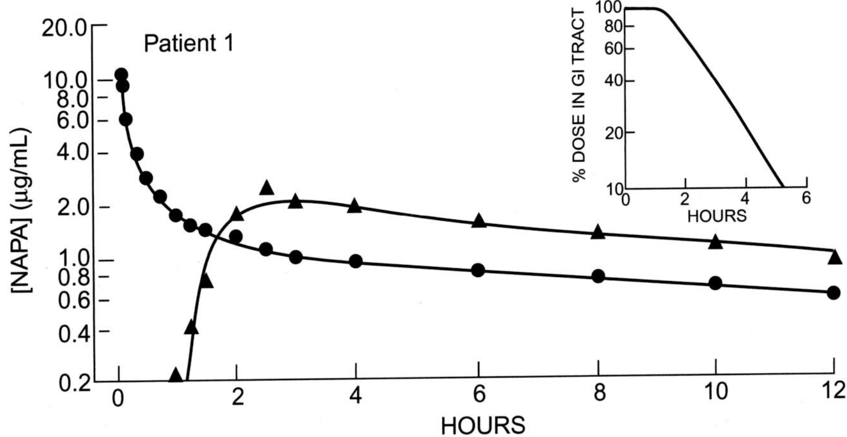

FIG. 4.5 Kinetic analysis of plasma concentrations resulting from the intravenous injection of NAPA-^{13}C (*circles*) and the simultaneous oral administration of a NAPA tablet (*triangles*). The *solid lines* are a least-squares fit of the measured concentrations shown by the data points. The calculated percentage of the oral dose remaining in the gastrointestinal (GI) tract is plotted in the insert. *(Reproduced with permission from Atkinson AJ Jr, Ruo TI, Piergies AA, Breiter HC, Connelly TJ, Sedek GS, et al. Pharmacokinetics of N-acetylprocainamide in patients profiled with a stable isotope method. Clin Pharmacol Ther 1989;46:182–189.)*

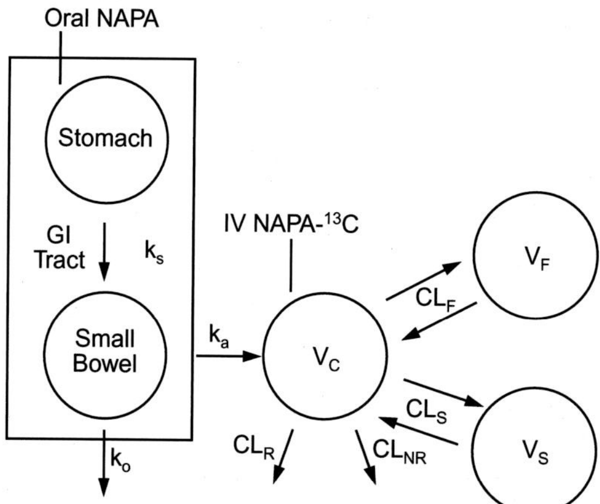

FIG. 4.6 Multicompartment system used to model the kinetics of NAPA absorption, distribution, and elimination. NAPA labeled with ^{13}C was injected intravenously (IV) to define the kinetics of NAPA disposition. NAPA distribution from intravascular space (V_C) to fast (V_F) and slow (V_S) equilibrating peripheral compartments is characterized by the intercompartmental clearances CL_F and CL_S. NAPA is cleared from the body by both renal (CL_R) and nonrenal (CL_{NR}) mechanisms. A NAPA tablet was administered orally with the intravenous dose to analyze the kinetics of NAPA absorption from the gastrointestinal (GI) tract. After an initial delay that consisted of a time lag (not shown) and presumed delivery of NAPA to the small bowel (k_s), the rate and extent of NAPA absorption were determined by k_a and k_o, as described in the text. *(Reproduced with permission from Atkinson AJ Jr, Ruo TI, Piergies AA, Breiter HC, Connelly TJ, Sedek GS, et al. Pharmacokinetics of N-acetylprocainamide in patients profiled with a stable isotope method. Clin Pharmacol Ther 1989;46:182–189.)*

In the study of *N*-acetylprocainamide (NAPA) pharmacokinetics in patients [44], a computer program employing a least-squares fitting algorithm was used to analyze that data in terms of the pharmacokinetic model shown in Fig. 4.6. The extent of NAPA absorption was calculated from model parameters representing the absorption rate (k_a) and nonabsorptive loss (k_o) from the gastrointestinal tract, as follows:

$$\% \text{Bioavailability} = \frac{k_a}{k_a + k_o} \times 100$$

The extent of absorption also was assessed by comparing the 12-h urine recovery of NAPA and NAPA-^{13}C. A correction was made to the duration of NAPA recovery to compensate for the lag in NAPA absorption that was observed after the oral dose was administered. The results of these two methods of assessing extent of absorption are compared in Table 4.3. The discrepancy was less than 2% for all but one of the patients.

TABLE 4.3 Comparison of bioavailability estimates.

Patient number	Kinetic analysis (%)	NAPA recovery in urine[a] (%)
1	66.1	65.9
2	92.1	92.1
3	68.1	69.9
4	88.2	73.1
5	75.7	75.6

[a] *Corrected for absorption lag time.*

Relative bioavailability

If the bioavailability comparison is made between two oral formulations of a drug, then their relative bioavailability is estimated. Two formulations generally are regarded as being *bioequivalent* if the 90% confidence interval of the ratios of the population average estimates of *AUC* and C_{max} for the test and reference formulations lie within a preestablished bioequivalence limit, usually 80%–125% [46]. Bioequivalence studies are needed during clinical investigation of a new drug product in order to ensure that different clinical trial formulations have similar performance characteristics. They also are required when significant manufacturing changes occur after drug approval. Following termination of marketing exclusivity, generic drugs that are introduced are expected to be bioequivalent to the innovator's product. Population average metrics of the test and reference formulations have traditionally been compared to calculate an *average bioequivalence*. However, more sophisticated statistical approaches continue to be evaluated [46].

The stable isotope method has also been used to increase the efficiency with which the relative bioavailability of two drug products can be assessed. Heck et al. [47] assessed the relative bioavailability of two imipramine tablet formulations by comparing the oral absorption of each of them with that of a coadministered stable isotope-labeled imipramine solution, used as a standard to represent optimal oral absorption. Although 12 subjects were studied, it was found that only 4–6 subjects would be required to detect a 20% difference in bioavailability, compared to the 28–36 subjects that would have been required using the conventional approach in which only the two test formulations would have been studied. Similarly, Eichelbaum et al. [48] estimated that more than 40 subjects would be required to assess the relative bioavailability of a new formulation of verapamil compared to the standard formulation, whereas only 6 subjects were needed when a solution of stable isotope labeled verapamil was coadministered as a reference standard.

Although *therapeutic equivalence* is assured if two formulations are bioequivalent, the therapeutic equivalence of two bioinequivalent formulations can be judged only within a specific clinical context [41]. Thus if we ordinarily treat streptococcal throat infections with a 10-fold excess of penicillin, a formulation having half the bioavailability of the usual formulation would be therapeutically equivalent since it still would provide a 5-fold excess of antibiotic. On the other hand, bioinequivalence of cyclosporine formulations, and of other drugs that have a narrow therapeutic index, could have serious therapeutic consequences.

In vitro prediction of bioavailability

Insufficient time and resources are available during drug discovery to conduct formal in vivo kinetic studies for each candidate compound that is screened. Consequently, there is a clear need to develop in vitro methods that can be integrated into biological screening processes as reliable predictors of bioavailability. For reformulation or generic formulations of some immediate-release compounds it even is possible that in vitro data will suffice and that the regulatory requirement for repeated in vivo studies can be waived [49].

The theoretical basis for waiving in vivo studies is a system of drug classification that focuses on three critical biopharmaceutical properties: the solubility and dissolution rate of the drug formulation, and the intestinal permeability of the drug [50]. A drug is considered to be *highly soluble* when the maximum strength drug dose can be completely dissolved in 250mL of water within a pH range of 1–6.8 at $37 \pm 1°C$ [49]. Dissolution is assessed in vitro using a standard apparatus and dissolution medium that are appropriately based on the physical chemistry of the drug and on the dosage form being evaluated [51]. For immediate-release products, a dissolution specification of at least 85% dissolved within 30min is considered sufficient to exclude dissolution-rate limitations to bioavailability [49]. Permeability is assessed either through studies of absolute bioavailability or mass balance after oral drug administration to humans. Drugs are considered highly permeable if the extent of oral absorption is $\geq$85% [49]. In some cases, in situ animal and in vitro cell culture methods can be used for this purpose. Based on these considerations, the following biopharmaceutic drug classification system (BCS) was established [49, 50].

Class 1—High solubility-high permeability drugs: Drugs in this class are well absorbed but their bioavailability may be limited either by first-pass metabolism or by P-gp-mediated efflux from the intestinal mucosa. In vitro-in vivo correlations of dissolution rate with the rate of drug absorption are expected if dissociation is slower than gastric emptying rate. If dissociation is sufficiently rapid, gastric emptying will limit absorption rate.

Class 2—Low solubility-high permeability drugs: Poor solubility may limit the extent of absorption of high drug doses. The rate of absorption is limited by dissolution rate and generally is slower than for drugs in Class 1. In vitro-in vivo correlations are tenuous in view of the many formulation and physiological variables that can affect the dissolution profile.

Class 3—High solubility-low permeability drugs: Intestinal permeability limits both the rate and extent of absorption for this class of drugs and intestinal reserve length may be marginal. Bioavailability is expected to be variable but, if dissolution is at least 85% complete within 30min, this variability will reflect differences in physiological variables such as intestinal permeability and intestinal transit time.

Class 4—Low solubility-low permeability drugs: Effective oral delivery of this class of drugs presents the most difficulties, and reliable in vitro-in vivo correlations are not expected.

As described in an account of the evolution of the BCS, the Food and Drug Administration (FDA) initially waived the need for repeated human bioavailability and bioequivalence testing of Class 1 drugs provided the drug product was rapidly dissolving [52]. A similar exception was subsequently made for Class 3 drugs with the added stipulation that excipients in these formulations be qualitatively the same and quantitatively similar to those in the original formulation [49].

Although the BCS was primarily developed for regulatory applications, it has increasingly been found useful in assisting the selection and development of new drug candidates [53]. The rapid evaluation of the intestinal membrane permeability of drugs represents a continuing challenge. Human intubation studies have been used to measure jejunal effective permeability of a number of drugs, and these measurements have been compared with the extent of drug absorption. It can be seen from Fig. 4.7 that the expected fraction absorbed exceeds 95% for drugs with a jejunal permeability of more than 2.4×10^{-4} cm/s [50]. Although human intubation studies are even more laborious than formal assessment of absolute bioavailability, they have played an important role in validating animal, in vitro, and in silico methods that have been developed [54]. In situ single pass and recirculating perfusion studies in rats gave results that agreed most closely with human permeability studies but do not lend themselves to high-throughput screening. The second best correlations were obtained with a commonly used in vitro method, based on measurement of drug transfer across a monolayer of cultured Caco-2 cells derived from a human colorectal carcinoma. Artursson and Karlsson [55] found that the apparent permeability of 20 drugs measured with the Caco-2 cell model was well correlated with the extent of drug absorption in human subjects, and that drugs with permeability coefficients exceeding 1×10^{-6} cm/s were completely absorbed (Fig. 4.8). However, Caco-2 cells, being derived from colonic epithelium, have less paracellular permeability than jejunal mucosa, and the activity of drug-metabolizing enzymes, transporters, and efflux mechanisms in these cells does not always reflect what is encountered in vivo. In addition, the Caco-2 cell model provides no assessment of the extent of hepatic first-pass metabolism. Despite these shortcomings, this in vitro model has been useful in high-throughput biological screening programs. Cabrera-Pérez et al. [54] found that current in silico estimates of permeability showed the poorest correlation with human permeability studies but improvements in this methodology can be expected and further discussion of this approach is provided in Chapter 31.

Several alternative methods have been proposed to characterize drug permeability. Thus Wu and Benet [56] observed that Class 1 and 2 drugs are mainly eliminated by metabolism, whereas Class 3 and 4 drugs are mainly eliminated by biliary or renal excretion of unchanged drug. On this basis they proposed an alternate biopharmaceutics drug disposition classification system (BDDCS) in which permeability is replaced by predominant route of elimination, initially defined as ≥70% but later ≥90% of an oral dose in humans [56,57]. Wu and Benet [56] also predicted that transporter effects would be minimal for BDDCS Class 1 drugs but would predominate for Class 2 drugs, that absorptive transporters would be necessary for Class 3

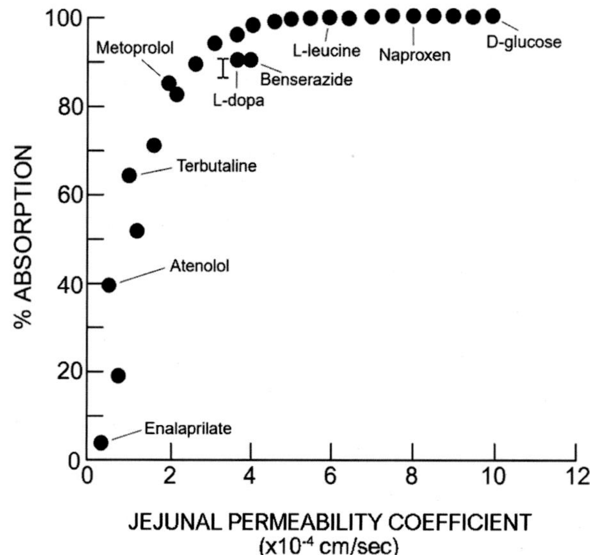

FIG. 4.7 Relationship between jejunal permeability measured by intestinal intubation and extent of absorption of a series of compounds. *(Reproduced with permission from Amidon GL, Lennernäs H, Shah VP, Crison JR. A theoretical basis for a biopharmaceutic drug classification: the correlation of* in vitro *drug product dissolution and* in vivo *bioavailability. Pharm Res 1995;12:413–420.)*

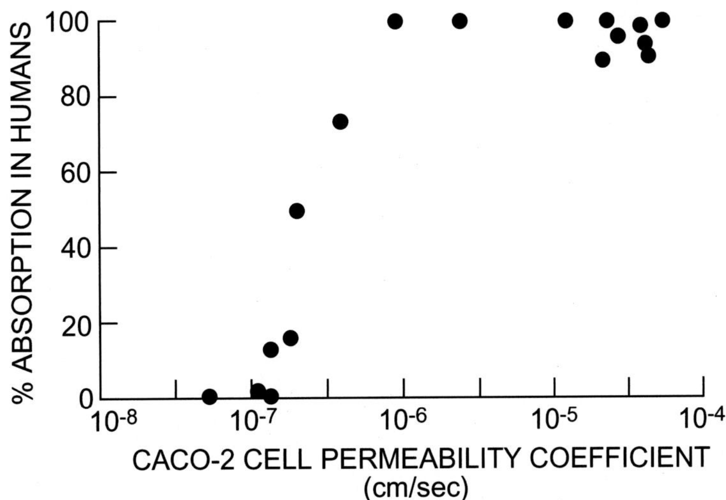

FIG. 4.8 Relationship for a series of 20 compounds between apparent permeability coefficients in a Caco-2 cell model and the extent of absorption after oral administration to humans. *(Reproduced with permission from Artursson P, Karlsson J. Correlation between oral drug absorption in humans and apparent drug permeability coefficients in human intestinal epithelial (Caco-2) cells. Biochem Biophys Res Commun 1991;175:880–885.)*

drugs, and that no Class 4 compounds would become effective drugs. Additional predictions also were made regarding the effects of food on the bioavailability of these different drug classes. The utility of the BDDCS classification stems from the fact that the extent to which a drug is metabolized is routinely assessed during the early course of drug development.

Kinetics of drug absorption after oral administration

Pharmacokinetic analysis of a continuous intravenous drug infusion is presented at the end of the chapter as a study problem and attention here is focused on oral administration. After an oral dose, some time passes before any drug appears in the systemic circulation. This lag time (t_{lag}) reflects the time required for disintegration and dissolution of the drug product, and the time for the drug to reach the absorbing surface of the small intestine. After this delay, the plasma-drug-concentration-vs.-time curve shown in Fig. 4.4 reflects the combined operation of the processes of drug absorption and of drug distribution and elimination. The peak concentration, C_{max}, is reached when drug entry into the systemic circulation no longer exceeds drug removal by distribution to tissues, metabolism, and excretion. Thus drug absorption is not completed when C_{max} is reached.

In Chapters 2 and 3 we analyzed the kinetic response to a bolus intravenous injection of a drug, an input that can be represented by a single impulse. Similarly, the input resulting from administration of an oral or intramuscular drug dose, or a constant intravenous infusion, can be regarded as a series of individual impulses, $G(\theta)d\theta$, where $G(\theta)$ describes the rate of absorption over a time increment between θ and $\theta+d\theta$. If the system is linear and the parameters are time invariant [58], we can think of the plasma response [$X(t)$] observed at time t as resulting from the sum or integral over each absorption increment occurring at prior time θ [$G(\theta)d\theta$ where $0 \leq \theta \leq t$] reduced by the fractional drug disposition that occurs between θ and t [$H(t-\theta)$], that is:

$$X(t) = \int_0^t G(\theta) \cdot H(t-\theta)d\theta$$

The function $H(t)$ describes drug disposition after intravenous bolus administration of a unit dose at time t. The interplay of these functions and associated physiological processes is represented schematically in Fig. 4.9. This expression for $X(t)$ is termed the *convolution* of $G(t)$ and $H(t)$ and can be represented as:

$$X(t) = G(t)*H(t)$$

where the operation of convolution is denoted by the symbol $*$. The operation of convolution in the time domain corresponds to multiplication in the domain of the subsidiary algebraic equation given by Laplace transformation. Thus in Laplace transform notation:

$$x(s) = g(s) \cdot h(s)$$

ABSORPTION | DISTRIBUTION & ELIMINATION | DRUG IN PLASMA

Absorption Function $G(t)$ → Disposition Function $H(t)$ → Output Function $X(t)$

FIG. 4.9 The processes of drug absorption and disposition (distribution and elimination) interact to generate the observed time course of drug in the body. Similarly, the output function can be represented as an interaction between absorption and disposition functions.

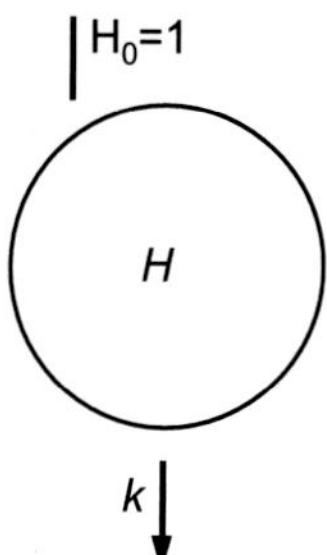

FIG. 4.10 Disposition model representing the elimination of a unit impulse drug dose ($H_0 = 1$) from a single body compartment. Drug in this compartment (H) is removed as specified by the first-order elimination rate constant k.

In the disposition model shown in Fig. 4.10, the kinetics of drug distribution and elimination are represented by a single compartment with first-order elimination as described by the equation:

$$dH/dt = -kH$$

Since:

$$\mathcal{L}F(t) = f(s)$$

and:

$$\mathcal{L}F'(t) = sf(s) - F_0$$

$$sh(s) - H_0 = -kh(s)$$

H_0 is a unit impulse function, so $h(s)$ is given by:

$$h(s) = \frac{1}{s+k} \tag{4.3}$$

Although the process of oral absorption is quite complex, it often follows simple first-order kinetics. To obtain the appropriate absorption function, consider absorption under circumstances where there is no elimination [59]. This can be diagrammed as shown in Fig. 4.11. In this absorption model, drug disappearance from the gut is described by the equation:

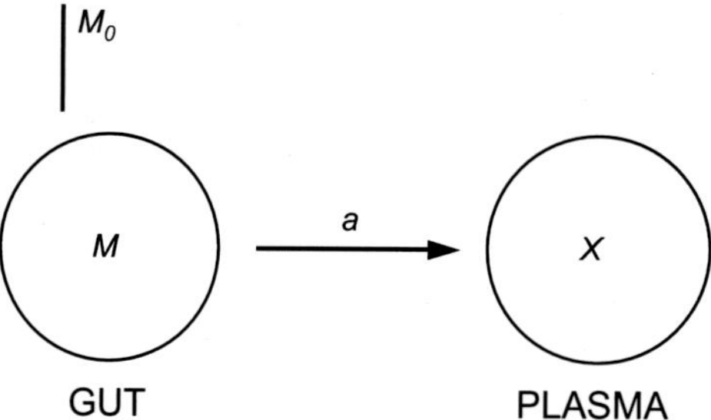

FIG. 4.11 Model representing the absorption of a drug dose (M_0) from a gut compartment to a plasma compartment. The first-order absorption constant a determines the rate at which drug remaining in the gut (M) is transferred to plasma (X).

$$\frac{dM}{dt} = -aM$$

So:

$$M = M_0 e^{-at}$$

But the rate of drug appearance in plasma is:

$$\frac{dX}{dt} = aM$$

The absorption function is defined as this appearance rate, so $G(t)$ is:

$$G(t) = aM_0 e^{-at}$$

By the definition in Appendix I, Table I.1:

$$g(s) = \int_0^\infty G(t)e^{-st}dt$$

So:

$$g(s) = aM_0 \int_0^\infty e^{-at}e^{-st}dt$$

$$g(s) = -\frac{aM_0}{s+a} e^{-(s+a)t} \Big|_0^\infty$$

Therefore:

$$g(s) = \frac{aM_0}{s+a} \tag{4.4}$$

Multiplication of Eq. (4.4) by Eq. (4.3) gives:

$$x(s) = g(s) \cdot h(s) = \frac{aM_0}{s+a} \cdot \frac{1}{s+k}$$

and

$$X(t) = \mathscr{L}^{-1} \frac{aM_0}{(s+a)(s+k)}$$

The table of inverse Laplace transforms (Appendix I, Table I.2) shows that there are two solutions for this equation. Usually, $a \neq k$ and:

$$X(t) = \frac{aM_0}{k-a}\left(e^{-at} - e^{-kt}\right) \tag{4.5}$$

In the special case, where $a = k$:

$$X(t) = aM_0 te^{-kt} \tag{4.6}$$

Time to peak level

The time needed to reach the peak level (t_{max}) can be determined by differentiating $X(t)$. For $a \neq k$:

$$X'(t) = \left[\frac{aM_0}{k-a}\right]\left(-ae^{-at} + ke^{-kt}\right)$$

At the peak level, $X'(t) = 0$. Therefore:

$$k e^{-kt_{max}} = a e^{-at_{max}} \tag{4.7}$$

$$a/k = e^{(a-k)t_{max}}$$

and

$$t_{max} = \frac{1}{a-k} \ln(a/k) \tag{4.8}$$

The absorption half-life is another kinetic parameter that can be calculated as $\frac{\ln 2}{a}$.

Value of peak level

The value of the peak level (C_{max}) can be estimated by substituting the value for t_{max} back into the equation for $X(t)$. For $a \neq k$, we can use Eq. (4.7) to obtain:

$$e^{-at_{max}} = \frac{k}{a} e^{-kt_{max}}$$

Substituting this result into Eq. (4.5):

$$X_{max} = \frac{aM_0}{k-a}\left(\frac{k}{a} - 1\right) e^{-kt_{max}}$$

Hence:

$$X_{max} = M_0 e^{-kt_{max}}$$

But from Eq. (4.8):

$$-kt_{max} = \frac{k}{k-a} \ln(a/k)$$

So:

$$e^{-kt_{max}} = (a/k)^{k/(k-a)}$$

Therefore:

$$X_{max} = M_0 (a/k)^{k/(k-a)} \tag{4.9}$$

The maximum plasma concentration would then be given by: $C_{max} = X_{max}/V_d$, where V_d is the distribution volume. It can be seen from Eqs. (4.8) and (4.9) that C_{max} and t_{max} are complex functions of both the absorption rate, a, and the elimination rate, k, of a drug.

Use of convolution/deconvolution to assess in vitro-in vivo correlations

Particularly for extended-release formulations, the simple characterization of drug absorption in terms of AUC, C_{max}, and t_{max} is inadequate and a more comprehensive comparison of in vitro test results with in vivo drug absorption is needed [60]. Both $X(t)$, the output function after oral absorption, and $H(t)$, the disposition function, can be obtained from experimental data and the absorption function, $G(t)$, estimated by the process of *deconvolution*. This process is the inverse of convolution and, in the Laplace domain, $g(s)$ can be obtained by dividing the transform of the output function, $x(s)$, by the transform of the disposition function, $h(s)$:

$$g(s) = \frac{x(s)}{h(s)}$$

Since this approach requires that $X(t)$ and $H(t)$ be defined by explicit functions, deconvolution is usually performed using numerical methods [61]. Alternatively, the absorption function can be obtained from a pharmacokinetic model, as shown by

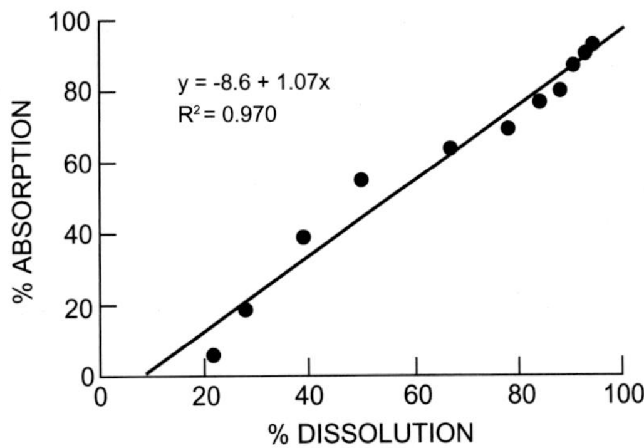

FIG. 4.12 Linear regression comparing the extent of drug dissolution and oral absorption at common time points. *(Reproduced with permission from Rackley RJ. Examples of* in vitro-in vivo *relationships with a diverse range of quality. In: Young D, Devane JG, Butler J, editors.* In vitro-in vivo *correlations. New York: Plenum Press; 1997, p. 1–15.)*

the insert in Fig. 4.5 [44]. Even when this approach is taken, numerical deconvolution methods may be helpful in developing the appropriate absorption model [43]. As a second step in the analysis, linear regression commonly is used to compare the time course of drug absorption with dissolution test results at common time points, as shown in Fig. 4.12 [62]. The linear relationship in this figure, with a slope and a coefficient of determination (R^2) of nearly one, would be expected primarily for Class 1 drugs. The nonzero intercept presumably reflects the time lag in gastric emptying.

Another approach is to convolute a function representing in vitro dissolution with the disposition function in order to predict the plasma-level-vs.-time curve following oral drug administration. Obviously, correlations will be poor if there is substantial first-pass metabolism of the drug or if in vivo conditions, such as rapid intestinal transit that results in inadequate reserve length, are not reflected in the dissolution test system.

References

[1] Hollander D, Dadugalza VD, Fairchild PA. Intestinal absorption of aspirin: influence of pH, taurocholate, ascorbate, and ethanol. J Lab Clin Med 1981;98:591–598.

[2] Meldrum SJ, Watson BW, Riddle HC, Sladen GE. pH profile of gut as measured by radiotelemetry capsule. Br Med J 1972;2:104–106.

[3] Estudante M, Morais JG, Soveral G, Benet LZ. Intestinal drug transporters: an overview. Adv Drug Deliv Rev 2013;65:1340–1356.

[4] Takano M, Yumoto R, Murakami T. Expression and function of efflux drug transporters in the intestine. Pharmacol Ther 2006;109:137–161.

[5] Dahan A, Amidon GL. Small intestinal efflux mediated by MRP2 and BCRP shifts sulfasalazine intestinal permeability from high to low, enabling its colonic targeting. Am J Physiol Gastrointest Liver Physiol 2009;297:G371–G377.

[6] Van Den Abeele J, Rubbens J, Brouwers J, Augustijns P. The dynamic gastric environment and its impact on drug and formulation behaviour. Eur J Pharm Sci 2017;96:207–231.

[7] Wilding IR, Coupe AJ, Davis SS. The role of γ-scintigraphy in oral drug delivery. Adv Drug Deliv Rev 1991;7:87–117.

[8] Kenyon CJ, Brown F, McClelland, Wilding IR. The use of pharmacoscintigraphy to elucidate food effects observed with a novel protease inhibitor (saquinavir). Pharm Res 1998;15:417–422.

[9] Nimmo J, Heading RC, Tothill P, Prescott LF. Pharmacological modification of gastric emptying: effects of propantheline and metoclopramide on paracetamol absorption. Br Med J 1973;1:587–589.

[10] Davis SS, Hardy JG, Fara JW. Transit of pharmaceutical dosage forms through the small intestine. Gut 1986;27:886–892.

[11] Higuchi WI, Ho NFH, Park JY, Komiya I. Rate-limiting steps in drug absorption. In: Prescott LF, Nimmo WS, editors. Drug absorption. Sydney: ADIS Press; 1981. p. 35–60.

[12] Manninen V, Melin J, Apajalahti A, Karesoja M. Altered absorption of digoxin in patients given propantheline and metoclopramide. Lancet 1973;1:398–399.

[13] Heizer WD, Smith TW, Goldfinger SE. Absorption of digoxin in patients with malabsorption syndromes. N Engl J Med 1971;285:257–259.

[14] Winne D. Influence of blood flow on intestinal absorption of drugs and nutrients. Pharmacol Ther 1979;6:333–393.

[15] Atkinson AJ Jr. The stable isotope method for determining absolute bioavailability. Transl Clin Pharmacol 2017;25:53–58.

[16] Schulz R, Winne D. Relationship between antipyrine absorption and blood flow rate in rat jejunum, ileum, and colon. Nauyn Schmiedebergs Arch Pharmacol 1987;335:97–102.

[17] Sousa T, Paterson R, Moore V, Carlsson A, Abrahamsson B, Basit AW. The gastrointestinal microbiota as a site for the biotransformation of drugs. Int J Pharm 2008;363:1–25.

[18] Klaassen CD, Cui JY. Review: mechanisms of how the intestinal microbiota alters the effects of drugs and bile acids. Drug Metab Dispos 2015;43:1505–1521.

[19] Gingell R, Bridges JW. Intestinal azo reduction and glucuronide conjugation of prontosil. Biochem J 1971;125:24P.

[20] Dobkin JF, Saha JR, Butler VP Jr, Neu HC, Lindenbaum J. Digoxin-inactivating bacteria: identification in human gut flora. Science 1983;220: 325–327.

[21] Haiser HJ, Seim KL, Balskus E, Turnbaugh PJ. Mechanistic insight into digoxin inactivation by *Eggerthella lenta* augments our understanding of its pharmacokinetics. Gut Microbes 2014;5:233–238.

[22] Okuda H, Ogura K, Kato A, Takubo H, Watabe T. A possible mechanism of eighteen patient deaths caused by interactions of sorivudine, a new antiviral drug, with oral 5-fluorouracil prodrugs. J Pharmacol Exp Ther 1998;287:791–799.

[23] Kao J, Kwak K, Das KM. Introducing and maintaining remission in ulcerative colitis: role of high-dose, extended-release mesalamine. J Clin Gastroenterol 2010;44:531–535.

[24] Paine MF, Haart HL, Ludington SS, Haining RL, Rettie AE, Zeldin DC. The human intestinal cytochrome P450 "pie". Drug Metab Dispos 2006;34:880–886.

[25] Doherty MM, Charman WN. The mucosa of the small intestine. How clinically relevant as an organ of drug metabolism? Clin Pharmacokinet 2002;41:235–253.

[26] Kolars JC, Merion RM, Awni WM, Watkins PB. First-pass metabolism of cyclosporine by the gut. Lancet 1991;338:1488–1490.

[27] Marzolini C, Paus E, Buclin T, Kim R. Polymorphisms in human MDR1 (P-glycoprotein): recent advances and clinical relevance. Clin Pharmacol Ther 2004;75:13–33.

[28] Thummel KE, Shen DD, Isoherranen N, Smith HE. Design and optimization of dosage regimens: pharmacokinetic data. In: Bruton LL, Lazo JS, Parker KL, editors. Goodman & Gilman's The pharmacological basis of therapeutics. 11th ed. New York: McGraw-Hill; 2006. p. 1787–1788.

[29] Cao X, Yu LX, Barbaciru C, Landowski CP, Shin H-C, Gibbs S, et al. Permeability dominates in vivo intestinal absorption of P-gp substrate with high solubility and high permeability. Mol Pharm 2005;4:329–340.

[30] Yeh KC, Stone JA, Carides AD, Rolan P, Woolf E, Ju WD. Simultaneous investigation of indinavir nonlinear pharmacokinetics and bioavailability in healthy volunteers using stable isotope labeling technique: study design and model-independent data analysis. J Pharm Sci 1999;88:568–573.

[31] Takano J, Maeda K, Bolger MB, Sugiyama Y. The prediction of the relative importance of CY3A/P-glycoprotein to the nonlinear intestinal absorption of drugs by advanced compartmental absorption and transit model. Drug Metab Dispos 2016;44:1808–1816.

[32] Porter JH, Trevaskis NL, Charman WN. Lipids and lipid-based formulations: optimizing the oral delivery of lipophilic drugs. Nat Rev Drug Discov 2007;6:231–248.

[33] Roberts MS, Magnusson BM, Burczynski FJ, Weiss M. Enterohepatic circulation. Clin Pharmacokinet 2002;41:751–790.

[34] Routledge PA, Shand DG. Presystemic drug elimination. Annu Rev Pharmacol Toxicol 1979;19:447–468.

[35] Lippman SB, Nash K. Monoamine oxidase inhibitor update. Potential adverse food and drug interactions. Drug Saf 1990;5:195–204.

[36] Welling PG. Interactions affecting drug absorption. Clin Pharmacokinet 1984;9:404–434.

[37] Dong J, Zhu X, Chen Z, Chun HF, Kwan HS, Wong CH, et al. A review of food-drug interactions on oral drug absorption. Drugs 2017;77:1833–1855.

[38] Lin JH. Drug-drug interaction mediated by inhibition and induction of P-glycoprotein. Adv Drug Deliv Rev 2003;55:53–81.

[39] Ogawa R, Echizen H. Clinically significant drug interactions with antacids: an update. Drugs 2011;21:1839–1864.

[40] Hanley MJ, Cancalon P, Widmer WW, Greenblatt DJ. The effect of grapefruit juice on drug disposition. Expert Opin Drug Metab Toxicol 2011;7:267–286.

[41] Koch-Weser J. Bioavailability of drugs. N Engl J Med 1974;291:233–237. 503–506.

[42] Yeh KC, Kwan KC. A comparison of numerical integrating algorithms by trapezoidal, Lagrange, and spline approximation. J Pharmacokinet Biopharm 1978;6:79–98.

[43] Strong JM, Dutcher JS, Lee W-K, Atkinson AJ Jr. Absolute bioavailability in man of N-acetylprocainamide determined by a novel stable isotope method. Clin Pharmacol Ther 1975;18:613–622.

[44] Atkinson AJ Jr, Ruo TI, Piergies AA, Breiter HC, Connelly TJ, Sedek GS, et al. Pharmacokinetics of N-acetylprocainamide in patients profiled with a stable isotope method. Clin Pharmacol Ther 1989;46:182–189.

[45] Fuglsang G, Hertz B, Holm EB, Borgström. Absolute bioavailability of terbutaline from a CR-granulate in asthmatic children. Biopharm Drug Dispos 1990;11:85–90.

[46] Cristofoletti R, Rowland M, Lesko LJ, Blume H, Rostami-Hodjegan A, Dressman JB. Past, present and future of bioequivalence: improving assessment and extrapolation of therapeutic equivalence for oral drug products. J Pharm Sci 2018;107:2519–2530.

[47] Heck Hd'A, Buttrill SE Jr, Flynn NW, Dyer RL, Anbar M, Cairns T, et al. Bioavailability of imipramine tablets relative to a stable isotope-labeled internal standard: increasing the power of bioavailability tests. J Pharmacokinet Biopharm 1979;7:233–247.

[48] Eichelbaum M, von Unruh GE, Somogy A. Application of stable isotope labeled drugs in clinical pharmacokinetic investigations. Clin Pharmacokinet 1982;7:490–507.

[49] Biopharmaceutic Classification Working Group, Biopharmaceutics Coordinating Committee, CDER. Waiver of *in vivo* bioavailability and bioequivalence studies for immediate-release solid oral dosage forms based on a biopharmaceutics classification system, In: Guidance for industry. Silver Spring, MD: FDA; 2017 Available from: http://www.fda.gov/downloads/Drugs/GuidanceComplianceRegulatoryInformation/Guidances/UCM070246.pdf.

[50] Amidon GL, Lennernäs H, Shah VP, Crison JR. A theoretical basis for a biopharmaceutic drug classification: the correlation of *in vitro* drug product dissolution and *in vivo* bioavailability. Pharm Res 1995;12:413–420.

[51] Rohrs BR, Skoug JW, Halstead GW. Dissolution assay development for *in vitro-in vivo* correlations: theory and case studies. In: Young D, Devane JG, Butler J, editors. *In vitro-in vivo* correlations. New York: Plenum Press; 1997. p. 17–30.

[52] Amidon GL, Shah VP. *Commentary on* G.L. Amidon, H. Lennernäs, V.P. Shah, and J.R. Crison. A theoretical basis for a biopharmaceutic drug classification: the correlation of *in vitro* drug product dissolution and *in vivo* bioavailability, Pharm Res 12,413-420, 1995 – backstory of BCS. AAPS J 2014;16:894–898.

[53] Lennernäs H, Abrahamsson B. The use of biopharmaceutic classification of drugs in drug discovery and development: current status and future extension. J Pharm Pharmacol 2005;57:273–285.

[54] Cabrera-Pérez MÁ, Pham-The H, Cervera MF, Hernández-Armengol R, Miranda-Pérez de Alejo C, Brito-Ferrer Y. Integrating theoretical and experimental permeability estimations for provisional biopharmaceutical classification: application to the WHO essential medicines. Biopharm Drug Dispos 2018;39:354–368.

[55] Artursson P, Karlsson J. Correlation between oral drug absorption in humans and apparent drug permeability coefficients in human intestinal epithelial (Caco-2) cells. Biochem Biophys Res Commun 1991;175:880–885.

[56] Wu C-Y, Benet LZ. Predicting drug disposition via application of BCS: transport/absorption/elimination interplay and the development of a biopharmaceutics drug disposition classification system. Pharm Res 2005;22:11–23.

[57] Benet LZ, Amidon GL, Barends DM, Lennernäs H, Polli JE, Shah VP, et al. The use of BDDCS in classifying the permeability of marketed drugs. Pharm Res 2008;52:483–488.

[58] Sokolnikoff IS, Redheffer RM. Mathematics of physics and modern engineering. 2nd ed. New York: McGraw-Hill; 1966. p. 224.

[59] Atkinson AJ Jr, Kushner W. Clinical pharmacokinetics. Annu Rev Pharmacol Toxicol 1979;19:105–127.

[60] Langenbucher F, Mysicka J. *In vitro* and *in vivo* deconvolution assessment of drug release kinetics from oxprenolol Oros preparations. Br J Clin Pharmacol 1985;19:151S–162S.

[61] Vaughan DP, Dennis M. Mathematical basis of point-area deconvolution method for determining *in vivo* input functions. J Pharm Sci 1978;67:663–665.

[62] Rackley RJ. Examples of *in vitro-in vivo* relationships with a diverse range of quality. In: Young D, Devane JG, Butler J, editors. *In vitro-in vivo* correlations. New York: Plenum Press; 1997. p. 1–15.

Study problems

1. An approach that has been used during drug development to estimate the absolute bioavailability of a drug is to administer an initial dose intravenously in order to calculate the area under the plasma-level-vs.-time curve from zero to infinite time (*AUC*). Subjects then are begun on oral therapy. When steady state is reached, the *AUC* during a dosing interval ($AUC_{0\rightarrow\tau}$) is calculated. The percent bioavailability of the oral formulation is determined from the following equation

$$\%\,\text{Bioavailability} = \frac{D_{IV} \cdot AUC_{0\rightarrow\tau\,(oral)}}{D_{oral} \cdot AUC_{IV}} \times 100$$

   This approach requires *AUC* to equal $AUC_{0\rightarrow\tau}$ if the same doses are administered intravenously and orally and the extent of absorption is 100%. Derive the proof for this equality.

2. When a drug is administered by constant intravenous administration, this zero-order input can be represented by a "step function." Derive the appropriate absorption function and convolute it with the disposition function to obtain the output function. (*Clue:* Remember that the absorption function is the *rate* of drug administration.)

3. A 70-kg patient is treated with an intravenous infusion of lidocaine at a rate of 2 mg/min. Assume a single-compartment distribution volume of 1.9 L/kg and an elimination half-life of 90 min.
   - **a.** Use the output function derived in Problem 2 to predict the expected steady-state plasma lidocaine concentration.
   - **b.** Use this function to estimate the time required to reach 90% of this steady-state level.
   - **c.** Express this 90% equilibration time in terms of number of elimination half-lives.

Chapter 5

Effect of kidney disease on pharmacokinetics

Thomas D. Nolin[a], Albert W. Dreisbach[b], Arthur J. Atkinson, Jr.[c], and Juan J.L. Lertora[d,e]

[a]*Department of Pharmacy and Therapeutics, and Department of Medicine, Renal-Electrolyte Division, University of Pittsburgh Schools of Pharmacy and Medicine, Pittsburgh, PA, United States,* [b]*Department of Internal Medicine, Division of Nephrology, University of Mississippi Medical Center, Jackson, MS, United States,* [c]*Department of Pharmacology, Feinberg School of Medicine, Northwestern University, Chicago, IL, United States,* [d]*Adjunct Professor, Division of Clinical Research, Pennington Biomedical Research Center, Louisiana State University, Baton Rouge, LA, United States,* [e]*Adjunct Professor, Department of Medicine, Duke University School of Medicine, Durham, NC, United States*

A 67-year-old man had been functionally anephric, requiring outpatient hemodialysis for several years. He was hospitalized for revision of his arteriovenous shunt and postoperatively complained of symptoms of gastroesophageal reflux. This complaint prompted institution of cimetidine therapy. In view of the patient's impaired kidney function, the usually prescribed dose was reduced by half. Three days later, the patient was noted to be confused. An initial diagnosis of dialysis dementia was made and the family was informed that dialysis would be discontinued. On teaching rounds, the suggestion was made that cimetidine be discontinued. Two days later the patient was alert and was discharged from the hospital to resume outpatient hemodialysis therapy.

Although drugs are developed to treat patients who have diseases, relatively little attention has been given to the fact that these diseases themselves exert important effects that impact patient response to drug therapy. Accordingly, the case presented earlier is an example from the past that illustrates a therapeutic problem that persists today. In the idealized scheme of contemporary drug development shown in Fig. 1.1 (Chapter 1), the pertinent information would be generated in pharmacokinetic/pharmacodynamic (PK/PD) studies in special populations that are carried out concurrently with Phase II and Phase III clinical trials. Additional useful information can be obtained by using population pharmacokinetic methods to analyze data obtained in the large-scale Phase III trials themselves [1]. However, a review of labeling in the *Physicians' Desk Reference* and other drug information resources indicates that there often is scant or contradictory information available to guide drug selection and dosing for individual patients [2–4].

Illness, aging, sex, and other patient factors may have important effects on *pharmacodynamic* aspects of patient response to drugs. For example, patients with advanced pulmonary insufficiency are particularly sensitive to the respiratory depressant effects of narcotic and sedative drugs. In addition, these patient factors may affect the *pharmacokinetic* aspects of drug elimination, distribution, and absorption. In this regard, kidney impairment has been estimated to account for one-third of the prescribing errors resulting from inattention to patient pathophysiology [5]. Even when the necessary pharmacokinetic and pharmacodynamic information is available, appropriate dose adjustments often were not made for patients with impaired kidney function because assessment of this function usually was based solely on serum creatinine measurements without concomitant estimation of creatinine clearance [6]. Fortunately, prescriber awareness of patients with impaired kidney function has improved since routine reporting of estimated glomerular filtration rate (eGFR) became standard clinical laboratory practice [7].

Because there is a large population of functionally anephric patients who are maintained in relatively stable condition by hemodialysis, a substantial number of pharmacokinetic studies have been carried out in these individuals. Patients with intermediate levels of impaired kidney function have not been studied to the same extent, but studies in these patients are recommended in current FDA guidelines [8].

Atkinson's Principles of Clinical Pharmacology. http://doi.org/10.1016/B978-0-12-819869-8.00003-3

Drug dosing in patients with impaired kidney function

The effects of decreased kidney function on drug elimination have been examined extensively. This is appropriate since only elimination clearance (CL_E) and drug dose determine the steady-state concentration of drug in the body (C_{ss}). This is true whether the drug is administered by continuous intravenous infusion (I), in which case

$$C_{ss} = I/CL_E \tag{5.1}$$

or by intermittent oral or parenteral doses, in which case the corresponding equation is:

$$\overline{C}_{ss} = \frac{Absorbed\ Dose/\tau}{CL_E} \tag{5.2}$$

where $\overline{C}_{ss}$ is the mean concentration during the dosing interval τ.

For many drugs, CL_E consists of additive renal (CL_R) and nonrenal (CL_{NR}) components, as indicated by the following equation:

$$CL_E = CL_R + CL_{NR} \tag{5.3}$$

Nonrenal clearance is usually equated with drug metabolism and/or transport by the liver, but also could include hemodialysis and other methods of drug removal. In fact, even the metabolic clearance of a drug frequently consists of additive contributions from several parallel metabolic pathways. The characterization of drug metabolism by a clearance term usually is appropriate, since the metabolism of most drugs can be described by first-order kinetics within the range of therapeutic drug concentrations.

Dettli [9] proposed that the additive property of *elimination rate constants* representing parallel elimination pathways provides a way of either using Eq. (5.3) or constructing nomograms to estimate the dose reductions that are appropriate for patients with impaired kidney function. This approach also can be used to estimate *elimination clearance*, as illustrated for cimetidine in Fig. 5.1 [10]. In implementing this approach, creatinine clearance (CL_{CR}) has been estimated in adults from the Cockcroft and Gault equation (Eq. 1.3) [11], and in pediatric patients from other simple equations (see Chapter 1) [12].

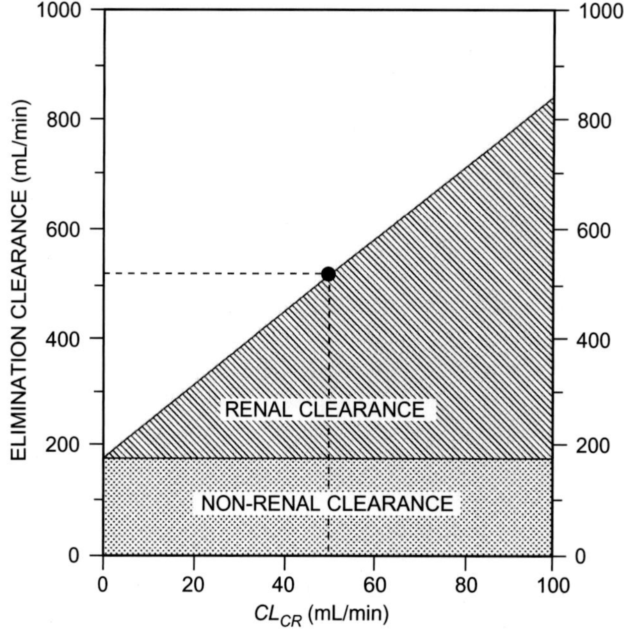

FIG. 5.1 Nomogram for estimating cimetidine elimination clearance (CL_E) for a 70-kg patient with impaired kidney function. The right-hand ordinate indicates cimetidine CL_E measured in young adults with normal kidney function, and the left-hand ordinate indicates expected cimetidine CL_E in a functionally anephric patient, based on the fact that 23% of an administered dose is eliminated by nonrenal routes in healthy subjects. The *heavy line* connecting these points can be used to estimate cimetidine CL_E from creatinine clearance (CL_{CR}). For example, a 70-kg patient with CL_{CR} of 50 mL/min (*large dot*) would be expected to have a cimetidine CL_E of 517 mL/min, and to respond satisfactorily to doses that are 60% of those recommended for patients with normal kidney function. *(Reproduced with permission from Atkinson AJ Jr, Craig RM. Therapy of peptic ulcer disease. In: Molinoff PB, editor. Peptic ulcer disease. Mechanisms and management. Rutherford, NJ: Healthpress Publishing Group, Inc.; 1990. pp. 83–112.)*

Since eGFR is widely reported and commonly used in clinical practice, it now provides clinicians an alternative for the purposes of drug dosing. Future FDA guidance will likely incentivize pharmaceutical manufacturers to generate eGFR-based dosing recommendations for inclusion in drug labels, which will facilitate use of eGFR for drug dosing in the clinical setting [13]. Calculations or nomograms for many drugs can be made after consulting drug information sources including the FDA-approved label (see Drugs@FDA; available at www.accessdata.fda.gov) to obtain values of CL_E and the fractional dose eliminated by renal excretion (percentage urinary excretion) in subjects with normal kidney function.

In the introductory case study, the cimetidine dose was reduced in accordance with the drug label which under "Dosage Adjustment for Patients with Impaired Renal Function," states that "Patients with creatinine clearance less than 30 cc/min who are being treated for prevention of upper gastrointestinal bleeding should receive half the recommended dose" [14]. However, under "Pharmacokinetics" the label indicates that "following I.V. or I.M. administration, approximately 75% of the drug is recovered from the urine after 24 h as the parent compound." Since only one-fourth of the dose is eliminated by nonrenal mechanisms, it can be expected, as illustrated by Fig. 5.1, that functionally anephric patients who receive half the usual cimetidine dose will have potentially toxic blood levels that are twice those recommended for patients with normal kidney function.

When dose adjustments are needed for patients with impaired function, they can be made by reducing the drug dose or by lengthening the dosing interval. Either approach, or a combination of both, may be employed in practice. For example, once the expected value for CL_E has been estimated, the daily drug dose can be reduced in proportion to the quotient of the expected clearance divided by the normal clearance. This will maintain the average drug concentration at the usual level, regardless of whether the drug is administered by intermittent doses or by continuous infusion. On the other hand, it is often convenient to administer doses of drugs that have a short elimination half-life at some multiple of their elimination half-life. The multiple that is used is determined by the therapeutic index of the drug. The expected half-life can be calculated from the following equation:

$$t_{1/2} = \frac{0.693 V_{d(area)}}{CL_E} \tag{5.4}$$

and the usual dose can be administered at an interval equal to the same multiple of the increased half-life. Dose-interval adjustment is usually necessary when safety and efficacy concerns specify a target range for both peak and trough plasma concentrations, or when selection of drug doses is limited.

The reliability of the Dettli method of predicting drug clearance depends on two critical assumptions:

1. The nonrenal clearance of the drug remains constant when kidney function is impaired.
2. CL_E declines in a linear fashion with CL_{CR}.

There are important exceptions to the first assumption that will be considered when the effect of impaired kidney function on nonrenal drug clearance is presented. Nonetheless, this approach is widely used for individualizing drug dosage for patients with impaired kidney function. In addition, Eqs. (5.3) and (5.4) provide a useful tool for hypothesis generation during drug development when pharmacokinetic studies are planned for subjects with impaired kidney function. Although the second assumption also has proved useful for many years in clinical practice, some exceptions to the intact nephron hypothesis have been described for drugs that have a large component of tubular handling [15]. In the future, measures of proximal tubular function may allow development of new renal dosing algorithms that take into account this phenomenon.

Effects of kidney disease on renal drug elimination mechanisms

Renal clearance of drugs is a net result of three important mechanisms of renal drug handing, namely glomerular filtration, tubular secretion, and reabsorption (Table 5.1).

Excretion mechanisms: Filtration and secretion

Glomerular filtration affects all drugs of small molecular size and is *restrictive* in the sense that it is limited by drug binding to plasma proteins. On the other hand, renal tubular secretion is *nonrestrictive* since both protein-bound and free drug concentrations in plasma are available for elimination. In fact, the proximal renal tubular secretion of *p*-aminohippurate is rapid enough that its elimination clearance is used to estimate renal blood flow. There are numerous proteins in renal tubular cells that actively transport compounds against a concentration gradient and contribute extensively to renal drug clearance. These include P-glycoprotein (P-gp), several multidrug resistance proteins, organic cation and organic anion transporters,

TABLE 5.1 Important mechanisms of renal elimination of drugs.

I. Glomerular filtration

- Affects all drugs and metabolites of appropriate molecular size
- Influenced by protein binding (f_u=free fraction)

II. Renal tubular secretion

- Not influenced by protein binding
- May be affected by competition with other drugs, etc.

Examples:
Active drugs: Acids—penicillin
Bases—procainamide
Metabolites: Glucuronides, hippurates, etc.

III. Reabsorption by nonionic diffusion

- Affects weak acids and weak bases
- Only important if excretion of free drug is major elimination path

Examples:
Weak acids: Phenobarbital
Weak bases: Quinidine

IV. Active reabsorption

- Affects ions, not proved for other drugs

Examples:
Halides: Fluoride, bromide
Alkaline metals: Lithium

along with a number of genetic variants [16, 17]. The transporters involved in drug secretion are located at both the basolateral membrane of renal tubule cells, where they transport drugs from blood into these cells, and the apical membrane, where they transport drugs from the intracellular space into proximal tubular lumen. Despite the progress that has been made in cloning these transporters and in establishing their binding affinities for various model substrates, which transporters are predominantly responsible for the renal secretion of individual drugs remains unclear.

Competition by drugs for renal tubular secretion is an important cause of drug-drug interactions [17]. Inhibitors of P-gp retard excretion by this pathway. Anionic drugs compete with other anionic drugs for these active transport pathways, as do cationic drugs for their pathways. When two drugs secreted by the same pathway are administered simultaneously, the renal clearance of each will be less than when either drug is given alone. For example, methotrexate is actively secreted by renal tubular cells, but its renal clearance is halved when salicylate is coadministered [18].

Reabsorption mechanisms

Net drug elimination also may be affected by drug reabsorption in the distal nephron, primarily by nonionic passive diffusion. Because only the nonionized form of a drug can diffuse across renal tubule cells, the degree of reabsorption of a given drug depends on its degree of ionization at a given urinary pH. For this reason, sodium bicarbonate is administered to patients with salicylate or phenobarbital overdose in order to raise urine pH, thereby increasing the ionization and minimizing the reabsorption of these acidic drugs. This therapeutic intervention also reduces reabsorption by increasing urine flow. Lithium and bromide are examples of drugs that are extensively reabsorbed by active transport mechanisms. Present evidence suggests that lithium is reabsorbed at the level of the proximal tubule by a Na^+/H^+ exchanger (NHE-3) at the brush border and extruded into the blood by sodium-potassium ATPase and the sodium bicarbonate cotransporter located at the basolateral membrane [19].

Proximal tubular endocytosis, mediated by the apical cell membrane receptors megalin and cipolin, plays an important role in removing proteins and peptides that pass through glomerular filtration pores [20]. This accounts for the daily elimination of only 100–300 mg of protein in normal urine, a fraction of the filtered load, and is responsible for the essential conservation of protein-carrier-bound vitamins and trace elements, which are thereby returned to the systemic circulation. However, the absorbed peptides and proteins are degraded by lysosomal proteases within the renal tubular cells. Aminoglycosides are freely filtered at the glomerulus and are nephrotoxic because of their subsequent active uptake by this endocytic receptor complex [21]. The fact that this uptake is saturable accounts for the fact that aminoglycosides are less nephrotoxic when administered as single daily doses rather than when one-third of that dose is given every 8 h, a phenomenon referred to as *dose-regimen dependency* [22].

Renal metabolism

The kidney plays a major role in the clearance of insulin from the systemic circulation, removing approximately 50% of endogenous insulin and a greater proportion of insulin administered to diabetic patients [23]. Insulin is filtered at the glomerulus, reabsorbed by the proximal tubule cell, and then degraded by lysosomal proteolytic enzymes. Consequently, insulin requirements are markedly reduced in diabetic patients with chronic kidney disease (CKD). Imipenem and other peptides and peptidomimetics are also filtered at the glomerulus, absorbed by endocytosis, then metabolized by proximal renal tubule cell proteases. Cilastatin, an inhibitor of proximal tubular dipeptidases, is coadministered with imipenem to enhance the clinical effectiveness of this antibiotic. Other examples of renal drug metabolism are provided in the comprehensive review by Lohr and colleagues [24].

Analysis and interpretation of renal excretion data

Renal tubular mechanisms of excretion and reabsorption can be analyzed by stop-flow and other standard methods used in renal physiology, but detailed studies are seldom performed. For most drugs, all that has been done is to correlate renal drug clearance with the reciprocal of serum creatinine or with creatinine clearance. Even though creatinine clearance primarily reflects GFR, it serves as a rough guide to the renal clearance of drugs that have extensive renal tubular secretion or reabsorption. This is a consequence of the glomerulo-tubular balance that is maintained in damaged nephrons by intrinsic tubule and peritubular capillary adaptations that parallel reductions in single nephron GFR [25]. For this reason, CL_R usually declines fairly linearly with reductions in CL_{CR}. However, some discrepancies can be expected. For example, with aging, renal secretion of some basic drugs declines more rapidly than GFR [26]. Also studies with *N*-1-methylnicotinamide, an endogenous marker of renal tubular secretion, have demonstrated some degree of glomerulo-tubular imbalance in patients with impaired kidney function [27].

Despite the paucity of detailed studies, it is possible to draw two general mechanistic conclusions from renal clearance values:

1. If renal clearance *exceeds* drug filtration rate (Table 5.1), there is net renal tubular secretion of the drug.
2. If renal clearance *is less than* drug filtration rate, there is net renal tubular reabsorption of the drug.

Effects of impaired kidney function on nonrenal clearance pathways

Most drugs are not excreted unchanged by the kidneys but first are biotransformed to metabolites that then are excreted. Kidney failure may not only retard the excretion of these metabolites, which may have important pharmacologic activity, but in some cases alters the nonrenal as well as the renal clearance of drugs [28–30]. Hepatic drug clearance (CL_H) is mediated by transporter uptake and excretion mechanisms, as well as by metabolism within hepatocytes and all of these processes may be impacted in the setting of impaired kidney function. For example, the expression and uptake function of hepatic organic anion transport polypeptides (OATPs) has been shown to be depressed in an animal model of chronic kidney failure; conversely, expression of the efflux transporter P-gp appeared to be increased [31].

Nonrenal metabolism

Impaired kidney function impacts the hepatic clearance of drugs that are metabolized by a number of enzymatic pathways, as indicated in Table 5.2. Both Phase I biotransformations (cytochrome P450 (CYP) and nonCYP enzymes) and Phase II

TABLE 5.2 Effect of kidney disease on drug metabolism.

I. Oxidations	Variably slowed[a]
	Example: CYP substrates
II. Reductions	Slowed
	Example: Hydrocortisone
III. Hydrolyses	
• Plasma esterase	Slowed
	Example: Procaine
• Plasma peptidase	Normal
	Example: Angiotensin
• Tissue peptidase	Slowed
	Example: Insulin
IV. Conjugations	
• Glucuronide formation	Reduced in some cases
	Example: Hydrocortisone
• Acetylation	Slowed
	Example: Procainamide
• Glycine conjugation	Slowed
	Example: Para-aminosalicylic acid
• O-Methylation	Normal
	Example: Methyldopa
• Sulfate conjugation	Normal
	Example: Acetaminophen

[a]*See Fig. 5.2.*

biotransformations (e.g., acetylation by NAT-2, glucuronidation by UGT2B) may be impaired to varying degrees, which are pronounced in patients with advanced CKD, particularly end-stage kidney disease (ESKD).

Recent attention has been focused primarily on the effects of impaired kidney function on the hepatic elimination of drugs that are substrates for CYP enzymes [28–30]. The effect on metabolism of moderate and severe kidney impairment for several CYP enzymes was previously estimated by back-calculating clinical estimates of CL_H to account for protein and erythrocyte binding for the following drug-CYP enzyme pairs: midazolam-CYP3A4, bufuralol-CYP2D6, bosentan-CYP2C9, theophylline-CYP1A2, omeprazole-CYP2C19, and rosiglitazone-CYP2C8 [32]. It can be seen from Fig. 5.2 that these enzymes may vary in their sensitivity to impaired kidney function, but that the extent of their impairment increases as kidney function deteriorates. Subsequent analysis of clinical pharmacokinetic data from the FDA database of kidney impairment studies using model-specific CYP and transport substrate drugs provides more clarity on this phenomenon [28–30]. Specifically, progression of CKD is correlated with a decline in OATP and CYP2D6 activity, but has no clear relationship with the activity of CYPs 1A2, 2C8, 2C9, 2C19, and 3A4/5 [28–30]. Relatively little information is available about the effects of impaired kidney function on Phase II metabolic pathways. In an early study, Gibson et al. [33] found that NAT2-mediated procainamide acetylation in hemodialysis-dependent patients was reduced by 61% in phenotypic slow

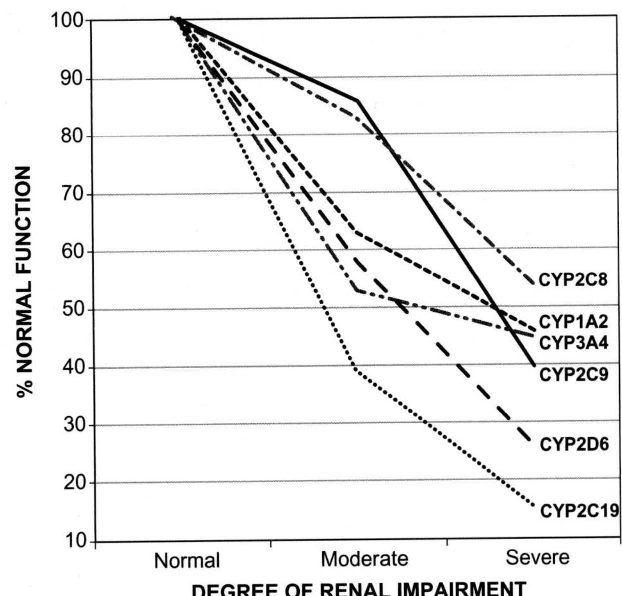

FIG. 5.2 Effect of increasing degrees of kidney impairment on hepatic clearance mediated by different CYP enzymes. Moderate impairment $= CL_{CR}$ 30–59 mL/min, Severe impairment $= CL_{CR} < 30$ mL/min, (— - - —) CYP3A4, (— — —) CYP2D6, (——) CYP2C9, (- - -) CYP1A2, (···) CYP2C19, (— - — - —) CYP2C8. *(Figure based on data from Rowland Yeo K, Aarabi M, Jamei M, Rostami-Hodjegan A. Expert Rev. Clin Pharmacol 2011;4:261–274.)*

acetylators and by 69% in rapid acetylators. Subsequently, Kim et al. [34] reported that isoniazid acetylation by NAT2 was decreased by 63% in ESKD slow acetylators but by only 23% in rapid acetylators. Phase II metabolism of morphine to form glucuronide conjugates is decreased by 48% in functionally anephric patients [35]. More importantly, these patients accumulated much higher concentrations of the morphine-6-glucuronide metabolite, which is a much more potent narcotic than morphine. Both of these factors account for the serious adverse events that have been reported in some patients with severely impaired kidney function who have been treated with morphine [36].

Nonrenal transport

Impaired kidney function also impacts the hepatic clearance of drugs that are transported in the liver. Sun et al. [37] found that CL_H of intravenously administered erythromycin, a drug in which metabolism accounts for <15% of CL_H, was markedly decreased in patients with end-stage kidney disease and suggested that this might have been the result of depressed OATP function. The most consistent finding of altered drug transporter activity in patients with kidney disease has been demonstrated using the transporter probe fexofenadine, which is minimally metabolized and minimally excreted in the urine. Unfortunately, fexofenadine is transported by multiple uptake (e.g., OATP1B1, OATP1B3, OATP2B1) and efflux (P-gp, MRP2, MRP3) transporters making it difficult to attribute altered pharmacokinetics to an individual transporter. Fexofenadine 120 mg was administered orally to healthy controls and ESKD patients on maintenance hemodialysis [38]. ESKD patients had a 2.8-fold increase in the fexofenadine AUC and a 63% decrease in clearance. In a separate study, patients with moderate to severe CKD (mean eGFR = 17 mL/min/1.73 m^2) and ESKD patients on maintenance hemodialysis and peritoneal dialysis were administered 120 mg fexofenadine orally [39]. The fexofenadine AUC in CKD, hemodialysis, and peritoneal dialysis patients was increased by 2.9-, 2.3-, and 2.1-fold with a corresponding 61%, 56%, and 49% decrease in CL/F, respectively. Together, these studies provide strong evidence that transporter activity is altered in humans with CKD.

Similar to fexofenadine, the HMG CoA reductase inhibitor rosuvastatin is minimally excreted in the urine (fractional excretion less than 6%) and has negligible hepatic metabolism. The drug is a substrate of multiple uptake (OATP1B1, OATP1B3, OATP2B1, OATP1A2, NTCP) and efflux (P-gp, BCRP, MRP2) transporters. Rosuvastatin plasma concentrations in patients with advanced CKD ($CL_{CR} < 30$ mL/min) are 3-fold higher than in individuals with normal kidney function, and steady-state plasma concentrations are 50% higher in ESKD patients on maintenance hemodialysis [40]. Although it is difficult to identify the specific pathway(s) responsible for altered rosuvastatin pharmacokinetics, it appears likely that its decreased hepatic clearance results from a decrease in OATP transporter activity.

FDA investigators recently assessed numerous studies of different OATP substrate drugs and corroborated earlier findings that OATP transporter function is impaired in humans with kidney disease [29, 30]. The OATP drug substrates included atorvastatin, bosentan, cerivastatin, erythromycin, fluvastatin, imatinib, pitavastatin, repaglinide, rosuvastatin, and torsemide and there was a clear trend of decreasing substrate clearance as kidney disease progressed. While none of the drugs studied is a "clean" OATP substrate (they all exhibit overlapping specificity with other transporters and/or metabolizing enzymes), this clear relationship, including a large number of drugs, strongly suggests that OATP-mediated clearance is decreased in humans with kidney disease.

Potential mechanisms of altered nonrenal clearance

The effects of impaired kidney function on hepatic drug elimination have been attributed to the accumulation of 3-carboxy-4-methyl-5-propyl-2-furan propanoic acid (CMPF), indoxyl sulfate, parathyroid hormone (PTH), cytokines, and perhaps other toxins that inhibit drug metabolism and transport [41, 42]. On the basis of experiments in rodent and in vitro models of chronic kidney failure it has been shown that impairment occurs in some cases at the level of gene transcription, as indicated by decreased levels of the mRNA that encodes OATP2, a number of CYP enzymes, and NAT2. In attempting to identify the toxin or toxins responsible for these effects, Sun et al. [37] documented that CMPF and indoxyl sulfate were increased in ESKD patients but found that plasma concentrations of these uremic toxins were not correlated with the extent to which erythromycin CL_H was decreased. On the other hand, Michaud et al. [43] showed that PTH antibodies could prevent the downregulation of CYP mRNA that was observed when rat hepatocytes were incubated with serum from ESKD patients. In subsequent studies, these investigators used this in vitro model to further demonstrate that this downregulation results from PTH stimulation of nuclear factor-κB (NF-κB), since it was prevented by adding andrographolide, an NF-κB inhibitor, to the incubation mixture [43]. This downregulation also was shown to be reversible by hemodialysis, since it did not occur when the hepatocytes were incubated with postdialysis patient serum. In this regard, it had previously been shown by Nolin et al. [44] that hemodialysis acutely increased hepatic clearance of erythromycin and by De Martin et al. [45] that the elimination clearance of lidocaine, a substrate for CYPs1A2 and 3A4, was impaired in ESKD patients not undergoing regular hemodialysis but was normal in dialyzed ESKD patients. However, the fact that the hepatic elimination of many drugs is not normalized by hemodialysis suggests the existence of other important inhibitory mechanisms, and there is a clear need for further study of the effects of impaired kidney function on drug metabolism and transport [40].

Effects of kidney disease on drug distribution

Impaired kidney function is associated with important changes in the binding of some drugs to *plasma proteins*. In some cases, the *tissue binding* of drugs is also affected.

Plasma protein binding of acidic drugs

Reidenberg and Drayer [46] have stated that protein binding in serum from uremic patients is decreased for every acidic drug that has been studied. Most acidic drugs bind to the bilirubin binding site on albumin, but there are also different binding sites that play a role. The reduced binding that occurs when kidney function is impaired has been variously attributed to reductions in serum albumin concentration, structural changes in the binding sites, or displacement of drugs from albumin binding sites by organic molecules that accumulate in uremia. As described in Chapter 3, reductions in the protein binding of acidic drugs result in increases in their distribution volume. In addition, the elimination clearance of *restrictively eliminated* drugs is increased. However, protein-binding changes do not affect distribution volume or clearance estimates when they are referenced to unbound drug concentrations. For restrictively eliminated drugs, the term *intrinsic clearance* is used to describe the clearance that would be observed in the absence of any protein-binding restrictions. As discussed in Chapter 7, CL_H for restrictively eliminated drugs, when referenced to total drug concentrations, simply equals the product of the unbound fraction of drug (f_u) and this intrinsic clearance (CL_{int}):

$$CL_H = f_u \cdot CL_{\text{int}} \tag{5.5}$$

Phenytoin is an acidic, restrictively eliminated drug that is classically used to illustrate some of the changes in drug distribution and elimination that occur in patients with impaired kidney function. In patients with normal kidney function, 92% of the phenytoin in plasma is protein bound. However, the percentage that is unbound or "free" rises from 8% in these individuals to 16% (or more) in hemodialysis-dependent patients. In a study comparing phenytoin pharmacokinetics in

TABLE 5.3 Effect of impaired kidney function on phenytoin kinetics.

	Healthy subjects ($n=4$)	Uremic patients ($n=4$)
Percent unbound (f_u)	12%	26%
Distribution volume ($V_{d(area)}$)	0.64 L/kg	1.40 L/kg
Hepatic clearance (CL_H)	2.46 L/h	7.63 L/h
Intrinsic clearance (CL_{int})	20.3 L/h	29.9 L/h

normal subjects and uremic patients, Odar-Cederlöf and Borgå [47] administered a single low dose of this drug so that first-order kinetics were approximated. The results presented in Table 5.3 can be inferred from their study.

The uremic patients had an increase in distribution volume that was consistent with the observed decrease in phenytoin binding to plasma proteins. The threefold increase in hepatic clearance that was observed in these patients also was primarily the result of decreased phenytoin protein binding. Although CL_{int} for this CYP2C9, CYP2C19, and P-gp substrate also appeared to be increased in the uremic patients, the difference did not reach statistical significance.

A major problem arises in clinical practice when only total (protein-bound+free) phenytoin concentrations are measured and used to guide therapy of patients with severely impaired kidney function. The decreases in phenytoin binding that occur in these patients result in commensurate decreases in total plasma concentrations (Fig. 5.3). Even though therapeutic and toxic pharmacologic effects are correlated with unbound rather than total phenytoin concentrations in plasma, the decrease in total concentrations can mislead physicians into increasing phenytoin doses inappropriately. Fortunately, rapid ultrafiltration procedures are now readily available and free phenytoin concentrations are routinely measured in these patients.

Plasma protein binding of basic and neutral drugs

The protein binding of basic drugs tends to be normal or only slightly reduced [46]. In some cases, this may reflect the facts that these drugs bind to α_1-acid glycoprotein and that concentrations of this glycoprotein are higher in hemodialysis-dependent patients than in patients with normal kidney function.

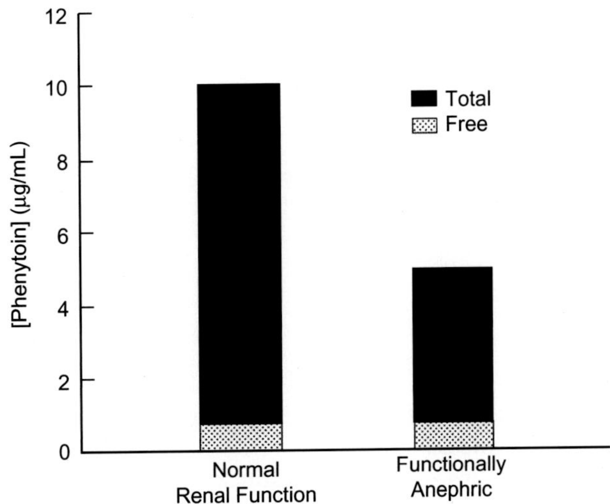

FIG. 5.3 Comparison of free and total plasma phenytoin concentrations in a patient with normal kidney function and a functionally anephric patient who are both treated with a 300-mg daily phenytoin dose and have identical CL_{int}. Although free phenytoin concentrations are 0.8 µg/mL in both patients, phenytoin is only 84% bound (16% free) in the functionally anephric patient, compared to 92% bound (8% free) in the patient with normal kidney function. For that reason, total phenytoin concentrations in the functionally anephric patient are only 5 µg/mL, whereas they are 10 µg/mL in the patient with normal kidney function.

Tissue binding of drugs

The distribution volume of some drugs also can be altered when kidney function is impaired. As described in Chapter 3, Sheiner et al. [48] have shown that impaired kidney function is associated with a decrease in digoxin distribution volume that is described by the following equation:

$$V_d\,(\text{in L}) = 3.84\,\text{weight}\,(\text{in kg}) + 3.12\,CL_{CR}\,(\text{in mL/min})$$

This presumably reflects a reduction in tissue levels of Na/K-ATPase, an enzyme that represents a major tissue-binding site for digoxin [49]. In other cases in which distribution volume is decreased in patients with impaired kidney function, the relationship between the degree of kidney impairment and decrease in distribution volume has not been characterized and neither have plausible mechanisms been proposed.

Effects of kidney disease on drug absorption

The bioavailability of most drugs that have been studied has not been found to be altered in patients with impaired kidney function. However, the absorption of D-xylose, a marker compound used to evaluate small intestinal absorptive function, was slowed (absorption rate constant: $0.555\,h^{-1}$ vs $1.03\,h^{-1}$) and less complete (% dose absorbed: 48.6% vs 69.4%) in patients with chronic kidney failure than in healthy subjects [50]. Although these results were statistically significant, there was considerable interindividual variation in both patients and healthy subjects. This primary absorptive defect may explain the fact that patients with impaired kidney function have *decreased* bioavailability of furosemide [51] and pindolol [52]. However, it also is possible that impaired kidney function will result in *increased* bioavailability of drugs exhibiting first-pass effects when the function of drug-metabolizing enzymes and/or transporters is compromised. In this regard, Sun et al. [37] observed a 36% increase in erythromycin bioavailability in ESKD patients that was attributed to decreased hepatic extraction rather than any change in gut availability.

The paucity of reliable bioavailability data in patients with impaired kidney function underscores the cumbersome nature of most absolute bioavailability studies in which oral and intravenous drug doses are administered on two separate occasions. The validity of this approach rests on the assumption that the kinetics of drug distribution and elimination remain unchanged in the interval between the two studies—an assumption that obviously is more tenuous for patients than for healthy subjects. As discussed in Chapter 4, these shortcomings can be overcome by conducting a single study in which an intravenous formulation of an isotope-labeled drug is administered simultaneously with the oral drug dose. Wood and colleagues [53] simultaneously administered radioisotopically labeled and unlabeled propranolol to healthy subjects and either hemodialyzed or nondialyzed ESKD patients and found no difference in bioavailability. Intravenous administration of a stable isotope-labeled drug would be preferred for absolute bioavailability studies in patients and subsequently has been used to demonstrate a modest decrease in cibenzoline absorption but no decrease in nitrendipine bioavailability in patients with kidney disease [54].

Study problem

The following pharmacokinetic data for *N*-acetylprocainamide (NAPA) were obtained in a Phase 1 study in which procainamide and NAPA kinetics were compared in volunteers with normal kidney function:

Elimination half-life: 6.2 h.
Elimination clearance: 233 mL/min.
% Renal excretion: 85.5%.

(a) Use these results to predict the elimination half-life of NAPA in functionally anephric patients, assuming that nonrenal clearance is unchanged in these individuals.

(b) Create a nomogram similar to that shown in Fig. 5.1 to estimate the elimination clearance of NAPA that would be expected for a patient with a creatinine clearance of 50 mL/min. Assume that a creatinine clearance of 100 mL/min is the value for individuals with normal kidney function.

(c) If the usual starting dose of NAPA is 1 g every 8 h in patients with normal kidney function, what would be the equivalent dosing regimen for a patient with an estimated creatinine clearance of 50 mL/min if the dose is decreased but the 8-h dosing interval is maintained?

(d) If the usual starting dose of NAPA is 1 g every 8 h in patients with normal kidney function, what would be the equivalent dosing regimen for a patient with an estimated creatinine clearance of 50 mL/min if the 1-g dose is maintained but the dosing interval is increased?

References

[1] Peck CC. Rationale for the effective use of pharmacokinetics and pharmacodynamics in early drug development. In: Yacobi A, Skelly JP, Shah VP, Benet LZ, editors. Integration of pharmacokinetics, pharmacodynamics, and toxicokinetics in rational drug development. New York, NY: Plenum; 1993. p. 1–5.

[2] Spyker DA, Harvey ED, Harvey BE, Harvey AM, Rumack BH, Peck CC, et al. Assessment and reporting of clinical pharmacology information in drug labeling. Clin Pharmacol Ther 2000;67:196–200.

[3] Mountford CM, Lee T, de Lemos J, Loewen PS. Quality and usability of common drug information databases. Can J Hosp Pharm 2010;63:130–7.

[4] Khanal A, Castelino RL, Peterson GM, Jose MD. Dose adjustment guidelines for medications in patients with renal impairment: how consistent are drug information sources? Intern Med J 2014;44:77–85.

[5] Lesar TS, Briceland L, Stein DS. Factors related to errors in medication prescribing. JAMA 1997;277:312–7.

[6] Piergies AA, Worwag EM, Atkinson AJ Jr. A concurrent audit of high digoxin plasma levels. Clin Pharmacol Ther 1994;55:353–8.

[7] Accetta NA, Gladstone EH, DiSogra C, Wright EC, Briggs M, Narva AS. Prevalence of estimated GFR reporting among US clinical laboratories. Am J Kidney Dis 2008;52:778–87.

[8] CDER, CBER. Pharmacokinetics in patients with impaired renal function—study design, data analysis, and impact on dosing and labeling. Draft Guidance for Industry, Rockville: FDA; 2010. (Internet at http://www.fda.gov/downloads/Drugs/Guidance ComplianceRegulatoryInformation/Guidances/UCM204959.pdf).

[9] Dettli L. Individualization of drug dosage in patients with renal disease. Med Clin North Am 1974;58:977–85.

[10] Atkinson AJ Jr, Craig RM. Therapy of peptic ulcer disease. In: Molinoff PB, editor. Peptic ulcer disease. Mechanisms and management. Rutherford, NJ: Healthpress Publishing Group, Inc.; 1990. p. 83–112.

[11] Cockcroft DW, Gault MH. Prediction of creatinine clearance from serum creatinine. Nephron 1976;16:31–41.

[12] Schwartz GJ, Munoz A, Schneider MF, Mak RH, Kaskel F, Warady BA, et al. New equations to estimate GFR in children with CKD. J Am Soc Nephrol 2009;20:629–37.

[13] Hudson JQ, Nolin TD. Pragmatic use of kidney function estimates for drug dosing: the tide is turning. Adv Chronic Kidney Dis 2018;25:14–20.

[14] Physician's Desk Reference. 59th ed. Montvale, NJ: Medical Economics; 2005. p. 1626–9.

[15] Chapron A, Shen DD, Kestenbaum BR, Robinson-Cohen C, Himmelfarb J, Yeung CK. Does secretory clearance follow glomerular filtration rate in chronic kidney diseases? Reconsidering the intact nephron hypothesis. Clin Transl Sci 2017;10:395–403.

[16] Yee SW, Brackman DJ, Ennis EA, Sugiyama Y, Kamdem LK, Blanchard R, et al. Influence of transporter polymorphisms on drug disposition and response: a perspective from the International Transporter Consortium. Clin Pharmacol Ther 2018;104:803–17.

[17] Ivanyuk A, Livio F, Biollaz J, Buclin T. Renal drug transporters and drug Interactions. Clin Pharmacokinet 2017;56:825–92.

[18] Liegler DG, Henderson ES, Hahn MA, Oliverio VT. The effect of organic acids on renal clearance of methotrexate in man. Clin Pharmacol Ther 1969;10:849–57.

[19] Ng LL, Quinn PA, Baker F, Carr SJ. Red cell Na+/Li+ countertransport and Na+/H+ exchanger isoforms in human proximal tubules. Kidney Int 2000;58:229–35.

[20] Christensen EI, Verroust PJ, Nielsen R. Receptor-mediated endocytosis in renal proximal tubule. Pflugers Arch 2009;458:1039–48.

[21] Quiros Y, Vicente-Vicente L, Morales AI, Lopez-Novoa JM, Lopez-Hernandez FJ. An integrative overview on the mechanisms underlying the renal tubular cytotoxicity of gentamicin. Toxicol Sci 2011;119:245–56.

[22] Freeman CD, Nicolau DP, Belliveau PP, Nightingale CH. Once-daily dosing of aminoglycosides: review and recommendations for clinical practice. J Antimicrob Chemother 1997;39:677–86.

[23] Duckworth WC, Bennett RG, Hamel FG. Insulin degradation: progress and potential. Endocr Rev 1998;19:608–24.

[24] Lohr JW, Willsky GR, Acara MA. Renal drug metabolism. Pharmacol Rev 1998;50:107–41.

[25] Brenner BM. Nephron adaptation to renal injury or ablation. Am J Physiol 1985;249:F324–37.

[26] Reidenberg MM, Camacho M, Kluger J, Drayer DE. Aging and renal clearance of procainamide and acetylprocainamide. Clin Pharmacol Ther 1980;28:732–5.

[27] Maiza A, Waldek S, Ballardie FW, Daley-Yates PT. Estimation of renal tubular secretion in man, in health and disease, using endogenous N-1-methylnicotinamide. Nephron 1992;60:12–6.

[28] Yoshida K, Sun B, Zhang L, Zhao P, Abernethy D, Nolin TD, et al. Systematic and quantitative assessment of the effect of chronic kidney disease on CYP2D6 and CYP3A4/5. Clin Pharmacol Ther 2016;100:75–87.

[29] Tan ML, Yoshida K, Zhao P, Zhang L, Nolin TD, Piquette-Miller M, et al. Effect of chronic kidney disease on nonrenal elimination pathways: a systematic assessment of CYP1A2, CYP2C8, CYP2C9, CYP2C19, and OATP. Clin Pharmacol Ther 2018;103:854–67.

[30] Tan ML, Zhao P, Zhang L, Ho YF, Varma MVS, Neuhoff S, et al. Use of physiologically based pharmacokinetic modeling to evaluate the eEffect of chronic kidney disease on the disposition of hepatic CYP2C8 and OATP1B drug substrates. Clin Pharmacol Ther 2019;105:719–29.

[31] Naud J, Michaud J, Lebond FA, Lefrancois S, Bonnardeaux A, Pichette V. Effects of chronic renal failure on liver drug transporters. Drug Metab Dispos 2008;36:124–8.

[32] Rowland Yeo K, Aarabi M, Jamei M, Rostami-Hodjegan A. Modeling and predicting drug pharmacokinetics in patients with renal impairment. Expert Rev Clin Pharmacol 2011;4:261–74.

[33] Gibson TP, Atkinson AJ Jr, Matusik E, Nelson LD, Briggs WA. Kinetics of procainamide and *N*-acetylprocainamide in renal failure. Kidney Int 1977;12:422–9.

[34] Kim YG, Shin JG, Shin SG, Jang IJ, Kim S, Lee JS, et al. Decreased acetylation of isoniazid in chronic renal failure. Clin Pharmacol Ther 1993;54:612–20.

[35] Osborne R, Joel S, Grebenik K, Trew D, Slevin M. The pharmacokinetics of morphine and morphine glucuronides in kidney failure. Clin Pharmacol Ther 1993;54:158–67.

[36] Lagas JS, Wagenaar JF, Huitema AD, Hillebrand MJ, Koks CH, Gerdes VE, et al. Lethal morphine intoxication in a patient with a sickle cell crisis and renal impairment: case report and a review of the literature. Hum Exp Toxicol 2011;30:1399–403.

[37] Sun H, Frassetto LA, Huang Y, Benet LZ. Hepatic clearance, but not gut availability, of erythromycin is altered in patients with end-stage renal disease. Clin Pharmacol Ther 2010;87:465–72.

[38] Nolin TD, Frye RF, Le P, Sadr H, Naud J, Leblond FA, et al. ESRD impairs nonrenal clearance of fexofenadine but not midazolam. J Am Soc Nephrol 2009;20:2269–76.

[39] Thomson BK, Nolin TD, Velenosi TJ, Feere DA, Knauer MJ, Asher LJ, et al. Effect of CKD and dialysis modality on exposure to drugs cleared by nonrenal mechanisms. Am J Kidney Dis 2015;65:574–82.

[40] Zhang Y, Zhang L, Abraham S, Apparaju S, Wu TC, Strong JM, et al. Assessment of the impact of renal impairment on systemic exposure of new molecular entities: evaluation of recent new drug applications. Clin Pharmacol Ther 2009;85:305–11.

[41] Yeung CK, Shen DD, Thummel KE, Himmelfarb J. Effects of chronic kidney disease and uremia on hepatic drug metabolism and transport. Kidney Int 2014;85:522–8.

[42] Prokopienko AJ, Nolin TD. Microbiota-derived uremic retention solutes: perpetrators of altered nonrenal drug clearance in kidney disease. Expert Rev Clin Pharmacol 2018;11:71–82.

[43] Michaud J, Naud J, Chouinard J, Desy F, Leblond FA, Desbiens K, et al. Role of parathyroid hormone in the downregulation of liver cytochrome P450 in chronic renal failure. J Am Soc Nephrol 2006;17:3041–8.

[44] Nolin TD, Appiah K, Kendrick SA, Le P, McMonagle E, Himmelfarb J. Hemodialysis acutely improves hepatic CYP3A4 metabolic activity. J Am Soc Nephrol 2006;17:2363–7.

[45] De Martin S, Orlando R, Bertoli M, Pegoraro P, Palatini P. Differential effect of chronic renal failure on the pharmacokinetics of lidocaine in patients receiving and not receiving hemodialysis. Clin Pharmacol Ther 2006;80:597–606.

[46] Reidenberg MM, Drayer DE. Alteration of drug-protein binding in renal disease. Clin Pharmacokinet 1984;9(Suppl. 1):18–26.

[47] Odar-Cederlöf I, Borgå O. Kinetics of diphenylhydantoin in uraemic patients: consequences of decreased plasma protein binding. Eur J Clin Pharmacol 1974;7:31–7.

[48] Sheiner LB, Rosenberg B, Marathe VV. Estimation of population characteristics of pharmacokinetic parameters from routine clinical data. J Pharmacokinet Biopharm 1977;5:445–79.

[49] Aronson JK, Grahame-Smith DG. Altered distribution of digoxin in renal failure—a cause of digoxin toxicity? Br J Clin Pharmacol 1976;3:1045–51.

[50] Craig RM, Murphy P, Gibson TP, Quintanilla A, Chao GC, Cochrane C, et al. Kinetic analysis of D-xylose absorption in normal subjects and in patients with chronic renal failure. J Lab Clin Med 1983;101:496–506.

[51] Huang CM, Atkinson AJ Jr, Levin M, Levin NW, Quintanilla A. Pharmacokinetics of furosemide in advanced renal failure. Clin Pharmacol Ther 1974;16:659–66.

[52] Chau NP, Weiss YA, Safar ME, Lavene DE, Georges DR, Milliez PL. Pindolol availability in hypertensive patients with normal and impaired renal function. Clin Pharmacol Ther 1977;22:505–10.

[53] Wood AJ, Vestal RE, Spannuth CL, Stone WJ, Wilkinson GR, Shand DG. Propranolol disposition in renal failure. Br J Clin Pharmacol 1980; 10:561–6.

[54] Atkinson AJ Jr. The stable isotope method for determining absolute bioavailability. Transl Clin Pharmacol 2017;25:53–8.

Chapter 6

Pharmacokinetics in patients requiring renal replacement therapy

Arthur J. Atkinson, Jr.[a], Thomas D. Nolin[b], and John M. Allen[c,d]

[a]*Department of Pharmacology, Feinberg School of Medicine, Northwestern University, Chicago, IL, United States,* [b]*Department of Pharmacy and Therapeutics, and Department of Medicine, Renal-Electrolyte Division, University of Pittsburgh Schools of Pharmacy and Medicine, Pittsburgh, PA, United States,* [c]*Department of Pharmacotherapy and Translational Research, College of Pharmacy, University of Florida, Orlando, FL, United States,* [d]*Department of Internal Medicine, College of Medicine, University of Central Florida, Orlando, FL, United States*

Although measurements of drug recovery in the urine enable reasonable characterization of the renal clearance of most drugs, analysis of drug elimination by the liver is hampered by the types of measurements that can be made in routine clinical studies. Hemodialysis and other extracorporeal dialytic modalities are considered at this point in the text because they provide an unparalleled opportunity to measure blood flow to the eliminating organ, drug concentrations in blood entering and leaving the eliminating organ, and recovery of eliminated drug in the dialysate or ultrafiltrate. The measurements that can be made in analyzing drug elimination by different routes are compared in Table 6.1. Unfortunately, few pharmacokinetic studies in patients undergoing intermittent hemodialysis or continuous renal replacement therapy (CRRT) have incorporated all of the measurements that are shown in the table. However, the US Food and Drug Administration [1] has issued draft guidance that specifies the essential measurements that should be made in these studies, and this approach will be emphasized in this chapter.

TABLE 6.1 Measurements made in assessing drug elimination by different routes.

Measurements	Renal elimination	Hepatic elimination	Hemodialysis
Blood flow	+[a]	+[a]	+
Afferent blood concentration	+	+	+
Efferent blood concentration	0	0	+
Recovery of eliminated drug	+	0	+

[a]*Not actually measured in routine pharmacokinetic studies.*

Hemodialysis is an area of long-standing interest to pharmacologists. In a landmark 1914 paper, the pioneer American pharmacologist, John Jacob Abel, and his colleagues described the construction of the first artificial kidney which they used in dogs to demonstrate its efficacy in removing poisons and drugs [2]. In 1924 European scientists started to apply this technique to humans but their results were hampered by inefficient dialysis membranes and the lack of a suitable anticoagulant [3, 4]. In 1943 Kolff and Berk began the modern era of hemodialysis by using repeated hemodialysis to treat a 29-year-old uremic woman who had chronic nephritis [5]. Unfortunately, vascular access problems limited her therapy to only 12 hemodialysis sessions. Successful long-term hemodialysis for treating patients with end-stage kidney disease finally was made possible in the 1960s when techniques were developed for establishing long-lasting vascular access. By the late 1970s, continuous peritoneal dialysis had become a therapeutic alternative for these patients and offered the advantages of simpler, nonmachine-dependent home therapy and less hemodynamic stress [6]. In 1977 continuous arteriovenous hemofiltration (CAVH) was introduced as a method for removing fluid from diuretic-resistant patients, whose hemodynamic instability made them unable to tolerate conventional intermittent

Atkinson's Principles of Clinical Pharmacology. https://doi.org/10.1016/B978-0-12-819869-8.00018-5

TABLE 6.2 Summary of selected renal replacement therapies.

Procedure	Abbreviation	Diffusion	Convection	Vascular access	Replacement fluid
Intermittent hemodialysis	HD	++++	+	Fistula or Vein-Vein	No
Intermittent high-flux dialysis	HFD	+++	++	Fistula or Vein-Vein	No
Short-duration daily hemodialysis	SDHD	++++	+	Fistula or Vein-Vein	No
Nightly hemodialysis	NHD	++++	+	Fistula or Vein-Vein	No
Sustained low-efficiency dialysis	SLED	++++	+	Fistula or Vein-Vein	No
Continuous ambulatory peritoneal dialysis	CAPD	++++	+	None	No
Continuous arteriovenous hemofiltration	CAVH	0	++++	Artery-Vein	Yes
Continuous venovenous hemofiltration	CVVH	0	++++	Vein-Vein	Yes
Continuous arteriovenous hemodialysis	CAVHD	++++	+	Artery-Vein	Yes
Continuous venovenous hemodialysis	CVVHD	++++	+	Vein-Vein	Yes
Continuous arteriovenous hemodiafiltration	CAVHDF	+++	+++	Artery-Vein	Yes
Continuous venovenous hemodiafiltration	CVVHDF	+++	+++	Vein-Vein	Yes

hemodialysis [7]. Since then, this and related CRRT modalities have become the preferred treatment option for critically ill patients with acute kidney injury.

Several variations of CRRT have been developed that use hemodialysis and/or hemofiltration to remove both solutes and fluid, and some of these are listed in Table 6.2 [8]. Also listed are three recently popularized hybrid dialytic modalities that differ from conventional hemodialysis in that they are administered daily in order to minimize the extent of intradialytic weight gain and changes in body fluid composition. Short-duration daily hemodialysis (SDHD) utilizes only the most productive initial 2 h during which most low molecular weight solutes are removed during conventional hemodialysis, whereas the 6–8 h duration of nocturnal hemodialysis (NHD) results in increased phosphate and middle molecule clearance [9]. Sustained low-efficiency dialysis (SLED) provides an alternative to CRRT for treating patients with acute kidney injury and has advantages in that it utilizes conventional dialysis machines, routine dialysate fluids, and affords some patient mobility since it lasts for only 6–12 h [10]. All of these methods can affect pharmacokinetics, but we will focus on conventional intermittent hemodialysis and selected aspects of CRRT in this chapter.

Kinetics of intermittent hemodialysis

Solute transfer across dialyzing membranes

In Abel's artificial kidney, blood flowed through a hollow cylinder of dialyzing membrane that was immersed in a bath of dialysis fluid. However, in modern hollow-fiber dialysis cartridges, there is a continuous countercurrent flow of dialysate along the outside of the dialyzing membrane that maximizes the concentration gradient between blood and dialysate. Mass transfer across the dialyzing membrane occurs by diffusion and ultrafiltration. The rate of transfer has been analyzed with varying sophistication by a number of investigators [11]. A simple approach is that taken by Eugene Renkin who likened

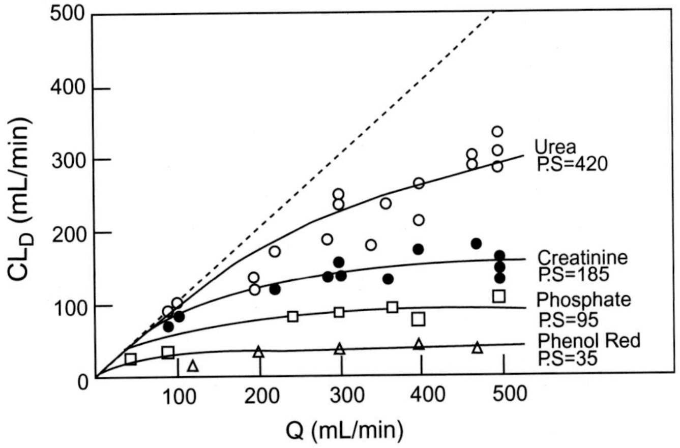

FIG. 6.1 Plot of dialysis clearance (CL_D) *vs* dialyzer blood flow (Q). The theoretical curves were fit to experimental data points to obtain estimates of the permeability coefficient-surface area product ($P{\cdot}S$) for each solute. Flow-limited clearance is indicated by the dashed line. The data were generated with a Kolff-Brigham type hemodialysis apparatus. *(Reproduced with permission from Renkin EM. Trans Am Soc Artif Intern Organs 1956;2:102–105.)*

this transfer process to mass transfer across capillary walls (see Chapter 3) [12]. Renkin expressed dialysis clearance (CL_D) as:

$$CL_D = Q\left(1 - e^{-P \cdot S/Q}\right) \tag{6.1}$$

where Q is blood flow through the dialyzer and $P{\cdot}S$ is the permeability coefficient-surface area product of the dialyzing membrane, defined by Fick's First Law of Diffusion as:

$$P \cdot S = DA/\lambda$$

In this equation, A is the surface area, λ is the thickness of the dialyzing membrane, and D is the diffusivity of a given solute in the dialyzing membrane. Solute diffusivity is primarily determined by molecular weight. Nonspherical molecular shape also may affect the diffusivity of larger molecules. This approach also neglects the effects of ultrafiltration, nonmembrane diffusive resistance, and drug binding to dialysis membranes.

Renkin used Eq. (6.1) to estimate $P{\cdot}S$ values for several solutes from flow and clearance measurements made on the Kolff-Brigham artificial kidney (Fig. 6.1). This theoretical analysis seems reasonably consistent with the experimental results. In the figure, the dashed line indicates a flow limitation to transport because clearance can never exceed dialyzer blood flow, a result that is obvious from inspection of Eq. (6.1) (i.e., $e^{-P \cdot S/Q}$ is never less than 0).

An analysis of relative dialysis clearance and dialyzer $P{\cdot}S$ values for the closely related compounds procainamide (PA) and N-acetylprocainamide (NAPA) is summarized in Table 6.3. Dialyzer clearance measurements of PA (CL_{PA}) and NAPA (CL_{NAPA}) made by Gibson et al. [13] were used together with Eq. (6.1) to calculate $P{\cdot}S$ values for PA ($P{\cdot}S_{PA}$) and NAPA ($P{\cdot}S_{NAPA}$). The ratio of these $P{\cdot}S$ values is also shown, since this ratio indicates the relative diffusivity of PA and NAPA. The utility of Renkin's approach is confirmed by the fact that the mean $P{\cdot}S$ ratio of 1.28 ± 0.23 ($\pm$SD) is in close agreement with the diffusion coefficient ratio of 1.23 that was obtained for PA and NAPA by the porous plate method of McBain and Liu [14]. The variation in dialyzer clearance estimates in Table 6.3 illustrates the problem encountered in transferring results between different dialyzers. However, the relative constancy of the $P{\cdot}S$ ratio estimates has prompted the suggestion that a reference compound, such as creatinine, be included in both in vitro and in vivo hemodialysis studies to facilitate extrapolation of dialysis clearance estimates from one dialyzer to another [15, 16].

Calculation of dialysis clearance

Currently, the efficiency of hemodialysis is expressed in terms of *dialysis clearance*. Dialysis clearance (CL_D) is commonly estimated from the Fick equation as follows:

$$CL_D = Q\left[\frac{A - V}{A}\right] \tag{6.2}$$

TABLE 6.3 Dialyzer permeability coefficient-surface area products for PA and NAPA.[a]

Column	CL_{PA} (mL/min)	CL_{NAPA} (mL/min)	$P{\cdot}S_{PA}$ (mL/min)	$P{\cdot}S_{NAPA}$ (mL/min)	Ratio $P{\cdot}S_{PA}/P{\cdot}S_{NAPA}$
Dow 4	79.9	55.3	102.0	64.7	1.58
Dow 5	114.6	89.9	170.2	119.4	1.43
Gambro 17	50.8	33.3	58.6	36.4	1.61
Ultra-Flow II	78.5	63.8	99.7	76.8	1.30
Ultra-Flow 145	63.4	50.4	76.3	58.1	1.31
Vivacell	37.1	27.8	41.0	29.9	1.37
Ex 23	50.4	50.4	58.1	58.1	1.00
Ex 25	71.6	62.6	88.6	75.1	1.18
Ex 29	81.4	78.0	104.5	98.9	1.06
Ex 55	51.8	53.9	60.0	62.8	0.93
Mean ± SD					1.28 ± 0.23

[a] *Clearance data obtained with dialyzer blood flow set at 200 mL/min and single pass dialysate flow at 400 mL/min (clearance data from Gibson TP, et al. Clin Pharmacol Ther 1976;20:720–726).*

where A is the solute concentration entering (arterial) and V the solute concentration leaving (venous) the dialyzer. This approach to calculating CL_D has been referred to as the *A-V difference* method [17]. The terms in brackets collectively describe what is termed the *extraction ratio* (E). As a general principle, clearance from an eliminating organ can be thought of as the product of organ blood flow and extraction ratio.

Single pass dialyzers are now standard for patient care and clearance calculations suffice for characterizing their performance. However, recirculating dialyzers were used in the early days of hemodialysis. Dialysis bath solute concentration (*Bath*) had to be considered in describing the performance of recirculating dialyzers and was included in the equation for calculating *dialysance* (D), as shown in the following equation [11]:

$$D = Q\left[\frac{A - V}{A - Bath}\right]$$

The currently preferred method for calculating dialysis clearance uses an equation that is analogous to the equation used to calculate renal clearance:

$$CL_P = \frac{R}{\overline{P} \cdot t} \tag{6.3}$$

where the amount of drug recovered by dialysis (R) is calculated as the product of the drug concentration in dialysate and total volume of dialysate collected during the dialysis time (t), and $\overline{P}$ is the average concentration of drug in plasma entering the dialyzer. The term *recovery clearance* has been coined for this clearance estimate, and Eq. (6.3) provides an estimate of dialysis plasma clearance (CL_P) that is *pharmacokinetically consistent* with estimates of elimination and intercompartmental clearance that are based on plasma concentration measurements [4, 16].

The recovery clearance is considered to be the "gold standard" estimate of dialysis clearance because it avoids the considerable confusion that surrounds proper calculation of dialysis clearance by the *A-V* difference method [4, 16, 18]. First, and contrary to the recommendation of some authors, either blood or plasma concentrations can be used in Eq. (6.2) because the ratio of red blood cell/plasma drug concentrations (RBC/P) is usually constant over a wide concentration range so the same estimate of extraction ratio is obtained regardless of whether plasma concentrations or blood concentrations are measured [4]. Second, although *blood clearance* is calculated correctly when Q is set equal to measured blood flow (Q_B), estimates of *plasma clearance* obtained by setting Q equal to plasma flow only are valid for those few solutes that are totally excluded from red blood cells because drug that partitions into erythrocytes is accessible to hemodialysis [19, 20]. When this partitioning occurs to the extent that plasma concentrations are less than blood concentrations, the value for Q needs to

METHOD	PLASMA CLEARANCE	BLOOD CLEARANCE
RECOVERY	$CL_p = \frac{R}{\overline{P} \bullet t}$	$CL_B = \frac{R}{\overline{B} \bullet t}$
A–V DIFFERENCE	$CL_p = Q_{EFF}\left(\frac{A-V}{A}\right)$	$CL_B = Q_B\left(\frac{A-V}{A}\right)$

FIG. 6.2 Equations for calculating whole blood and plasma dialysis clearance by the recovery *(top row)* and *A-V* difference *(bottom row)* methods. For the recovery method, *R* represents total drug recovery from the dialysis bath fluid, $\overline{B}$ and $\overline{P}$ are the respective average blood and plasma concentrations of solute entering the dialyzer, and τ is the dialysis time. Dialyzer blood clearance (CL_B) calculated by the *A-V* difference method equals that calculated by the recovery method when Q_B represents blood flow through the dialyzer. However, when plasma concentrations are less than blood concentrations, plasma clearance (CL_P) calculated by the recovery method is greater than CL_B *(upper left)*. So Q_{EFF} in the *A-V* difference equation for CL_P (lower left) needs to be greater than Q_B in order to obtain the recovery method result. As described in the text, erroneous dialysis clearance values would be obtained in this case if either measured blood flow or estimated plasma flow through the dialyzer were used to calculate CL_P.

be *greater* than Q_B if the recovery and *A-V* difference methods of estimated dialysis plasma clearance are to agree (Fig. 6.2). For example, in one study it was found that NAPA partitions preferentially from plasma into erythrocytes, so a value 223 mL/min was needed for *Q* in order to give *A-V* clearance method estimates that were consistent with those calculated by the recovery method [19]. This exceeded both the calculated plasma flow of 148 mL/min and the measured blood flow of 195 mL/min. Eq. (6.2) can provide a closer approximation to plasma clearance results obtained by the recovery method when an estimated effective dialyzer blood flow Q_{EFF} is used that takes red cell partitioning and hematocrit (Hct) into account:

$$Q_{EFF} = [(1 - \text{Hct}) + (\text{RBC/P})\,\text{Hct}]\,Q_{MEAS} \tag{6.4}$$

However, an important caveat in using the recovery method is to ensure that adsorption of the dialyzed drug does not impair the extent of drug recovery [21].

As shown in Fig. 6.3, pharmacokinetic models can be constructed that incorporate all the measurements that are readily accessed during hemodialysis [19]. When this is done, a pharmacokinetically derived estimate (Q_{PK}) of Q_{EFF} can be calculated by rearranging Eq. (6.2) as follows:

$$V = [(Q_{PK} - CL_D)/Q_{PK}] \cdot A$$

$$Q_{PK} = \frac{CL_D}{1 - V/A} \tag{6.5}$$

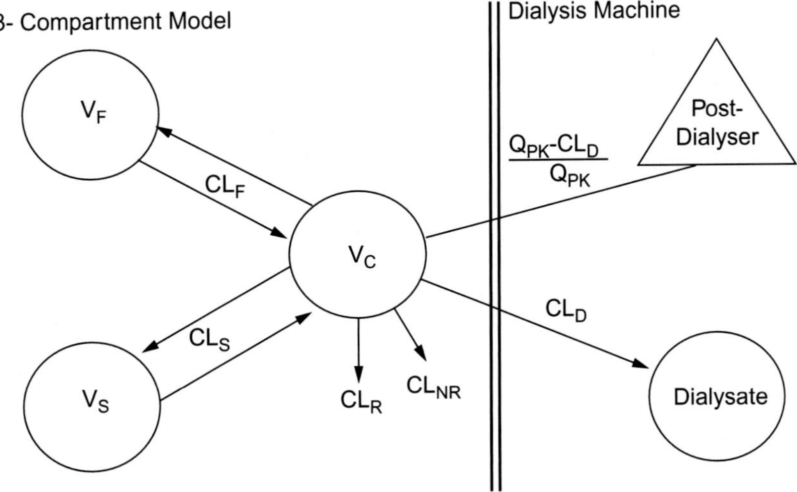

FIG. 6.3 Multicompartmental system for modeling pharmacokinetics during hemodialysis. Drug is delivered to the dialysis machine from the central compartment (V_C) and represents *A* in the Fick Equation. The dialysis machine is modeled by a compartment representing drug recovery in dialysis bath fluid and a proportionality *(triangle)* representing the drug concentration in blood returning to the patient (Eq. 6.5).

Since CL_D is calculated directly from the recovery of drug in dialysis bath fluid, and the V/A ratio is incorporated in the model, this estimate of Q_{EFF} is internally consistent with all the available data. Unfortunately, most hemodialysis studies have not incorporated the full range of readily available measurements in an integrated pharmacokinetic analysis of this type.

Patient factors affecting hemodialysis of drugs

Because elimination clearances are additive, total solute clearance during hemodialysis (CL_T) can be expressed as the sum of dialysis clearance (CL_D), and the patient's renal clearance (CL_R) and nonrenal clearance (CL_{NR}):

$$CL_T = CL_D + CL_R + CL_{NR} \tag{6.6}$$

When CL_D is small relative to the sum of CL_R and CL_{NR}, hemodialysis can be expected to have little impact on the overall rate of drug removal. The extent of drug binding to plasma proteins is the most important patient factor affecting dialysis clearance of most drugs, and in that sense dialysis clearance is restrictive. However, partitioning into erythrocytes enhances rather than retards dialytic clearance and Eq. (6.4) has been used in some studies to correct Eq. (6.2) for this. A large distribution volume also reduces the fraction of total body stores of a drug that can be removed by hemodialysis and limits the effect of hemodialysis on shortening drug elimination half-life since:

$$t_{1/2} = \frac{0.693V_d}{CL_T}$$

An assumption made in the analysis of most hemodialysis studies is that drug distribution and elimination kinetics remain unchanged during this procedure. However, Nolin et al. [22] used the erythromycin breath test to show that hepatic clearance of that drug increases by 27% as early as 2h after hemodialysis, presumably reflecting the dialytic removal of low molecular weight uremic toxins that inhibit cytochrome P450 (CYP) 3A4 and/or transporter activity. Finally, there are significant hemodynamic changes during hemodialysis that not only may affect the extent of drug removal by this procedure but also may have an important impact on patient response.

Hemodynamic changes during Dialysis

Few studies of pharmacokinetics during hemodialysis have used a compartmental model to evaluate the impact of hemodynamic changes that may affect the efficiency of this procedure. The fall in both A and V drug concentrations that occurs during hemodialysis is generally followed by a postdialysis rebound, as shown in Fig. 6.4. However, if no change in drug distribution is assumed, two discrepancies are likely to be encountered when the recovery method is incorporated in an integrated analysis of hemodialysis kinetics:

1. The total amount of drug recovered from the dialysis fluid is less than would be expected from the drop in plasma concentrations during hemodialysis.
2. The extent of the rebound in plasma concentrations is less than would be anticipated.

The only single pharmacokinetic parameter change that can resolve these discrepancies is a reduction in the intercompartmental clearance for the slowly equilibrating large peripheral compartment (CL_S). This is illustrated in the bottom panel of Fig. 6.4, and in this study the extent of reduction in CL_S was found to average 77% during hemodialysis [19]. This figure also shows that a reduction in CL_S persisted for some time after hemodialysis was completed.

The hemodynamic basis for these changes in CL_S was investigated subsequently in a dog model [23]. Urea and inulin were used as probes and were injected simultaneously 2h before dialysis. The pharmacokinetic model shown in Fig. 6.3 was used for data analysis and representative results are shown in Fig. 6.5. During hemodialysis, CL_S for urea and inulin fell on average to 19% and 63% of their respective predialysis values and it was estimated that the efficiency of urea removal was reduced by 10%. In the 2h after dialysis, urea CL_S averaged only 37% of predialysis values but returned to its predialysis level for inulin. Compartmental blood flow and permeability coefficient-surface area products of the calculated intercompartmental clearances were calculated as described in Chapter 3 from the permeability-flow equation derived by Renkin [24]. During and after dialysis, blood flow to the slow equilibrating compartment (Q_S) on average was reduced to 10% and 20%, respectively, of predialysis values. The permeability coefficient-surface area product did not change significantly. There were no changes in either fast compartment blood flow or permeability

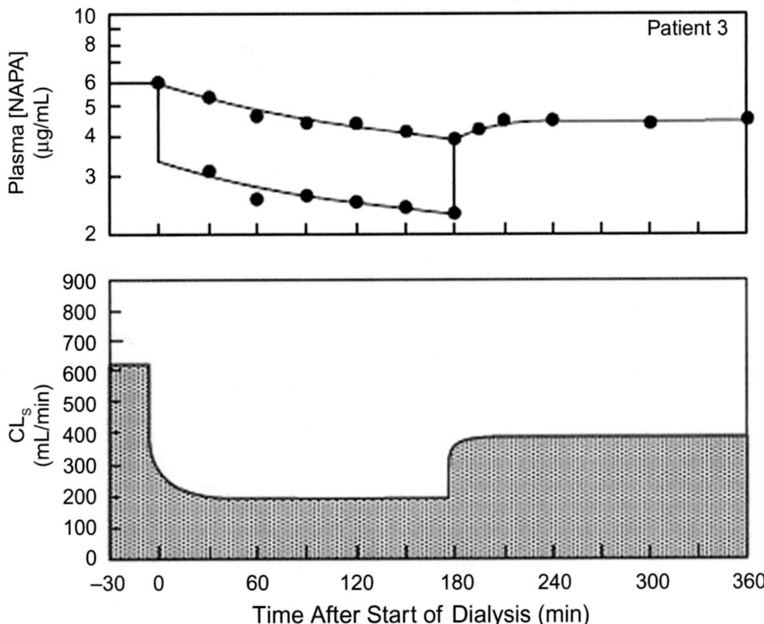

FIG. 6.4 Computer-fitted curves from pharmacokinetic analysis of NAPA plasma concentrations (●) measured before, during, and after hemodialysis. NAPA plasma concentrations entering (*A*) and leaving (*V*) the artificial kidney are shown during dialysis. The bottom panel shows changes occurring in slow compartment intercompartmental clearance (CL_S) during and after dialysis. *(Reproduced with permission from Stec GP, Atkinson AJ Jr, Nevin MJ, Thenot J-P, Gibson TP, Ivanovich P, del Greco F. Clin Pharmacol Ther 1979;26:618–628.)*

coefficient-surface area product. Measurements of plasma renin activity during and after hemodialysis of dogs with intact kidneys (lower panel of Fig. 6.5) suggest that this hemodynamic change was mediated at least in part by the renin-angiotensin system.

Since the slow equilibrating peripheral compartment in this model is largely composed of skeletal muscle, it is not surprising that the hemodynamic changes associated with hemodialysis result in the skeletal muscle cramps that have been estimated to complicate more than 20% of hemodialysis sessions [25]. Plasma volume contraction appears to be the initiating event which triggers blood pressure homeostatic responses. Those patients who are particularly prone to cramps appear to have a sympathetic nervous system response to this volume stress that is not modulated by activation of a normal renin-angiotensin system [26]. Because this hemodynamic change also reduces the intradialytic and post-dialytic transfer of drug from the periphery to the intravascular space, it acts as a pharmacokinetic tourniquet to sequester drug in peripheral sites that are pharmacologically inert. In this way it can be of therapeutic benefit by reducing a drug's apparent distribution volume for several hours, thus enhancing the efficacy of hemodialysis when it is used to treat drug intoxications [27].

Kinetics of CRRT and sustained renal replacement therapy

While the use of hemodialysis is considered optimal renal replacement therapy for most patients, a subset of critically ill patients may not tolerate the substantial hemodynamic effects associated with hemodialysis. Specifically, patients with profound hypotension, in whom increasing hypotension could have a deleterious impact on organ perfusion, and traumatic brain injured patients, in whom intracerebral shifts of serum proteins can lead to cerebral edema and intracranial hypertension, may benefit from other renal replacement modalities. In these instances, CRRT or SLED may be utilized. Hemofiltration is a prominent feature of many CRRT modalities (Table 6.2). However, continuous hemodialysis can also be employed to accelerate solute removal, albeit at a much slower rate than during traditional intermittent hemodialysis [28]. The contribution of both processes to extracorporeal drug clearance will be considered separately in the context of CRRT.

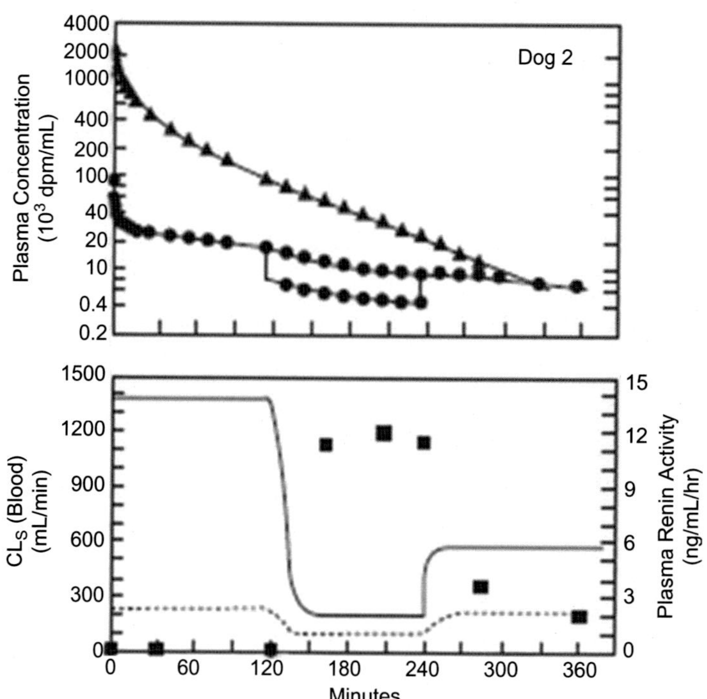

FIG. 6.5 Kinetic analysis of urea ^{14}C (●) and inulin ^{3}H (▲) plasma concentrations *(upper panel)*. Although inulin was not dialyzable, its plasma concentration fell throughout the study because renal function was preserved. The *lower panel* shows CL_S estimates for urea (—) and inulin (- - -), and measured plasma renin activity (■). *(Reproduced with permission from Bowsher DJ, Krejcie TC, Avram MJ, Chow MJ del Greco F, Atkinson AJ Jr. J Lab Clin Med 1985;105:489–497.)*

Clearance by continuous hemofiltration

Hemofiltration removes solutes by convective mass transfer down a hydrostatic pressure gradient [29, 30]. As plasma water passes through the hemofilter membrane, solute is carried along by solvent drag. Convective mass transfer thus mimics the process of glomerular filtration. The pores of hemofilter membranes are larger than those of dialysis membranes and permit passage of solutes having a molecular weight of up to 50 kDa. Accordingly, a wider range of compounds will be removed by hemofiltration than by hemodialysis. Since large volumes of fluid are removed, fluid replacement solutions need to be administered at rates exceeding 10 L/day [31]. This fluid can be administered either before (predilution mode) or after (postdilution mode) the hemofilter. In contemporary practice, roller pumps are used to generate the hydrostatic driving force for ultrafiltration, and the need for arterial catheterization has been obviated by the placement of double-lumen catheters into a large vein [28].

Albumin and other drug-binding proteins do not pass through the filtration membrane, so only unbound drug in plasma water is removed by ultrafiltration. In addition, albumin and other negatively charged plasma proteins exert a Gibbs-Donnan effect that retards the transmembrane convection of some polycationic drugs such as gentamicin [32, 33]. The situation with regard to erythrocyte drug binding is less clear. Although predilution reduces the efficiency of solute removal because solute concentrations in the hemofilter are less than in plasma water [34], it has been reported that net urea removal is enhanced when replacement fluid is administered in the predilution mode, because it can diffuse down its concentration gradient from red blood cells into the diluted plasma water before reaching the hemofilter [31].

The extent to which a solute is carried in the ultrafiltrate across a membrane is characterized by its *sieving coefficient*. An approximate equation for calculating sieving coefficients (SC) is as follows:

$$SC = \frac{UF}{A} \tag{6.7}$$

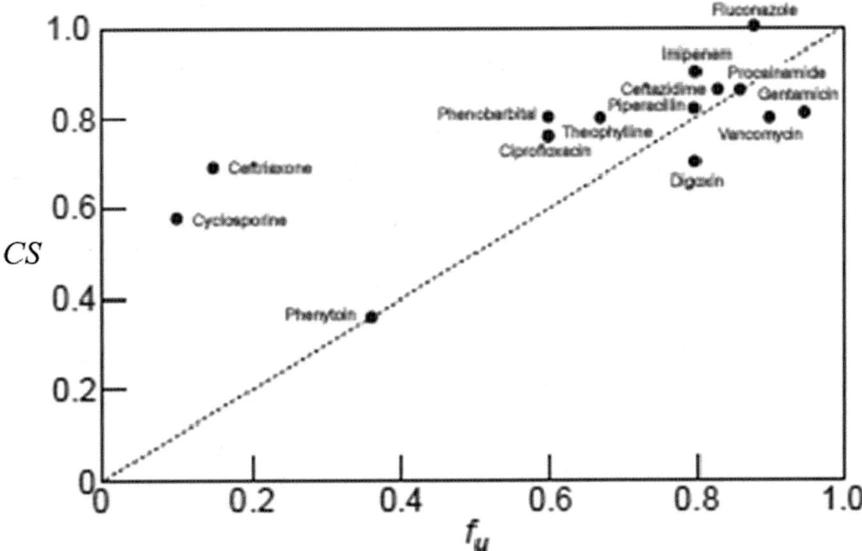

FIG. 6.6 Relationship between free fraction (f_u) and hemofiltration sieving coefficient (*SC*) for selected drugs. The line of identity *(dotted line)* indicates what would be expected if *SC* were equal to f_u (see text for further details).

where *UF* is the solute concentration in the ultrafiltrate and *A* is the solute concentration in plasma water entering the hemofilter [35]. The convective clearance of solute across an ultrafilter (CL_{UF}) is given by the product of *SC* and the rate at which fluid crosses the ultrafilter (*UFR*):

$$CL_{UF} = SC \cdot UFR \tag{6.8}$$

Since *UFR* cannot exceed blood flow through the hemofilter, that establishes the theoretical upper limit for CL_{UF}. The major determinants of *SC* are molecular size and the unbound fraction of a compound in plasma water. Values of *SC* may range from 0 for macromolecules that do not pass through the pores of the hemofilter membrane to 1 for small molecule drugs that are not protein bound, and have unrestricted transport across the hemofilter membrane. Although less information has been accumulated about the ultrafiltration clearance of drugs than about their dialysis clearance, in many cases the unbound fraction of drug in plasma water can be used to approximate *SC*.

Measured values of *SC* and fraction of unbound drug in plasma (f_u) are compared for several drugs in Fig. 6.6 which is largely based on data published by Golper and Marx [33]. However, measurements of f_u for a number of drugs are much higher in hemodialyzed patients than in normal subjects [36]. Accordingly, uremic patient values for f_u in the figure were chosen for theophylline [36], phenytoin [37], ceftazidime [38], ceftriaxone [39], ciprofloxacin [40], and cyclosporine [41]. On the other hand, SC values for cyclosporine and ceftriaxone are considerably higher than expected from f_u measurements. So it is likely that factors other than plasma protein binding may affect the sieving of some drugs during hemofiltration [42].

Clearance by continuous hemodialysis and SLED

Some of the renal replacement therapies listed in Table 6.2 incorporate continuous hemodialysis, or a combination of continuous hemofiltration and hemodialysis. Continuous hemodialysis differs importantly from conventional intermittent hemodialysis and SLED in that the flow rate of dialysate is much lower than countercurrent blood flow through the dialyzer. As a result, concentrations of many solutes in dialysate leaving the dialyzer (C_D) will have nearly equilibrated with their plasma concentrations in blood entering the dialyzer (C_P) [28, 43]. The extent to which this equilibration is complete is referred to as the dialysate saturation (S_D) and is calculated as the following ratio:

$$S_D = \frac{C_D}{C_P}$$

Under conditions of minimal ultrafiltration, diffusive drug clearance (CL_D) is calculated from the following equation in which Q_D equals dialysate flow:

$$CL_D = Q_D \cdot S_D \tag{6.9}$$

Because $Q_D = V_D/t$, where V_D is the volume of dialysate produced during time t, Eq. (6.9) can be rewritten as follows:

$$CL_D = \frac{C_D \cdot V_D}{C_P \cdot t} \tag{6.10}$$

which is identical to Eq. (6.3). Both Eqs. (6.10) and (6.3) are nonmechanistic descriptions of clearance that do not incorporate the factors of molecular size or protein binding that account for incomplete equilibration of plasma and dialysate solute concentrations. However, in contrast with intermittent hemodialysis, in which dialyzer blood flow is rate limiting, diffusive drug clearance during CRRT is limited by Q_D, which typically is only 25 mL/min. Another important characteristic of dialysate saturation is that it becomes progressively less complete as dialysate flow approaches blood flow [28]. Few studies have been conducted in which SLED is compared with other modalities, but the *SC* of linezolid during SLED is similar to CVVH, but higher than with intermittent hemodialysis [44].

Extracorporeal clearance during continuous renal replacement therapy

Extracorporeal clearance during CRRT (CL_{EC}) can be regarded as the sum of convective and hemodialytic clearance [28, 43]:

$$CL_{EC} = SC \cdot UFR + Q_D \cdot S_D \tag{6.11}$$

Because solute diffusivity decreases with increasing molecular weight, diffusion becomes relatively inefficient even with large-pore hemofilter membranes and convection becomes the primary mechanism involved in the extracorporeal clearance of vancomycin (MW: 1448 Da) and other high molecular weight drugs [34]. Unfortunately, *UFR* tends to decrease with time, falling rather rapidly during the first 6 h of therapy and reaching about half of its original value in approximately 20 h [28]. Conversely, drug adsorption to the dialyzer membrane may decrease during therapy, resulting in an increase in the *SC* [45]. For these reasons, estimates of extracorporeal drug clearance during CRRT are most reliable when based on drug recovery in dialysate, as discussed for conventional clearance. Thus where V_{UF} is the volume of ultrafiltrate:

$$CL_{EC} = \frac{C_D \cdot V_{UF}}{C_P \cdot t} \tag{6.12}$$

By analogy with Eq. (6.6), the contribution of CL_{EC} to total solute clearance during CRRT is given by:

$$CL_T = CL_{EC} + CL_R + CL_{NR} \tag{6.13}$$

Clinical considerations

From the clinical standpoint, the two main pharmacokinetic considerations regarding renal replacement therapy deal with the use of these therapeutic modalities to treat drug toxicity and, more frequently, the need to administer supplemental drug doses to patients whose impaired kidney function necessitates intervention. The factors that determine the extent of drug removal by renal replacement therapy are summarized in Table 6.4. As yet, it has been difficult to analyze the interaction of all these factors with sufficient rigor to formulate generally applicable guidelines for clinical practice. A major problem in applying past studies of dialysis pharmacokinetics has been the transition from conventional low-flux (e.g., cuprophan or cellulose acetate) to high-flux (e.g., polysulfone) dialyzing membranes [46]. Whereas only 5% of patients were treated with high-flux dialyzers in 1987, 46% of patients received high-flux dialysis in 1997, and that percentage is probably higher at this time [47]. Current clinical practice guidelines formulated by a Work Group of the National Kidney Foundation recommend that either high-flux or low-flux hemodialysis can be used as there is no difference in survival benefit [48]. However, the Work Group found in a metaanalysis that cardiovascular mortality was reduced when high-flux dialyzers were used. So if their higher cost is not a constraint, the conclusion of the Work Group was that high-flux dialyzers are preferable. From the standpoint of drug therapy, the transition to high-flux hemodialysis has had a particularly significant impact on the hemodialytic removal of larger molecular weight drugs like vancomycin (MW = 1449 Da) that required no supplementary dosing during low-flux hemodialysis but require additional doses to replace drug lost through high-flux dialyzers [49].

TABLE 6.4 Factors affecting the extent of drug removal by renal replacement therapy.

Characteristics of hemodialysis or hemofiltration
• Low-flux *vs* high-flux membrane
• Dialyzer blood flow and ultrafiltration rate
• Dialysate flow
• Duration of hemodialysis or hemofiltration
Drug and patient characteristics
• Molecular weight of drug
• Drug binding to plasma proteins
• Distribution volume of drug
• Drug partitioning into erythrocytes
• Reduction in intercompartmental clearance

Dialysis clearance during hemodialysis is limited by and can never exceed dialyzer blood flow, whereas clearance during continuous renal replacement therapy is limited by dialysate flow [50]. Extensive binding to plasma proteins is another factor that limits the extent to which drugs can be removed by hemodialysis or hemofiltration. Phenytoin is approximately 90% protein bound in patients with normal kidney function. However, phenytoin is only 70%–80% protein bound in hemodialysis patients with end-stage kidney disease, raising the possibility that significant hemodialytic removal of phenytoin might occur in these patients [50]. Despite this, the hemodialytic removal of phenytoin was found to be negligible when low-flux dialyzers were used [51]. On the other hand, Frenchie and Bastani [52] recently reported that some of their patients have experienced grand mal seizures at the end of dialysis or in the early postdialysis period when high-flux dialyzers were used. These investigators then used the recovery method to estimate in one of their patients that approximately 48% of total body phenytoin stores were removed during 4 h of high-flux hemodialysis. Patients who present with toxicity following phenytoin ingestion usually have normal kidney function and phenytoin binding to plasma proteins. However, high-flux dialyzers have shown some promise in treating these patients [53]. Particularly impressive results were obtained in one study in which a high cut-off dialyzer removed an estimated 1.1 g of phenytoin over an 8-h dialysis period, achieving a clearance that exceeded that reported with standard high-flux dialyzers [54]. The authors attributed this to the larger surface area of their dialysis filter and to the high blood and dialysate flows that were used.

Large distribution volume is another important factor that limits the extent to which drugs can be removed by hemodialysis or hemofiltration. Drugs with a distribution volume less than 1 L/kg are more easily dialyzed and hemodialytic removal of drugs generally is not clinically significant for drugs whose distribution volume exceeds 2 L/kg [55]. Accordingly, neither conventional intermittent hemodialysis nor CRRT will significantly enhance the removal of digoxin or digitoxin. Fortunately, digoxin-specific antibody fragments (Fab) now are available for treating severe intoxication with these drugs [56]. This obviates even the need for hemodialysis as initial improvement is observed within 1 h of Fab administration and toxicity is resolved completely within 4 h in most patients.

Reductions in the intercompartmental clearance between the intravascular space and the periphery can have important effects during and for some time after hemodialysis. This tourniquet-like action effectively sequesters a substantial amount of drug in skeletal muscle and other pharmacologically inert tissues, thus reducing the amount of drug removed during hemodialysis. However, this also causes an apparent reduction in the drug's distribution volume so that there is a greater than expected decrease in drug concentrations in plasma and in rapidly equilibrating tissues that may be of clinical utility in treating patients with central nervous system or cardiovascular toxic reactions to drugs [27]. The reduced intercompartmental clearance that persists after hemodialysis also attenuates the rebound in plasma drug concentrations that typically occurs. Although intercompartmental clearance has not been studied during CRRT or SLED, these modalities produce less hemodynamic instability and would be expected to provoke a smaller cardiovascular homeostatic response.

Drug dosing guidelines for patients requiring renal replacement therapy

Given the complexity of integrating the impact of the separate factors listed in Table 6.4 empirical criteria have been proposed for assessing *dialyzability*, the ability of extracorporeal methods to remove a clinically significant percentage of the total body content of a drug [57]. Traditionally, dialyzability sufficient to warrant increasing or supplementing drug doses for patients requiring renal replacement therapy has been assessed by comparing CL_{EC}, representing extracorporeal clearance from either intermittent hemodialysis or CRRT, with the sum of the nondialytic clearances. Levy [58] has proposed that supplementation is needed only for drugs whose CL_{EC} is greater than 30% of $CL_R + CL_{NR}$. On the other hand, the preferred assessment of dialyzability used to evaluate the efficacy of hemodialysis in treating drug intoxications is based on the percentage of the drug in the body that is removed in 6h of hemodialysis [57].

Several approaches will be considered that can be used to make appropriate drug dose adjustments for patients requiring renal replacement therapy. Perhaps the simplest approach is to guide dosage using standard reference tables, such as those published by Aronoff and colleagues [59]. These tables are based on published literature and suggest drug dose adjustments for adult and pediatric patients with various levels of impaired kidney function, as well as for patients requiring conventional hemodialysis, chronic ambulatory peritoneal dialysis, and CRRT. Unfortunately, no distinction is made between data obtained with low-flux and high-flux dialyzers. Even within a single dialyzer class, estimates of CL_D obtained with any one dialyzer usually do not reflect the performance of other dialyzers. For this reason, it has been proposed that a suitable standard compound could be selected for in vitro studies, such as that described by Gibson et al. [13], so that Eq. (6.1) could be used to facilitate the extrapolation of results to different dialyzers [15, 16].

Although fewer data are available for patients treated with CRRT than with conventional intermittent hemodialysis, CRRT generally provides clearances of approximately 30–50mL/min depending on a number of factors that include dialysate flow rate, age of dialysis filter, and remaining intrinsic kidney function. As a result, some drugs may require an increase in dosing during CRRT as compared to intermittent hemodialysis.

A second approach is to calculate supplemental doses to replace drug lost during hemodialysis or continuous renal replacement therapy by directly measuring drug loss by extracorporeal removal or by estimating this loss from drug concentrations measured in plasma. It is relatively easy to use these measurements to refine supplemental dose estimates and replacement doses are indicated particularly for antibiotic, anticonvulsant, and some antiarrhythmic drugs. The most reliable approach would be to base a supplemental dose on the amount of drug actually removed. However, this method is usually implemented by estimating the supplemental dose (D_{sup}) from a plasma concentration measured at the conclusion of hemodialysis, or at a convenient interval during continuous renal replacement therapy ($C_{measured}$):

$$D_{sup} = \left(C_{target} - C_{measured}\right)V_d \tag{6.14}$$

In the setting of conventional intermittent hemodialysis, caution is warranted when using this method to estimate supplemental doses of drugs that have a narrow therapeutic index because drug redistribution to the intravascular space from the periphery is slowed by the marked hemodynamic changes that occur during and for some time after hemodialysis, so Eq. (6.14) is likely to overestimate the supplemental dose that is needed [19]. For example, Pollard et al. [60] reported that the postdialysis rebound in serum vancomycin concentrations following high-flux hemodialysis ranged from 19% to 60% of the intradialytic concentration drop and did not peak for an average of 6h (range: 1–12h). On the other hand, Eq. (6.14) provides a reasonably reliable guide to drug dosing during continuous renal replacement therapy and SLED because hemodynamic changes are minimized and the rate of drug removal by these modalities is usually less than the rate of drug redistribution from the periphery. For example, postdialysis rebound in patients on SLED has been reported to be $<4\%$ for gentamicin [61] and $<10\%$ for vancomycin [62]. Thus serum trough concentrations should be measured immediately after SLED to determine if post-SLED supplemental doses are needed [63]. For medications that are significantly removed during dialysis, specifically antimicrobials administered every 24h, the daily dose or a supplemental dose should be administered immediately after SLED. For dialyzable agents that require administration every 12h, supplemental doses should be administered after SLED and 12h later [63].

An exception to this approach is that *postdialysis* dosing is suboptimal for therapy with gentamicin and other drugs that exhibit concentration-dependent antibiotic efficacy, a prolonged postantibiotic effect, and increased toxicity when trough concentrations are elevated [64, 65]. Doses of these drugs should be administered 2–6h *before* intermittent hemodialysis in order to achieve optimally effective peak concentrations. Subsequent dialysis then acts to minimize trough antibiotic concentrations.

A third approach is to use the principles discussed before to calculate a maintenance dose multiplication factor (*MDMF*) that can be used to augment the dose that would be appropriate in the absence of renal replacement therapy [45]. For continuous renal replacement therapy, *MDMF* is given simply by the following ratio of clearances:

$$MDMF = \frac{CL_{EC} + CL_R + CL_{NR}}{CL_R + CL_{NR}} \tag{6.15}$$

The relative time on (t_{ON}) and off (t_{OFF}) extracorporeal therapy during a dosing interval also must be taken into account for conventional hemodialysis and other intermittent interventions such as SLED. In this situation:

$$MDMF = \frac{(CL_{EC} + CL_R + CL_{NR})t_{ON} + (CL_R + CL_{NR})t_{OFF}}{(CL_R + CL_{NR})(t_{ON} + t_{OFF})}$$

$$MDMF = \left(\frac{CL_{EC}}{CL_R + CL_{NR}}\right)\left(\frac{t_{ON}}{t_{ON} + t_{OFF}}\right) + 1 \tag{6.16}$$

Estimates of *MDMF* for several drugs are listed in Table 6.5 in which the abbreviations used for treatment modality are defined in Table 6.2. In addition, more extensive tables are presented by Reetze-Bonorden et al. [45]. With the exception of vancomycin, baseline drug clearance values for functionally anephric patients ($CL_{aneph.}$) given in Table 6.2 are taken from either the intermittent hemodialysis or the continuous renal replacement references that are cited. In the first 2 weeks after the onset of acute kidney injury, vancomycin $CL_{aneph.}$ falls from approximately 40 mL/min to the value of 6.0 mL/min that is found in patients with end-stage kidney disease [79]. This latter value is included in Table 6.5. Eq. (6.16) was used to estimate *MDMF* for a hemodialysis time of 4 h during a single 24-h period. A 4-h dialysis time also was used to calculate the MDMF value for SLED to facilitate comparison of the extent of drug removal by the two techniques. The CL_{EC} values for ceftazidime [38], ciprofloxacin [40], and gentamicin [71] during continuous renal replacement therapy all were obtained with a dialysate flow rate of 1 L/h and estimates of MDMF were made from Eq. (6.15).

As in treating other patients with impaired kidney function, maintenance drug doses for patients receiving renal replacement therapy can be adjusted by increasing the dosing interval as well as by reducing the drug dose. An estimate of the increased dosing interval (τ') can be made by dividing the maintenance dosing interval (τ) by *MDMF* [45].

Extracorporeal therapy of patients with drug toxicity

Intensive supportive therapy is all that is required for most patients suffering from dose-related drug toxicity and drug removal by extracorporeal methods generally is indicated only for those patients whose condition deteriorates despite institution of these more conservative measures [80]. However, a decision to intervene with extracorporeal therapy may be prompted by other clinical and pharmacologic considerations that are listed in Table 6.6. For example, most intoxications with phenobarbital can be managed by a combination of supportive care and minimization of renal tubular reabsorption of this drug by forced diuresis and urine alkalinization. However, extracorporeal therapy is indicated for patients who are severely hypotensive or exhibit depression or deep and prolonged coma [81].

The same factors that determine the extent of drug removal by renal replacement therapy (Table 6.4) during the course of usual care are applicable to patients with drug toxicity. That is, the physicochemical and pharmacokinetic properties of a drug in the setting of toxicity (i.e., *toxicokinetics*) may be used to predict whether extracorporeal therapy is likely to enhance total body clearance and effectively remove the toxin, thereby lowering the total amount in the body. The primary determinants of effective toxin removal by extracorporeal therapy are molecular weight, distribution volume, lipophilicity, protein binding, and ongoing systemic clearance.

The molecular weight of a toxin strongly influences CL_{EC}. Toxins with molecular weight <500 Da are efficiently cleared by diffusive extracorporeal modalities such as hemodialysis [64]. Although contemporary high-flux filters are capable of clearing larger toxins in the middle molecular weight range (i.e., up to 5000 Da) when used with diffusive modalities, convective modalities, such as hemofiltration, permit clearance of even larger solutes in excess of 15,000 Da.

Distribution volume is the most important determinant of effective toxin removal by extracorporeal therapy. Hydrophilic toxins exhibit a small distribution volume and are more readily removed by extracorporeal therapies. This is because toxins with a small distribution volume (<1 L/kg) have a substantial exposure to the dialysis filter and are typically removed

TABLE 6.5 Estimated drug dosing requirements for patients requiring renal replacement therapy.

	$CL_{aneph.}$ (mL/min)	Intermittent hemodialysis				Continuous renal replacement therapy							
		Mode	CL_D (mL/min)	*MDMF*	Ref.	Mode	*SC*	*UFR* (mL/min)	CL_{UF} (mLmin)	CL_{HD} (mL/min)	CL_{EC} (mL/min)	*MDMF*	Ref.
Ceftazidime	11.2	HD	43.6	1.6	[66]	CAVHD	0.86	7.5	6.5	6.6	13.1	2.2	[38]
Ceftriaxone	7.0	HD	11.8	1.0	[67]	CVVH	0.69	24.1	16.6		16.6	3.4	[39]
Ciprofloxacin	188[a]	HD	40	1.0	[68]	CAVHD/ CVVHD	0.76	7.2	4.8	7.3	12.1	2.4	[40]
Cyclosporine	463	HD	0.31	1.0	[69]	CAVH	0.58	4.4	2.6		2.6	1.0	[41]
Gentamicin	15.3	HFD	116	2.0	[70]	CAVHD					5.2	1.3	[71]
Levetiracetam	10.9	HD	127	3.1	[72]								
Levofloxacin	37	SLED	49	1.4	[73]	CVVH	0.96	21.7	21		21	1.6	[74]
Linezolid	76	SLED	33	1.2	[44]	CVVH	0.69	40	31		31	1.4	[75]
Phenytoin	83[b]	HD	12	1.2	[51]	CAVH	0.36	2.8	1.0		1.0	1.0	[37]
		HFD	160	1.5	[52]								
Sotalol	26.7	HD	78	1.7	[76]								
Vancomycin	6	HFD	106	4.1	[77]	CVVH	0.88	25	23		23	4.8	[78]
		SLED	35	1.1	[62]								

[a]*Calculated from CL/F with F assumed to be 60% as in normals.*
[b]*Elimination of this drug follows Michaelis-Menten kinetics. Apparent clearance will be lower when plasma levels are higher than those obtained in this study.*

TABLE 6.6 Considerations for extracorporeal treatment of drug intoxications.

General clinical considerations
• Clinical deterioration despite intensive supportive therapy
• Severe intoxication indicated by depression of midbrain function or measured plasma or serum level
• Condition complicated by pneumonia, sepsis, or other coexisting illness
Pharmacologic considerations
• Extracorporeal intervention can increase drug elimination significantly
• Drug clearance is slow due to pharmacologic properties of intoxicant or patient's impaired renal or hepatic function
• Intoxicant has a toxic metabolite or has toxic effects that are delayed

more effectively by extracorporeal therapy [82]. Conversely, lipophilic toxins are able to cross cellular membranes and distribute throughout body tissues, leading to a large distribution volume. The larger the distribution volume, the greater the fraction of toxin that is peripheral to the intravascular space and not exposed to the dialysis filter, leading to dramatically decreased and often negligible removal of total body stores [83]. Importantly, even if the toxin is able to be cleared from the blood by a dialysis filter, if the toxin exhibits a large distribution volume (>2 L/kg), then the efficacy of extracorporeal therapy generally will be low. However, hemodynamic changes during hemodialysis temporarily decrease the apparent distribution volume of at least some drugs [27]. On the other hand, CRRT modalities have been useful in clearing some toxins with a large distribution volume. They are not associated with the same hemodynamic changes as hemodialysis, so postdialysis redistribution (rebound) is attenuated [84].

The degree of plasma protein binding of a toxin inversely relates to its CL_{EC}. Toxins with high protein binding are associated with low unbound concentrations (free fraction) in plasma. Only unbound toxin is likely to be removed by extracorporeal therapies. The molecular weight of a toxin-protein complex often exceeds 60,000 Da and is too large to be filtered, so also leads to decreased CL_{EC} of highly protein-bound drugs. In general, toxins that are >80% protein bound are poorly removed by extracorporeal therapy.

The patient's underlying systemic clearance (i.e., sum of renal and nonrenal clearance) must be considered when assessing the potential benefit of extracorporeal therapy for drug toxicity. Extracorporeal therapy can exert a clinically beneficial effect on the amount of toxin in the body if CL_{EC} is similar to, or greater than, systemic clearance. In other words, if systemic clearance is high, then extracorporeal therapy is unlikely to significantly increase clearance enough to justify its use [57, 83].

In some instances, alternative approaches for treating intoxications have been developed that are even more efficient than extracorporeal therapy. For example, methanol and ethylene glycol are low molecular weight alcohols that are converted to toxic metabolites. Methanol is metabolized by hepatic alcohol dehydrogenase (ADH) to formaldehyde and formic acid, which causes metabolic acidosis and, after a 12–18-h latent period, retinal injury and blindness [85]. Ethylene glycol is also metabolized by ADH to glycoaldehyde and further oxidized to glycolic and oxalic acid. Formation of glycolic acid causes metabolic acidosis, whereas calcium oxalate precipitation results in severe kidney damage. Ethyl alcohol has traditionally been used to treat both of these intoxications because it competitively inhibits ADH. However, ethyl alcohol exhibits Michaelis-Menten elimination kinetics that make appropriate drug dosing difficult, must be infused continuously in large fluid volumes that may be deleterious, and depresses the central nervous system, thus complicating patient evaluation. Fomepizole (4-methylpyrazole) is a more effective inhibitor of ADH than ethyl alcohol [86]. It can be administered at a convenient interval and does not depress the central nervous system. Accordingly, it has replaced ethyl alcohol as the standard of care in managing patients who have ingested either methanol or ethylene glycol. Although some patients with high concentrations of these alcohols have been treated successfully with fomepizole alone, hemodialysis effectively reduces exposure risk from both these alcohols and their toxic metabolites. Therefore hemodialysis remains an important adjunctive therapy, particularly for patients in whom treatment is only begun several hours after ingestion.

Therapy with drug-specific antibody fragments (Fab) represents a possible strategy for rapidly treating intoxications for which extracorporeal therapy is ineffective. For example, digoxin can be removed by extracorporeal methods despite its large molecular weight but its large V_d limits their efficacy [87]. However, digoxin-specific Fab are effective in treating patients with severe intoxication with either digoxin or digitoxin [56]. The use of Fab to treat toxicity with tricyclic antidepressants and colchicine has also been demonstrated but their commercial development has not been feasible [88].

References

[1] CDER. Pharmacokinetics in patients with impaired renal function—Study design, data analysis, and impact on dosing. Draft guidance for industry, Silver Spring: FDA; September, 2020.http://www.fda.gov/downloads/Drugs/Guidance ComplianceRegulatoryInformation/Guidances/UCM204959.pdf.

[2] Abel JJ, Rowntree LG, Turner BB. On the removal of diffusible substances from the circulating blood of living animals by dialysis. J Pharmacol Exp Ther 1914;5:275–317.

[3] Wizemann V. Hemodialysis: 70 years. Clin Investig 1994;72:720–721.

[4] Atkinson AJ Jr. Pitfalls in the calculation of hemodialysis clearance and in the assessment of dialysis efficacy. Transl Clin Pharmacol 2016;24:153–165.

[5] Kolff WJ, Berk HTJ. The artificial kidney: a dialyzer with a great area. Acta Med Scand 1944;117:121–134.

[6] Baillie GR, Eisele G. Continuous ambulatory peritoneal dialysis: a review of its mechanics, advantages, complications, and areas of controversy. Ann Pharmacother 1992;26:1409–1420.

[7] Kramer P, Wigger W, Rieger J, Matthaei D, Scheler F. Arteriovenous haemofiltration: a new and simple method for the treatment of overhydrated patients resistant to diuretics. Klin Wochenschr 1977;55:1121–1122.

[8] Ronco C, Bellomo R. Continuous renal replacement therapies: the need for a standard nomenclature. Contrib Nephrol 1995;116:28–33.

[9] Blagg CR, Ing TS, Berry D, Kjellstrand CM. The history and rationale of daily and nightly hemodialysis. Contrib Nephrol 2004;145:1–9.

[10] Tolwani AJ, Wheeeler TS, Wille KM. Sustained low efficiency dialysis. Contrib Neprhol 2007;156:320–324.

[11] Henderson LW. Hemodialysis: rationale and physical principles. In: Brenner BM, Rector FC Jr, editors. The kidney. Philadelphia: WB Saunders; 1976. p. 1643–1671.

[12] Renkin EM. The relation between dialysance, membrane area, permeability and blood flow in the artificial kidney. Trans Am Soc Artif Intern Organs 1956;2:102–105.

[13] Gibson TP, Matusik E, Nelson LD, Briggs WA. Artificial kidneys and clearance calculations. Clin Pharmacol Ther 1976;20:720–726.

[14] McBain JW, Liu TH. Diffusion of electrolytes, non-electrolytes and colloidal electrolytes. J Am Chem Soc 1931;53:59–74.

[15] Atkinson AJ Jr, Umans JG. Pharmacokinetic studies in hemodialysis patients. Clin Pharmacol Ther 2009;86:548–552.

[16] Matzke GR, Aronoff GR, Atkinson AJ Jr, Bennett WM, Decker BS, Eckardt K-U, et al. Drug dosing consideration in patients with acute and chronic kidney disease—a clinical update from Kidney Disease: Improving Global Outcomes (KDIGO). Kidney Int 2011;80:1122–1137.

[17] Lee CS, Marbury TC. Drug therapy in patients undergoing haemodialysis. Clinical pharmacokinetic considerations. Clin Pharmacokinet 1984;9:42–66.

[18] Gibson TP. Problems in designing hemodialysis drug studies. Pharmacotherapy 1985;5:23–29.

[19] Stec GP, Atkinson AJ Jr, Nevin MJ, Thenot J-P, Ruo TI, Gibson TP, et al. N-Acetylprocainamide pharmacokinetics in functionally anephric patients before and after perturbation by hemodialysis. Clin Pharmacol Ther 1979;26:618–628.

[20] Lee CS, Marbury TC, Benet LZ. Clearance calculations in hemodialysis: application to blood, plasma, and dialysate measurements for ethambutol. J Pharmacokinet Biopharm 1980;8:69–81.

[21] Dahlke M, Halabi A, Canadi J, Tsubouchi C, Machineni S, Pang Y. Pharmacokinetics of serelaxin in patient with severe renal impairment or end-stage renal disease requiring hemodialysis: a single-dose, open-label, parallel-group study. J Clin Pharmacol 2016;56:474–483.

[22] Nolin TD, Appiah K, Kendrick SA, Le P, McMonagle E, Himmelfarb J. Hemodialysis acutely improves hepatic CYP3A4 metabolic activity. J Am Soc Nephrol 2006;17:2363–2367.

[23] Bowsher DJ, Krejcie TC, Avram MJ, Chow MJ, del Greco F, Atkinson AJ Jr. Reduction in slow intercompartmental clearance of urea during dialysis. J Lab Clin Med 1985;105:489–497.

[24] Renkin EM. Effects of blood flow on diffusion kinetics in isolated perfused hindlegs of cats: a double circulation hypothesis. Am J Physiol 1953;183:125–136.

[25] Bregman H, Daugirdas JT, Ing TS. Complications during hemodialysis. In: Daugirdas JT, Ing TS, editors. Handbook of dialysis. Boston: Little, Brown; 1988. p. 106–120.

[26] Atkinson AJ Jr. Elucidation of the pathophysiology of intradialytic muscle cramps: pharmacokinetics applied to translational research. Transl Clin Pharmacol 2019;27:119–122.

[27] Atkinson AJ Jr, Krumlovsky FA, Huang CM, del Greco F. Hemodialysis for severe procainamide toxicity. Clinical and pharmacokinetic observations. Clin Pharmacol Ther 1976;20:585–592.

[28] Sigler MH, Teehan BP, Van Valceknburgh D. Solute transport in continuous hemodialysis: a new treatment for acute renal failure. Kidney Int 1987;32:562–571.

[29] Bressolle F, Kinowski J-M, de la Coussaye JE, Wynn N, Eledjam J-J, Galtier M. Clinical pharmacokinetics during continuous haemofiltration. Clin Pharmacokinet 1994;26:457–471.

[30] Meyer MM. Renal replacement therapies. Crit Care Clin 2000;16:29–58.

[31] Golper TA. Continuous arteriovenous hemofiltration in acute renal failure. Am J Kidney Dis 1985;6:373–386.

[32] Golper TA, Saad A-MA. Gentamicin and phenytoin in vitro sieving characteristics through polysulfone hemofilters: effect of flow rate, drug concentration and solvent systems. Kidney Int 1986;30:937–943.
[33] Golper TA, Marx MA. Drug dosing adjustments during continuous renal replacement therapies. Kidney Int 1998;53(Suppl. 66):S165–S168.
[34] Clark WR, Ronco C. CRRT efficiency and efficacy in relation to solute size. Kidney Int 1999;56(Suppl. 72):S3–S7.
[35] Golper TA, Wedel SK, Kaplan AA, Saad A-M, Donta ST, Paganini EP. Drug removal during continuous arteriovenous hemofiltration: theory and clinical observations. Int J Artif Organs 1985;8:307–312.
[36] Vanholder R, Van Landschoot N, De Smet R, Schoots A, Ringoir S. Drug protein binding in chronic renal failure: evaluation of nine drugs. Kidney Int 1988;33:996–1004.
[37] Lau AH, Kronfol NO. Effect of continuous hemofiltration on phenytoin elimination. Ther Drug Monit 1994;16:53–57.
[38] Davies SP, Lacey LF, Kox WJ, Brown EA. Pharmacokinetics of cefuroxime and ceftazidime in patients with acute renal failure treated by continuous arteriovenous haemodialysis. Nephrol Dial Transplant 1991;6:971–976.
[39] Kroh UF, Lennartz H, Edwards DJ, Stoeckel K. Pharmacokinetics of ceftriaxone in patients undergoing continuous veno-venous hemofiltration. J Clin Pharmacol 1996;36:1114–1119.
[40] Davies SP, Azadian BS, Kox WJ, Brown EA. Pharmacokinetics of ciprofloxacin and vancomycin in patients with acute renal failure treated by continuous haemodialysis. Nephrol Dial Transplant 1992;7:848–854.
[41] Cleary JD, Davis G, Raju S. Cyclosporine pharmacokinetics in a lung transplant patient undergoing hemofiltration. Transplantation 1989;48:710–712.
[42] Lau AH, Pyle K, Kronfol NO, Libertin CR. Removal of cephalosporins by continuous arteriovenous ultrafiltration (CAVU) and hemofiltration (CAVH). Int J Artif Organs 1989;12:379–383.
[43] Schetz M, Ferdinande P, Van den Berghe G, Verwaest C, Lauwers P. Pharmacokinetics of continuous renal replacement therapy. Intensive Care Med 1995;21:612–620.
[44] Fiaccadori E, Maggiore H, Rotelli C, Giacosa R, Parenti E, Picetti E, et al. Removal of linezolid by conventional intermittent hemodialysis, sustained low-efficiency dialysis, or continuous venovenous hemofiltration in patients with acute renal failure. Crit Care Med 2004;32:2437–2442.
[45] Reetze-Bonorden P, Böhler J, Keller E. Drug dosage in patients during continuous renal replacement therapy: pharmacokinetic and therapeutic considerations. Clin Pharmacokinet 1993;24:362–379.
[46] Ronco C, Clark WR. Hemodialysis membranes. Nat Rev Nephrol 2018;14:394–410.
[47] Finelli L, Miller JT, Tokars JI, Alter MJ, Arduino MJ. National surveillance of dialysis-associated disease in the United States, 2002. Semin Dial 2000;13:75–85.
[48] National Kidney Foundation. KDOQI clinical practice guideline for hemodialysis adequacy: 2105 update. Am J Kidney Dis 2015;66:884–930.
[49] Meyer CC, Calis KA. New hemodialysis membranes and vancomycin clearance. Am J Health Syst Pharm 1995;52:2794–2796.
[50] Gotta V, Dao K, Rodieux F, Buclin, Livio F, Pfister M. Guidance to develop individual dose recommendations for patients on chronic hemodialysis. Expert Rev Clin Pharmacol 2017;10:737–752.
[51] Martin E, Gambertoglio JG, Adler DS, Tozer TN, Roman LA, Grausz H. Removal of phenytoin by hemodialysis in uremic patients. JAMA 1977;238:1750–1753.
[52] Frenchie D, Bastani B. Significant removal of phenytoin during high flux dialysis with cellulose triacetate dialyzer. Nephrol Dial Transplant 1998;13:817–818.
[53] Anseeuw K, Mowry JB, Burdmann EA, Ghannoum M, Hoffman RS, Gosselin S, et al. Extracorporeal treatment in phenytoin poisoning: systematic review and recommendations from the EXTRIP (Extracorporeal Treatments in Poisoning) workgroup. Am J Kidney Dis 2016;67:187–197.
[54] Cormier MJ, Desmeules S, St-Onge M, Ghannoum M. Phenytoin overdose treated with hemodialysis using a high cut-off dialyzer. Hemodial Int 2017;21:E13–E17.
[55] Ghannoum M, Hoffman RS, Gosselin S, Nolin TD, Lavergne V, Roberts DM. Use of extracorporeal treatments in the management of poisonings. Kidney Int 2018;94:682–688.
[56] Chan BSH, Buckley NA. Digoxin-specific antibody fragments in the treatment of digoxin toxicity. Clin Toxicol 2014;52:824–836.
[57] Lavergne V, Nolin TD, Hoffman RS, Roberts D, Gosselin S, Goldfarb DS, et al. The EXTRIP (Extracorporeal Treatments In Poisoning) workgroup: guideline methodology. Clin Toxicol 2012;50:403–413.
[58] Levy G. Pharmacokinetics in renal disease. Am J Med 1977;62:461–465.
[59] Aronoff GR, Bennett WM, Berns JS, Brier ME, Kasbekar N, Mueller BA, et al. Drug prescribing in renal failure: Dosing guidelines for adults and children. 5th ed. Philadelphia: American College of Physicians; 2007.
[60] Pollard TA, Lampasona V, Akkerman S, Tom K, Hooks MA, Mullins RE, et al. Vancomycin redistribution: dosing recommendations following high-flux hemodialysis. Kidney Int 1994;45:232–237.
[61] Manley HJ, Bailie GR, McClaran ML, Bender WL. Gentamicin pharmacokinetics during slow daily home hemodialysis. Kidney Int 2003;63:1072–1078.
[62] Kielstein JT, Czock D, Schöpke T, Hafer C, Bode-Böger SM, et al. Pharmacokinetics and total elimination of meropenem and vancomycin in intensive care unit patients undergoing extended daily dialysis. Crit Care Med 2006;34:51–56.
[63] Mushatt DM, Mihm LB, Dreisbach AW, Simon EE. Antibiotic dosing in slow extended daily dialysis. Clin Infect Dis 2009;49:433–437.
[64] Decker BS, Mueller BA, Sowinski KM. Drug dosing considerations in alternative hemodialysis. Adv Chronic Kidney Dis 2007;14:17–25.
[65] O'Shea S, Duffull S, Johnson DW. Aminoglycosides in hemodialysis patients: is the current practice of post dialysis dosing appropriate? Semin Dial 2009;22:225–230.
[66] Ohkawa M, Nakashima T, Shoda R, Ikeda A, Orito M, Sawaki M, et al. Pharmacokinetics of ceftazidime in patients with renal insufficiency and in those undergoing hemodialysis. Chemotherapy 1985;31:410–416.

[67] Ti T-Y, Fortin L, Kreeft JH, East DS, Ogilvie RI, Somerville PJ. Kinetic disposition of intravenous ceftriaxone in normal subjects and patients with renal failure on hemodialysis or peritoneal dialysis. Antimicrob Agents Chemother 1984;25:83–87.
[68] Singlas E, Taburet AM, Landru I, Albin H, Ryckelinck JP. Pharmacokinetics of ciprofloxacin tablets in renal failure; influence of haemodialysis. Eur J Clin Pharmacol 1987;31:589–593.
[69] Venkataramanan R, Ptachcinski RJ, Burckart GJ, Yang SL, Starzl TE, van Theil DH. The clearance of cyclosporine by hemodialysis. J Clin Pharmacol 1984;24:528–531.
[70] Amin NB, Padhi ID, Touchette MA, Patel RV, Dunfee TP, Anandan JV. Characterization of gentamicin pharmacokinetics in patients hemodialyzed with high-flux polysulfone membranes. Am J Kidney Dis 1999;34:222–227.
[71] Ernest D, Cutler DJ. Gentamicin clearance during continuous arteriovenous hemodiafiltration. Crit Care Med 1992;20:586–589.
[72] Baltez E, Coupez R. Levetiracetam dose adjustment for patients on hemodialysis. Epilepsia 2000;42(S4):254 (abstract).
[73] Czock D, Husig-Linde C, Langhoff A, Schopke T, Hafer C, de Groot K, et al. Pharmacokinetics of moxifloxacin and levofloxacin in intensive care unit patients who have acute renal failure and undergo extended daily dialysis. Clin J Am Soc Nephrol 2006;1:1263–1268.
[74] Hansen E, Bucher M, Jakob W, Lemberger P, Kees F. Pharmacokinetics of levofloxacin during continuous veno-venous hemofiltration. Intensive Care Med 2001;27:371–375.
[75] Meyer B, Kornek GV, Nikfardjam M, Delle Karth G, Heinz G, Locker GJ, et al. Multiple-dose pharmacokinetics of linezolid during continuous venovenous haemofiltration. J Antimicrob Chemother 2005;56:172–179.
[76] Blair AD, Burgess ED, Maxwell BM, Cutler RE. Sotalol kinetics in renal insufficiency. Clin Pharmacol Ther 1981;29:457–463.
[77] Touchette MA, Patel RV, Anandan JV, Dumler F, Zarowitz BJ. Vancomycin removal by high-flux polysulfone hemodialysis membranes in critically ill patients with end-stage renal disease. Am J Kidney Dis 1995;26:469–474.
[78] Boereboom FTJ, Verves FFT, Blankestijn PJ, Savelkoul TJF, van Dijk A. Vancomycin clearance during continuous venovenous hemofiltration in critically ill patients. Intensive Care Med 1999;25:1100–1104.
[79] Macias WL, Mueller BA, Scarim KS. Vancomycin pharmacokinetics in acute renal failure: preservation of nonrenal clearance. Clin Pharmacol Ther 1991;50:688–694.
[80] Winchester JF. Active methods for detoxification. In: Haddad LM, Shannon MW, Winchester JF, editors. Clinical management of poisoning and drug overdose. 3rd ed. Philadelphia, PA: WB Saunders; 1998. p. 175–188.
[81] de Pont A-C. Extracorporeal treatment of intoxications. Curr Opin Crit Care 2007;13:668–73.
[82] Lam YW, Banerji S, Hatfield C, Talbert RL. Principles of drug administration in renal insufficiency. Clin Pharmacokinet 1997;32:30–57.
[83] Roberts DM, Buckley NA. Pharmacokinetic considerations in clinical toxicology: clinical implications. Clin Pharmacokinet 2007;46:897–939.
[84] Singh T, Maw TT, Henry BL, Pastor-Soler NM, Unruh ML, Hallows KR, et al. Extracorporeal therapy for dabigatran removal in the treatment of acute bleeding: a single center experience. Clin J Am Soc Nephrol 2013;8:1533–1539.
[85] Brent J. Fomepizole for ethylene glycol and methanol poisoning. N Engl J Med 2009;360:2216–2223.
[86] McMartin K, Jacobsen D, Hovda KE. Antidotes for poisoning by alcohols that form toxic metabolites. Br J Clin Pharmacol 2015;81:505–515.
[87] Mowry JB, Burdmann EA, Anseeuw K, Ayoub P, Ghannoum M, Hoffman RS, et al. Extracoporeal treatment for digoxin poisoning: systematic review and recommendations from the EXTRIP Workgroup. Clin Toxicol 2016;54:103–114.
[88] Flanagan RJ, Jones AL. Fab antibody fragments: some applications in clinical toxicology. Drug Saf 2004;27:1115–1133.

Chapter 7

Effect of liver disease on pharmacokinetics

Nathalie K. Zgheib[a], Juan J.L. Lertora[b,d], and Robert A. Branch[c]

[a]*Department of Pharmacology and Toxicology, American University of Beirut Faculty of Medicine, Beirut, Lebanon,* [b]*Adjunct Professor, Division of Clinical Research, Pennington Biomedical Research Center, Louisiana State University, Baton Rouge, LA, United States,* [c]*Orenda Health, Pittsburgh, PA, United States,* [d]*Adjunct Professor, Department of Medicine, Duke University School of Medicine, Durham, NC, United States*

Liver disease in humans encompasses a wide range of pathological disturbances that can lead to a reduction in liver blood flow, extrahepatic or intrahepatic shunting of blood, hepatocyte dysfunction, quantitative and qualitative changes in serum proteins, and changes in bile flow. Different forms of hepatic disease may produce different alterations in drug absorption, disposition, and pharmacologic effect. The pharmacokinetic or pharmacodynamic consequences of a specific hepatic disease may differ between individuals or even within a single individual over time. Each of the major determinants of hepatic clearance, blood flow to the liver (Q), the fraction of drug not bound to plasma proteins (f_u), and intrinsic clearance (CL_{int}), and vascular architecture may be independently altered.

Although there are numerous causes of hepatic injury, it appears that the hepatic response to injury is a limited one and that the functional consequences are determined more by the extent of the injury than by the cause. At this time there is no generally available test that can be used to correlate changes in drug absorption and disposition with the degree of hepatic impairment. In this chapter, we summarize the known effects of liver disease on drug disposition and provide some guidance for modification of drug therapy in patients with liver disease. We make the case that more research and collaborative efforts are needed in the field for more precise drug use in these patients.

Physiologic determinants of hepatic drug clearance

Hepatic elimination of drugs

Hepatic clearance (CL_H) may be defined as the volume of blood perfusing the liver that is cleared of drug per unit time. Usually, hepatic clearance is equated with nonrenal clearance and is calculated as total body clearance (CL_E) minus renal clearance (CL_R).

$$CL_H = CL_E - CL_R \tag{7.1}$$

Accordingly, these estimates may include a component of extrahepatic nonrenal clearance.

The factors that affect hepatic clearance include blood flow to the liver (Q), the fraction of drug not bound to plasma proteins (f_u), and intrinsic clearance (CL_{int}) [1, 2]. Intrinsic clearance is simply the hepatic clearance that would be observed in the absence of blood flow and protein binding restrictions. As discussed in Chapter 2, hepatic clearance usually can be considered to be a first-order process. In those cases, intrinsic clearance represents the ratio of V_{max}/K_m, and this relationship has been used as the basis for correlating in vitro studies of drug metabolism with in vivo results [3]. However, for phenytoin and several other drugs the Michaelis-Menten equation is needed to characterize intrinsic clearance.

The well-stirred model, shown in Fig. 7.1, is the model of hepatic clearance that is used most commonly in pharmacokinetics. If we apply the Fick Equation (see Chapter 6) to this model, hepatic clearance can be defined as follows [2]:

$$CL_H = Q\left[\frac{C_a - C_v}{C_a}\right] \tag{7.2}$$

The ratio of concentrations defined by the terms within the brackets is termed the *extraction ratio* (*ER*). An expression for the extraction ratio also can be obtained by applying the following mass balance equation to the model shown in Fig. 7.1:

$$V\frac{dC_a}{dt} = QC_a - QC_v - f_u CL_{int} C_v$$

 https://doi.org/10.1016/B978-0-12-819869-8.00005-7

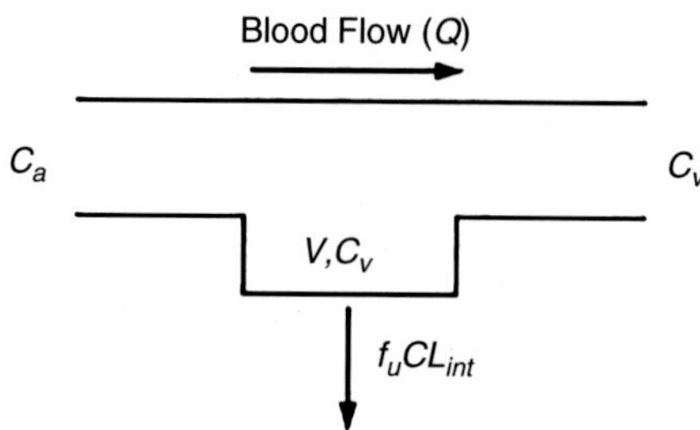

FIG. 7.1 The well-stirred model of hepatic clearance, in which the liver is viewed as a single compartment having a volume (V) and blood flow (Q). Drug concentrations reaching the liver via the hepatic artery and portal vein are designated by C_a, and those in emergent hepatic venous blood by C_v. Drug concentrations within the liver are considered to be in equilibrium with those in emergent venous blood. Intrinsic clearance (CL_{int}) acts to eliminate the fraction of drug not bound to plasma proteins (f_u).

At steady state,

$$Q(C_a - C_v) = f_u CL_{int} C_v \tag{7.3}$$

Also,

$$QC_a = (Q + f_u CL_{int}) C_v \tag{7.4}$$

since

$$ER = \frac{C_a - C_v}{C_a}$$

Eq. (7.3) can be divided by Eq. (7.4) to define extraction ratio in terms of Q, f_u, and CL_{int}:

$$ER = \frac{f_u CL_{int}}{Q + f_u CL_{int}} \tag{7.5}$$

By substituting this expression for extraction ratio into Eq. (7.2), hepatic clearance can be expressed as follows:

$$CL_H = Q\left[\frac{f_u CL_{int}}{Q + f_u CL_{int}}\right] \tag{7.6}$$

Two limiting cases arise when $f_u CL_{int} << Q$ and when $f_u CL_{int} >> Q$ [2]. In the former instance Eq. (7.5) can be simplified to

$$CL_H = f_u CL_{int} \tag{7.7}$$

Hepatic clearance is termed *restrictive* in this case, since it is limited by protein binding. This situation is analogous to the elimination of drugs by glomerular filtration. Drugs that are restrictively eliminated have extraction ratios <0.3.

When $f_u CL_{int} >> Q$, Eq. (7.5) can be reduced to:

$$CL_H = Q \tag{7.8}$$

In this case, hepatic clearance is *flow limited*, similar to the renal tubular excretion of *p*-aminohippurate. Because protein binding does not affect their clearance, drugs whose hepatic clearance is flow limited are said to be *nonrestrictively* eliminated and have extraction ratios >0.7.

Yang et al. [4] point out that the well-stirred model equates whole blood clearance, rather than plasma clearance, to liver blood flow because the liver is capable of extracting drug from both plasma and red blood cells. This situation is similar to that encountered for drugs removed by hemodialysis (see Chapter 6). So if plasma drug clearance is to be estimated from plasma concentration measurements, then Eq. (7.6) must be modified as follows by including the total blood to plasma drug concentration ratio (B/P):

$$CL_H = Q\left[\frac{f_u CL_{int}}{Q + f_u CL_{int}/(B/P)}\right] \tag{7.9}$$

In addition to this modification of the well-stirred model, several other kinetic models of hepatic clearance have been developed [5]. However, the following discussion will be based on the relationships defined by Eq. (7.6), and the limiting cases represented by Eqs. (7.7) and (7.8).

Restrictively metabolized drugs ($ER < 0.3$)

The product of f_u and CL_{int} is small relative to liver blood flow (usually about 1500 mL/min) for drugs that are restrictively metabolized. Although the extraction ratio of these drugs is less than 0.3, hepatic metabolism often constitutes their principal pathway of elimination and they frequently have long elimination-phase half-lives (e.g., diazepam: $t_{1/2} = 43$ h). The hepatic clearance of these drugs is affected by changes in their binding to plasma proteins, by induction or inhibition of hepatic drug-metabolizing enzymes, and by age, nutrition, and pathological factors. However, as indicated by Eq. (7.7), their hepatic clearance is not affected significantly by changes in hepatic blood flow.

Effect of changes in protein binding on hepatic clearance

It usually is assumed that the free drug concentration in blood is equal to the drug concentration to which hepatic drug-metabolizing enzymes are exposed. Although protein binding would not be anticipated to change hepatic clearance significantly for restrictively metabolized drugs that have $f_u > 80\%$, displacement of highly bound ($f_u < 20\%$) drugs from their plasma protein-binding sites will result in a significant increase in their hepatic clearance. However, steady-state concentrations of unbound drug will be unchanged as long as there is no change in CL_{int}. This occurs in some drug interactions, as diagrammed in Fig. 7.2 [6]. This situation also is encountered in pathological conditions in which plasma proteins or plasma protein binding is decreased, as described in Chapter 5 for phenytoin kinetics in patients with impaired renal function. Since pharmacological effects are related to concentrations of unbound drug, pure displacement-type drug interactions put patients at risk for only a brief period of time. Similarly, dose adjustments are not needed for patients whose protein binding is impaired. In fact, as pointed out in Chapter 5, measurement of total rather than unbound drug levels in these patients actually may lead to inappropriate dose increases.

Effect of changes in intrinsic clearance on hepatic drug clearance

Both hepatic disease and drug interactions can alter the intrinsic clearance of restrictively eliminated drugs. Drug interactions will be considered in more detail in Chapter 15. The effects of liver disease on drug elimination will be discussed in the following sections. Although a number of probe drugs have been used to characterize hepatic clearance, analysis of the factors influencing the intrinsic clearance of drugs is hampered by the fact that, in contrast to the use of creatinine clearance to assess renal function, there are no simple measures that can be applied on a routine clinical basis to assess hepatic

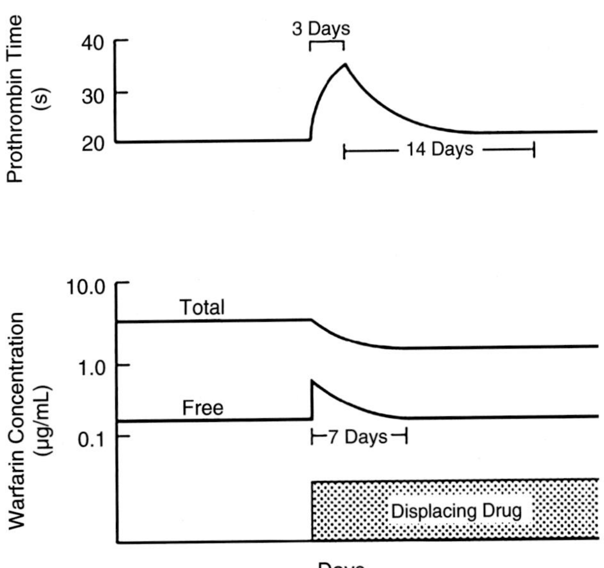

FIG. 7.2 Time course of an interaction in which warfarin, a restrictively metabolized drug, is displaced from its plasma protein-binding sites. Although free warfarin concentrations rise initially as a result of the interaction, they subsequently return to preinteraction levels. As a result, the increase in prothrombin time is only transient. Because f_u is increased, total (bound plus free) warfarin levels remain depressed as long as treatment with the displacing drug is continued. *(Reproduced with permission from Atkinson AJ Jr, Reidenberg MM, Thompson WL. Clinical pharmacology. In: Greenberger N, editor. MKSAP VI syllabus. Philadelphia, PA: American College of Physicians; 1982. p. 85–96 [6].)*

clearance: a fact that is further complicated by evidence that liver dysfunction can have a differential effect on different drug-metabolizing enzymes [7].

Drugs with an intermediate extraction ratio ($0.3 < ER < 0.7$)

Few drugs exhibit an intermediate extraction ratio. Evaluation of the hepatic clearance of these drugs requires consideration of all of the parameters included in Eq. (7.6). Disease-associated or drug-induced alterations in protein binding, hepatic blood flow, or intrinsic clearance may alter hepatic clearance significantly.

Nonrestrictively metabolized drugs ($ER > 0.70$)

The product of f_u and CL_{int} is large relative to liver blood flow for drugs that are nonrestrictively metabolized. These drugs characteristically have short elimination-phase half-lives (e.g., propranolol: $t_{1/2} = 3.9$ h), and changes in hepatic blood flow have a major effect on their hepatic clearance (Eq. 7.8). Accordingly, hemodynamic changes, such as congestive heart failure, that reduce liver blood flow will reduce the hepatic clearance of these drugs and may necessitate appropriate adjustments in intravenous dosage.

Biliary excretion of drugs

Relatively few drugs, usually large molecular weight substrates, are taken up by the liver and without further metabolism excreted into bile which, as an aqueous solution, generally favors excretion of more water-soluble compounds [8]. On the other hand, many polar drug metabolites, such as glucuronide conjugates, undergo biliary excretion, with the added complexity of deconjugation in the gut and creation of an enterohepatic circulation of the parent drug [9]. In order for compounds to be excreted in bile they must pass through the fenestrated endothelium that lines the hepatic sinusoids, then cross both the luminal and canalicular membrane surfaces of hepatocytes. Passage across these two hepatocyte membrane surfaces often is facilitated by active transport systems that will be discussed in Chapter 14. Consequently, chemical structure, polarity, and molecular weight are important determinants of the extent to which compounds are excreted in bile. In general, polar compounds with a molecular weight range of 500–600 Da are excreted in bile, whereas those with a lower molecular weight tend to be eliminated preferentially by renal excretion. However, 5-fluorouracil has a molecular weight of only 130 Da, yet is excreted in bile with a bile/plasma concentration ratio of 2.0 [10]. Nonetheless, biliary excretion of parent drug and metabolites accounts for only 2%–3% of the elimination of an administered 5-fluorouracil dose in patients with normal renal function [11].

Compounds that enhance bile production stimulate biliary excretion of drugs normally eliminated by this route, whereas biliary excretion of drugs will be decreased by compounds that decrease bile flow or pathophysiologic conditions that cause cholestasis [12]. Route of administration may also influence the extent of drug excretion into bile. Oral administration may cause a drug to be extracted by the liver and excreted into bile to a greater degree than if the intravenous route were used.

Enterohepatic circulation

Drugs excreted into bile traverse the biliary tract to reach the small intestine where they may be reabsorbed [8]. Drug metabolites that reach the intestine also may be converted back to the parent drug and be reabsorbed. This is particularly true for some glucuronide conjugates that are hydrolyzed by β-glucuronidase present in intestinal bacteria [9]. The term *enterohepatic circulation* refers to this cycle in which a drug or metabolite is excreted in bile and then reabsorbed from the intestine either as the metabolite or after conversion back to the parent drug. Thus enterohepatic cycling of a drug increases its bioavailability, as assessed from the area under the plasma-level vs time curve, and prolongs its elimination-phase half-life. Interestingly cholecystectomy, a commonly performed surgery, was shown to affect the intestinal bile flow and the enterohepatic circulation of bile acids, phenomena that may be associated with alteration in the gut microbiota potentially impacting bacterial deconjugation of drug metabolites [13].

Studies in different animal species with collection of peripheral blood, feces, bile, and urine have demonstrated that biliary clearance actually may exceed plasma clearance for some drugs and species with extensive enterohepatic circulation [14]. Interruption of enterohepatic circulation reduces the area under the plasma-level vs time curve. Enterohepatic circulation also increases the total exposure of the intestinal mucosa to potentially toxic drugs. Thus the intestinal toxicity of indomethacin is most marked in those species such as the dog that have a high ratio of biliary to renal drug excretion [14].

Enterohepatic circulation may result in a second peak in the plasma-level vs time curve, as shown in Fig. 7.3A. The occurrence of this second peak in plasma drug concentrations appears to reflect intermittent gallbladder contraction and pulsatile delivery of drug-containing bile to the intestine, because this double peak phenomenon is not encountered in animal species that lack a gallbladder [15]. Realistic pharmacokinetic modeling of this process entails incorporation of a variable lag-time interval that can reflect intermittent gallbladder emptying, as in Fig. 7.3B. Cimetidine is typical of many drugs that undergo enterohepatic circulation, in that secondary plasma concentration peaks occur after oral but not intravenous administration [15]. These secondary peaks were seen after meals in individuals who were given cimetidine while fasting but were allowed subsequent food intake that presumably triggered gallbladder contraction and the discharge of drug-containing bile into the small intestine. Secondary peaks were not seen when cimetidine was administered intravenously or coadministered orally with food. On the other hand, ranitidine differs from cimetidine and is unusual in that secondary peaks occur after both intravenous and oral administration to fasting patients who subsequently were fed, as shown in Fig. 7.3A [16]. This difference reflects the fact that cimetidine reaches the bile from the liver primarily during first-pass transit via the portal circulation (k_1 in Fig. 7.3B), whereas there is substantial hepatic uptake of ranitidine from the systemic circulation (k_2 in Fig. 7.3B).

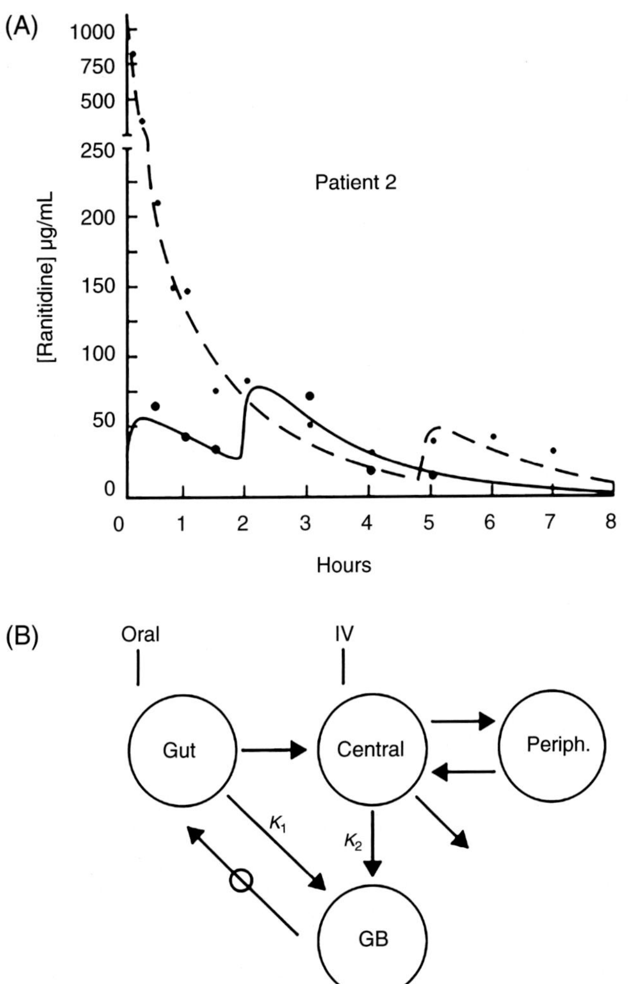

FIG. 7.3 (A) Pharmacokinetic analysis of secondary plasma concentration peaks following the oral and intravenous administration of single 20-mg doses of ranitidine to a healthy subject. The lines are based on the pharmacokinetic model shown in (B) and represent a least-squares fit of the plasma concentrations measured after the intravenous *(dashed line)* and oral *(solid line)* doses. (B) Pharmacokinetic model used for the analysis of the enterohepatic cycling of cimetidine and ranitidine. Drug enters the gallbladder via the liver, for which a separate compartment is not required, either during first-pass transit from the gut via the portal circulation (k_1) or directly from the systemic circulation (k_2). The irregular discharge of drug-containing bile from the gallbladder is indicated by the arrow going from gallbladder (GB) to gut. Drug distribution within the body is modeled as a two-compartment system. *(Reproduced with permission from Miller R. J Pharm Sci 1984;73:1376–1379 [16].)*

Effects of liver disease on pharmacokinetics

Although there are numerous causes of hepatic injury, it appears that the hepatic response to injury is a limited one and that the functional consequences are determined more by the extent of the injury than by the cause.

Acute hepatitis

Acute hepatitis is an inflammatory condition of the liver that is caused by viruses or hepatotoxins. In acute viral hepatitis, inflammatory changes in the hepatocyte are generally mild and transient, although they can be chronic (chronic active hepatitis) and severe, resulting in cirrhosis or death. Blaschke and Williams and their colleagues [17–20] have conducted informative studies of the effects of acute viral hepatitis on drug disposition. These investigators used a longitudinal study design in which each of a small number of patients was studied initially during the time that they had acute viral hepatitis and subsequently after recovery (Table 7.1). The drugs that were administered included phenytoin [17], tolbutamide [18], warfarin [19], and lidocaine [20]. The most consistent significant finding was that the plasma protein binding of both phenytoin and tolbutamide was reduced during acute hepatitis. For both drugs, this was partly attributed to drug displacement from protein-binding sites by elevated bilirubin levels. As a result of these changes, the distribution volume of phenytoin increased slightly during hepatitis (see Chapter 3). Although no significant change was noted in the average values of either phenytoin CL_H or CL_{int}, CL_{int} was reduced by approximately 50% in the two patients with the greatest evidence of hepatocellular damage. On the other hand, the reduction in tolbutamide binding to plasma proteins had no observable effect on distribution volume or CL_{int} but did result in an increase in CL_H. No consistent changes were observed in warfarin kinetics during acute viral hepatitis. However, prothrombin time was prolonged in two of the five patients, but remained within normal limits in all five participants during the recovery period, reflecting impaired synthesis of Factor VII in the acute disease stage. Lidocaine kinetics also was not altered consistently during acute viral hepatitis, although clearance decreased in four of the six patients that were studied.

In general, drug elimination during acute viral hepatitis is either normal or only moderately impaired. Observed changes tend to be variable and related to the extent of hepatocellular damage incurred. If the acute hepatitis resolves, drug disposition returns to normal. Drug elimination is likely to be impaired most significantly in patients who develop chronic hepatitis B virus-related liver disease, but even then only late in the evolution of this disease [21]. This stands in marked contrast to the severity of acute hepatitis that can be caused by hepatotoxins. For example, Prescott and Wright [22] found that liver damage can occur within 2–3 h after ingestion of an acetaminophen overdose. The elimination-phase half-life of acetaminophen averaged only 2.7 h in patients without liver damage, but ranged from 4.3 to 7.7 h (mean = 5.8 h) in four patients with liver damage and from 4.3 to 13.9 h (mean = 7.7 h) in three patients with both liver and kidney damage resulting from acetaminophen toxicity. These authors observed that a fatal outcome was likely in patients whose acetaminophen elimination half-life exceeded 10–12 h.

TABLE 7.1 Pharmacokinetics of some drugs during and after acute viral hepatitis.

	f_u		V_d		CL_H		CL_{int}		
	During	After	During (L/kg)	After (L/kg)	During (mL/h/kg)	After (mL/h/kg)	During (mL/h/kg)	After (mL/h/kg)	References
Phenytoin[a]	0.126[b]	0.099	0.68[b]	0.63	0.0430	0.0373	0.352	0.385	[17]
Tolbutamide	0.087[b]	0.068	0.15	0.15	26[b]	18	300	260	[18]
Warfarin	0.012	0.012	0.09	0.21	6.1	6.1	519	514	[19]
Lidocaine	0.56	0.49	3.1	2.0	13.0	20.0	23.2[c]	40.8[c]	[20]

[a]A low dose of phenytoin was administered so that first-order kinetics would be approximated.
[b]Difference in studies during and after recovery from acute viral hepatitis was significant at $P < 0.05$ by paired t-test.
[c]Protein binding results for individual patients were not given so CL_{int} was estimated from average values.

Chronic liver disease and cirrhosis

Chronic liver disease is usually secondary to chronic alcohol abuse or chronic viral hepatitis. Alcoholic liver disease is most common and begins with the accumulation of fat vacuoles within hepatocytes and hepatic enlargement. There is a decrease in cytochrome P450 content per weight of tissue, but this is compensated for by the increase in liver size so that drug metabolism is not initially impaired [23]. Alcoholic fatty liver may be accompanied or followed by alcoholic hepatitis, in which hepatocyte degeneration and necrosis become evident. In neither of these conditions is there significant diversion of blood flow past functioning hepatocytes by functional or anatomic shunts. Notably over the past couple of decades, and because of the increased prevalence of obesity and associated metabolic syndrome, nonalcoholic fatty liver disease (NAFLD) and nonalcoholic steatohepatitis (NASH) emerged as common causes of chronic liver disease. A number of pathological events are triggered starting with fat deposition and metabolic stress, followed by oxidative stress, inflammation, and apoptosis, and ultimately liver fibrosis, all of which may be associated with consequences for drug disposition [24].

Chronic liver disease is associated with decreased expression of CYP enzymes and drug transporters probably because they are most susceptible to the reduced availability of oxygen [25]. Nevertheless, this may also be due to the underlying inflammatory state associated with chronic liver disease [26, 27]. For example in chronic hepatitis C, high concentrations of inflammatory mediators such as cytokines and interferons are paralleled with reduced mRNA expression of *CYP1A2*, *CYP2E1*, *CYP3A4*, *OATP1B1*, and *OATP2B1* [26, 28].

Cirrhosis represents the final common pathway of most chronic liver diseases. The development of cirrhosis is characterized by the appearance of fibroblasts and collagen deposition. This is accompanied by a reduction in liver size and the formation of nodules of regenerated hepatocytes. As a result, total liver content of cytochrome P450 is reduced in these patients. Initially, fibroblasts deposit collagen fibrils in the sinusoidal space, including the space of Disse [23]. Collagen deposition not only produces characteristic bands of connective scar tissue but also forms a basement membrane devoid of microvilli along the sinusoidal surface of the hepatocyte. This process thickens and defenestrates the endothelial barrier between the sinusoid and the hepatocytes, a process referred to as *capillarization* [29]. This process, in conjunction with alterations in the sinusoidal membrane of the hepatocyte, results in functional shunting of blood past the remaining hepatocyte mass. These changes can interfere significantly with the function of hepatic transporters and the hepatic uptake of oxygen, nutrients, and plasma constituents, including drugs and metabolites [27].

The deposition of fibrous bands also disrupts the normal hepatic vascular architecture and increases vascular resistance and portal venous pressure. This reduces portal venous flow that normally accounts for 70% of total liver blood flow [30]. However, the decrease in portal venous flow is compensated for by an increase in hepatic artery flow, so that total blood flow reaching the liver is maintained at the normal value of 18 mL/min kg in patients with either chronic viral hepatitis or cirrhosis [31]. The increase in portal venous pressure also leads to the formation of extrahepatic and intrahepatic shunts. Extrahepatic shunting occurs through the extensive collateral network that connects the portal and systemic circulations [30]. Important examples include collaterals at the gastroesophageal junction, which can dilate to form varices, the umbilical vein, and retroperitoneal vascular connections that can now be observed with high resolution imaging. In a study of cirrhotic patients with bleeding esophageal varices, an average of 70% of mesenteric and 95% of splenic blood flow was found to be diverted through extrahepatic shunts [32]. Intrahepatic shunting results both from intrahepatic vascular anastomoses that bypass hepatic sinusoids and from the functional sinusoidal barrier caused by collagen deposition. Iwasa et al. [31] found that the combination of anatomic and functional intrahepatic shunting averaged 25% of total liver blood flow in normal subjects, but was increased to 33% in patients with chronic viral hepatitis and to 52% in cirrhotic patients. The maintenance of intrahepatic flow with increasing shunts may explain the high cardiac output failure associated with advanced liver disease.

Pharmacokinetic consequences of liver cirrhosis

The net result of chronic hepatic disease that leads to cirrhosis is that pathophysiologic alterations may cause both decreased hepatocyte function, with as much as a 50% decrease in cytochrome P450 content, and/or shunting of blood away from optimally functioning hepatocytes. Accordingly, cirrhosis affects drug metabolism more than any other form of liver disease does. In fact, cirrhosis may decrease the clearance of drugs that are nonrestrictively eliminated in subjects with normal liver function to the extent that it no longer approximates hepatic blood flow but is influenced to a greater extent by hepatic intrinsic clearance [33]. By reducing first-pass hepatic metabolism, cirrhosis also may cause a clinically significant increase in the extent to which nonrestrictively eliminated drugs are absorbed.

Influence of portosystemic shunting on nonrestrictively metabolized drugs

When portosystemic shunting is present, total hepatic blood flow (Q) equals the sum of perfusion flow (Q_p) and shunt flow (Q_s). Portocaval shunting will impair the efficiency of hepatic extraction and reduce the extraction ratio, as indicated by the following modification of Eq. (7.5) [34].

$$ER = \frac{f_u CL_{int}}{Q + f_u CL_{int}} \cdot \frac{Q_p}{Q} \tag{7.10}$$

The corresponding impact on hepatic clearance is given by the following equation:

$$CL_H = Q_p \left[\frac{f_u CL_{int}}{Q + f_u CL_{int}} \right] \tag{7.11}$$

Because Q and Q_p are both reduced in patients with severe cirrhosis, in whom portocaval shunting is most pronounced, hepatic clearance will be reduced more for nonrestrictively than for restrictively metabolized drugs.

Similarly, restrictively metabolized drugs exhibit little first-pass metabolism even in subjects with normal liver function, so portocaval shunting will have little impact on drug bioavailability. On the other hand, portocaval shunting will decrease the extraction ratio and increase the bioavailability of nonrestrictively metabolized drugs as follows:

$$F = 1 - \frac{f_u CL_{int}}{Q + f_u CL_{int}} \cdot \frac{Q_p}{Q} \tag{7.12}$$

For nonrestrictively metabolized drugs, and if there is no loss of drug due to degradation or metabolism within the gastrointestinal tract or to incomplete absorption, the relationship between bioavailability (F) and extraction ratio is given by the following equation:

$$F = 1 - ER \tag{7.13}$$

Because Eq. (7.8) implies that $ER = 1$ for nonrestrictively metabolized drugs, yet the oral route of administration can be used for many drugs in this category (e.g., $F > 0$ for morphine and propranolol), it is apparent that Eq. (7.13) represents only a rough approximation. By using Eq. (7.5) to substitute for ER in Eq. (7.13), we obtain a more precise estimate of the impact of first-pass metabolism on bioavailability:

$$F = \frac{Q}{Q + f_u CL_{int}} \tag{7.14}$$

Considering the case in which a drug is eliminated only by hepatic metabolism, Eq. (4.2) from Chapter 4 can be rewritten as follows:

$$D_{oral} \cdot F = CL_H \cdot AUC_{oral}$$

Using Eqs. (7.6) and (7.14) to substitute, respectively, for CL_H and F yields the result that

$$D_{oral} = f_u CL_H \cdot AUC_{oral} \tag{7.15}$$

It can be seen from Eq. (7.15) that oral doses of nonrestrictively metabolized drugs should not need to be adjusted in response to changes in hepatic blood flow. Eq. (7.15) also forms the basis for using AUC_{oral} measurements to calculate so-called "oral clearance" as an estimate of $f_u CL_{int}$. However, if renal excretion contributes to drug elimination, it will reduce AUC_{oral} and lead to overestimation of $f_u CL_{int}$ unless the contribution of renal clearance is accounted for [2].

If the extraction ratio of a completely absorbed but nonrestrictively metabolized drug falls from 0.95 to 0.90, the bioavailability will double from 0.05 to 0.10. Because this increase in absorption is accompanied by a decrease in elimination clearance, total exposure following oral administration of nonrestrictively eliminated drugs will increase to an even greater extent than will the increase in bioavailability, as presented in Table 7.2 for meperidine [35], pentazocine [35], and propranolol [36]. Cirrhosis also is associated with a reduction in propranolol binding to plasma proteins, so this also contributes to increased exposure following either intravenous or oral doses of this drug (see the following section). Accordingly, the relative exposure estimates for propranolol in Table 7.2 are based on comparisons of area under the plasma-level vs time curve of nonprotein-bound plasma concentrations. The increase in drug exposure resulting from these changes may cause unexpected increases in intensity of pharmacologic response or in toxicity when the usual doses of these drugs are prescribed for patients with liver disease.

TABLE 7.2 Impact of cirrhosis[a] on bioavailability and relative exposure to doses of nonrestrictively eliminated drugs.

	Sample size		Absolute bioavailability		Relative exposure (cirrhotics/controls)		
	Controls (N)	Cirrhotics (N)	Controls (%)	Cirrhotics (%)	IV	Oral	References
Meperidine	4	8	48	87	1.6	3.1	[35]
Pentazocine	4	8	18	68	2.0	8.3	[35]
Propranolol	9	7	38	54	1.5[b]	2.0[b]	[36]

[a]*Compensated cirrhosis.*
[b]*These estimates also incorporate the 55% increase in propranolol free fraction that was observed in cirrhotic patients as more of the drug was found in the unbound form in these patients.*

Consequences of decreased protein binding

Hypoalbuminemia frequently accompanies chronic liver disease and may reduce drug binding to plasma proteins [37]. In addition, endogenous substances such as bilirubin and bile acids accumulate and may displace drugs from protein-binding sites. Reductions in protein binding will tend to increase the hepatic clearance of restrictively metabolized drugs. For drugs that have low intrinsic clearance and tight binding to plasma proteins, it is possible that liver disease results in a decrease in CL_{int} but also an increase in f_u. The resultant change in hepatic clearance will depend on changes in both these parameters. Thus hepatic disease generally produces no change in warfarin clearance, a decrease in diazepam clearance, and an increase in tolbutamide clearance. However, as discussed in Chapter 5, unbound drug concentrations will not be affected by decreases in the protein binding of restrictively metabolized drugs. Therefore no dosage alterations are required for these drugs when protein binding is the only parameter that is changed.

Although reduced protein binding will not affect the clearance or total (bound plus free) plasma concentration of non-restrictively eliminated drugs, it will increase the plasma concentration of free drug. This may increase the intensity of pharmacological effect that is observed at a given total drug concentration [37]. Therefore, even in the absence of changes in other pharmacokinetic parameters, a reduction in the plasma protein binding of nonrestrictively eliminated drugs will necessitate a corresponding reduction in drug dosage.

As previously discussed in the context of renal disease (Chapter 5), reduced protein binding will increase the distribution volume referenced to total drug concentrations and this will tend to increase elimination-phase half-life [37].

Consequences of hepatocellular changes

Intrinsic clearance depends on the activity of sinusoidal and canalicular transporters and hepatocyte metabolic enzymes [38, 39]. The liver content of cytochrome P450 enzymes is decreased in patients with cirrhosis. In these patients, intrinsic clearance is the main determinant of the systemic clearance of lidocaine and indocyanine green, two drugs that have non-restrictive metabolism in subjects with normal liver function. In general, enzyme activities and drug binding protein concentrations are progressively reduced as disease severity increases. However, cirrhosis does not reduce the function of different drug-metabolizing enzymes uniformly [39, 40]. CYP enzymes content is selectively altered in the presence of liver disease depending on disease severity and etiology being cholestatic or noncholestatic [41–48]. In addition, the expression of basolateral and canalicular drug transporters has also been extensively evaluated in vitro in cholestatic and noncholestatic liver diseases with variable results [27]. As can be seen from the results of representative in vitro studies summarized in Table 7.3, CYP1A2 content is consistently reduced in cirrhosis, while significant reductions in CYP2E1 and CYP3A also have been found by some investigators. In vitro results for CYP2C8, CYP2C9, and CYP2C19 enzymes are less clear, a fact that is compounded by the use of nonspecific antibodies in some of the studies [42, 45]. Notably, in the evaluation of CYP expression (mRNA and protein levels in relation to GAPDH) and activity (using marker substrates) in microsomes isolated from livers of normal subjects and patients with NAFLD, expression and activity of CYP1A2, CYP2C19, CYP2D6, and CYP3A4 tend to decrease with increasing severity of NAFLD, while the activity of CYP2A6 and CYP2C9 tends to increase with progressive disease [47].

TABLE 7.3 Representative studies of in vitro evaluations of CYP protein content in human liver samples.

		Enzyme						
Liver diseases/cirrhosis	**N**	**1A1**	**2C8**	**2C9**	**2C19**	**2E1**	**3A4**	**References**
Cholestatic	18	↓						[41]
Noncholestatic	13	↓						
Not defined	42	↓	↔[a]	↔[a]		↓	↔	[42]
Noncholestatic	9	↓	↔	↓		↔	↔	[43]
Mixed	42	↔				↔		[44]
Cholestatic	18	↓	↓[a]	↓[a]		↓	↔	[45]
Noncholestatic	32	↓	↔[a]	↔[a]		↔	↓	
Cholestatic	6						↓	[46]
Noncholestatic	6						↔	
Noncholestatic	32	↓	↓	↔	↓	↓	↓	[47]

[a] *The antibody used in these studies was not specific and likely represents a summation of many CYP2C proteins (CYP2C8, CYP2C9, and CYP2C10).*
Based on Zgheib NK, Branch RA. Drug metabolism and liver disease: a drug-gene-environment interaction. Drug Metab Rev 2017;49:35–55 [48].

In vivo studies showed similar results to in vitro findings. For example, a study in patients with liver disease, in whom the presence or absence of cholestasis was not noted, indicated that clearance of S-mephenytoin, a CYP2C19 probe, was decreased by 63% in cirrhotic patients with mild cirrhosis and by 96% in patients with moderate cirrhosis [49]. Importantly in a more recent study, although activities of CYP2E1 and CYP1A2 were significantly decreased with increased severity of liver disease, there was no evidence of a differential effect of liver disease etiology on neither enzyme activity in patients with mild cholestatic liver cirrhosis compared to noncholestatic disease; CYP2C19 was not evaluated in this study [50]. Interestingly, inconsistent results were seen in patients with hepatocellular carcinoma (HCC) on top of liver cirrhosis or fibrosis. For instance, the evaluation of CYPs in microsomes from normal and HCC liver tissues showed that, while CYP1A2, CYP2C8, and CYP2C19 enzyme activities (using probe drugs) were decreased, those of CYP3A were unchanged, and those of CYP2C9, CYP2D6, and CYP2E1 were higher when compared to controls [51, 52].

Of note, glucuronide conjugation of morphine and other drugs is relatively well preserved in patients with mild and moderate cirrhosis [40], but morphine clearance was 59% reduced in patients whose cirrhosis was severe enough to have caused previous hepatic encephalopathy [53]. Therefore, although glucuronidation may be spared in patients with mild to moderate liver disease, it has been shown to be reduced in patients with severe liver disease [54]. The story may however be more complex based on early evidence from dogs in whom the blood concentration time profiles of morphine and its glucuronide were comparable. So the reported differential effect of liver disease severity on glucuronidation actually may reflect a change in the balance of drug conjugation and deconjugation [55].

Use of therapeutic drugs in patients with liver disease

A number of clinical classification schemes and laboratory measures have been proposed as a means of guiding dose adjustments in patients with liver disease, much as creatinine clearance has been used to guide dose adjustments in patients with impaired renal function.

Classification schemes for liver function

The Pugh modification of Child's classification of liver disease severity (Table 7.4) is the classification scheme that is used most commonly in studies designed to formulate drug dosing recommendations for patients with liver disease [56, 57]. Another classification scheme, the model for end-stage liver disease (MELD), is based on serum bilirubin, serum creatinine, the international normalized prothrombin time ratio (INR), and the underlying cause of liver disease [58]. Unfortunately, these classification schemes are unable to precisely quantify the effect that liver disease has on the drug-metabolizing capability of individual patients.

TABLE 7.4 Pugh modification of child's classification of liver disease severity.

Assessment parameters	Assigned score		
	1 point	2 points	3 points
Encephalopathy Grade	0	1 or 2	3 or 4
Ascites	Absent	Slight	Moderate
Bilirubin (mg/dL)	1–2	2–3	>3
Albumin (g/dL)	>3.5	2.8–3.5	<2.8
Prothrombin time (seconds > control)	1–4	4–10	>10
Classification of clinical severity			
Clinical Severity	Mild	Moderate	Severe
Total Points	5–6	7–9	>9
Encephalopathy grade			
Grade 0	Normal consciousness, personality, neurological examination, EEG		
Grade 1	Restless, sleep disturbed, irritable/agitated, tremor, impaired hand writing, 5 cps waves on EEG		
Grade 2	Lethargic, time-disoriented, inappropriate, asterixis, ataxia, slow triphasic waves on EEG		
Grade 3	Somnolent, stuporous, place-disoriented, hyperactive reflexes, rigidity, slower waves on EEG		
Grade 4	Unarousable coma, no personality/behavior, decerebrate, slow 2–3-cps delta waves on EEG		

Based on Pugh RNH, Murray-Lyon IM, Dawson JL, et al. Br J Surg 1973;60:646–649 [56], and CDER, CBER. Guidance for Industry. Rockville: FDA; 2003. www.fda.gov/downloads/Drugs/GuidanceComplianceRegulatoryInformation/Guidances/ucm072123.pdf [57].)

FDA guidance for industry on pharmacokinetic studies in patients with impaired hepatic function

The updated 2003 FDA guidance for industry on pharmacokinetic studies in patients with impaired liver function was designed to facilitate the conduct of the studies by industry, rather than to guide drug prescribing in patients with severe disease. [57]. It proposes using the Child-Pugh classification to assess hepatic impairment, and recommends pharmacokinetic studies for drugs with narrow therapeutic ranges or those that are extensively metabolized in the liver. The proposed sample size is eight controls and eight patients with no more than moderate liver disease. Therefore only patients with mild or moderately severe liver disease are enrolled in these studies; there are hence relatively few data from patients with severe liver disease, in whom both pharmacokinetic changes and altered pharmacologic response are expected to be most pronounced. Uncertainty is further compounded by the large intersubjects variability in phenotypic measures of drug disposition in both controls and subjects with variable liver disease. In addition, the guidance does not ask for the pharmacokinetics of renally excreted drugs to be evaluated in patients with decompensated liver disease and associated *hepatorenal syndrome*.

Other tools for the assessment of liver function

Prediction of pharmacokinetic alterations resulting from varying degrees of hepatic dysfunction remains a challenge, given the multiple factors that may impact the hepatic clearance of drugs. The use of "probe" drugs to obtain phenotypic measures of metabolizing enzyme activities in human subjects has been advocated for several decades [59]. Nevertheless, the method is relatively cumbersome and there are no clinically relevant probes for the evaluation of drug transporters; hence there is a need for other platforms or models for evaluating hepatic drug clearance.

Whole-body *physiologically based* pharmacokinetic modeling has been proposed by Edgington and Willman [60] and, more recently, by Johnson et al. [61]. These approaches are based on the "well-stirred" model of hepatic drug clearance and incorporate in vitro-in vivo extrapolation of the intrinsic metabolic clearance for each enzymatic pathway, with corrections for estimated abundance of individual specific enzymes and liver weight, and utilize the Monte Carlo method to generate *virtual populations* of individuals with varying physiologic and pathophysiologic characteristics [61]. Reasonable predictions were generated for orally administered midazolam, oral caffeine, oral and intravenous theophylline, oral and intravenous metoprolol, oral nifedipine, oral quinidine, oral diclofenac, oral sildenafil, and oral omeprazole, but not for intravenous omeprazole [61]. However, the clinical applicability of these predictive modeling approaches remains to be determined. In addition to these modeling approaches, recent evidence supports the "facilitation dissolution model" to predict in vivo albumin-mediated hepatic uptake and clearance of OATP substrates based on in vitro studies with isolated hepatocytes [62, 63]. Furthermore, engineered human liver platforms are gradually becoming an integral part of drug metabolism studies in drug development, especially for the preclinical evaluation of drug-induced hepatotoxicity [64]; they also have been used to determine the effect of liver disease on drug metabolism, though further efforts are needed to better mimic the disease phenotype over a longer period of time [65]. In addition, improved physiological cell culture microenvironments with three-dimensional liver microphysiological systems (MPS) may enhance the potential for predicting and evaluating drug effects in liver disease [66].

With advances in molecular biology and sequencing techniques, there has been an active quest for peripheral blood biomarkers for all pathologic conditions, including liver disease [67]. We have previously advocated the use of peripheral white blood cell mRNA expression of the *CYP2D6* enzyme as a marker of liver CYP2D6 enzyme activity in healthy subjects and recipients of liver transplants [68, 69]. More recently, peripheral blood extracellular vesicles and circulating nucleic acids have been included, in what have been termed "liquid biopsies," especially in patients with HCC [70]. This has been coupled with epigenetic measurements of cell-free DNA methylation modifications and cell-free noncoding microRNA levels in various liver disease etiologies. The predictive and prognostic potential of these liquid biopsy tools is encouraging and may replace invasive liver biopsies [67, 71–73]. For example, a promoter region in the peroxisome proliferator-activated receptor gamma (PPAR-γ) was shown to be hypermethylated in plasma of subjects with NAFLD and hepatitis B and C fibrosis [74, 75]. In addition, a variety of miRNAs such as miR-122 and miR-155 are downregulated in plasma of patients with viral hepatitis, alcoholic liver disease, and NAFLD, while others such as miR-762 that are potentially involved in liver fibrosis are upregulated and enter the systemic circulation. More extensive information is provided in the recent review by Mann et al. [70].

Effects of liver disease on the hepatic elimination of drugs

Eq. (7.14) emphasizes the central point that changes in perfusion and protein binding, as well as intrinsic clearance, will affect the hepatic clearance of a number of drugs. The intact hepatocyte theory has been proposed as a means of simplifying this complexity [76]. This theory is analogous to the intact nephron theory (see Chapter 5) in that it assumes that the increase in portocaval shunting parallels the loss of functional cell mass, and that the reduced mass of normally functioning liver cells is perfused normally. Nevertheless, the compelling in vitro and in vivo evidence for an effect of liver disease that influences different mechanisms of drug metabolism differentially as the disease process progresses, later labeled as the "sequential progressive model of liver disease," challenges the intact hepatocyte theory (Fig. 7.5) [7]. Other theories have also been proposed to account for the effects of chronic liver disease on hepatic drug clearance and it currently is not clear which, if any, of these theories is most appropriate [77]. However, what is apparent from studies in patients with significantly impaired liver function is that the intrinsic clearance of some drugs that normally are nonrestrictively metabolized is reduced to the extent that $f_u CL_{int}$ now becomes rate limiting and clearance is no longer approximated by hepatic perfusion rate [33]. It also is apparent from Eq. (7.14) that the presence of portosystemic shunting and hepatocellular damage will significantly increase the bioavailability of drugs that normally have extensive first-pass hepatic metabolism.

Correlation of laboratory tests with drug metabolic clearance

Bergquist et al. [78] presented examples in which several laboratory tests that are commonly used to assess liver function provide a more reliable indication of impaired drug metabolic clearance than the Child-Pugh clinical classification scheme (Table 7.5). Reduction in serum albumin concentrations that occur relatively late in disease progression was of greatest predictive value for two of the drugs shown in the table. However, this marker was not correlated with the hepatic clearance of lansoprazole, and a combination of all three laboratory tests was better correlated with hepatic clearance of atorvastatin than serum albumin alone. Serum concentrations of aspartate aminotransferase (AST) or alanine aminotransferase (ALT) were not correlated with hepatic drug clearance, as might be expected from the fact that these enzymes reflect hepatocellular damage rather than hepatocellular function.

Use of probe drugs to characterize hepatic drug clearance

A number of probe drugs have been administered to normal subjects and to patients to evaluate hepatic clearance. Quantitative liver function tests using probe drugs can be categorized either as specific for a given metabolic pathway or as more

TABLE 7.5 Correlation of laboratory test results with impaired hepatic clearance.

		Laboratory test		
Drug	Enzyme(s)	Albumin	PT[a]	Bilirubin
"A"	CYP2C9	X		
"B"	Not given	X		
Atorvastatin	CYP3A4	X	X	X
Lansoprazole	CYP3A4+CYP2C19		X	

[a]*Prothrombin time.*
Data from Bergquist C, Lindergård J, Salmonson T. Clin Pharmacol Ther 1999;66:201–204 [78].

generally reflective of hepatic metabolism, perfusion, or biliary function. An example of the latter category is the *aminopyrine breath test*, which is a broad measure of hepatic microsomal drug metabolism, since aminopyrine is metabolized by at least six cytochrome P450 enzymes [79]. Other tests in this category are the *galactose elimination test*, to measure cytosolic drug metabolism; *sorbitol clearance*, to measure liver parenchymal perfusion; and *indocyanine green clearance*, reflecting both parenchymal perfusion and biliary secretory capacity. Fig. 7.4 illustrates the relationship between the degree of impairment in these tests and Child-Pugh class of liver disease severity in patients with chronic hepatitis B and C [80]. These results indicate that hepatic metabolic capacity is impaired before portosystemic shunting becomes prominent in the pathophysiology of chronic viral hepatitis. However, these nonspecific tests are, by their nature, of limited value in predicting the clearance of a specific drug in an individual patient.

The monoethylglycinexylidide (MEGX) test is an example of a test that specifically evaluates the function of a single metabolic pathway. In this test, a 1-mg/kg dose of lidocaine is administered intravenously and plasma concentrations of its N-dealkylated metabolite, MEGX, are measured either 15 or 30 min later. Testa et al. [81] found that a 30-min postdose MEGX concentration of 50 ng/mL provided the best discrimination between chronic hepatitis and cirrhosis (sensitivity, 93.5%; specificity, 76.9%). These authors concluded that both hepatic blood flow and the enzymatic conversion of lidocaine to MEGX, initially thought to be mediated by CYP3A4 but subsequently shown to be due primarily to CYP1A2 [82], were well preserved in patients with mild and moderate chronic hepatitis. However, MEGX levels fell significantly in patients with cirrhosis and were well correlated with the clinical stage of cirrhosis, as shown in Fig. 7.5. Muñoz et al. [83] subsequently reported that serum lidocaine levels measured 120–180 min after administering a 5-mg/kg oral lidocaine dose had greater sensitivity (100%) than serum bilirubin (57%), serum albumin (62%), prothrombin concentrations (43%), or MEGX serum concentrations (57%) in differentiating cirrhotic patients from healthy controls, and suggested that this approach would be better than either standard liver function tests or the MEGX test for evaluating liver function in cirrhotic patients.

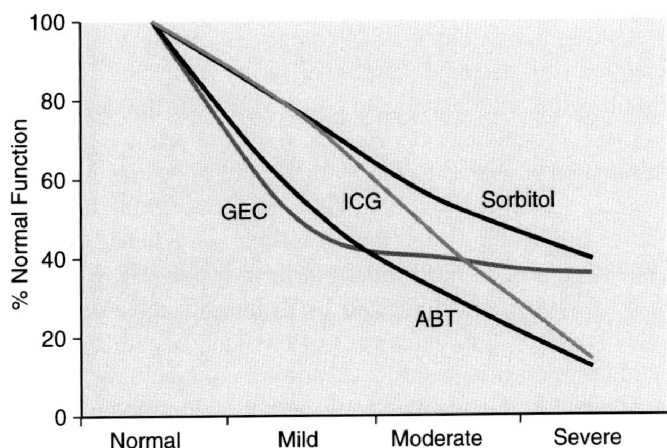

FIG. 7.4 Relationship between Child-Pugh stages of liver disease severity and extent of impairment in antipyrine breath test (ABT), galactose elimination capacity (GEC), sorbitol clearance, and indocyanine green clearance (ICG). *(Based on data published by Herold C, Heinz R, Niedobitek G, et al. Liver 2001;21:260–265 [80].)*

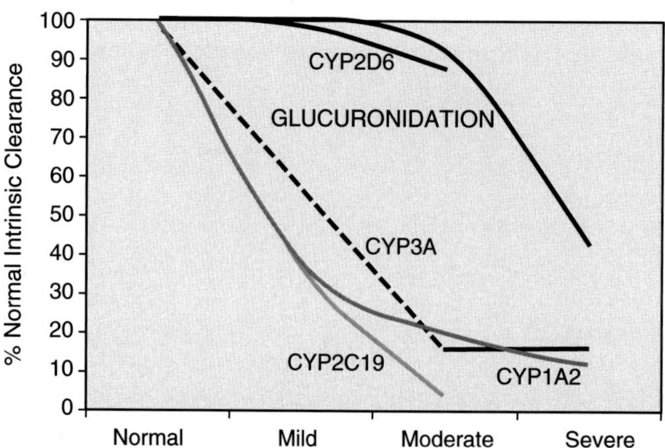

FIG. 7.5 Schematic diagram showing the relationship between Child-Pugh stages of liver disease severity and the intrinsic clearance of drugs mediated by specific cytochrome P450 metabolic pathways. Estimates for glucuronidation [47], CYP2D6 [49], CYP1A2 [78], CYP3A4 [79], and CYP2C19 [49] pathways are based on the literature sources indicated ibetween brackets. The erythromycin breath test was used to assess hepatic CYP3A in a study in which no patients with mild liver disease were included and results in patients with moderate and severe liver disease were combined.

Morphine, S-mephenytoin, debrisoquine, and erythromycin also have been used as selective probes to evaluate, respectively, glucuronidation and the CYP2C19, CYP2D6, and CYP3A4 metabolic pathways in patients with different Child-Pugh classes of liver disease severity, and these results are included in Fig. 7.5. Also see Table 7.6 for representative studies of in vivo evaluations of CYP activity using probe drugs in patients with liver disease compared to healthy controls [48, 49, 59, 82, 84–100].

To increase the efficiency of evaluating specific drug metabolic pathways, the strategy has been developed of simultaneously administering a combination of probes [101]. As many as five probe drugs have been administered in this fashion to provide a profile of CYP1A2, CYP2E1, CYP3A, CYP2D6, CYP2C19, and *N*-acetyltransferase activity using a single gas chromatography-mass spectrometry assay from one blood sample to measure all parent drugs and metabolites to generate a phenotype [59, 102]. The method was evaluated to exclude the possibility of a significant metabolic interaction between the individual probes. Although a number of different versions of the cocktail approach have been described, these all are too cumbersome for routine clinical use [103]. In addition, even when the metabolic pathway for a given drug is known, prediction of hepatic drug clearance in individual patients is complicated by the effects of drug interactions and pharmacogenetic variation [51, 95].

Effects of liver disease on the renal elimination of drugs

Drug therapy in patients with advanced cirrhosis is further complicated by the fact that renal blood flow and glomerular filtration rate are frequently depressed in these patients in the absence of other known causes of renal failure. Renal hemodynamics are compromised long before cirrhosis is categorized as severe because even moderate portal hypertension triggers increased production of nitric oxide and other factors that cause arterial vasodilation in the splanchnic circulation [104]. Initially, cardiac output can increase to compensate for the decrease in systemic vascular resistance. However, in advanced cirrhosis, the sympathetic nervous system, the renin-angiotensin system, and the nonosmotic release of arginine vasopressin must be activated to maintain arterial pressure. Activation of these additional compensatory mechanisms causes intrarenal vasoconstriction and hypoperfusion that adversely affect renal sodium excretion and solute-free water retention, leading to the formation of ascites and edema, and ultimately results in renal failure. This etiology of renal failure has been termed the *hepatorenal syndrome* (HRS) and has been subdivided into Type I HRS, which presents as acute renal failure characterized by a doubling of a previously measured serum creatinine, or a 50% reduction in creatinine clearance, within 2 weeks of an acute hepatotoxic event; and Type II HRS, in which refractory ascites is prominent and progression to serum creatinine concentrations of 1.5–2.5 mg/dL occurs more gradually over a period of weeks to months [105]. However, a number of factors, including administration of certain drugs or spontaneous bacterial peritonitis resulting from the bacterial translocation from the intestine to the peritoneum, can precipitate acute renal failure in patients with Type II HRS.

Ginès et al. [106] monitored 234 patients with cirrhosis, ascites, and a glomerular filtration rate (GFR) of more than 50 mL/min. These authors found that HRS developed within 1 year in 18%, and within 5 years in 39%, of these patients.

TABLE 7.6 Representative studies of in vivo evaluations of CYP activity in patients with liver disease compared to healthy controls.

		Enzyme activity			
Isozyme	**Probe drug**	**Mild cirrhosis**	**Moderate cirrhosis**	**Severe cirrhosis**	**References**
CYP1A2	Lidocaine	↓	↓↓	↓↓	[87]
	Caffeine			↓↓↓	[88]
	Caffeine	↓	↓↓	↓↓↓	[59]
CYP2A6	Coumarin	↔	↓	↓↓	[87]
CYP2C8	Repaglinide			↓↓↓	[88]
CYP2C9	Tolbutamide	↔	↓↓		[89]
	Diclofenac	↔	↔		[90]
	Ibuprofen	↔	↔		[91]
CYP2C19	Mephenytoin	↓↓	↓↓↓		[49]
	Esomeprazole	↓	↓	↓↓	[92]
	Omeprazole	↓	↓	↓↓	[93]
	Aminopyrine	↓			[94]
	Omeprazole	↓↓↓			[95]
	Mephenytoin	↓↓	↓↓↓	↓↓↓	[59]
CYP2D6	Debrisoquine	↓	↓		[49]
	Atomoxetine		↓	↓↓	[96]
	Debrisoquine	↓	↓↓	↓↓↓	[59]
CYP2E1	Chlorzoxazone	↔	↓	↓↓	[59]
CYP3A4	Nifedipine		↓↓		[82]
	Lidocaine	↓	↓	↓↓↓	[87]
	Midazolam		↓↓		[97]
	Ranolazine	↔	↓		[98]
	Cortisol	↓			[95]
	Levetiracetam	↔	↔	↓↓	[99]
	Midazolam	↔	↓↓	↓↓↓	[100]

Based on Zgheib NK, Branch RA. Drug metabolism and liver disease: a drug-gene-environment interaction. Drug Metab Rev 2017;49:35–55 [48].

Although the Pugh score was of no prognostic value, high plasma renin activity, low serum sodium concentrations, small liver size, and baseline estimates of renal function were independent predictors of the onset of this syndrome. However, conventional assessment of renal function in patients with advanced liver disease is complicated by the fact that GFR is overestimated when it is based on serum creatinine concentration measurements. Thus many patients with cirrhosis and ascites have a normal serum creatinine concentration with a GFR <60 mL/min and serum creatinine concentrations may remain within the normal range even when inulin clearance falls as low as 10 mL/min [107]. This occurs because creatinine production is reduced, due to the reduced skeletal muscle mass that occurs in patients with advanced liver disease, and renal tubular secretion of creatinine increases as glomerular filtration rate is reduced. Consequently, both the Cockcroft and Gault and MDRD equations [108], and even the actual measurement of creatinine clearance based on timed urine collections, provide an inaccurate guide to the status of renal function in these patients [109]. Until a better routine approach is developed for evaluating renal function in liver disease patients, the current version of the MDRD equation is recommended as most suitable for routine clinical use [105]. New biomarkers of glomerular filtration rate such as cystatin C may improve the prognostic stratification of patients with kidney injury in cirrhosis. Other emerging markers may also be useful to differentiate *hepatorenal syndrome* from acute tubular necrosis [110].

The need for caution in estimating drug dosage for patients with *hepatorenal syndrome* is exemplified by carbenicillin, an antipseudomonal, semisynthetic penicillin that is excreted primarily by the kidneys, with biliary excretion normally accounting for less than 20% of total elimination. The decline in renal function that is associated with severe liver disease prolongs the elimination half-life of this drug from 1 h in subjects with normal renal and liver function to approximately 24 h [111]. Although studies in patients with *hepatorenal syndrome* were not reported, similar half-life prolongations have been described in patients with combined renal and hepatic functional impairment who were treated with the newer but pharmacokinetically similar antipseudomonal penicillins piperacillin [112] and mezlocillin [113]. Aminoglycosides are other relevant antimicrobials that are primarily excreted by the kidneys and commonly prescribed for gram-negative infections in patients with advanced cirrhosis, and it has been proposed to measure urinary β_2-microglobulin as a marker of acute renal damage in order to differentiate aminoglycoside nephrotoxicity from functional renal failure [114]. As a general rule, it is advisable to consider reducing doses even for drugs that are eliminated to a significant extent by renal excretion when treating patients with cirrhosis that is severe enough to be accompanied by ascites.

Effects of liver disease on patient response

The relationship between drug concentration and response also can be altered in patients with advanced liver disease. Of greatest concern is the fact that customary doses of sedatives may precipitate the confusion, disorientation, and eventual coma that are characteristic of portal-systemic or hepatic encephalopathy that frequently occurs in the terminal phase of advanced liver disease [115]. Hepatic encephalopathy is primarily caused by the synergistic effects of excess ammonia production and inflammation that together result in astrocyte swelling and brain edema. Specific measures to treat patients with hepatic encephalopathy include oral administration of lactulose and the poorly absorbed antibiotic rifaximin to reduce ammonia formation by intestinal bacteria. However, experimental hepatic encephalopathy also is associated with increased γ-aminobutyric acid-mediated inhibitory neurotransmission, and there has been some success in using the benzodiazepine antagonist flumazenil to reverse this syndrome [116]. This provides the rationale for using flumazenil to treat patients who fail to respond to ammonia-reduction therapy, as well as those whose hepatic encephalopathy is triggered by exogenous benzodiazepines [117]. It provides a theoretical basis for the finding that brain hypersensitivity, together with impaired drug elimination, is responsible for the exaggerated sedative response to diazepam that is exhibited by some patients with chronic liver disease [118]. Changes in the cerebrospinal fluid/serum concentration ratio of cimetidine have been reported in patients with liver disease, suggesting an increase in blood-brain barrier permeability that also could make these patients more sensitive to the adverse central nervous system effects of a number of other drugs [119].

Although cirrhotic patients frequently are treated with diuretic drugs to reduce ascites, they exhibit a reduced responsiveness to loop diuretics that cannot be overcome by administering larger doses. This presumably is related to the pathophysiology of increased sodium retention that contributes to the development of ascites [120]. In addition, decreases in renal function, which is often unrecognized in these patients [107], may lead to decreased delivery of loop diuretics to their renal tubular site of action. Because hyperaldosteronism is prevalent in these patients and spironolactone is not dependent on glomerular filtration for efficacy, it should be the mainstay of diuretic therapy in this clinical setting [121].

When diuretic therapy does result in effective fluid removal in cirrhotic patients, it is associated with a very high incidence of adverse reactions. In one study of diuretic therapy in cirrhosis, furosemide therapy precipitated HRS in 12.8%, and hepatic coma in 11.6%, of the patients [122]. Although daily doses of this drug did not differ, patients who had adverse drug reactions received total furosemide doses that averaged 1384 mg, whereas patients without adverse reactions received lower total doses that averaged 743 mg. Accordingly, when spironolactone therapy does not provide an adequate diuresis, only small frequent doses of loop diuretics should be added to the spironolactone regimen [121]. Cirrhotic patients also appear to be at an increased risk of developing acute renal failure after being treated with angiotensin-converting enzyme inhibitors and nonsteroidal antiinflammatory drugs [123].

Modification of drug therapy in patients with liver disease

It is advisable to avoid using certain drugs in patients with advanced liver disease. For example, angiotensin-converting enzyme inhibitors and nonsteroidal antiinflammatory drugs should be avoided because of their potential to cause acute renal failure. Paradoxically, administration of captopril to cirrhotic patients with ascites actually impairs rather than promotes sodium excretion [124]. Since coagulation disorders are common in patients with advanced cirrhosis, alternatives should be sought for therapy with β-lactam antibiotics that contain the *N*-methylthiotetrazole side chain (e.g., cefotetan) that inhibits γ-carboxylation of vitamin K-dependent clotting factors [123].

It also is prudent to reduce the dosage of a number of other drugs that frequently are used to treat patients with liver disease [38, 125–127]. Delcò and colleagues [126] recommend that although drug conjugation pathways also may be impaired in patients with liver failure, drugs that are mainly metabolized by these pathways are preferred because only one metabolic pathway usually is involved. Particular attention has been focused on drugs whose clearance is significantly impaired in patients with moderate hepatic impairment, as assessed using the Child-Pugh classification scheme presented in Table 7.4. Even greater caution should be exercised in using these drugs to treat patients with severely impaired liver function. Table 7.7 lists several drugs whose dose should be reduced in treating patients with moderate hepatic impairment. Most of the drugs in this table have first-pass metabolism that is greater than 50% in normal subjects but is substantially reduced when liver function is impaired [35, 47, 125–138].

Although initial and maintenance oral drug doses may need to be reduced in patients with moderate to severe liver disease, the extent of reduction cannot be accurately predicted since neither the extent of portosystemic shunting nor the actual hepatic blood flow usually is known in a given patient [126]. Given this uncertainty, maintenance doses need to be adjusted empirically to achieve the desired pharmacologic effect while avoiding toxicity. When medications are administered intravenously, a normal initial or loading dose may be administered, but the maintenance dose should be lowered to reflect the reduction in hepatic clearance [126]. Although not routinely evaluated in most studies of patients with liver disease, drug binding to plasma proteins also may be reduced in these patients and may contribute to exaggerated responses to nonrestrictively metabolized drugs. Formation of pharmacologically active metabolites is another complicating factor that deserves consideration. For example, losartan has an active metabolite, EXP3174, which is primarily responsible for the extent and duration of pharmacological effect in patients treated with this drug [133]. Although standard doses produce plasma concentrations of losartan that are four to five times higher in patients with cirrhosis than those observed in normal subjects, plasma levels of EXP3174 are only increased by a factor of 1.5–2.0 [135]. This provided the rationale for reducing the usual losartan dose by only half in a trial in which this drug was used to reduce portal pressure in patients with cirrhosis and esophageal varices [139].

When no drug-specific recommendations are available, Delcò et al. [126] recommend using the Child-Pugh classification as a guide to reduce normal maintenance drug doses by 50% in patients with mild, and by 75% in patients with

TABLE 7.7 Some drugs where there is evidence to support a dose reduction in patients with moderate cirrhosis.

		Parameter values or changes in cirrhosis			
	F (%)	*F* (%)	Clearance	f_u	References
Analgesic drugs:					
Morphine	47	100	↓ 59%		[47]
Meperidine	47	91	↓ 46%		[35]
Pentazocine	17	71	↓ 50%		[35]
Cardiovascular drugs:					
Propafenone	21	75	↓ 24%	↑ 213%	[125]
Verapamil	22	52	↓ 51%	No change	[126]
Nifedipine	51	91	↓ 60%	↑ 93%	[127]
Nitrendipine	40	54	↓ 34%	↑ 43%	[128]
Nisoldipine	4	15	↓ 42%		[129]
Losartan	33	66	↓ 50%		[130–135]
Other:					
Omeprazole	56	98	↓ 89%		[132, 136]
Tacrolimus	27	36	↓ 72%		[133, 134, 137, 138]

TABLE 7.8 Dosage adjustments in patients with liver disease.[a]

Clinical setting	Recommendation
Drugs with a relatively high extraction ratio (>70%)	The dose should be reduced because the oral bioavailability can be significantly increased
Drugs with a low hepatic extraction ratio (<30%) and high plasma protein binding (>90%)	Pharmacokinetic evaluations should be based on the unbound blood/plasma concentrations because the unbound fraction of drug may be significantly increased. Dosage adjustments may be necessary even though total blood/plasma concentrations are within the normal range
Drugs with a low hepatic extraction ratio (<30%) and low plasma protein binding (<90%)	Dosage adjustment may be necessary and should be targeted at maintaining normal total (bound plus unbound) plasma concentrations
The elimination of drugs partly excreted unchanged by the kidneys will be impaired in patients with hepatorenal syndrome	Consider that creatinine clearance significantly overestimates glomerular filtration rate in these patients
The distribution volume of hydrophilic drugs may be increased in patients with edema or ascites	The loading dose may have to be increased if a rapid and complete response to the drug is required. Many of these drugs are eliminated by the kidneys so renal function should be taken into consideration
Drug selection and dosing in patients with severe liver disease (Child-Pugh classification)	Use caution when administering drugs with narrow therapeutic indices to patients with liver disease and any drug to patients with severe liver disease

[a]Recommendations from Verbeeck RK. Eur J Clin Pharmacol 2008;64:1147–1161 [38].

moderate, liver disease. In patients with severe liver disease, they recommend using drugs whose safety is known, or whose pharmacokinetics is not affected by liver disease, or for which therapeutic drug monitoring is available. Verbeeck [38] has provided the more detailed guidelines, listed in Table 7.8, for adjusting drug dosage in patients with liver failure. None of these guidelines obviates the need to monitor patient response closely and to make the further dose adjustments that may be required to both achieve the desired therapeutic response and avoid toxicity.

Because there are currently limited recommendations for specific drug dose modification in patients with liver disease, more research and collaborative efforts are needed in this field. We have previously advocated the development and compilation of a database coupled with a web-based resource to provide health care practitioners with evidence-based prescribing guidelines for patients with liver disease [48]. Such an initiative has already started in the Netherlands by Weersink et al. [140] who describe a six-step protocol for evaluating the safety and dosing of drugs in patients with liver cirrhosis. They plan to evaluate a preselected list of drug classes and will classify them according to a safety classification scheme in which the evaluated drugs would be assigned to one of the following six categories: safe, no additional risks known, additional risks known, unsafe, unknown, and not yet classified.

References

[1] Rowland M, Benet LZ, Graham GG. Clearance concepts in pharmacokinetics. J Pharmacokinet Biopharm 1973;1:123–136.

[2] Wilkinson GR, Shand DG. A physiological approach to hepatic drug clearance. Clin Pharmacol Ther 1975;18:377–390.

[3] Rane A, Wilkinson GR, Shand DG. Prediction of hepatic extraction ratio from *in vitro* measurement of intrinsic clearance. J Pharmacol Exp Ther 1977;200:420–424.

[4] Yang J, Jamei M, Yeo KR, Rostami-Hodjegan A, Tucker GT. Misuse of the well-stirred model of hepatic drug clearance. Drug Metab Dispos 2007;35:501–502.

[5] Roberts MS, Donaldson JD, Rowland M. Models of hepatic elimination: comparison of stochastic models to describe residence time distributions and to predict the influence of drug distribution, enzyme heterogeneity, and systemic recycling on hepatic elimination. J Pharmacokinet Biopharm 1988;16:41–83.

[6] Atkinson AJ Jr, Reidenberg MM, Thompson WL. Clinical pharmacology. In: Greenberger N, editor. MKSAP VI syllabus. Philadelphia, PA: American College of Physicians; 1982. p. 85–96.

[7] Branch RA. Drugs in liver disease. Clin Pharmacol Ther 1998;64:462–465.

[8] Roberts MS, Magnusson BM, Burczynski FJ, Weiss M. Enterohepatic circulation: physiological, pharmacokinetic and clinical implications. Clin Pharmacokinet 2002;41:751–790.

[9] Klaassen CD, Cui JY. Review: mechanisms of how the intestinal microbiota alters the effects of drugs and bile acids. Drug Metab Dispos 2015;43:1505–1521.
[10] Rollins DE, Klaassen CD. Biliary excretion of drugs in man. Clin Pharmacokinet 1979;4:368–379.
[11] Heggie GD, Sommadossi J-P, Cross DS, Huster WJ, Diasio RB. Clinical pharmacokinetics of 5-fluorouracil and its metabolites in plasma, urine, and bile. Cancer Res 1987;47:2203–2206.
[12] Siegers C-P, Bumann D. Clinical significance of the biliary excretion of drugs. Prog Pharmacol Clin Pharmacol 1991;8:537–549.
[13] Yoon WJ, Kim HN, Park E, Ryu S, Chang Y, Shin H, et al. The impact of cholecystectomy on the gut microbiota: a case-control study. J Clin Med 2019;8:E79. https://doi.org/10.3390/jcm8010079.
[14] Duggan DE, Hooke KF, Noll RM, Kwan KC. Enterohepatic circulation of indomethacin and its role in intestinal irritation. Biochem Pharmacol 1975;24:1749–1754.
[15] Veng Pedersen P, Miller R. Pharmacokinetics and bioavailability of cimetidine in humans. J Pharm Sci 1980;69:394–398.
[16] Miller R. Pharmacokinetics and bioavailability of ranitidine in humans. J Pharm Sci 1984;73:1376–1379.
[17] Blaschke TF, Meffin PJ, Melmon KL, Rowland M. Influence of acute viral hepatitis on phenytoin kinetics and protein binding. Clin Pharmacol Ther 1975;17:685–691.
[18] Williams RL, Blaschke TF, Meffin PJ, Melmon KL, Rowland M. Influence of acute viral hepatitis on disposition and plasma binding of tolbutamide. Clin Pharmacol Ther 1977;21:301–309.
[19] Williams RL, Schary WL, Blaschke TF, Meffin PJ, Melmon KL, Rowland M. Influence of acute viral hepatitis on disposition and pharmacologic effect of warfarin. Clin Pharmacol Ther 1976;20:90–97.
[20] Williams RL, Blaschke TF, Meffin PJ, Melmon KL, Rowland M. Influence of viral hepatitis on the disposition of two compounds with high hepatic clearance: lidocaine and indocyanine green. Clin Pharmacol Ther 1976;20:290–299.
[21] Villeneuve JP, Thibeault MJ, Ampelas M, Fortunet-Fouin H, LaMarre L, Côtè J, et al. Drug disposition in patients with HB_sAg-positive chronic liver disease. Dig Dis Sci 1987;32:710–714.
[22] Prescott LF, Wright N. The effects of hepatic and renal damage on paracetamol metabolism and excretion following overdosage. A pharmacokinetic study. Br J Pharmacol 1973;49:602–613.
[23] Sotaniemi EA, Niemelä O, Risteli L, Stenbäck F, Pelkonen RO, Lahtela JT, et al. Fibrotic process and drug metabolism in alcoholic liver disease. Clin Pharmacol Ther 1986;40:46–55.
[24] Albhaisi S, Sanyal A. Recent advances in understanding and managing non-alcoholic fatty liver disease. F1000Research 2018;7:389–391.
[25] Morgan DJ, McLean AJ. Therapeutic implications of impaired hepatic oxygen diffusion in chronic liver disease. Hepatology 1991;14:1280–1282.
[26] Nakai K, Tanaka H, Hanada K, Ogata H, Suzuki F, Kumada H, et al. Decreased expression of cytochromes P450 1A2, 2E1, and 3A4 and drug transporters Na+-taurocholate-cotransporting polypeptide, organic cation transporter 1, and organic anion-transporting peptide-C correlates with the progression of liver fibrosis in chronic hepatitis C patients. Drug Metab Dispos 2008;36:1786–1793.
[27] Thakkar N, Slizgi JR, Brouwer KLR. Effect of liver disease on hepatic transporter expression and function. J Pharm Sci 2017;106:2282–2294.
[28] Hanada K, Nakai K, Tanaka H, Suzuki F, Kumada H, Ohno Y, et al. Effect of nuclear receptor downregulation on hepatic expression of cytochrome P450 and transporters in chronic hepatitis C in association with fibrosis development. Drug Metab Pharmacokinet 2012;27:301–306.
[29] Le Couteur DG, Fraser R, Hilmer S, Rivory LP, McLean AJ. The hepatic sinusoid in aging and cirrhosis. Clin Pharmacokinet 2005;44:187–200.
[30] Boyer TD, Henderson JM. Portal hypertension and bleeding esophageal varices. In: Zakim D, Boyer TD, editors. Hepatology: A textbook of liver disease. 4th ed. Philadelphia, PA: Saunders; 2003. p. 581–629.
[31] Iwasa M, Nakamura K, Nakagawa T, Watanabe S, Katoh H, Kinosada Y, et al. Single photon emission computed tomography to determine effective hepatic blood flow and intrahepatic shunting. Hepatology 1995;21:359–365.
[32] Lebrec D, Kotelanski B, Cohn JN. Splanchnic hemodynamics in cirrhotic patients with esophageal varices and gastrointestinal bleeding. Gastroenterology 1976;70:1108–1111.
[33] Huet P-M, Villeneuve J-P. Determinants of drug disposition in patients with cirrhosis. Hepatology 1983;3:913–918.
[34] McLean A, du Souich P, Gibaldi M. Noninvasive kinetic approach to the estimation of total hepatic blood flow and shunting in chronic liver disease—a hypothesis. Clin Pharmacol Ther 1979;25:161–166.
[35] Neal EA, Meffin PJ, Gregory PB, Blaschke TF. Enhanced bioavailability and decreased clearance of analgesics in patients with cirrhosis. Gastroenterology 1979;77:96–102.
[36] Wood AJJ, Kornhauser DM, Wilkinson GR, Shand DG, Branch RA. The influence of cirrhosis on steady-state blood concentrations of unbound propranolol after oral administration. Clin Pharmacokinet 1978;3:478–487.
[37] Blaschke TF. Protein binding and kinetics of drugs in liver diseases. Clin Pharmacokinet 1977;2:32–44.
[38] Verbeeck RK. Pharmacokinetics and dosage adjustment in patients with hepatic dysfunction. Eur J Clin Pharmacol 2008;64:1147–1161.
[39] Kusuhara H, Sugiyama Y. *In vitro–in vivo* extrapolation of transporter-mediated clearance in the liver and kidney. Drug Metab Pharmacokinet 2009;24:37–52.
[40] Elbekai RH, Korashy HM, El-Kadi AOS. The effect of liver cirrhosis on the regulation and expression of drug metabolizing enzymes. Curr Drug Metab 2004;5:157–167.
[41] Iqbal S, Vickers C, Elias E. Drug metabolism in end-stage liver disease. In vitro activities of some phase I and phase II enzymes. J Hepatol 1990;11:37–42.
[42] Guengerich FP, Turvy CG. Comparison of levels of several human microsomal cytochrome P-450 enzymes and epoxide hydrolase in normal and disease states using immunochemical analysis of surgical liver samples. J Pharmacol Exp Ther 1991;256:1189–1194.
[43] Lown K, Kolars J, Turgeon K, Merion R, Wrighton SA, Watkins PB. The erythromycin breath test selectively measures P450IIIA in patients with severe liver disease. Clin Pharmacol Ther 1992;51:229–238.

[44] Lucas D, Berthou F, Dreano Y, Lozac'h P, Volant A, Menez JF. Comparison of levels of cytochromes P-450, CYP1A2, CYP2E1, and their related monooxygenase activities in human surgical liver samples. Alcohol Clin Exp Res 1993;17:900–905.

[45] George J, Murray M, Byth K, Farrell GC. Differential alterations of cytochrome P450 proteins in livers from patients with severe chronic liver disease. Hepatology 1995;21:120–128.

[46] Yang LQ, Li SJ, Cao YF, Man XB, Yu WF, Wang HY, et al. Different alterations of cytochrome P450 3A4 isoform and its gene expression in livers of patients with chronic liver diseases. World J Gastroenterol 2003;9:359–363.

[47] Fisher CD, Lickteig AJ, Augustine LM, Ranger-Moore J, Jackson JP, Ferguson SS, et al. Hepatic cytochrome p450 alterations in humans with progressive stages of nonalcoholic fatty liver disease. Drug Metab Dispos 2009;37:2087–2094.

[48] Zgheib NK, Branch RA. Drug metabolism and liver disease: a drug-gene-environment interaction. Drug Metab Rev 2017;49:35–55.

[49] Adedoyin A, Arns PA, Richards WO, Wilkinson GR, Branch RA. Selective effect of liver disease on the activities of specific metabolizing enzymes: investigation of cytochromes P450 2C19 and 2D6. Clin Pharmacol Ther 1998;64:8–17.

[50] Zgheib NK, Buch S, Steele A, Shaw-Stiffel TA, Zacharia L, Romkes M, et al. Cholestasis does not induce selective regulation in patients with liver disease [abstract]. Clin Pharmacol Ther 2007;81:S75.

[51] Zhou J, Wen Q, Li SF, Zhang YF, Gao N, Tian X, et al. Significant change of cytochrome P450s activities in patients with hepatocellular carcinoma. Oncotarget 2016;7:50612–50623.

[52] Gao J, Zhou J, He XP, Zhang YF, Gao N, Tian X, et al. Changes in cytochrome P450s-mediated drug clearance in patients with hepatocellular carcinoma in vitro and in vivo: a bottom-up approach. Oncotarget 2016;7:28612–28623.

[53] Hasselström J, Eriksson S, Persson A, Rane A, Svensson O, Säwe J. The metabolism and bioavailability of morphine in patients with severe liver cirrhosis. Br J Clin Pharmacol 1990;29:289–297.

[54] Hoyumpa AM, Schenker S. Is glucuronidation truly preserved in patients with liver disease? Hepatology 1991;13:786–795.

[55] Jacqz E, Ward S, Johnson R, Schenker S, Gerkens J, Branch RA. Extrahepatic glucuronidation of morphine in the dog. Drug Metab Dispos 1986;14:627–630.

[56] Pugh RNH, Murray-Lyon IM, Dawson JL, Pietroni MC, Williams R. Transection of the oesophagus for bleeding oesophageal varices. Br J Surg 1973;60:646–649.

[57] CDER, CBER. Pharmacokinetics in patients with impaired hepatic function: Study design, data analysis, and impact on dosing and labeling. Guidance for industry, Rockville, MD: FDA; 2003.www.fda.gov/downloads/Drugs/GuidanceComplianceRegulatoryInformation/Guidances/ucm072123.pdf2003.

[58] Wieisner R, Edwards E, Freeman R, Harper A, Kim R, Kamath P, et al. United Network for Organ Sharing Liver Disease Severity Score Committee. Model for end-stage liver disease (MELD) and allocation of donor livers. Gastroenterology 2003;124:91–96.

[59] Frye RF, Zgheib NK, Matzke GR, Chaves-Gnecco D, Rabinovitz M, Shaikh OS, et al. Liver disease selectively modulates cytochrome P450–mediated metabolism. Clin Pharmacol Ther 2006;80:235–245.

[60] Edginton AN, Willman S. Physiology-based simulations of a pathological condition. Prediction of pharmacokinetics in patients with liver cirrhosis. Clin Pharmacokinet 2008;47:743–752.

[61] Johnson TN, Boussery K, Rowland-Yao K, Tucker GT, Rostami-Hodjegan A. A semi-mechanistic model to predict the effects of liver cirrhosis on drug clearance. Clin Pharmacokinet 2010;49:189–206.

[62] Kim SJ, Lee KR, Miyauchi S, Sugiyama Y. Extrapolation of in vivo hepatic clearance from in vitro uptake clearance by suspended human hepatocytes for anionic drugs with high binding to human albumin: improvement of in vitro-to-in vivo extrapolation by considering the "albumin-mediated" hepatic uptake mechanism on the basis of the "facilitated-dissociation model". Drug Metab Dispos 2019;47:94–103.

[63] Miyauchi S, Masuda M, Kim SJ, Tanaka Y, Lee KR, Iwakado S, et al. The phenomenon of albumin-mediated hepatic uptake of organicanion transport polypeptide substrates: prediction of the in vivo uptake clearance from the in vitro uptake by isolated hepatocytes using a facilitated-dissociation model. Drug Metab Dispos 2018;46:259–267.

[64] Underhill GH, Khetani SR. Advances in engineered human liver platforms for drug metabolism studies. Drug Metab Dispos 2018;46:1626–1637.

[65] Kostrzewski T, Cornforth T, Snow SA, Ouro-Gnao L, Rowe C, Large EM, et al. Three-dimensional perfused human in vitro model of non-alcoholic fatty liver disease. World J Gastroenterol 2017;23:204–215.

[66] Ribeiro AJS, Yang X, Patel V, Madabushi R, Strauss DG. Liver microphysiological systems for predicting and evaluating drug effects. Clin Pharmacol Ther 2019;106:139–147.

[67] Nallagangula KS, Nagaraj SK, Venkataswamy L, Chandrappa M. Liver fibrosis: a compilation on the biomarkers status and their significance during disease progression. Future Sci OA 2017;4:FSO250. https://doi.org/10.4155/fsoa-2017-0083.

[68] Carcillo JA, Parise RA, Adedoyin A, Frye R, Branch RA, Romkes M. CYP2D6 mRNA expression in circulating peripheral blood mononuclear cells correlates with in vivo debrisoquine hydroxylase activity in extensive metabolizers. Res Commun Mol Pathol Pharmacol 1996;91:149–159.

[69] Carcillo JA, Adedoyin A, Burckart GJ, Frye RF, Venkataramanan R, Knoll C, et al. Coordinated intrahepatic and extrahepatic regulation of cytochrome p4502D6 in healthy subjects and in patients after liver transplantation. Clin Pharmacol Ther 2003;73:456–467.

[70] Mann J, Reeves HL, Feldstein AE. Liquid biopsy for liver diseases. Gut 2018;67:2204–2212.

[71] Szabo G, Bala S. MicroRNAs in liver disease. Nat Rev Gastroenterol Hepatol 2013;10:542–552.

[72] Murphy SK, Yang H, Moylan CA, Pang H, Dellinger A, Abdelmalek M, et al. Relationship between methylome and transcriptome in patients with nonalcoholic fatty liver disease. Gastroenterology 2013;145:1076–1087.

[73] Pogribny IP, Beland FA. Role of microRNAs in the regulation of drug metabolism and disposition genes in diabetes and liver disease. Expert Opin Drug Metab Toxicol 2013;9:713–724.

[74] Hardy T, Zeybel M, Day CP, Dipper C, Masson S, McPherson S, et al. Plasma DNA methylation: a potential biomarker for stratification of liver fibrosis in non-alcoholic fatty liver disease. Gut 2017;66:1321–1328.

[75] Yigit B, Boyle M, Ozler O, Erden N, Tutucu F, Hardy T, et al. Plasma cell-free DNA methylation: a liquid biomarker of hepatic fibrosis. Gut 2018;67:1907–1908.

[76] Wood AJJ, Villeneuve JP, Branch RA, Rogers LW, Shand DG. Intact hepatocyte theory of impaired drug metabolism in experimental cirrhosis in the rat. Gastroenterology 1979;76:1358–1362.

[77] Tucker GT. Alteration of drug disposition in liver impairment. Br J Clin Pharmacol 1998;46:355.

[78] Bergquist C, Lindergård J, Salmonson T. Dosing recommendations in liver disease. Clin Pharmacol Ther 1999;66:201–204.

[79] Engel G, Hofmann U, Heidemann H, Cosme J, Eichelbaum M. Antipyrine as a probe for human oxidative drug metabolism: identification of the cytochrome P450 enzymes catalyzing 4-hydroxyantipyrine, 3-hydroxymethylantipyrine, and norantipyrine formation. Clin Pharmacol Ther 1996;59:613–623.

[80] Herold C, Heinz R, Niedobitek G, Schneider T, Hahn EG, Schuppan D. Quantitative testing of liver function in relation to fibrosis in patients with chronic hepatitis B and C. Liver 2001;21:260–265.

[81] Testa R, Caglieris S, Risso D, Arzani L, Campo N, Alvarez S, et al. Monoethylglycinexylidide formation measurement as a hepatic function test to assess severity of chronic liver disease. Am J Gastroenterol 1997;92:2268–2273.

[82] Orlando R, Piccoli P, De Martin S, Padrini R, Floreani M, Palatini P. Cytochrome P50 1A2 is a major determinant of lidocaine metabolism *in vivo*: effects of liver function. Clin Pharmacol Ther 2004;75:80–88.

[83] Muñoz AE, Miguez C, Rubio M, Bartellini M, Levi D, Podesta A, et al. Lidocaine and monoethylglycinexylidide serum determinations to analyze liver function of cirrhotic patients after oral administration. Dig Dis Sci 1999;44:789–795.

[84] Anderson GD, Hakimian S. Pharmacokinetic of antiepileptic drugs in patients with hepatic or renal impairment. Clin Pharmacokinet 2014;53:29–49.

[85] Thummel KE, Lin YS. Sources of interindividual variability. Methods Mol Biol 2014;1113:363–415.

[86] Villeneuve JP, Pichette V. Cytochrome P450 and liver diseases. Curr Drug Metab 2004;5:273–282.

[87] Sotaniemi EA, Rautio A, Backstrom M, Arvela P, Pelkonen O. CYP3A4 and CYP2A6 activities marked by the metabolism of lignocaine and coumarin in patients with liver and kidney diseases and epileptic patients. Br J Clin Pharmacol 1995;39:71–76.

[88] Hatorp V, Walther KH, Christensen MS, Haug-Pihale G. Single-dose pharmacokinetics of repaglinide in subjects with chronic liver disease. J Clin Pharmacol 2000;40:142–152.

[89] Nelson E. Rate of metabolism of tolbutamide in test subjects with liver disease or with impaired renal function. Am J Med Sci 1964;248:657–659.

[90] Zimmerer J, Tittor W, Degen P. Anti-rheumatic therapy in patients with liver diseases. Plasma levels of diclofenac and elimination of diclofenac and metabolites in urine of patients with liver disease. Fortschr Med 1982;100:1683–1688.

[91] Juhl RP, Van Thiel DH, Dittert LW, Albert KS, Smith RB. Ibuprofen and sulindac kinetics in alcoholic liver disease. Clin Pharmacol Ther 1983;34:104–109.

[92] Sjövall H, Björnsson E, Holmberg J, Hasselgren G, Röhss K, Hassan-Alin M. Pharmacokinetic study of esomeprazole in patients with hepatic impairment. Eur J Gastroenterol Hepatol 2002;14:491–496.

[93] Pique JM, Feu F, de Prada G, Röhss K, Hasselgren G. Pharmacokinetics of omeprazole given by continuous intravenous infusion to patients with varying degrees of hepatic dysfunction. Clin Pharmacokinet 2002;41:999–1004.

[94] Giannini E, Fasoli A, Chiarbonello B, Malfatti F, Romagnoli P, Botta F, et al. 13C-aminopyrine breath test to evaluate severity of disease in patients with chronic hepatitis C virus infection. Aliment Pharmacol Ther 2002;16:717–725.

[95] Ohnishi A, Murakami S, Akizuki S, Mochizuki J, Echizen H, Takagi I. In vivo metabolic activity of CYP2C19 and CYP3A in relation to CYP2C19 genetic polymorphism in chronic liver disease. J Clin Pharmacol 2005;45:1221–1229.

[96] Chalon SA, Desager JP, Desante KA, Frye RF, Witcher J, Long AJ, et al. Effect of hepatic impairment on the pharmacokinetics of atomoxetine and its metabolites. Clin Pharmacol Ther 2003;73:178–191.

[97] Gorski JC, Chalasani N, Patel N, Galinsky RE, Craven R, Hall SD. Hepatic and intestinal CYP3A activity in cirrhotics with transjugular intrahepatic portosystemic shunts (TIPS) [abstract]. Clin Pharmacol Ther 2001;69:37.

[98] Abdallah H, Jerling M. Effect of hepatic impairment on the multiple-dose pharmacokinetics of ranolazine sustained-release tablets. J Clin Pharmacol 2005;45:802–809.

[99] Brockmöller J, Thomsen T, Wittstock M, Coupez R, Lochs H, Roots I. Pharmacokinetics of levetiracetam in patients with moderate to severe liver cirrhosis (Child-Pugh classes A, B, and C): characterization by dynamic liver function tests. Clin Pharmacol Ther 2005;77:529–541.

[100] Albarmawi A, Czock D, Gauss A, Ehehalt R, Lorenzo Bermejo J, Burhenne J, et al. CYP3A activity in severe liver cirrhosis correlates with Child-Pugh and model for end-stage liver disease (MELD) scores. Br J Clin Pharmacol 2014;77:160–169.

[101] Breimer DD, Schellens JHM. A "cocktail" strategy to assess *in vivo* oxidative drug metabolism in humans. Trends Pharmacol Sci 1990;11:223–225.

[102] Frye RF, Matzke GR, Adedoyin A, Porter JA, Branch RA. Validation of the five-drug "Pittsburgh cocktail" approach for assessment of selective regulation of drug-metabolizing enzymes. Clin Pharmacol Ther 1997;62:365–376.

[103] Tanaka E, Kurata N, Yasuhara H. How useful is the "cocktail approach" for evaluating human hepatic drug metabolizing capacity using cytochrome P450 phenotyping probes *in vivo*? J Clin Pharm Ther 2003;28:157–165.

[104] Ginès P, Schrier RW. Renal failure in cirrhosis. N Engl J Med 2009;361:1279–1290.

[105] Wong F, Nadim MK, Kellum JA, Salerno F, Bellomo R, Gerbes A, et al. Working Party proposal for a revised classification system of renal dysfunction in patients with cirrhosis. Gut 2011;60:702–709.

[106] Ginès A, Escorsell A, Ginès P, Saló J, Jiménez W, Inglada L, et al. Incidence, predictive factors, and prognosis of the hepatorenal syndrome in cirrhosis with ascites. Gastroenterology 1993;105:229–236.
[107] Papadakis MA, Arieff AI. Unpredictability of clinical evaluation of renal function in cirrhosis: prospective study. Am J Med 1987;82:945–952.
[108] MacAulay J, Thompson K, Kiberd BA, Barnes DC, Peltekian KM. Serum creatinine in patients with advanced liver disease is of limited value for identification of moderate renal dysfunction: are the equations for estimating renal function better? Can J Gastroenterol 2006;20:521–526.
[109] Proulx NL, Akbari A, Garg AX, Rostom A, Jaffey J, Clark HD. Measured creatinine clearance from timed urine collections substantially overestimates glomerular filtration rate in patients with liver cirrhosis: a systematic review and individual patient meta-analysis. Nephrol Dial Transplant 2005;20:1617–1622.
[110] Piano S, Brocca A, Angeli P. Renal function in cirrhosis: a critical review of available tools. Semin Liver Dis 2018;38:230–241.
[111] Hoffman TA, Cestero R, Bullock WE. Pharmacodynamics of carbenicillin in hepatic and renal failure. Ann Intern Med 1970;73:173–178.
[112] Green L, Dick JD, Goldberger SP, Anelopulos CM. Prolonged elimination of piperacillin in a patient with renal and liver failure. Drug Intell Clin Pharm 1985;19:427–429.
[113] Cooper BE, Nester TJ, Armstrong DK, Dasta JF. High serum concentrations of mezlocillin in a critically ill patient with renal and hepatic dysfunction. Clin Pharm 1986;5:764–766.
[114] Cabrera J, Arroyo V, Ballesta AM, Rimola A, Gual J, Elena M, et al. Aminoglycoside nephrotoxicity in cirrhosis. Value of urinary beta 2-microglobulin to discriminate functional renal failure from acute tubular damage. Gastroenterology 1982;82:97–105.
[115] Prakash R, Mullen KD. Mechanisms, diagnosis and management of hepatic encephalopathy. Nat Rev Gastroenterol Hepatol 2010;7:515–525.
[116] Ferenci P, Grimm G, Meryn S, Gangl A. Successful long-term treatment of portal-systemic encephalopathy by the benzodiazepine antagonist flumazenil. Gastroenterology 1989;96:240–243.
[117] Romero-Gómez M. Pharmacotherapy of hepatic encephalopathy in cirrhosis. Expert Opin Pharmacother 2010;11:1317–1327.
[118] Branch RA, Morgan MH, James J, Read AE. Intravenous administration of diazepam in patients with chronic liver disease. Gut 1976;17:975–983.
[119] Schentag JJ, Cerra FB, Calleri GM, Leising ME, French MA, Bernhard H. Age, disease, and cimetidine disposition in healthy subjects and chronically ill patients. Clin Pharmacol Ther 1981;29:737–743.
[120] Brater DC. Resistance to loop diuretics: why it happens and what to do about it. Drugs 1985;30:427–443.
[121] Brater DC. Use of diuretics in cirrhosis and nephrotic syndrome. Semin Nephrol 1999;19:575–580.
[122] Naranjo CA, Pontigo E, Valdenegro C, González G, Ruiz I, Busto U. Furosemide-induced adverse reactions in cirrhosis of the liver. Clin Pharmacol Ther 1979;25:154–160.
[123] Westphal J-F, Brogard J-M. Drug administration in chronic liver disease. Drug Saf 1997;17:47–73.
[124] Daskalopoulos G, Pinzani M, Murray N, Hirschberg R, Zipser RD. Effects of captopril on renal function in patients with cirrhosis and ascites. J Hepatol 1987;4:330–336.
[125] Rodighiero V. Effects of liver disease on pharmacokinetics: an update. Clin Pharmacokinet 1999;37:399–431.
[126] Delcò F, Tchambaz L, Schlienger R, Drewe J, Krähenbühl S. Dose adjustment in patients with liver disease. Drug Saf 2005;28:529–545.
[127] Nguyen HM, Cutie AJ, Pham DQ. How to manage medications in the setting of liver disease with the application of six questions. Int J Clin Pract 2010;64:858–867.
[128] Lee JT, Yee Y-G, Dorian P, Kates RE. Influence of hepatic dysfunction on the pharmacokinetics of propafenone. J Clin Pharmacol 1987;27:384–389.
[129] Somogyi A, Albrecht M, Kliems G, Schäfer K, Eichelbaum M. Pharmacokinetics, bioavailability and ECG response of verapamil in patients with liver cirrhosis. Br J Clin Pharmacol 1981;12:51–60.
[130] Kleinbloesem CH, van Harten J, Wilson JPH, Danhof M, van Brummelen P, Breimer DD. Nifedipine: kinetics and hemodynamic effects in patients with liver cirrhosis after intravenous and oral administration. Clin Pharmacol Ther 1986;40:21–28.
[131] Dylewicz P, Kirch W, Santos SR, Hutt HJ, Mönig H, Ohnhaus EE. Bioavailability and elimination of nitrendipine in liver disease. Eur J Clin Pharmacol 1987;32:563–568.
[132] van Harten J, van Brummelen P, Wilson JHP, Lodewijks MTM, Breimer DD. Nisoldipine: kinetics and effects on blood pressure in patients with liver cirrhosis after intravenous and oral administration. Eur J Clin Pharmacol 1988;34:387–394.
[133] Lo M-W, Goldberg MR, McCrea JB, Lu H, Furtek CI, Bjornsson TD. Pharmacokinetics of losartan, an angiotensin II receptor antagonist, and its active metabolite EXP3174 in humans. Clin Pharmacol Ther 1995;58:641–649.
[134] Goa KL, Wagstaff AJ. Losartan potassium. A review of its pharmacology, clinical efficacy and tolerability in the management of hypertension. Drugs 1996;51:820–845.
[135] McIntyre M, Caffe SE, Michalak RA, Reid JL. Losartan, an orally active angiotensin (AT_1) receptor antagonist: a review of its efficacy and safety in essential hypertension. Pharmacol Ther 1997;74:181–194.
[136] Andersson T, Olsson R, Regårdh C-G, Skänberg I. Pharmacokinetics of [^{14}C]omeprazole in patients with liver cirrhosis. Clin Pharmacokinet 1993;24:71–78.
[137] Venkataramanan R, Jain A, Cadoff E, Warty V, Iwasaki K, Nagase K, et al. Pharmacokinetics of FK 506: preclinical and clinical studies. Transplant Proc 1990;22(Suppl. 1):52–56.
[138] Jain AB, Venkataramanan R, Cadoff E, Fung JJ, Todo S, Krajack A, et al. Effect of hepatic dysfunction and T tube clamping on FK 506 pharmacokinetics and trough concentrations. Transplant Proc 1990;22(Suppl. 1):57–59.
[139] Schneider AW, Kalk JF, Klein CP. Effect of losartan, and angiotensin II receptor antagonist, on portal pressure in cirrhosis. Hepatology 1999;29:334–339.
[140] Weersink RA, Bouma M, Burger DM, Drenth JP, Hunfeld NG, Kranenborg M, et al. Evaluating the safety and dosing of drugs in patients with liver cirrhosis by literature review and expert opinion. BMJ Open 2016;6:e012991. https://doi.org/10.1136/bmjopen-2016-012991.

Chapter 8

Noncompartmental and compartmental approaches to pharmacokinetic data analysis

David M. Foster[a] and Paolo Vicini[b]

[a]*Department of Bioengineering, University of Washington, Seattle, WA, United States,* [b]*Confo Therapeutics NV, Ghent, Belgium*

Introduction

From previous chapters, it is clear that the evaluation of pharmacokinetic parameters is an essential part of understanding how drugs function in the body. To estimate these parameters, studies are undertaken in which time-dependent measurements are collected. These studies can be conducted in animals at the preclinical level, through all stages of clinical trials, and can be data rich or sparse. No matter what the situation, there must be some common means by which to communicate the experimental results and summarize key features of a drug's properties. Pharmacokinetic parameters serve this purpose. It is essential that these parameters be precisely defined to minimize any chance of misunderstanding. Thus, in the field of pharmacokinetics, the definitions and formulas for the parameters must be agreed upon, and the methods used to calculate them understood. This understanding includes assumptions and domains of validity, for the utility of the parameter values depends upon them. This chapter examines the assumptions and domains of validity for the two commonly used methods of pharmacokinetic modeling analysis—noncompartmental and compartmental. Compartmental models have been presented in earlier chapters. This chapter will expand upon this and compare the two methods.

Pharmacokinetic parameters fall basically into two categories. One category is qualitative or descriptive, in that the parameters are observational and require no formula for calculation. Examples would include the maximal observed concentration of a drug or the amount of drug excreted in the urine during a given time period. The other category is quantitative. Quantitative parameters require a mathematical formalism for calculation. Examples here would include mean residence times, clearance rates, and volumes of distribution. Estimation of terminal slopes would also fall into this category.

The quantitative parameters require not only data from which to estimate them, but also a mathematical formalism. As noted, the two most common methods used for pharmacokinetic estimation are noncompartmental and compartmental analysis. Gillespie [1] has compared the two methods as applied to pharmacokinetics. Comparisons regarding the two methodologies as applied to metabolic studies have been provided by DiStefano [2] and Cobelli and Toffolo [3]. Covell et al. [4] have made an extensive theoretical comparison of the two methods. It is worth noting that in the literature the term "noncompartmental" has been used in two different contexts: not only to indicate methods based on the statistical analysis (i.e., averaging or integration) of time-dependent drug concentration profiles, but also to describe modeling formalisms (i.e., distributed systems [5] or recirculatory models [6]) that essentially relax the assumption of "lumping" (i.e., combining processes with similar space-time characteristics) that is inherent in the compartmental models used both in pharmacokinetics and tracer kinetics. We will not be concerned with these latter classes of models but will focus on the commonly used moment-based method of noncompartmental pharmacokinetic data analysis.

The use of compartment- and moment-based methods for determining pharmacokinetic parameters has been the subject of intense discussion in the literature and various clarifications have been proposed to deal with some of the issues we will cover here [7, 8]. Despite this, questions remain regarding the circumstances under which these two methods can be used to estimate the pharmacokinetic parameters of interest. To begin to formulate an answer, one must start with a definition of kinetics, since it is through this definition that one can rigorously introduce the mathematical and statistical analyses needed to study the dynamic characteristics of a system and proceed to define specific parameters of interest that can be estimated

Atkinson's Principles of Clinical Pharmacology. http://doi.org/10.1016/B978-0-12-819869-8.00035-5

from the experimental data. From the definition of kinetics, the types of equations that can be used to provide a mathematical description of the system can be given. The assumptions underlying noncompartmental analysis and estimation techniques for the different parameters for different experimental input-output configurations can then be discussed. One then moves to compartmental analysis with the understanding that models set in full generality are very difficult to practically solve. With appropriate assumptions that are commonly made in pharmacokinetic studies, a simpler set of compartmental models will evolve. These models are easy to solve, and it will be seen that all parameters estimated using noncompartmental analysis can be recovered from these compartmental models. Under conditions when the two methods should, in theory, yield the same estimates, differences can be attributed to the numerical techniques used (e.g., sums of exponentials or differential equations fitted to data vs. trapezoidal or log-trapezoidal integration). With this knowledge, the circumstances under which the two methods will provide the same or different estimates of the pharmacokinetic parameters can be discussed. Thus it is not the point of this chapter to favor one method over another; rather, the intent is to describe the assumptions and consequences of using either method.

Most often, estimating pharmacokinetic parameters requires some approach to matching the predictions of the required formulas to data (curve fitting), which will be discussed in the next sections. An interesting facet of our discussion is that estimating parameters from data provides a vehicle for communicating information about a drug (e.g., summarizing the pharmacokinetics of a drug by way of its residence time, half-life, or apparent volume of distribution) to what may be a diverse audience. Noncompartmental parameters are usually easy to grasp in their implication and fit this role very well. Our purpose here is to discuss the implications of different parameter estimation methods, all the while describing a reliance on conceptual models that has stimulated much debate in both the pharmacokinetic [9] and integrative physiology [2] literature.

Most of the theoretical details of the material covered in this chapter can be found in Covell et al. [4], Jacquez and Simon [10], and Jacquez [11]. Of particular importance to this chapter is the material covered in Covell et al. [4] in which the relationship between the calculation of kinetic parameters from statistical moments and the same parameters calculated from the rate constants of a linear, constant-coefficient compartmental model are derived. Jacquez and Simon [10] discuss in detail the mathematical properties of systems that depend upon local mass balance; this forms the basis for understanding compartmental models and the simplifications that result from certain assumptions about a system under study. Berman [12] gives examples using metabolic turnover data, while the pharmacokinetic examples provided in Gibaldi and Perrier [13] and Rowland and Tozer [14] are more familiar to clinical pharmacologists.

Kinetics, pharmacokinetics, and pharmacokinetic parameters

Kinetics and the link to mathematics

Substances being processed in a biological system are constantly undergoing change. These changes can include transport (e.g., transport via the circulation or transport into or out from a cell) or transformation (e.g., biochemically changing from one substance to another). These changes and the concomitant outcomes form the basis for the system in which the substance interacts. How can one formalize these changes, and once formalized, how can one describe their quantitative nature? Dealing with these questions involves an understanding and utilization of concepts related to kinetics.

The *kinetics* of a substance in a biological system are its spatial and temporal distribution in that system. Kinetics is the result of several complex events, including entry into the system, subsequent distribution (which may entail circulatory dynamics and transport into and from cells), and elimination (which usually requires biochemical transformations). Taken together these events characterize both the transformations undergone by the substance and the system in which it resides.

In this chapter, the substance will be assumed to be a drug that is not normally present in the system (exogenous), but in other contexts it could be an element such as calcium or zinc, or a compound such as an amino acid, protein, or sugar that exists normally in the body (endogenous). Thus, in this chapter, *pharmacokinetics* is defined as the spatial and temporal distribution of a drug in a system. Unlike endogenous substances which are normally present, input of drugs into the system normally occurs from exogenous sources. In addition, unless otherwise noted, the system under consideration will be the whole body. When the therapeutic drug is an endogenous substance (e.g., recombinant endogenous proteins or hormones such as insulin), then more general considerations apply. It should be noted that this definition of pharmacokinetics differs somewhat from the more conventional definition given in Chapter 1. The reason for this is seen in the following section.

Our definition of pharmacokinetics contains a spatial component, so location of the substance in the biological system is important. From the temporal component of the definition, it follows that the amount of substance at a specific location is changing with time. Mathematically, the combination of these temporal and spatial components leads to partial derivatives,

$$\frac{\partial}{\partial t}, \frac{\partial}{\partial x}, \frac{\partial}{\partial y}, \frac{\partial}{\partial z} \tag{8.1}$$

which, mathematically, reflect rates of change in time and space. Here t is time, and a three-dimensional location in the system is represented by the spatial coordinates (x, y, z).

If one chooses to use partial derivatives to describe drug kinetics in the body, then expressions for each of $\frac{\partial}{\partial t}$, $\frac{\partial}{\partial x}$, $\frac{\partial}{\partial y}$, and $\frac{\partial}{\partial z}$ must be explicitly written. That is, a system of partial differential equations must be specified. Conceptually, writing these equations involves knowledge of physical chemistry, irreversible thermodynamics, and circulatory dynamics, specific to the substance at hand. Such equations will incorporate parameters that can be either deterministic (known) or stochastic (contain statistical uncertainties). Although such equations can sometimes be written for specific systems, defining, and then estimating the unknown parameters is in most cases impossible because of the difficulty in obtaining measurements at a resolution sufficient to resolve the spatial components of the system. In pharmacokinetic applications, partial differential equations are sometimes used to describe distributed systems models [15, 16].

How does one resolve the difficulty associated with partial differential equations? The most common way is to reduce the system into a finite number of components. This can be accomplished by lumping together processes based upon time, location, or a combination of the two. One thus moves from partial derivatives to ordinary derivatives, where space is not taken directly into account. This reduction in complexity results in the compartmental models discussed later in this chapter. The same lumping process also forms the basis for the noncompartmental models discussed in the next section, although the resulting models are conceptually much simpler than compartmental models in that they have a less explicitly defined structure.

One can now appreciate why conventional definitions of pharmacokinetics are a little different from the definition given here. The conventional definitions make references to events other than temporal and spatial distribution (e.g., absorption, distribution, metabolism, and excretion). These events are, in fact, consequences of a drug's own kinetics, and thus the two should be conceptually separated. The processes of drug absorption, distribution, metabolism, and elimination relate to quantitative parameters that can only be estimated from a mathematical model describing the kinetics of the drug. The point is that, to understand the mathematical basis of pharmacokinetic parameter estimation, it is necessary to keep in mind the separation between the general concepts of kinetics per se and the use of data to estimate pharmacokinetic parameters of practical interest.

Using the general definition of pharmacokinetics given in terms of spatial and temporal distribution and transformation processes, one can easily progress to a description of the underlying assumptions and mathematics of noncompartmental and compartmental analysis, and, from there, proceed to the processes involved in estimating the pharmacokinetic parameters. This will permit a better understanding of the domain of validity of noncompartmental vs. compartmental parameter estimation.

The pharmacokinetic parameters

What is desired from the pharmacokinetic parameters is a quantitative measure of how a drug behaves in the system. To estimate these parameters, one must design an experiment to collect transient data that can then be used, in combination with an appropriate mathematical formalism, to estimate the parameters of interest. These fundamental concepts have been reviewed in the past from a variety of viewpoints [17].

To design such an experiment, the system must contain at least one *accessible pool*, that is, the system must contain a "site" that is available for drug input and data collection. As we will see, this site must have certain properties. If the system contains an accessible pool, this implies that other parts of the system are not accessible for test input and/or data collection. This divides the system into accessible and nonaccessible pools. A drug (or drug metabolite) in each pool interacts with other components of the system. The only difference between noncompartmental and compartmental models is the way in which the nonaccessible portion of the system is described.

The pharmacokinetic parameters defined in the following section can be used to characterize both the accessible pool and the system (i.e., the totality of accessible and nonaccessible pools), although accessible pool and system parameters are usually distinct. This situation is illustrated by the two models shown in Fig. 8.1. For example, Fig. 8.1A could describe the situation where plasma is the accessible pool and is used for both drug input and sampling. Fig. 8.1B accommodates extravascular input (e.g., oral dosing or intramuscular injection) followed by the collection of serial blood samples, but it can also accommodate the situation where the input is intravascular and only urine samples are collected. Thus the schematic in Fig. 8.1 describes the experimental situation for most pharmacokinetic studies. The case with a single accessible pool

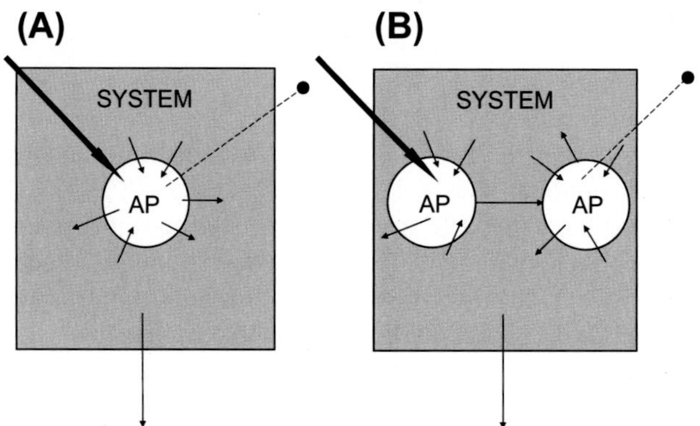

FIG. 8.1 (A) A system in which an accessible pool (AP) is available for test input (*bold arrow*) and sampling (*dashed line with bullet*). Loss of material from the system is indicated by the arrow leaving the system box. Material exchanging between the accessible pool and the rest of the system is indicated by the small arrows leaving and entering the accessible pool. The pharmacokinetic parameters estimated from kinetic data characterize the accessible pool and the system in which the accessible pool is embedded. (B) A system in which there are two accessible pools, one of which is available for test input (*bold arrow*) and a second which is available for sampling (*dashed line with bullet*); the test input is transported to the second accessible pool as indicated by the transfer arrow. Other transfer arrows are as explained in (A).

is of most frequent interest, while the case with two accessible pools has been studied in the context of substances involved in intermediary metabolism and studied with multiple-input, multiple-output experiments.

Accessible pool parameters

The pharmacokinetic parameters descriptive of the accessible pool are given as follows (these definitions apply both to noncompartmental and compartmental models; how they relate to the situation where there are two accessible pools will be discussed for the individual cases):

- *Volume of distribution*: V_a (units: volume). The volume of the accessible pool is the volume in which the drug, upon introduction into the system, intermixes uniformly (kinetically homogeneous) and instantaneously.
- *Clearance rate*: CL_a (units: volume/time). This is the rate at which the accessible pool is irreversibly cleared of drug per unit time. The fundamental concept of clearance rate is perhaps one of the most important in pharmacokinetics and has been recently reviewed in the context of the original considerations that brought about its definition [18].
- *Elimination rate constant*: k_e (units: 1/time, or inverse time). This is the fraction of drug that is irreversibly cleared from the accessible pool per unit time. (In some literature, this is referred to as the fractional clearance or fractional catabolic rate.)
- *Mean residence time*: MRT_a (units: time). This is the average time a drug spends in the accessible pool during all passages through the system before being irreversibly cleared. A useful commentary on mean residence time determination has been provided by Landaw and Katz [19].

System parameters

The pharmacokinetic parameters descriptive of the system are as follows (although these definitions apply both to the noncompartmental and compartmental models, some modification will be needed for two accessible pool models as well as compartmental models):

- *Total equivalent volume of distribution*: V_{tot} (units: volume). This is the total volume of the system seen from the accessible pool; it is the volume in which the total amount of drug would be distributed, assuming the concentration of material throughout the system is uniform and equal to the concentration in the accessible pool. As in Chapter 3, this is also often referred to as the apparent volume of distribution at steady state, $V_{d(ss)}$.
- *System mean residence time*: MRT_s (units: time). This is the average time the drug spends in the system before leaving the system for the last time.
- *Mean residence time outside the accessible pool*: MRT_o (units: time). This is the average time the drug spends outside the accessible pool before leaving the system for the last time.
- *Extent of absorption*: F (units: dimensionless, or percent). This is the fraction of drug that appears in a second accessible (to measurement, but not test input) pool following administration in a first accessible (to test input, but not to measurement) pool.

- *Absorption rate constant*: k_a (units: 1/time, or inverse time). This is the fraction of drug that appears per unit time in a second accessible (to measurement, but not test input) pool following administration in a first accessible (to test input, but not to measurement) pool. As discussed in Chapter 4, both F and k_a are components of *bioavailability*.

Moments

Moments are the weighted integrals of a function and play an essential role in estimating specific pharmacokinetic parameters. The modern use of moments in the analysis of pharmacokinetic data and the notions of noncompartmental or integral equation analysis can be traced to Yamaoka et al. [20], although these authors correctly point out that the formulas were known since the pioneering effort of Torsten Teorell [21] in the late 1930s. Beal [7] places the method of moments as early as the work of Karl Pearson [22] in 1902. In other areas of kinetics, specifically tracer (indicator) kinetics, seminal references on the theory of moments are provided by Zierler [23] and Perl [24], with considerations that extend to nonsteady-state conditions [25].

The moments of a function are defined as follows; how they are used will be described later. Suppose $C(t)$ is a time-dependent function defined on the time interval $[0, \infty]$, where $C(t)$ is used to denote a functional description of a set of pharmacokinetic measurement data. The zeroth and first-order moment of $C(t)$, denoted S_0 and S_1 are defined as:

$$S_0 = \int_0^\infty C(t)dt = AUC \tag{8.2}$$

$$S_1 = \int_0^\infty t \cdot C(t)dt = AUMC \tag{8.3}$$

In these equations, S_0 and S_1 are also defined, respectively, as AUC, "area under the curve," and $AUMC$, "area under the first moment curve." AUC was introduced in the discussion of bioavailability in Chapter 4. AUC and $AUMC$ are quite common expressions in pharmacokinetics and will be used in the following discussions. Higher order moments are rarely used in our context of interest.

The following discussion will describe how AUC and $AUMC$ are estimated, how they are used to estimate specific pharmacokinetic parameters (including related assumptions), and what their relationship is to specific pharmacokinetic parameters estimated from compartmental models. Both moments, however, are used for other purposes that relate to model building. For example, AUC acts as a surrogate for drug exposure, and values of AUC from different dose levels of a drug are used to justify assumptions of pharmacokinetic linearity. Analyses, including limitations, of moment-based noncompartmental analysis have been described, both with reference to pharmacokinetics [26] and more general biological systems [27], and against other formalisms such as those incorporated in circulatory models [28].

Noncompartmental analysis

Noncompartmental model

The noncompartmental model provides a framework to introduce and use statistical moment analysis to estimate pharmacokinetic parameters. There are basically two forms of the noncompartmental model: the single accessible pool model and the two accessible pool model. These are schematized in Fig. 8.2.

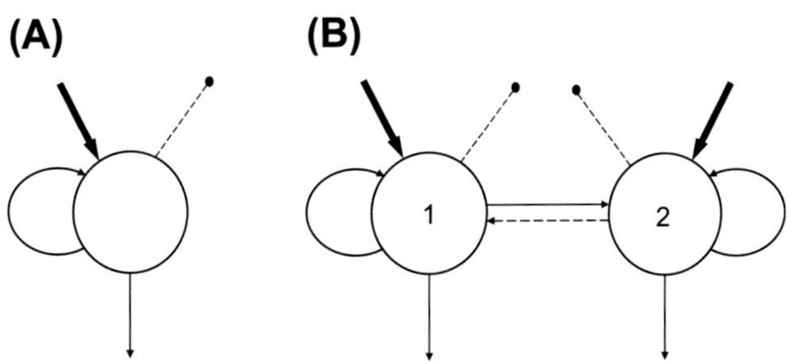

FIG. 8.2 The single (A) and two (B) accessible pool models. See text for explanation.

What is the relationship between the situation described in Fig. 8.1 and the two models shown in Fig. 8.2? Consider first the single accessible pool model shown in Fig. 8.2A. The accessible pool here, denoted by the circle into which drug is input (*bold arrow*) and from which samples are taken (*dotted line with bullet*), is the same as that shown in Fig. 8.1A. The entire interaction of the accessible pool with the rest of the system is indicated by the arrow leaving and returning to the accessible pool. This so-called *recirculation-exchange* arrow encompasses all interactions the drug undergoes in the system outside of the accessible pool. Notice that a drug introduced into this pool has two routes by which it can leave the accessible pool. One is via recirculation-exchange, and the other is via irreversible loss, denoted by the arrow leaving the accessible pool. As indicated in Fig. 8.2A, the drug molecules can only enter and leave the system via the accessible pool. Drug can neither enter nor leave the system along the recirculation-exchange arrow. This is called the equivalent sink and source constraint and is fundamental in understanding the domain of validity of the pharmacokinetic parameters estimated from this model (2). The single accessible pool model is used primarily when the accessible pool is plasma, and the drug is administered directly into plasma.

In the case of more involved experimental designs, including extravascular administration and measurements, the two accessible pool model depicted in Fig. 8.2B may apply. This model is derived from the model shown in Fig. 8.1B in a similar fashion as seen for the single accessible pool model. The difference between the single and two accessible pool models is as follows: while both accessible pools have recirculation-exchange arrows, as can be seen from the figure, material can flow from pool 1 to pool 2. Thus this model is suitable for describing oral or other extravascular drug input, or the situation in which either plasma concentrations of a drug and its metabolite are measured or both plasma and urine data are collected, for example.

Note that there is a dashed arrow from pool 2 to pool 1 in Fig. 8.2B. This indicates that exchange can occur in this direction also. Although analysis of this exchange is frequently incorporated in metabolic kinetic studies, there are relatively few examples in pharmacokinetics in which this has been studied. It is essential to note that this dashed arrow is not equivalent to an arrow in a multicompartmental model! This arrow represents transfer of material from pool 2 to pool 1 by whatever routes exist and can be a composite of many activities including delays.

The two accessible pool model accommodates even more complex experimental formats. For example, one could have inputs into both pools, and samples from both as well. However, in most pharmacokinetic studies with the two accessible pool model, pool 2 is plasma and input is only into pool 1, as with oral dosing. In this situation, the pharmacokinetic parameters depend on bioavailability and can only be estimated up to a proportionality constant, as is the case with so-called *oral clearance* (*CL*/*F*), referred to as *relative clearance* in this chapter and elsewhere sometimes referred to as *apparent clearance*.

Kinetic parameters of the noncompartmental model

The kinetic parameters of the noncompartmental model are those defined before for the accessible pool and system. However, the formulas depend upon the experimental protocol, especially on the mode of drug administration. In this chapter, only the canonical inputs will be considered, such as an intravenous bolus (or multiple boluses) or constant infusion (or multiple constant infusions). References will be given for those interested in more complex protocols.

The relationships among the *accessible pool* parameters in the noncompartmental model are given in the following equations.

$$k_e = \frac{CL_a}{V_a} \tag{8.4}$$

$$MRT_a = \frac{1}{k_e} = \frac{V_a}{CL_a} \tag{8.5}$$

Note that $V_a = \frac{d}{C(0)}$, where $C(0)$ is the concentration of drug in the system at time zero and d is the amount of drug injected, for a pulse input in the accessible pool. Eq. (8.5) can be rearranged to yield.

$$k_e \cdot V_a = CL_a \tag{8.6}$$

In addition, Eqs. (8.5) and (8.6) can be combined to yield the more familiar.

$$V_a = MRT_a \cdot CL_a \tag{8.7}$$

The relationships among the *system* parameters for the noncompartmental model are:

$$V_{tot} = MRT_s \cdot CL_a \tag{8.8}$$

$$MRT_o = MRT_s - MRT_a \tag{8.9}$$

Other commonly used noncompartmental parameters include T_{max} (the time at which the concentration in the accessible pool reaches its observed maximum) and C_{max} (the observed maximum of the concentration in the accessible pool). These descriptive parameters are often reported based on inspection of the measured pharmacokinetic data.

The single accessible pool model

Assume now either a single bolus injection of drug whose amount is denoted by d or a constant infusion of drug whose infusion rate is u over the time interval [0, t]. Then, the pharmacokinetic parameters of interest can be calculated from features of the measurements (including moments) and the test input as:

Bolus	Infusion	
$V_a = \frac{d}{C(0)}$	$V_a = \frac{u}{\dot{C}(0)}$	(8.10)
$CL_a = \frac{d}{AUC}$	$CL_a = \frac{u}{\overline{C}}$	(8.11)
$MRT_s = \frac{AUMC}{AUC}$	$MRT_s = \frac{\int_0^\infty \left[\overline{C} - C(t)\right] dt}{\overline{C}}$	(8.12)

In these formulas, $C(0)$ is the concentration of drug in the system at time zero, $\dot{C}(0)$ is the first derivative of $C(t)$ evaluated at time zero, and $\overline{C}$ is the steady-state value for the concentration of drug in the accessible pool following a constant infusion into that pool. The remaining single accessible pool parameters, k_e, V_{tot}, and MRT_o can be calculated for either test input format using Eqs. (8.4), (8.8), and (8.9). For example, the mean residence time outside the accessible pool is calculated for a bolus injection as $MRT_o = MRT_s - MRT_a = \frac{AUMC}{AUC} - \frac{V_a}{CL_a} = \frac{AUMC}{AUC} - \frac{AUC}{C(0)}$.

Although these formulas are for a single-input format, formulas also exist for generic inputs including multiple boluses or infusions. If $u(t)$ is a generic input function, the formulas for V_a, CL_a, and MRT_s are:

$$V_a = \frac{u(0)}{\dot{C}(0)} \tag{8.13}$$

$$CL_a = \frac{\int_0^\infty u(t)\,dt}{AUC} \tag{8.14}$$

$$MRT_s = \frac{\int_0^\infty t \cdot C(t)\,dt}{AUC} - \frac{\int_0^\infty t \cdot u(t)\,dt}{\int_0^\infty u(t)\,dt} \tag{8.15}$$

What is the origin of these formulas? That is, how are Eqs. (8.10)–(8.12), and (8.13)–(8.15) obtained? The answer is not obvious, although the various definitions of mean residence time can be intuitively interpreted as "weighted averages" (with respect to concentration values) of times. In an excellent description of mean residence times, Weiss [29] points out that, besides an accessible pool that must be available for test input and measurement, the system must be linear and time invariant for the equations to be valid. Veng-Pedersen [30] has reviewed the concept of linearity with reference to noncompartmental and compartmental formalisms, and we will discuss the notions of linearity and time invariance later. For a formal derivation of these equations, the reader is referred to Weiss [29], Cobelli et al. [31], or the already cited Covell et al. [4], or Gibaldi and Perrier [13]. In practice, *AUC* and *AUMC* are calculated from concentration measurements in the accessible pool. However, an understanding of the derivation of these equations is essential to understanding the domain of validity of the pharmacokinetic parameters obtained by noncompartmental methods, no matter what numerical method of evaluating the required integrals or extrapolations is employed.

The two accessible pool model

The two accessible pool model presents problems in estimating the pharmacokinetic parameters characterizing this situation. This is largely because the desired parameters such as clearance, volumes, and residence times cannot be uniquely estimated from a single-input-single-output experiment with input into the first pool and samples from the second pool. To deal with this situation, recall first the notion of absolute bioavailability discussed in Chapter 4. Let D_{oral} be the total dose of drug input into the first accessible pool and let D_{iv} be the dose into the second accessible pool, assumed to be intravascular space. Let $AUC[2]$ be the area under the concentration-time curve in the second accessible pool following the dose D_{oral} (this is AUC_{oral} in the notation of Chapter 4), and let AUC_{iv} be the area under the concentration-time curve in the second accessible pool following the bolus dose D_{iv} (in a separate experiment). Since the amounts of D_{oral} and D_{iv} are usually different, the absolute bioavailability is defined as

$$F = \frac{AUC[2]}{AUC_{iv}} \cdot \frac{D_{iv}}{D_{oral}} \tag{8.16}$$

The following parameters can be calculated from data following a bolus injection into the first accessible pool. Let $CL[2]$ and $V[2]$, respectively, be the clearance from and volume of the second accessible pool, and let $CL[2,rel]$ and $V[2,rel]$ be the relative clearance (oral clearance) from and volume of the second accessible pool. Then.

$$MRT[2,1] = \frac{\int_0^\infty tC[2](t)\,dt}{\int_0^\infty C[2](t)\,dt} \tag{8.17}$$

$$CL[2,rel] = \frac{CL[2]}{F} = \frac{D_{oral}}{AUC[2]} \tag{8.18}$$

$$V[2,rel] = \frac{V[2]}{F} = CL[2,rel] \cdot MRT[2,1] \tag{8.19}$$

$MRT[2,1]$ is the mean residence time of drug in the second accessible pool following introduction of drug into the first accessible pool.

Clearly this situation is not as rich in information as the single accessible pool situation. Of course the parameters $CL[2]$ and $V[2]$ can be calculated in the event that F is independently known or when a separate intravenous dose is administered. Information on other input formats or the situation when there is a two-input-four-output experiment can be found in Cobelli et al. [31].

Estimating the kinetic parameters of the noncompartmental model

For the canonical input of drug, what information is needed? For the bolus input, an estimate of the drug concentration at time zero, $C(0)$, is needed in order to estimate V_a. For a constant infusion of drug, an estimate of $\dot{C}(0)$ is needed to estimate V_a, and an estimate of the plateau concentration, $\overline{C}$, is needed to estimate clearance and the system mean residence time.

The most important estimates, however, involve *AUC* and *AUMC*. These integrals are supposed to be calculated from time zero to time infinity, whereas a real experiment is only carried out over a finite time domain $[0, t_n]$, where t_n is the time of the last measurement. In addition, it is rarely the case that the first measurement is obtained at time zero. Consequently, accurate calculation of the integrals requires extrapolation both to time zero and to infinite time. Hence, assuming that the time of the first measurement is t_1, one must partition the integral as follows to numerically estimate AUC and $AUMC$:

$$AUC = \int_0^\infty C(t)dt = \int_0^{t_1} C(t)dt + \int_{t_1}^{t_n} C(t)dt + \int_{t_n}^\infty C(t)dt \tag{8.20}$$

$$AUMC = \int_0^\infty t \cdot C(t)dt = \int_0^{t_1} t \cdot C(t)dt + \int_{t_1}^{t_n} t \cdot C(t)dt + \int_{t_n}^\infty t \cdot C(t)dt \tag{8.21}$$

The first and third integrals in either equation require extrapolation beyond the experimental start and end times, while the middle integral only requires interpolation of existing data. One approach to solve these issues is to fit the available data to suitable functions of time that can automatically provide the needed extrapolations. Clearly, the use of such functional descriptors also implies that noncompartmental analysis is not truly "model-independent" as has been sometimes claimed [9]. This characteristic is in addition to the other limitations that arise from incomplete knowledge of elimination routes.

Estimating AUC and AUMC using sums of exponentials

For the single accessible pool model, following a bolus injection of amount D into the pool, the pharmacokinetic data can usually be described by a sum of exponentials equation of the general form shown in Eq. (8.22).

$$C(t) = A_1 e^{-\lambda_1 t} + \cdots + A_n e^{-\lambda_n t} \tag{8.22}$$

In this, and subsequent equations, the A_i are called *coefficients* and the λ_i are *exponentials* (in mathematical parlance, they are called *eigenvalues*). Following a constant infusion into the accessible pool, Eq. (8.22) changes to Eq. (8.23) with the additional restriction that the sum of the coefficients equals zero, reflecting the fact that no drug is present in the system at time zero.

$$C(t) = A_0 + A_1 e^{-\lambda_1 t} + \cdots + A_n e^{-\lambda_n t} \tag{8.23}$$

$$A_0 + A_1 + \cdots + A_n = 0$$

What is the advantage of using sums of exponentials to describe pharmacokinetic data in the situation of the single accessible pool model following a bolus injection or constant infusion? The reason is that the integrals required to estimate the pharmacokinetic parameters are very easy to calculate!

Assuming the data can be fit (for example, by using weighted nonlinear regression techniques) to exponential functions, the coefficients and the exponentials can be used to calculate AUC and $AUMC$ and, hence, the pharmacokinetic parameters. For the bolus injection, from Eq. (8.22),

$$AUC = \int_0^\infty C(t)dt = \frac{A_1}{\lambda_1} + \cdots + \frac{A_n}{\lambda_n} \tag{8.24}$$

$$AUMC = \int_0^\infty t \cdot C(t)dt = \frac{A_1}{\lambda_1^2} + \cdots + \frac{A_n}{\lambda_n^2} \tag{8.25}$$

In addition, for the bolus injection,

$$C(0) = A_1 + \cdots + A_n \tag{8.26}$$

provides an estimate for $C(0)$. Thus, with knowledge of the amount of drug in the bolus dose, D, all pharmacokinetic parameters can be estimated.

For a constant infusion, the steady-state concentration, $\overline{C}$, can be seen from Eq. (8.23) to equal A_0. An estimate for $\dot{C}(0)$ can be obtained.

$$\dot{C}(0) = -A_1\lambda_1 - \cdots - A_n\lambda_n \tag{8.27}$$

and since the estimate for $\overline{C}$ is A_0,

$$\int_0^\infty \left[\overline{C} - C(t)\right] dt = \frac{A_1}{\lambda_1} + \cdots + \frac{A_n}{\lambda_n} \tag{8.28}$$

Thus all the pharmacokinetic parameters for the constant infusion case can be estimated in a straightforward manner from the coefficients and the exponentials.

An advantage of using sums of exponentials is that error estimates (precisions) for all the pharmacokinetic parameters can also be obtained as part of the process of fitting the calculated curves to the observed data. As discussed in the following section, this is not the case for most of the so-called numerical (i.e., based on direct interpolation) techniques for calculating *AUC* and *AUMC*, for which calculation of precision is not straightforward. In addition, for multiple inputs (i.e., multiple boluses or infusions) sums of exponentials can be used over each experimental temporal period for a specific bolus or infusion, recognizing that the exponentials λ_i remain the same (i.e., assuming the system is linear and time invariant) across dosing intervals. The reason is that the exponentials are system parameters and do not depend on a particular mode of introducing drug into the system [32].

Estimating AUC and AUMC using other functions

While sums of exponentials may seem a logical choice of function to use to describe $C(t)$ and hence estimate *AUC* and *AUMC*, the literature is full of other recommendations for estimating AUC and AUMC (see, for example, Yeh and Kwan [33] or Purves [34]). These include the trapezoidal rule, the log-trapezoidal rule, combinations of the two, splines, and Lagrangians, among others. All result in formulas for calculations over the available time domain of the data, and one is then left with the problem of estimating the integrals $\int_{t_n}^{\infty} C(t)dt$ and $\int_{t_n}^{\infty} t \cdot C(t)\,dt$. The problem of estimating $\int_0^{t_1} C(t)\,dt$ and $\int_0^{t_1} t \cdot C(t)\,dt$, and estimating a value for $C(0)$, $\dot{C}(0)$, or $\overline{C}$, is rarely discussed in the context of these methods.

There are two problems with this approach. First, estimating *AUMC* is very difficult. While one hopes that the experiment has been designed so that $\int_{t_n}^{\infty} C(t)\,dt$ contributes 5% or less to the overall *AUC*, $\int_{t_n}^{\infty} t \cdot C(t)\,dt$ can contribute as much as 50% or more to *AUMC* if the drug is cleared relatively slowly. Hence estimates of *AUMC* can be subject to large errors. The second problem is that it can be difficult to obtain error estimates for *AUC* and *AUMC* that will translate into error estimates for the pharmacokinetic parameters derived from them. For example, there are interesting statistical considerations to be made when circumstances dictate that only a single time point can be obtained in each experimental subject, thus making it difficult to separate measurement noise and biological variability between subjects. [35]. As a result, it is normal practice in individual studies to ignore error estimates for these parameters, and hence the pharmacokinetic parameters that rely upon them. One attempt to circumvent this statistical problem entails conducting studies in several subjects and basing statistical analysis on averages and standard errors of the mean, although this approach includes biological variation among subjects. This distinction is particularly important in population pharmacokinetic studies, such as those described in Chapter 9.

Estimating $\int_{t_1}^{t_n} C(t)\,dt$ and $\int_{t_1}^{t_n} t \cdot C(t)\,dt$

In what follows, some comments will be made on the commonly used functional approaches to estimating $\int_{t_1}^{t_n} C(t)dt$ and $\int_{t_1}^{t_n} t \cdot C(t)dt$ (i.e., the trapezoidal rule or a combination of the trapezoidal and log-trapezoidal rule) [15, 18]. Other methods such as splines and Lagrangians will not be discussed. The interested reader is referred to Yeh and Kwan [33] or Purves [34].

Suppose $[(y_{obs}(t_i), t_i]_{i=1}^{n}$ is a set of pharmacokinetic data. For example, this can be n plasma samples starting with the first measurable sample obtained at time t_1 and the last measurable sample at time t_n. If $[t_{i-1}, t_i]$ is the ith interval, then the *AUC* and *AUMC* for this interval calculated using the trapezoidal rule are

$$AUC_{i-1}^{i} = \frac{1}{2}\left(y_{obs}(t_i) + y_{obs}(t_{i-1})\right)(t_i - t_{i-1}) \tag{8.29}$$

$$AUMC_{i-1}^{i} = \frac{1}{2}\left(t_i \cdot y_{obs}(t_i) + t_{i-1} \cdot y_{obs}(t_{i-1})\right)(t_i - t_{i-1}) \tag{8.30}$$

For the log-trapezoidal rule, the formulas are

$$AUC_{i-1}^{i} = \frac{1}{\ln\left(\frac{y_{obs}(t_i)}{y_{obs}(t_{i-1})}\right)}\left(y_{obs}(t_i) + y_{obs}(t_{i-1})\right)(t_i - t_{i-1}) \tag{8.31}$$

$$AUMC_{i-1}^{i} = \frac{1}{\ln\left(\frac{y_{obs}(t_i)}{y_{obs}(t_{i-1})}\right)}\left(t_i \cdot y_{obs}(t_i) + t_{i-1}.y_{obs}(t_{i-1})\right)(t_i - t_{i-1}) \tag{8.32}$$

One method by which AUC and $AUMC$ can be estimated from t_1 to t_n is to use the trapezoidal rule and add up the individual terms AUC_{i-1}^{i} and $AUMC_{i-1}^{i}$. If one chooses this approach, then it is possible to obtain an error estimate for AUC and $AUMC$ using the quadrature method proposed by Katz and D'Argenio [36]. Some software systems use a combination of the trapezoidal and log-trapezoidal formulas to estimate AUC and $AUMC$, and the formulas resulting from them. The idea here is that the trapezoidal approximation is a good approximation when $y_{obs}(t_i) \geq y_{obs}(t_{i-1})$ (i.e., when the data are rising), and the log-trapezoidal rule is a better approximation when $y_{obs}(t_i) < y_{obs}(t_{i-1})$ (i.e., the data are falling). The rationale is that the log-trapezoidal formula takes into account some of the curvature in the falling portion of the curve. However, the method of Katz and D'Argenio cannot be used with this combination of formulas to obtain an error estimate for AUC and $AUMC$ from t_1 to t_n.

Extrapolating from t_n to infinity

One now has to deal with estimating $\int_{t_n}^{\infty} C(t)\,dt$ and $\int_{t_n}^{\infty} t \cdot C(t)\,dt$. The most common way to estimate these integrals is to assume that the data decay monoexponentially beyond the last measurement at time t_n. Such a function can be written.

$$y(t) = A_z e^{-\lambda_z t} \tag{8.33}$$

Here the exponent λ_z characterizes the terminal rate of concentration decay that is observed over the time course of the pharmacokinetic study, and is used in practice to calculate the half-life of the terminal decay, or terminal half-life,

$$t_{z,1/2} = \frac{\ln(2)}{\lambda_z} \tag{8.34}$$

If it is assumed that this single exponential decay remains applicable from the last observation onward, estimates for $\int_{t_n}^{\infty} C(t)\,dt$ and $\int_{t_n}^{\infty} t \cdot C(t)\,dt$ can be based on the last available measurement:

$$AUC_{extrap-dat} = \int_{t_n}^{\infty} C(t)\,dt = \frac{y_{obs}(t_n)}{\lambda_z} \tag{8.35}$$

$$AUMC_{extrap-dat} = \int_{t_n}^{\infty} t \cdot C(t)\,dt = \frac{t_n \cdot y_{obs}(t_n)}{\lambda_z} + \frac{y_{obs}(t_n)}{\lambda_z^2} \tag{8.36}$$

or from the model-predicted value at the last measurement time:

$$AUC_{extrap-calc} = \int_{t_n}^{\infty} C(t)\,dt = \frac{A_z e^{-\lambda_z t_n}}{\lambda_z} \tag{8.37}$$

$$AUMC_{extrap-calc} = \int_{t_n}^{\infty} t \cdot C(t)\,dt = \frac{t_n \cdot A_z e^{-\lambda_z t_n}}{\lambda_z} + \frac{A_z e^{-\lambda_z t_n}}{\lambda_z^2} \tag{8.38}$$

There are a variety of ways that one can use to estimate λ_z. Most rely on the fact that the last two or three data points often appear to decrease monoexponentially, and thus Eq. (8.33) can be fitted to these data. Various options for including or excluding other data have been proposed (e.g., Gabrielsson and Weiner [37], Marino et al. [38]) but will not be discussed here. What is certain is that all parameters and area estimates will in principle have statistical (precision) information, since they are obtained by fitting Eq. (8.33) to the data.

It is of interest to note that an estimate for λ_z could differ from λ_n, the terminal slope of a multiexponential function describing the totality of the pharmacokinetic data over the experimental time interval. The reason is that all data are considered in estimating λ_n as opposed to a finite (terminal) subset used to estimate λ_z. Thus a researcher using both methods to test robustness of the estimates should not be surprised if there are slight differences.

Estimating AUC and AUMC from 0 to infinity

Estimating *AUC* and *AUMC* from zero to infinity is now simply a matter of adding the two components (i.e., the *AUC* and *AUMC*) over the time domain of the data and the extrapolation from the last measurement to infinity. The zero-time value can be handled in several ways. For the bolus injection, it can be estimated using a modification of the methodology used to estimate λ_z, where extrapolation is from the first measurements back to time zero. In this way, statistical information on C (0) would be available. Otherwise, if an arbitrary value is assigned, no such information is available.

Error estimates for the pharmacokinetic parameters will be available only if error estimates for *AUC* and *AUMC* are calculated. In general, this will not be the case when numerical formulas are used over the time domain of the data. As mentioned previously, the error estimates we are referring to here pertain to a single subject (precision) and are not the same as those that are obtained from studies on several individuals (variability). Unfortunately, sums of exponentials are not used as the function of choice as often as they could be, especially since the canonical inputs, boluses and infusions, are the most common ways to introduce a drug into the system. Possible reasons for this include the sensitivity of exponential estimates to noise in the data, which often allows quantifying reliably only a relatively small number of exponential functions in the sum (up to two or three in practice). However, this potential limitation has to be considered on a case-by-case basis that should explicitly take into account experimental design considerations [39].

Compartmental analysis

Definitions and assumptions

As noted earlier in this chapter, it is very difficult to use partial differential equations to describe the kinetics of a drug. A convenient way to deal with this situation is to lump portions of the system into discrete entities and then discuss movement of material among these entities. These lumped portions of the system essentially contain subsets of the material whose kinetics share a similar time frame. Thus the act of lumping portions of a system together for the purpose of kinetic analysis is based on a combination of known system physiology and biochemistry on the one hand, and the time frame of a particular experiment on the other. Lumping based on a priori known organ physiology, as opposed to empirical temporal and spatial kinetic characteristics, forms the basis of *physiologically based pharmacokinetic models*. These models, which embody an integrated, bottom-up approach which starts from the individual physiological components needed to predict pharmacokinetic time courses, are described in Chapter 31 and have been reviewed in [40, 41] and more recently in [42, 43].

Compartmental models can be seen as the mathematical result of such lumping. Whereas compartments can in some cases be referenced to *physiological spaces* as in Chapter 3, in this chapter we will define a *compartment* simply as an amount of *material* that is kinetically homogeneous. *Kinetic homogeneity* means that material introduced into a compartment mixes instantaneously, and that each particle in the compartment has the same probability as all other particles in the compartment of leaving the compartment along the various exit pathways from that compartment. A *compartmental model* consists of a finite number of compartments with specified interconnections, inputs, and losses. In addition, a compartmental model specifies the interactions occurring among accessible and inaccessible portions of the system in more (mechanistic) detail than the noncompartmental formalism.

Let $X_i(t)$ be the mass of a drug in the ith compartment. The notation for input, loss, and transfers is summarized in Fig. 8.3. In Fig. 8.3, the rate constants describe mathematically the mass transfer of material among compartments interacting with the ith compartment (F_{ji} is transfer of material from compartment i to compartment j, F_{ij} is the transfer of material from compartment j to compartment i), the new input F_{i0} (this corresponds to X_0 in Chapter 4), and loss to the environment F_{0i} from compartment i. The careful reader will have noticed that we are using (engineering) matrix notation here as opposed to the more common pharmacokinetic notation, where F_{ij} would be the transfer of material from compartment i to compartment j. The notation in this chapter, the same as that used in Chapter 3, describes the compartment in full generality, making it easier to transition to linear compartmental models and to write some of the equations that we will discuss. The mathematical expression describing the rate of change for $X_i(t)$ is derived from the mass balance equation:

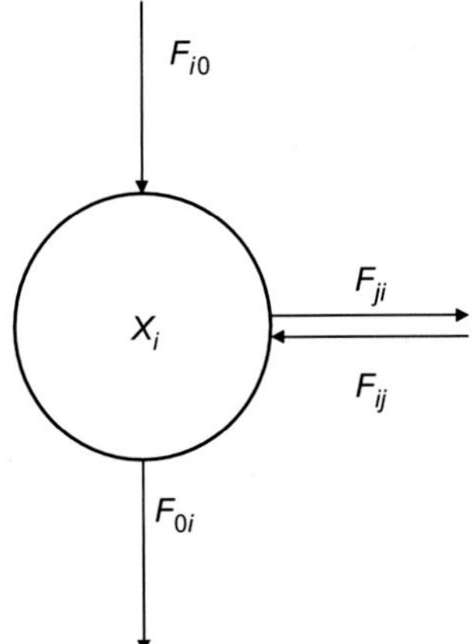

FIG. 8.3 The *i*th compartment of an *n*-compartment model. See text for explanation.

$$\frac{dX_i(t)}{dt} = \frac{dX_i}{dt} = \sum_{\substack{j=0 \\ j\neq i}}^{n} F_{ij} - \sum_{\substack{j=0 \\ j\neq i}}^{n} F_{ji} \tag{8.39}$$

There are several important features to understand about the fluxes F_{ij} that derive from the fact that the compartmental model is being used to describe a biological system, and hence conservation of mass must be obeyed. First, the F_{ij} must be nonnegative for all times t (assumed to be between time zero and infinity). In fact, the F_{ij} can be either stochastic (have uncertainly associated with them) or deterministic (known exactly). In this chapter, the F_{ij} will be assumed to be deterministic but can be functions of the X_i and/or time t. (Readers interested in stochastic compartmental models can find references to numerous articles in Covell et al. [4], and Macheras et al. [44].) Second, as pointed out by Jacquez and Simon [10], if $X_i = 0$, then $F_{ji} = 0$ for all $j \neq i$ and hence $\frac{dX_i}{dt} \geq 0$. An important consequence of this, as shown by these authors, is that the F_{ji}, with the exception of F_{i0}, which remains unchanged, can be written:

$$F_{ji}\left(\vec{X}, \vec{p}, t\right) = k_{ji}\left(\vec{X}, \vec{p}, t\right) \cdot X_i(t) \tag{8.40}$$

The function F_{i0} is either a constant or a function of t alone. The k_{ji} written in this format are called the *fractional transfer functions*. $\vec{X} = (X_1, \cdots, X_n)$ is a notation for compartmental masses (mathematically called a vector); $\vec{p}$ is a descriptor of other elements (parameters) that control the system, such as blood flow, pH, and temperature; and t is time. We are using vector notation here (as in $\vec{X}$) to signify that, in general, the fluxes can be functions of any $X_i(t)$ (the vector $\vec{X}$ contains all of them) and especially a set of (most often unknown) parameters $\vec{p}$.

Eq. (8.40) is a subtle but important step in moving from the general compartmental model to the linear, constant-coefficient model, because it shows explicitly that the fractional transfers can be functions of time and other system entities, not necessarily constants, and that, as functions, the mass terms can be split out from the fractional transfer term. Written in this format, Eq. (8.39) becomes.

$$\frac{dX_i}{dt} = -\left(\sum_{\substack{j=0 \\ j\neq i}}^{n} k_{ji}\left(\vec{X}, \vec{p}, t\right)\right) X_i(t) + \sum_{\substack{j=0 \\ j\neq i}}^{n} k_{ji}\left(\vec{X}, \vec{p}, t\right) X_j(t) + F_{i0} \tag{8.41}$$

Define

$$k_{ii}\left(\vec{X}, \vec{p}, t\right) = -\left(\sum_{\substack{j=0 \\ j\neq i}}^{n} k_{ji}\left(\vec{X}, \vec{p}, t\right)\right) \tag{8.42}$$

and write

$$K\left(\vec{X}, \vec{p}, t\right) = \begin{bmatrix} k_{11} & k_{12} & \cdots & k_{1n} \\ k_{21} & k_{22} & \cdots & k_{2n} \\ \vdots & \vdots & \ddots & \vdots \\ k_{n1} & k_{n2} & \cdots & k_{nn} \end{bmatrix} \tag{8.43}$$

where in Eq. (8.43) the individual terms of the matrix, for convenience, do not contain the $\left(\vec{X}, \vec{p}, t\right)$. The matrix $K\left(\vec{X}, \vec{p}, t\right)$ is called the *compartmental matrix*. This matrix is key to deriving many kinetic parameters, and in making the conceptual link between compartmental and noncompartmental analysis.

There are several reasons for starting at this level of mathematical generality for introducing the n-compartment model.

- First, this approach clearly points out that the theories underlying noncompartmental and compartmental models are very different. While the theory underlying noncompartmental models relies more on statistical (moments) theory and data-based approaches, especially in developing residence time concepts (see, for example, Weiss [29]), the theory underlying compartmental models is really the theory of ordinary, first-order differential equations, with some special features due to the nature of the biological applications. These are reviewed in detail in Jacquez and Simon [10] and in many other texts and research articles written on the subject.
- Second, these ideas demonstrate the complexity involved in postulating the structure of a compartmental model to describe the kinetics of a particular drug. As illustrated by the presentation in Chapter 3, it is seldom possible to postulate a model structure in which the model compartments have physiological relevance as opposed to simply being a mathematical construct, especially when one is dealing with a single-input-single-output experiment and the limited amount of information it provides. Although the most general compartmental model must be appreciated in its potential application to the interpretation of kinetic data, the fact is that such complex models are not often used. Thus the most common models are the linear, constant-coefficient compartmental models described in the next section. In this discussion, it also will be assumed that all systems are open (i.e., drug introduced into the system will eventually irreversibly leave the system). This means that some special situations discussed by Jacquez and Simon [10] do not have to be considered (i.e., compartmental models with submodels—called traps—from which material cannot escape).

Linear, constant coefficient compartmental models

Suppose the compartmental matrix is a constant matrix (i.e., all k_{ij} are constants). In this situation, one can write K instead of $K\left(\vec{X}, \vec{p}, t\right)$ to indicate that the elements of the matrix no longer depend on $\left(\vec{X}, \vec{p}, t\right)$. As will be seen, there are several important features of the K matrix that will be used in recovering pharmacokinetic parameters of interest. In addition, as described several times in the kinetic analysis literature, the solution to the compartmental equations, which in this case are a system of linear, constant coefficient equations, involves sums of exponentials.

What is needed for the compartmental matrix to be constant? Recall that the individual elements of the matrix $k_{ij}\left(\vec{X}, \vec{p}, t\right)$ can be functions of several variables. For the $k_{ij}\left(\vec{X}, \vec{p}, t\right)$ to be constant, $\vec{X}$ and $\vec{p}$ must be constant (this assumption can be relaxed but for purposes of this discussion, constancy will be assumed), and the $k_{ij}\left(\vec{X}, \vec{p}, t\right)$ cannot depend explicitly on time (i.e., the elements $k_{ij}\left(\vec{X}, \vec{p}, t\right)$ are time invariant). Notice with this concept that the time invariant $k_{ij}\left(\vec{X}, \vec{p}, t\right)$ can assume different values depending upon the constant values for both $\vec{X}$ and $\vec{p}$. This leads naturally to the steady-state concepts that have been historically so useful in tracer kinetics.

Under what circumstances are compartmental models linear, constant coefficient? This normally depends upon features of the drug being studied and a particular experimental design, and should be consistently tested and verified in practice. The reason is that most biological systems, including those in which drugs are analyzed, are inherently nonlinear. However, if the assumption of linearity holds reasonably well over the dose range studied, and studies can be carried out under stable conditions of minimal physiological perturbation, these assumptions can hold in practice. Otherwise, more complex modeling formalisms are needed. An example is shown in Chapter 6, where the dialysis kinetics of urea and inulin in a dog model [45] were studied. Compartmental methods were required in this case to account for the totality of pharmacokinetic data available, and the conclusion was that skeletal muscle blood flow (which correlated with the slow equilibrating compartment in the model) decreased by 90% during dialysis, contributing to adverse events (e.g., muscle cramps) sometimes seen in patient hemodialysis sessions.

Parameters estimated from compartmental models

Experimenting on compartmental models: Input and measurements

In postulating a compartmental model such as that shown in Fig. 8.4A, one is actually making a statement concerning how the system is believed to behave. To know if a particular model structure can predict the behavior of a drug in the body, one must be able to obtain kinetic data from which the parameters characterizing the system of differential equations can be estimated; the model predictions can then be compared against the data. Experiments are designed to generate the data, so the experimental design must then be reproduced on the model. This is done by specifying inputs and samples, as shown in Fig. 8.4B, which reflect the actual conduct of the experiment. More specifically, the input specifies the F_{i0} terms in the differential equations, and the samples provide the measurement equations that link the model's predictions, which are normally in units of drug mass, with the samples, that are usually measured in concentration units.

To emphasize this point, once a model structure is postulated, the compartmental matrix can be estimated in principle, since it depends only upon the defined arrangement of compartments and their transfers and losses. The input, the F_{i0}, represents the experimental perturbation and thus is determined by the investigator. In addition, the units of the differential equation (i.e., the units of the X_i) are determined by the units of the input. In practical terms, if the data obtained from a particular experimental design permit the parameters of the postulated compartmental model to be estimated, then the specific form of the input is not important, as long as it is informative on the model structure and parameters (concepts and applications of a priori identifiability have been extensively reviewed by Cobelli and DiStefano [46]). In theory, data arising from a bolus injection or constant infusion should be equally rich from an information point of view, although extracting this information would require different practical experimental designs involving different sampling frequencies.

The final point to make in dealing with experiments on the model relates to the measurement variable(s). The units of the X_i are determined by the experimental input units and are usually in units of mass (e.g., grams or moles). The units of the data are normally concentration. No matter what the units of the data, there must be an appropriately dimensioned measurement equation linking the X_i with the data. For example, if the measurement was taken from compartment 1 and the units of the data are concentration, one would need to write the measurement equation.

$$C_1(t) = \frac{X_1(t)}{V_1} \tag{8.44}$$

Here V_1 is the volume of compartment 1 and is a parameter to be estimated from the data.

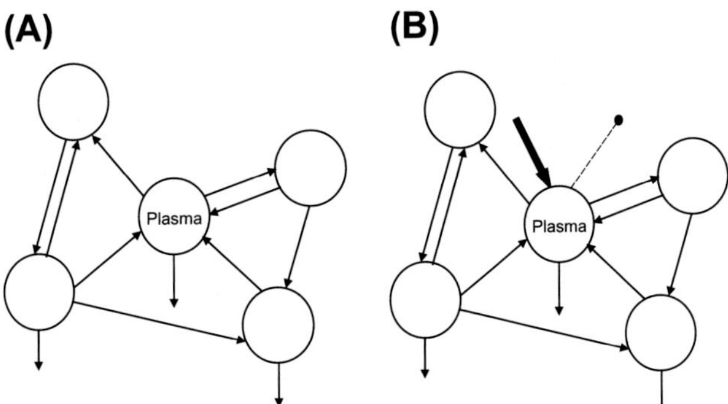

FIG. 8.4 (A) A compartmental model of drug behavior in the body. (B) An experimental protocol on (A) showing drug administration (*bold arrow*) and plasma sampling (*dashed line with bullet*).

Clearly, once a compartmental structure is postulated, there are many experimental protocols and measurement variables that can be accommodated. One just needs to be sure that the parameters characterizing the compartmental matrix, K, and the parameters characterizing the measurement variables can be reliably estimated from the data generated by the experiment, since they may provide important physiological insight which is otherwise unobtainable. In Chapter 4, it is described how bioavailability of NAPA in healthy subjects appeared reduced when intercompartmental clearance to the fast-equilibrating compartment was reduced. It was proposed that this model-based estimate of clearance relates to splanchnic blood flow.

Nonlinearities in compartmental models

Some fractional transfer functions of compartmental models may actually be functions of compartmental masses or concentrations (i.e., the model may actually be nonlinear). The most common example is when a transfer or loss is saturable. Here, a Michaelis-Menten type of transfer function can be defined, as was shown in Chapter 2 for the elimination of phenytoin. In this case, loss from compartment 1 is concentration dependent and saturable, and one can write.

$$CL_1 = k_{01} \cdot V_1 = \frac{V_{\max}}{K_m + C_1} \cdot V_1 \tag{8.45}$$

where V_{max} (in units of concentration per unit time) and K_m (having units of concentration) are parameters that can be estimated from the pharmacokinetic data. The concentration in the accessible compartment is still defined as in Eq. (8.44), $C_1(t) = \frac{X_1(t)}{V_1}$. The corresponding differential equation $\frac{dX_1}{dt}$ can then be written:

$$\frac{dX_1(t)}{dt} = -k_{01} \cdot X_1(t) = -\frac{V_{\max}}{K_m + C_1(t)} \cdot X_1(t) \tag{8.46}$$

Another example of a function-dependent transfer function is given in Chapter 6, in which hemodynamic changes during and after hemodialysis reduce intercompartmental clearance between the intravascular space and a peripheral compartment, as shown in Fig. 6.3.

If one has pharmacokinetic data and knows that the situation calls for nonlinear kinetics, then compartmental models, no matter how difficult to postulate, are really required. Noncompartmental models cannot deal with the time-varying situation and estimates derived from them will be prone to varying degrees of error. However, noncompartmental analysis can be

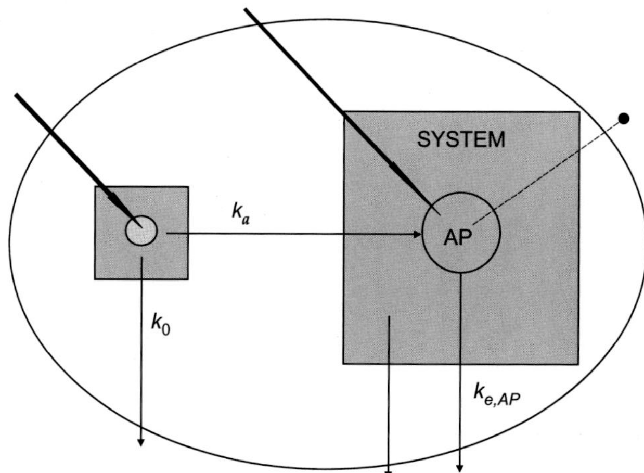

FIG. 8.5 The system model shown on the right contains an accessible pool (AP) embedded in an arbitrary multicompartmental model indicated by the shaded box. The drug can be introduced directly into this pool, as indicated by the bold arrow. The drug can also be introduced into a second compartment, indicated by the circle in the small, shaded box on the left. Drug can move from this compartment, as denoted by the arrow passing through the shaded small box and large box, into the accessible pool at a rate denoted by k_a. Material also can be lost from the second compartment; this is denoted k_0. Finally, material has two ways by which it can leave the system. One is directly from the accessible pool, $k_{e,AP}$, and the other is from nonaccessible pools, denoted by the arrow leaving the large box. That both small and large boxes exist in the context of a larger system is denoted by the ellipse surrounding the individual components of the system. See text for additional explanation.

useful to investigate the presence or absence of nonlinearities, e.g., by calculating AUC at various doses and checking that linearity holds.

Calculating pharmacokinetic parameters from a compartmental model

Realizing the full generality of the compartmental model, consider now only the limited situation of linear, constant-coefficient models. What parameters can be calculated from a model? The answer to this question can be addressed in the context of Fig. 8.5.

Model parameters

Once a specific multicompartmental structure has been developed to explain the pharmacokinetics of a particular drug, the parameters characterizing this model are the components of the compartmental matrix, K, and the distribution space (volume) parameters associated with the individual measurements. The components of the compartmental matrix are the rate constants k_{ij}. Together, these comprise the primary *mathematical* parameters of the model. The parameters of clearance and distribution volume, which are of primary physiological relevance, are secondary from a mathematical standpoint. For this reason, the mathematical parameters of compartmental models often must be reparametrized to recover the physiological parameters of interest (e.g., see Fig. 3.8). Although this works relatively well for simple models, it can be a difficult exercise once one moves to more complex models.

The next question is whether the parameters characterizing a model can be estimated from a set of pharmacokinetic data. The answer to the question has two parts. The first is called a priori *identifiability*. This answers the question, "given a particular model structure and experimental design, if the data are 'perfect' can the model parameters be estimated?" The second is a posteriori *identifiability*. This answers the question, "given a particular model structure and experimental design and a set of pharmacokinetic data, can the model parameters be estimated with a reasonable degree of statistical precision?"

A priori identifiability is a critical part of model development. While the answer to the question for many of the simpler models used in pharmacokinetics is well known, the general answer, even for linear, constant-coefficient models, is more difficult. Fig. 8.6 illustrates the situation with some specific model structures (A–F); the interested reader is referred to Cobelli et al. [31] for precise details. Model A is a standard two-compartment model with input and sampling from a "plasma" compartment. There are three k_{ij} and a volume term to be estimated. This model can be shown to be a priori identifiable. Model B has four k_{ij} and a volume term to be estimated. The parameters for this model cannot be estimated from a single set of pharmacokinetic data, no matter how information rich they are. In fact, there are an infinite number of

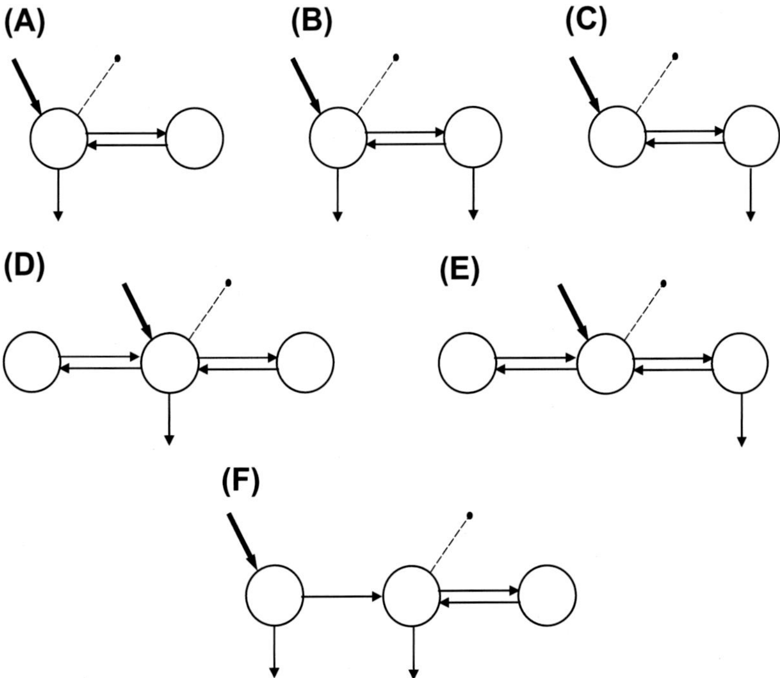

FIG. 8.6 Examples of multicompartmental models. See text for explanation.

values for the k_{ij} and volume term that will fit the data equally well. If one insists on using this model structure (e.g., for reasons of biological plausibility), then some independent constraint will have to be placed on the parameters, such as e.g., defining a relationship among the k_{ij}. Model C, while a priori identifiable, will have a different compartmental matrix from that of Model A, and hence, some of the pharmacokinetic parameters will be different between the two models.

Two commonly used three-compartment models are shown in Fig. 8.6D and E. Of the two peripheral compartments, one exchanges rapidly and one slowly with the central compartment. Model D is a priori identifiable while Model E is not, since it will have two different compartmental matrices that will produce the same fit to the data. The reason is that the loss in Model E is from a peripheral compartment. Finally, Model F, a model very commonly used to describe the pharmacokinetics of drug absorption, is not a priori identifiable. Again, there are two values for the compartmental K matrix that will produce the same fit to the data, one resulting in slow elimination and fast absorption, and the other reversing the two.

A posteriori identifiability is linked to the theory of optimization in mathematics and statistics because one normally uses a software package that has an optimization (data-fitting) capability in order to estimate parameter values for a multi-compartmental model from a set of pharmacokinetic data. Typically, one obtains an estimate for the parameter values, an estimate for their errors, and a value for the correlation (or covariance) matrix of the estimates via data-fitting algorithms such as weighted least squares. The details of optimization and how to deal with the output from an optimization routine are beyond the scope of this chapter, but they have been discussed extensively with reference to compartmental models. The point to be made here is that the output from these routines is crucial in assessing the goodness-of-fit—that is, how well the model performs when compared to the data—since inferences about a drug's pharmacokinetics will be made from these parameter values. Most often, inference about model selection—i.e., the desired level of model complexity—can also be made based on the performance of such fitting routines.

Residence time calculations

As we have discussed in the context of noncompartmental analysis, the notion of residence times can be important in assessing the pharmacokinetics of a drug. The information about residence times available from a linear, constant coefficient compartmental model is rich, and will be reviewed in the following comments.

Residence time calculations are a direct result of manipulating the compartmental matrix K. Let $\Theta = -K^{-1}$ be the negative inverse of the compartmental matrix, and let ϑ_{ij} be the ijth element of Θ. The matrix Θ is called the mean residence time matrix and has units of time (since the rates in K have units of inverse time). The following information given concerning the interpretation of this matrix comes from the original reference of Covell et al. [4] and Cobelli et al. [31]. Further detail is beyond the scope of this chapter, and the interested reader is directed to these two references.

The elements of the mean residence time matrix have important probabilistic interpretations for linear, constant-coefficient models. First, the generic element ϑ_{ij} represents the average time a drug particle entering the system in compartment j spends in compartment i before irreversibly leaving the system by any route. Second, the ratio $\frac{\vartheta_{ij}}{\vartheta_{ii}}$, $i \neq j$, equals the probability that a drug particle in compartment j will eventually reach compartment i. Finally, if a compartmental model has loss from a single compartment only, say compartment 1, then it can be shown that $k_{01} = \frac{1}{\vartheta_{11}}$. Clearly if one is analyzing pharmacokinetic data using compartmental models in which the K matrix is constant, this information can be critical in assessing the behavior of a particular drug in various nonaccessible pools.

However, more can be said about the ϑ_{ij} that is important in comparing compartmental and noncompartmental models. Suppose there is a generic input into compartment 1 only, F_{10} (remember in this situation F_{10} can be a function). Then it can be shown that the area under $X_i(t)$, the drug mass in the ith compartment, equals:

$$\int_0^\infty X_i(t)\,dt = \vartheta_{i1} \int_0^\infty F_{10}\,dt \tag{8.47}$$

whence

$$\vartheta_{i1} = \frac{\int_0^\infty X_i(t)\,dt}{\int_0^\infty F_{10}\,dt} \tag{8.48}$$

More generally, suppose F_{j0} is an arbitrary input into compartment j, and $X_i^j(t)$ is the amount of drug in compartment i following an initial administration in compartment j. Then:

$$\vartheta_{ij} = \frac{\int_0^{\infty} X_i^j(t)\,dt}{\int_0^{\infty} F_{j0}\,dt} \tag{8.49}$$

This equation shows that ϑ_{ij} equals the area under the model predicted drug mass curve in compartment i resulting from an input compartment j, normalized to the dose. An example of the application of these concepts is provided by a study of monoclonal immunoglobulin kinetics in mice [47].

The use of the mean residence time matrix can be a powerful tool in pharmacokinetic analysis with a compartmental model, especially if one is dealing with a model of the system in which physiological and/or anatomical correlates are being assigned to specific compartments [2]. Information about the mean residence time matrix is usually available from the compartmental matrix, which can be obtained from many commonly used modeling software tools.

Noncompartmental versus compartmental models

In comparing noncompartmental with compartmental models, it should now be clear that this is not a question of declaring one method better than the other. It is a question of considering: (1) what information about the system is desired from the data and (2) what is the most appropriate method to obtain this information. It is hoped that the reader of this chapter will be enabled to make an informed decision on this issue, and especially to grasp the limitations and implications of each method, since they are both used in practice.

This discussion will rely heavily on the following sources. First, the publications of DiStefano and Landaw [39, 48] deal with issues related to compartmental versus single accessible pool noncompartmental models. Second, Cobelli and Toffolo [3] discuss the two accessible pool noncompartmental model. Finally, Covell et al. [4] provide the theory to demonstrate the link between noncompartmental and compartmental models in estimating the pharmacokinetic parameters.

Models of data vs. models of system

Suppose one has a set of pharmacokinetic data. The question is how to obtain information from the data related to the disposition of the drug under investigation. DiStefano and Landaw [48] deal with this question by making the distinction between models of data and models of system. Understanding this distinction is useful in understanding the differences between compartmental and noncompartmental models. As discussed, the noncompartmental model divides the system into two components: an accessible pool and nonaccessible pools. The kinetics of the nonaccessible pools are lumped into the recirculation-exchange process. From this, as has been discussed, we can estimate pharmacokinetic parameters describing the accessible pool and system.

What happens in the compartmental model framework? A common way to deal with pharmacokinetic data is by fitting a sum of exponential functions to them, taking advantage of the fact that in a linear, constant-coefficient system, the number of exponential phases seen in the plasma concentration vs. time curve equals the number of compartments in the model.

Consider the situation in which plasma data are obtained following a bolus injection of the drug. Suppose that the data can be described by:

$$C(t) = A_1 e^{-\lambda_1 t} + A_2 e^{-\lambda_2 t} \tag{8.50}$$

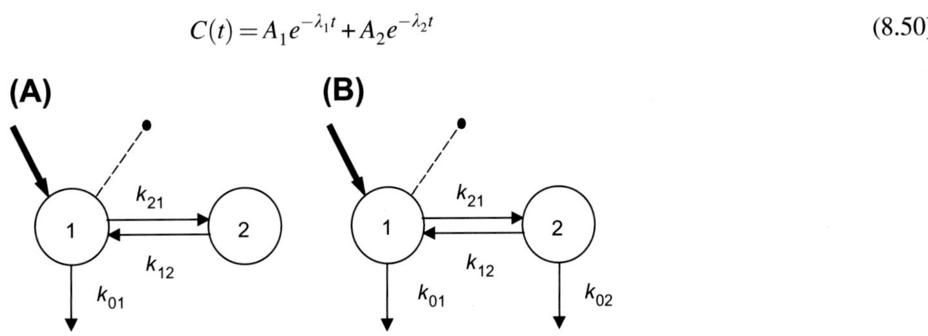

FIG. 8.7 Two two-compartment models in which drug is administered intravenously into compartment 1; samples are taken from this compartment. See text for explanation.

While the presence of two exponential functions in this equation supports the presence of two distinct compartments, the data could be modeled equally well by the model in Fig. 8.7A, whose solution is a sum of two exponential functions. In this case, both the exponential equation and the compartmental model serve only to describe the data and to allow extrapolation of the pharmacokinetic time course beyond the experimental boundaries. That is, no comment is being made about a physiological, biochemical, and/or anatomical significance to the extravascular compartment 2. This is what DiStefano and Landaw [48] would call a *model of data* because little to nothing is being said about the system into which the drug is administered. Incidentally, if the model in Fig. 8.7A were physiologically the most appropriate for the drug, the noncompartmental formulas would be valid.

Suppose, on the other hand, additional information is known about the disposition of the drug. For example, suppose it is known that a major extravascular tissue in the body is where virtually all of the drug is taken up, and that the approximate fraction of the drug metabolized in that compartment is known from independent experiments. Now, given that the plasma data can be fitted by a sum of two exponentials, one can start to develop a *model of system* for the drug, and the mechanistically most appropriate model seems to be the one in Fig. 8.7B. While this model is not a priori identifiable, one can write an equation in which the irreversible loss rate constants k_{01} and k_{02} are related through knowledge of how much of the drug is metabolized in the tissue; compartment 2 can thus be conceptually associated with this tissue.

Such modeling techniques have been the subject of intense debate. First, one has used the fact that the data support a two-compartment model, and the fact that a relationship between the irreversible loss rate constants can be written based upon a priori knowledge. Some physiological significance can thus be associated with the compartments and the k_{ij} that goes beyond the descriptive model of data just discussed. Atkinson et al. [49, 50] list some examples of physiological insight which can be provided by these models, despite their being relatively simple when compared to physiologically based pharmacokinetic models. In some cases, physiological insight may be provided by conducting a study in which marker compounds for known physiological spaces are coadministered with the study drug [51]. A criticism of such an approach is that these models do not contain all elements of the system in which the drug is known to interact. If this limitation is critical, then one must design a new experiment to uncover information on those more relevant parts of the system. One may have to change the sampling schedule to resolve more components in the data or design a different series of input-output experiments.

This is not a shortcoming of the modeling approach but illustrates how knowledge of compartmental modeling can be a powerful tool for understanding the pharmacokinetics of a drug. Such an understanding is not often available from noncompartmental models or when compartmental models are used only as models of data, except that these can be used as preliminary data analysis approaches to uncover more detailed information. Thus predicting detailed events in nonaccessible portions of the system model is the underlying rationale for developing models of systems—remembering, of course, that such predictions are only as good as the assumptions in the model.

The equivalent sink and source constraints

When are the parameter estimates from the noncompartmental model equal to those from a linear, constant coefficient compartmental model? As DiStefano and Landaw [48] explain, they are equal when the equivalent sink and source constraints are valid. The equivalent source constraint means that all drugs enter the same accessible pools; this is almost universally the case in pharmacokinetic studies. The equivalent sink constraint means that irreversible loss of drug can occur only from the accessible pools. If any irreversible loss occurs from the nonaccessible part of the system, this constraint is not valid. For the single accessible pool model, for example, the system mean residence time and the total equivalent volume of distribution will be underestimated [2].

The equivalent sink constraint is illustrated in Fig. 8.8. In Fig. 8.8A, the constraint holds and hence the parameters estimated either from the noncompartmental model (*left*) or multicompartmental model (*right*) will be equal. If the multicompartmental model is a model of the system, then, of course, the information about the drug's disposition will be much richer, since many more specific parameters can be estimated to describe each compartment.

In Fig. 8.8B, the constraint is not satisfied, and the noncompartmental model is not appropriate. As previously described, if used, it will underestimate certain parameters. On the other hand, the multicompartmental model shown on the right can account for sites of loss from nonaccessible compartments, providing a richer source of information about the drug's disposition.

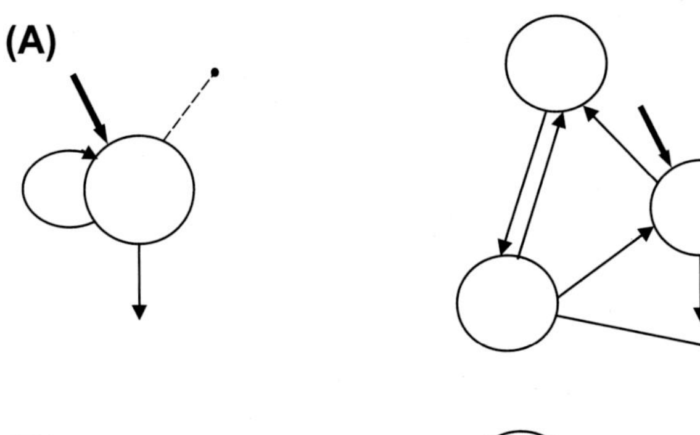

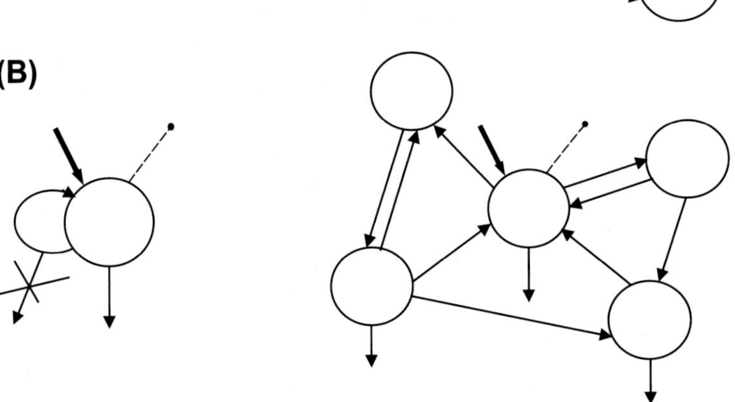

FIG. 8.8 (A) A single accessible pool model (*left*) and a multicompartmental model showing a structure for the recirculation-exchange arrow (*right*). (B) A single accessible pool model with an irreversible loss from the recirculation-exchange arrow (*left*) and a multicompartmental model showing a structure for the recirculation-exchange arrow that includes loss from peripheral compartments (*right*). See text for additional explanation.

Linearity and time invariance

If the system cannot be adequately described by a linear, constant-coefficient model, then linearity and time invariance cannot be assumed. In this case, noncompartmental parameters do not provide an adequate description of the pharmacokinetics and can be at times misleading. Studying the pharmacokinetics over an adequate dose range usually uncovers these situations and other areas where noncompartmental hypotheses may not apply and provides insight for the definition of nonlinear models of the system from which parameters of interest can be determined [52]. Such models, when mechanistically appropriate, can be a generalization of the compartmental framework that, for example, can account for extravascular drug removal or for nonlinear disposition of both drug and drug target. These issues have been studied in detail to describe the disposition of antibody drugs [53].

Recovering pharmacokinetic parameters from compartmental models

We will now use a simple example to demonstrate how noncompartmental and compartmental approaches can be studied together. Assume a linear, constant coefficient compartmental model in which compartment 1 is the accessible compartment into which the drug is administered and from which samples are taken. Following a bolus injection of the drug, the volume V_1 will be estimated as a parameter of the model. V_1 thus will correspond to V_a for the noncompartmental model. The clearance rate from compartment 1, CL_1, is equal to the product of V_1 and k_{01}:

$$CL_1 = V_1 \cdot k_{01} \tag{8.51}$$

If the only loss is from compartment 1, then k_{01} equals k_e, and one has.

$$CL_a = CL_1 = V_1 \cdot k_{01} = V_a \cdot k_e \tag{8.52}$$

showing the equivalence of the two methods. From the residence time matrix,

$$\vartheta_{11} = \frac{\int_0^{\infty} X_1(t)\,dt}{d} = k_{01} \tag{8.53}$$

hence, the mean residence time in compartment 1, MRT_1, equals the reciprocal of k_{01}. Again if the only loss from the system is via compartment 1, then MRT_1 equals MRT_a.

Similar results hold for the constant infusion or generic input. In other words, the parameters can be shown to be equal if the equivalent sink and source constraints are valid. Again, the interested reader is referred to the bibliography for details and for consideration of the situation in which the equivalent source and sink constraints are not valid.

Conclusion

In conclusion, noncompartmental models and linear, constant-coefficient models have different domains of validity. When the domains are identical, then the pharmacokinetic parameters estimated by either method should, in theory, be equivalent. If they are not, then differences are due to the methods used to estimate them. When linearity and time invariance cannot be assumed, then more complex system models are required for pharmacokinetic analysis.

The information provided in this chapter should make it easier for a researcher to choose a particular method and to have greater confidence in evaluating reported results of pharmacokinetic analyses.

References

[1] Gillespie WR. Noncompartmental versus compartmental modelling in clinical pharmacokinetics. Clin Pharmacokinet 1991;20:253–62.
[2] DiStefano III JJ. Noncompartmental vs. compartmental analysis: some bases for choice. Am J Physiol 1982;243:R1–6.
[3] Cobelli C, Toffolo G. Compartmental vs. noncompartmental modeling for two accessible pools. Am J Physiol 1984;247:R488–96.
[4] Covell DG, Berman M, Delisi C. Mean residence time—theoretical development, experimental determination, and practical use in tracer analysis. Math Biosci 1984;72:213–44.
[5] Norwich K. Noncompartmental models of whole-body clearance of tracers: a review. Ann Biomed Eng 1997;25:421–39.
[6] Weiss M, Förster W. Pharmacokinetic model based on circulatory transport. Eur J Clin Pharmacol 1979;16:287–93.
[7] Beal SL. Some clarifications regarding moments of residence times with pharmacokinetic models. J Pharmacokinet Biopharm 1987;15:75–92.
[8] Mordenti J, Rescigno A. Estimation of permanence time, exit time, dilution factor, and steady-state volume of distribution. Pharm Res 1992;9:17–25.
[9] Wagner JG. Linear pharmacokinetic equations allowing direct calculation of many needed pharmacokinetic parameters from the coefficients and exponents of polyexponential equations which have been fitted to the data. J Pharmacokinet Biopharm 1976;4:443–67.
[10] Jacquez JA, Simon CP. Qualitative theory of compartmental systems. SIAM Rev 1993;35:43–79.
[11] Jacquez JA. Compartmental analysis in biology and medicine. 3rd ed. Ann Arbor, MI: BioMedware; 1996.
[12] Berman M. Kinetic analysis of turnover data. Prog Biochem Pharmacol 1979;15:67–108.
[13] Gibaldi M, Perrier D. Pharmacokinetics. 2nd ed. New York: Marcel Dekker; 1982.
[14] Rowland M, Tozer TN. Clinical pharmacokinetics: concepts and applications. 3rd ed. Baltimore, MD: Williams & Wilkins; 1995.
[15] Morrison PF, Dedrick RL. Transport of cisplatin in rat brain following microinfusion: an analysis. J Pharm Sci 1986;75:120–8.
[16] Morrison PF, Bungay PM, Hsiao JK, Ball BA, Mefford IN, Dedrick RL. Quantitative microdialysis: analysis of transients and application to pharmacokinetics in brain. J Neurochem 1991;57:103–19.
[17] Rescigno A. Fundamental concepts in pharmacokinetics. Pharmacol Res 1997;35:363–90.
[18] Benet L. Clearance (née Rowland) concepts: a downdate and an update. J Pharmacokinet Pharmacodyn 2010;37:529–39.
[19] Landaw EM, Katz D. Comments on mean residence time determination. J Pharmacokinet Biopharm 1985;13:543–7.
[20] Yamaoka K, Nakagawa T, Uno T. Statistical moments in pharmacokinetics. J Pharmacokinet Biopharm 1978;6:547–58.
[21] Teorell T. Kinetics of distribution of substances administered to the body. Arch Intern Pharmacodyn Ther 1937;57:205–25.
[22] Pearson K. On the systematic fitting of curves to observations and measurements. Biometrika 1902;1:265–303.
[23] Zierler KL. Theory of use of indicators to measure blood flow and extracellular volume and calculation of transcapillary movement of tracers. Circ Res 1963;12:464–71.
[24] Perl W, Effros RM, Chinard FP. Indicator equivalence theorem for input rates and regional masses in multi-inlet steady-state systems with partially labeled input. J Theor Biol 1969;25:297–316.
[25] Zierler KL. Theory of the use of arteriovenous concentration differences for measuring metabolism in steady and non-steady states. J Clin Invest 1961;40:2111–25.
[26] Rescigno A. The rise and fall of compartmental analysis. Pharm Res 2001;44:337–42.
[27] DiStefano III JJ. Concepts, properties, measurement, and computation of clearance rates of hormones and other substances in biological systems. Ann Biomed Eng 1976;4:302–19.
[28] Mari A. Circulatory models of intact-body kinetics and their relationship with compartmental and non-compartmental analysis. J Theor Biol 1993;160:509–31.
[29] Weiss M. The relevance of residence time theory to pharmacokinetics. Eur J Clin Pharmacol 1992;43:571–9.
[30] Veng-Pedersen P. Noncompartmentally-based pharmacokinetic modeling. Adv Drug Deliv Rev 2001;48:265–300.
[31] Cobelli C, Foster D, Toffolo G. Tracer kinetics in biomedical research: from data to model. New York: Kluwer Academic/Plenum Publishers; 2000.
[32] Berman M, Schoenfeld R. Invariants in experimental data on linear kinetics and the formulation of models. J Appl Phys 1956;27:1361–70.

[33] Yeh KC, Kwan KC. A comparison of numerical integrating algorithms by trapezoidal, Lagrange, and spline approximation. J Pharmacokinet Biopharm 1978;6:79–98.

[34] Purves RD. Optimum numerical integration methods for estimation of area-under-the-curve (AUC) and area-under-the-moment-curve (AUMC). J Pharmacokinet Biopharm 1992;20:211–26.

[35] Bailer AJ. Testing for the equality of area under the curves when using destructive measurement techniques. J Pharmacokinet Biopharm 1988;16:303–9.

[36] Katz D, D'Argenio DZ. Experimental design for estimating integrals by numerical quadrature, with applications to pharmacokinetic studies. Biometrics 1983;39:621–8.

[37] Gabrielsson J, Weiner D. Pharmacokinetic/pharmacodynamic data analysis: concepts and applications. 2nd ed. Stockholm: Swedish Pharmaceutical Press; 1997.

[38] Marino AT, DiStefano III JJ, Landaw EM. DIMSUM: an expert system for multiexponential model discrimination. Am J Physiol 1992;262:E546–56.

[39] Landaw EM, DiStefano III JJ. Multiexponential, multicompartmental, and noncompartmental modeling. II. Data analysis and statistical considerations. Am J Physiol 1984;246:R665–77.

[40] Pang KS, Weiss M, Macheras P. Advanced pharmacokinetic models based on organ clearance, circulatory, and fractal concepts. AAPS J 2007; 9:E268–83.

[41] Nestorov I. Whole body pharmacokinetic models. Clin Pharmacokinet 2003;42:883–908.

[42] Rowland M, Peck C, Tucker G. Physiologically-based pharmacokinetics in drug development and regulatory science. Annu Rev Pharmacol Toxicol 2011;51:45–73.

[43] Jones HM, Chen Y, Gibson C, Heimbach T, Parrott N, Peters SA, Snoeys J, Upreti VV, Zheng M, Hall SD. Physiologically based pharmacokinetic modeling in drug discovery and development: a pharmaceutical industry perspective. Clin Pharmacol Ther 2015;97:247–62.

[44] Macheras P, Iliadis A. Stochastic compartmental models. In: Modeling in biopharmaceutics, pharmacokinetics, and pharmacodynamics. New York: Springer; 2006. p. 205–87.

[45] Bowsher DJ, Avram MJ, Frederiksen MC, Asada A, Atkinson AJ Jr. Urea distribution kinetics analyzed by simultaneous injection of urea and inulin: demonstration that transcapillary exchange is rate limiting. J Pharmacol Exp Ther 1984;230:269–74.

[46] Cobelli C, DiStefano III JJ. Parameter and structural identifiability concepts and ambiguities: a critical review and analysis. Am J Physiol 1980;239: R7–24.

[47] Covell DG, Barbet J, Holton OD, Black CD, Parker RJ, Weinstein JN. Pharmacokinetics of monoclonal immunoglobulin G1, F(ab')2, and Fab' in mice. Cancer Res 1986;46:3969–78.

[48] JJ III DS, Landaw EW. Multiexponential, multicompartmental, and noncompartmental modeling. I. Methodological limitations and physiological interpretations. Am J Physiol 1984;246:R651–64.

[49] Atkinson AJ Jr, Ruo TI, Frederiksen MC. Physiological basis of multicompartmental models of drug distribution. Trends Pharmacol Sci 1991; 12:96–101.

[50] Atkinson AJ Jr. Physiological spaces and multicompartmental pharmacokinetic models. Transl Clin Pharmacol 2015;23:38–41.

[51] Belknap SM, Nelson JE, Ruo TI, Frederiksen MC, Worwag EM, Shin S-G, Atkinson AJ Jr. Theophylline distribution kinetics analyzed by reference to simultaneously injected urea and inulin. J Pharmacol Exp Ther 1987;287:963–9.

[52] Mager DE. Target-mediated drug disposition and dynamics. Biochem Pharmacol 2006;72:1–10.

[53] Lobo ED, Hansen RJ, Balthasar JP. Antibody pharmacokinetics and pharmacodynamics. J Pharm Sci 2004;93:2645–68.

Chapter 9

Population pharmacokinetics

Ophelia Yin and Raymond Miller

Advanced Pharmacometrics, Quantitative Clinical Pharmacology, Daiichi Sankyo Inc, Basking Ridge, NJ, United States

Introduction

The aim of pharmacokinetic modeling is to define mathematical models to describe and quantify drug behavior in individuals. The development of a successful pharmacokinetic model allows one to summarize large amounts of data into a few values that describe the whole dataset. The general procedure used to develop a pharmacokinetic model is outlined in Table 9.1. Certain aspects of this procedure have also been described in Chapters 3 and 8. For example, the technique of curve peeling frequently is used to indicate the number of compartments that are included in a compartmental model. In any event, the eventual outcome should be a model that can be used to interpolate or extrapolate to other conditions. Pharmacokinetic studies in patients have led to the appreciation of the large degree of variability in pharmacokinetic parameter estimates that exist across patients. Such a variability can be attributed to intrinsic factors, such as age, gender, the presence and extent of liver or renal impairment, or extrinsic factors, such as food intake or concomitant medications that may interact with the administered drug. Many studies have quantified the effects of these intrinsic and extrinsic factors, with the purpose of accounting for the interindividual variability. Finding a population model that adequately describes the data may have important implications for clinical management strategies in that the dose regimen for a specific patient may need to be individualized based on relevant physiological information. This is particularly important for drugs with a narrow therapeutic range.

Population pharmacokinetic analysis is an extension of the previously mentioned modeling procedure and can be defined as the study of the variability in plasma drug concentrations among individuals. Drug concentrations can vary significantly among individuals when the same dose or dosing regimen is administered. The purpose of population pharmacokinetic analysis is summarized in Table 9.2. The term population pharmacokinetics has been commonly associated with the analysis of sparse data (few observations per subject with unstructured sampling time schedules) collected under the circumstances that conventional pharmacokinetic study with multiple samples taken at fixed intervals is not feasible, such as late stage clinical trials, studies in young children, or patients in intensive care. However, this approach can be applied equally well to conventional pharmacokinetic studies. Recently there is a trend of increased use of population pharmacokinetic analysis to integrate all relevant information from studies with rich or sparse pharmacokinetic sampling, after a single dose or at steady state, and from healthy individuals or the patient population, to inform clinical management strategies or further clinical development.

Analysis of pharmacokinetic data

Structure of pharmacokinetic models

As discussed in Chapters 3 and 8, it is often found that the relationship between drug concentrations and time may be described by a sum of exponential terms. This lends itself to compartmental pharmacokinetic analysis in which the pharmacokinetics of a drug are characterized by representing the body as a system of well-stirred compartments with the rates of transfer between compartments following first-order kinetics. The required number of compartments is equal to the number of exponents in the sum of exponentials equation that best fits the data. In the case of a drug that seems to be distributed homogeneously in the body, a one compartment model is appropriate, and this relationship can be described in a single individual by the following monoexponential equation:

$$A = \text{Dose} \cdot e^{-kt} \tag{9.1}$$

Atkinson's Principles of Clinical Pharmacology. https://doi.org/10.1016/B978-0-12-819869-8.00032-X

TABLE 9.1 Steps in developing a pharmacokinetic model.

Step	Activity
1	Design an experiment
2	Collect the data and compile an analysis dataset
3	Develop a model based on the observed characteristics of the data
4	Express the model mathematically
5	Analyze the data in terms of the model
6	Evaluate the fit of the data to the model
7	If necessary revise the model in step 3 to eliminate inconsistencies in the data fit and repeat the process until the model provides a satisfactory description of the data

TABLE 9.2 The purpose of pharmacokinetic analysis.

Estimate the population mean of parameters of interest
Identify and investigate sources of variability that influence drug pharmacokinetics
Estimate the magnitude of intersubject variability
Estimate the random residual variability

This equation describes the typical time course of amount of drug in the body (A) as a function of initial dose, time (t), and the first-order elimination rate constant (k). As described in Eq. (2.14), this rate constant equals the ratio of the elimination clearance (CL) relative to the distribution volume of the drug (V_d), so that Eq. (9.1) can then be expressed in terms of concentration in plasma (Cp).

$$Cp = \frac{\text{Dose}}{V_d} \cdot e^{-\frac{CL}{V_d} \cdot t} \tag{9.2}$$

Therefore if one has an estimate of clearance and volume of distribution, the plasma concentration can be predicted at different times after administration of any selected dose. The quantities that are known because they are either measured or controlled, such as dose and time, are called "fixed effects", in contrast to effects that are not known and are regarded as random. The parameters CL and V_d are called fixed effect parameters because they quantify the influence of the fixed effects on the dependent variable, Cp.

Fitting individual data

Assuming that we have measured a series of concentrations over time, we can define a model structure and obtain initial estimates of the model parameters. The objective is to determine an estimate of the parameters (Cl, V_d) such that the differences between the observed and predicted concentrations are comparatively small. Three of the most commonly used criteria for obtaining a best fit of the model to the data are ordinary least squares (OLS), weighted least squares (WLS), and extended least squares (ELS), which is a maximum likelihood procedure. These criteria are achieved by minimizing the following quantities, which are often called the objective function (O).

Ordinary least squares (OLS) (where $\hat{C}_i$ denotes the predicted value of C_i based on the model):

$$O_{OLS} = \sum_{i=1}^{n} (C_i - \hat{C}_i)^2 \tag{9.3}$$

Weighted least squares (WLS) (where W is typically 1/the observed concentration):

$$O_{WLS} = \sum_{i=1}^{n} W_i (C_i - \hat{C}_i)^2 \tag{9.4}$$

Extended least squares (ELS):

$$O_{ELS} = \sum_{i=1}^{n} \left[W_i (C_i - \hat{C}_i)^2 + \text{In}\,\text{var}(\hat{C}_i) \right] \tag{9.5}$$

The correct criterion for best fit depends upon the assumption underlying the functional form of the variances (var) of the dependent variable C. The model that fits the data from an individual minimizes the differences between the observed and the model predicted concentrations (Fig. 9.1).

What one observes is a measured value which differs from the model-predicted value by some amount called a residual error (also called intrasubject error or within-subject error). There are many reasons why the actual observation may not correspond to the predicted value. The structural model may only be approximate, or the plasma concentrations may have been measured with error. It is too difficult to model all the sources of error separately so the simplifying assumption is made that each difference between an observation and its prediction is random. When the data are from an individual, and the error model is the additive error model, the error is denoted by ε.

$$C = \frac{\text{Dose}}{V_d} \cdot e^{-\frac{CL}{V_d} \cdot t} + \varepsilon \tag{9.6}$$

Population pharmacokinetics

Corresponding to the purpose of population pharmacokinetic analysis outlined in Table 9.2, a population pharmacokinetic model consists of the following three main components: structural model, covariate model, and statistical model (Fig. 9.2). The covariate model describes predictable sources (fixed effects) of variability via defining the quantitative relationships between pharmacokinetic parameters and covariates. The statistical model describes variability (random effects) around the structural model. There are two primary sources of variability in any population pharmacokinetic model: between-subject variability (intersubject variability), which is the variance of a parameter across individuals; and residual variability, which is unexplained variability after controlling for other sources of variability. Some datasets also support the estimation of interoccasion variability, where a drug is administered on two or more occasions in each subject, and there is sufficient time interval for the underlying kinetics to vary between occasions.

Obtaining the above-mentioned information is necessary to design a dosage regimen for a drug. If all patients were identical, the same dose would be appropriate for all. However, since patients vary, it may be necessary to individualize

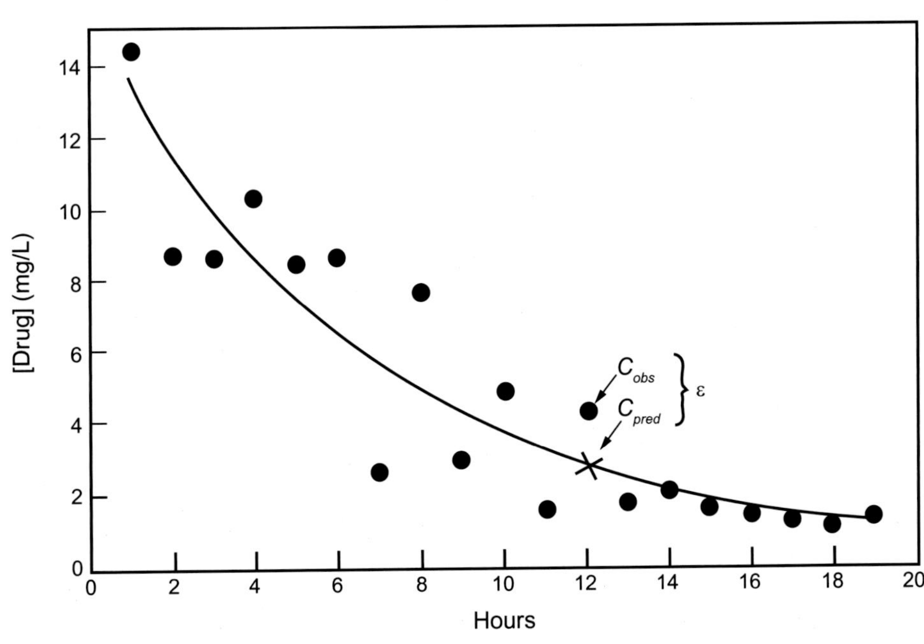

FIG. 9.1 Fit obtained using a one-compartment model (see Eq. 9.6) to fit plasma concentration vs time data observed following intravenous bolus administration of a drug: C_{obs} designates the actual measured concentrations and C_{pred} represents the concentrations predicted by the pharmacokinetic model. *(Based on Grasela TH Jr, Sheiner LB. Pharmacostatistical modeling for observational data. J Pharmacokinet Biopharm 1991;19(Suppl):25S–36S.)*

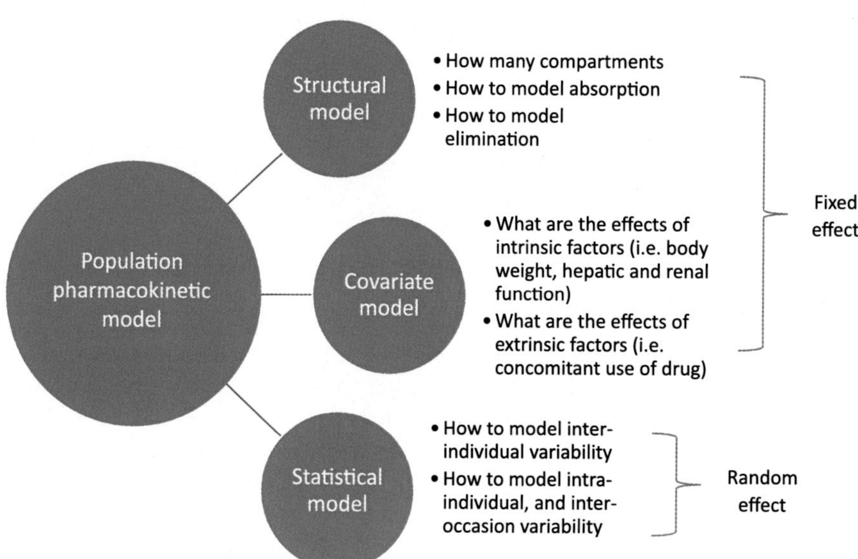

FIG. 9.2 Key components of a population pharmacokinetic model.

a dose depending on how large the between-subject variation is. For example, to choose an initial dose, one needs to know the relationship between the administered dose and the concentration achieved and thus pharmacological response anticipated in a patient. This is the same as knowing the typical pharmacokinetics of individuals of similar sex, age, weight, and function of elimination organs. This information is available if one knows the fixed effect pharmacokinetic parameters governing the relationship of the pharmacokinetics to sex, age, weight, renal function, liver function, and so on. Large unexplained variability in pharmacokinetics in an apparently homogeneous population can lead to an investigation as to the reason for the discrepancy, which in turn may lead to an understanding of fundamental principles.

A well-known application is antimicrobial dosing and clinical management of critically ill patients with severe infections. The pharmacokinetics and pharmacodynamics of antimicrobials in critically ill patients differ significantly from the patient groups from whose data the conventional dosing regimens were developed. Therefore individualized dosing, based on population pharmacokinetic models and patient factors (e.g., renal function and weight) known to influence antimicrobial pharmacokinetics, can lead to better patient outcomes by increasing the probability of achieving therapeutic drug exposures while at the same time avoiding toxic concentrations.

Population analysis methods

Assume an experiment in which a group of subjects selected to represent a spectrum of severity of some condition (e.g., renal insufficiency) are given a dose of drug and drug concentrations are measured in blood samples collected at intervals after dosing. The structural kinetic models used when performing a population analysis do not differ at all from those used for analysis of data from an individual patient. One still needs a model for the relationship of concentration to dose and time, and this relationship does not depend on whether the fixed effect parameter changes from individual to individual or with time within an individual. The population pharmacokinetic parameters can be determined in a number of ways of which only a few will be described.

The naïve pooled data method

If interest focuses entirely on the estimation of population parameters then the simplest approach is to combine all the data as if they came from a single individual [1]. The doses may need to be normalized so that the data are comparable. Eq. (9.6) would be applicable if an intravenous bolus dose were administered. The minimization procedure is similar to that described in Fig. 9.1.

The advantages of this method are its simplicity, familiarity, and the fact that it can be used with sparse data and differing numbers of data points per individual. The disadvantages are that it is not possible to determine the fixed effect sources of interindividual variability. It also cannot distinguish between variability within and between individuals, and an imbalance between individuals results in biased parameter estimates.

Although pooling has the risk of masking individual behavior, it might still serve as a general guide to the mean pharmacokinetic parameters. If this method is used, it is recommended that a spaghetti plot be made to visually determine if any individual or group of individuals deviates from the central tendency with respect to absorption, distribution, or elimination.

The two-stage method

The two-stage method is so called because it proceeds in two steps [1]. The first step is to use OLS to estimate each individual patient's parameters assuming a model such as Eq. (9.6). The minimization procedure described in Fig. 9.1 is repeated for each individual independently (Fig. 9.3).

The next step is to estimate the population parameters across the subjects by calculating the mean of each parameter, its variance and covariance. The relationship between fixed effect parameters and covariates of interest can be investigated by regression techniques. To investigate the relationship between drug clearance (CL) and creatinine clearance (CL_{CR}) one could try a variety of models depending on the shape of the relationship. As described in Chapter 5, in case of a linear relationship, Eq. (9.7) can be applied (Fig. 9.4):

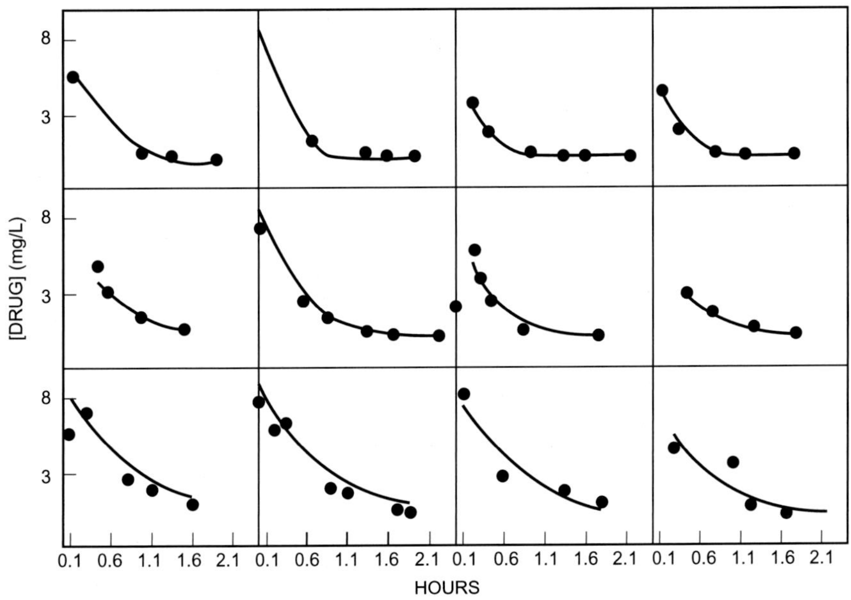

FIG. 9.3 Fit obtained using a one-compartment model to fit plasma concentration vs time data observed following intravenous bolus administration of a drug. Each panel represents an individual subject.

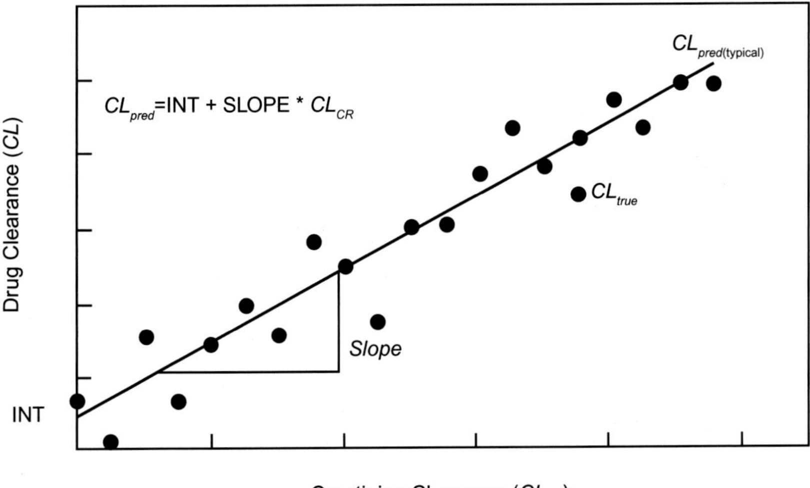

FIG. 9.4 Linear regression analysis of drug clearance (CL) vs creatinine clearance (CL_{CR}). Typical values of drug clearance are generated for an individual or group of individuals with a given creatinine clearance. The discrepancy between the true value for drug clearance (CL_{true}) and the typical value (CL_{pred}) necessitates the use of a statistical model for interindividual variability. INT denotes the intercept of the regression line. *(Based on Grasela TH Jr, Sheiner LB. Pharmacostatistical modeling for observational data. J Pharmacokinet Biopharm 1991;19 (Suppl):25S–36S.)*

$$CL = \text{INT} + \text{SLOPE} \cdot CL_{CR} \tag{9.7}$$

The intercept in this equation provides an estimate of nonrenal clearance.

The advantages of this method are that it is easy and most investigators are familiar with it. Because parameters are estimated for each individual, these estimates have little or no bias. Pharmacokinetic-pharmacodynamic models can be applied since individual differences can be considered. Covariates can be included in the model. Disadvantages of the method are that variance-covariance of parameters across subjects is biased and contains elements of interindividual variability, intraindividual variability, assay error, time error, model misspecification, and variability from the individual parameter estimation process. In addition, the same structural model is required for all subjects, and numerous blood samples must be obtained at appropriate times to obtain accurate estimates for Step 1.

Nonlinear mixed effects modeling method

This method is depicted in Fig. 9.5 and will be described using the conventions of the NONMEM software [2] and the description by Vozeh et al. [3]. It is based on the principle that the individual pharmacokinetic parameters of a patient population arise from a distribution that can be described by the population mean and the interindividual variance. Each individual pharmacokinetic parameter can be expressed as a population mean and a deviation, typical for that individual. The deviation is the difference between the population mean and the individual parameter, explaining biological variability of the population. The clearance and volume of distribution for subject j using the structural pharmacokinetic model described in Eq. (9.6) are represented by the following equations.

$$C_{ij} = \frac{\text{Dose}}{V_{dj}} \cdot e^{\frac{CL_j}{V_{dj}} \cdot t_{ij}} + \varepsilon_{ij} \tag{9.8}$$

where,

$$CL_j = \overline{CL} + \eta_j^{CL} \tag{9.9}$$

and,

$$V_{dj} = \overline{V_d} + \eta_j^{V_d} \tag{9.10}$$

where $\overline{CL}$ and $\overline{V_d}$ are the population mean of clearance and volume of distribution, respectively, and η_j^{CL} and $\eta_j^{V_d}$ are the differences between the population mean and the clearance (CL_j) and volume of distribution (V_{dj}) of subject j. Each η is assumed to be a random variable with an expected mean of zero and variance ω^2. These equations can be applied to subject k by substituting a k for j in the equations, and so on for each subject. There are, however, two levels of random effects. The first level is needed in the parameter model to help model unexplained interindividual differences in the parameters.

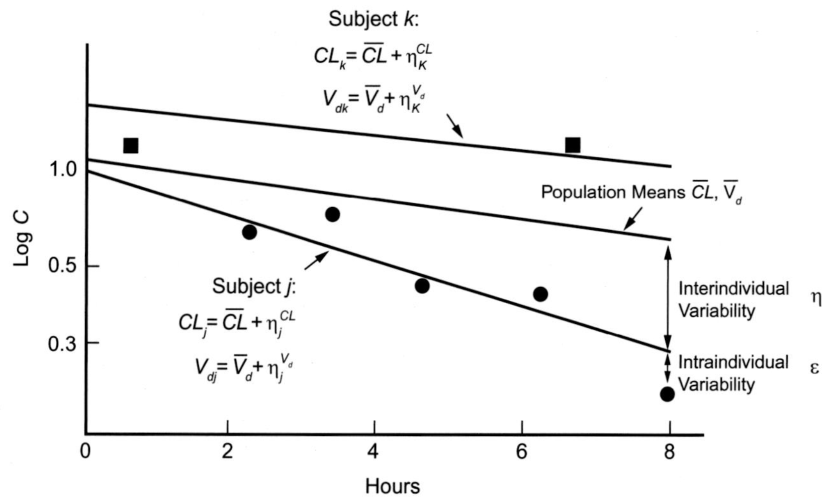

FIG. 9.5 Graphical illustration of the statistical model used in NONMEM for the special case of a one-compartment model following intravenous bolus administration of a drug. •, Subject j; ▪, subject k. *(Based on Vozeh S, Katz G, Steiner V, Follath F. Population pharmacokinetic parameters in patients treated with oral mexiletine. Eur J Clin Pharmacol 1982;23:445–451.)*

The second level represents a random error (ε_{ij}), familiar from classical pharmacokinetic analysis, which expresses the deviation of the expected plasma concentration in subject j from the measured value. Each ε variable is assumed to have a mean zero and a variance denoted by σ^2. Each pair of elements in η has a covariance which can be estimated. A covariance between two elements of η is a measure of statistical association between these two random variables.

NONMEM is a one-stage analysis that simultaneously estimates mean parameters, fixed effect parameters, interindividual variability, and residual random effects. The fitting routine makes use of the ELS method. A global measure of goodness of fit is provided by the objective function value based on the final parameter estimates, which, in the case of NONMEM, is minus twice the log likelihood of the data [1]. Any improvement in the model fit would be reflected by a decrease in the objective function value. The purpose of adding independent variables to the model, such as CL_{CR} in Eq. (9.7), is usually to explain kinetic differences between individuals. This means that such differences were not explained by the model prior to adding the variable and were part of random interindividual variability. Therefore inclusion of additional variables in the model is often accompanied by a decrease in the estimates of the intersubject variance, and under certain circumstances intrasubject variance.

The advantages of the one-stage analysis are that interindividual variability of the parameters can be estimated, random residual error can be estimated, covariates can be included in the model, parameters for individuals can be estimated, and pharmacokinetic/pharmacodynamic models can be used. Since allowance can be made for individual differences, this method can be used with routine data, sparse data, and unbalanced number of data points per patient [4, 5]. The models are also much more flexible. For example, a number of studies can be pooled into one analysis while accounting for differences between study sites, and all fixed effect covariate relationships and any interindividual or residual error structure can be investigated.

Disadvantages arise mainly from the complexity of the statistical algorithms and the fact that fitting models to data is time consuming. For example, the maximum likelihood estimation methods in NONMEM include the first-order (FO), the first-order conditional estimation (FOCE), and second-order conditional estimation (Laplace) methods. The FO method is fast, but sometimes results in inaccurate assessments, especially when the distribution of interindividual variability is specified incorrectly, or the residual error or intersubject variability is large. The FOCE method is more accurate but is more time consuming and sometimes fails to converge. The Laplace approach was even more accurate than FOCE for sparse data, but it has decreased efficiency and robustness. Newer algorithms, such as Monte Carlo importance sampling (IMP), expectation maximization (EM), and stochastic approximation expectation maximization (SAEM), have been introduced to recent version of NONMEM (version 7.2 and above). These algorithms are useful for complex pharmacokinetic-pharmacodynamic models or very sparse data, but their execution requires a higher level of expertise.

Model comparison

In the maximum likelihood approach, the objective function value (OFV) is minimized. The minimum OFV is important for comparing and ranking models. When comparing candidate models, it is necessary to compensate for improvements of fit due to increased model complexity, since generally complex models with more parameters are better able to describe a given dataset. The Akaike information criterion (AIC) and Bayesian information criterion (BIC) are useful for comparing structural models [6, 7]:

$$AIC = OFV + 2 \cdot n_p \tag{9.11}$$

$$BIC = OFV + n_p \cdot Ln(N) \tag{9.12}$$

where n_p is the total number of parameters in the model, and N is the number of data observations. Both can be used to rank models based on goodness of fit. BIC penalizes the.

OBJ for model complexity more than AIC and may be preferable when data are limited. A drop in AIC or BIC by ≥ 2 may be used for considering one model over another. However, mechanistic plausibility and utility should be taken into consideration for model selection.

The likelihood ratio test (LRT) can be used to compare the OFV of two models that are nested, such as covariate models selection. For nested models the difference of two log likelihoods is asymptotically chi-squared distributed. Hence with one parameter difference (one degree of freedom) a decrease in OFV by ≥ 3.84, 6.63, and 10.83 corresponds to the significance level of $P \leq .05$, .01, and .001, respectively.

Model evaluation

The most common prediction based graphical diagnostics are goodness-of-fit plots, used as part of model evaluation to detect potential bias or issues with the structural model or random effects. They typically include some or all of the following: population prediction (PRED) versus observations or time, individual prediction (IPRED) versus observations or time, conditional weighted residual (CWRES) versus PRED or time, and individual weighted residual (IWRES) versus IPRED or time [8]. An example is shown in Fig. 9.6. To make such plots as informative as possible, a combination of the use of logscales, faceting, and/or conditioning on explanatory variables is commonly applied.

The most common simulation-based diagnostics are visual predictive checks (VPC) or prediction-corrected visual predictive check (pcVPC) [9, 10]. The principle of the VPC is to assess graphically whether simulations from the selected model are able to reproduce both the central trend and overall distribution of the observed data. A VPC is based on multiple simulations with the model and observed data structure (i.e., dosing, timing, and number of samples). Percentiles of the simulated data are then compared to the corresponding percentiles of the observed data, typically the median and 2.5th and 97.5th percentiles. The interpercentile range between the outer percentiles of all the simulated data is often referred to as a prediction interval. For example, 2.5th to 97.5th percentile corresponds to 95% prediction interval. By calculating the percentiles of interest for each of the simulated replicates of the original dataset, a nonparametric confidence interval can also be generated for the predicted percentiles. The size of the confidence intervals acts as a reference to better judge what is likely to be a true deviation between model predictions and observations. This is thought to make the interpretation of VPCs less subjective (see illustration in Fig. 9.7). VPC plots stratified by dose and relevant covariates are commonly constructed to demonstrate model performance in these subsets. pcVPC normalizes the observed and simulated data based on the PRED

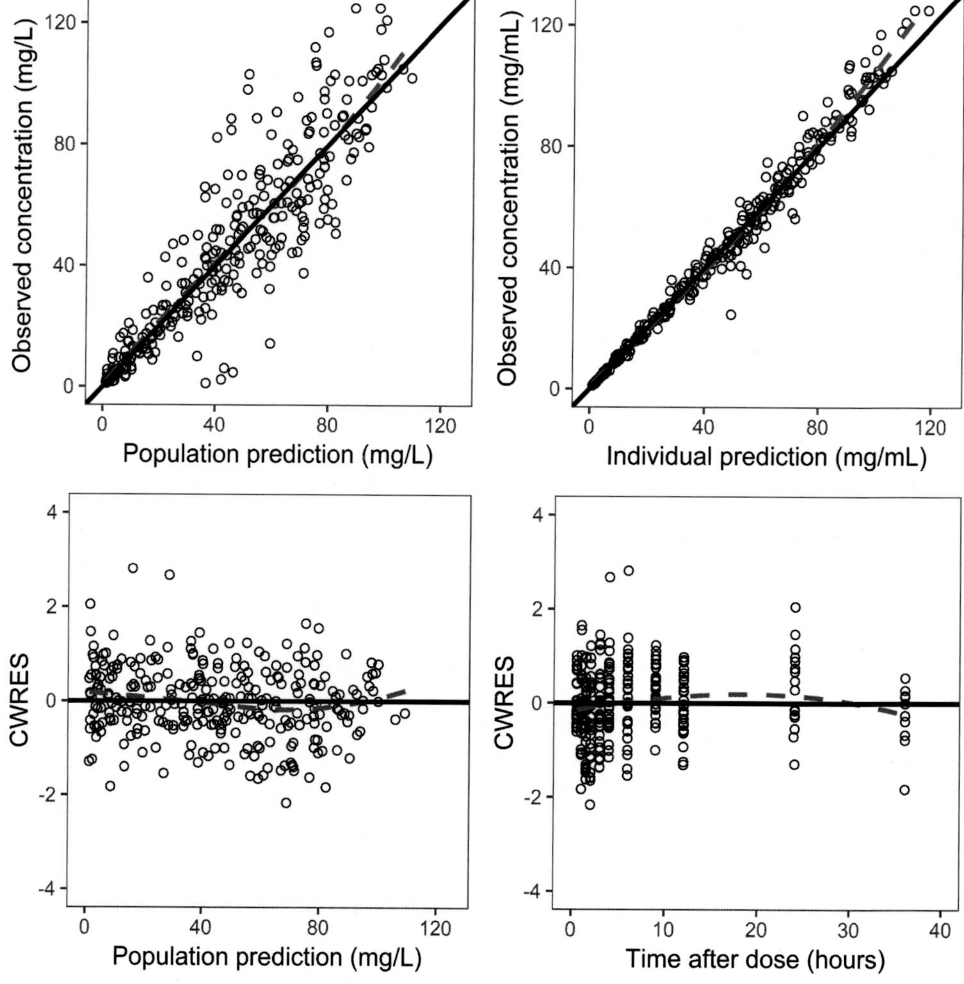

FIG. 9.6 Basic goodness-of-fit plot. Upper panel: Observed concentrations versus population predicted or individual predicted concentrations. Lower panel: Conditional weighted residuals versus population predictions or versus time after dose. *Solid lines* represent lines of identity (upper panel) or null value (lower panel), and *dotted lines* are loess smooth through the data.

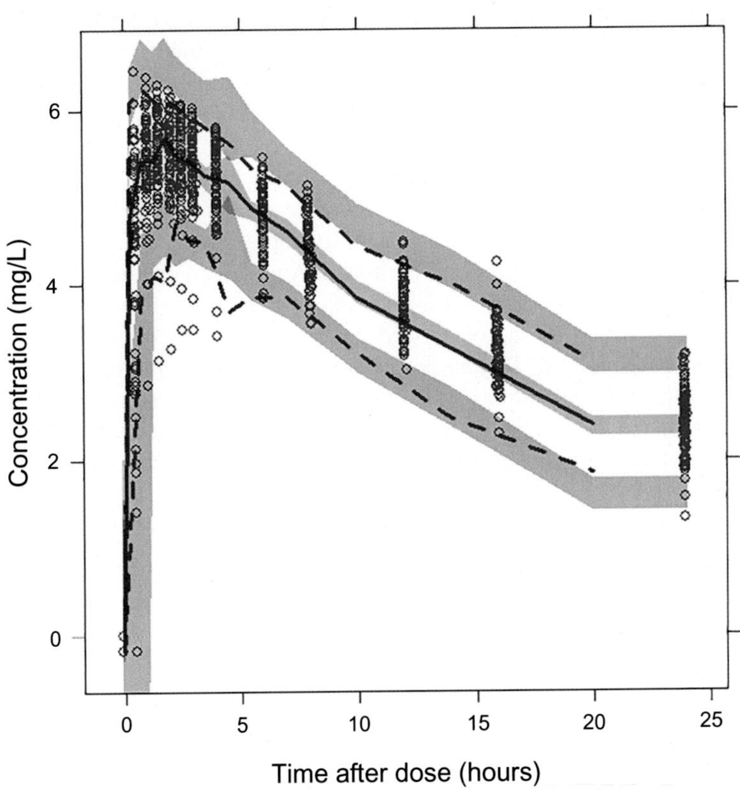

FIG. 9.7 Prediction-corrected visual predictive check (pcVPC) plot. *Blue dots* represent prediction-corrected observed data. *Solid line* is observed median; *dashed lines* are 2.5th and 97.5th percentiles of prediction-corrected observations; *shaded areas* are 95% confidence intervals of the median, and 2.5th and 97.5th percentile values from 1000 simulations.

value, which is thought to overcome the potential bias and model misspecification with VPC, when there is considerable variability due to the differences in design or important covariate influences. In a very simple case of linear pharmacokinetics, with a fixed sampling schedule that is identical for all subjects and a model without any covariate relationships, this would be equivalent to performing a VPC based on dose-normalized plasma concentrations.

The precision of parameter estimates is another important aspect of model evaluation, because it serves as an indicator of model reliability. Precision can be expressed as relative standard of error (SE), or 95% confidence intervals (CI) calculated as:

$$95\%\,\mathrm{CI} = \text{Parameter value} \pm 1.96 \cdot \mathrm{SE} \tag{9.13}$$

The level of precision that is acceptable depends on the size of the dataset. For most pharmacokinetic datasets, <30% SE for fixed effects and <50% SE for random effects are usually achievable (SE for random effects are generally higher than for fixed effects).

CIs calculated from SE of the parameter estimates are associated with the assumption of normal distribution. Bootstrapping provides an alternative for estimating parameter precision without the assumption of normal distribution. Therefore such a nonparametric approach is commonly applied to verify the robustness of standard approximations for parameter uncertainty in population pharmacokinetic analyses [11]. Bootstrapping involves generating replicate datasets where individuals are randomly drawn from the original dataset and can be drawn multiple times or not drawn at all for each replicate. Typically, at least 500 replicates are generated and evaluated using the final model, and replicate parameter estimates are tabulated. The 95% CI are constructed by taking the 2.5th and 97.5th percentile values of each parameter estimate from model runs.

Model applications

One of the common applications of population pharmacokinetic analyses is to identify covariates that significantly impact pharmacokinetic variability and to inform dosing regimens for evaluation in clinical trials, with the ultimate goal to minimize the variability of treatment response in patients. Population pharmacokinetic models can be used to simulate drug exposures that are expected to occur following doses or dosing regimens that have not been directly investigated in prior clinical studies, or in certain specific patient subgroups. Such information, together with the understanding of the exposure-response relationship for clinical efficacy and safety, can be used to support dose recommendation in special populations, or evaluation of alternate dose regimen in later trials during drug development. This will be illustrated in the case studies of mirogabalin and milademetan later.

When appropriately justified, population pharmacokinetic analyses, in conjunction with the exposure-response data, may be used to approve dosing regimens that have not been directly evaluated in the clinical trials. For example, avelumab, an anti-PD-L1 monoclonal antibody, was initially approved with a dose regimen of 10mg/kg every 2weeks, for the treatment of metastatic Merkel cell carcinoma and platinum-treated urothelial carcinoma. A population pharmacokinetic analysis was conducted based on the data from 1827 patients enrolled in 3 clinical studies, where avelumab was administered at doses of 1, 3, 10, or 20mg/kg every 2 weeks. Based on the developed population pharmacokinetic model, simulations were conducted to compare avelumab exposure metrics for the dosing regimens of 10mg/kg and 800mg. The simulated exposure metrics were also used to compare the probability of objective response, and the probability of experiencing an adverse event of special interest between the two dosing regimens. Results suggested that one fixed dose (flat dosing) was predicted to provide similar exposure to weight-based dosing, with slightly lower variability. Benefit and risk profiles were also predicted to be similar for the two dosing regimens. These analyses provided the basis for the US Food and Drug Administration approval of a flat dose of avelumab 800mg every 2weeks in approved indications [12].

Mirogabalin case study

Mirogabalin (Tarlige) is an orally administered gabapentinoid, approved in Japan for the treatment of peripheral neuropathic pain (PNP), including diabetic PNP and postherpetic neuralgia. Mirogabalin is predominantly eliminated in the urine and undergoes minimal metabolism, therefore renal function is expected to play an important role in its disposition. In this context, a population pharmacokinetic analysis was conducted to quantify the impact of varying degrees of kidney function on mirogabalin exposure and to explore a dose-adjustment scheme for subjects with renal impairment [13].

The analysis dataset included a total of 32 subjects with normal renal function or with mild, moderate, or severe renal impairment. All subjects received a single oral dose of 5mg mirogabalin, and pharmacokinetic samples were collected up to 72h postdose. A nonlinear mixed-effects modeling was implemented in NONMEM software (version 7.2), using FOCE method.

A two-compartment model with first-order absorption was used to describe the observed concentration-time profiles of mirogabalin. Interindividual variability was modeled as an exponential error term on the absorption rate constant (K_a), lag-time for absorption (T_{lag}), renal clearance (CL_R), nonrenal clearance (CL_{NR}), and volume of distribution of the central compartment (V_2). The residual variability was modeled using a proportional residual error term on the normal scale of plasma concentrations of mirogabalin.

Following the development of a base model, the effects of subject demographic and clinical factors on all parameters were assessed in a single stepwise evaluation, where a significance level of $P \leq .01$ (OFV $\geq$6.63) and $P \leq .001$ (OFV $\geq$10.83) was used in the forward addition and backward deletion step, respectively. Creatinine clearance (CL_{CR}) was found to significantly affect CL_R, and body weight (WT) significantly affected V_2. CL_R value decreases with decreasing CL_{CR}, whereas V_2 decreases in subjects with lower WT:

$$CL_R = 6.93 \cdot \left(CL_{CR}/55.4\right)^{1.26}$$

$$V_2 = 48.7 \cdot (WT/75.0)^{0.924}$$

In addition, it was noted that incorporating a CL_{CR} effect on CL_{NR} was necessary to further improve the overall model fit (i.e., without the addition of CL_{CR} effect on CL_{NR}, there was an apparent underprediction for the severe renal impairment group, as well as an overprediction for the normal renal function or mild renal impairment groups). The relationship was described as follows:

$$CL_{NR} = 1.94 + 0.0418 \cdot CL_{CR}$$

$$\text{If } CL_{CR} \geq 50\text{mL/min} : CL_{NR} = 1.94 + 0.0418 \cdot 50$$

Thus CL_{NR} remains constant when $CL_{CR} \geq 50$ mL/min, but decreases with decreasing CL_{CR} when $CL_{CR} < 50$ mL/min. This refinement is also supported by emerging literature data, suggesting renal impairment can lead to alterations in nonrenal clearance via affecting drug-metabolizing enzymes and/or transporters.

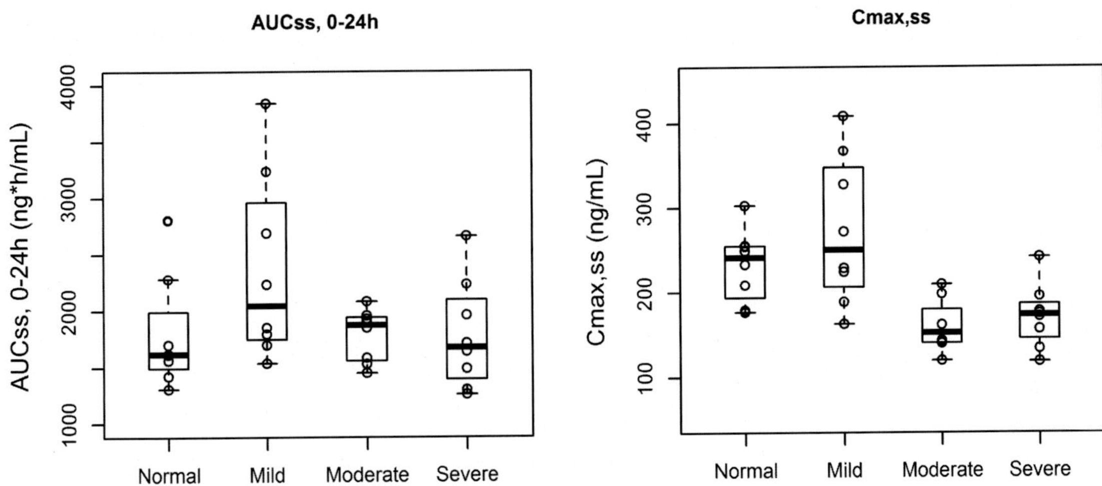

FIG. 9.8 Simulated steady-state exposure measures when mirogabalin is given as 15mg BID to subjects with normal renal function or mild renal impairment, 7.5mg BID to subjects with moderate renal impairment, and 7.5mg QD to subjects with severe renal impairment. Box refers to the first (Q1) to third quartiles (Q3), and horizontal line within the box is median or second quartile (Q2). Whisker is 1.5 × IQR [1.5 × (Q3 − Q1)] extended from the upper or lower end of the box, and open circles are simulated individual values. $AUC_{ss,0-24h}$, area under the plasma concentration-time curve (0–24h) at steady state; $C_{max,ss}$, maximum plasma concentration at steady state. *(Based on Yin OQ, Merante D, Truitt K, Miller R. Population pharmacokinetic modeling and simulation for assessing renal impairment effect on the pharmacokinetics of mirogabalin. J Clin Pharmacol 2016;56(2):203–212. doi:10.1002/jcph.584.)*

After adding the covariate relationships into the final model, intersubject variability in V_2, CL_R, and CL_{NR} were notably reduced as compared to the base model. Intersubject variability of V_2 was 24.1% in the base model and 17.4% in the final model. Intersubject variability was reduced from 89.5% to 24.6%, and 34.5% to 28.5%, for CL_R and CL_{NR}, respectively.

Upon confirmation of the model performance by goodness-of-fit and VPC plots, as well as evaluation of model robustness by nonparametric bootstrapping, simulation was conducted to estimate the steady-state C_{max} ($C_{max,ss}$) and AUC (AUC_{ss}) of mirogabalin, with various dose-adjustment scenarios in subjects with renal impairment. Fig. 9.8 shows simulated $C_{max,ss}$ and AUC_{ss} of mirogabalin, for the following scenario: mirogabalin is given as 15mg twice daily (BID) to subjects with normal renal function or mild renal impairment, 7.5mg BID to subjects with moderate renal impairment, and 7.5mg once daily (QD) to subjects with severe renal impairment. Simulation results showed that in comparison with the normal renal function group receiving mirogabalin 15mg BID, dose reduction by 50% or 75% in subjects with moderate or severe renal impairment would produce similar AUC_{ss}, but 37% or 28% lower $C_{max,ss}$ of mirogabalin. Predicted mirogabalin AUC_{ss} is 26% higher, while $C_{max,ss}$ is similar in subjects with mild renal impairment compared with those having normal renal function taking the same dose. Based on these, together with the knowledge that mirogabalin effect on chronic pain reduction is likely to be driven by the overall systemic exposure (i.e., AUC_{ss} or average concentration over a dosing interval) rather than $C_{max,ss}$, a recommendation was made for a dose reduction by 50% or 75% in subjects with moderate or severe renal impairment, and no dose adjustment for subjects with mild renal impairment [13].

Milademetan case study

Milademetan is a novel small-molecule inhibitor of murine double minute 2 (MDM2) that is in clinical development for the treatment of solid tumors and leukemia. In Phase 1 studies where milademetan was administered as escalating doses of 15–240mg QD in 21 out of 28days per cycle (QD 21/28), high incidences of thrombocytopenia were observed at the maximum tolerated dose of 120mg QD 21/28. Subsequently, population pharmacokinetic and pharmacodynamic modeling was conducted to explore alternative dosing regimens that may mitigate the risk of thrombocytopenia [14].

In the first step, data from two Phase 1 studies in patients with solid tumor ($n = 87$) and one Phase 1 study in patients with leukemia ($n = 37$) were used to develop a population pharmacokinetic model for milademetan. The pharmacokinetic profile of milademetan was described by a two-compartment model with zero-order input into an intermediate depot compartment followed by a first-order input into the central compartment.

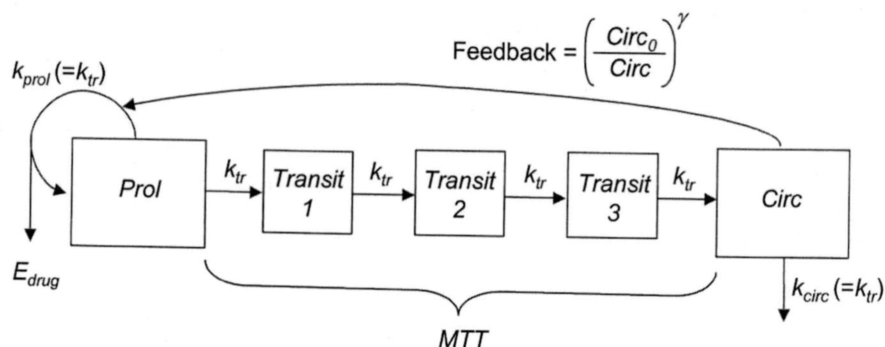

FIG. 9.9 Semimechanistic platelet model. Transit, transit compartment; MTT, mean transit time; *Circ*, circulating platelet; $Circ_0$, baseline value of circulating platelet; γ, feedback term; *Prol*, proliferative cells; K_{prol}, proliferation rate constant; K_{tr}, transit rate constant; K_{circ}, circulation rate constant. *(Based on Friberg LE, Henningsson A, Maas H, Nguyen L, Karlsson MO. Model of chemotherapy-induced myelosuppression with parameter consistency across drugs. J Clin Oncol 2002;20:4713–4721.)*

In the second step, Empirical Bayesian estimates of individual pharmacokinetic parameters from the population pharmacokinetic model were then used to model platelet profiles. A semimechanistic longitudinal model, previously proposed by Friberg et al. [15], was adopted with some modifications to capture the observed platelet count profiles across different doses. As illustrated in Fig. 9.9, the number of cells in the proliferation compartment was determined by the proliferation rate constant (K_{prol}) and a feedback mechanism from the circulating cells $\left(\frac{Circ_0}{Circ}\right)^\gamma$. The feedback loop was included to describe the rebound of cells, with which a mixture model was found to be necessary to account for the heterogeneity in the observed data. That is, different exponent of feedback (γ) was estimated for three subpopulations categorized as weak, moderate, and strong feedback groups. A maturation chain, with transit compartments and transit rate constant (K_{tr}), allowed the description of a time delay between administration and observed effect. Drug effect was modeled as a reduction of K_{prol} by a linear function. At steady state, $K_{prol}=K_{tr}$. Therefore the estimated structural model parameters were baseline platelet count ($Circ_0$), mean transit time (MTT, defined as $MTT=4/K_{tr}$), slope of drug effect, γ, and the corresponding proportion for each subpopulation. Interindividual variability was modeled as an exponential error term on MTT and slope of drug effect. The residual variability was modeled using an additive error model on the log scale of platelet count.

Lastly, based on the developed pharmacokinetic and pharmacodynamic models, simulation was conducted to predict platelet profiles and the risk of thrombocytopenia for various doses and dose regimens of milademetan. Results suggested that less frequent and higher doses, such as 200–340mg 1 week on and 3 weeks off, or on days 1–3 and 15–17, are associated with lower incidence of ≥grade 2 or ≥grade 3 thrombocytopenia, as compared to 120mg QD 21/28 (Table 9.3). Representative simulated profiles for the doses of 120 and 260mg are shown in Fig. 9.10. These alternative dosing regimens were subsequently incorporated into the clinical study, and further evaluation showed consistent results with the model predictions [15–17].

TABLE 9.3 Model-predicted probability (%) of thrombocytopenia with various milademetan dosing regimens.

	Dosing regimen	Grade ≥2	Grade ≥3
120mg	3 Weeks on, 1 week off (QD 21/28)	40.1	29.1
200mg	1 Week on, 3 weeks off	19.9	13.1
	Days 1–3 and 15–17 only	15.7	8.7
260mg	1 Week on, 3 weeks off	27.9	19.9
	Days 1–3 and 15–17 only	24.2	15.3
340mg	1 Week on, 3 weeks off	34.3	28.0
	Days 1–3 and 15–17 only	31.4	26.1

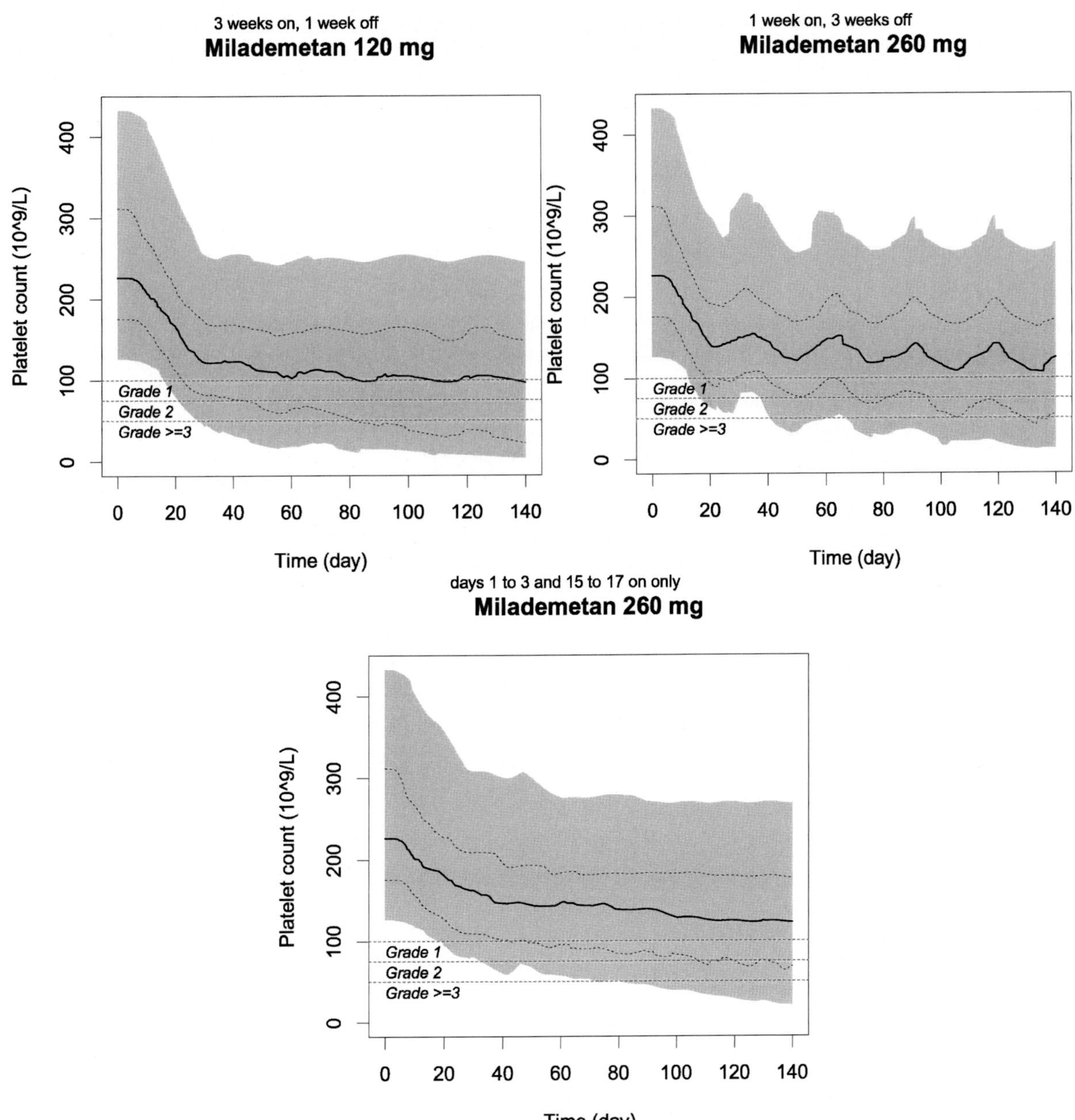

FIG. 9.10 Simulated platelet profiles and risk of thrombocytopenia at milademetan doses of (A) 120mg 3 weeks on and 1 week off, (B) 260mg 1 week on and 3 weeks off, and (C) 260mg on days 1–3 and 15–17 only. *Solid line* corresponds to median, *dashed lines* correspond to the 20th and 80th percentiles of simulated profiles; *shaded areas* correspond to 90% prediction interval ($n = 1000$). *Horizontal red dashed lines* indicate the threshold for grade 1, 2, or 3 thrombocytopenia.

Conclusions

Population pharmacokinetics describes the typical relationships between physiology and pharmacokinetics, the interindividual variability in these relationships, and their residual intraindividual variability. Knowledge of population kinetics can help one choose initial drug dosage, modify dosage appropriately in response to observed drug levels, make rational decisions regarding certain aspects of drug regulation, and elucidate certain research questions in pharmacokinetics. Patients with the disease for which the drug is intended are probably a better source of pharmacokinetic data than healthy subjects. However, this type of data is contaminated by varying quality, accuracy, and precision, as well as by the fact that generally only sparse data is collected from each patient.

Although population pharmacokinetic parameters have been estimated either by fitting all individuals' data together as if there were no kinetic differences, or by fitting each individual's data separately and then combining the individual parameter estimates, these methods have certain theoretical problems which can only be aggravated when the deficiencies of typical clinical data are present. The nonlinear mixed effect analysis avoids many of these deficiencies and provides a flexible means of estimating population pharmacokinetic parameters. Therefore the nonlinear mixed effect modeling approach has gained a lot of popularity and is more commonly used in recent years.

References

[1] Sheiner LB. The population approach to pharmacokinetic data analysis: rationale and standard data analysis methods. Drug Metab Rev 1984;15:153–171.

[2] Beal SL, Sheiner LB. NONMEM user's guides, NONMEM Project Group. San Francisco, CA: University of California; 1989.

[3] Vozeh S, Katz G, Steiner V, Follath F. Population pharmacokinetic parameters in patients treated with oral mexiletine. Eur J Clin Pharmacol 1982;23:445–451.

[4] Sheiner LB, Rosenberg B, Marathe VV. Estimation of population characteristics of pharmacokinetics parameters from routine clinical data. J Pharmacokinet Biopharm 1997;5:445–479.

[5] Grasela TH Jr, Sheiner LB. Pharmacostatistical modeling for observational data. J Pharmacokinet Biopharm 1991;19(Suppl):25S–36S.

[6] Schwartz G. Estimating the dimension of a model. Ann Stat 1978;6:461–464.

[7] Akaike H. A new look at the statistical model identification. IEEE Trans Autom Control 1974;19:716–723.

[8] Karlsson MO, Savic RM. Diagnosing model diagnostics. Clin Pharmacol Ther 2007;82:17–20.

[9] Bergstrand M, Hooker AC, Wallin JE, Karlsson MO. Prediction-corrected visual predictive checks for diagnosing nonlinear mixed effects models. AAPS J 2011;13:143–151.

[10] Nguyen THT, Mouksassi MS, Holford N, Al-Huniti N, Freedman I, Hooker AC, et al. Model evaluation of continuous data pharmacometric models: metrics and graphics. CPT Pharmacometrics Syst Pharmacol 2017;6:87–109.

[11] Yafune A, Ishiguro M. Bootstrap approach for constructing confidence intervals for population pharmacokinetic parameters. I: a use of bootstrap standard error. Stat Med 1999;18:581–599.

[12] Novakovic AM, Wilkins JJ, Dai H, Wade JR, Neuteboom B, Brar S, et al. Changing body weight-based dosing to a flat dose for avelumab in metastatic merkel cell and advanced urothelial carcinoma. Clin Pharmacol Ther 2020;107:588–596.

[13] Yin OQ, Merante D, Truitt K, Miller R. Population pharmacokinetic modeling and simulation for assessing renal impairment effect on the pharmacokinetics of mirogabalin. J Clin Pharmacol 2016;56:203–212.

[14] Kang D, Kumar P, Zernovak O, Song S, Xiong Y, Bergsma T, et al. Population pharmacokinetics and exposure-response analyses of an MDM2 inhibitor milademetan. J Pharmacokinet Pharmacodyn 2018;45(1_Suppl)M-045.

[15] Friberg LE, Henningsson A, Maas H, Nguyen L, Karlsson MO. Model of chemotherapy-induced myelosuppression with parameter consistency across drugs. J Clin Oncol 2002;20:4713–4721.

[16] Bauer TC, Gounder MM, Weise AM, Schwartz GK, Carvajal RD, Kumar P, et al. A Phase 1 study of MDM2 inhibitor DS-3032b in patients with well/de-differentiated liposarcoma (WD/DD LPS), solid tumors (ST) and lymphomas (L). J Clin Oncol 2018;36(15_Suppl):11514.

[17] Gounder M.M, Bauer T.M., Schwartz G.K., LoRusso P., Kumar P., Kato K., et al., Milademetan, an oral MDM2 inhibitor, in well-differentiated/dedifferentiated liposarcoma: results from a Phase 1 study in patients with solid tumors or lymphomas. Euro J Cancer 2020; 138 (2_Suppl): S3–S4.

Chapter 10

Pathways of drug metabolism

R. Scott Obach[a] **and Nina Isoherranen**[b]

[a]*ADME Sciences Group, Medicinal Sciences, Pfizer Inc., Groton, CT, United States,* [b]*Department of Pharmaceutics, School of Pharmacy, University of Washington, Seattle, WA, United States*

Introduction

The major routes of drug elimination are metabolism in the liver, and excretion by the kidneys into urine and by the liver into bile. In addition, drugs can be metabolized to some degree in other organs such as the intestines, lungs, and kidneys. As drug metabolism and excretion are the two processes that together define the clearance of drugs from the body, they are of major interest in assessing dose–exposure relationships and duration of action of medicinal compounds. Differences in drug metabolism between patients are a main contributor to interindividual variability in drug exposures and ultimately clinical response. Therefore understanding the processes that contribute to drug metabolism is of utmost importance to clinical pharmacologists.

The pharmacological action of drugs and other xenobiotics is generally terminated by irreversible biotransformation to metabolites or by direct elimination from the body via excretion and active transport. As discussed in Chapter 5, the renal elimination of drugs, their metabolites, and other xenobiotics is governed by glomerular filtration of the unbound drug and active secretion and passive reabsorption by the tubular cells of the nephron. Hepatic elimination of xenobiotics can involve metabolism by a panel of enzymes and biliary secretion by various transporters. Of these processes, drug metabolism in the liver is responsible for eliminating the majority of therapeutic compounds from the body. The efficient hepatic removal of drugs and other xenobiotics is largely due to the high blood perfusion of the liver, which enables their efficient hepatic delivery, and the high expression of enzymes in hepatocytes, which enable their efficient metabolic transformation. However, other organs can also contribute to drug metabolism. The gut mucosa and metabolic enzymes in the enterocytes are a particularly important site of drug metabolism during the oral absorption of drugs (see Chapter 4), and several drug-metabolizing enzymes such as cytochrome P450 CYP3A4 and glucuronosyl transferases (UGTs) are often highly expressed in the small intestine [1, 2]. As discussed in Chapters 4 and 36, the gut microbiome also makes a potentially important contribution to drug metabolism and xenobiotic transformations. A classic reaction catalyzed by the gut microbiome is the cleavage of glucuronide conjugates by bacterial β-glucuronidase, a key step in enterohepatic recycling of conjugated metabolites.

In addition to being the major route of detoxication and elimination of xenobiotics, drug metabolism can also result in the formation of active metabolites that are important either in the desired pharmacological effects of the drug or in the toxic side effects of the drug [3]. It is increasingly common for pharmacologically inactive *prodrugs* to be developed that have good absorption characteristics but require enzymatic biotransformation to form the active entity. For example, ester drugs such as enalapril are hydrolyzed to their active metabolites, such as enalaprilat. Prasugrel is also hydrolyzed by esterases and then requires oxidation by P450 enzymes to yield its active metabolite. Similarly, several drugs such as tenofovir and 5-fluorouracil require phosphorylation to be activated. Many other examples exist for presence of active metabolites that contribute to the pharmacological action of the drug, such as formation of morphine from codeine, norfluoxetine from fluoxetine, or paliperidone from risperidone. Some of the classic examples of metabolites that contribute to the toxicity of the drug of interest include NAPQI as the metabolite of acetaminophen (Fig. 10.1) [4] and Δ4-ene-valproic acid as the hepatotoxic metabolite of valproic acid [5]. Notably, in both of these cases the major elimination pathway of these drugs is glucuronidation, and the formation of the toxic metabolite is quantitatively a minor pathway in the overall elimination of the drug.

Overall, the complement of metabolic enzymes, the metabolic reactions that they catalyze, and the rate and extent to which metabolites are formed establish the foundation for the sojourn of drugs in the body. As the activity and expression of the drug-metabolizing enzymes is largely controlled by genetic and environmental factors, including coadministered drugs

Atkinson's Principles of Clinical Pharmacology. https://doi.org/10.1016/B978-0-12-819869-8.00001-X

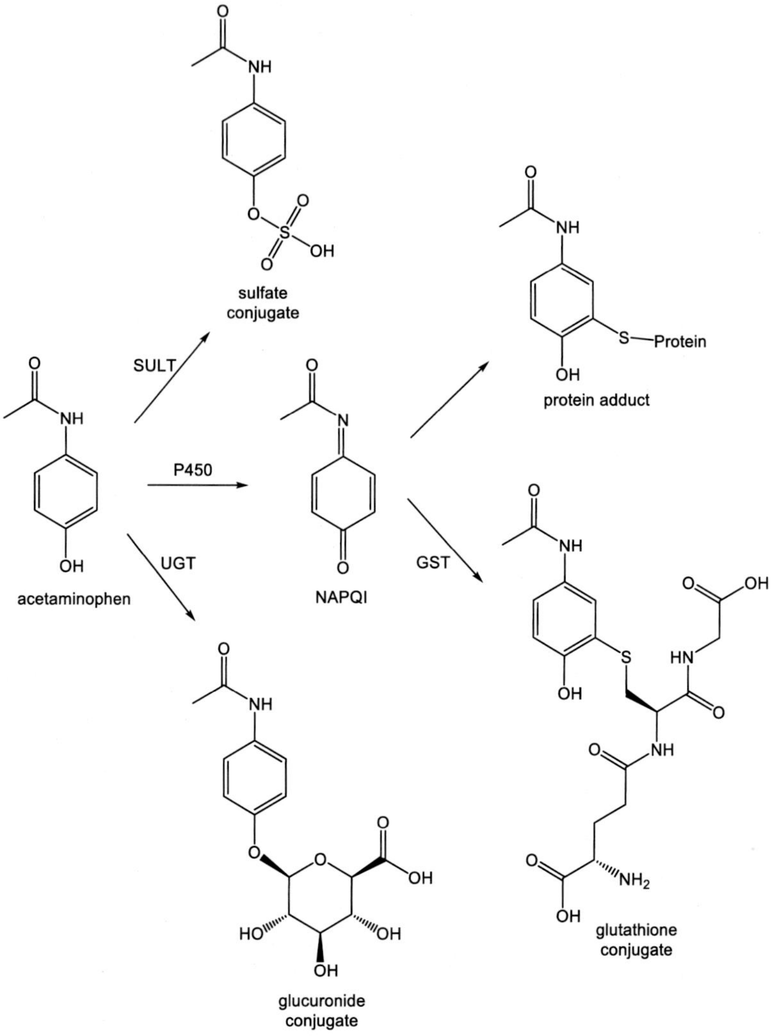

FIG. 10.1 The metabolic pathway for acetaminophen. While most acetaminophen is metabolized by conjugation reactions to form nontoxic glucuronide and sulfate metabolites, a portion is metabolized oxidatively to N-acetylparaquinonimine (NAPQI) which can react with tissue nucleophiles to cause toxicity or be conjugated with glutathione to be detoxicated.

that can alter the expression or activity of metabolic enzymes, knowledge of the biochemistry of drug metabolism is integral for fully understanding the basis for interindividual variability in clinical pharmacology.

The chemistry and enzymology of drug metabolism

Many drugs and xenobiotics are lipophilic compounds that can readily penetrate lipid bilayer membranes and penetrate tissues. Removal of these compounds is facilitated by chemically converting them to more hydrophilic metabolites that are better substrates for transporters that pump them into urine and bile. Clearly this capability evolved long before medicinal chemists designed drugs and it is hypothesized that what we now refer to as the drug-metabolizing enzymes arose to handle the entry of foreign compounds to which we are exposed through the diet, such as plant natural products. So, unlike the enzymes that are involved in the metabolism of endogenous compounds, the drug-metabolizing enzymes must be able to handle a wide variety of chemicals. This requires entire families of drug-metabolizing enzymes that can catalyze reactions on a wide array of foreign compounds. Substrate binding pockets of each of these enzymes are such that they exhibit considerable substrate promiscuity, albeit there can be some trends in substrate types that are handled by individual drug-metabolizing enzymes (e.g., CYP2D6 preference for amines, CYP2C8 preference for large anionic compounds, etc.). In fact, the ability of these enzymes to metabolize drugs is so good that considerable research is required to design new drugs that have a metabolic clearance that is not too high to provide efficacious exposures.

Drug metabolism reactions can be considered to be of two types: functionalization reactions (such as oxidations) and conjugation reactions. In the past, these have also been referred to as "Phase 1 and Phase 2" to indicate that a drug would first be hydroxylated and then the hydroxy substituent could be conjugated with a hydrophilic entity such as glucuronic acid or sulfuric acid. However, this terminology, while common, is a misnomer as there are many drugs that undergo "Phase 2" conjugation reactions directly, and there have even been rare instances where a conjugated metabolite undergoes subsequent "Phase 1" oxidation. Also, xenobiotic and drug metabolism has sometimes been referred to as "detoxication" but this is also a misnomer as it can be the case that the metabolite generated is more toxic than the parent compound. Thus it is best to keep in mind that, with few exceptions, the central theme of drug metabolism is to convert lipophilic membrane permeable drugs into hydrophilic membrane impermeable metabolites that are more readily excreted from the body.

Oxidations and nonconjugation reactions

Cytochrome P450 monooxygenases

In synthetic chemistry, it is extremely difficult to carry out reactions selectively at unactivated C—H bonds. Yet, this is what cytochrome P450 enzymes are capable of doing, and considerable research has been carried out for more than 60 years to understand how these enzymes catalyze their reactions. Common drug metabolism reactions catalyzed by P450 enzymes include hydroxylations, epoxidations, N-dealkylations, O-dealkylations, desaturations, N-oxidations, oxidative ester cleavages, and others (Fig. 10.2) [6]. Two very important concepts must be kept in mind to appreciate how all of these different chemistries can be catalyzed by one group of enzymes:

(1) Irrespective of the reaction that ultimately occurs, all P450s have a common basic mechanism.
(2) The type of reaction catalyzed for a given drug depends on the chemical substituent of the drug that is presented to the active center of the enzyme. This is dictated by the binding orientation of the drug to the enzyme.

Some other important facts essential to understanding cytochrome P450-catalyzed drug metabolism are as follows:

(1) A drug can be a substrate for more than one P450 enzyme, and this is the case more often than not.
(2) A drug can be converted to more than one metabolite by the same enzyme; if so, the reaction types can be the same or different.

Thus there is a massive array of possible drug metabolism reactions catalyzed by P450 enzymes for any drug. Whereas some drugs, especially ones that are larger in size (e.g., MW > 500 Da), have multiple drug metabolism pathways, others

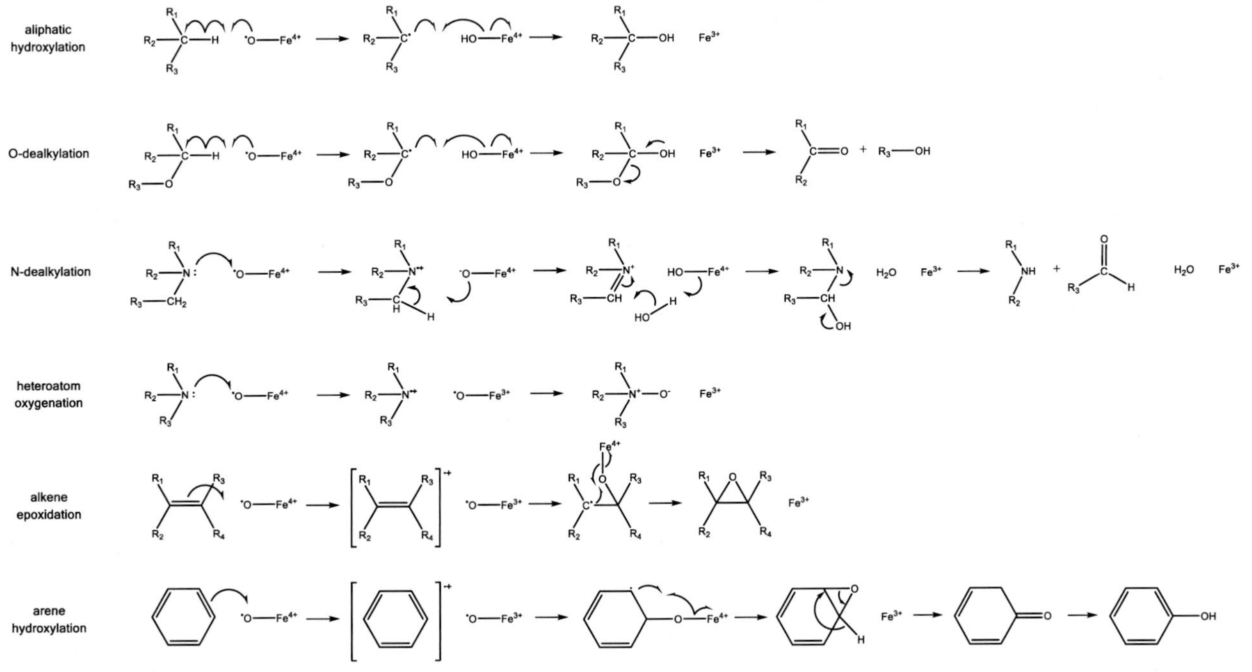

FIG. 10.2 Common drug metabolism reactions catalyzed by P450 enzymes. The reactions all utilize the iron-oxo radical but the nature of the reactions differs depending on the structure of the substrate.

may have fewer or even just one. If a drug is hydrophilic, it is less likely to be a substrate of P450 enzymes and may already be able to be excreted in urine or bile directly without metabolism.

The chemical mechanism of P450 catalysis can be best understood in terms of its general catalytic cycle [7]. Cytochrome P450 is a heme-containing protein in which the iron of the heme is coordinated to four pyrrole nitrogens of the porphyrin with a cysteine sulfhydryl that serves as the fifth ligand to the heme iron atom. (Fig. 10.3) [8]. As opposed to other hemoproteins, it is this fifth ligand that affords the enzyme its unique ability to catalyze drug oxidation reactions and also allows it, when the iron is reduced, to be liganded to carbon monoxide which is the basis for its name because this species absorbs visible light with a wavelength maximum at 450nm (hence "pigment 450"). As shown in Fig. 10.3, the catalytic cycle commences with substrate binding to the enzyme in its oxidized Fe^{3+} state by displacing water which is the sixth ligand of the iron [9]. When this occurs, an electron can be transferred to the iron center from P450 oxidoreductase (POR) using NADPH as the source of the electron, and the iron center is reduced to the Fe^{2+} oxidation state. Oxygen can then bind to the iron yielding an Fe^{3+}-OOH or other equivalent state. A second electron is donated from a second molecule of NADPH via POR (or cytochrome b_5), the O—O bond is broken and water is lost, yielding the highly reactive Fe^{4+}–$O^{\bullet}$ radical. This is the species that is responsible for the reactions that result in drug metabolism.

The chemical reaction that occurs between the drug and the Fe^{4+}–$O^{\bullet}$ species is highly dependent on the chemical substituent of the drug that is oriented closest to the reactive center. The conceptually simplest reaction is carbon hydroxylation (Fig. 10.2). In this reaction, the Fe^{4+}–$O^{\bullet}$ species abstracts a hydrogen atom from the drug leaving a carbon-centered radical. This carbon radical then recombines with the oxygen radical and the iron–oxygen bond is broken, yielding the hydroxylated metabolite which dissociates from the enzyme, is replaced by water, returning the enzyme back to its initial Fe^{3+} state. If the Fe^{4+}–$O^{\bullet}$ species is presented with an aromatic ring or alkene, then the radical abstracts a π electron to initiate the reaction sequence. For amine substrates, the Fe^{4+}–$O^{\bullet}$ species will abstract an electron from the lone pair of the nitrogen to initiate the metabolic transformation. A summary of the mechanisms of the most common P450-catalyzed drug metabolism reactions is shown in Fig. 10.2. There are also numerous unusual reactions catalyzed by these enzymes that are beyond the scope of this chapter. The overall stoichiometry of P450-catalyzed reactions is the consumption of oxygen, two NADPH, and substrate to yield the oxidized metabolite, two NADP, and water. The final metabolite formed depends on the stability of the immediately formed product and subsequent spontaneous rearrangements will determine the structure of the final metabolite.

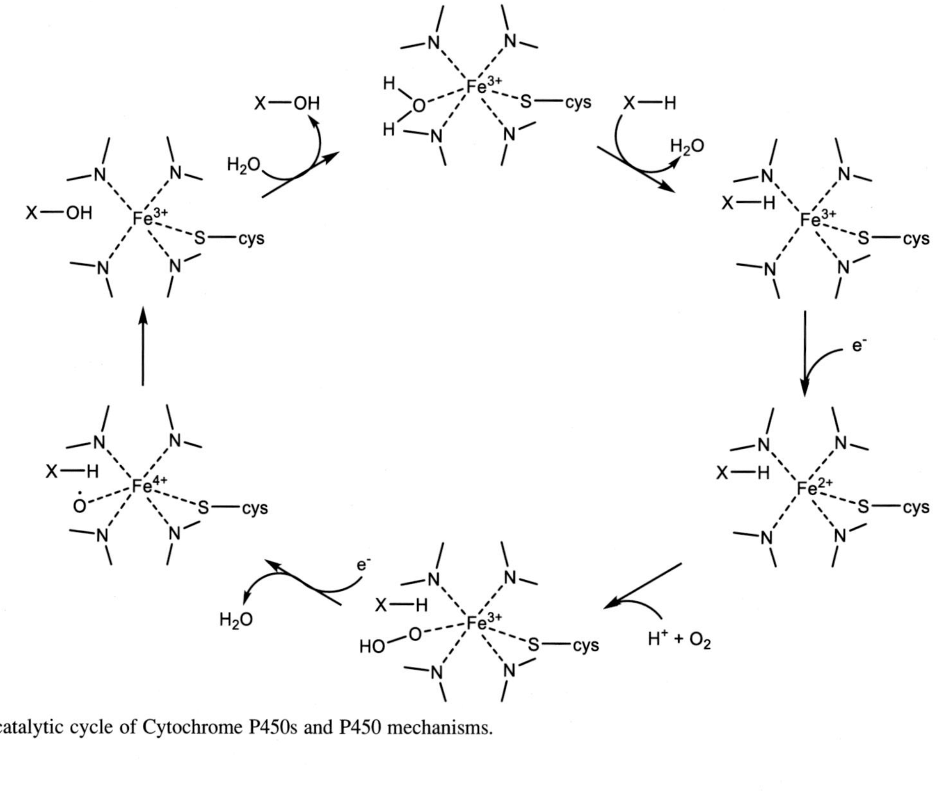

FIG. 10.3 The catalytic cycle of Cytochrome P450s and P450 mechanisms.

Cytochrome P450 families

P450 enzymes are generally considered to be responsible for more than half of all drug metabolism. While P450s are a large family of enzymes all sharing the same general mechanism, only a subset of P450 enzymes are believed to participate in drug metabolism reactions. In general, drug-metabolizing CYPs are all in the 1, 2, and 3 families and include CYP1A, CYP2C, CYP2D, and CYP3A enzymes which are all expressed in the human liver (Table 10.1) [9–11]. Of these, enzymes CYP3A4 and CYP3A5 account for approximately 30% of total hepatic P450 expression and 80% of intestinal P450 expression, and CYP3A4 often contributes to intestinal first pass metabolism of xenobiotics [12].

The CYP3A family

CYP3A enzymes are generally believed to be the most important drug-metabolizing enzymes because they participate in the metabolism of the majority of drugs. Several of the sensitive index substrates (ie drugs that demonstrate an increase in AUC of ≥5-fold with strong inhibitors of a given metabolic pathway in clinical drug–drug interaction studies) of CYP3A4 are listed in Table 10.1 but the complete list of drugs that are metabolized by CYP3A is much more extensive. The most well-characterized examples include midazolam; several statins such as simvastatin, lovastatin, and atorvastatin; various HIV medications such as nelfinavir, ritonavir, and maraviroc; immunosuppressants such as cyclosporin and tacrolimus; and endogenous substrates such as cholesterol, cortisol, steroids, and vitamin D metabolites.

As described in Chapter 12, the expression of CYP3A5 is polymorphic and only a fraction of the population expresses this CYP, with different ethnic groups showing different distributions of the polymorphisms. In contrast, no loss-of-function genetic polymorphisms have as yet been identified in CYP3A4 and this enzyme is considered a promiscuous P450 that is present in all humans. CYP3A4 expression is highly inducible by several mechanisms that involve ligand-activated nuclear receptors such as pregnane X receptor (PXR), glucocorticoid receptor, constitutive androgen receptor (CAR), and vitamin D receptor (VDR) [13]. Furthermore, different mechanisms may be involved in the induction of hepatic and intestinal CYP3A4. The expression levels of CYP3A4 vary considerably between individuals due to constitutive regulation of CYP3A4 expression and within an individual upon exposure to inducers. The most common and well

TABLE 10.1 Common drug-metabolizing enzymes and their sensitive in vivo and in vitro marker substrates.

Enzyme	Common in vivo markers	Common in vitro reactions
CYP1A1/ CYP1A2	caffeine, melatonin, duloxetine, ramelteon, tizanidine	phenacetin O-deethylation, ethoxyresorufin O-dethylation, tacrine 1-hydroxylation
CYP2B6	bupropion, efavirenz	bupropion hydroxylation
CYP2C8	dasabuvir, repaglinide	paclitaxel 6a-hydroxylation, amodiaquine N-deethylation
CYP2C9	tolbutamide, (*S*)-warfarin, ibuprofen, lornoxicam	warfarin 7-hydroxylation, diclofenac 4′-hydroxylation, tolbutamide 4-methyl hydroxylation
CYP2C19	omeprazole, lansoprazole	S-mephenytoin 4′hydroxylation, omeprazole 5-hydroxylation
CYP2D6	atomoxetine, codeine, desipramine, dextromethorphan, metoprolol	dextromethorphan *O*-demethylation, bufuralol 1′-hydroxylation
CYP2E1	chlorzoxazone	chlorzoxazone 6-hydroxylation
CYP3A4	midazolam, lovastatin, simvastatin, alfentanil, tacrolimus, lopinavir, sildenafil	midazolam 1′hydroxylation, testosterone 6β-hydroxylation
AOX		phthalazine oxidation
CES	clopidogrel, oseltamivir, enalapril	
UGT1A1	bilirubin, irinotecan, buprenorphine	bilirubin glucuronidation, ethinyl estradiol glucuronidation
UGT1A4	lamotrigine, olanzapine	lamotrigine N-glucuronidation
UGT2B7	morphine, zidovudine, mycophenolic acid	zidovudine glucuronidation

characterized inducers of CYP3A4 include rifampicin, carbamazepine, and phenobarbital. Dietary components and natural products are also well known to modulate CYP3A4 expression and activity, and one of the well-known dietary inhibitors of CYP3A4 is grapefruit juice. Extensive investigations have shown that grapefruit juice, especially when taken at high quantities, inactivates the intestinal CYP3A4 due to the furanocoumarins present in grapefruit juice. Similar effects are not seen with some other fruit juices such as orange or apple juice.

Another member of the CYP3A family is CYP3A7 which is expressed predominantly in the fetal liver. CYP3A7 appears to have generally lower catalytic activity than CYP3A4 and CYP3A5 but does appear to contribute to the fetal metabolism of some drugs such as glyburide and retinoic acid. While CYP3A4 and CYP3A5 are not expressed in the fetal liver, their expression becomes detectable after birth while CYP3A7 activity disappears at this time.

The CYP2C family

The enzymes in the CYP2C family include CYP2C8, CYP2C9, and CYP2C19. The CYP2C family of P450 enzymes accounts for 20–30% of overall hepatic P450 enzyme expression with CYP2C9 being the most abundant and CYP2C19 the least abundant enzyme in this family [14]. CYP2C9 and CYP2C19 also are subject to genetic variation and polymorphisms that are described in detail in Chapter 12. The enzymes in the CYP2C family appear to be inducible by typical P450 inducers such as phenobarbital but the magnitude of both in vitro and in vivo induction is usually much smaller than is observed with CYP3A4. Despite their high sequence similarity, the three CYP2C enzymes have different substrate preferences and limited substrate overlap. CYP2C9 appears to prefer acidic drugs, and its classic substrates include (*S*)-warfarin and nonsteroidal antiinflammatory drugs such as diclofenac and ibuprofen. The hydroxylation of (*S*)-warfarin by CYP2C9 is of particular clinical interest, as those CYP2C9 genetic polymorphisms that result in reduced activity have been linked to increased bleeding events after warfarin dosing. Similarly, inhibition of CYP2C9 by coadministered drugs also remains a concern with warfarin dosing. CYP2C9 is also the critical enzyme clearing phenytoin, and the nonlinear kinetics and saturable elimination of phenytoin described in Chapter 2 is due to the Michaelis–Menten kinetics exhibited by CYP2C9 metabolism. The classic substrate of CYP2C19 has been (*S*)-mephenytoin but, as (*S*)-mephenytoin is no longer available for clinical therapy, it is only used currently as an in vitro probe. The best characterized index substrates of CYP2C19 that are in current clinical use are some of the proton pump inhibitors, including omeprazole, esomeprazole, and pantoprazole. CYP2C19 also metabolizes many of the selective serotonin reuptake inhibitors (SSRIs) such as citalopram and fluoxetine. The role of CYP2C19 in the bioactivation of clopidogrel is clinically significant because genetic polymorphisms that decrease CYP2C19 activity have been shown to decrease the anticoagulant efficacy of clopidogrel. CYP2C19 genetic polymorphisms are relatively common, so considerable interindividual variability can be expected in the clearance of drugs that have significant CYP2C19 elimination pathways.

CYP2C8 was identified as a drug-metabolizing enzyme later than CYP2C9 and CYP2C19 and there is still a lack of specific in vivo index substrates for CYP2C8, partially due to the substrate overlap between CYP2C8 and OATP transporters. Dasabuvir and repaglinide are considered sensitive in vivo substrates of CYP2C8 but both compounds are also eliminated by other P450 enzymes, so drug interactions with these two substrates need to be considered in this context. Amodiaquine *N*-demethylation has been identified as a selective reaction for CYP2C8 that is useful as an in vitro marker [15]. In addition, CYP2C8 seems to accept some unusual substrates such as gemfibrozil glucuronide which has been shown to be a time-dependent inhibitor of CYP2C8 that increases the exposure of CYP2C8 substrates in vivo.

The CYP2D6 family

CYP2D6 is one of the best characterized P450 enzymes largely due to the extensive genetic polymorphisms that affect its activity (see Chapter 12 for details). Classic marker substrates of CYP2D6 include debrisoquine and sparteine, and the variability in the metabolism of these two substrates originally led to the discovery of CYP2D6 genetic variability [16]. A large number of drugs in current use are substrates of CYP2D6 and include opioid analgesics such as dextromethorphan, codeine, and oxycodone, β-blockers such as metoprolol, antiarrhythmics, and many antidepressants, including tricyclics like desipramine, and SSRIs like fluoxetine, paroxetine, and venlafaxine. Due to the extensive variation in CYP2D6 activity within a population, several phenotyping markers of CYP2D6 activity have been developed that are widely used to assess the overall CYP2D6 status of an individual and to differentiate poor metabolizers from extensive, intermediate, and ultrarapid metabolizers. CYP2D6 does not appear to be inducible by classic CYP inducers such as rifampicin or carbamazepine. However, as described in Chapter 23, a striking increase in CYP2D6 expression occurs during pregnancy suggesting that constitutive CYP2D6 expression is under transcriptional regulation, and some variability in CYP2D6 expression within a population can be expected due to transcriptional regulation.

The CYP 1A family

CYP1A2 usually prefers planar compounds as substrates, and typical substrates of CYP1A2 include caffeine, theophylline, tizanidine, and ramelteon and endogenous melatonin. CYP1A2 is fairly abundant in the liver but its role in drug clearance is rather limited relative to the CYP2C, CYP2D, and CYP3A enzymes. On the other hand, CYP1A2 is one of the key enzymes involved in the elimination of many environmental pollutants and pesticides. While CYP1A2 appears to be mainly expressed in the liver, the second member of the CYP1A family CYP1A1 has significant extrahepatic expression and is present in the lung, intestine, and the placenta. Both CYP1A1 and CYP1A2 are induced by aryl hydrocarbon receptor (AhR) mediated mechanisms [17]. The most pronounced manifestation of this mechanism is the induction of CYP1A2 by tobacco smoking. CYP1A2 also has been shown to be induced in vitro by omeprazole but the mechanism of this induction is still unclear. In contrast, oral contraceptives and estrogen replacement therapy appear to decrease CYP1A2 expression and CYP1A2 activity is known to be significantly reduced during pregnancy. CYP1A2 activity is also decreased by inflammation and infection and that can result in considerable variability in exposure to CYP1A2 substrates.

Non-CYP oxidations

Flavin-containing monooxygenases

Flavin-containing monooxygenase (FMO) enzymes catalyze the oxygenation of drugs with nucleophilic heteroatoms (e.g., nitrogen and sulfur) [18]. For N-oxygenations, a rule of thumb is that if the nitrogen is not basic (as in an aniline, pyridine, or pyrimidine) an N-oxygenation is catalyzed by P450 but if it is basic (as in an alkylamine) then the reaction can be catalyzed by FMO, P450, or both. Although both enzymes use NADPH as their cofactor, FMOs are very heat labile, so heat inactivation has been used to differentiate FMO from P450 contributions to microsomal drug metabolism. FMO-catalyzed reactions are equivalent to using hydrogen peroxide or a peracid to N or S-oxygenate as a reactant in chemical synthesis. The mechanism of FMO catalysis diagrammed in Fig. 10.4 begins with reduction of the FAD cofactor to $FADH_2$ [19]. This then reacts with molecular oxygen to yield the C(4a) peroxide and it is this intermediate that oxygenates the substrate. The nucleophilic heteroatom, N or S, attacks the electrophilic peroxo oxygen to form the oxygenated metabolite and hydroxy FADH. The latter then loses water to regenerate the FAD.

The family of FMOs includes five members of which FMO1, FMO3, and FMO5 are of interest for drug metabolism. FMO3 and FMO5 are expressed in the liver with FMO3 being the main hepatic FMO [20]. FMO1 is present in the kidney, intestines, and fetal liver and FMO3 is also expressed in the kidney and lungs. Classic substrates of FMOs include nicotine and voriconazole which both undergo N-oxidation by FMOs. Another FMO substrate of interest is trimethylamine which undergoes N-oxidation by FMO to form TMAO and genetic mutations in FMO3 that yield an inactive enzyme cause inherited trimethylaminuria (fish odor syndrome). Interestingly, it also appears that FMO3 expression is sexually dimorphic with FMO3 expression being higher in females. Testosterone appears to repress FMO3 expression and estrogen potentially upregulates FMO3 via an estrogen receptor binding element in the FMO promoter.

Monoamine oxidases

Monoamine oxidases (MAO-A and MAO-B) are ordinarily associated with the metabolism of endogenous neurotransmitters and inhibitors of these enzymes have been used to treat psychiatric conditions. They are also expressed in the liver as well as the brain where they can metabolize some drugs, such as sumatriptan, selegiline, and sertraline. Amines are the specific substrates of these enzymes and they catalyze N-dealkylation and deamination reactions.

The chemical mechanism, shown as reaction 1 in Fig. 10.5, begins with oxidation of the amine to an imine intermediate and the reduction of a flavin adenine dinucleotide (FAD) cofactor in the enzyme to $FADH_2$. The imine is hydrolyzed to the amine and aldehyde, much like in the N-dealkylation reactions catalyzed by P450. If the amine substrate is cyclic, the imine may be the ultimate product and if it is a tertiary cyclic amine, the cyclic iminium ion is likely the stable metabolite. The reaction completes by reoxidation of the $FADH_2$ to FAD using molecular oxygen which yields hydrogen peroxide. Thus the overall stoichiometry is the generation of H_2O_2 and imine product from O_2 and amine substrate, with the imine product either staying as an imine or spontaneously hydrolyzing to a carbonyl and an amine that has one less alkyl group. If the substrate is a primary amine, then ammonia is the product and the overall reaction is a deamination. An alternate nucleophilic mechanism has also been proposed (Fig. 10.5, reaction 2) wherein the amine substrate actually attacks the flavin directly followed by abstraction of a proton from the alpha carbon, transfer of the electron pair to the amine nitrogen which subsequently reduces the flavin yielding the reduced $FADH_2$ and the imine product [21].

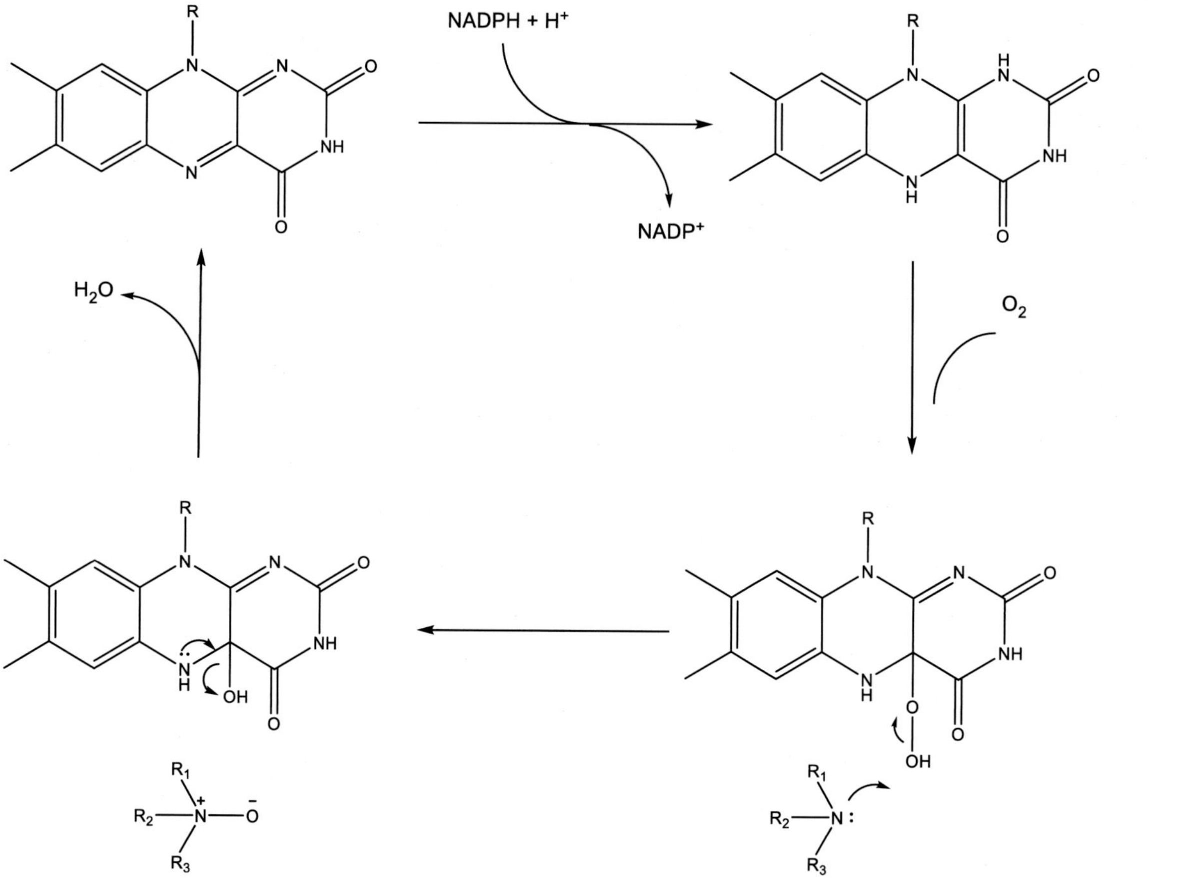

FIG. 10.4 The mechanism of FMO catalysis. The 4a peroxo intermediate is attached by the nucleophilic atom on a drug, like an amine, to generate the oxide product.

Molybdenum-containing oxidases

The molybdenum cofactor containing enzymes, aldehyde oxidase (AO) and xanthine oxidase (XO), catalyze nucleophilic oxidation reactions by adding oxygen to an electrophilic carbon, such as an aldehyde (AO only) or imine bond (AO and XO), to yield carboxylic acids from aldehydes and amides from imines [22]. For AO and XO, the oxidation of the C=N imine is frequently a bond within an azaaromatic structure, such as is present in pyridines, pyrimidines, pyrazines, cinnolines, and their fused multicyclic counterparts. AO and XO are both expressed in the liver but they can also be found in the lung, kidney (AO), small intestine (AO), and adipose tissue (XO). However, the extent of contribution of the extrahepatic expression to drug metabolism is unknown. It is established that XO contributes to the metabolism of mercaptopurine, and coadministration of the XO inhibitor allopurinol can cause an important drug interaction. The contribution of AO to the metabolism of drugs has garnered more recent attention, yet examples of the importance of this enzyme have been known for older examples such as famciclovir, carbazeran, and zaleplon. While inhibitors of AO have been identified in vitro, there are no established drug–drug interactions caused by affecting the activity of AO.

As shown in Fig. 10.6, the oxidation reaction catalyzed by AO and XO begins with the attack of an electrophilic carbon alpha to the nitrogen in an imine or azaaromatic by the nucleophilic oxyanion of the molybdenum cofactor, with transfer of the hydrogen to the sulfur of the molybdenum and displacement of the electron pair in the Mo=S double bond into the molybdenum center to form a putative covalent intermediate and the molybdenum reduced to the 4+ oxidation state [23]. The newly formed C—O bond is hydrolyzed by water to the oxidized metabolite and the molybdenum cofactor. The cofactor is regenerated by oxidation, with oxygen as the terminal acceptor of electrons to yield hydrogen peroxide. The oxygen does not interact directly with the molybdenum cofactor but initiates the flow of electrons through a cascade of flavin and iron–sulfur centers on the enzyme. It should be noted that other electron acceptors, including some drugs, can serve in place of oxygen when oxygen tension is low, thus AO can also catalyze reduction reactions of xenobiotics.

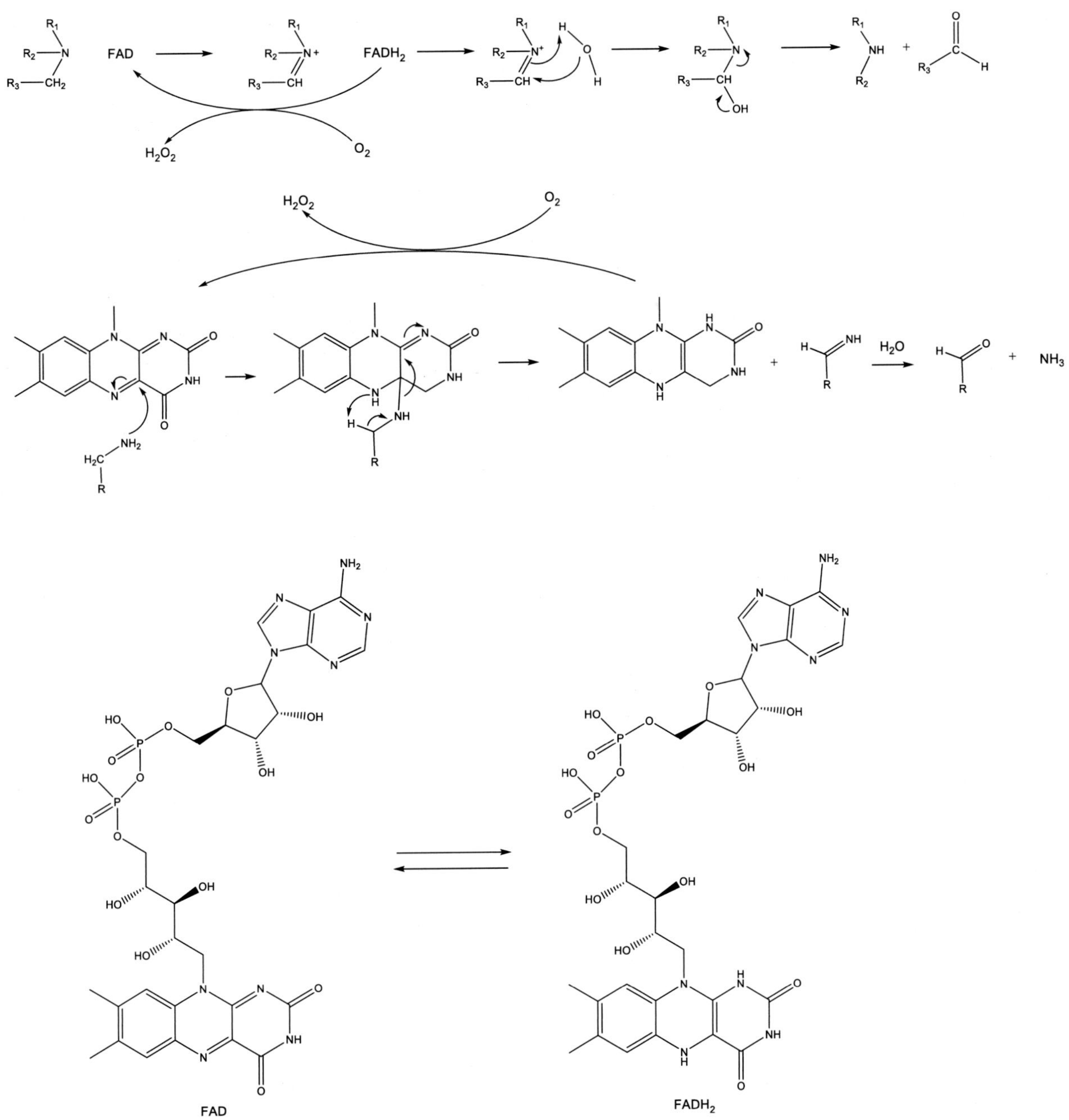

FIG. 10.5 Two proposed reaction mechanisms for monoamine oxidase catalyzed amine oxidations. Reaction 1 is the electron abstraction mechanism and reaction 2 is a nucleophilic attack on FAD by the amine substrate.

In addition, XO can utilize NAD as the terminal acceptor of electrons and in this way act as a dehydrogenase under such conditions, perhaps being how this enzyme actually works in vivo.

Esterases

Ester groups are common in prodrugs and carboxyesterases are the enzymes most likely to be involved in their hydrolysis to the active drug (alcohol or carboxylic acid, depending on the drug). Classic carboxyesterase substrates include dabigatran, oseltamivir, and prasugrel, all of which require ester hydrolysis for activation, as well as methylphenidate and cocaine [24]. The carboxyesterase enzymes important for human drug metabolism include CES1 and CES2. They are expressed in the cytosol and in the endoplasmic reticulum of the liver and small intestine. However, CES1 and CES2 do have different tissue expression patterns. In the liver CES1 appears to be the predominant enzyme, while in the intestine CES2 appears to be the

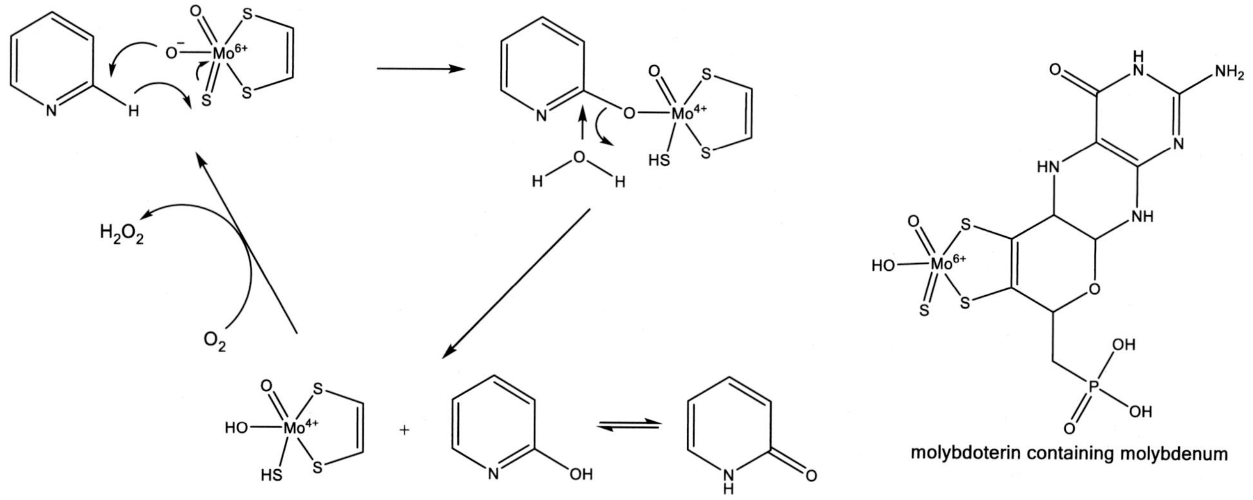

FIG. 10.6 Aldehyde oxidase and xanthine oxidase reaction mechanisms. The reaction begins by nucleophilic attack by the molybdate oxygen on the electrophilic imine-like carbon, followed by hydrolysis by water and reoxidation of the molybdenum center.

main carboxyesterase and there is little CES1 expression. Although substrate specificity is typically low for carboxyesterase, the two enzymes do have some differences in their substrate preference. CES1 prefers esters with small alcohol groups and large acyl groups while CES2 prefers substrates with small acyl groups. Besides CES1 and CES2, there are other esterases known to contribute to drug metabolism. For example, butyrylcholinesterase converts bambuterol to its active β-agonist metabolite terbutyline through hydrolysis of two carbamate bonds.

Carboxyesterases act via a covalent mechanism (Fig. 10.7) wherein an active site serine hydroxyl group, in concert with a close-by histidine imidazole, serves as a nucleophile that transesterifies the substrate [24]. This releases the alcohol portion of the ester and forms a new ester bond between the carboxylic acid portion of the drug and the enzyme. The imidazole then serves as a general base catalyst to activate an active site water to hydrolyze the covalent intermediate, thereby releasing the acid product and restoring the enzyme.

Epoxide hydrolases

Ordinarily epoxide hydrolase (EH) is not considered as an enzyme that can metabolize drugs directly but instead will catalyze the hydrolytic ring opening of epoxide metabolites that have arisen due to P450-catalyzed oxidation of alkenes and aromatic rings. Recent demonstrations of the EH-catalyzed hydrolysis of 4-membered ring analogues, oxetanes, also place this enzyme among those that can be important in metabolic clearance of drugs. Classic examples of epoxide hydrolysis are the hydrolysis of styrene oxide or carbamazepine epoxide [25]. Notably, carbamazepine epoxide is stable enough to circulate in humans and has been evaluated as possible carbamazepine replacement therapy for patients with epilepsy and trigeminal neuralgia [26]. As discussed in Chapter 15, some drugs are metabolized to more chemically reactive epoxide

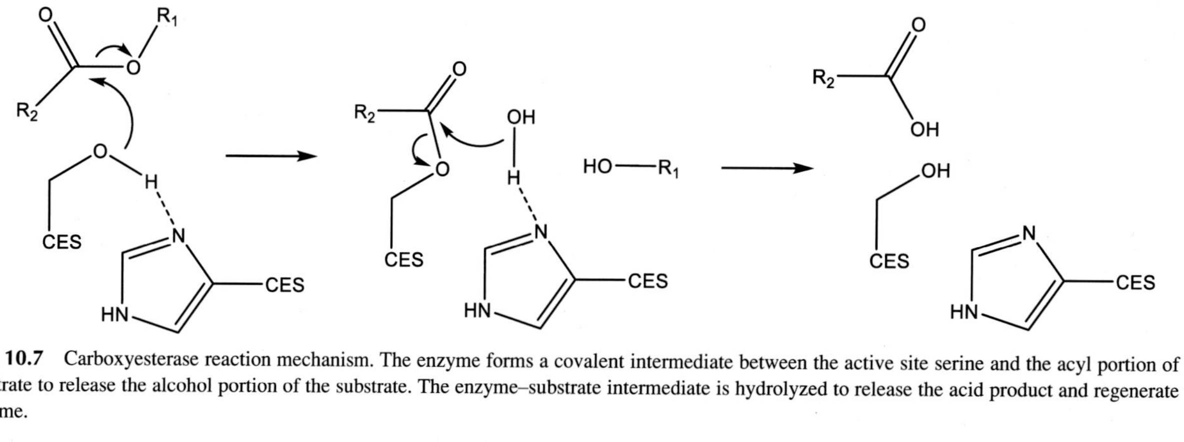

FIG. 10.7 Carboxyesterase reaction mechanism. The enzyme forms a covalent intermediate between the active site serine and the acyl portion of the substrate to release the alcohol portion of the substrate. The enzyme–substrate intermediate is hydrolyzed to release the acid product and regenerate the enzyme.

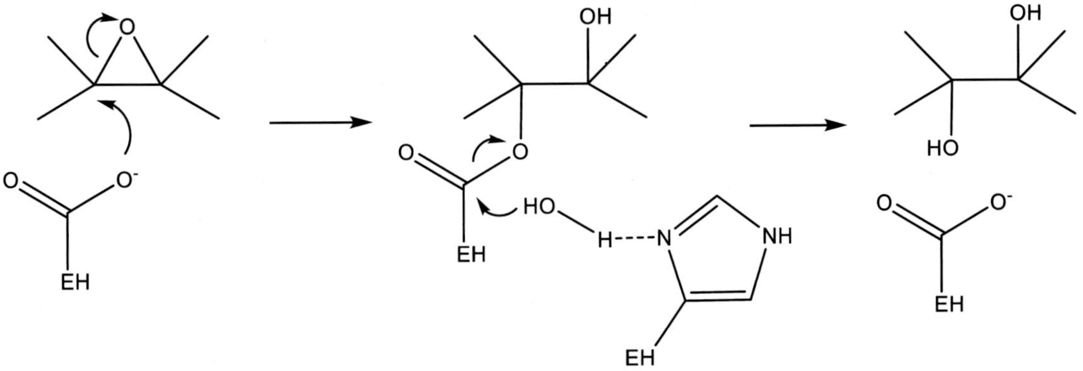

FIG. 10.8 Epoxide hydrolase reaction mechanism. An active site aspartate in the enzyme attacks the epoxide to open the strained ring and generate an enzyme–substrate intermediate. Hydrolysis of the intermediate regenerates the enzyme and releases the diol product.

metabolites that have been implicated in drug toxicity. In either case, EH constitutes an important epoxide clearance pathway. Because of their inherent reactivity, epoxides are rarely a substituent present in drugs (e.g., scopolamine).

Like the previously described carboxyesterases, the mechanism of EH involves a covalent intermediate (Fig. 10.8) [27]. An aspartate residue in EH attacks one of the oxirane carbons of the epoxide (most likely the least sterically hindered carbon), displacing the pair of electrons to the epoxide oxygen. The ester intermediate is hydrolyzed by water in a general base-catalyzed reaction with an imidazole of a histidine residue of the protein serving as the base, to release the diol product.

Conjugation reactions

Glucuronosyl transferases

Glucuronidation is probably the most common of the conjugation reactions. A general theme among the conjugation reactions is that they utilize a high energy cofactor that possesses a good leaving group that is easily displaced by a nucleophile on the drug. Glucuronidation is no exception to this—the glucuronic acid that is added to the drug comes from uridine diphosphoglucuronic acid (UDPGA) as the cosubstrate wherein the leaving group is the phosphodiester UDP. Phosphate is an excellent leaving group since it can maintain a negative charge at neutral pH. The nucleophiles on the drug can be relatively weak such as alcohols and carboxylic acids, or stronger such as phenols, amines, and thiols. The glucuronic acid is attached to UDP in an α configuration. The reaction (Fig. 10.9) proceeds via an S_N2 mechanism which conjugates the drug to the glucuronic acid in the β configuration [28]. Ether, amine, N-carbamoyl, and thio glucuronides are stable metabolites; however, acyl glucuronides can undergo rearrangement or react with tissue nucleophiles.

Humans have a number of UGT enzymes that catalyze glucuronidation reactions but UGT1A and UGT2B are the two main UGT enzyme subfamilies that are important for drug metabolism [29]. Many of the UGT enzymes are not only expressed in the liver and intestines but also in the kidney and throughout the GI tract [30]. The UGT1A enzymes are typically highly inducible and their expression varies considerably in the population because their expression is regulated by a variety of dietary factors, environmental exposures, and endogenous regulators [31]. Classic P450 inducers such as rifampicin induce UGT1A enzymes and drug–drug interactions involving UGT substrates are a concern. In addition, many dietary factors such as resveratrol are known effective regulators of UGT expression. Hormones such as progesterone and estradiol also have been shown to induce UGT1A expression and the activity of the enzymes in the UGT1A family is typically increased during human pregnancy. Notably, it appears that UGT2B enzymes such as UGT2B4 and UGT2B10 are the predominant UGT enzymes in human fetal liver and UGT1A1 expression is absent. UGT2B enzymes constitute $>50\%$ of the total liver UGTs in the adult liver with UGT2B7 being the most abundant ($\sim 28\%$ of total liver UGTs) followed by UGT2B4 (13%) and UGT2B15 (12%). Of the UGT1A enzymes, UGT1A1 and UGT1A4 constitute $\sim 14\%$ of the total liver UGTs each with UGT1A3, UGT1A6, and UGT1A9 each contributing $<10\%$ of total adult liver UGTs [32].

A curious characteristic of the UGT1A enzymes is that they all share exons 2–5 and the different members of this family result from variation in the sequence of exon 1 (i.e., each of the UGT1A family enzymes has its own unique exon 1). Genetic polymorphisms that impact the activity and/or expression of UGT1A enzymes are all within exon 1 with the best characterized polymorphism being UGT1A1*28, which is in the UGT1A1 promoter and affects the transcription of UGT1A1. This polymorphism decreases the expression of UGT1A1 and is associated with the decreased clearance of endogenous

FIG. 10.9 The reaction mechanism for glucuronic acid conjugation by glucuronosyl transferases. The UDPGA cosubstrate is in the alpha configuration. Bimolecular nucleophilic substitution (SN2 attack) by the substrate results in a glucuronide conjugate in the beta configuration with the release of UDP.

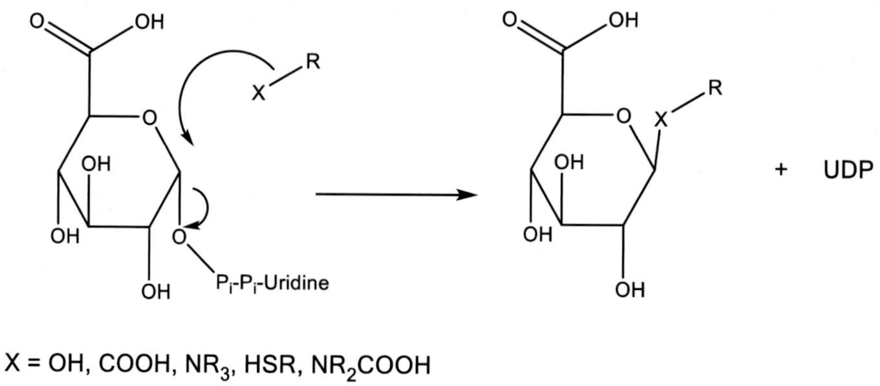

X = OH, COOH, NR_3, HSR, NR_2COOH

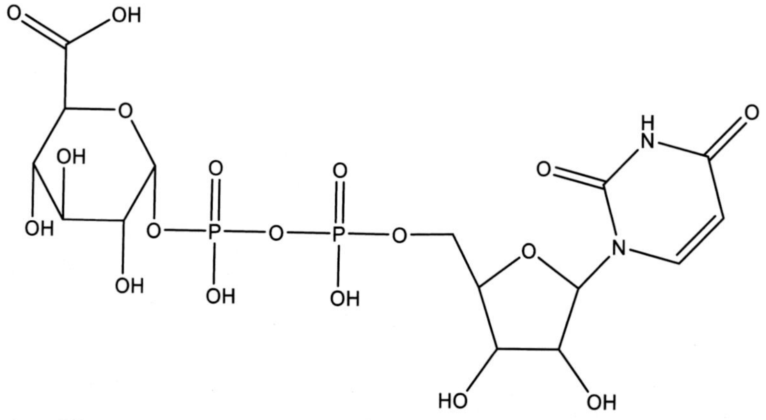

Uridine-5'-diphosphoglucuronic acid (UDPGA)

bilirubin that results in Gilbert's syndrome. UGT1A1*28 polymorphism also increases the risk of toxicity in patients treated with the antineoplastic drug irinotecan. The active metabolite of irinotecan SN-38 is cleared predominantly by UGT1A1 and dosage reduction of irinotecan is recommended in subjects with the UGT*28/*28 genotype. The metabolic pathway of irinotecan is shown in Fig. 10.10.

While UGT enzymes often share substrates and tend to be promiscuous in drug metabolism, some UGTs have very specific substrate preferences. For example, UGT1A4 appears to be the predominant catalyst for N-glucuronidation of lamotrigine, this drug being one of the classic substrates for this enzyme [33]. On the other hand, UGT1A1 conjugates several critical endogenous substrates such as bilirubin and estradiol, UGT1A3 and UGT1A6 metabolize valproic acid, acetaminophen, and some planar aromatics, UGT1A9 conjugates propofol, mycophenolic acid, β-blockers such as labetalol and propranolol, and several nonsteroidal antiinflammatory drugs (NSAIDs) such as ibuprofen and naproxen. UGT2B7 is perhaps the best characterized member of the UGT2B family as zidovudine, and most opioids including morphine, codeine, and naloxone are all glucuronidated by this enzyme. In addition, UGT2B7 conjugates oxazepam and number of NSAIDs. UGT2B15 is known for its activity toward oxazepam, lorazepam, and androgens. Yet, the quantitative importance of specific UGT2B enzymes in drug clearance is sometimes difficult to discern because multiple UGT2B enzymes often appear to accept these drugs as substrates.

Sulfotransferases

Sulfonation of phenols, alcohols, and amines yields arylsulfates, alkylsulfates, and sulfamates, respectively [34]. The high energy cosubstrate used by the sulfotransferase (SULT) enzymes is 3′-phosphoadenosine-5′-phosphosulfate [35]. A nucleophilic atom on a drug attacks the phosphosulfate mixed ester and displaces 3′-phosphoadenosine monophosphate (3'phosphoAMP) as the leaving group (Fig. 10.11). Humans have a large number of sulfotransferases and of those the SULT1,

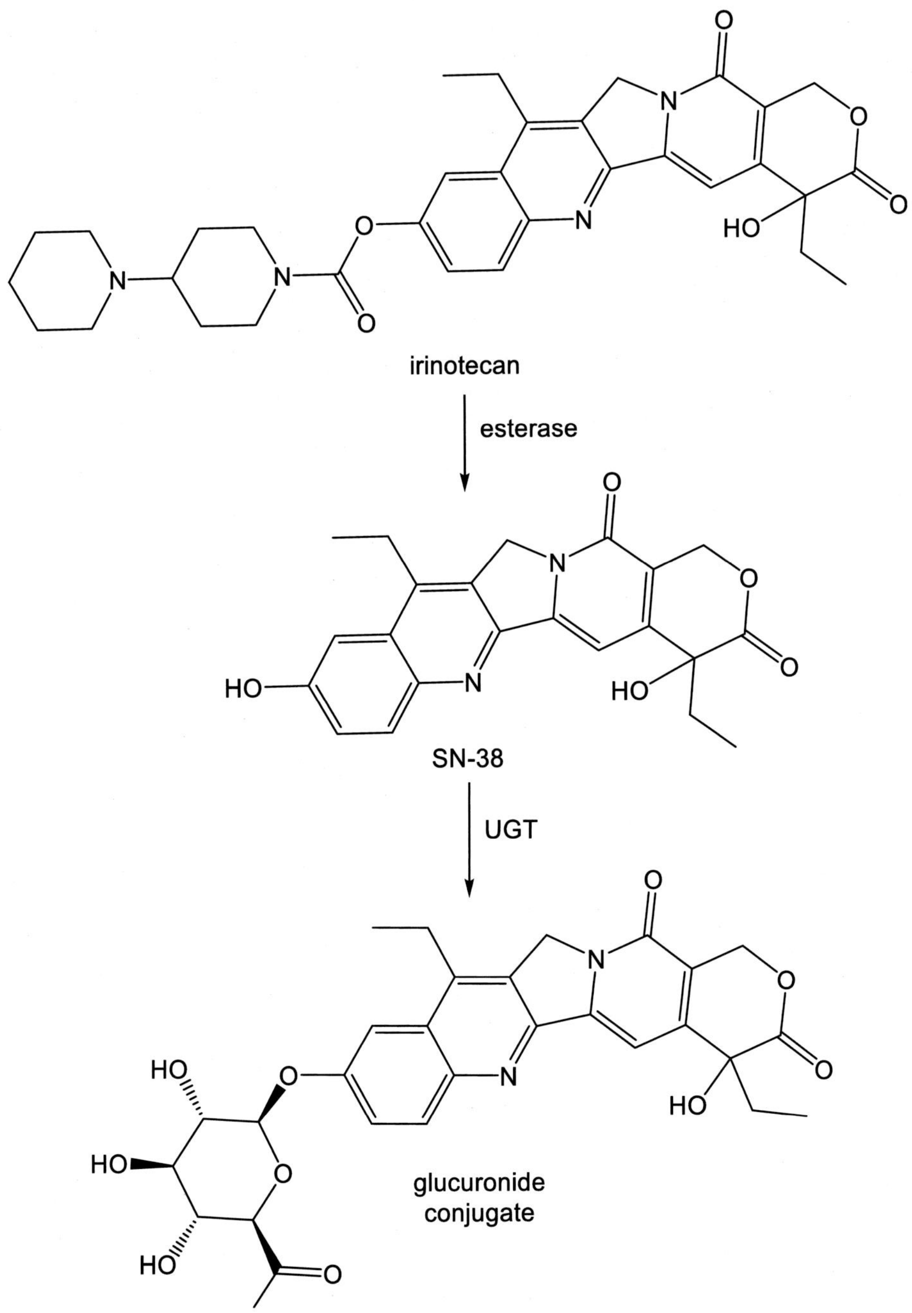

FIG. 10.10 The metabolic pathway for irinotecan. Esterases cleave the carbamate bond releasing the active (and toxic) metabolite SN-38. Glucuronidation of SN-38 renders it inactive and nontoxic. Patients with deficient UGT1A1 can be exposed to higher levels of SN-38 and suffer toxic reactions.

SULT2, and SULT4 families are of greatest interest [36]. Although there are a plethora of SULT substrates, such as ethinylestradiol, acetaminophen, and salbutamol, knowledge is limited regarding the substrate specificity and role of individual SULTs in drug metabolism and conjugation reactions.

Acetyl transferases

N-acetyltransferases (NATs) are cytosolic enzymes that were some of the earliest enzymes characterized for pharmacogenetic variation. The antituberculosis agent isoniazid is a well characterized NAT substrate [37]. The distinct distribution of isoniazid pharmacokinetics led to the discovery of pharmacogenetic variability in the NAT2 enzyme. NAT2 has a large number of genetic polymorphisms and individuals are typically classified on the basis of their phenotype as slow or rapid

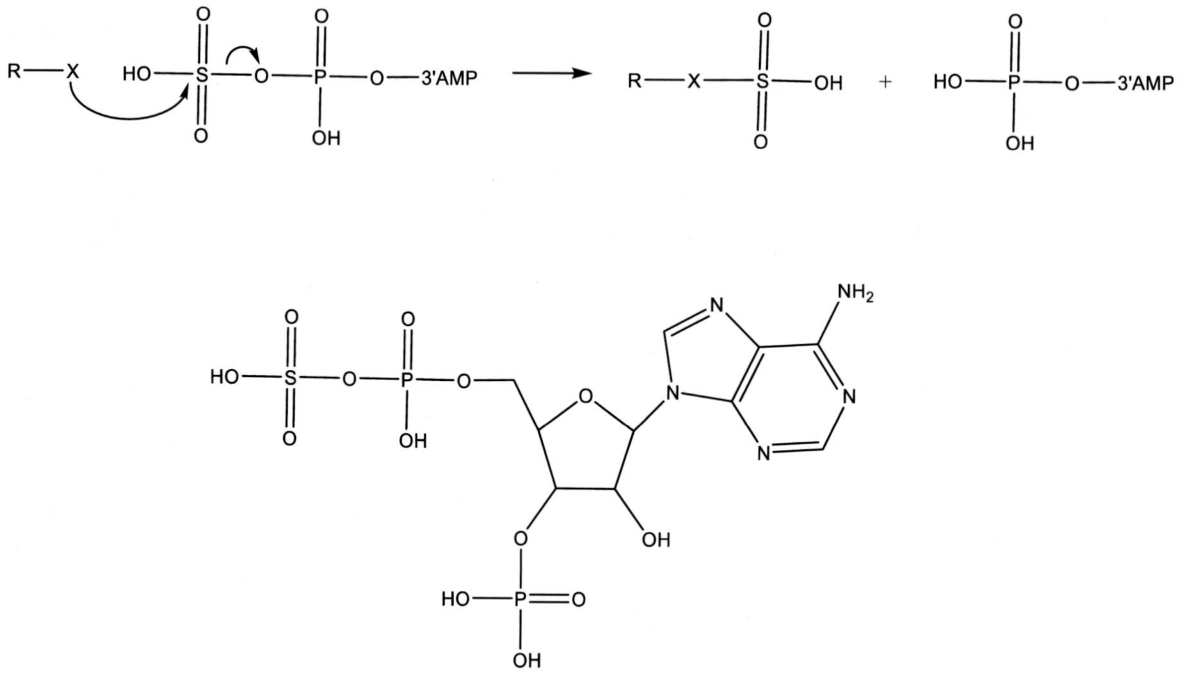

3'-Phosphoadenosine-5'-phosphosulfate

FIG. 10.11 The reaction mechanisms by sulfotransferases. The high energy phosphosulfate ester shown at the bottom of the figure is attacked by weak nucleophiles of substrates (alcohols, phenols, amines) to generate the sulfate ester product, as shown at the top.

acetylators (see Chapter 12). As discussed in Chapter 15, slow acetylators may have a greater risk of developing hepatotoxic reactions from isoniazid than rapid acetylators [38]. Other important NAT2 substrates include procainamide and sulfamethazine. Notable substrates of NAT1 are p-aminosalicylic acid and p-aminobenzoic acid.

Acetylation chemistry takes advantage of a high-energy thioester cosubstrate acetyl-coenzyme A. The thiolate is displaced by the enzyme itself to generate an acetylated enzyme intermediate. This is subsequently attacked by the amine drug to form an amide metabolite and regenerate the enzyme (Fig. 10.12) [37]. This is one of the few instances where the metabolism of a drug yields a metabolite that is more lipophilic than the drug itself. But the nature of the drug is changed considerably since the weakly basic amine group is now a neutral amide group.

Methyltransferases

N-Methyltransferases (NMT), thiomethyltransferase (TMT), thiopurine methyltransferase (TPMT), and catechol *O*-methyltransferase (COMT) catalyze methylation of azaaromatic nitrogen, thiol, thiophenol, or phenolic oxygen, respectively. The methylation reaction utilizes sulfonium chemistry irrespective of which atom type is being methylated. S-Adenosylmethionine contains an electrophilic sulfonium ion that can readily transfer a methyl to a nucleophilic atom on a drug to relieve the cationic character of S-adenosylmethionine to form S-adenosylhomocysteine and a methylated drug as the products (Fig. 10.13) [39]. In some cases, the product is also a cation, such as a pyridinium arising from *N*-methylation of pyridine. In this case, the metabolite is more hydrophilic by virtue of its quaternary ammonium ion character. In others, the product is an ether or thioether and this is another instance in which the metabolite is more hydrophobic than the drug. For *O*-methyl transfer, the reaction involves an oxygen on an aromatic ring and not an alkyl alcohol. Methyltransferases are expressed in the fetal and adult liver as well as in the lung, kidney, and small intestine. Some well-known substrates of methyltransferases include 6-mercaptopurne, 6-thioguanine, and azathioprine.

Glutathione transferases

Glutathione transferase (GST) metabolizes drugs by conjugating them, or usually an oxidized metabolite, with glutathione (GSH). The reaction mechanism is simple nucleophilic attack of the thiol of GSH at the electrophilic center of the drug or

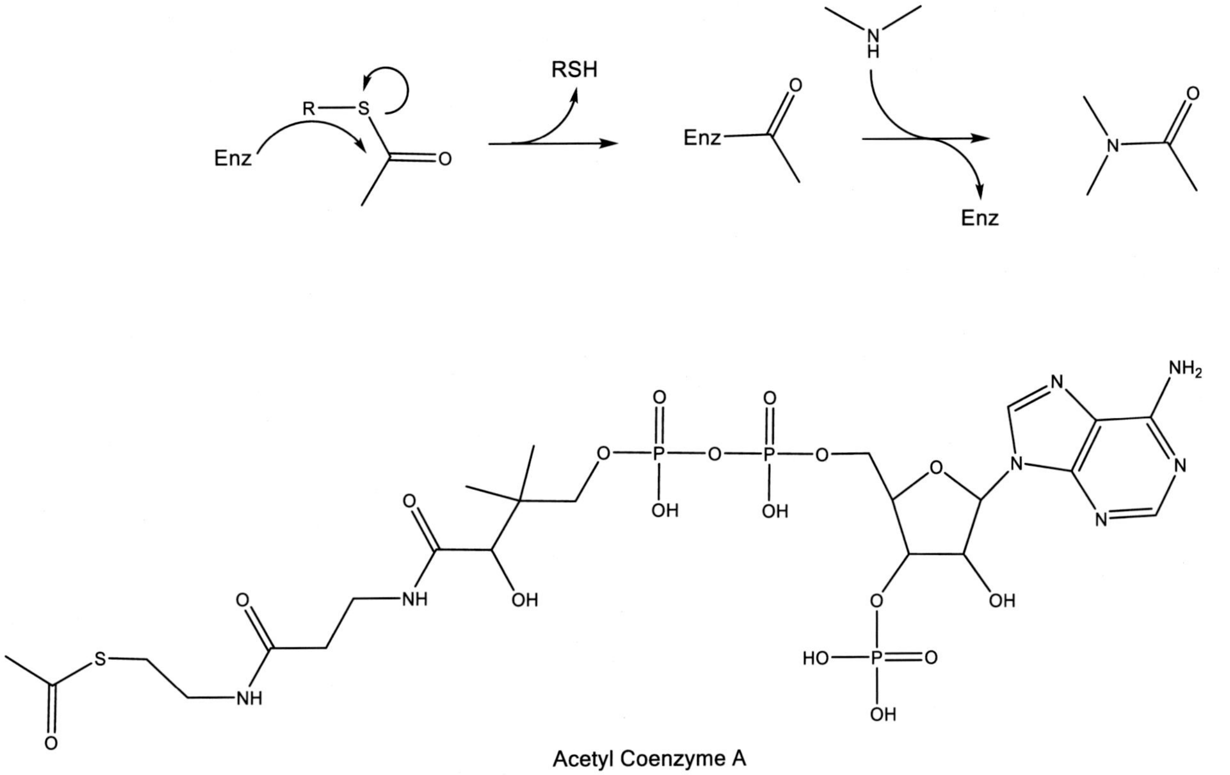

Acetyl Coenzyme A

FIG. 10.12 Acetyltransferase reaction mechanism. The amine or aniline nucleophile attacks the high energy thioester carbonyl to generate the amide product and release coenzyme A.

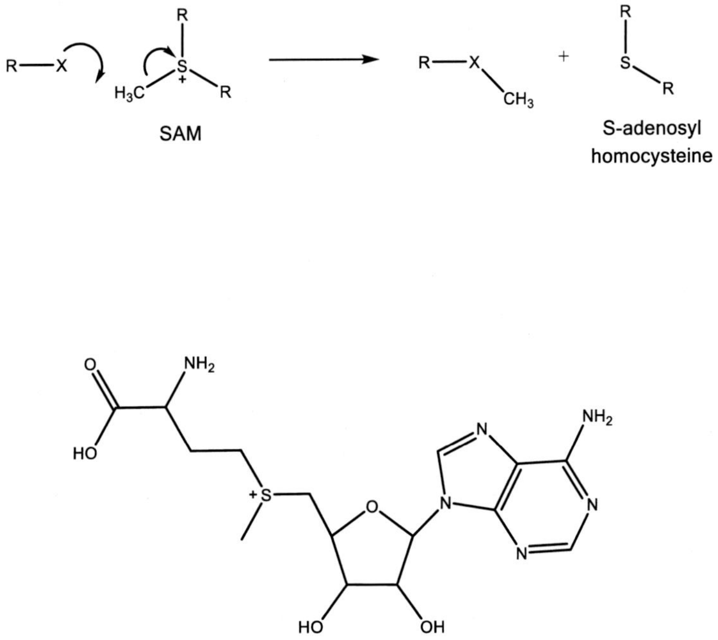

SAM

S-adenosyl homocysteine

S-Adenosylmethionine (SAM)

FIG. 10.13 Mechanism of methylation by methyltransferases. The sulfonium ion of SAM readily transfers the methyl substituent to a nucleophilic atom sulfur, oxygen, or nitrogen in the substrate thereby relieving the positive charge to generate homocysteine.

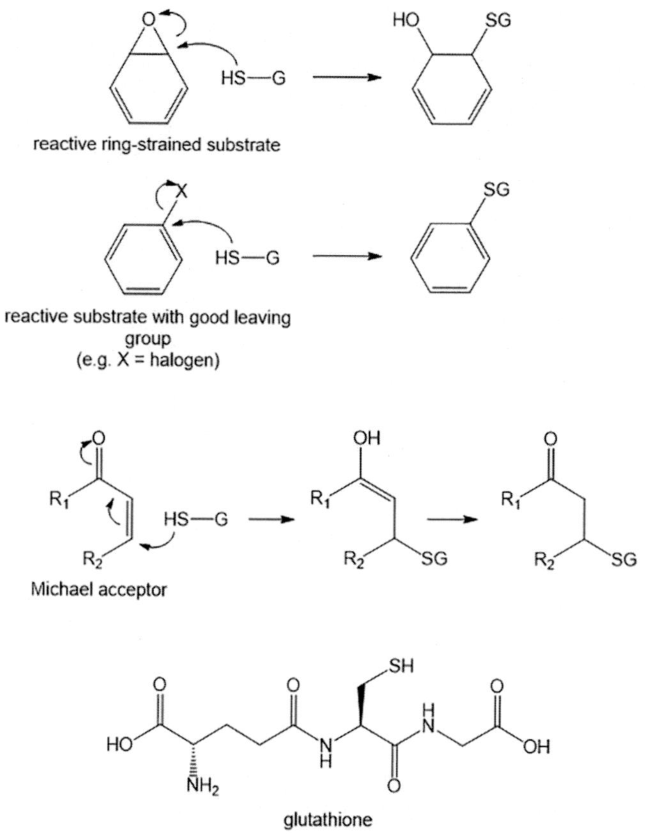

FIG. 10.14 GST reaction mechanism. The thiol (or thiolate) of the cysteine in glutathione serves as a nucleophile that can attack various electrophilic centers of xenobiotics (e.g., aryl halides and Michael acceptors) and reactive metabolites (e.g., epoxides).

metabolite (Fig. 10.14) [40]. Most drugs do not possess electrophiles themselves but these are introduced through oxidative metabolism that in some cases forms a chemically reactive and potentially toxic metabolite, as described in Chapter 15. The transfer of GSH to this metabolite quenches its reactivity and prevents it from adducting to important macromolecules, thereby detoxicating it. In this way, transfer of GSH can be thought of as a drug clearance pathway. However, more recently, some new drugs for oncology indications are intentionally designed with electrophilic centers that can form reversible covalent bonds with their pharmacological targets.

GSTs catalyze reactions that can occur in the absence of enzyme if the substrate and GSH are incubated together at high concentration and weakly alkaline pH. In contrast to the other drug-metabolizing enzymes described where enzyme catalysis requires high energy cosubstrates and/or complex multistep reactions, GSTs are marginal catalysts and may serve mostly to bring the substrates in close proximity for reaction. The thiol substituent of glutathione is nucleophilic and if deprotonated the thiolate anion is highly nucleophilic. Substituents on xenobiotics that can be substrates for adduction by glutathione include epoxides, acrylamides, α,β-unsaturated carbonyl compounds (Michael acceptors), and electrophilic alkyl and aryl halides.

There are several classes of GST enzymes (with nomenclature using Greek letters) but several are more involved in the metabolism of endogenous substances (e.g., prostaglandins and leukotrienes) than drugs. The families associated with the metabolism of foreign compounds such as electrophilic drugs and metabolites mostly include the alpha, mu, and pi classes, each containing one enzyme (pi) or multiple enzymes. Dominant sites of expression include the liver for some (alpha and mu classes) and extrahepatic sites such as blood for others (pi class). This can lead to a complex situation for GST metabolized drugs and as the research tools to evaluate GST metabolism are not as well developed as the CYPs or UGTs, uncertainties can exist in understanding the quantitative roles that each enzyme can contribute to overall drug clearance [41,42]. For example, the cancer drug busulfan is conjugated by several GSTs [43], and this, compounded with known pharmacogenetic variation of GST expression, complicates the clinical use of the drug which usually requires therapeutic drug monitoring guidance [44].

References

[1] Paine MF, Hart HL, Ludington SS, Haining RL, Rettie AE, Zeldin DC. The human intestinal cytochrome P450 "pie". Drug Metab Dispos 2006;34:880–886.

[2] Shen DD, Kunze KL, Thummel KE. Enzyme-catalyzed processes of first-pass hepatic and intestinal drug extraction. Adv Drug Deliv Rev 1997;27:99–127.

[3] Nelson SD. Mechanisms of the formation and disposition of reactive metabolites that can cause acute liver injruy. Drug Metab Rev 1995;27:147–177.

[4] Holtzman JL. The role of covalent binding to microsomal proteins in the hepatotoxicity of acetaminophen. Drug Metab Rev 1995;27:277–297.

[5] Rettie AE, Rettenmeier AW, Howald WN, Baillie TA. Cytochrome P-450-catalyzed formation of delta 4-VPA, a toxic metabolite of valproic acid. Science 1987;235:890–893.

[6] Guengerich FP. Common and uncommon cytochrome P450 reactions related to metabolism and chemical toxicity. Chem Res Toxicol 2001;14:611–650.

[7] Guengerich FP. Mechanisms of cytochrome P450-catalyzed oxidations. ACS Catal 2018;8:10964–10976.

[8] Ortiz de Montellano PR, De Voss JJ. Oxidizing species in the mechanism of cytochrome P450. Nat Prod Rep 2002;19:477–493.

[9] Guengerich FP. Mechanisms of cytochrome P450 substrate oxidation: MiniReview. J Biochem Mol Toxicol 2007;21:163–168.

[10] Seliskar M, Rozman D. Mammalian cytochromes P450—importance of tissue specificity. Biochim Biophys Acta 1770;2007:458–466.

[11] Zhang H, Wang H, Gao N, Wei J, Tian X, Zhao Y, et al. Physiological content and intrinsic activities of 10 cytochrome P450 isoforms in human normal liver microsomes. J Pharmacol Exp Ther 2016;358:83–93.

[12] Paine MF, Shen DD, Kunze KL, Perkins JD, Marsh CL, McVicar JP, et al. First-pass metabolism of midazolam by the human intestine. Clin Pharmacol Ther 1996;60:14–24.

[13] Gibson GG, Plant NJ, Swales KE, Ayrton A, El-Sankary W. Receptor-dependent transcriptional activation of cytochrome P4503A genes: induction mechanisms, species differences and interindividual variation in man. Xenobiotica 2002;32:165–206.

[14] Enayetallah AE, French RA, Thibodeau MS, Grant DF. Distribution of soluble epoxide hydrolase and of cytochrome P450 2C8, 2C9, and 2J2 in human tissues. J Histochem Cytochem 2004;52:447–454.

[15] Li XQ, Björkman A, Andersson TB, Ridderström M, Masimirembwa CM. Amodiaquine clearance and its metabolism to N-desethylamodiaquine is mediated by CYP2C8: a new high affinity and turnover enzyme-specific probe substrate. J Pharmacol Exp Ther 2002;300:399–407.

[16] Eichelbaum M, Gross AS. The genetic polymorphism of debrisoquine/sparteine metabolism—clinical aspects. Pharmacol Ther 1990;46:377–394.

[17] Li W, Harper PA, Tang BK, Okey AB. Regulation of cytochrome P450 enzymes by aryl hydrocarbon receptor in human cells: CYP1A2 expression in the LS180 colon carcinoma cell line after treatment with 2,3,7,8-tetrachlorodibenzo-p-dioxin or 3-methylcholanthrene. Biochem Pharmacol 1998;56:599–612.

[18] Krueger SK, Williams DE. Mammalian flavin-containing monooxygenases: structure/function, genetic polymorphisms and role in drug metabolism. Pharmacol Ther 2005;106:357–387.

[19] Ziegler DM. Flavin-containing monooxygenases: catalytic mechanism and substrate specificities. Drug Metab Rev 1988;19:1–32.

[20] Cashman JR. Human flavin-containing monooxygenase (form 3): polymorphisms and variations in chemical metabolism. Pharmacogenomics 2002;3:325–339.

[21] Edmondson DE, Mattevi A, Binda C, Li M, Hubalek F. Structure and mechanism of monoamine oxidase. Curr Med Chem 2004;11:1983–1993.

[22] Pryde DC, Dalvie D, Hu Q, Jones P, Obach RS, Tran T. Aldehyde oxidase: an enzyme of emerging importance in drug discovery. J Med Chem 2010;53:8441–8460.

[23] Alfaro JF, Jones JP. Studies on the mechanism of aldehyde oxidase and xanthine oxidase. J Org Chem 2008;73:9469–9472.

[24] Yao J, Chen X, Zheng F, Zhan C. Catalytic reaction mechanism for drug metabolism in human carboxylesterase-1: cocaine hydrolysis pathway. Mol Pharm 2018;15:3871–3880.

[25] Kitteringham NR, Davis C, Howard N, Pirmohamed M, Park BK. Interindividual and interspecies variation in hepatic microsomal epoxide hydrolase activity: studies with cis-stilbene oxide, carbamazepine 10,11-epoxide and naphthalene. J Pharmacol Exp Ther 1996;278:1018–1027.

[26] Tomson T, Almkvist O, Nisson BY, Svensson J-O, Bertilsson L. Carbamazepine-10,11 epoxide in epilepsy—a pilot study. Arch Neurol 1990;471:888–892.

[27] Armstrong RN. Kinetic and chemical mechanism of epoxide hydrolase. Drug Metab Rev 1999;31:71–86.

[28] Kasper CB, Henton D. Glucuronidation. In: Jakoby WB, editor. Enzymatic basis of detoxication. vol. 1. New York: Academic Press; 1980. p. 3–36.

[29] Tukey RH, Strassburg CP. Human UDP-glucuronosyltransferases: metabolism, expression, and disease. Annu Rev Pharmacol Toxicol 2000;40:581–616.

[30] Nakamura A, Nakajima M, Yamanaka H, Fujiwara R, Yokoi T. Expression of UGT1A and UGT2B mRNA in human normal tissues and various cell lines. Drug Metab Dispos 2008;36:1461–1464.

[31] McCarver DG, Hines RN. The ontogeny of human drug-metabolizing enzymes: phase II conjugation enzymes and regulatory mechanisms. J Pharmacol Exp Ther 2002;300:361–366.

[32] Margaillan G, Rouleau M, Klein K, Fallon JK, Caron P, Villeneuve L, et al. Multiplexed targeted quantitative proteomics predicts hepatic glucuronidation potential. Drug Metab Dispos 2015;43:1331–1335.

[33] Hawes EM. N+-glucuronidation, a common pathway in human metabolism of drugs with a tertiary amine group. Drug Metab Dispos 1998;26:830–837.

[34] Kauffman FC. Sulfonation in pharmacology and toxicology. Drug Metab Rev 2004;36:823–843.

[35] Jakoby WB, Sekura RD, Lyon ES, Marcus CJ, Wang J-L. Sulfotransferases. In: Jakoby WB, editor. Enzymatic basis of detoxication. New York: Academic Press; 1980. p. 199–228.
[36] Gamage N, Barnett A, Hempel N, Duggleby RG, Windmill KF, Martin JL, et al. Human sulfotransferases and their role in chemical metabolism. Toxicol Sci 2006;90:5–22.
[37] Steinberg MS, Cohen SN, Weber WW. Isotope exchange studies on rabbit liver N-acetyltransferase. Biochim Biophys Acta 1971;235:89–98.
[38] Dickinson DS, Bailey WC, Hirschowitz BL, Soong S-J, Eidus L, Hodgkin MM. Risk factors for isoniazid (INH)-induced liver dysfunction. J Clin Gastroenterol 1981;3:271–279.
[39] Hegazi MF, Borchardt RT. Schowen RL α-deuterium and carbon-13 isotope effects for methyl transfer catalyzed by catechol-*O*-methyl-transferase: S_N2-like transition state. J Am Chem Soc 1979;101:4359–4365.
[40] Keen JH, Habig WH, Jakoby WB. Mechanism for the several activities of the glutathione S-transferases. J Biol Chem 1976;251:6183–6188.
[41] Leung L, Yang X, Strelevitz TJ, Montgomery J, Brown MF, Zientek MA, et al. Clearance prediction of targeted covalent inhibitors by in vitro-in vivo extrapolation of hepatic and extrahepatic clearance mechanisms. Drug Metab Dispos 2017;45:1–7.
[42] Shibata Y, Chiba M. The role of extrahepatic metabolism in the pharmacokinetics of the targeted covalent inhibitors afatinib, ibrutinib, and neratinib. Drug Metab Dispos 2015;43:375–384.
[43] Czerwinski M, Gibbs JP, Slattery JT. Busulfan conjugation by glutathione S-transferases alpha, mu, and pi. Drug Metab Dispos 1996;24:1015–1019.
[44] Myers AL, Kawedia JD, Champlin RE, Kramer MA, Nieto Y, Ghose R, et al. Clarifying busulfan metabolism and drug interactions to support new therapeutic drug monitoring strategies: a comprehensive review. Expert Opin Drug Metab Toxicol 2017;13:901–903.

Chapter 11

Bioanalytical methods: Technological platforms and method validation

Mark E. Arnold[a] and Brian Booth[b]

[a]Labcorp Drug Development, Westampton, NJ, United States, [b]Office of Clinical Pharmacology, Office of Translational Sciences, Center for Drug Evaluation and Research, US Food and Drug Administration, Silver Spring, MD, United States

The science of clinical pharmacology has applications in clinical practice and drug development. From the use of therapeutic drug monitoring in clinical practice to adjust a patient's drug dose to the selection of a safe and effective dose for developing a new pharmaceutical, clinical pharmacology-based decisions are dependent upon the accurate and reliable measurement of drug, metabolite, and/or biomarker concentrations in the applicable biological matrix. Without reliable assays, the application of clinical pharmacology to patient treatment or drug development is quite limited, if not altogether impossible. Thus it is fundamental that these assays must be properly developed and thoroughly vetted in order to assure that the science of clinical pharmacology can be applied to make sound decisions.

Bioanalytical methods have many important uses in clinical pharmacology. Assays are developed to measure drug concentrations for pharmacokinetic and metabolic analyses, as well as to generate quantitative data from biological matrices for biomarkers. Assay-based biomarkers include a variety of physiological entities such as soluble proteins, systemic organic compounds, RNA or DNA fragments, and even radiological images. The types of bioanalytical platforms used for these applications can vary quite widely. These varied methodologies cannot all be covered in this chapter. Nevertheless, proving the reliability of these assays, or validating them, has become a science unto itself. So this chapter will not only discuss a number of currently used technological platforms but will include a discussion of the principles of assay validation.

One further point needs to be mentioned. In broad terms, assays for drugs can be thought of in terms as developmental (pre-FDA approval) and "patient practice." In drug development, assays are developed to generate data to help understand the behavior of the new drug and support its approval for the US market. Once the drug is approved by the FDA, these assays are essentially "retired"; they are generally no longer used by the drug company. In this setting the FDA Guidance for Industry Bioanalytical Method Validation [1] describes the expectations for ensuring the reliability of bioassays used to measuring analyte concentrations in both nonclinical and clinical studies of drug metabolism and pharmacokinetics. The principles described are also generally applicable to biomarker assays used to support drug development.

On the other hand, assays sometimes are developed during drug development for application and marketing with the drug in clinical practice. These are often termed companion diagnostics or complementary diagnostic assays. Included in this group are "standalone" diagnostic assays that are developed to identify, diagnose, or provide an action point for a clinical intervention. They are used by health care providers to guide patient treatment. The development of these assays is governed by the Center for Devices and Radiological Health (CDRH) at the US FDA, in the form of 510k [2] and/or Premarket Approval (PMA) [3] applications. In addition, the Clinical Laboratory Improvement Amendments (CLIA), as promulgated by the Centers for Medicare and Medicaid Services in the United States, are also applicable to assays developed to inform treatment of patients [4]. Readers who are interested in drug and/or diagnostic development should research official documents published by the appropriate US government agency.

Technological platforms of bioassays

Many different technologies are exploited as the basis for measuring drugs or biomarkers. For small drug molecules, chromatographic methods have generally been employed. Larger therapeutics, e.g., proteins, have been predominantly measured by immunoassays. Newer therapeutic modalities (e.g., gene therapy) are stimulating the development of yet newer approaches. A brief introduction to these techniques is fundamental to understanding the strategy of method validation.

Atkinson's Principles of Clinical Pharmacology. https://doi.org/10.1016/B978-0-12-819869-8.00030-6

High performance/pressure liquid chromatography

Chromatographic methods have been used extensively to measure small molecule drug products. High performance/pressure liquid chromatography (HPLC) is a technique in which a liquid stream (mobile phase) is passed through or over a solid adsorbent and interactions of the analytes in the liquid stream with the adsorbent in the chromatographic column result in the separation of the analytes. The eluent from the column is directed to the detector and the output from the detector is recorded to form a chromatogram in which the analyte and interferences are represented by different chromatographic peaks. HPLC systems are made up of several modules that may be standalone instruments or may be combined within a single housing (Fig. 11.1). One or more liquid pumps are used to deliver the mobile phases from their reservoirs into the system. An autosampler can be used to take a small volume of the sample and inject it into the liquid stream of mobile phase which is directed to the column. The separation of the analytes from other components within the sample occurs on the column and is based on differences in the interactions, i.e., mass transfer, of the analytes in the mobile phase with the column packing material, where the solvation power of the mobile phase is greater than the interaction with the stationary phase and moves the analyte and interferences in the sample through the column at different rates. The differences in the interactions of the analyte and interfering compounds with the stationary phase result in the separation (resolution) of their chromatographic peaks. During method development, the experimental conditions (column packing, mobile phase makeup, linear or gradient mobile phase conditions) are fine tuned to optimize peak separation and peak shape.

Chromatographic column

Inside the HPLC column is the solid adsorbent, also known as the *stationary phase* or packing. Stationary phases are predominantly particulate in nature with some examples using porous solids or string-like polymers. The particles are typically spherical in shape and made of a variety of materials, including silica, polymers, and agarose. Through modification of the surface by the binding of specific molecules, a variety of surface chemistries are generated that provide the different retention properties that are needed to separate molecules as the sample passes through the column in the *mobile phase*. The stationary phase particles are tightly packed into the columns (typically stainless steel). Based on the nature of the bonded molecule (e.g., 2-carbon chains, 18-carbon chains, carboxylic acid) on the particle surface, interactions with the molecules in the sample differ; allowing for the selection of the stationary phase best suited for the analytes of interest [5]. Mobile phases are tailored to the chemistry of the selected stationary phase in order to optimize the separation of the interferences from the analytes of interest. The liquid stream may consist of aqueous or organic solvents in various mixtures and may be combined with different additives which alter the chemistry of the liquid stream to achieve an optimal separation of the analytes of interest from components of the samples that are not of interest (interferences) [5].

Mobile phase

Depending on the type of chromatography (see later), the mobile phase may consist of a single consistent mixture of components (isocratic) or a mixture of components that varies (gradient) over the course of the sample separation which is then recorded in a chromatogram. Mobile phases for reverse phase and hydrophilic interaction liquid chromatography (HILIC)

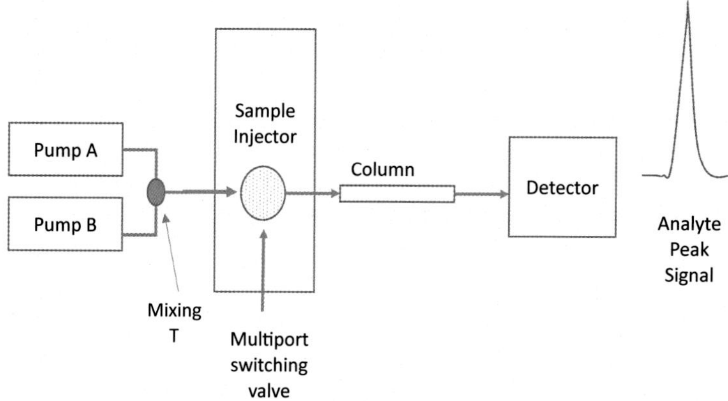

FIG. 11.1 Diagram of HPLC components. Mobile phase pumps A and B provide a consistent flow (isocratic) or variable flow (gradient) of solvents. The mixing T blends the two mobile phases. The mobile phases go to the sample injector, where the sample is introduced into the liquid stream. The sample is carried to the column and based on the interactions of the analyte with the other matrix components, the analyte is resolved prior to going to the detector to be measured as an electronic signal that can be integrated and either the peak height or area is used as the measure of analyte presence.

chromatography use a mixture of water and water-miscible organic solvents (e.g., methanol, acetonitrile) and may include buffers of various strength to maintain consistent pH, as well as other solvents with particular properties that aid in resolution or peak shape (tetrahydrofuran). In normal phase chromatography, only organic miscible solvents and modifiers are used.

Reverse phase chromatography is the most widely used approach for analyzing small molecule drugs and metabolites. It is also used for peptide and protein drug analysis. Stationary phases are nonpolar and mobile phases are mixtures of water and water-miscible solvents that may be modified to have different pH values or solute molarity. The most polar molecules elute first from the column and progress to the least polar compounds. Depending on the strength of the mobile phase, some interfering compounds from the sample may be highly retained and take extensive time to elute, in some cases, eluting in subsequent chromatograms. When a consistent mixture of mobile phase components is used, it is called linear chromatography. If the percentages of two or more components are changed in the final delivered mobile phase over the duration of the chromatographic run, it is considered gradient chromatography and is performed from the lowest concentration of organic solvents to higher concentrations. These higher concentrations must be returned to the lower concentrations and the column conditions stabilized prior to the next injection to ensure consistent retention of the analytes between injections. Gradients that have a high organic content are often used to drive highly retained interferences off the column quickly to prevent their impacting subsequent chromatograms.

Normal phase chromatography uses nonpolar solvents and a polar stationary phase to achieve separation of the sample components. Here, the least polar components elute first while the most polar components are retained and elute later. Ion exchange chromatography uses stationary phases with bonded phases that contain a charge opposite that of the compounds of interest. Thus, interferences that are neutral or have a charge that is opposite to the analyte of interest pass through the column whereas the analyte and similarly charged molecules are retained. However, since the spatial charge of the analyte and similarly charged molecules differs, the interactions with the stationary phase differ and result in separation. Other chromatographic approaches used less frequently in bioanalysis include hydrophilic interaction chromatography (HILIC) and chiral, flash, affinity, size exclusion, and partition chromatography.

Ultra-high performance/pressure liquid chromatography (UPLC) achieves faster separations by using higher flow rates at pressures that are many times higher than those used in HPLC. Under reverse phase conditions, UPLC typically is performed with lower amounts of organic solvent in the mobile phase. The advantages of UPLC are improved sample throughput, reduced solvent cost, and a more environmentally friendly approach (reduced organic solvent consumption and disposal) and has resulted in many adherents. Technical changes in instrumentation (pump designs, seals, and fittings) have been required to deal with pressures.

In contrast to ULPC, a growing trend in chromatography is the use of smaller columns and lower flow rates. Flow rates in the low microliter/min to low nanoliter/min, and even picoliter/min have been shown to improve sensitivities for mass spectrometer detection. In an odd juxtaposition, the reduced flow rate, containing less actual extracted analyte, produces equivalent or superior sensitivity. This is a result of more effective evaporation (of the lower volumes of column eluate) in the MS source, which results in more analyte ions being ejected and drawn to source inlet.

Detectors

Optical detectors have been historically used to detect analytes in the column eluate. These detectors measure light at a wavelength that is absorbed by the analyte (e.g., ultraviolet light) and the reduction in light passing through the liquid stream hitting the sensor is recorded, or the light absorbed by the analyte causes light to be generated at a different wavelength (fluorescence) with higher amounts of the analyte causing the signal to increase. For ultraviolet absorbance assays, specificity is often a problem as the extracted sample may have other components or metabolites present that may also absorb light at the same wavelength. Only by developing an extraction method to purify the sample, and chromatography conditions that separate the drug from its metabolites and other interferences, can specificity be established. Fluorescence assays typically benefit from fewer matrix component interferences and have better specificity because the absorbance and fluorescence wavelengths can both be specified. Currently, mass spectrometers have become the HPLC detectors of choice for the assay of most small molecule drugs (e.g., LC-MS/MS).

Alternative chromatographic approaches

Gas chromatography

Gas chromatography systems use an inert carrier gas (e.g., nitrogen, helium, argon) under pressure flowing past the high-temperature sample inlet to move the vaporized sample through the column to the detector. Some chemicals are not readily volatile and require chemical derivatization to add functional groups that improve volatility. Derivatization may also be required to improve the chromatographic peak shape of the analyte. GC columns sit in temperature-controlled ovens, and isocratic or thermal gradients may be used to aid the separation of the analytes in the column. Modern columns are typically capillary columns with the stationary phases bonded chemically to the inner surfaces of the column. It is the difference in the strength of the interaction of the sample components with the stationary phase versus the carrier gas, and the temperature conditions that determine the rate at which the analyte moves along the column [6].

The use of gas chromatography (GC) with different detectors (e.g., flame ionization detector (FID), flame photometric detector (FPD), nitrogen phosphorus detector (NPD), mass spectrometric detector (MS)) for bioanalysis has waned over the years as LC-MS/MS simplified the analysis of small molecule drugs by eliminating the need for derivatization of the analytes. However, there are some drugs that are easily assayed on that platform. In addition, GC-MS utilization is undergoing a resurgence with the need to analyze the broad array of biomarkers. In particular, the chromatographic power of GC-MS permits separation of related lipids but has the drawback that many lipids need derivatization to improve their volatility [7].

LC-MS/MS and high resolution mass spectrometry (HRMS)

As with any technology, advances have reduced the size of LC-MS instruments from bed-sized to bench top and, at the same time, have improved their sensitivity by orders of magnitude. These changes also came along with improved accuracy in specifying the mass/charge (*m*/*z*) ratio of molecular and fragment mass spectral ions. Although magnetic sector mass spectrometers coupled to a gas chromatograph (GC-MS) were first used for pharmacologic research, quadrupole mass spectrometers are preferred at this time. These mass spectrometers are termed "quadrupole" (quad) because the original designs employed four charged rods (poles) to which alternating or direct current voltages were applied to create electrical fields that can focus ions in the sample with selected mass to charge ratio (*m*/*z*) on the detector at the end of the quadrupole. The types of instruments that fall under the LC-MS category include single quad, triple quad (also known as tandem or QQQ), time of flight (ToF), and orbitraps (ion trap). In addition, some hybrids have been developed that offer the advantages of triple quad instruments and HRMS systems.

LC-interfaced mass spectrometers (Fig. 11.2) take the LC column effluent into them and must first transition the analyte of interest from liquid into the gas phase. There are several probe and ionization chamber (ion source) designs in common use that vary in how the liquid stream is converted into droplets that are then reduced in size and result in the ejection of the analyte into the gas phase (desolvation). In doing so, the ion source provides a positive or negative charge to the analyte. The analyte is drawn to the curtain plate that operates under the opposite charge to the analyte and from there into the mass spectrometer. Excess gas (vaporized mobile phase) is drawn off by a rough vacuum pump. It is sometimes necessary to split the flow going from the chromatograph column to the ion source so as to permit adequate desolvation and ionization of the analytes without overwhelming the source. As the ions pass the curtain plate, they may traverse a space where a curtain gas, typically high purity nitrogen, is used to separate the gasses in the ion source from the very low pressure required by the quadrupole space deeper within the instrument. Ions that transition the curtain gas zone are drawn through one or more small holes in a "skimmer."

Selected ion monitoring (SIM), also known as selected reaction monitoring (SRM), is used in most LC-MS/MS methods, to direct ions of the selected *m*/*z* into the instrument [8]. Because ion monitoring is based on *m*/*z*, it is possible for multiple coeluting compounds to be selected, even if they cannot be separated chromatographically. For example, a compound with a mass of 342 and a single charge would have an *m*/*z* of 342. A similar *m*/*z* would be observed for compounds with a mass of 684 with 2 charges ($m/z = 342 = 684/2$) and for a molecule with a molecular weight of 1026 having 3

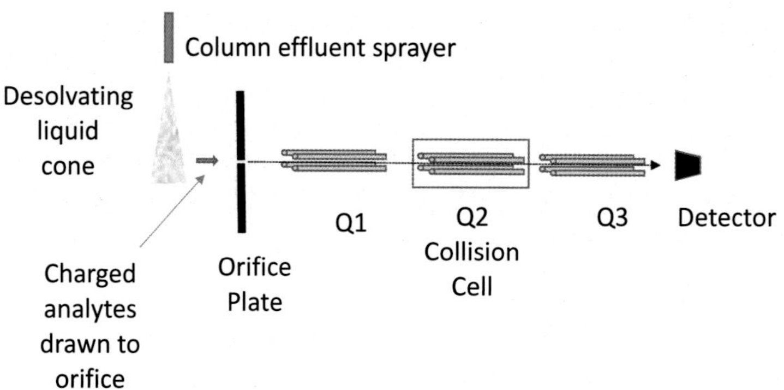

FIG. 11.2 Path of the analytes of interest through a triple quadrupole mass spectrometer. The *dashed line* shows the precursor ions of the analyte once they have entered the source and then through to the second quadrupole (collision cell) where the product ions are formed prior to their being selected in the third quadrupole and sent to the detector.

charges ($m/z = 342 = 1026/3$). However, with LC-MS/MS, ions with the appropriate *m/z* selected in the first quad are passed into the second quadrupole (Q2) which is used as a collision cell to split the compounds into two or more fragments through collisions with a neutral gas. The incoming analyte is designated as the precursor ion and the fragments are known as product ions. Compounds with similar molecular weights but different chemical structures rarely produce product ions with the same *m/z*. The additional electromagnetic fields in the second quadrupole transmit the produced (product) ions into the third quadrupole (Q3), where further electrical fields are used to discard most ions and select the product ion of specific *m/z* related to the analyte. Whether it is the most abundant product ion (providing the best sensitivity) or the one with the least interference, the chosen product ion is transmitted to the detector. This dual selection of the precursor ion and product ion with specific *m/z* provides a powerful selectivity of only ions related to the analyte of interest and reduces the potential for interferences. Modern triple quads have electronics capable of rapid changes in the electrical field strength within the quadrupoles allowing for millisecond changes in the precursor and product ions selected for measurement. This permits multiple analytes (drugs and their metabolites) to be simultaneously measured in the same injection, as well as internal standards (analog or stable isotope labeled).

Internal standards

In all chromatographic methods, the amount of analyte measured can be significantly affected by a number of factors which can have a profound effect on measurement accuracy. Variability or errors in sample handling, sample extraction, injection volumes, solvent evaporation, etc., can lead to inaccuracies in the measurement of the sample. These issues are addressed by the addition of an internal standard (IS) to all the standards and samples in the analysis in the first step of sample preparation in the analytical laboratory. The IS needs to be a compound that is chemically similar to the analyte. Adding the internal standard to all calibrators, quality control samples (QCs) and study samples permit normalization of the drug response in each sample so that concentrations can be generated from calibrator regression curves using the ratio of the drug response to that of the internal standard on the *Y*-axis and the concentration of the drug in the calibrators on the *X*-axis.

For methods using optical detectors the IS should be easily resolved from the drug by the chromatographic procedure. For LC-MS, although the mass spectrometers are highly selective in measuring the drug in the presence of matrix components, those matrix components may enhance or suppress the ionization of the drug in the source, and therefore, the IS should coelute or elute close to the analyte while maintaining good chromatographic properties. In LC-MS methods, internal standards may be structurally similar analogs of the drug or versions of the drug that incorporate stable labeled isotopes of some atoms in the drug. Deuterium, ^{13}C, and ^{15}N are the most common. When a structural analog is used, the further away that it separates chromatographically from the drug, the less likely the same matrix interferences will be present and the analog and drug may not see the same extent of enhanced or suppressed ionization. It also is generally desirable to include three or more stable isotope labels in these internal standards to avoid interference from the natural abundance of stable isotopes in the test drug [9]. The advantage of a stable labeled version of the drug is that it is structurally identical which results in it chromatographing with the drug, thus the ionization enhancement or suppression will be the same. The molecular weight difference between the drug and the stable isotope labeled internal standard is detected by monitoring different *m/z* selections in the mass spectrometer. This makes the stable labeled internal standard the preferred approach for drug measurements by LC-MS methods.

Accelerator mass spectrometry

Accelerator mass spectrometers (AMS) have been used for microdosing pharmacokinetic and metabolism studies (see Chapter 31). The value of AMS is the extreme sensitivity of the measurement and the ability to use a stable labeled drug rather than a radiolabeled drug as a tracer. The shortcoming of AMS is the complex sample preparation that requires both chromatographic fractionation and graphitization prior to introducing the sample into the AMS. Due to its extreme sensitivity, a low specific-activity radiolabeled analog of a drug at the normal dose amount or a microdose of a high specific activity radiolabel is used. In the absence of an internal standard, the sample preparation steps must be carefully undertaken to maintain accuracy and precision as the AMS measures the ^{14}C vs total ^{12}C content. With the introduction of Exploratory IND studies (Phase 0 studies) [10], the use of a radiolabeled subtherapeutic microdose enabled human pharmacokinetic assessments to be conducted prior to obtaining investigational new drug (IND) approval. It also laid the groundwork for other post-IND uses of subtherapeutic microdoses, including their use with AMS in determining absolute bioavailability of an oral drug formulation [11]. These studies represent an extension to AMS and microdosing technology of a more generally available approach that, as described in Chapter 4, used stable isotope-labeled drugs and either GC-MS or LC-MS technology [12, 13].

Immunoassays

Immunoassays (ligand binding assays; LBA) have been developed and are extensively used to measure large molecules such as proteins (e.g., monoclonal antibody drugs). Immunoassays rely on the specific molecular interaction recognition of antibodies (i.e., binding) to capture, detect, and measure an analyte. Immunoassays may use a single molecular interaction or even multiple interactions to achieve analyte detection and measurement. Depending on the reagent molecules used to interact with the analyte, different levels of specificity and sensitivity are achieved. Reagents have historically been receptors, ligands, or antibodies from a variety of species. Currently other motifs also are being used, including small proteins (affimers) or oligonucleotides (aptamers).

At the unimolecular interaction level, the assays are typically based on the competitive assay format. In this format, using a variety of chemistries, there is a ligand, receptor, or antibody to the analyte that is used as the capture reagent and is bound to a substrate surface (e.g., to the bottom of a well in a 96-well plate) in the first step of the assay. The capture molecule must have a surface structure to which a specific, complementary structure (epitope) on the analyte will bind. For antibody drugs, the receptor or ligand to which the antibody binds to achieve activity is frequently chosen as the capture reagent, due to the relative specificity of the reaction. However, due to the potential for endogenous compounds to also bind to the capture reagent, antibodies generated against specific epitopes of the analyte are used to improve assay specificity. The second step of the assay requires mixing the sample containing the analytes with a fixed amount of the analyte that is labeled with a characteristic that permits its detection. To obtain the best sensitivity, the earliest assays used radioactive or chromogenic labels but more recent labels support chromogenic, fluorescent, or electrochemiluminescent readouts. Once mixed and added to the reaction tube or well containing the capture molecule, the two forms of the analyte (from the sample and labeled) compete to bind to the capture molecule (Fig. 11.3). In most assays, the excess labeled analyte and matrix are washed away prior to taking a measurement of the detection reagent. Thus, in competitive assays at low analyte concentrations, the ratio of the bound analyte to bound labeled analyte is small and the measured signal from the labeled analyte is high. As the concentration of the analyte increases, the ratio increases and less labeled analyte is bound resulting in a lower measured signal. When a calibration curve is prepared with known ratios of the analyte and labeled analyte, it, like many immunoassays, is sigmoidal in nature as shown in Fig. 11.4 and like most immune assays typically uses a 4- or 5-parameter logistic regression [14]. A deficiency of the competitive format is that molecules that are not the analyte (interferences) can bind to the capture reagent and compete with the analyte and the labeled analyte detection reagent, thus causing less detection reagent to be bound with the result being biased (high) measured analyte concentration.

Early detection reagents bonded with gamma or beta emitting radioactive molecules and were known as radio immunoassays (RIAs) [15]. While extremely sensitive, the need for special handling precautions in the laboratory, as well as

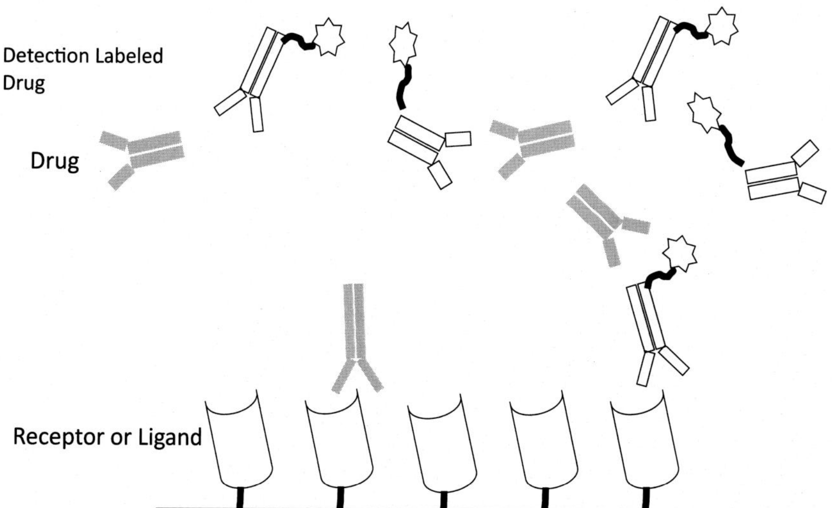

FIG. 11.3 Competitve formatted immunoassay. Fixed amounts of the detection labeled drug are spiked into the patient sample and compete with the drug to bind with the receptor or ligand that acts as the capture reagent. When the drug concentration is low, more detection reagent binds and a larger signal is measured. As the drug concentration increases, less detection reagent binds and the measured signal decreases. Depending on the detection scheme, the detection reagent may have a chromophore, enzyme to generate a chromogenic measured compound, or be part of an electrochemiluminescent signal generation.

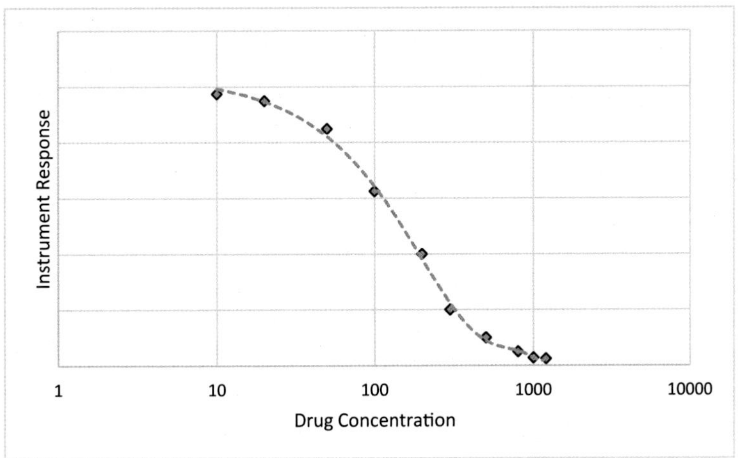

FIG. 11.4 The calibration curve for a competitive formatted immunoassay.

disposal needs, caused a shift toward other detection methods. A common method used today involves attaching an enzyme (e.g., alkaline phosphatase, β-galactosidase, horse radish peroxidase) to the detection reagent and using the enzyme to produce a chromogenic product. These assays are known as enzyme-linked immunosorbent assays (ELISA) [16]. Incubating horseradish peroxidase in the presence of hydrogen peroxide and a suitable substrate (e.g., 3,3′,5,5′-tetramethylbenzidine (TMB)) generates a reduced product (tetramethylbenzidine diimine) with UV absorbance. When used in assays with a calibration curve and fixed incubation times, it is necessary to stop the incubation with a stopping reagent (e.g., acid). The level of reduced TMB can then be compared to a regression line produced from the calibration curve to determine the amount of drug in a study sample. If sulfuric acid is used to stop the reduction of TMB, the reduced product turns yellow and can be measured colorimetrically at 450nm [17]. The value of an enzymatic detection scheme is that each bound enzyme can produce multiple product molecules, thus amplifying the signal to be measured and producing a more sensitive assay. An alternative detection scheme, electrochemiluminescence (ECL), uses an electrical current to drive an oxidative-reduction cycle to produce a radical cation which excites the ruthenium-labeled detection reagent, and as the ruthenium returns to its ground state, it emits a photon of light which is measured by traditional photomultiplier tubes or CCD cameras [18].

Immunoassays may also be based on bimolecular interactions. Two common formats are the sandwich and bridging assays. Similar to the competitive format, in a sandwich assay, a capture molecule is bound to a surface and the sample containing the analyte is added. Here, however, no labeled analyte is used during the capture step and only the analyte binds to the capture molecule. Once binding is completed, the sample matrix is washed away. Then, a buffer is added that contains the detection reagent that will bind to the analyte. After allowing time for binding, excess unbound detection reagent is washed away and an enzyme substrate is added and incubated to produce the chromogen. As the amount of analyte bound increases, there is an increase in bound detection reagent that produces an increase in the amount of chromogen that is measured. As noted for some unimolecular assays, a stopping chemical is typically added to stop further product formation prior to the samples being measured. The format of the assay is presented in Fig. 11.5 and the structure of the curve is presented in Fig. 11.6. A bridging assay is possible for antibody drugs having identical Fab regions or any drug with similar divalency. In this format the capture and detection reagents are designed to bind to the two Fab regions, thus the antibody drug bridges between the two reagents. The advantage of the bridging assay is that only a single reagent is needed to create both the capture and detection reagents. Bridging assays are, however, more prone to endogenous interferences that may bind to the drug [19].

In contrast to the competitive assay, the sandwich assay provides improved specificity by using two molecular interactions with the two different molecular recognition sites to measure the analyte. However, there is still the potential for molecules to interfere with the assay. For instance, if a soluble target molecule is present, it may be bound to the analyte in such a way that the analyte cannot bind to the capture or detection reagents. Advances in generating antibodies to biologic drugs and the development of improved screening practices for them have resulted in antibody reagents that are better characterized and less prone to interferences as compared to the use of ligand or receptor reagents. It is still incumbent on the method developer to be aware of endogenous molecules that might be capable of interfering with the binding of the drug to the reagent and to challenge the assays appropriately.

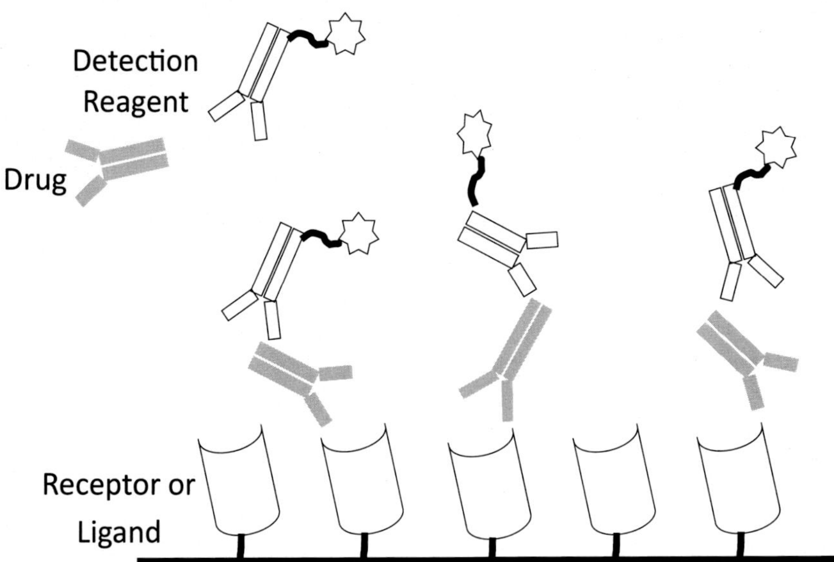

FIG. 11.5 Sandwich assay formatted immunoassay. The drug is first bound to the capture reagent and nonbinding matrix components are washed away. The detection reagent is then added and allowed to bind. Depending on the detection scheme, the detection reagent may have a chromophore, enzyme to generate a chromogenic measured compound, or be part of an electrochemiluminescent signal generation.

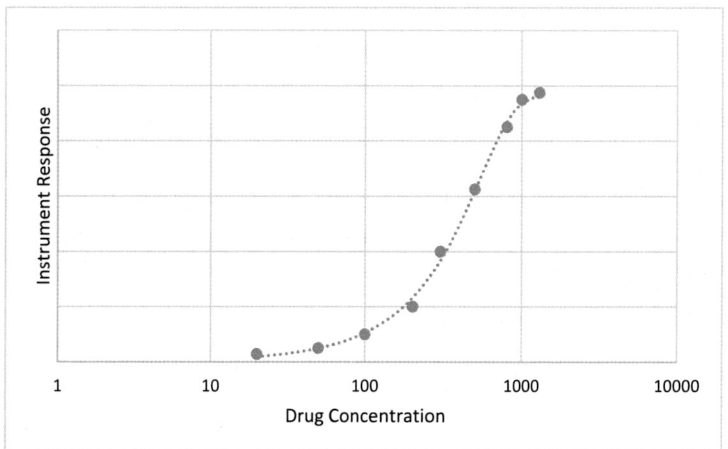

FIG. 11.6 The calibration curve for a sandwich-formatted immunoassay.

Recent advances in technology have expanded the form for the capture surface to utilize beads instead of a well bottom. The bead format has the advantage of being able to be mixed well with the sample or any reagents and provides comparatively more reaction surface area. This allows greater interaction between the bound molecules and those in solution, as well as greater effectiveness of washing steps. The increased surface area also permits greater binding capacity which can translate into more bound drug and greater sensitivity. Additionally, some beads have iron particle cores that allow the beads to be held to the bottom of wells by a magnetic field during aspiration steps, thereby reducing their potential loss.

To achieve in vivo efficacy, biologic drugs are designed to interact with endogenous receptors or ligands which are sometimes free and in circulation. Central to immunoassays are the molecular interactions. The capture and detection reagents are chosen for their specificity to the analyte and binding characteristics (affinity). The more specific the capture or detection reagent is to the analyte, the less risk there is for endogenous molecules to interfere with the assay. When the drug-target receptor or ligand is free in circulation, it may be present in the serum/plasma along with the drug and may be complexed with the drug. These complexes may block the capture or detection reagent if the binding complex sterically blocks the binding of the reagent to the drug. The selection of the capture and detection reagents must, therefore, take into account the potential for such competition. However, since the levels of the circulating receptor or ligand may be higher in patients, the interference may not be apparent until patient study samples are tested. Beyond the binding recognition, the strength of the binding affinity is important with strong binders allowing more aggressive washing conditions to be applied to eliminate interferences. Another factor of the binding affinity is the duration of the binding event—a fast on-rate and slow off-rate are optimal [20]. Antibodies raised against the analyte have the potential to provide better specificity and binding characteristics and may be used for both capture and detection reagents.

Antibodies against the whole analyte molecule or a fragment are generated by dosing animal species to which the analyte or its fragment is seen as a foreign molecule to which an immune response is stimulated. These responses produce a polyclonal set of antibodies (i.e., the various antibodies produced do not bind to the same epitope on the analyte). Multiple challenges with the analyte are used to increase the immune response and improve the specificity of the antibodies against the analyte. Serums from the animals are screened to identify the nature of these polyclonal antibodies to see if they have the correct specificity and binding characteristics. Each animal will have antibodies that may bind at the same epitope or different ones. Multiple dosings are used to challenge the animal's immune system and produce the highest circulating titers. Once the desired characteristics are achieved, multiple blood draws are taken and the polyclonal antibodies are harvested and purified. Since the immune response changes over time, subsequent samples and harvested lots of antibodies must be tested within the assay to demonstrate comparable results. Since the changes typically result in minor performance differences, use of the new lots must frequently include minor changes to the amounts used in each well. To overcome that issue and improve the reagent specificity, antibody clones (i.e., monoclonal antibodies) with high specificity are generated through the culture of hybridoma cell lines.

The polyclonal or monoclonal antibody, affimer or aptamer reagents cannot be used directly in the assay as they do not bind to the well surface or contain the label necessary to act as the detection reagent. Most antibodies used for capture reagents are biotinylated through a chemical reaction that attaches biotin to the antibody. The well bottom for the experiment is coated with streptavidin which has a high affinity to bind the biotin on the antibody, thus securing the antibody capture reagent to the well surface. The same process is used to secure the antibody to beads in bead-formatted assays, or when using aptamers or affirmers as capture reagents. Depending on the detection label, a variety of chemistries may be used to attach the label to the detection reagent. Because of differences in the lot to lot preparations of the biotinylated capture and detection-labeled reagents, they must be titered and compared to prior lots to ensure a consistent performance of the assay [21].

To improve on the sensitivity and performance of immunoassays, a number of technologies have been implemented. An automated, microfluidic device utilizes microchannels etched into compact discs and nanoliter volumes of samples and reagents are used to achieve greater sensitivity and larger dynamic range. As the reagents or samples are added, the discs are spun and centrifugal force drives the liquid through the channels to effect the same process used in well or bead-based approaches. Other technologies that have been implemented to achieve greater sensitivity and larger dynamic range include incorporation of digital camera technologies for greater sensitivity and larger dynamic ranges. Another approach, single molecule counting (SMC), claims further improvements in sensitivity by adding several steps to a sandwich immunoassay. In SMC, after the detection reagent has been bound to the analyte and excess reagent washed away, the detection antibody is dissociated from the analyte and, using fluidics, is passed across a detection laser. The laser excites the fluorescent tag on the detection reagent molecule and the resulting fluorescent photons are individually measured [22]. While these and other technologies are being used to improve the sensitivity of the assay, the specificity of the assays is still reliant on the quality of the capture and detection reagents.

Polymerase chain reaction assays

With the increasing numbers of cell and gene therapies in development and being approved, additional assay technologies are being utilized to answer key questions about the pharmacokinetics of these moieties. For genetic-based therapeutics (RNA- or DNA-based), polymerase chain reaction (PCR) assays are now the method of choice. Two primary technologies are currently used for PCR: quantitative PCR (qPCR) and digital droplet PCR (ddPCR). For DNA, a number of standard procedures are used to rapidly extract all DNA from the sample. Using the UV absorbance of the sample at 260λ, the total DNA concentration is determined. This total DNA is a combination of the genomic DNA and the administered therapeutic. Note that the administered therapeutic is a minute percentage of the total DNA, so that the total DNA is treated as the genomic DNA content in later calculations. Based on the total concentration, an appropriate volume is used for the analysis. After using heat to split any double stranded DNA, a small segment of complementary DNA (cDNA) to the administered therapeutic DNA (drug) is annealed to the drug and then the temperatures adjusted to allow the added DNA polymerase to complete the creation of the cDNA to the full length of the drug. Multiple cycles of this amplification process are used, with each cycle designed to create a copy of the drug DNA. In this way, the number of copies of the drug DNA is doubled in each cycle. The detection process is based on dyes that fluoresce when intercalated within double stranded DNA at the end of each amplification cycle [23].

For a sample being measured by qPCR, once its fluorescence signal achieves the detection limit signal (i.e., the number of cycles required to achieve a reliable signal), its cycle number is compared with a calibration curve in which the number of cycles needed to reach this threshold is plotted against a range of spiked analyte copies that was put through the replication process. This backcalculation determines the initial numbers of copies of drug DNA per μg genomic DNA. For RNA drugs, after the extraction of the genetic material, the RNA must be reverse transcribed into its complementary DNA. The sample is then processed using the procedures for DNA amplification [24]. Based on FDA guidance, assay sensitivity is expected to achieve a limit of quantitation of <50 copies/μg genomic DNA [25]. The advantage of PCR assays is their sensitivity can be increased to a high level by using additional replication cycles to amplify the amount of DNA that is generated to achieve the detection threshold. Most assays are run to ~40 cycles. Samples with high numbers of drug DNA copies need fewer cycles (e.g., 28) to achieve the detection threshold, while samples with low drug concentrations require a higher number of cycles (e.g., 37–40).

ddPCR is a newer technology that has only been available commercially since 2011. It does not require a calibration curve because it can detect the presence of each copy of the drug DNA by using microetched chips to create a lipid microemulsion of the sample with the amplification reagents and a lipid. The remainder of the amplification experiment may be maintained as a microemulsion or with the microemulsion is spread across a surface having depressions large enough to capture just one lipid emulsion particle. The liquid emulsion droplet reaction volume is in the nanoliter range. Each approach creates thousands of microreaction vessels. Any particular droplet may or may not hold a drug molecule. Using the polymerase amplification process described earlier, copies are made of the drug DNA within each drop and the presence of a fluorescent drug signal measured. With the microfluidic approach, the sample is maintained as a microemulsion in solution and droplets are passed in a single file stream through a microfluidic detector to detect positive and negative reaction droplets. Using the microwell approach, a charge-coupled device (CCD) camera is used to measure the numbers of positive and negative microwell reactions. For both approaches, the fraction of reactions with a positive signal is used to calculate the drug DNA concentration using a Poisson distribution [26, 27].

Method validation

Regardless of the analytical platform selected, a process of validation is necessary to demonstrate the reliability of the assay to reproducibly produce accurate data. There are three phases to this process, method development, method validation, and study sample analysis. Method development consists of selecting the analytical platform and deriving the conditions necessary for a workable assay. Method validation then follows, and it is the process of proving that the assay generates accurate, reliable data for its intended purpose. The validation results describe the reliability of the assay within a specific set of parameters. Any measurements outside these parameters would not be considered reliable and should not be used. For instance, an assay is validated to measure drug concentrations within a specified range, e.g., 5–1000 ng/mL. Any measurement beyond 1000 ng/mL cannot be assured and should be rejected (although you can do other things to bring the sample within the validated range of the assay).

The specific parameters that require validation may differ depending on the analytical platform, and sometimes, the particular application. Technically, these differences produce a very complex situation, even for bioanalytical scientists who may be very highly trained in one or a couple of methodologies, e.g., LC-MS. However, when switching to a new methodology, it may not always be clear to them which parameters may need to be assessed during validation, and perhaps more frequently, what acceptance criteria are appropriate for each parameter. Generally in LC-MS, accuracy is assessed within +/− 15% of nominal concentration. But is that performance what is required to validate flow cytometry assay to assess white cell counts? Perhaps not. Each analytical platform has its own unique characteristics.

With respect to chromatographic assays and ligand binding assays, which have long been reliably used to assess drug concentrations, the FDA Guidance for Industry "Bioanalytical Method Validation" [1] has evolved over time and with significant input from industry scientists. The Guidance provides the specific parameters and acceptance criteria for these parameters. But these criteria may not adequately address the needs of other analytical methodologies, especially ones that rely on significantly different physicochemical principles. Delving into the details of each methodology is not possible here, but it is perhaps more important to understand the common strategy that underlies method validation.

For every assay, regardless of how different they are from each other, the same questions need to be addressed. These questions are as follows:

- Does the method measure the intended analyte?
- What is the variability associated with these measurements?
- What is the range of the assay that provides reliable data?
- How does sample handling, storage, and collection affect the reliability of the assay?

Answering these questions provides the required level of assurance about the reliability and utility of the assay.

Does the method measure the intended analyte? Fundamentally, we need an assay that provides concentration data solely for the analyte of interest. We need to assure ourselves that no other compounds or entities interfere with that measurement, because this would produce higher or lower analyte concentrations than those that truly exist and might lead to erroneous conclusions and treatment actions with patients. This assessment is often referred to as the selectivity and/or specificity of the assay. Generally, chemically similar compounds are measured simultaneously with the moiety of interest to assess if they interfere with the assay. Upon discovery of an interference, steps need to be taken to modify the assay and mitigate the interference. With chromatographic assays, this generally is achieved by altering the mobile phase, the mobile phase rate, the column solid phase, or the selected ion monitoring of the mass spectrometer.

What is the variability associated with these measurements? In other words, how good is the measurement? Usually, the variability of the assay is reported in terms of accuracy and precision, although how these parameters are assessed differs depending on the analytical platform. In general, the accuracy and precision of LC-MS assays are each within +/− 15% of the nominal concentration. In other words, these assays can provide very accurate and precise drug concentration data. However, with new types of assays, e.g., biomarkers, a more fundamental question needs to be addressed; how much variability can you live with in your data? This answer depends upon the purpose of the assay. For instance, if you were monitoring platelet counts as a biomarker of activity, very large changes are needed before they become clinically meaningful, so perhaps an assay with accuracy and precision of ± 30 might suffice for its purpose. Understanding the pharmacological need will greatly aid in developing an assay that is appropriate.

What is the range of the assay that provides reliable data? Every assay has finite limits within which it can provide reliable data. Interpolation between the highest and lowest ends of the range is generally acceptable, whereas extrapolation beyond the ends of the range generally is not acceptable. The lowest end of the range is often termed the lower limit of quantitation (LLOQ). It is closely associated with the sensitivity of an assay; the analytical system is incapable of measuring lower quantities of the analyte. Any analyte concentrations below that point cannot be reliably assessed. The highest concentration is often termed the upper limit of quantitation (ULOQ). Sometimes, the ULOQ is defined by the highest concentration tested, although the analytical platform may be capable of assaying even higher concentrations. In other cases, the ULOQ is the physical limit of the assay. Regardless, concentrations above this point cannot be reliably measured. Often in these cases, samples can be diluted with sample matrix (e.g., human plasma), and then remeasured within the validated range of the assay.

How does sample handling, storage, and collection affect the reliability of the assay? The various manipulations involved in the collection and storage of patient samples can have a serious impact on the stability of the drug analyte, leading to degradation and erroneously low quantitation of the analyte. Sample collection at the clinical site, sample storage at the clinical site, transport of the samples (sometimes from locations across the globe), receipt of the samples, storage, and sample thawing and processing in the analytical laboratory have been known to impact sample integrity. Understanding the chemistry and metabolic fate of the analyte is fundamental to establishing effective sample storage and transport practices. Appropriate processes must be developed during method development, and validated so that the user can know that the samples are reliable for analysis, and when to question the integrity of the samples because the samples were exposed to conditions that may have led to analyte degradation. Consequently, analytical methodologies will provide an appropriate plan for sample collection, transport, and storage. Further, the analytical laboratory must assess benchtop stability to determine the conditions needed to manipulate samples safely as they are prepared for analysis (e.g., storage on ice on the benchtop maintains stability for 2 h), and to assess how long samples are stable during longer-term storage. The latter is referred to as long-term storage stability, and samples that are stored beyond the time of documented stability would be considered unusable and data from such samples must be rejected. There are many examples of methodologic failures in sample collection (e.g., samples left on benchtop at the site of collection for 2 h unattended; samples left in a hot airport hangar over a weekend during transport to the analytical site). Therefore, understanding how the analyte behaves under these various conditions is crucial to establishing the procedures necessary to ensure their storage integrity. Deviations from these procedures should be cause for suspecting sample degradation and rejection.

Sample analysis

Once the assay is validated, it is ready to be used to analyze samples from nonclinical or clinical studies with the assurance that the data will be reliable. During sample analysis, a standard curve is also analyzed with the samples each time an analytical run is performed. Use of standard curve from a prior run to interpret the results of the current run is unacceptable and would lead to a rejection of the data. In addition, quality control samples (QCs) are included in each analytical run. These are samples made up of known quantities of the analyte in matrix, typically stored under the same conditions as the samples, and are used to assess the performance of each analytical run. If the QCs once measured are within the prescribed accuracy and precision of the assay, the run is acceptable. If the QCs fail those criteria, it is an indication that the assay did not perform as designed, the data is considered unreliable, and steps may be needed to correct the analytical problems before continuing the analysis of study samples. Another practice is to reassay some study samples at a later time. This is termed incurred sample reanalysis (ISR). By reanalyzing some study samples, one assesses the robustness of the assay. Failed ISR reveals weakness in the assay procedures that requires attention. Most of the ISR failures reported in the literature were due to analyst errors (e.g., poor sampling thawing/mixing practices) or sample instability (e.g., acyl glucuronide metabolites back converting to parent because the storage conditions were not appropriate). So ISR represents a postvalidation check of the method, as well as the operator. Sometimes an unanticipated exigency occurs during sample analysis. For example, additional QCs are needed, or a slightly different concentration range is needed. These occurrences are not uncommon, and they are addressed by amending the method, and then performing a partial validation of the change. Depending on the nature of the change, partial validation can range from a short accuracy and precision determination, to almost a complete revalidation of the assay. This practice demonstrates that the changes made to the assay are reliable.

Cross-validation

Sometimes, more than one assay is developed to measure the drug concentrations in a study. As there are always some inherent differences between assays, different results might be provided for the same drug concentration, which can lead to confusion or misinterpretation of the study results. The fundamental question that arises is which assay is the right one? There is no way to ascertain which method provides a truer value. These discrepancies are generally revealed by a cross-validation, which is a process in which a number of study samples and/or laboratory prepared samples are analyzed by both assays and the results are statistically compared by means of a regression analysis. Generally, 10% differences from the mean would generally be considered acceptable. But what happens if the differences are greater? Bioanalysts generally work to revise assays when possible to minimize assay differences, which is the most pragmatic solution. However, it is arguably more important to understand how the two assays relate to each other and to understand if the bias of one assay to another is consistent across the required concentration range. If this is the case, it may be reasonable for the pharmacokineticist to make an appropriate mathematical adjustment to the data as needed to bring conformity. This is the process that has generally been applied to the pediatric development of new drugs. In these cases, the pharmacokinetic, safety, and efficacy data generated in adult studies is the knowledge base that is used to interpret the pharmacokinetic outcomes in pediatric studies. In some examples where this approach was used, the adult data was generated with an assay that employed plasma samples, whereas in the pediatric studies, an assay was used that relied on dried blood spot sampling. Cross-validation of the two assays led to an understanding of the methodological bias and allowed for appropriate data adjustment to interpret the study outcomes appropriately [28].

Case examples

Interference

Avoiding interference in the quantitation of the analyte is a fundamental consideration in developing and validating an assay. With early HPLC-UV assays, interferences could easily be viewed on the chromatogram (Fig. 11.7). Although the more general use of LC-MS/MS has greatly reduced analytical interference, it still remains a fundamental consideration. Early adopters of LC-MS/MS technology felt that the extreme selectivity of the triple quad mass spectrometers for specific *m/z* would eliminate the need for optimized chromatography and eliminate interferences. Many scientists adopted methods with chromatographic runs of less than 1 or 2 min using an extremely rapid mobile phase gradient (ballistic) to have high-throughput assays. In theory, the approach was valid, but as a relatively new technology at the time, not all of the characteristics of the instrument were fully understood. Specifically, the impact of the conditions within the source, where electrical charges and heat were applied to cause desolvation of the nebulized liquid stream, was not well understood. With the lack of chromatographic separation, it was found that under these highly energetic conditions some drug-related molecules could be chemically changed to the drug and thereby, increase its measured concentration. Five drugs and their known or predicted metabolites were tested for their interference potential when a rapidly changing (ballistic) gradient was used. The five drugs included (1) a lactone drug, with its open-ring metabolite; (2) a phenolic drug and its prodrug; (3) an *E*-isomer methyloxime drug and its *Z*-isomer as the potential biotransformation product; (4) a carboxylic acid drug and acylglucuronide metabolite; and (5) a thiol drug, with its disulfides. In each case, the metabolite or drug-related product was shown to undergo a chemical change in the source to generate the analyte drug. Fig. 11.8 shows the selected ion monitoring mass spectrometer chromatograms of an unnamed lactone drug in panel A and in panel B of its acid form that converted to the lactone in the source [29]. As shown in Panel C, resolution of these chromatographic

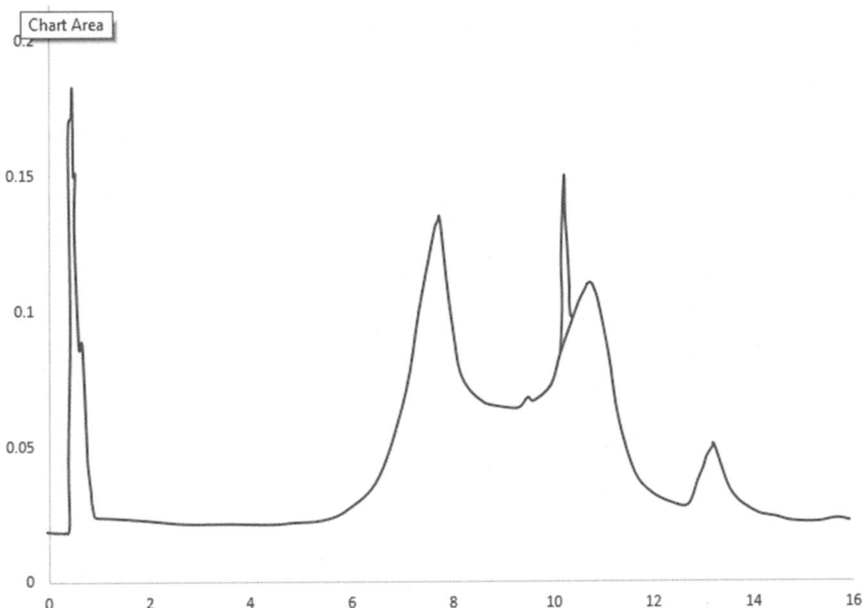

FIG. 11.7 Chromatographic demonstration of interference. The retention time of the analyte is just over 10 min (sharp peak), coincidental with a very large, broad interference which renders appropriate quantitation unreliable.

peaks was obtained when the chromatographic procedure was modified by using a different mobile phase. Subsequently, bioanalysts paid closer attention to the chromatography and, as needed, revised their methods when metabolites were later identified that were shown to have in-source conversions to the drug.

Even though the mass spectrometer is highly specific and is only measuring the *m/z* that are specified for the drug and its internal standard, the extent to which matrix components interfere with drug measurements by LC-MS/MS varies considerably and is influenced by factors such as the drug chemical properties and similarity to endogenous molecules, the extraction's ability to remove matrix components, and the chromatography used. However, the conditions in the source are highly energetic and, depending on the sample cleanup and chromatography that is utilized, some matrix components are likely to remain within the extracted sample and elute at the same time as the drug. Furthermore, these other chemicals and the analyte are competing in the source for ionization from the applied charge and desolvation. Some of these matrix components have been shown to actually enhance ionizations, but others have more frequently been shown to suppress ionization of the drug. As these components may have diurnal cycles or be derived from dietary intake, their presence may vary sample to sample. To explore a class of known suppressors, Ye et al. [30] tested 14 drugs, a hormone and caffeine for the impact of phospholipids within extracted samples. Using the *m/z* for the parent and daughter ions of choline-containing phospholipids, they were able to observe phospholipid elution from the LC column at the same time as the model drug compounds that they were measuring. However, LC conditions could be changed so that the chromatogram peaks of the model drug compounds and phospholipids could be completely resolved. Preventing coelution of the model compounds with phospholipids resulted in instrument responses very similar to that generated with reference solutions of the model compounds that contained no matrix components. Fig. 11.9 shows superimposed chromatograms for midazolam (M), tamoxifen (T), and the phospholipids (PC) under various chromatographic conditions that provide partial resolution to complete resolution. Thus, a search for phospholipids and other endogenous compounds residual in sample extracts should be part of a robust method development approach to prevent interference problems during sample analysis.

In immunoassays, the specificity of the reagents used for capture and detection is critical to the quality of the data. Soluble ligands or shed receptors in circulation may bind to the drug at the same epitope as the capture or detection reagent and affect the measurement of the drug. In a sandwich-style ELISA, the presence of soluble ligand interfered by binding to the Fab portion of the antibody, and resulted in noncomplexed on both Fab, complexed on one Fab, or potentially on both [29]. Obviously, antibody therapeutics with no bound ligand would be measured appropriately, those with one Fab bound would be captured by the assay but not detected and those with both Fabs bound to ligand would not even be captured. A variety of approaches have been developed to disrupt the drug-ligand interactions and permit capture and subsequent detection of the drug. Partridge et al. [31] found for one of their antibody drugs that treatment of the sample to a mildly acidic pH prior to the sample being added to the 96-well plate was sufficient to disrupt the drug-ligand complexes, which resulted in significantly higher measured drug concentration. Fig. 11.10 presents the results of both the initial assay and of

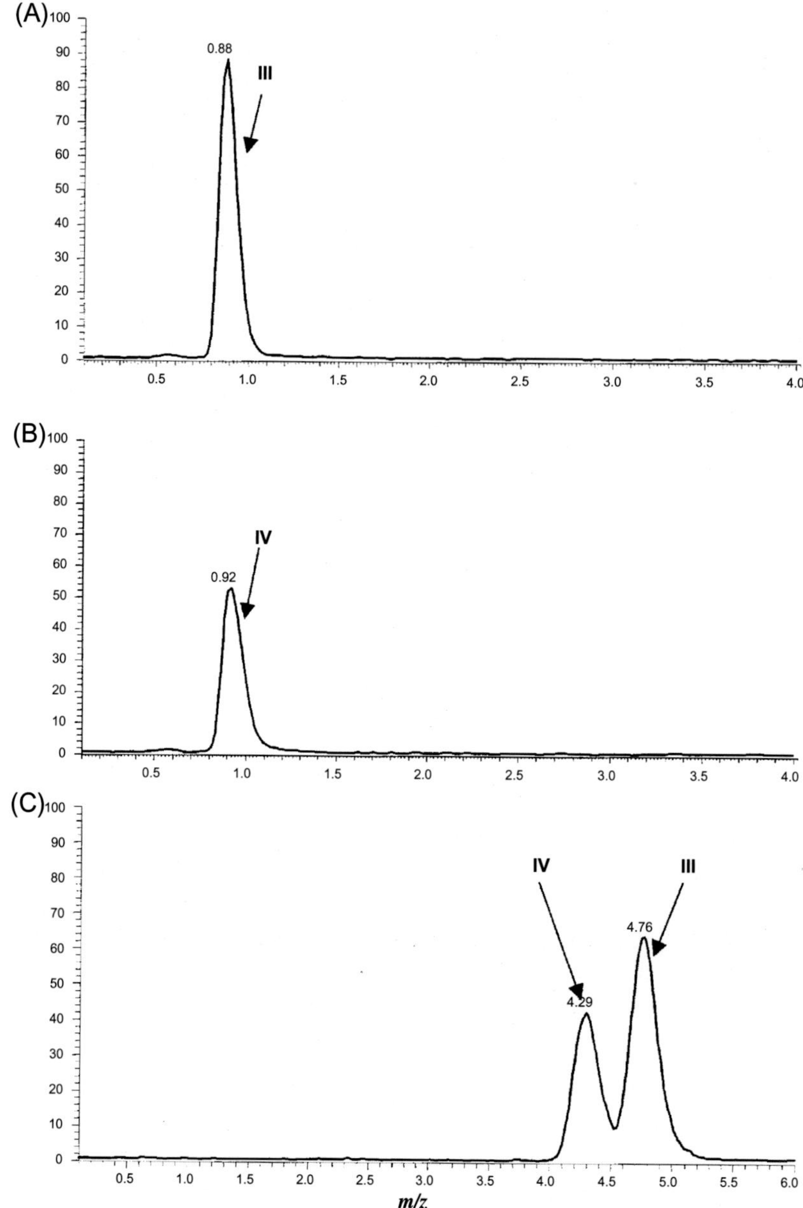

FIG. 11.8 In-source formation of a lactone drug from its open ringed form. Selected reaction monitoring ion chromatograms using the mass transition of the lactone drug (*m/z* 363 to *m/z* 285) (A) the chromatogram of the lactone drug (B) the chromatogram of the open-ring form of the drug that elutes with the same retention time as the drug because it lactonizes in the source to produce the same precursor and product spectra and (C) chromatogram in which both compounds are separated because a different isocratic mobile phase was used for chromatography. *(Reproduced with permission from Jemal M, Xia YQ. The need for adequate chromatographic separation in the quantitative determination of drugs in biological samples by high performance liquid chromatography with tandem mass spectrometry. Rapid Commun Mass Spectrom 1999;13:97–106.)*

the optimized assay in which acid treatment was shown to eliminate the interference from concentrations of the ligand (target) up to 2280 ng/mL.

Establishing assay range

Each instrument platform and assay has a range of reliable measurements that is based on a variety of factors related to the structure of the molecule and the performance of the platform and the assay. In animal safety studies, the drug is administered at doses higher than those expected for clinical use to identify likely toxicities and establish safe maximal doses for

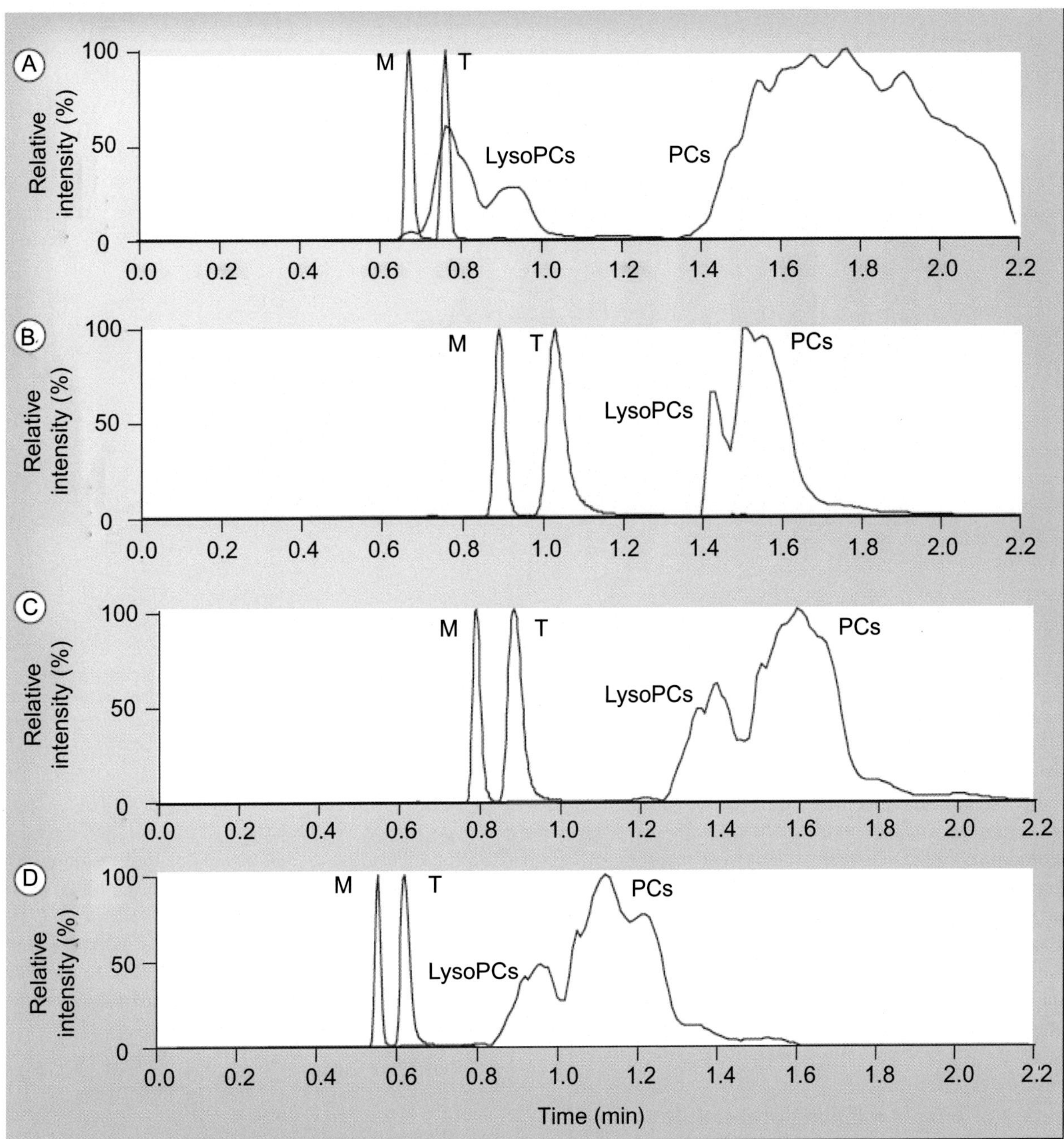

FIG. 11.9 Relative separation of midazolam (M) and tamoxifen (T) from phospholipids (PCs and LysoPCs) under various chromatographic conditions (panels A–D). *(Reproduced with permission from Ye Z, Tsao H, Gao H. Minimizing matrix effects while preserving throughput in LC–MS/MS bioanalysis. Bioanalysis 2011;3:1587–1601.)*

humans. Therefore, bioanalytical methods for these studies rarely have difficulty in being sensitive enough, but because the repeated doses produce extremely high circulating levels, samples at the highest doses are frequently diluted into the range of the assays. For example, an LC-MS method may have a range of 5–5000 ng/mL but concentrations observed at the highest dose may exceed 40,000–60,000 ng/mL. For many ELISA immunoassays, the typical range for the assays is two orders of magnitude, so samples frequently must be diluted into the range of the assay in order to measure concentration at the C_{max} of even the lowest dose. Animal pharmacokinetic and toxicokinetic study data, along with data obtained with in vitro studies on human hepatocytes, are used to model the expected clinical pharmacokinetic profiles for the first-in-human studies. Most of the predictions are relatively reliable; however, situations are known in which they can be wildly off, either overpredicting or underpredicting human exposure. In a case that one of the chapter authors experienced, the

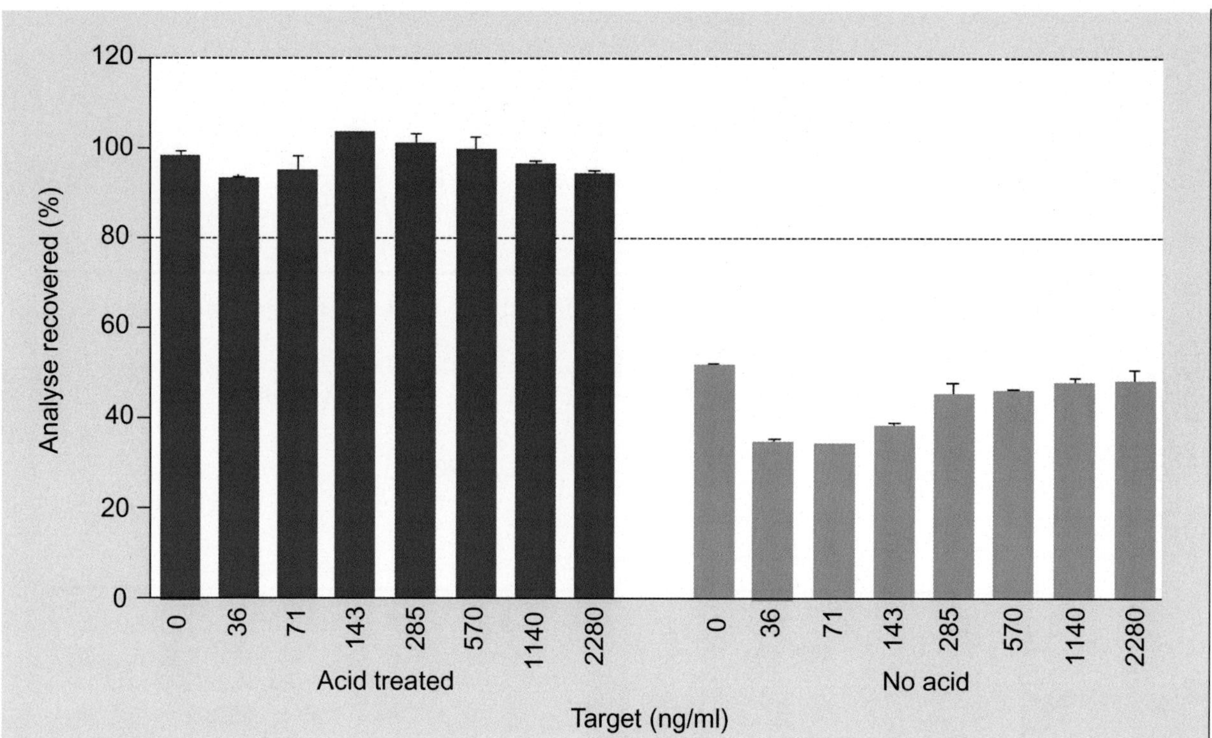

FIG. 11.10 Eliminating target Interferences in Immunoassays. In this example, acid treatment of the samples optimized conditions and eliminated matrix interference from the ligand (target) assay up to concentrations of 2280 ng/mL. *(Reproduced with permission from Partridge M, Pham J, Dziadiv O, Luong O, Rafique A, Sumner G, et al. Minimizing target interference in PK immunoassays: new approaches for low-pH-sample treatment. Bioanalysis 2013;5:1897–1910.)*

prediction indicated that the C_{max} of the first dose in humans would be 50 pg/mL and an assay with a LLOQ of 1–2 pg/mL was requested. The laboratory spent several months developing an assay but its LLOQ was only 10 pg/mL and the LC-MS method was predicted to lack sensitivity to measure lower concentrations. The dose escalations in this first-in-human study were planned weekly and the clinical team wanted data prior to moving forward with the next dose. Upon analysis of samples from the first dose, a number of samples were found to have concentrations in excess of the assay ULOQ of 2500 ng/mL and reanalysis of diluted samples was required to measure their concentration. Both the laboratory and the clinical team were shocked when the C_{max} from the first dose was 100 times higher than predicted. Due to the weekly timeline for dose escalation, there was no time to revalidate the method with a higher calibration range and when subsequent doses were administered most samples had to be diluted into the range of the assay.

Impact of sample handling or instability

Inadequate sample handing (e.g., sample collection, transport, benchtop handling, sample thawing) can create conditions that lead to degradation of the analyte in the sample. Similarly, inadequate storage conditions (e.g., samples that are not sufficiently stable when stored at −20°C) can lead to the loss of the analyte over time. In these cases, the assay produces results that are lower than the true values, which may lead to a misinterpretation of the study outcome and could lead one to make erroneous patient decisions or dose adjustments.

For example, testosterone suppression by gonadotropin inhibitors is a therapeutic approach that is used to treat patients with advanced prostate cancer. The clinical endpoint, which is the basis of FDA marketing approval for a number of these agents, is suppression of testosterone concentrations below 50 ng/dL for an extended period. Any excursions in the plasma concentrations above 50 ng/dL indicate a therapeutic failure. A sensitive, well-validated assay is necessary to accurately and reliably measure testosterone plasma concentrations in patients. A successful outcome is depicted in the left panel of Fig. 11.11 in which plasma concentrations of testosterone are maintained below 50 ng/dL. However, the assay shown in the right panel of Fig. 11.11 was conducted on degraded samples after poor sample handling or storage practices had been observed. The impact of these shortcomings was to produce plasma concentrations that were erroneously low and lead

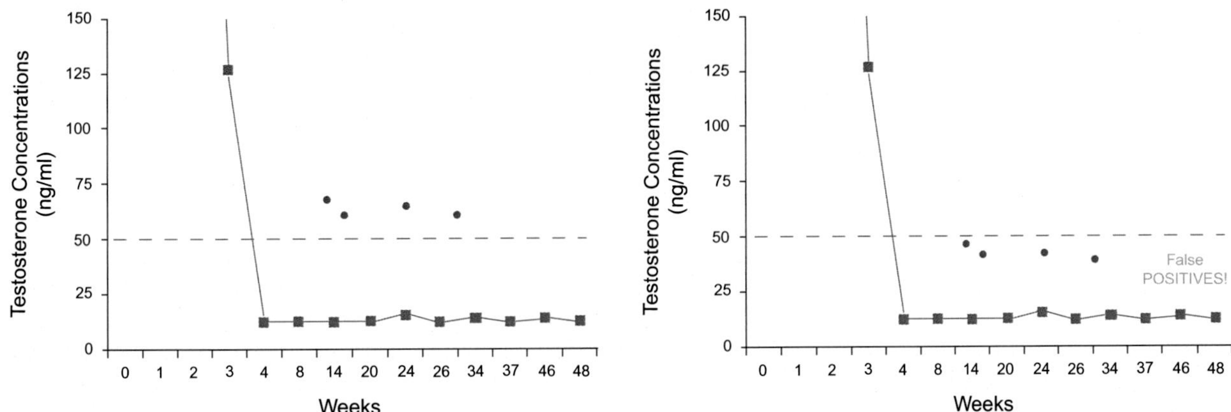

FIG. 11.11 The impact of sample instability on plasma concentrations of drugs. The *left panel* shows plasma concentrations of testosterone that occasionally exceed the 50ng/dL limit, indicating the failure of the drug at these times. The *right panel* shows plasma concentrations of testosterone measured after sample degradation. As a result, these plasma concentrations could be interpreted as successful therapy because they are below the 50ng/dL limit defined as a clinical endpoint.

to a false positive impression of therapeutic success for the drug being tested. When poor practices such as these occur in clinical trials, the assay and data will both be judged unreliable and the study results will be rejected, which may lead to the nonapproval of the drug.

Assessing results from two assays: Cross-validation

In drug development, multiple assays frequently are developed for different reasons and at different times. Generally, only one assay for the drug is ultimately used during clinical development but that is not always the case. So the question arises as to whether the results from both assays are interchangeable. Often they are not and different assays then generate different concentrations for the same amount of drug. A situation that occurs with some frequency in drug development is that an assay is developed that uses dried blood spot sampling (DBS) for pediatric studies of the drug. The pediatric pharmacokinetic data will be compared against the pharmacokinetic, safety, and efficacy data generated from the whole blood or plasma samples that were obtained in the adult population. Therefore, understanding how the data from the different assays compare is important to interpreting the experimental results obtained in the two populations. Most frequent, a set of samples is analyzed with both assays and the results are plotted against each other, as shown in the left panel of Fig. 11.12. Assessing the bias of one assay vs the other allows for appropriate adjustment of the data. However, if the bias is not consistent over the concentration range needed, a simple comparison of regression plots may not be sufficient. In other cases, the data has been plotted as plasma concentration vs. time curves, as shown in right panel of Fig. 11.12. In this case, the inconsistent bias resulted in differing assayed concentrations of the same samples over time. The area under the drug concentration vs time curves for the plasma and DBS assays differed by almost 40%. If the DBS assay alone had been used, the data may have prompted the study sponsors to recommend an increase in dose for pediatric patients, which might have resulted in dangerous toxicity for these patients.

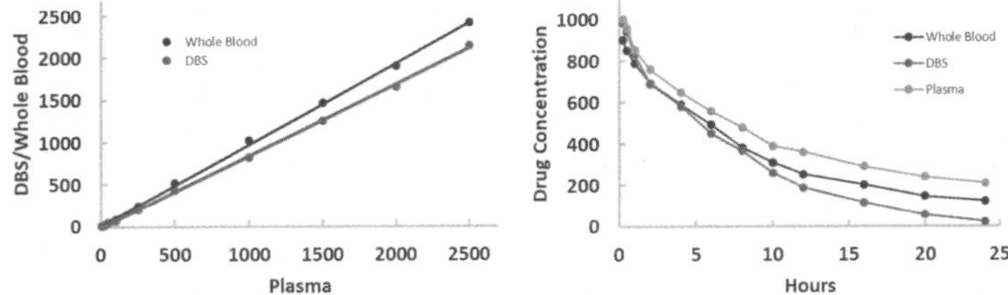

FIG. 11.12 Cross-validation comparison of a dried blood spot (DBS) method with plasma and whole blood sampling assays. The *left panel* shows the approach of regressing the results of a set of whole blood (*whol*) and DBS samples. In the *right panel*, a whole blood assay and a DBS assay were tested against the plasma assay for the drug and data were plotted as concentration-vs.-time plots. Note that the data from the DBS assay and the plasma assay increasingly diverge as time progresses.

Conclusion

Method development and validation are critically important to clinical pharmacology. For the measurement of drugs, there are well-developed procedures for method development and validation, but in more recent times interest has grown immensely in the development of assays for biomarkers which can be used to indicate drug response or disease response in patients. Lack of data limits the use of clinical pharmacology tools to develop new drugs and to help individualize patient treatment, and inaccurate data can lead to mistaken interpretations of study results, and may lead one to recommend unwarranted dosing changes, potentially causing unnecessary toxicity, or reducing therapeutic effectiveness. The examples given here demonstrate, to some extent, the complexity of bioanalytical development. For example, the technical issues associated with a chromatographic assay differ from those of a ligand binding assay, and all of the considerations for a LC-MS assay may not be applicable to flow cytometry. In fact, the technical issues will differ with each type of analytical platform, generally because they operate on different scientific principles. However, we have described the questions one should ask with respect to developing and validating an assay. The questions would generally be true of all assays (although, for a specific technology, you may have additional questions). These questions need to be addressed in order to have assays available that provide reliable data. A perennial question that arises is what acceptance criteria should be used for different validation parameters? Again, these will differ based on the type of analytical platform and the intended use of the analytical results. Accuracy and precision criteria for an LC-MS assay of a drug are likely to be different than those used for an LBA assay of a soluble biomarker used to support early development dose selection. In the former case, a higher degree of accuracy and precision is required to support the approval of a generic drug for instance. Whereas in the latter case, the biomarker may provide information that supports interpretation of clinical outcome data, such as a response rate to an oncology drug. This brings up the concept of Fit-for-Purpose. Tailoring the capability of the assay to the task for which it is needed is sometimes a tricky proposition. Nevertheless, regardless of the platform or the purpose of the assay, the four method validation questions we described serve as an underlying development guide for most assays.

Acknowledgments

The authors wish to thank Dr. Guoxiang George Shen for his help in preparation of this chapter.

References

[1] CDER. Bioanalytical method validation. Guidance for industry. Silver Spring, MD: FDA; 2018. Available from: https://www.fda.gov/media/70858/download.

[2] CDRH. Premarket notification 510 (k). Silver Spring, MD: FDA; 2020. Available from: https://www.fda.gov/medical-devices/premarket-submissions/premarket-notification-510k.

[3] CDRH. Premarket approval (PMA). Silver Spring, MD: FDA; 2019. Available from: https://www.fda.gov/medical-devices/premarket-submissions/premarket-approval-pma.

[4] CMS. Clinical Laboratory Improvement Amendments (CLIA). Baltimore, MD: CMS; 2020. Available from: https://www.cms.gov/Regulations-and-Guidance/Legislation/CLIA.

[5] Unger S, Weng N. Best practice in liquid chromatography for LC-MS bioanalysis. In: Li W, Zhang J, Tse FLS, editors. Handbook of LC-MS bioanalysis: best practices, experimental protocols, and regulations. Hoboken, NJ: John Wiley and Sons; 2013. p. 185–204 [chapter 15].

[6] Barry E. Columns: packed and capillary; column selection in gas chromatography. In: Grob R, Barry E, editors. Modern practice of gas chromatography. 4th ed. Hoboken, NJ: John Wiley & Sons; 2004. p. 65–142.

[7] Jumhawan UY. Simultaneous profiling of 17 steroid hormones for the evaluation of endocrine-disrupting chemicals in H295R cells. Bioanalysis 2016;9:67–79.

[8] van Breeman R, Martinez E. Best practice in mass spectrometry for LC-MS. In: Li W, Zhang J, Tse FLS, editors. Handbook of LC-MS bioanalysis: best practices, experimental protocols, and regulations. Hoboken, NJ: John Wiley and Sons; 2013. p. 205–16 [chapter 16].

[9] Dutcher JS, Strong JM, Lee W-K, Atkinson AJ Jr. Stable isotope methods for pharmacokinetic studies in man. In: Klein R, editor. Proceedings of the second international conference on stable isotopes. Washington, DC: US Govt Printing Office; 1976 [CONF-751027].

[10] CDER. Exploratory IND studies. Guidance for industry. Rockville, MD: FDA; 2006. Available from: https://www.fda.gov/media/72325/download.

[11] Boulton D, Kasichayanula S, Keung CF, Arnold ME, Christopher LJ, Xu XS, et al. Simultaneous oral therapeutic and intravenous 14C-microdoses to determine the absolute oral bioavailability of saxagliptin and dapagliflozin. Br J Clin Pharmacol 2013;75:763–8.

[12] Jiang H, Zeng J, Li W, Bifano M, Gu H, Titsch C, et al. Practical and efficient strategy for evaluating oral absolute bioavailability with an intravenous microdose of a stable isotopically-labeled drug using a selected reaction monitoring mass spectrometry assay. Anal Chem 2012;84:10031–7.

[13] Atkinson AJ Jr. The stable isotope method for determining absolute bioavailability. Transl Clin Pharmacol 2017;25:53–8.

[14] Findlay J, Dillard R. Appropriate calibration curve fitting in ligand binding assays. AAPS J 2007;9:E260–7.

[15] Berson S, Yalow RS, Bauman A, Rothschild MA, Newerly K. Insulin-I^{131} metabolism in human subjects: demonstration of insulin binding globulin in the circulation of insulin treated subjects. J Clin Invest 1956;35:170–90.

[16] Engvall E, Perlmann P. Enzyme-linked immunosorbent assay (ELISA): quantitative assay of immunoglobulin G. Immunochemistry 1971;8:871–4.

[17] Thermo Scientific. Tech tip #33. Guide to enzyme substrates for ELISA. Rockford, IL: Pierce Biotechnology; 2011. Available from: https://tools.thermofisher.com/content/sfs/brochures/TR0033-Substrates-ELISA.pd).f.

[18] Meso Scale Discovery. Electrochemiluminescence. Rockville, MD: Meso Scale Discovery; 2020. Available from: https://www.mesoscale.com/en/technical_resources/our_technology/ecl.

[19] Thway T. Fundamentals of large-molecule protein therapeutic bioanalysis using ligand-binding assays. Bioanalysis 2016;8:11–7.

[20] O'Hara E. Ligand binding assays in the 21st century laboratory: recommendations for characterization and supply of critical reagents. AAPS J 2012;14:316–28.

[21] King L. Ligand binding assay critical reagents and their stability: recommendations and best practices from the global bioanalysis consortium harmonization team. AAPS J 2014;13:504–15.

[22] Fischer S. Emerging technologies to increase ligand binding assay sensitivity. AAPS J 2015;17:93–101.

[23] Primerdesign. Beginner's guide to real-time PCR. Chandlers Ford, UK: Primerdesign; 2019. Available from: http://www.primerdesign.co.uk/assets/files/beginners_guide_to_real_time_pcr.pdf.

[24] ThermoFisher. Introduction to gene expression. Getting started guide. Publication No. 4454239, Waltham, MA: ThermoFisher Scientific; 2018. Available from: https://assets.thermofisher.com/TFS-assets/LSG/manuals/4454239_IntrotoGeneEx_GSG.pdf.

[25] CBER. Long term follow-up after administration of human gene therapy products. Guidance for industry. Silver Spring, MD: FDA; 2020. Available from: https://www.fda.gov/media/113768/download.

[26] Hindson CM, Chevillet JR, Briggs HA, Gallichotte EN, Ruf IK, Hindson BJ, et al. Absolute quantification by droplet digital PCR versus analog real-time PCR. Nat Methods 2013;10:1003–5.

[27] Hindson BJ, Ness KD, Masquelier DA, Belgrader P, Heredia NJ, Makarwics AJ, et al. High-throughput droplet digital PCR system for absolute quantitation of DNA copy number. Anal Chem 2011;83:8604–10.

[28] Kothare PA, Bateman KP, Dockendorf M, Stone J, Xu Y, Woolf E, et al. An integrated summary for implementation of dried blood spots in clinical development programs. AAPS J 2016;18:519–27.

[29] Jemal M, Xia YQ. The need for adequate chromatographic separation in the quantitative determination of drugs in biological samples by high performance liquid chromatography with tandem mass spectrometry. Rapid Commun Mass Spectrom 1999;13:97–106.

[30] Ye Z, Tsao H, Gao H, Brummel CL. Minimizing matrix effects while preserving throughput in LC–MS/MS bioanalysis. Bioanalysis 2011;3:1587–601.

[31] Partridge M, Pham J, Dziadiv O, Luong O, Rafique A, Sumner G, et al. Minimizing target interference in PK immunoassays: new approaches for low-pH-sample treatment. Bioanalysis 2013;5:1897–910.

Chapter 12

Clinical pharmacogenetics

Anuradha Ramamoorthy[a], Tristan Sissung[b], and Michael Pacanowski[a]
[a]*Office of Clinical Pharmacology, Office of Translational Sciences, Center for Drug Evaluation and Research, US Food and Drug Administration, Silver Spring, MD, United States,* [b]*Clinical Pharmacology Program, National Cancer Institute, National Institutes of Health, Bethesda, MD, United States*

Introduction

The juxtaposition in time of the human genome sequencing with the realization that medication errors constitute one of the leading causes of death in the United States led many to believe that *pharmacogenetics* may be able to improve pharmacotherapy. As a result, a fairly uncritical series of hopes and predictions have led not only physicians and scientists but also venture capitalists and Wall Street to believe that genomics will lead to a new era of *personalized medicine* (also referred to at times as *precision medicine* or *targeted therapy*). If this is to occur, it will require accurate and reliable genetic tests that will allow physicians to predict clinically relevant outcomes with confidence. In addition, if medicine is to become more personalized, further consideration needs to be given to the evidence required to support the *clinical utility* of various genetic tests [1] and the means for developing these genetic markers in a way that facilitates their reliable clinical implementation [2, 3]. Genomic education for healthcare professionals is a critical first step toward the integration of genomic discoveries into clinical application [4]. Using pertinent examples to emphasize important underlying concepts, we hope that this chapter will provide a useful group of principles, and constitute a brief primer to the rapidly evolving field of *clinical pharmacogenetics.*

General principles

Pharmacogenetics and pharmacogenomics

Pharmacogenetics is the study of the relationship of variations in DNA sequence to drug response [5]. It is a subset of *pharmacogenomics*, which is the study of variations of DNA and RNA characteristics as related to drug response [5]. These terms tend to be used rather interchangeably; in this chapter, *pharmacogenetics* is used to refer to any of the genetic variations that affect drug exposure and/or response.

Human genetics

Progress in pharmacogenetics in large part can be attributed to the Human Genome Project, through which the blueprint of the human genome was built [6]. The human genome consists of about 4.5 billion base pairs arranged into 23 pairs of chromosomes. It contains about 20,000 coding and 24,000 noncoding genes, including over 675 million short variants and 6 million structural variants [7]. *Genetic variations*, i.e., differences in DNA sequences, can occur between individuals and can occur either in germline (heritable) or in somatic cells. These genetic variations can be broadly classified as: (1) single nucleotide polymorphisms (SNPs), (2) indels (insertions and/or deletions), or (3) structural variations (Fig. 12.1). Apart from these broad categories of genetic variation, other types of variations such as *epigenetic variations*, defined as heritable changes in gene expression without changes to the underlying DNA sequence, can also have a profound impact on the resulting phenotype.

SNPs are the most common type of genetic variation. SNPs can be present in the exons, introns, regulatory regions, or intergenic regions. Most research efforts have focused on exon-based changes as those were considered most likely to result in a clinical effect, but there are good examples of changes in introns, regulatory regions, or intergenic regions that result in expressed changes. Through a wide range of laboratory techniques, the variants can be expressed and tested to assess whether the activity is changed in vitro. The information hierarchy for SNPs is illustrated in Fig. 12.2. Synonymous SNPs do not result in a change in amino acid coding, whereas nonsynonymous SNPs do result in a coding change. The substitution

Atkinson's Principles of Clinical Pharmacology. https://doi.org/10.1016/B978-0-12-819869-8.00016-1

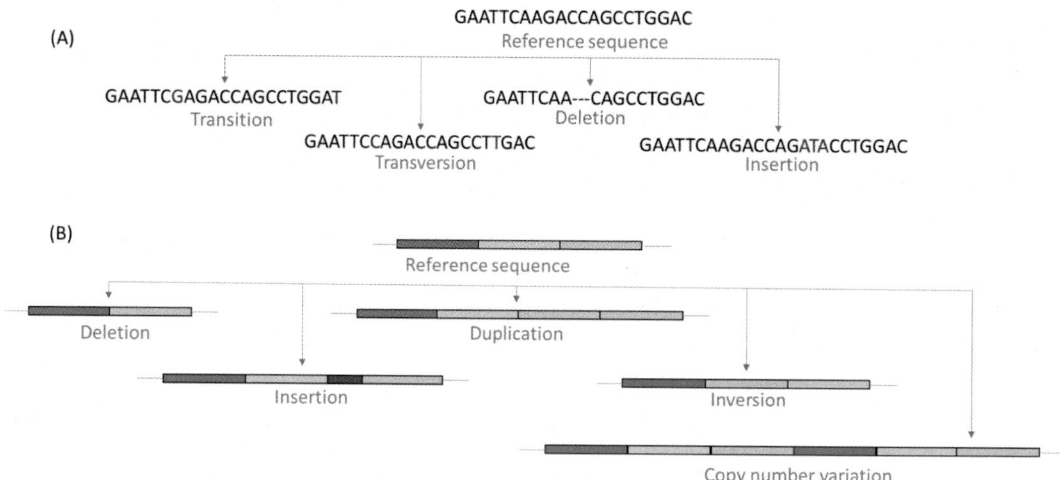

FIG. 12.1 Common types of genetic variations. (A) Single nucleotide polymorphisms (SNPs) can result from nucleic acid substitution and can be either transitions (interchange of purine (adenine/guanine) or pyrimidine (thymine/cytosine)) or transversions (interchange of purine with pyrimidine or vice versa). Short insertions and deletions (indels) are also a very frequent source of genetic variation. (B) Structural variations are typically used to describe genetic variation that occurs simultaneously over a larger DNA sequence (several genes or large areas of a chromosome).

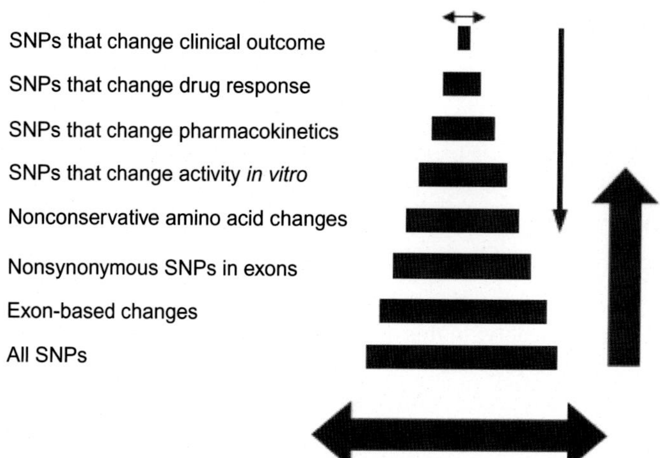

FIG. 12.2 The hierarchy of pharmacogenetic information from single nucleotide polymorphisms (SNPs). The pyramid becomes dramatically thinner as data on nonsynonymous SNPs, nonconservative amino acid changes, and SNPs that change activity in vitro, pharmacokinetics, drug response, or eventually, clinically important outcomes become progressively smaller. A similar hierarchy could equally be constructed for deletions, insertions, duplications, splice variants, copy number variations, and other types of genetic variations.

is termed nonconservative when the two amino acids have different physicochemical properties and therefore have a greater chance of changing the structure or activity of the protein they code for. SNPs in receptors, transporters, or drug-metabolizing enzymes can result in statistically significant changes in pharmacokinetics or pharmacodynamics. However, very few of these result in clinically significant changes in drug response and clinical outcomes.

Fig. 12.2 also makes clear the long scientific route from the discovery of an individual SNP to the actual demonstration of a clinically important outcome. This is particularly pertinent in view of the simple fact that the vast majority of individual polymorphisms in human DNA likely have no dynamic consequence. As a result, a number of clinical pharmacologists and scientists with expertise in pharmacology, genetics, and medicine have elected to start at the top of the pyramid. By searching for outliers in populations that demonstrate aberrant clinical responses and by focusing on these polymorphisms, they hope to elicit valuable genetic, mechanistic, and clinical lessons. With respect to drug response, population outliers can be very broadly categorized as nonresponders and responders (including exceptional responders). A number of intrinsic and extrinsic factors can explain the variability; genetics is one such intrinsic factor that can explain some of the variability in drug response. When an outlier phenotype is identified, the next step is to demonstrate that this phenotype is mediated by genetic variation. Pharmacogenetic studies aim to determine if genetic variations in nonresponders and responders can explain at least some of the variation in drug exposure and/or response.

Indications for performing pharmacogenetic studies

Pharmacogenetic evaluations become particularly important and valuable for drugs that exhibit a highly variable pharmacokinetic, safety, and/or efficacy profile [8]. The situations in which pharmacogenetics can provide additional information to understand variability include: (1) highly variable pharmacokinetics or response with significant outliers or a multimodal distribution; (2) extensive metabolism by a polymorphic enzyme or transport by a polymorphic transporter; (3) racial or ethnic variability in pharmacokinetics, efficacy, or safety; (4) poor tolerability; (5) narrow therapeutic index; and (6) idiosyncratic adverse events.

A variety of approaches can be used to begin the search for genetic predictors of drug pharmacokinetic or response. The two basic categories of research study designs are as follows:

(1) **Candidate-gene approach**—this approach can be used when the target and/or target pathways impacted by the drug are known to have functional polymorphisms or when the drug is subject to metabolism or transport by a protein encoded by a polymorphic gene. Even with such a targeted approach, it is important to confirm the association with experimental and clinical evidence. A good example of this approach is provided by the pharmacogenetic studies of clopidogrel that are described later in this chapter.

(2) **Hypothesis-free approach**—this approach can be used when limited information is available about the pharmacology of the drug, including its mechanism of action or metabolism and transport, and no prior knowledge or specific genetic hypothesis exists. In such cases, genome-wide association studies (GWAS) can be performed using high-throughput platforms (e.g., drug-metabolizing enzyme and transporter gene panels, genome-wide arrays, high-throughput sequencing) to compare the frequency of genetic variations between responders and nonresponders or between individuals with or without drug toxicity [9]. As high-throughput technologies may generate a higher rate of false positives, it is important to confirm the role of a newly identified genetic marker with experimental and clinical evidence. A pharmacogenetic study that identified the association of *SLCO1B1* variant (rs4363657) with statin-induced myopathy is a good example of this approach [10].

Irrespective of the approach used, it is important to conduct validation and replication studies to ensure that the associations are indeed true and can be generalized to both the individual and to diverse populations.

Examples of genes with variations that have important clinical consequences include those which: (1) affect drug metabolism and transport (e.g., *CYP2D6*, *CYP2C9*, and CYP2C19); (2) affect the drug target or pathway (e.g., *EGFR* and *VKORC1*); and (3) affect drug safety/immunological reactions (e.g., *HLA-B*) (discussed in Chapter 16). Selecting only those alleles that are more frequent in one population may lead to incorrect interpretation for other populations because relevant alleles might be overlooked. So, frequency differences in genetic variation across racial/ethnic populations should also be considered while performing genetic analysis [11].

Genetic analysis techniques and informatics

A number of genetic analysis methods and techniques can be utilized in pharmacogenetic analysis. Method or technique selection will depend on factors such as the purpose of the genetic analysis; considerations regarding the cost, time, sample quantity, quality, and number of samples; and the maturity of the selected technology.

Molecular genetic techniques are the most commonly used tools to identify genetic variations like SNPs or changes in RNA expression. These can include analysis of DNA or RNA, using a broad range of techniques such as polymerase chain reaction (PCR), reverse transcription PCR (RT-PCR), sequencing, and microarrays. Microarrays can be used to genotype multiple regions of the genome or to perform gene expression analysis. Sequencing can be performed on short or long sequences or even the entire exome (whole-exome sequencing or WES) or entire genome (whole-genome sequencing or WGS). The rapid pace of progress in genome sequencing technologies has resulted in a lower cost of genetic analysis as well as an increase in the diversity of genomes that have been sequenced [12].

Cytogenetic techniques can be used for detecting larger genomic changes (e.g., deletions, duplications, translocations) using methods such as karyotyping, fluorescence in situ hybridization (FISH), and comparative genomic hybridization (CGH).

The rapid advance in genetic analysis technologies has been paralleled by the advance in bioinformatics and computational analysis that is needed to interpret and obtain clinically useful insight from the wealth of data, so-called big data, that is being rapidly generated. A number of publicly available databases have been built to house genetic and other relevant information. For example, the Entrez System is a publicly available data hub provided by the National Center for Biotechnology Information (NCBI) that currently contains billions of records within an integrated system of over 35 databases devoted to the curation of scientific literature, health, genomes, genes, proteins, and chemicals [13]. Table 12.1 highlights some of the more commonly used databases, tools, and resources that can be helpful in understanding the interactions between genes and therapeutics.

Examples of clinically relevant genetic polymorphisms

Some genetic variations can lead to interindividual differences in pharmacokinetics by causing changes in drug absorption, distribution, metabolism, and elimination, which can consequently affect therapeutic response. Individual genetic variants and haplotypes (consisting of two or more variants that tend to be inherited together rather than randomly) are commonly referred to by the *star allele* nomenclature system [29]. This standardized nomenclature has provided laboratory and clinical scientists with a framework for cataloging the biological consequences of genetic variation in cytochrome P450 (CYP) drug-metabolizing enzymes and transporters across numerous laboratories in several countries. Moreover, this nomenclature system has been used in therapeutic product labeling approved by the Food and Drug Administration (FDA) and clinical practice guidelines provided by other organizations, such as the Clinical Pharmacogenetic Implementation Consortium (CPIC) [27] and the Dutch Pharmacogenomics Working Group (DPWG) [28] to establish recommendations for the translation of pharmacogenetic information into specific drug administration guidelines. Since a patient's germline DNA sequence does not change, genotype information must be portable over time and readily interpretable between clinics. So, the star allele nomenclature is also useful for reporting and sharing of pharmacogenetic information across unaffiliated clinical laboratories and different institutions' electronic medical records (EMRs). Phenotype interpretation nomenclature has also been standardized for many CYPs. Such standardization of allele and phenotype nomenclature is important since the number of medications for which metabolic genotypes can be used to tailor doses is growing.

Gene-drug interactions: Gene-drug interactions (*GDIs*) involving certain polymorphic pharmacogenes (e.g., CYP2C9, CYP2C19, CYP2D6) can lead to high interindividual variability in drug metabolism [30]. In such instances, GDIs are somewhat analogous to *drug-drug interactions* (*DDIs*), described in Chapter 15, that can occur when one drug affects the pharmacokinetics and/or the pharmacodynamics of a concomitantly administered drug or its active metabolites by altering its absorption, metabolism, distribution, or elimination. During drug development, in vitro, in vivo, and in silico DDI studies are routinely conducted to provide appropriate recommendations (e.g., dose adjustments, warnings, contraindications) in the approved therapeutic product labeling [31, 32]. During drug development, DDI evaluations are performed more routinely than GDI evaluations. When information from GDI studies is not available, DDI studies may inform clinical management. Conversely, in some instances, such as when a high fraction of the substrate drug is metabolized by a single CYP enzyme that has loss-of-function alleles, GDI studies may also substitute a prospective DDI study [31]. For example, results from DDI studies can be used to predict GDIs for CYP2D6 substrates, but predictions for CYP2C9 and CYP2C19 substrates are more complex [33]. In addition, DDIs may not always reliably predict GDIs because of the involvement of multiple metabolic enzymes or transporters. When drug labeling includes DDI information, it increasingly includes analogous GDI information [30].

Transporter pharmacogenetics: As discussed in Chapter 13, genetic polymorphisms in membrane transporters can affect absorption and elimination of some drugs, and consequently the response to a number of clinically important therapeutics.

Metabolism pharmacogenetics: Metabolism of drugs by polymorphic drug-metabolizing Phase I and II enzymes is an important contributor to significant variability in exposure, which consequently may lead to variability in clinical response. Some important Phase I and II pharmacogenes are described in detail as follows.

Genetic variation in Phase I metabolic pharmacogenes

Some of the clinically relevant Phase I drug metabolizing enzymes are listed in Table 12.2, together with their clinically relevant star alleles and their phenotypic consequences. The frequencies of their genotypes/phenotypes, some of which may

TABLE 12.1 Examples of common databases, tools, and resources used in pharmacogenetic analysis.

Selected resources	Selected use/information available	Ref.
Genome data		
Nucleotide	Collates genomic data from GenBank, RefSeq, TPA, and PDB	[14]
1000 Genomes Project	Provides genotype frequencies and haplotype structures from specific world populations	[15]
Sequence analysis tools		
BLAST (Basic Local Alignment Search Tool)	Searches specific sequences within Entrez Nucleotide	[14]
PharmCAT (Pharmacogenomics Clinical Annotation Tool)	Analyses sequencing and genotyping technologies to assign haplotypes and extract genomic variants	[16]
Gene and variant analysis		
Entrez Gene	Provides information on gene geography, publications, links	[13, 17]
dbSNP (Database of Short Genetic Variation/SNP)	Provides information on SNPs including accession numbers (rsID), basic genotype frequency, chromosomal position, molecular consequences	[18]
OMIM (Online Mendelian Inheritance in Man)	Provides basic scientific information about genes and variants obtained in vitro and in vivo	[19]
Translational		
dbGaP (Database of Genotypes and Phenotypes)	Collates results from genotype-phenotype studies, cohort studies, clinical trials, and others	[20]
GTR (Genetic Testing Registry)	Provides information on genetic tests to providers and researchers	[21]
ClinVar, ClinGen	Provides reports of the relationships among variations and phenotypes to support interpretation of clinical significance of variants	[22, 23]
Pharmacogenetics		
PharmGKB (Pharmacogenomics Knowledgebase)	Collates information on pharmacogene variation, literature curation, and integration of several resources	[24]
PharmVar (Pharmacogene Variation)	Provides information on allelic variation, haplotype structure, and star nomenclature system for select pharmacogenes	[25]
DGIdb (Drug-Gene Interaction Database)	Provides gene-drug interaction information	[26]
Clinical pharmacogenetics practice guidelines		
CPIC (Clinical Pharmacogenetics Implementation Consortium)	Provides clinical practice guidelines for 47 pharmacogene-drug pairs (as of 2019)	[27]
DPWG (Dutch Pharmacogenetics Working Group)	Provides clinical practice guidelines for 54 pharmacogene-drug pairs (as of 2019)	[28]

Note: *PDB*, protein data bank; *rsID*, reference SNP ID; *TPA*, Third Party Annotation sequence from peer reviewed data.

vary across different populations, are detailed in resources such as PharmGKB [24] and/or CPIC [27]. In Table 12.3, CYP2C19 is used as an example to illustrate how standardized phenotype interpretation is derived from genotype information. This terminology also has been applied for CYP2C9, CYP2D6, CYP3A5, thiopurine methyltransferase (TPMT), dihydropyrimidine dehydrogenase (DPYD), and UDP-glucuronosyltransferase (UGT) 1A1 (UGT1A1). Of note, the proposed *CYP2D6* activity score conversion to phenotype shown in Fig. 12.3 is based on a continuum of metabolic activity scores and lacks a specifically designated rapid metabolizer phenotype [34].

TABLE 12.2 Select examples of clinically relevant star alleles and their consequence.[a,b]

Allele	rsID	Select base or amino acid change	Primary molecular consequence	Phenotype consequence[c]
CYP2B6				
**4*	rs2279343	K262R	Altered catalysis	Increased function
**5*	rs3211371	R487C	N/A	Normal function
**6*	rs3745274 rs2279343	Q172H K262R	Decreased catalysis, splicing defect	Decreased function
**9*	rs3745274	Q172H	Splicing defect	Decreased function
**18*	rs28399499	I328T	Temperature lability	No function
**22*	rs34223104	-82T>C	CAAT enhancer	Increased function
CYP2C9				
**2*	rs1799853	R144C	Decreased catalysis	Decreased function
**3*	rs1057910	I359L	Decreased catalysis	Decreased function
**6*	rs9332131	10601delA	Frameshift	No function
**25*	rs1304490498	3531delAGAAATGGAA	Frameshift	No function
CYP2C19				
**2*	rs4244285	P227P	Premature stop codon	No function
**3*	rs4986893	W212X	Premature stop codon	No function
**4*	rs28399504	M1V	Start codon variant	No function
**5*	rs56337013	R433W	Decreased catalysis	No function
**6*	rs72552267	R132Q	Decreased catalysis	No function
**7*	rs72558186	24319T>A	Splicing defect	No function
**8*	rs41291556	W120R	Decreased catalysis	No function
**9*	rs17884712	R144H	Decreased catalysis	Decreased function
**17*	rs12248560	-806C>T	Transcription factor binding site	Increased function
CYP2D6				
**1xN*		Duplication	Copy number increase	Increased function
**2*	rs16947 rs1135840	R296C S486T	Normal	Normal function
**2xN*		Duplication	Copy number increase	Increased function
**3*	rs35742686	2549delA	Frameshift	No function
**4*	rs1065852 rs3892097 rs1135840	P34S 1846C>A S486T	Splicing defect	No function
**4xN*		Duplication	Splicing defect	No function
**5*		Whole gene deletion		No function
**9*	rs5030656	2616delAAG	Small deletion	Decreased function
**10*	rs1065852 rs1135840	P34S S486T	Decreased catalysis	Decreased function
**13*		Deletions and tandem rearrangements	CYP2D7/CYP2D6 hybrid	No function

TABLE 12.2 Select examples of clinically relevant star alleles and their consequence.[a,b]—cont'd

Allele	rsID	Select base or amino acid change	Primary molecular consequence	Phenotype consequence
**17*	rs28371706 rs16947 rs1135840	T107I R296C S486T	Decreased catalysis	Decreased function
**41*	rs16947 rs28371725 rs1135840	R296C Splicing defect S486T	Splicing defect	Decreased function
CYP3A5				
**3*	rs776746	6986A>G	Splicing defect	Severely decreased function
**6*	rs10264272	14690G>A	Splicing defect	None or severely decreased

[a]*The present table is not comprehensive; rather, it addresses alleles that have clear phenotypic consequences and are commonly tested in populations.*
[b]*Information derived from PharmGKB [24], PharmVar [25], and CPIC [27].*
[c]*Substrate specificity reported for some alleles.*

TABLE 12.3 Standardized phenotype interpretation using genotype information using CYP2C19 as an example.

Standard term	Functional definition	Genetic definition	Examples of *CYP2C19* diplotypes
Ultrarapid metabolizer (UM)	Increased enzyme activity compared to RMs	Two increased function alleles, or more than two normal function alleles	**17/*17*
Rapid metabolizer (RM)	Increased enzyme activity compared to NMs but less than UMs	Combinations of normal function and increased function alleles	**1/*17*
Normal metabolizer (NM)	Fully functional enzyme activity	Two normal function alleles	**1/*1*
Intermediate metabolizer (IM)	Decreased enzyme activity (activity between NMs and PMs)	Combinations of normal function, decreased function, and/or no function alleles	**1/*2, *2/*17, *1/*3, *3/*17*
Poor metabolizer (PM)	Little to no enzyme activity	Combination of no function alleles and/or decreased function alleles	**2/*2, *2/*3, *3/*3*

Table modified from Caudle KE, Dunnenberger HM, Freimuth RR, Peterson JF, Burlison JD, Whirl-Carrillo M, et al. Standardizing terms for clinical pharmacogenetic test results: consensus terms from the Clinical Pharmacogenetics Implementation Consortium (CPIC). Genet Med 2017;19:215–223 and Relling MV, Klein TE, Gammal RS, Whirl-Carrillo M, Hoffman JM, Caudle KE. The Clinical Pharmacogenetics Implementation Consortium: 10 years later. Clin Pharmacol Ther 2020;107:171–175 to represent phenotype consensus terms for CYP2C19.

CYP2B6

More than three dozen distinct star *CYP2B6* alleles have been described [29]. Several in vitro functional studies have characterized the effects of SNPs that alter the expression or catalytic activity of the gene (Table 12.2) [35–39]. The *CYP2B6*4* allele is a nonsynonymous SNP that has substrate-dependent effects, reducing the rate of metabolism of some drugs (e.g., cyclophosphamide) but increasing metabolic activity toward others (e.g., efavirenz) [35]. Thus it is considered both a reduced and increased function allele depending on the substrate. *CYP2B6*6* and *CYP2B6*9* variants are considered to

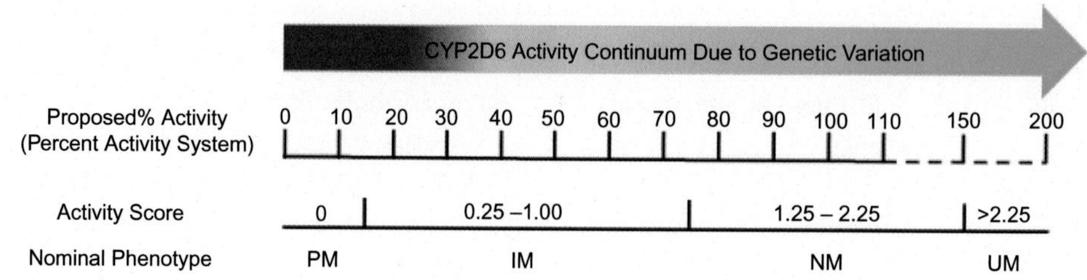

FIG. 12.3 The CYP2D6 activity score is based on a continuum of CYP2D6 activity as determined through assays determining CYP2D6 catalytic function (e.g., metabolism assays conducted in cells or cellular materials). Phenotype categories represent a distribution of different activity scores. *(Modified from Caudle KE, Sangkuhl K, Whirl-Carrillo M, Swen JJ, Haidar CE, Klein TE, et al. Standardizing CYP2D6 genotype to phenotype translation: consensus recommendations from the Clinical Pharmacogenetics Implementation Consortium and Dutch Pharmacogenetics Working Group. Clin Transl Sci 2020;13:116–124.)*

have decreased function, primarily due to their splicing defect [40]. The *CYP2B6*6* allele is the most frequently inherited variant in CYP2B6, with an approximate 15%–60% minor allele frequency, depending on ancestry. Predominantly observed in subjects with African ancestry, the *CYP2B6*18* allele demonstrates low expression and low function; it is thus considered to be a null allele. *CYP2B6*22* encodes a base change in the *CYP2B6* promoter leading to increased *CYP2B6* expression; this causes greater inducibility in the presence of chemical inducers (e.g., rifampicin) and consequently, increased *CYP2B6* activity [38, 41–43]. Several other variants have been characterized, particularly in more recently studied populations [38]. In addition, several nongenetic factors may confound associations between *CYP2B6* variants and drug metabolism rate [44, 45].

CYP2C9

CYP2C9 is highly polymorphic with over 60 cataloged star alleles [29], of which 4 star alleles are presented in Table 12.2. Of these, *CYP2C9*2* and *CYP2C9*3* are the most studied alleles since they each decrease the catalytic activity of CYP2C9 and are commonly inherited in different world populations. Rarer variants, including *CYP2C9*6*and **25*, are responsible for loss of enzyme function [46]. CYP2C9 phenotypes are classified as normal metabolism (NM), intermediate metabolism (IM), or poor metabolism (PM), based on whether the patient carries 0, 1, or 2 copies of a gene with a decreased function polymorphism [46]. Drugs like warfarin, prasugrel, and phenytoin are metabolized by CYP2C9.

CYP2C19

Approximately three dozen star alleles have been described for *CYP2C19* [29]. Several genetic variants in *CYP2C19* that can significantly affect gene expression and activity are presented in Table 12.2. For example, *CYP2C19*2* is characterized by an aberrant splice site in exon 5 that results in a truncated protein with no function. Similarly, *CYP2C19*3* has a premature stop codon in exon 4, resulting in a truncated protein with no function [47, 48]. Less frequent loss-of-function or reduced-activity alleles include: *CYP2C19*4*, **5*, **6*, **7*, and **8* [49]. A consensus binding site for the GATA transcription factor family is located within the promoter of *CYP2C19*17* and increases the expression of *CYP2C19*, thus increasing its activity [50]. An amino acid change in the *CYP2C19*9* allele confers decreased function and results in "likely intermediate" metabolism status (e.g., *CYP2C19*1/*9*, **9/*9*, **9/*17*) [51, 52]. While numerous combinations are possible, some combinations of CYP2C19 star alleles that result in ultrarapid metabolism (UM), rapid metabolism (RM), NM, IM, and PM status are listed in Table 12.3. Several drugs like clopidogrel, voriconazole, and many of the selective serotonin reuptake inhibitors (SSRIs) and tricyclic antidepressants (TCAs) are metabolized by CYP2C19.

CYP2D6

CYP2D6 is a highly polymorphic gene with over 130 star alleles reported. CYP2D6 metabolizes about 20% of clinically used small molecular drugs [29, 53]. CYP2D6 demonstrates significant phenotypic variability, a substantial portion of which can be attributed to genetic variability (Table 12.2). The metabolism status resulting from each allele initially was determined using the rate of transformation of dextromethorphan, a CYP2D6 probe substrate, in a large number of human subjects [54]. Although this approach to phenotypic classification is not ideal [55], significant progress has been made recently to assign metabolic phenotype based on genotype-predicted activity scores to CYP2D6. These activity scores are quanta used to describe the activity of *CYP2D6* based on the percent increase or decrease in activity conferred by the different *CYP2D6* alleles (Fig. 12.3) [34]. There is significant evidence that *CYP2D6* phenotype prediction from genotype is useful for guiding dosing regimens for certain drugs and drug classes. Not surprisingly, *CYP2D6* information is included in several drug labels [56] and also constitutes the largest proportion of pharmacogenetic content in the current pharmacogenetic guidelines published by the CPIC [27] and DPWG [28]. Examples include drugs such as atomoxetine, codeine, tamoxifen, SSRIs, TCAs, eliglustat, metoprolol, pimozide, and propafenone.

A gene deletion (*CYP2D6*5*) and several gene duplications (*CYP2D6*1xN*, **2xN*, **4xN*, and **41xN*) are observed for *CYP2D6* [57, 58]. There are now well-documented examples that illustrate that duplicated *CYP2D6* gene copies (e.g., *CYP2D6*4xN*) do not always lead to increased activity [59]. Gene deletions and tandem rearrangements are also responsible for several *CYP2D7/CYP2D6* hybrids (*CYP2D6*13*), the entire series of which contains a *CYP2D7*-derived exon 1 with a T-insertion that results in a nonfunctional protein. *CYP2D6* is also subject to splicing defects (e.g., *CYP2D6*4*) and frameshift mutation (e.g., *CYP2D6*3*) that inactivate *CYP2D6*. Several nonsynonymous polymorphisms also reduce CYP2D6 catalytic activity toward several substrates including *CYP2D6*10* (highly prevalent in Asia), *CYP2D6*14*, and *CYP2D6*17* (predominantly in individuals with African ancestry). Numerous other genetic variants affect CYP2D6 phenotype [57] but are beyond the scope of this chapter.

CYP3A4 *and* CYP3A5

CYP3A4 and CYP3A5 are expressed abundantly in liver and gut, and are responsible for metabolizing the highest proportion (~30%) of clinically used small molecular drugs [53]. Genetic variants in CY3A are often found to have uncertain significance, limiting their utility (particularly, for CYP3A4) in pharmacogenetics-guided treatment decisions. Numerous nongenetic factors confound prediction of CYP3A4 phenotype from genotype, including coadministered medications, hormonal status, age, gender, and inflammatory processes [60]. CYP3A5 has approximately 85% sequence similarity to CYP3A4 and highly similar substrate selectivity [61]. CYP3A5 has several genetic variants that significantly affect gene expression and activity (Table 12.2). The *CYP3A5*3* allele encodes a splice junction variant that results in nonsense-mediated decay of *CYP3A5* mRNA and a lack of CYP3A5 protein expression [62]. *CYP3A5*6* encodes a SNP that results in exon skipping and truncated protein, resulting in null activity [63]. *CYP3A5*7* results in a frameshift mutation that likely eliminates the expression of CYP3A5 [64].

Genetic variation in Phase II metabolic pharmacogenes

Phase II metabolizing enzymes mediate biotransformation via conjugation. They are mainly transferases such as UGTs, sulfotransferases (SULTs), *N*-acetyltransferases (NATs), methyl transferases, and glutathione S-transferases (GSTs). Genetic variants in the genes encoding these variants can affect metabolism and clearance of many drugs, consequently leading to variability in drug response [65]. Select examples of Phase II pharmacogenes are described as follows.

Thiopurine S-*methyltransferase (TPMT)*

Thiopurine *S*-methyltransferase (TPMT) is a cytosolic enzyme whose precise physiological role is unknown. The *TPMT* gene is polymorphic, and a trimodal distribution of enzyme activity is observed [66]. The frequency with which TPMT activity is lost varies in different racial/ethnic populations. The *TPMT* variants, **3A*, **3B*, *3C, and **2*, are the most common inactivating alleles and account for over 90% of low activity phenotypes [66]. TPMT catalyzes the *S*-methylation of the thiopurine agents azathioprine, 6-mercaptopurine, and 6-thioguanine [67]. *TPMT* genetic polymorphisms are attributed to serious adverse drug reactions (myelosuppression) in patients treated with thiopurines (discussed in Chapter 16) and may also contribute to interindividual variability in efficacy [66, 68].

N-*Acetyltransferase 2 (NAT2)*

Genetic variations in *N*-acetyltransferase 2 (*NAT2*) are very common with over 100 *NAT2* alleles described [69]. Genetic variations in *NAT*2 can affect enzyme activity by decreasing enzyme stability or altering affinity for a substrate. Based on enzyme activity or genotype, individuals can be grouped into three different phenotypes: slow acetylator (two slow alleles), intermediate acetylator (1 slow and 1 rapid allele), and rapid (or fast) acetylator (2 rapid alleles) [70]. Frequency differences in NAT2 genotype/phenotype exist among racial/ethnic populations. The NAT2 slow acetylator phenotype is more common among Caucasians and Africans (40%–70%) than Asians (10%–30% among Japanese, Chinese, Korean, and Thai), though a wide range of variability in the frequencies have been reported in the literature [70]. Although a number of studies have attempted to associate this polymorphism with the risk for xenobiotic-induced cancers, there are very limited examples where phenotyping data can be used to personalize drug treatment. See Chapter 16 for more information.

Target/efficacy pharmacogenetics

Vitamin K epoxide reductase complex, subunit 1 (VKORC1)

VKORC1 encodes a multifunctional enzyme that converts vitamin K epoxide into its reduced, hydroquinone form [71] and is the rate-limiting step of vitamin K recycling [72]. Reduced vitamin K acts as a cosubstrate of γ-glutamyl carboxylase (GGCX) during the conversion of glutamate to γ-carboxyglutamate (Gla) [73, 74]. In response to vascular injury, Gla residues are formed on coagulation factors (e.g., factors II, VII, IX, and X), enabling these factors to bind calcium ions and promote coagulation [74]. Warfarin inhibits VKORC1, thereby blocking efficient reduction of vitamin K and preventing clotting factor activation [75, 76]. Variants in *VKORC1* lead to variability in warfarin response. A promoter variant (-*1639G>A*; rs9923231) in *VKORC1* is thought to be located in a transcription factor binding site and is associated with a 44% decreased expression of the enzyme in a cellular assay [77, 78]. This variant is in linkage disequilibrium with other variants (rs2359612, rs8050894, rs9934438, and rs7196161), and either rs9923231 or rs9934438 (*1173C>T*) are recommended markers for prediction of VKORC1 phenotype [79]. Other rare genetic variants also associated with decreased VKORC1 function are V29L (rs104894539), N36Y (rs61742245), V45A (rs104894540), R58G (rs104894541), R98W (rs72547528), and L128R (rs104894542) [80, 81].

Epidermal growth factor receptor (EGFR) and genes of the EGFR-signaling pathway

Lung cancer continues to be a leading cause of death in the United States [82]. The identification of driver somatic mutations, particularly in nonsmall cell lung cancer (NSCLC), has led to the development of several molecularly targeted therapies. The advent of tyrosine kinase inhibitors (TKIs) such as gefitinib brought about a new approach in treatment, albeit for a very small population of patients with lung cancer. Gefitinib was first approved in the United States for use in patients with advanced NSCLC in 2003. However, the lack of benefit resulted in the drug being withdrawn from the market in 2005. It was clear from the start that only a few patients appeared to benefit from gefitinib, and development of other TKIs during this time showed that somatic mutations in the epidermal growth factor receptor (EGFR) appeared to identify a subpopulation of patients who respond well to this and other TKIs [83]. These *EGFR* gene mutations are present in approximately 10% of patients with NSCLC in the United States and 35% in East Asia. They result in a "gain of function" within the tumors of these patients but appear to enhance their responsiveness to TKIs. Based on this understanding, gefitinib was reapproved in 2015 for patients with select EGFR mutations (exon 19 deletions or exon 21 L858R substitution).

EGFR activation also is linked with downstream events that regulate cell growth, proliferation, and survival via the *KRAS* gene that codes for K-Ras protein. Retrospective studies of cetuximab, a monoclonal antibody targeted against EGFR that is approved for treating patients with metastatic colorectal cancer and head and neck cancers, showed that patients with colorectal cancer bearing activating mutations of *KRAS* did not benefit from cetuximab treatment [84] (Fig. 12.4). Subsequently, the FDA revised the indication section of the cetuximab labeling to limit its use when the results of the *Ras* mutation tests are unknown. However, there are still patients with "wildtype" *KRAS* who do not respond to EGFR-blocking drugs, so additional genomic or other biomarkers are needed to select only those patients who would benefit from treatment with this drug.

Cystic fibrosis transmembrane conductance regulator (CFTR)

The *CFTR* gene encodes for a chloride channel that mediates conduction of chloride ion across the apical membrane of epithelial cells. Variants in the *CFTR* gene result in cystic fibrosis (*CF*), an autosomal recessive genetic disorder with abnormal chloride conductance that affects a number of organs (e.g., lung airways, pancreas, sweat glands). Nearly 2000 *CFTR* variants have been identified and about 350 are known to be pathogenic. There is a range in severity of *CF*: from absence of the protein to a near normal amount of protein production and cell surface localization, but with altered channel-gating mechanisms [85]. CFTR modulators have been developed that can improve the function of the defective CFTR protein. Thus far, four CFTR modulators (ivacaftor and three other ivacaftor combinations) have FDA approval for treating patients with specific *CFTR* variants. One of the approvals even brought about a paradigm change in the drug approval process. After initial approval in 2012, approval for an extended patient population in 2017 was based on clinical trial data as well as in vitro cell-based assay data for certain variants (even in the absence of correlating clinical data) demonstrating increased chloride ion transport across cells in response to ivacaftor [86].

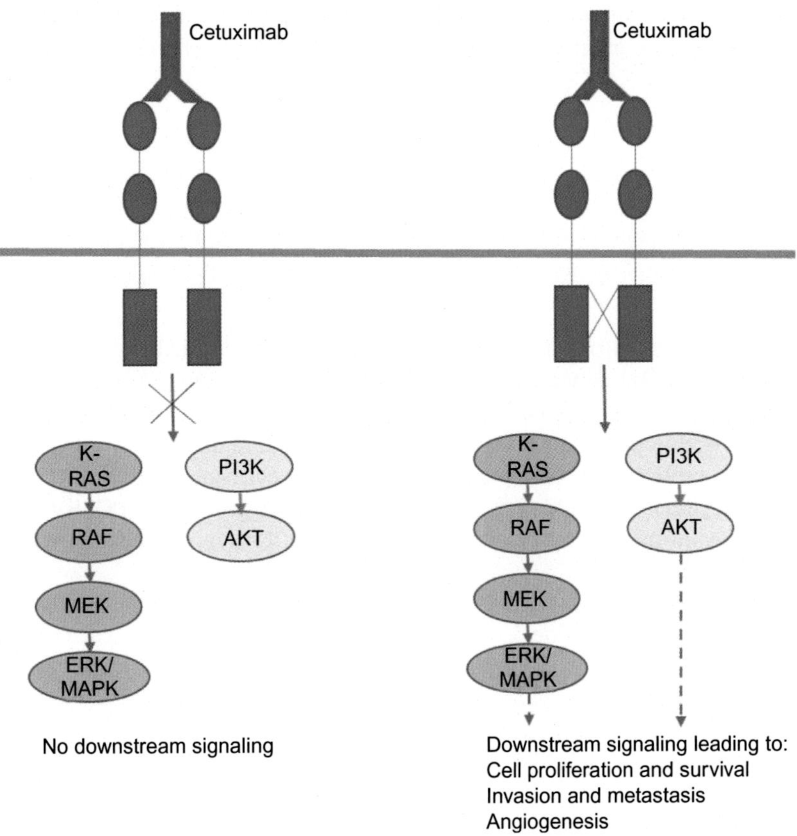

FIG. 12.4 Cetuximab mechanism of action and downstream signaling. In the wild-type state of *KRAS* (*left panel*), the binding of cetuximab to EGFR can shut down receptor-mediated signaling. In the variant *KRAS* state (*right panel*), the system is in an active state that is not responsive to cetuximab, so there is persistent signaling.

Safety pharmacogenetics

As discussed in Chapter 16, pharmacogenetics is one of many factors that can explain adverse drug response. For example, carbamazepine labeling contains a boxed warning about toxic epidermal necrosis (TEN) and Stevens-Johnson Syndrome (SJS) in Asian patients with *HLA-B*1502* allele. Similarly, for abacavir, patients with *HLA-B*5701* allele are at high risk for experiencing a hypersensitivity reaction.

Combined variants in drug metabolism and target genes: The value of drug pathway analysis

Each drug has a pharmacokinetic pathway of absorption, distribution, metabolism, and elimination that is ultimately linked to an effect pathway involving receptor targets and downstream signaling pathways. It is possible that many of the proteins in both these pathways may be genetically polymorphic and a patient's response may be affected by variants in a gene involved in drug metabolism and transport as well as by variants in a receptor. As exemplified by warfarin, considering the combination of both these factors provides greater predictive power than when either is considered alone.

Pharmacogenetics in drug discovery, development, regulation, and utilization

The rate of attrition of candidate drugs during development continues to be high, with an overall success rate of about 10% from Phase 1 entry to marketing approval [87, 88]. Even after the approval of a drug, individual patient response rates are abysmal as estimated response rates for the 10 highest-grossing marketed drugs range from 4% to 25% [89]. This highlights a need to take into account the factors that cause interindividual variability in both exposure and response during drug development and utilization. As a result, human genetics and pharmacogenetics have come to play increasingly important roles in the discovery, development, regulation, and utilization (DDRU) of novel therapeutics.

Drug discovery and development

Human genetics has become an integral driver of drug discovery strategies. Population genomic resources are increasingly utilized to identify new drug targets in the expectation that they should improve the likelihood of successful drug development [90–94]. Particularly in oncology, clinical development programs more commonly target the molecular pathology of disease, leading to the approval of numerous treatments that were developed through highly targeted clinical trials.

More specifically, human genetics and pharmacogenetics can be used for:

(1) **Target validation:** genetics can inform drug discovery and development by helping to identify drug targets that will be relevant for a given disease [91]. Since completion of the Human Genome Project, increasingly large amounts of human genomic data have been generated from epidemiologic research studies and large biobanks that are linked to EMRs (Table 12.1). Additionally, molecular diagnosis of some rare diseases or conditions can be used to characterize the loss of a given protein, and consequently identify therapeutic interventions that could be useful. The availability of this information has led to the identification of novel drug targets such as PCSK9 that resulted in development of monoclonal antibodies to treat dyslipidemia, as well as identification of a number of additional potential targets (e.g., ANGPTL3 for dyslipidemia).

(2) **Guiding clinical trial designs:** genetics can be leveraged to inform clinical trial design features such as:

  (a) *Enriched and adaptive clinical trial designs:* during drug development, the clinical trial population can be enriched by selecting a subset of patients in whom the potential effect of a drug can more readily be demonstrated [95]. Predictive enrichment strategies to choose patients who are more likely to respond can be used to provide a larger effect size and to obtain statistically significant results with a smaller study population. Based on interim results from a biomarker-defined subpopulation, the design (e.g., eligibility criteria, enrollment) of a clinical trial can be adaptively modified [96]. Including biomarker testing as part of the study inclusion criteria to select patients has been associated with a higher likelihood of approval—from about 10% without biomarker-based selection to about 25% with biomarker-based selection [94].

  (b) *Master protocols:* genomically driven master protocols that test one or more interventions in one or more diseases can be used to study biomarker-defined population or disease subtypes. For example, NCI-MATCH trial is a *basket master protocol* in which patients with any cancer type (e.g., colon, breast, lung, and others) sharing the same genetic abnormality (e.g., *EGFR*, neurotrophic tyrosine receptor kinase (*NTRK*)) are treated [97]. Similarly, Lung-Map is a type of *umbrella master protocol* in which patients receive genomic profiling to determine the genomic alterations that drives their lung cancer and the patients are then matched to a treatment that is being tested in the protocol [98].

(3) **Identifying sources of concentration or response variability:** after clinical trials have been completed, it is possible to analyze stored specimens to identify sources of concentration or response variability. When clinical trials uncover variability that cannot be explained by other demographic or clinical factors, genomic studies like GWAS may reveal clearance pathways or response mechanisms that were not anticipated from other routine drug development experiments. Such studies have been instrumental in finding sources of variability for drugs, like interferon-alfa 2b in the setting of chronic hepatitis C virus infection [99]. In situations where a strong hypothesis can be formulated, such as known metabolism via polymorphic pathway, retrospective studies can be conducted to compare concentration or response endpoint distributions across genetic subgroups. However, it is also possible to prospectively conduct pharmacogenetic studies by balancing enrollment of certain genotypic or phenotypic subgroups such as PMs and NMs. In cases where there may be a single metabolism or transport pathway, it can even be possible to extrapolate genetic findings to anticipate possible DDIs.

(4) **PD response:** biomarkers, such as gene expression patterns, may be used as an endpoint to determine if the drug modulates the target and has the potential to cause a downstream effect. This information can be used for internal decision-making during drug development and sometimes as endpoints in clinical trials.

Human genetics and pharmacogenetics have revolutionized drug development and treatment for diseases such as cancers and some rare diseases, and have brought about a paradigm change in patient care. In the past, cancer drugs were approved to treat specific tumor types that were located in a single anatomic site (e.g., kidney, skin, lung). Following the discovery that genetic markers can act to predict tumor response, drug development efforts for certain cancers were directed toward specific targets (e.g., EGFR or anaplastic lymphoma kinase (ALK) fusion-positive NSCLC) as listed in Table 12.4. Many of

TABLE 12.4 Select examples of drug-device coapprovals in oncology.

Drug	Cancer/mechanism	Indicated subset	Diagnostic name
Gefitinib	NSCLC/EGFR inhibitor	EGFR exon 19 deletions or exon 21 L858R substitution	therascreen EGFR RGQ PCR Kit, cobas EGFR Mutation Test v2, FoundationOne CDx, Oncomine Dx Target Test
Osimertinib	NSCLC/EGFR inhibitor	EGFR exon 19 deletions or exon 21 L858R substitution or T790M	cobas EGFR Mutation Test v2, FoundationOne CDx
Cetuximab[a]	CRC/EGFR inhibitor	KRAS wild-type	FoundationOne CDx, cobas KRAS Mutation Test, therascreen KRAS RGQ PCR Kit, Dako EGFR pharmDx Kit
Olaparib	Ovarian/PARP inhibitor	Deleterious or suspected deleterious germline BRCA mutation	BRACAnalysis CDx, FoundationOne CDx, Myriad myChoice CDx

Select information on the disease, subsets, and diagnostics are included in the Table. Refer to [100] and [101] for more information on drugs and devices, respectively. *CRC*, colorectal cancer; *EGFR*, epidermal growth factor receptor; *KRAS*, Kirsten rat sarcoma viral oncogene homolog; *NSCLC*, nonsmall cell lung cancer; *PARP*, poly (ADP-ribose) polymerase.
[a]*Narrowing of indication and companion diagnostic approval occurred postmarketing.*

these drugs were developed along with *companion diagnostics* that were used to identify patients who would benefit from these therapies [101]. These companion diagnostics are medical devices which provide information that is essential for the safe and effective use of a corresponding drug or biological product and often are coapproved with the therapeutic product [102]. Some examples are listed in Table 12.4. In a few instances, drugs have been approved with *complementary diagnostics* which may bear on improving the benefit/risk ratio of a drug without restricting access to it [103]. More recently, genetics has been leveraged to develop and approve cancer drugs that are "tissue agnostic" in that they are based on a common genetic marker across different tumor types (e.g., microsatellite instability-high (MSI-H) or mismatch repair deficient (dMMR), *NTRK* gene fusion) rather than the anatomic location where the tumor originated [104].

Use of pharmacogenetics in drug regulation

To support development of personalized medicines, regulatory agencies including FDA, European Medicines Agencies (EMA), and Japanese Pharmaceuticals and Medical Devices Agency (PMDA) provide regulatory advice and review therapeutic product applications to support the use of pharmacogenetics to facilitate rational drug development and therapeutic individualization. To this end, regulatory agencies across the globe have developed guidances to identify emergent pharmacogenetic issues and to facilitate the development of both drugs and diagnostics. Some common issues that regulatory agencies have offered: recommendations on when and how to conduct pharmacogenetic studies as part of a drug development program [105, 106], how to develop in vitro diagnostic tests [102, 107], and how to harmonize genomic sampling and management of genomic data in clinical studies [108].

About a decade ago, when pharmacogenetic information was included in the product labeling, this was mostly based on research conducted after the approval of the drug. *Retrospective analyses* (e.g., as in the case of warfarin, clopidogrel, carbamazepine) were utilized to explain variable responses to therapeutic products, identify responders, and identify patients at risk for serious drug reactions. However, with better understanding of the role of genetics and pharmacogenetics in disease and drug development, over the course of the 2010s, drug developers have increasingly incorporated prospective genetic analysis early in the drug development process in order to predict drug exposure, minimize variability, and select responders, nonresponders, or even toxic responders. These *prospective analyses* have led to the development of increasing numbers of personalized medicines. In fact, 42% of the new molecular entities approved by the FDA in 2018 were considered personalized medicines in that the product labeling included reference to specific biological markers, identified by diagnostic tools, that help guide decisions for their use [109]. This is an increase from the past years when 27%–34% of approved medicines could be considered personalized [109].

In general, therapeutic product labeling contains information on pharmacogenetic biomarkers to inform prescribers about the impact or lack of impact of patient genotype or phenotype and to indicate whether a test is available, and if the test is to be considered, is recommended, or is necessary. Product labeling can include information on genetic biomarkers (including frequencies of alleles, genotypes, haplotypes) and can describe the expected impact on drug exposure

TABLE 12.5 Select examples of drugs with pharmacogenetic information in the US-approved product labeling.

Drug	Gene	Select recommendations[a]
Metabolism pharmacogenetics		
Belinostat	*UGT1A1*	Reduce the starting dose to 750 mg/m^2 in patients known to be homozygous for *UGT1A1*28* allele
Clobazam	*CYP2C19*	In known CYP2C19 PMs, starting dose should be 5 mg/day and dose titration should proceed slowly
Eliglustat	*CYP2D6*	Select patients using an FDA-cleared test for determining *CYP2D6* genotype; Recommended Dosage Regimen by CYP2D6 Metabolizer Status: EMs (84 mg twice daily), IMs (84 mg twice daily), and PMs (84 mg once daily). Limitations of Use: CYP2D6 UMs and IMs
Tetrabenazine	*CYP2D6*	Patients requiring doses above 50 mg/day should be genotyped for *CYP2D6* to determine if PM or EM.
Target/efficacy pharmacogenetics		
Afatinib	*EGFR*	Select patients based on the presence of nonresistant *EGFR* mutations as detected by an FDA-approved test
Cobimetinib with vemurafenib	*BRAF*	Confirm the presence of *BRAF V600E/K* mutation as detected by an FDA-approved test
Crizotinib	*ALK, ROS1*	Select patients on the presence of *ALK* or *ROS1* positivity as detected by an FDA-approved test
Ivacaftor	*CFTR*	Indicated for patients who have specific mutation in the *CFTR* gene that is responsive to ivacaftor potentiation based on clinical and/or in vitro assay data
Safety pharmacogenetics		
Codeine[b]	*CYP2D6*	Contraindication in children (select age groups) based on risk of respiratory depression and death in CYP2D6 UMs
Phenytoin	*HLA-B*	Warning regarding *HLA-B*1502* and risk of toxic epidermal necrolysis (TEN) and Stevens-Johnson syndrome (SJS)
Carbamazepine	*HLA-B, HLA-A*	Information regarding *HLA-B*1502* (testing required) and *HLA-A*3101* and risk of SJS and TEN
Valproic acid	*POLG*	Warnings and Contraindication for select patients because of increased risk of valproate-induced acute liver failure and resultant deaths in patients with mitochondrial *POLG* gene mutations

[a]*For detailed recommendations for the different genotype or phenotype groups, refer to the latest labeling available at Drugs@FDA [100].*
[b]*Metabolism related.*

(e.g., altered drug pharmacokinetics because of reduced CYP enzyme activity caused by genetic variation) and clinical response, risk for adverse events, genotype- or phenotype-specific dosing, mechanisms of drug action, and clinical trial design features (e.g., patient selection). Table 12.5 contains examples of drugs that include pharmacogenetic information in the product labeling. A more extensive list of FDA-approved therapeutic products with pharmacogenetic information (both actionable and informative) in the product labeling can be found in the Table of Pharmacogenomic Biomarkers in Drug Labeling [110] and other resources like PharmGKB [24].

Incorporation of pharmacogenetics in therapeutic guidelines

Advances in pharmacogenetics have encouraged a movement away from a one-size-fits-all population-based treatment approach to a more personalized and individualized treatment paradigm. The clinical implementation of pharmacogenetics has grown substantially in recent years and pharmacogenetic data are now increasingly used to guide treatment with certain drugs. Apart from actionable recommendations included in the FDA-approved product labeling (Table 12.5), organizations such CPIC [27] and DPWG [28] have been providing clinical guidelines for managing clinically important pharmacogenetic interactions and creating resources to support clinical testing. In the first 10 years after the formation of the CPIC, guidelines were developed for 47 gene-drug pairs. From its formation in 2005 until 2019, the DPWG has developed guidelines for 54 gene-drug pairs. The goal of these guidelines is to facilitate translation of genetic laboratory test results into information that can be used to guide prescribing decisions for specific drugs. Some examples of clinically important gene-drug interactions for which guidelines have been issued are listed as follows.

CYP2B6 *genotype for the use of efavirenz*

Efavirenz is a nonnucleoside reverse transcriptase inhibitor that is extensively prescribed worldwide to treat HIV/AIDS. Many CYPs and UGTs are involved in efavirenz metabolism. CYP2B6 initially converts efavirenz to its inactive major metabolite, 8-hydroxy-efavirenz, which then undergoes glucuronidation and renal clearance [111]. Interestingly, efavirenz also induces *CYP2B6*, thereby augmenting its own metabolism. The extent of such autoinduction depends on the duration of an individual's exposure to efavirenz, as well on as several demographic and environmental factors. *CYP2B6*6* is significantly less inducible, resulting in steadier but still higher efavirenz plasma concentrations over time [112]. Virologic failure is observed in many patients whose plasma concentrations are lower than 1 μg/mL, whereas CNS side effects are more likely to develop in patients with plasma concentrations above 4 μg/mL [113]. Higher plasma concentrations are more likely in patients who are CYP2B6 PM (**6/*6*, **18 /*18*, and **6/*18*) or IM (**1/*6*, **1/*18*, **4/*6*, **4/*18*, **6/*22*, and **18/*22*), resulting in drug toxicity and treatment discontinuation [114]. Thus the CPIC guideline for this drug recommends reducing the usual adult efavirenz starting dose (600 mg) to at least 400 mg for PMs [114]. In pediatric patients, the FDA-approved efavirenz starting dose is age- and weight-dependent, and use of genotype-guided dosing or therapeutic drug monitoring (TDM) is recommended [115, 116].

CYP2C19 *genotype for the use of clopidogrel*

Clopidogrel, an antiplatelet agent, has been a mainstay of treatment to reduce the rate of myocardial infarction and stroke in patients with cardiovascular disease [117]. Clopidogrel is a prodrug that requires hepatic metabolism by CYP2C19 in order to generate its pharmacologically active metabolite. Carboxylesterases hydrolyze approximately 85% of clopidogrel in the systemic circulation and CYP2C19 bioactivates the remaining 15%. Individuals who carry *CYP2C19* loss-of-function alleles have consistently been shown to have reduced concentrations of the active metabolite and, correspondingly, reduced platelet inhibition that may result in higher rates of stent thrombosis and potentially fatal cardiovascular events [118, 119]. It was subsequently demonstrated that treating *CYP2C19*2* heterozygotes with 225 mg/day clopidogrel reduced their platelet reactivity to the same level as observed in noncarriers who received the standard 75 mg/day dose [118]. However, even doses as high as 300 mg/day did not provide *CYP2C19*2* homozygotes with comparable levels of platelet inhibition. A subsequent meta-analysis of data from several clinical trials showed that patients with only one reduced-function allele of *CYP2C19* have reduced clinical efficacy or increased stent thrombosis during clopidogrel treatment [120]. In patients undergoing percutaneous coronary intervention, a real-world observational study demonstrated a higher risk for cardiovascular events in patients with a *CYP2C19* loss-of-function allele when clopidogrel, rather than alternative therapy, was prescribed [121]. In addition, a prospective study demonstrated that a *CYP2C19* genotype-guided strategy for selection of oral P2Y12 inhibitor therapy was noninferior to standard treatment with ticagrelor or prasugrel at 12 months with respect to thrombotic events and resulted in a lower incidence of bleeding [122]. However, not all studies have agreed on a relationship between *CYP2C19* status and outcome in patients treated with clopidogrel [123, 124]. The FDA added a warning to the clopidogrel label indicating that alternative treatments should be considered for PMs. The CPIC guideline recommends that in patients with acute coronary syndromes undergoing consideration for percutaneous intervention should be given alternative antiplatelet therapy (e.g., prasugrel, ticagrelor) for both *CYP2C19* IMs (**1/*2*, **1/*3*, **2/*17*) and PMs (**2/*2*, **2/*3*, **3/*3*) [125].

CYP2D6 *genotype for the use of codeine and tamoxifen*

The analgesic activity of codeine depends on its metabolic conversion to morphine, which has a 200-fold greater affinity for the μ-opioid receptor [126, 127]. CYP2D6 NMs convert approximately 5%–10% of the codeine dose to morphine, while UMs convert a greater proportion of the dose to morphine and PMs have impaired conversion [128]. Codeine is also extensively converted to inactive metabolites through glucuronidation and *N*-demethylation via CYP3A4 [126]. Though codeine conversion to morphine is a minor pathway among the several competing metabolic routes, variation in CYP2D6 activity significantly influences the plasma concentration of morphine, and therefore patient response to codeine therapy. Consequently, individuals harboring UM phenotypes have the potential to experience toxicity whereas those harboring PM phenotypes are at risk for experiencing insufficient pain relief. For both UMs and PMs, tramadol and, to a lesser extent, hydrocodone and oxycodone are not considered alternatives since these medications also are metabolized by CYP2D6

[128]. The FDA provides specific recommendations, both contraindication and warning, for different specific populations including children, adolescents, and breast-feeding mothers [100].

Tamoxifen is a selective estrogen receptor modulator for the treatment of estrogen receptor-positive breast cancers and is frequently used to treat early stage breast cancer in premenopausal women. Like codeine, tamoxifen is a prodrug that is metabolized by polymorphic CYP2D6 to metabolites 4-hydroxy tamoxifen and endoxifen that have approximately 100-fold greater potency than tamoxifen itself. Recent publications have reported conflicting results with respect to the influence of *CYP2D6* genotype on tamoxifen outcomes [129–134]. However, a meta-analysis demonstrated a relationship between *CYP2D6* genotype and outcome in patients who received 20 mg/day tamoxifen for 5 years as adjuvant therapy [135]. Other studies have demonstrated low endoxifen concentrations (<14 nM) were associated with recurrence or death when compared with high concentrations (>35 nM) [136, 137]. Current CPIC guidelines recommend that UMs and NMs with an activity score of 1.5–2.0 receive standard-of-care tamoxifen dosing, whereas 40 mg/day tamoxifen or considerations for other hormone therapies are recommended for NMs with an activity score of 1.0 and IMs [138]. The CPIC guideline recommends that PMs receive alternate hormone therapy or a higher dose of tamoxifen (40 mg/day) which increases but does not normalize endoxifen concentrations.

CYP2C9, CYP4F2, *and* VKORC1 *genotype for the use of warfarin*

Warfarin is an anticoagulant that is widely used for prophylaxis and treatment of venous thrombosis, pulmonary embolism, thromboembolic complications associated with atrial fibrillation and/or cardiac valve replacement, recurrent myocardial infarction, and thromboembolic events such as stroke, or systemic embolization after myocardial infarction [100]. Warfarin has a narrow therapeutic window and exhibits wide response variability in that the same dose can result in low or high international normalized ratio (INR) in different individuals, putting some at risk for either rethrombosis or potentially fatal hemorrhagic complications [139]. Thus proper use requires using the INR to monitor both the starting and maintenance dose. Based on population averages, the initial adult dose of warfarin is about 4–5 mg/day, and the dose subsequently is titrated based on INR measurements. However, it can sometimes take weeks to months to reach as stable dosing regimen, during which patients are at risk of over- or undercoagulation [140].

Numerous factors have been identified that can help estimate what an individual's warfarin starting dose and stable maintenance doses. Age, weight, diet, liver function, comorbidities (e.g., chronic kidney disease), lifestyle factors (e.g., alcohol consumption), and concomitant therapies (e.g., antiplatelet agents and CYP inducers) have all been associated with needed warfarin dose adjustments, as well as bleeding risk, and are particularly important to consider during warfarin dose selection [141, 142]. Similarly, variant *CYP2C9* alleles significantly influence the clearance of the pharmacologically active *S*-enantiomer of warfarin, affecting not only its concentrations, but also the time needed to reach a stable INR. *VKORC1* has been identified as a gene responsible for warfarin's pharmacodynamic effects and also accounts for a significant proportion of warfarin dose variance [75, 81, 143]. The myriad determinants of warfarin dose have been studied for many years to identify approaches for predicting an individual's dose. A number of complex algorithms, accounting for both clinical factors and genotypes, have been developed to optimize an individual's warfarin dose. Two of these algorithms have even been evaluated in randomized trials that have shown that patients for whom genotype was used to inform the starting dose reached therapeutic INR and stable warfarin doses earlier than a control group in which only clinical factors were used [141, 142]. Table 12.6 gives the ranges of expected warfarin doses based on select *CYP2C9* and *VKORC1* genotypes as listed in the therapeutic product labeling.

Although the specifics of the various algorithms are beyond the scope of the present chapter, CPIC has developed guidelines using an algorithm for patients who self-identify as having non-African ancestry and have *CYP2C9*2*, *CYP2C9*3*,

TABLE 12.6 Ranges of expected maintenance COUMADIN daily doses based on *CYP2C9* and *VKORC1* genotypes.[a]

VKORC1	CYP2C9					
	*1/*1	*1/*2	*1/*3	*2/*2	*2/*3	*3/*3
GG	5-7 mg	5-7 mg	3-4 mg	3-4 mg	3-4 mg	0.5-2 mg
AG	5-7 mg	3-4 mg	3-4 mg	3-4 mg	0.5-2 mg	0.5-2 mg
AA	3-4 mg	3-4 mg	0.5-2 mg	0.5-2 mg	0.5-2 mg	0.5-2 mg

[a]*Ranges are derived from multiple published clinical studies.* VKORC1 − 1639G>A *(rs9923231) variant is used in this table. Other coinherited* VKORC1 *variants may also be important determinants of warfarin dose.*

Based on FDA-approved product labeling. US Food and Drug Administration. Drugs@FDA: FDA-approved drugs; 2020. Available from: https://www.accessdata.fda.gov/scripts/cder/daf/index.cfm. [Accessed 2 January 2020].

and *VKORC1 -1639G>A* genotypes available [140]. The dose can be refined using *CYP2C9*5*, **6*, **8*, **11*, and the *CYP4F2* rs2108622 T allele, if available [144]. However, these genotypes are considered optional. Patients self-identifying with African ancestry must have *CYP2C9*5*, **6*, **8*, and **11* genotypes in order to proceed with the algorithm [140]. Additionally, these patients should also have been tested for the *CYP2C* cluster variant (rs12777823) [145]. These recommendations are considered to have "moderate" evidence supporting them and patients without genotype information are recommended to be dosed using clinical criteria [140]. An online warfarin dosing algorithm, WarfarinDosing (http://www.warfarindosing.org/Source/InitialDose.aspx), is also available to assist in dose selection. Although this algorithm currently contains a slightly different set of genotypes than does CPIC, it accounts for several clinical factors as well as genotype information.

For the use of genotype-based algorithms, prospective genotyping results must be available prior to initiating warfarin treatment. Unfortunately, very few individuals have this information available to them at the time of a warfarin prescription, since fewer than 10% of hospitals offer pharmacogenetic testing [146], and what testing is available is typically reactive rather than preemptive [147, 148].

Genetic testing in clinical practice

If implementation of pharmacogenetics in clinical practice is to become successful, it will require accurate and reliable genetic tests that allow physicians to predict clinically relevant outcomes with confidence. Currently, an individual may obtain genetic testing results in a variety of ways, one being physician-ordered tests that address specific gene–drug interactions such as those listed in Table 12.5. Reimbursement for genetic tests has been a major challenge in the implementation of pharmacogenetic testing and has commonly been limited to those interactions where evidence of clinical utility is available, that is, performing the test influences health outcomes. While organizations such as CPIC focus on how to manage a pharmacogenetic interaction when the result is available, various professional societies have offered advice on whether and when to perform certain genetic tests [149–151]. However, as the cost of testing decreases and throughput increases, access to genomic testing will be more widespread. In fact, many academic institutions have established preemptive genetic testing programs so that results could be integrated into the healthcare record to be available on-demand [152]. In addition to physician-ordered tests, direct-to-consumer tests have grown in popularity and can be ordered from a variety of vendors. Regardless of the sources and test methods, specific alleles should be tested are not standardized across laboratories, pointing to the need for more comprehensive practice standards to be developed, as has been done for CYP2C9 [153, 154].

The evidence supporting the clinical utility of any test will necessarily need to be diverse and will not only consist of data generated from randomized clinical trials. Alternative and credible study designs will inevitably be required to translate new tests and into practice. Indeed, many complementary sources of evidence (mechanistic, pharmacological, and observational studies) can all contribute to establishing clinical utility [155]. Coordinated efforts such as the Precision Medicine Initiative and "All of Us" are expected to drive translation of genetic (and other) discoveries into patient care and in turn inform research [156]. Large-scale biobanks are proving to be valuable resources for use in research. For example, the UK Biobank, a biorepository that stores human biological samples and is linked to population health data, is being used to research into the most common and life-threatening diseases. Similarly, BioVU is an EMR-linked biorepository that has been used to perform comprehensive genome-wide phenome-wide scans to uncover genetic risk factors for many diseases [157]. Large-scale activities such as the "Electronic MEdical Records and Genomics" (eMERGE) network that has been organized and funded by the National Human Genome Research Institute (NHGRI, NIH) is a national network that combines DNA biorepositories with EMR systems for large-scale, high-throughput genetic research to support implementation of genomic medicine [158]. These combined biorepositories also support efforts such as "All of Us" that aims to collect and study data over many years from one million or more people, with a goal to speed up health research breakthroughs, enabling new kinds of individualized healthcare [159]. Additionally, the focus on generating real-world evidence (RWE) from the real-world data (RWD) sources outside of the traditional clinical trials [160] will continue to see concerted efforts toward building real-world clinico-genomic databases to inform patient care [161]. In the future, this will assist regulatory agencies, professional societies, and healthcare reimbursement agencies to provide guidances and guidelines that allow approval and access to appropriately characterized groups of patients.

Conclusions and future directions

Some key pharmacogenetic principles discussed in this chapter are outlined in Table 12.7. Pharmacologically significant genetic variations have been described at every point of the hierarchy shown in Fig. 12.2, and lead to interindividual

TABLE 12.7 Key pharmacogenetic principles.

- Rapid advances in genetic analysis technologies and parallel advances in bioinformatics and computational analysis have helped develop new insights into the genetic underpinning of human health and disease as well as the exposure and response to therapeutics.
- Pharmacogenetics and human genetics are increasingly used to support rational drug development and treatment.
- Pharmacogenetic variations can affect drug pharmacokinetics and/or response.
- It is critical to replicate pharmacogenetic findings in relatively large datasets consisting of diverse patients.
- Pharmacogenetic testing is of most clinical value when there is great variability in drug effect. However, the clinical utility of these tests should be established.

differences in pharmacokinetics, because of changes in absorption, distribution, metabolism, and elimination as well as pharmacodynamics, because of direct or indirect action on drug targets. Drug metabolism by polymorphic enzymes or transportation of drugs or metabolites by polymorphic transporters are important contributors to variability in exposure. This exposure variability may consequently lead to response variability. In this way, polymorphic drug pathways or targets contribute to a variability that can result in a suboptimal therapeutic response or toxic response.

Since the completion of the Human Genome Project and the rise of genome-wide association studies and whole-exome/-genome sequencing studies, there has been rapid progress in identifying the contribution of human genetics to health and disease. Large-scale genomic and other -omic (e.g., proteomic, metabolomic, phenomic) repositories are increasingly utilized to develop knowledge that can improve efficiency of healthcare delivery. However, translating the knowledge to insights and then to action has been one of the biggest challenges in implementing pharmacogenetics.

The hyperbole that surrounded many pharmacogenetics studies before they were replicated had resulted in an initially inappropriately high level of expectation of clinically meaningful results. A full understanding of drug effect continues to elude us in many situations. A single study or studies designed using single candidate gene approaches may miss important associations. On the other hand, looking at thousands of loci may generate false-positive results. It is important to conduct validation and replication studies to confirm that the associations and inferences drawn from pharmacogenetic studies are reliable and can be generalized at the individual level and at the population level. Studies across diverse populations are also needed to ensure that the associations and inferences are valid for different racial and ethnic populations.

There are many potential pitfalls on the route from the discovery of genetic variations to the development of a clinically useful pharmacogenetic test. Beyond ensuring that a pharmacogenetic interaction is indeed real, understanding the clinical utility of genomic tests is critical for their practical use. If implementation of pharmacogenetics in clinical practice is to become successful, it will require accurate and reliable genetic tests that allow physicians to predict clinically relevant outcomes with confidence. It can also be anticipated that access to genomic testing will be more widespread as the cost of testing decreases and throughput increases. Consequently, it stands to reason that genetic test results, whether related specifically to drugs or not, will be more ubiquitous in medical records, and more routinely incorporated in clinical decision-making. Organizations such CPIC [27] and DPWG [28] have aided in bolstering implementation of pharmacogenetics in clinical practice by providing guidelines for the use of specific biomarkers/tests with individual drug therapies.

To achieve successful implementation of pharmacogenetics, research must be carried from the clinic to the laboratory, and back. To that end, multidisciplinary and cross-functional collaborations among various stakeholders including physicians, pharmacologists, bioinformaticians, statisticians, epidemiologists, molecular biologists, and geneticists will continue to be important in order to increase the efficiency of drug development and patient care. Broader education of all stakeholders in genomics and pharmacogenomics will also be essential.

Dedication

This chapter is dedicated to Dr. David Flockhart, a pioneer and a leader in the field of pharmacogenetics.

References

[1] Lesko LJ, Zineh I, Huang SM. What is clinical utility and why should we care? Clin Pharmacol Ther 2010;88:729–733.
[2] Hamburg MA, Collins FS. The path to personalized medicine. N Engl J Med 2010;363:301–304.
[3] Zineh I, Huang SM. Biomarkers in drug development and regulation: a paradigm for clinical implementation of personalized medicine. Biomark Med 2011;5:705–713.
[4] Feero WG, Green ED. Genomics education for health care professionals in the 21st century. JAMA 2011;306:989–990.

[5] International Conference on Harmonisation. E15: Pharmacogenomics definitions and sample coding, Available from:https://www.fda.gov/media/71389/download; 2008. [Accessed 31 March 2021].
[6] The Human Genome Project. Available from: https://www.genome.gov/human-genome-project/What. [Accessed 31 March 2021].
[7] Ensembl release 100. April 2020. Available from: http://useast.ensembl.org/Homo_sapiens/Location/Genome?r=Y:1-1000. [Accessed 1 July 2020].
[8] Pacanowski MA, Leptak C, Zineh I. Next-generation medicines: past regulatory experience and considerations for the future. Clin Pharmacol Ther 2014;95:247–249.
[9] Crowley JJ, Sullivan PF, McLeod HL. Pharmacogenomic genome-wide association studies: lessons learned thus far. Pharmacogenomics 2009;10:161–163.
[10] SEARCH Collaborative Group. Link E, Parish S, Armitage J, Bowman L, Heath S, et al. SLCO1B1 variants and statin-induced myopathy—a genomewide study. N Engl J Med 2008;359:789–799.
[11] Ramamoorthy A, Pacanowski MA, Bull J, Zhang L. Racial/ethnic differences in drug disposition and response: review of recently approved drugs. Clin Pharmacol Ther 2015;97:263–273.
[12] Goodwin S, McPherson JD, McCombie WR. Coming of age: ten years of next-generation sequencing technologies. Nat Rev Genet 2016;17:333–351.
[13] Sayers EW, Beck J, Brister JR, Bolton EE, Canese K, Comeau DC, et al. Database resources of the National Center for Biotechnology Information. Nucleic Acids Res 2019;47:D23–D28.
[14] Clark K, Karsch-Mizrachi I, Lipman DJ, Ostell J, Sayers EW. GenBank. Nucleic Acids Res 2016;44:D67–D72.
[15] Auton A, Brooks LD, Durbin RM, Garrison EP, Kang HM, et al. A global reference for human genetic variation. Nature 2015;526:68–74.
[16] Sangkuhl K, Whirl-Carrillo M, Whaley RM, Woon M, Lavertu A, Altman RB, et al. Pharmacogenomics clinical annotation tool (PharmCAT). Clin Pharmacol Ther 2020;107:203–210.
[17] Maglott D, Ostell J, Pruitt KD, Tatusova T. Entrez Gene: gene-centered information at NCBI. Nucleic Acids Res 2007;35:D26–D31.
[18] Sherry ST, Ward MH, Kholodov M, Baker J, Phan L, Smigielski EM, et al. dbSNP: the NCBI database of genetic variation. Nucleic Acids Res 2001;29:308–311.
[19] Amberger JS, Hamosh A. Searching online Mendelian inheritance in man (OMIM): a knowledgebase of human genes and genetic phenotypes. Curr Protoc Bioinformatics 2017;58:1.2.1–12.
[20] Wong KM, Langlais K, Tobias GS, Fletcher-Hoppe C, Krasnewich D, Leeds HS, et al. The dbGaP data browser: a new tool for browsing dbGaP controlled-access genomic data. Nucleic Acids Res 2017;45:D819–D826.
[21] Rubinstein WS, Maglott DR, Lee JM, Kattman BL, Malheiro AJ, Ovetsky M, et al. The NIH genetic testing registry: a new, centralized database of genetic tests to enable access to comprehensive information and improve transparency. Nucleic Acids Res 2013;41:D925–D935.
[22] Landrum MJ, Kattman BL. ClinVar at five years: delivering on the promise. Hum Mutat 2018;39:1623–1630.
[23] Rehm HL, Berg JS, Brooks LD, Bustamante CD, Evans JP, Landrum MJ, et al. ClinGen-the clinical genome resource. N Engl J Med 2015;372:2235–2242.
[24] Barbarino JM, Whirl-Carrillo M, Altman RB, Klein TE. PharmGKB: a worldwide resource for pharmacogenomic information. Wiley Interdiscip Rev Syst Biol Med 2018;10. https://doi.org/10.1002/wsbm, e1417.
[25] Gaedigk A, Sangkuhl K, Whirl-Carrillo M, Twist GP, Klein TE, Miller NA, et al. The evolution of PharmVar. Clin Pharmacol Ther 2019;105:29–32.
[26] Cotto KC, Wagner AH, Feng YY, Kiwala S, Coffman AC, Spies G, et al. DGIdb 3.0: a redesign and expansion of the drug-gene interaction database. Nucleic Acids Res 2018;46:D1068–D1073.
[27] Relling MV, Klein TE, Gammal RS, Whirl-Carrillo M, Hoffman JM, Caudle KE. The Clinical Pharmacogenetics Implementation Consortium: 10 years later. Clin Pharmacol Ther 2020;107:171–175.
[28] Dutch Pharmacogenomics Working Group (DPWG). Available from: https://www.knmp.nl/patientenzorg/medicatiebewaking/farmacogenetica/pharmacogenetics-1/pharmacogenetics. [Accessed 29 December 2019].
[29] PharmVar: Pharmacogene Variation Consortium. Available from: https://www.pharmvar.org/. [Accessed 29 December 2019].
[30] Conrado DJ, Rogers HL, Zineh I, Pacanowski MA. Consistency of drug-drug and gene-drug interaction information in US FDA-approved drug labels. Pharmacogenomics 2013;14:215–223.
[31] US Food and Drug Administration. Clinical drug interaction studies—Cytochrome P450 Enzyme- and transporter-mediated drug interactions. Guidance for industry, Available from:https://www.fda.gov/media/134581/download; 2020. [Accessed 31 March 2021].
[32] US Food and Drug Administration. In vitro metabolism- and transporter-mediated drug-drug interaction studies. Guidance for industry, Available from:https://www.fda.gov/media/134582/download; 2020. [Accessed 31 March 2021].
[33] Lagishetty CV, Deng J, Lesko LJ, Rogers H, Pacanowski M, Schmidt S. How informative are drug-drug interactions of gene-drug interactions? J Clin Pharmacol 2016;56:1221–1231.
[34] Caudle KE, Sangkuhl K, Whirl-Carrillo M, Swen JJ, Haidar CE, Klein TE, et al. Standardizing CYP2D6 genotype to phenotype translation: consensus recommendations from the Clinical Pharmacogenetics Implementation Consortium and Dutch Pharmacogenetics Working Group. Clin Transl Sci 2020;13:116–124.
[35] Ariyoshi N, Ohara M, Kaneko M, Afuso S, Kumamoto T, Nakamura H, et al. Q172H replacement overcomes effects on the metabolism of cyclophosphamide and efavirenz caused by CYP2B6 variant with Arg262. Drug Metab Dispos 2011;39:2045–2048.
[36] Radloff R, Gras A, Zanger UM, Masquelier C, Arumugam K, Karasi JC, et al. Novel CYP2B6 enzyme variants in a Rwandese population: functional characterization and assessment of in silico prediction tools. Hum Mutat 2013;34:725–734.

[37] Xu C, Ogburn ET, Guo Y, Desta Z. Effects of the CYP2B6*6 allele on catalytic properties and inhibition of CYP2B6 in vitro: implication for the mechanism of reduced efavirenz metabolism and other CYP2B6 substrates in vivo. Drug Metab Dispos 2012;40:717–725.
[38] Zanger UM, Klein K. Pharmacogenetics of cytochrome P450 2B6 (CYP2B6): advances on polymorphisms, mechanisms, and clinical relevance. Front Genet 2013;4:24. https://doi.org/10.3389/fgene.2013.00024.
[39] Zhang H, Sridar C, Kenaan C, Amunugama H, Ballou DP, Hollenberg PF. Polymorphic variants of cytochrome P450 2B6 (CYP2B6.4-CYP2B6.9) exhibit altered rates of metabolism for bupropion and efavirenz: a charge-reversal mutation in the K139E variant (CYP2B6.8) impairs formation of a functional cytochrome p450-reductase complex. J Pharmacol Exp Ther 2011;338:803–809.
[40] Hofmann MH, Blievernicht JK, Klein K, Saussele T, Schaeffeler E, Schwab M, et al. Aberrant splicing caused by single nucleotide polymorphism c.516G>T [Q172H], a marker of CYP2B6*6, is responsible for decreased expression and activity of CYP2B6 in liver. J Pharmacol Exp Ther 2008;325:284–292.
[41] Li H, Ferguson SS, Wang H. Synergistically enhanced CYP2B6 inducibility between a polymorphic mutation in CYP2B6 promoter and pregnane X receptor activation. Mol Pharmacol 2010;78:704–713.
[42] Rotger M, Tegude H, Colombo S, Cavassini M, Furrer H, Decosterd L, et al. Predictive value of known and novel alleles of CYP2B6 for efavirenz plasma concentrations in HIV-infected individuals. Clin Pharmacol Ther 2007;81:557–566.
[43] Zukunft J, Lang T, Richter T, Hirsch-Ernst KI, Nussler AK, Klein K, et al. A natural CYP2B6 TATA box polymorphism (– 82T- -> C) leading to enhanced transcription and relocation of the transcriptional start site. Mol Pharmacol 2005;67:1772–1782.
[44] Lamba V, Lamba J, Yasuda K, Strom S, Davila J, Hancock ML, et al. Hepatic CYP2B6 expression: gender and ethnic differences and relationship to CYP2B6 genotype and CAR (constitutive androstane receptor) expression. J Pharmacol Exp Ther 2003;307:906–922.
[45] Ferguson CS, Tyndale RF. Cytochrome P450 enzymes in the brain: emerging evidence of biological significance. Trends Pharmacol Sci 2011;32:708–714.
[46] Caudle KE, Rettie AE, Whirl-Carrillo M, Smith LH, Mintzer S, Lee MT, et al. Clinical pharmacogenetics implementation consortium guidelines for CYP2C9 and HLA-B genotypes and phenytoin dosing. Clin Pharmacol Ther 2014;96:542–548.
[47] de Morais SM, Wilkinson GR, Blaisdell J, Nakamura K, Meyer UA, Goldstein JA. The major genetic defect responsible for the polymorphism of S-mephenytoin metabolism in humans. J Biol Chem 1994;269:15419–15422.
[48] De Morais SM, Wilkinson GR, Blaisdell J, Meyer UA, Nakamura K, Goldstein JA. Identification of a new genetic defect responsible for the polymorphism of (S)-mephenytoin metabolism in Japanese. Mol Pharmacol 1994;46:594–598.
[49] Scott SA, Sangkuhl K, Shuldiner AR, Hulot JS, Thorn CF, Altman RB, et al. PharmGKB summary: very important pharmacogene information for cytochrome P450, family 2, subfamily C, polypeptide 19. Pharmacogenet Genomics 2012;22:159–165.
[50] Sim SC, Risinger C, Dahl ML, Aklillu E, Christensen M, Bertilsson L, et al. A common novel CYP2C19 gene variant causes ultrarapid drug metabolism relevant for the drug response to proton pump inhibitors and antidepressants. Clin Pharmacol Ther 2006;79:103–113.
[51] Blaisdell J, Mohrenweiser H, Jackson J, Ferguson S, Coulter S, Chanas B, et al. Identification and functional characterization of new potentially defective alleles of human CYP2C19. Pharmacogenetics 2002;12:703–711.
[52] Moriyama B, Obeng AO, Barbarino J, Penzak SR, Henning SA, Scott SA, et al. Clinical Pharmacogenetics Implementation Consortium (CPIC) guidelines for CYP2C19 and voriconazole therapy. Clin Pharmacol Ther 2017;102:45–51.
[53] Zanger UM, Schwab M. Cytochrome P450 enzymes in drug metabolism: regulation of gene expression, enzyme activities, and impact of genetic variation. Pharmacol Ther 2013;138:103–141.
[54] Gaedigk A, Simon SD, Pearce RE, Bradford LD, Kennedy MJ, Leeder JS. The CYP2D6 activity score: translating genotype information into a qualitative measure of phenotype. Clin Pharmacol Ther 2008;83:234–242.
[55] Hicks JK, Swen JJ, Gaedigk A. Challenges in CYP2D6 phenotype assignment from genotype data: a critical assessment and call for standardization. Curr Drug Metab 2014;15:218–232.
[56] Food and Drug Administration. Table of pharmacogenomic biomarkers in drug labeling. Available from: https://www.fda.gov/drugs/science-and-research-drugs/table-pharmacogenomic-biomarkers-drug-labeling, [Accessed 31 March 2021]
[57] Gaedigk A. Complexities of CYP2D6 gene analysis and interpretation. Int Rev Psychiatry 2013;25:534–553.
[58] Hicks JK, Bishop JR, Sangkuhl K, Muller DJ, Ji Y, Leckband SG, et al. Clinical Pharmacogenetics Implementation Consortium (CPIC) guideline for CYP2D6 and CYP2C19 genotypes and dosing of selective serotonin reuptake inhibitors. Clin Pharmacol Ther 2015;98:127–134.
[59] PharmVar: CYP2D6 reference gene locus. Available from: https://www.pharmvar.org/gene/CYP2D6. [Accessed 20 December 2019].
[60] Klein K, Zanger UM. Pharmacogenomics of cytochrome P450 3A4: recent progress toward the "missing heritability" problem. Front Genet 2013;4:12. https://doi.org/10.3389/fgene.2013.00012.
[61] Williams JA, Ring BJ, Cantrell VE, Jones DR, Eckstein J, Ruterbories K, et al. Comparative metabolic capabilities of CYP3A4, CYP3A5, and CYP3A7. Drug Metab Dispos 2002;30:883–891.
[62] Busi F, Cresteil T. CYP3A5 mRNA degradation by nonsense-mediated mRNA decay. Mol Pharmacol 2005;68:808–815.
[63] Kuehl P, Zhang J, Lin Y, Lamba J, Assem M, Schuetz J, et al. Sequence diversity in CYP3A promoters and characterization of the genetic basis of polymorphic CYP3A5 expression. Nat Genet 2001;27:383–391.
[64] Hustert E, Haberl M, Burk O, Wolbold R, He YQ, Klein K, et al. The genetic determinants of the CYP3A5 polymorphism. Pharmacogenetics 2001;11773–11779.
[65] Crettol S, Petrovic N, Murray M. Pharmacogenetics of phase I and phase II drug metabolism. Curr Pharm Des 2010;16:204–219.
[66] Relling MV, Schwab M, Whirl-Carrillo M, Suarez-Kurtz G, Pui CH, Stein CM, et al. Clinical Pharmacogenetics Implementation Consortium guideline for thiopurine dosing based on TPMT and NUDT15 genotypes: 2018 update. Clin Pharmacol Ther 2019;105:1095–1105.

[67] Krynetski EY, Tai HL, Yates CR, Fessing MY, Loennechen T, Schuetz JD, et al. Genetic polymorphism of thiopurine S-methyltransferase: clinical importance and molecular mechanisms. Pharmacogenetics 1996;6:279–290.

[68] Stanulla M, Schaeffeler E, Flohr T, Cario G, Schrauder A, Zimmermann M, et al. Thiopurine methyltransferase (TPMT) genotype and early treatment response to mercaptopurine in childhood acute lymphoblastic leukemia. JAMA 2005;293:1485–1489.

[69] The arylamine N-acetyltransferase Gene Nomenclature Committee. Available from: http://nat.mbg.duth.gr/Human%20NAT2%20alleles_2013.htm. [Accessed 27 December 2019].

[70] McDonagh EM, Boukouvala S, Aklillu E, Hein DW, Altman RB, Klein TE. PharmGKB summary: very important pharmacogene information for N-acetyltransferase 2. Pharmacogenet Genomics 2014;24:409–425.

[71] Chu PH, Huang TY, Williams J, Stafford DW. Purified vitamin K epoxide reductase alone is sufficient for conversion of vitamin K epoxide to vitamin K and vitamin K to vitamin KH2. Proc Natl Acad Sci U S A 2006;103:19308–19313.

[72] Wajih N, Hutson SM, Owen J, Wallin R. Increased production of functional recombinant human clotting factor IX by baby hamster kidney cells engineered to overexpress VKORC1, the vitamin K 2,3-epoxide-reducing enzyme of the vitamin K cycle. J Biol Chem 2005;280:31603–31607.

[73] Brenner B, Sanchez-Vega B, Wu SM, Lanir N, Stafford DW, Solera J. A missense mutation in gamma-glutamyl carboxylase gene causes combined deficiency of all vitamin K-dependent blood coagulation factors. Blood 1998;92:4554–4559.

[74] Wu SM, Cheung WF, Frazier D, Stafford DW. Cloning and expression of the cDNA for human gamma-glutamyl carboxylase. Science 1991;254:1634–1636.

[75] Li T, Chang CY, Jin DY, Lin PJ, Khvorova A, Stafford DW. Identification of the gene for vitamin K epoxide reductase. Nature 2004;427:541–544.

[76] Whitlon DS, Sadowski JA, Suttie JW. Mechanism of coumarin action: significance of vitamin K epoxide reductase inhibition. Biochemistry 1978;17:1371–1377.

[77] Pfister A, Osman A. The VKORC1 promoter is occupied by c-Myc transcription factor in HepG2 cells. Thromb Res 2010;126:e150–e151. https://doi.org/10.1016/j.thromres.2010.01.050.

[78] Yuan HY, Chen JJ, Lee MT, Wung JC, Chen YF, Charng MJ, et al. A novel functional VKORC1 promoter polymorphism is associated with inter-individual and inter-ethnic differences in warfarin sensitivity. Hum Mol Genet 2005;14:1745–1751.

[79] Limdi NA, Beasley TM, Crowley MR, Goldstein JA, Rieder MJ, Flockhart DA, et al. VKORC1 polymorphisms, haplotypes and haplotype groups on warfarin dose among African-Americans and European-Americans. Pharmacogenomics 2008;9:1445–1458.

[80] Loebstein R, Dvoskin I, Halkin H, Vecsler M, Lubetsky A, Rechavi G, et al. A coding VKORC1 Asp36Tyr polymorphism predisposes to warfarin resistance. Blood 2007;109:2477–2480.

[81] Rost S, Fregin A, Ivaskevicius V, Conzelmann E, Hortnagel K, Pelz HJ, et al. Mutations in VKORC1 cause warfarin resistance and multiple coagulation factor deficiency type 2. Nature 2004;427:537–541.

[82] American Cancer Society. Cancer facts and figures 2019, Atlanta, GA: American Cancer Society; 2019. Available from:https://www.cancer.org/content/dam/cancer-org/research/cancer-facts-and-statistics/annual-cancer-facts-and-figures/2019/cancer-facts-and-figures-2019.pdf. [Accessed 2 January 2020].

[83] Lynch TJ, Bell DW, Sordella R, Gurubhagavatula S, Okimoto RA, Brannigan BW, et al. Activating mutations in the epidermal growth factor receptor underlying responsiveness of non-small-cell lung cancer to gefitinib. N Engl J Med 2004;350:2129–2139.

[84] Karapetis CS, Khambata-Ford S, Jonker DJ, O'Callaghan CJ, Tu D, Tebbutt NC, et al. K-ras mutations and benefit from cetuximab in advanced colorectal cancer. N Engl J Med 2008;359:1757–1765.

[85] Ivanov M, Matsvay A, Glazova O, Krasovskiy S, Usacheva M, Amelina E, et al. Targeted sequencing reveals complex, phenotype-correlated genotypes in cystic fibrosis. BMC Med Genomics 2018;11(Suppl 1):13. https://doi.org/10.1186/s12920-018-0328-z.

[86] Durmowicz AG, Lim R, Rogers H, Rosebraugh CJ, Chowdhury BA. The U.S. Food and Drug Administration's experience with ivacaftor in cystic fibrosis. Establishing efficacy using in vitro data in lieu of a clinical trial. Ann Am Thorac Soc 2018;15:1–2.

[87] Arrowsmith J, Miller P. Trial watch: phase II and phase III attrition rates 2011-2012. Nat Rev Drug Discov 2013;12:569.

[88] Calcoen D, Elias L, Yu X. What does it take to produce a breakthrough drug? Nat Rev Drug Discov 2015;14:161–162.

[89] Schork NJ. Personalized medicine: time for one-person trials. Nature 2015;520:609–611.

[90] Nelson MR, Tipney H, Painter JL, Shen J, Nicoletti P, Shen Y, et al. The support of human genetic evidence for approved drug indications. Nat Genet 2015;47:856–860.

[91] Plenge RM, Scolnick EM, Altshuler D. Validating therapeutic targets through human genetics. Nat Rev Drug Discov 2013;12:581–594.

[92] Hurle MR, Nelson MR, Agarwal P, Cardon LR. Trial watch: impact of genetically supported target selection on R&D productivity. Nat Rev Drug Discov 2016;15:596–597.

[93] Cook D, Brown D, Alexander R, March R, Morgan P, Satterthwaite G, et al. Lessons learned from the fate of AstraZeneca's drug pipeline: a five-dimensional framework. Nat Rev Drug Discov 2014;13:419–431.

[94] Carroll A. Utilizing selection biomarkers in clinical trials: is this the future of drug development? Biomark Med 2016;10:939–941.

[95] US Food and Drug Administration. Enrichment strategies for clinical trials to support determination of effectiveness of human drugs and biological products. Guidance for industry, Available from:https://www.fda.gov/media/121320/download; 2019. [Accessed 31 March 2021].

[96] US Food and Drug Administration. Adaptive designs for clinical trials of drugs and biologics. Guidance for industry, Available from:https://www.fda.gov/media/78495/download; 2019. [Accessed 31 March 2021].

[97] National Cancer Institute. NCI-MATCH trial (Molecular Analysis for Therapy Choice). Available from: https://www.cancer.gov/about-cancer/treatment/clinical-trials/nci-supported/nci-match. [Accessed 31 March 2021]

[98] Steuer CE, Papadimitrakopoulou V, Herbst RS, Redman MW, Hirsch FR, Mack PC, et al. Innovative clinical trials: the LUNG-MAP study. Clin Pharmacol Ther 2015;97:488–491.

[99] Ge D, Fellay J, Thompson AJ, Simon JS, Shianna KV, Urban TJ, et al. Genetic variation in IL28B predicts hepatitis C treatment-induced viral clearance. Nature 2009;461:399–401.

[100] US Food and Drug Administration. Drugs@FDA: FDA-approved drugs. Available from: https://www.accessdata.fda.gov/scripts/cder/daf/index.cfm. [Accessed 31 March 2021]

[101] US Food and Drug Administration. List of cleared or approved companion diagnostic devices (in vitro and imaging tools). Available from: https://www.fda.gov/medical-devices/vitro-diagnostics/list-cleared-or-approved-companion-diagnostic-devices-vitro-and-imaging-tools. [Accessed 31 March 2021]

[102] US Food and Drug Administration. In vitro companion diagnostic devices. Guidance for industry and food and drug administration staff, Available from:https://www.fda.gov/media/81309/download; 2014. [Accessed 31 March 2021].

[103] Scheerens H, Malong A, Bassett K, Boyd Z, Gupta V, Harris J, et al. Current status of companion and complementary diagnostics: strategic considerations for development and launch. Clin Transl Sci 2017;10:84–92.

[104] Flaherty KT, Le DT, Lemery S. Tissue-agnostic drug development. Am Soc Clin Oncol Educ Book 2017;37:222–230.

[105] US Food and Drug Administration. Clinical pharmacogenomics: premarket evaluation in early-phase clinical studies and recommendations for labeling. Guidance for industry, Available from:https://www.fda.gov/media/84923/download; 2013. [Accessed 31 March 2021].

[106] US Food and Drug Administration. Developing targeted therapies in low-frequency molecular subsets of a disease. Guidance for industry, Available from:https://www.fda.gov/media/117173/download; 2018. [Accessed 31 March 2021].

[107] US Food and Drug Administration. Principles for codevelopment of an in vitro companion diagnostic device with a therapeutic product. Draft guidance for industry and food and drug administration staff, Available from:https://www.fda.gov/media/99030/download; 2016. [Accessed 31 March 2021].

[108] US Food and Drug Administration. E18 genomic sampling and management of genomic data. Guidance for industry, Available from:https://www.fda.gov/regulatory-information/search-fda-guidance-documents/e18-genomic-sampling-and-management-genomic-data-guidance-industry; 2018 [Accessed 31 March 2021].

[109] Personalized Medicine Coalition (PMC). Personalized medicine at FDA: a progress & outlook report, Available from:http://www.personalizedmedicinecoalition.org/Userfiles/PMC-Corporate/file/PM_at_FDA_A_Progress_and_Outlook_Report.pdf; 2018. [Accessed 31 March 2021].

[110] US Food and Drug Administration. Table of pharmacogenomic biomarkers in drug labeling. Available from: https://www.fda.gov/drugs/science-and-research-drugs/table-pharmacogenomic-biomarkers-drug-labeling. [Accessed 31 March 2021]

[111] McDonagh EM, Lau JL, Alvarellos ML, Altman RB, Klein TE. PharmGKB summary: Efavirenz pathway, pharmacokinetics. Pharmacogenet Genomics 2015;25:363–376.

[112] Ngaimisi E, Mugusi S, Minzi OM, Sasi P, Riedel KD, Suda A, et al. Long-term efavirenz autoinduction and its effect on plasma exposure in HIV patients. Clin Pharmacol Ther 2010;88:676–684.

[113] Marzolini C, Telenti A, Decosterd LA, Greub G, Biollaz J, Buclin T. Efavirenz plasma levels can predict treatment failure and central nervous system side effects in HIV-1-infected patients. AIDS 2001;15:71–75.

[114] Desta Z, Gammal RS, Gong L, Whirl-Carrillo M, Gaur AH, Sukasem C, et al. Clinical Pharmacogenetics Implementation Consortium (CPIC) guideline for CYP2B6 and efavirenz-containing antiretroviral therapy. Clin Pharmacol Ther 2019;106:226–233.

[115] US Department of Health and Human Services. Guidelines for the use of antiretroviral agents in pediatric HIV infection, Available from:https://aidsinfo.nih.gov/guidelines/html/2/pediatric-arv/123/efavirenz; 2021. [Accessed 13 April 2021].

[116] Bolton Moore C, Capparelli EV, Samson P, Bwakura-Dangarembizi M, Jean-Philippe P, Worrell C, et al. CYP2B6 genotype-directed dosing is required for optimal efavirenz exposure in children 3-36 months with HIV infection. AIDS 2017;31:1129–1136.

[117] Levine GN, Bates ER, Bittl JA, Brindis RG, Fihn SD, Fleisher LA, et al. 2016 ACC/AHA guideline focused update on duration of dual antiplatelet therapy in patients with coronary artery disease: a report of the American College of Cardiology/American Heart Association Task Force on clinical practice guidelines. J Thorac Cardiovasc Surg 2016;152:1243–1275.

[118] Mega JL, Hochholzer W, Frelinger III AL, Kluk MJ, Angiolillo DJ, Kereiakes DJ, et al. Dosing clopidogrel based on CYP2C19 genotype and the effect on platelet reactivity in patients with stable cardiovascular disease. JAMA 2011;306:2221–2228.

[119] Mega JL, Close SL, Wiviott SD, Shen L, Hockett RD, Brandt JT, et al. Cytochrome P-450 polymorphisms and response to clopidogrel. N Engl J Med 2009;360:354–362.

[120] Mega JL, Simon T, Collet JP, Anderson JL, Antman EM, Bliden K, et al. Reduced-function CYP2C19 genotype and risk of adverse clinical outcomes among patients treated with clopidogrel predominantly for PCI: a meta-analysis. JAMA 2010;304:1821–1830.

[121] Cavallari LH, Lee CR, Beitelshees AL, Cooper-DeHoff RM, Duarte JD, Voora D, et al. Multisite investigation of outcomes with implementation of CYP2C19 genotype-guided antiplatelet therapy after percutaneous coronary intervention. JACC Cardiovasc Interv 2018;11:181–191.

[122] Claassens DMF, Vos GJA, Bergmeijer TO, Hermanides RS, van't Hof AWJ, van der Harst P, et al. A genotype-guided strategy for oral P2Y12 inhibitors in primary PCI. N Engl J Med 2019;381:1621–1631.

[123] Bhatt DL, Pare G, Eikelboom JW, Simonsen KL, Emison ES, Fox KA, et al. The relationship between CYP2C19 polymorphisms and ischaemic and bleeding outcomes in stable outpatients: the CHARISMA genetics study. Eur Heart J 2012;33:2143–2150.

[124] Pare G, Mehta SR, Yusuf S, Anand SS, Connolly SJ, Hirsh J, et al. Effects of CYP2C19 genotype on outcomes of clopidogrel treatment. N Engl J Med 2010;363:1704–1714.

[125] Scott SA, Sangkuhl K, Stein CM, Hulot JS, Mega JL, Roden DM, et al. Clinical Pharmacogenetics Implementation Consortium guidelines for CYP2C19 genotype and clopidogrel therapy: 2013 update. Clin Pharmacol Ther 2013;94:317–323.
[126] Thorn CF, Klein TE, Altman RB. Codeine and morphine pathway. Pharmacogenet Genomics 2009;19:556–558.
[127] Volpe DA, McMahon Tobin GA, Mellon RD, Katki AG, Parker RJ, Colatsky T, et al. Uniform assessment and ranking of opioid mu receptor binding constants for selected opioid drugs. Regul Toxicol Pharmacol 2011;59:385–390.
[128] Crews KR, Gaedigk A, Dunnenberger HM, Leeder JS, Klein TE, Caudle KE, et al. Clinical Pharmacogenetics Implementation Consortium guidelines for cytochrome P450 2D6 genotype and codeine therapy: 2014 update. Clin Pharmacol Ther 2014;95:376–382.
[129] Goetz MP, Rae JM, Suman VJ, Safgren SL, Ames MM, Visscher DW, et al. Pharmacogenetics of tamoxifen biotransformation is associated with clinical outcomes of efficacy and hot flashes. J Clin Oncol 2005;23:9312–9318.
[130] Goetz MP, Suman VJ, Hoskin TL, Gnant M, Filipits M, Safgren SL, et al. CYP2D6 metabolism and patient outcome in the Austrian Breast and Colorectal Cancer Study Group trial (ABCSG) 8. Clin Cancer Res 2013;19:500–507.
[131] Rae JM, Drury S, Hayes DF, Stearns V, Thibert JN, Haynes BP, et al. CYP2D6 and UGT2B7 genotype and risk of recurrence in tamoxifen-treated breast cancer patients. J Natl Cancer Inst 2012;104:452–460.
[132] Regan MM, Leyland-Jones B, Bouzyk M, Pagani O, Tang W, Kammler R, et al. CYP2D6 genotype and tamoxifen response in postmenopausal women with endocrine-responsive breast cancer: the breast international group 1-98 trial. J Natl Cancer Inst 2012;104:441–451.
[133] Schroth W, Antoniadou L, Fritz P, Schwab M, Muerdter T, Zanger UM, et al. Breast cancer treatment outcome with adjuvant tamoxifen relative to patient CYP2D6 and CYP2C19 genotypes. J Clin Oncol 2007;25:5187–5193.
[134] Schroth W, Goetz MP, Hamann U, Fasching PA, Schmidt M, Winter S, et al. Association between CYP2D6 polymorphisms and outcomes among women with early stage breast cancer treated with tamoxifen. JAMA 2009;302:1429–1436.
[135] Province MA, Goetz MP, Brauch H, Flockhart DA, Hebert JM, Whaley R, et al. CYP2D6 genotype and adjuvant tamoxifen: meta-analysis of heterogeneous study populations. Clin Pharmacol Ther 2014;95:216–227.
[136] Madlensky L, Natarajan L, Tchu S, Pu M, Mortimer J, Flatt SW, et al. Tamoxifen metabolite concentrations, CYP2D6 genotype, and breast cancer outcomes. Clin Pharmacol Ther 2011;89:718–725.
[137] Saladores P, Murdter T, Eccles D, Chowbay B, Zgheib NK, Winter S, et al. Tamoxifen metabolism predicts drug concentrations and outcome in premenopausal patients with early breast cancer. Pharmacogenomics J 2015;15:84–94.
[138] Goetz MP, Sangkuhl K, Guchelaar HJ, Schwab M, Province M, Whirl-Carrillo M, et al. Clinical Pharmacogenetics Implementation Consortium (CPIC) guideline for CYP2D6 and tamoxifen therapy. Clin Pharmacol Ther 2018;103:770–777.
[139] Harter K, Levine M, Henderson SO. Anticoagulation drug therapy: a review. West J Emerg Med 2015;16:11–17.
[140] Johnson JA, Caudle KE, Gong L, Whirl-Carrillo M, Stein CM, Scott SA, et al. Clinical Pharmacogenetics Implementation Consortium (CPIC) guideline for pharmacogenetics-guided warfarin dosing: 2017 update. Clin Pharmacol Ther 2017;102:397–404.
[141] Gage BF, Eby C, Johnson JA, Deych E, Rieder MJ, Ridker PM, et al. Use of pharmacogenetic and clinical factors to predict the therapeutic dose of warfarin. Clin Pharmacol Ther 2008;84:326–331.
[142] International Warfarin Pharmacogenetics Consortium, Klein TE, Altman RB, Eriksson N, Gage BF, Kimmel SE, et al. Estimation of the warfarin dose with clinical and pharmacogenetic data. N Engl J Med 2009;360:753–764.
[143] Rieder MJ, Reiner AP, Gage BF, Nickerson DA, Eby CS, McLeod HL, et al. Effect of VKORC1 haplotypes on transcriptional regulation and warfarin dose. N Engl J Med 2005;352:2285–2293.
[144] Caldwell MD, Awad T, Johnson JA, Gage BF, Falkowski M, Gardina P, et al. CYP4F2 genetic variant alters required warfarin dose. Blood 2008;111:4106–4112.
[145] Perera MA, Cavallari LH, Limdi NA, Gamazon ER, Konkashbaev A, Daneshjou R, et al. Genetic variants associated with warfarin dose in African-American individuals: a genome-wide association study. Lancet 2013;382:790–796.
[146] Johnson JA, Weitzel KW. Advancing pharmacogenomics as a component of precision medicine: how, where, and who? Clin Pharmacol Ther 2016;99:154–156.
[147] Cavallari LH, Beitelshees AL, Blake KV, Dressler LG, Duarte JD, Elsey A, et al. The IGNITE Pharmacogenetics Working Group: an opportunity for building evidence with pharmacogenetic implementation in a real-world setting. Clin Transl Sci 2017;10:143–146.
[148] Luzum JA, Pakyz RE, Elsey AR, Haidar CE, Peterson JF, Whirl-Carrillo M, et al. The Pharmacogenomics Research Network Translational Pharmacogenetics Program: outcomes and metrics of pharmacogenetic implementations across diverse healthcare systems. Clin Pharmacol Ther 2017;102:502–510.
[149] National Comprehensive Cancer Network clinical practice guidelines in oncology (NCCN guidelines): Breast cancer version 4. Available from: http://www.nccn.org/. [Accessed 31 March 2021]
[150] Levine GN, Bates ER, Blankenship JC, Bailey SR, Bittl JA, Cercek B, et al. 2011 ACCF/AHA/SCAI guideline for percutaneous coronary intervention: a report of the American College of Cardiology Foundation/American Heart Association Task Force on practice guidelines and the Society for Cardiovascular Angiography and Interventions. J Am Coll Cardiol 2011;58:e44–122. https://doi.org/10.1016/j.jacc.2011.08.007.
[151] National Comprehensive Cancer Network clinical practice guidelines in oncology (NCCN guidelines): acute lymphoblastic leukemia. Available from: http://www.nccn.org/. [Accessed 31 March 2021]
[152] Dunnenberger HM, Crews KR, Hoffman JM, Caudle KE, Broeckel U, Howard SC, et al. Preemptive clinical pharmacogenetics implementation: current programs in five US medical centers. Annu Rev Pharmacol Toxicol 2015;55:89–106.
[153] Pratt VM, Cavallari LH, Del Tredici AL, Hachad H, Ji Y, Moyer AM, et al. Recommendations for clinical CYP2C9 genotyping allele selection: a joint recommendation of the Association for Molecular Pathology and College of American Pathologists. J Mol Diagn 2019;21:746–755.

[154] Pratt VM, Zehnbauer B, Wilson JA, Baak R, Babic N, Bettinotti M, et al. Characterization of 107 genomic DNA reference materials for CYP2D6, CYP2C19, CYP2C9, VKORC1, and UGT1A1: a GeT-RM and Association for Molecular Pathology collaborative project. J Mol Diagn 2010;12:835–846.

[155] Woodcock J. Assessing the clinical utility of diagnostics used in drug therapy. Clin Pharmacol Ther 2010;88:765–773.

[156] The Precision Medicine Initiative. Available from: https://ghr.nlm.nih.gov/primer/precisionmedicine/initiative. [Accessed 31 March 2021].

[157] Ritchie MD, Denny JC, Crawford DC, Ramirez AH, Weiner JB, Pulley JM, et al. Robust replication of genotype-phenotype associations across multiple diseases in an electronic medical record. Am J Hum Genet 2010;86:560–572.

[158] McCarty CA, Chisholm RL, Chute CG, Kullo IJ, Jarvik GP, Larson EB, et al. The eMERGE Network: a consortium of biorepositories linked to electronic medical records data for conducting genomic studies. BMC Med Genomics 2011;4:13. https://doi.org/10.1186/1755-8794-4-13.

[159] All of Us. Available from: https://allofus.nih.gov/about. [Accessed 31 March 2021].

[160] US Food and Drug Administration. Real-world evidence program. Available from: https://www.fda.gov/science-research/science-and-research-special-topics/real-world-evidence. [Accessed 31 March 2021]

[161] Agarwala V, Khozin S, Singal G, O'Connell C, Kuk D, Li G, et al. Real-world evidence in support of precision medicine: clinico-genomic cancer data as a case study. Health Aff 2018;37:765–772.

Chapter 13

Mechanisms and genetics of drug transport

Lei Zhang[a], Osatohanmwen J. Enogieru[b], Sook Wah Yee[b], Shiew-Mei Huang[c], and Kathleen M. Giacomini[b]

[a]*Office of Research and Standards, Office of Generic Drugs, Center for Drug Evaluation and Research, U.S. Food and Drug Administration, Silver Spring, MD, United States,* [b]*Department of Bioengineering and Therapeutic Sciences, University of California, San Francisco, CA, United States,* [c]*Office of Clinical Pharmacology, Office of Translational Sciences, Center for Drug Evaluation and Research, U.S. Food and Drug Administration, Silver Spring, MD, United States*

Introduction

The processes of drug absorption, distribution, metabolism, and excretion (ADME) include transport steps that are mediated by membrane-bound carriers or transporters [1]. Over 400 membrane transporters have been annotated in the human genome, belonging to two major superfamilies: ATP-binding cassette (ABC) and solute carrier (SLC). Most of the membrane transporters have been cloned, characterized, and localized to tissues and within epithelial tissues, to polarized membrane domains (apical or basolateral) in the human body. The physiological roles of transporters include supplying nutrients, removing waste products, maintaining cell homeostasis, and participating in signal transduction and energy production. Although more than 400 transporters are identified in the human genome, approximately 30 appear to be important in drug absorption and disposition [2]. Numerous preclinical and clinical studies now suggest that drug transport is an important determinant of pharmacokinetics (PK) and pharmacodynamics (PD) because transport mechanisms control the access of many drugs to the systemic circulation as well as to various tissues and to their sites of action. In some instances, membrane transporters may represent the rate-limiting step in the processes of drug absorption, distribution, and elimination, and are involved in many drug-drug interactions (Chapter 14).

There is growing appreciation that it is important to examine the role of membrane transporters during drug development, including evaluating their contributions to drug efficacy and toxicity outcomes. Transporter evaluation is recommended in regulatory guidances [3–6] and is an integral part of drug development strategy [7, 8]. The first Transporter White Paper from the International Transporter Consortium (ITC) (https://www.itc-transporter.org/) was published in 2010 [9] following a DIA-FDA Critical Path Initiative [9]-sponsored transporter workshop [10]. The White Paper provided an overview of key transporters that play a role in drug absorption and disposition, and clinical drug interactions, and described examples of various technologies used to study drug transporter-based interactions, including computational methods for constructing models to predict drug transporter interactions. Furthermore, it provided criteria based on in vitro assessment along with decision trees that can be used by drug developers and regulatory scientists to decide if clinical studies of transporter-mediated drug-drug interaction are warranted. The White Paper and subsequent whitepapers illustrate how government, industry, and academic scientists have collaborated to develop and apply innovative, predictive tools to enhance the safety and efficacy of medical therapies. Two subsequent transporter workshops organized by the ITC in 2012 and 2017 led to additional whitepapers [11, 12]. The incorporation of these scientific advances in drug development and their rapid regulatory adoption are both critical to the development of novel medical products.

Mechanisms of transport across biological membranes

After oral administration, there are multiple membrane barriers that a drug must traverse to reach its cellular target. Research over many years has defined mechanisms by which drugs are transported across biological membranes (Fig. 13.1). Some drugs cross membranes by simple diffusion, by either a paracellular or transmembrane mechanism. Their transfer obeys Fick's law of diffusion and is driven by the cross-membrane concentration gradient. As described in Chapter 3, physicochemical properties of drugs that can affect simple diffusion include molecular weight, charge and polarity, and lipophilicity (e.g., octanol:buffer partition ratio). However, transmembrane transport can be mediated by carrier proteins, known as transporters, that help solutes cross hydrophobic membranes. This process, called *carrier-mediated* transport, can be either facilitated (passive) or active. Mechanistically, the molecule binds to the transporter,

Atkinson's Principles of Clinical Pharmacology. https://doi.org/10.1016/B978-0-12-819869-8.00010-0

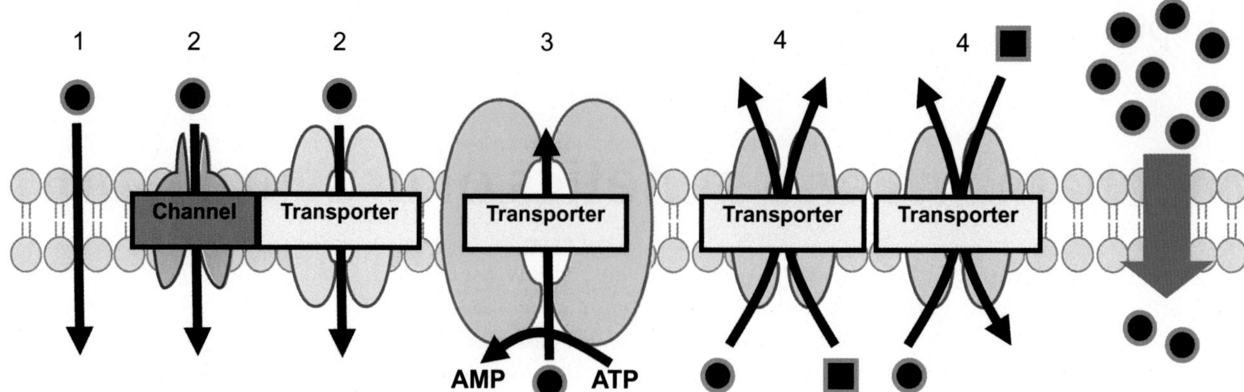

FIG. 13.1 Energy-based classification of drug transport across membranes. (1) Simple diffusion; (2) facilitated diffusion; (3) primary active transport; (4) secondary active transport. Note that *two arrows* in the same direction show a symport or cotransport process, whereas *two arrows* in opposite directions show an antiport or exchange process. (The authors acknowledge Dr. Naoki Ishiguro, Boehringer Ingelheim, for this figure.)

is translocated across the membrane, and is then released on the other side of the membrane. The process is usually specific to substrates with similar chemical properties, saturable, inhibitable, temperature sensitive, and, if applicable, inducible. Carrier-mediated transport processes are categorized as follows:

1. Facilitated passive diffusion (driven by a concentration gradient)
2. Active transport (i.e., via energy linked transporters)
   a. Primary active
   b. Secondary active
      i. Symport (cotransporters)
      ii. Antiport (exchangers).

Facilitative transporters are not energy dependent and are often uniporters that move substrates down an electrical-chemical gradient. Examples of facilitative transporters in the SLC superfamily include the organic cation transporters (OCTs). Active transporters that move solutes against a concentration gradient are energy dependent. Primary active transporters generate energy themselves (e.g., by ATP hydrolysis) and include transporters in the ABC families, such as P-gp (P-glycoprotein) and BCRP (breast cancer resistance protein). Secondary active transporters utilize energy stored in a voltage or ion gradient that is generated by a primary active transporter (e.g., Na^+/K^+-ATPase). Symporters, such as the Na^+-glucose transporter (SLC5A1 encoding SGLT1), transport glucose molecules against a concentration gradient in the same direction as the driving ion, Na^+, which moves downhill in accordance with its transmembrane gradient. Antiporters or counter-porters, such as the Na^+/H^+-exchanger, or multidrug and toxin extrusion transport proteins (MATEs) transport molecules against a concentration gradient in the opposite direction of the counterion. Some transporters are considered tertiary active such as the organic anion transporters, OAT1 and OAT3. Here, the sodium gradient created by Na^+/K^+-ATPase is used by dicarboxylate transporters (SLC13 family) to import dicarboxylates such as alpha-ketoglutarate against their concentration gradients. Intracellular dicarboxylates then move down their concentration gradient via OAT1 or OAT3 providing the energy for OAT-mediated uptake of organic anions such a para-aminohippurate.

Nomenclature, genetic classification, and function of selected membrane transporters

The physiological or pharmacological functions of a substantial number of transporters have been defined in various tissues, and have been associated with specific genes, mRNA, and deduced protein sequences. However, relatively few have been isolated and fully characterized biochemically. In humans, the ABC superfamily includes about 50 transporters that contain an ATP-binding cassette and function as primary active transporters. Their Human Genome Organization (HUGO) [13] gene nomenclature, which frequently differs from their protein names, begins with "ABC," which is followed by a letter and a number. For example, P-gp is *ABCB1*, BCRP is *ABCG2*, MRP2 (multidrug-resistance related protein 2) is *ABCC2*. The SLC superfamily contains more transporters than the ABC superfamily, and currently includes more than 400 transporters and 65 families (http://slc.bioparadigms.org/) [14]. They are either facilitated passive transporters or secondary or tertiary active transporters.

A transporter is assigned to a specific SLC family if it has at least 20%–25% amino acid sequence identity to other members of that family [15–17]. Most of the HUGO nomenclature for gene names begins with SLC, followed by a number, a letter, and another number, with an exception being the OATPs (SLC family 21). For example, OCT2 is the protein encoded by *SLC22A2* and OAT1 is encoded by *SLC22A6*. For organic anion transporting polypeptides, the HUGO nomenclature begins with SLCO (solute carrier organic anion transporter family), followed by a family number, subfamily letter, and member number (e.g., 1A2, 1B1). For example, OATP1A2 is encoded by *SLCO1A2* (also known as *SLC21A3*) and OATP1B1 is *SLCO1B1* (also known as *SLC21A6*). Recently, many of the gene names are being substituted for the protein names to avoid confusion. Table 13.1 provides a partial listing of membrane transporter families.

The ATP-binding cassette (ABC) superfamily

ABC transporters, such as P-gp, BCRP, and multidrug resistance related proteins (MRPs), are expressed in multiple tissues, including intestine, liver, kidney, and brain.

P-glycoprotein

The most extensively studied drug transporter of the ABC superfamily is P-glycoprotein (P-gp, *ABCB1*), a member of the multidrug resistance (MDR) family of transporters and the product of the multidrug resistance 1 (*ABCB1*) gene [24]. P-gp mediates the ATP-dependent export of drugs from cells and has a wide tissue distribution, being expressed in the luminal membrane of the small intestine and capillary endothelial cells of the blood-brain barrier, and in the apical membranes of excretory cells such as hepatocytes and kidney proximal tubule epithelia. P-gp is an important determinant of intestinal absorption and of biliary and urinary excretion of many drugs, but also limits the entry of various drugs into the central nervous system (CNS). The level of expression and functionality of P-gp can be modulated by inhibition and induction, which can affect the PK, efficacy, and safety of P-gp substrate drugs [25–29].

Initially discovered as a result of its interaction with multiple anticancer drugs, P-gp is responsible for the efflux across biological membranes of a broad range of different drugs [30]. Digoxin is a notable substrate of P-gp and altered activity of this transporter can have clinically important consequences because of the narrow therapeutic range of this drug (Table 13.1). Recently, dabigatran etexilate (DE), a pro-drug of dabigatran, has been identified as a clinical substrate of P-gp and can be used as a probe to study intestinal P-gp inhibition [31]. Because many drugs are inhibitors of P-gp, their coadministration may cause a two- to threefold increase in the systemic exposure of P-gp substrates such as DE, digoxin, or fexofenadine. However, not all potent in vitro inhibitors of P-gp produce clinically meaningful changes in the PK of digoxin or other P-gp substrates, and changes in tissue exposure to these substrates may not be detected by monitoring their plasma concentrations [32]. Potent P-gp inhibitors include itraconazole and dronedarone. Many drugs have been identified as substrates and/or inhibitors of P-gp (Table 13.2) [33, 34].

Multidrug resistance-related protein

The multidrug resistance-related protein (MRP, *ABCC*) family of transporters is closely related and structurally similar to the MDR family (*ABCB*). MRP transporters constitute nine members of the ATP-binding cassette C subfamily (*ABCC1-6, 10-12*). Cloning, functional characterization, and cellular localization of most MRP subfamily members have identified them as ATP-dependent efflux pumps that transport a broad spectrum of endogenous and xenobiotic anionic substances across cellular plasma membranes [35–37]. ABCC subfamily members, which are not considered traditional transporters, include cystic fibrosis transmembrane conductance regulator (*ABCC7*) and two sulfonylurea receptor isoforms (*ABCC8* and *-9*) [35–37].

MRP1 (*ABCC1*), MRP2 (*ABCC2*), and MRP4 (*ABCC4*) have been the most widely studied members of the MRP family in the context of PK and drug response. MRP1 was initially identified in lung cells and pumps anionic compounds, in contrast to the cations pumped by P-gp [38]. Substrates for MRP1 include anionic natural products; glutathione, glucuronosyl, and sulfate conjugates; and, in some cases, unconjugated neutral molecules coupled to glutathione transport. MRP2 (*ABCC2*) is similar to MRP1 except in its tissue distribution and localization. It is expressed on the canalicular membrane of hepatocytes and was formerly known as the canalicular multispecific organic anion transporter (cMOAT). The hepatobiliary and renal elimination of many drugs and their metabolites is mediated by MRP2 in the hepatocyte canalicular membrane and by MRP4 as well as MRP2 in the luminal membrane of proximal renal tubules. Therefore inhibition of these efflux pumps may affect PK or intrahepatocyte substrate levels unless compensation is provided by other efflux transporters with overlapping substrate specificities. Genetic mutations in MRP2 cause Dubin-Johnson syndrome, a disease characterized by hyperbilirubinemia resulting from reduced transport of conjugated bilirubin into bile [39]. Drug-induced

TABLE 13.1 Selected transporter-mediated clinically significant drug-drug interactions.[a]

Gene	Aliases[b]	Tissue	Function	Interacting drug	Substrate (affected drug)	Changes in substrate plasma AUC (AUC ratios)
ABC transporters of clinical importance in the absorption, disposition, and excretion of drugs						
ABCB1	P-gp, MDR1	Intestinal enterocyte, kidney proximal tubule, hepatocyte (canalicular), brain endothelia	Efflux	Verapamil	Dabigatran	2.4-fold
				Dronedarone	Digoxin	2.6-fold
				Quinidine	Digoxin	1.7-fold
				Ranolazine	Digoxin	1.6-fold
				Verapamil	Simvastatin	4.6-fold
				Cyclosporine	Paclitaxel	8.5-fold
				Verapamil	(*R*)-Fexofenadine	2.9-fold
				Tipranavir/ritonavir	Loperamide	0.5-fold
				Tipranavir/ritonavir	Saquinavir/ritonavir	0.2-fold
ABCG2	BCRP	Intestinal enterocyte, hepatocyte (canalicular), kidney proximal tubule, brain endothelia, placenta, stem cells, mammary gland (lactating)	Efflux	Rolapitant	Sulfasalazine	2.3-fold
				Elacridar/GF120918	Topotecan	2.4-fold
				Curcumin	Sulfasalazine	3.2-fold
				Lopinavir/Ritonavir	Rosuvastatin	2.1-fold[c,d]
				Cyclosporine	Rosuvastatin	7.1-fold[c,d]
				Atazanavir/Ritonavir	Rosuvastatin	3.13-fold[c,d]
				Fostamatinib/R406	Rosuvastatin	1.8- to 2.2-fold[c,d]
				Eltrombopag	Rosuvastatin	1.6- to 2.3-fold[c,e]

SLC transporters of clinical importance in the disposition and excretion of drugs						
SLCO1B1	OATP1B1, OATP-C, OATP2, LST-1	Hepatocyte (sinusoidal)	Uptake	Lopinavir/ritonavir	Bosentan	5- to 48-fold[f]
				Cyclosporine	Pravastatin	9.9-fold
				Rifampin (single dose)	Glyburide	2.3-fold
				Lopinavir/ritonavir	Rosuvastatin	2.1-fold
SLCO1B3	OATP1B3, OATP-8	Hepatocyte (sinusoidal)	Uptake	Cyclosporine	Rosuvastatin	7.1-fold[g]
				Cyclosporine	Pitavastatin	4.6-fold[c]
				Lopinavir/ritonavir	Rosuvastatin	2.1-fold[c]
SLC22A2	OCT2	Kidney proximal tubule	Uptake	Cimetidine	Dofetilide	1.5-fold
				Cimetidine	Pindolol	1.5-fold
				Cimetidine	Metformin	1.4-fold[h]
				Dolutegravir	Metformin	2.4-fold
SLC47A1	MATE-1	Kidney proximal tubule, hepatocytes (canalicular)	Efflux	Pyrimethamine	Metformin	2.7-fold[h]
SLC47A2	MATE-2K	Kidney proximal tubule	Efflux	Pyrimethamine	Metformin	2.7-fold[h]
SLC22A6	OAT1	Kidney proximal tubule, placenta	Uptake	Probenecid	Cephradin	3.6-fold
				Trimethoprim/sulfamethoxazole	Apricitabine	1.7-fold
				Probenecid	Cidofovir	1.5-fold
				Probenecid	Acyclovir	1.4-fold
SLC22A8	OAT3	Kidney proximal tubule, choroid plexus, brain endothelia	Uptake	Probenecid	Furosemide	2.9-fold[i]

[a]*Abbreviations:* BCRP, *breast cancer resistance protein;* LST, *liver-specific transporters;* MDR, *multidrug resistance;* OATP, *organic anion transporting polypeptide;* OCT, *organic cation transporter;* OAT, *organic anion transporter;* P-gp, *p-glycoprotein.*
[b]*Implicated transporter refers to the likely transporter; however, because the studies are in vivo, it is not possible to assign definitively specific transporters to these interactions.*
[c]*Interaction could be partly mediated by OATP1B1.*
[d]*These studies are obtained from Refs. [18–22]*
[e]*Fold change is lower in Asian vs Non-Asian healthy volunteers based on Ref. [23].*
[f]*Minimum predose plasma level (C_{trough}) data from Day 4 (48-fold), Day 10 (5-fold) after coadministration.*
[g]*Interaction could be partly mediated by BCRP.*
[h]*Interaction could be partly mediated by MATE-1/MATE-2K.*
[i]*Interaction could be partly mediated by OAT1.*
Reproduced from the FDA Drug Interaction Website (https://www.fda.gov/drugs/drug-interactions-labeling/drug-development-and-drug-interactions-table-substrates-inhibitors-and-inducers#table5-1); University of Washington Drug Interaction Solutions (https://www.druginteractionsolutions.org/); UCSF-FDA TransPortal website (http://transportal.compbio.ucsf.edu/); Morrissey KM, et al. The UCSF-FDA TransPortal: a public drug transporter database. Clin Pharmacol Ther 2012;92(5):545–6.

TABLE 13.2 Partial list of drugs that are substrates, inhibitors, or inducers of transporters.[a]

Transporter	Substrate	Inhibitor
ABC transporters		
P-gp	Aliskiren, ambrisentan, ***boceprevir***, ***cabazitaxel***, colchicine, ***crizotinib***, ***cyclosporine***, dabigatran etexilate, ***eribulin***, ***everolimus***, ezogabine (metabolite), fexofenadine, fidaxomicin, ***lapatinib***, ***maraviroc***, ***nilotinib***, pazopanib, posaconazole, propranolol, ***ranolazine***, rivaroxaban, saxagliptin, silodosin, sirolimus, sitagliptin, ***ticagrelor***, ***tipranavir***,[b] ***tolvaptan***, topotecan, ***vemurafenib***	***Boceprevir***, ***cabazitaxel***, clarithromycin, conivaptan, ***crizotinib***, ***cyclosporine***, dronedarone, etravirine, ***eribulin***, ***everolimus***, ***lapatinib***, ***maraviroc***, ***nilotinib***, paliperidone, ***ranolazine***, sorafenib, ***ticagrelor***, ***tipranavir***,[b] ***tolvaptan***, ***vemurafenib***
BCRP	***Eltrombopag***, sulfasalazine, ***lapatinib***, rosuvastatin, pazopanib, pralatrexate, topotecan, lamivudine, methotrexate, nitrofurantoin, pemetrexed, pitavastatin, sildenafil, vardenafil, ethinyl estradiol, pantoprazole, glyburide, edaravone sulfate	Cabazitaxel, ***eltrombopag***, ***lapatinib***, elacridar/GF120918, sulfasalazine, fumitremorgin C, Ko134, Ko143, novobiocin, erlotinib, fostamatinib, dehydroaripiprazole, sunitinib, leflunomide, teriflunomide
MRP2	Mycophenolate, ***pralatrexate***, valsartan	***Pralatrexate***
SLC transporters		
OATP1B1	Ambrisentan, atorvastatin, valsartan, pravastatin	Cyclosporine,[c] dronedarone, eltrombopag,[d] lapatinib, pazopanib, telithromycin, rifampicin
OATP1B3	Ambrisentan, telmisartan	Dronedarone, telithromycin, rifampicin
OAT1	Adefovir, cidofovir, tenofovir, *p*-aminohippurate, furosemide	Probenecid, *p*-aminohippuric acid (PAH), teriflunomide
OAT3	Sitagliptin, methotrexate, pravastatin	Dronedarone, probenecid
OCT2	Metformin, gabapentin, pramipexole, varenicline, atenolol, salbutamol	Dronedarone, vandetanib, cimetidine
MATE-1/ MATE2-K	Metformin	Famotidine, pyrimethamine, trimethoprim, cimetidine

Note that when the drug names are *italicized* and *bolded*, they are both substrates and inhibitors.

[a]*Abbreviations:* BCRP, *breast cancer resistance protein;* MRP, *multidrug resistance-associated protein;* OAT, *organic anion transporter;* OATP, *organic anion transporting polypeptide;* OCT, *organic cation transporter;* P-gp, *P-glycoprotein.*

[b]*Tipranavir is also a P-gp inducer.*

[c]*Cyclosporine is stated as an inhibitor in the labeling for other drugs.*

[d]*In eltrombopag labeling, the following were mentioned as OATP1B1 substrates: benzylpenicillin, atorvastatin, fluvastatin, pravastatin, rosuvastatin, methotrexate, nateglinide, repaglinide, rifampin.*

Based on in vitro or in vivo data available from Huang SM, Zhang L, Giacomini KM. The International Transporter Consortium: a collaborative group of scientists from academia, industry, and the FDA. Clin Pharmacol Ther 2010;87(1):32–36; U.S. Food and Drug Administration. Drug development and drug interactions: table of substrates, inhibitors and inducers; 2020. Available from: https://www.fda.gov/drugs/drug-interactions-labeling/drug-development-and-drug-interactions-table-substrates-inhibitors-and-inducers#major. [cited 2020]; University of Washington Drug Interaction Solutions (https://www.druginteractionsolutions.org/) and UCSF-FDA TransPortal website (http://transportal.compbio.ucsf.edu/); Morrissey KM, et al. The UCSF-FDA TransPortal: a public drug transporter database. Clin Pharmacol Ther 2012;92(5):545–546.

conjugated hyperbilirubinemia, in patients or in preclinical species, may be caused by inhibition of MRP2. In hepatocytes, MRP3 and MRP4 are localized to the basolateral (sinusoidal) membrane and mediate efflux of several substrates, particularly glucuronides and glutathione conjugates, into sinusoidal blood and play a compensatory role in cholestasis. For example, MRP3 has been shown to transport phenolic glucuronide conjugates of acetaminophen, etoposide, methotrexate, and morphine from the apical surface of hepatocytes into blood [40, 41]. MRP3 also transports endogenous substances, particularly bilirubin monoglucuronide and bilirubin bisglucuronide. MRP4 (*ABCC4*) has been shown to transport a number of endogenous substrates, such as eicosanoids, urate, conjugated steroids, folate, bile acids, and glutathione, as well as many drug substrates, including cephalosporins, methotrexate, and nucleotide analog reverse transcriptase inhibitors [42, 43].

Breast cancer resistance protein

Breast cancer resistance protein (BCRP, *ABCG2*) is a "half ABC transporter," consisting of 655 amino acids and 6 transmembrane domains, and forming a homodimer for functional activity [44]. BCRP was identified originally as a determinant of in vitro multidrug resistance in cancer cell lines [45, 46]. Similar to P-gp, BCRP is expressed in the gastrointestinal tract, liver, kidney, brain endothelium, mammary tissue, testis, and placenta. It has a role in limiting the oral absorption and subsequent transport of substrates across the blood-brain barrier, blood-testis barrier, and maternal-fetal barrier [47, 48]. Similar to P-gp, BCRP has a wide variety of substrates and inhibitors. Although there is considerable overlap between BCRP and P-gp substrates and inhibitors, a quantitative structure-activity relationship (QSAR) analysis has been used to identify key structural elements that enable a molecule to interact with BCRP or P-gp and is thus able to differentiate some substrates and inhibitors of BCRP from those of P-gp [49–51].

BCRP function can contribute to variable bioavailability, exposure, and pharmacological response to BCRP substrate drugs. The most clinically significant effects are likely to be for drugs that have a low bioavailability and a narrow therapeutic range. Recent studies also have demonstrated that patients with reduced BCRP function, associated with the Q141K (*ABCG2* c.421C > A) variant, are at increased risk for gefitinib-induced diarrhea [52] and have altered irinotecan, rosuvastatin, sulfasalazine, and topotecan PK [53–57]. Furthermore, large clinical studies using a genome-wide association study (GWAS) approach showed that Q141K is significantly associated with a suboptimal response to rosuvastatin and allopurinol [58–60]. Based on in vitro data, several drugs (e.g., eltrombopag, lapatinib, pazopanib, sulfasalazine, topotecan, rosuvastatin, allopurinol, and oxypurinol) have been found to be substrates, while eltrombopag, GF-120918, and lapatinib are inhibitors of BCRP (Table 13.2). A clinical study has shown that eltrombopag increased rosuvastatin exposure by approximately twofold [23], possibly due to inhibition of BCRP and OATP1B1. Exposure to sulfasalazine administered as an immediate release oral formulation (suspension or tablet) was significantly increased in healthy volunteers who harbored the Q141K variant [56, 61]. These findings are consistent with studies in *Bcrp1*$^{-/-}$ mice that also demonstrated increased oral bioavailability and reduced systemic clearance of sulfasalazine [62, 63]. However, a clinical study with a delayed release formulation (enteric-coated tablets) of sulfasalazine failed to show an effect of the *ABCG2* c.421C > A polymorphism on plasma exposure [64]. On the contrary, a PK interaction study by Kusuhara et al. [65] in healthy subjects evaluated the impact of curcumin as an in vivo inhibitor of BCRP and found that curcumin could increase sulfasalazine exposure 2.0- and 3.2-fold after administration of 100 μg and 2 g of sulfasalazine, respectively. These authors concluded that curcumin is a useful inhibitor of BCRP in vitro and in vivo, but further work is needed to validate the utility of sulfasalazine as an in vivo probe of BCRP. The same authors reported that sulfasalazine uptake and efflux in the small intestine is dose dependent and is mediated by OATP2B1, which functions as a high-affinity, low-capacity uptake transporter, and by BCRP, respectively [65].

Bile salt export pump

Enterohepatic circulation of bile acids is mediated by specific transporters in hepatocytes and enterocytes [36]. Bile salt export pump (BSEP, *ABCB11*) is a transporter that is expressed exclusively on the canalicular side of hepatocytes and is involved in the biliary efflux of monovalent bile acids, whereas MRP2 exports divalent and sulfated and/or glucuronidated bile acids and other conjugated anions including Phase II drug metabolites. Although BSEP primarily transports bile acids, it can also transport drugs such as pravastatin [66].

BSEP has no functional redundant protein (i.e., no other known proteins that perform the same function as BSEP), and impairment of BSEP function may lead to liver disease as evidenced by increased plasma bile salt concentrations and liver enzymes. Altered bile-acid transporter expression or function can be either a cause or a consequence of cholestasis. Progressive familial intrahepatic cholestasis type 2 (PFIC2) is caused by mutations in the *ABCB11* gene, which encodes BSEP [67, 68]. Mutations in the *ABCB11* gene can lead to a rapid progressive hepatic dysfunction in early infancy. In such patients, the bile salt levels in the bile duct can be reduced to less than 1% of that in normal subjects. These defects or inhibition of BSEP may contribute to increased susceptibility to drug-induced cholestasis or other liver injury [69–71], but further research is needed to best determine how drugs can be studied early in their development to assess their BSEP-related safety liabilities [72]. A number of BSEP inhibitors have been identified (e.g., troglitazone, cyclosporine A, rifampicin, and glibenclamide) [73–76] and their relevance to drug-induced liver injury has been widely assessed using various methodologies, including 3D culture and modeling [77, 78]. Besides BSEP inhibition, drug-induced BSEP repression (reduction in BSEP expression) or the combination of inhibition and repression has emerged as important alternative mechanisms leading to drug-induced cholestasis [79, 80].

Solute carriers (SLCs)

Organic anion transporting polypeptides

Organic anion transporting polypeptides (OATPs, *SLCOs*) are a family of important membrane transport proteins within the solute carrier (SLC) superfamily and mediate the sodium-independent transport of a diverse range of amphiphilic organic compounds [81–83]. These include bile acids, steroid conjugates, thyroid hormones, anionic peptides, and drugs. OATP1B1 and OATP1B3 are the major OATPs expressed on the sinusoidal side of hepatocytes and, though they are reversible mediating both influx and efflux, they function primarily as uptake transporters that transport molecules from blood into hepatocytes. Recently, a new member of the OATP1B family, OATP1B3-1B7 (gene name LST-3TM12), was functionally characterized and shares similar OATP1B1 and OATP1B3 substrates, such as dehydroepiandrosterone sulfate (DHEAS) and bile acids [84, 85]. OATP1B3-1B7 is a splice variant of OATP1B3 and OATP1B7, and is expressed in the endoplasmic reticulum (ER) of hepatocytes. When heterologously expressed in HeLa cells, this transporter was shown to be expressed on the plasma membrane as well as in the ER [84, 85].

OATP2B1 exhibits broad tissue expression relative to OATP1B1 and OTAP1B3, and is expressed in the liver, intestine, and brain [86]. It is the main intestinal OATP isoform and is responsible for DDIs previously attributed to OATP1A2, whereas recent proteomic data suggest that OATP1A2 is expressed only in the kidney, brain, and retina [87, 88]. OATP2B1 has broad substrate specificity and transports many drugs, including atorvastatin and rosuvastatin. In vivo evidence that supports intestinal OATP2B1 as a mediator of DDIs comes largely from drug-fruit juice interactions [89–91]. For example, the C_{max} and AUC of several OATP2B1 substrates (including fexofenadine, aliskiren, and celiprolol) were decreased 1.5–2-fold by grapefruit, apple, and orange juice. A study showed that ronacaleret, an inhibitor of OATP2B1, decreased rosuvastatin plasma exposure by 50% without altering its terminal half-life. Intestinal OATP2B1 may need to be considered if there are observed decreases in the absorption of substrate drugs or possible excipient effects on drug absorption [89, 92–94].

OATP4C1 (SLCO4C1) is localized to the basolateral membrane of renal proximal tubule cells [95]. Substrates of OATP4C1 include digoxin, ouabain, and sitagliptin [96]. However, the contribution of OATP4C1 to renal elimination of drugs and DDIs has not been well established beyond its role in the tubular secretion of digoxin [97].

Link et al. [98] conducted a GWAS of patients with simvastatin-induced myopathy and demonstrated that polymorphisms in the *SLCO1B1* gene that encodes for OATP1B1 play an important role in predisposing individuals to simvastatin-induced myopathy (see Chapter 16). Since the study by Link et al., multiple GWAS have identified polymorphisms in *SLCO1B1*, including OATP1B1-Val174Ala (*SLCO1B1*, c.521T>C), associated with multiple phenotypes affecting drug response (e.g., statin toxicity and response) [99, 100] and drug disposition (e.g., methotrexate clearance) [101, 102]. In addition, clinically relevant drug interactions have been noted for certain OATPs, such as OATP1B1 and OATP1B3 (Table 13.1). Inhibition of OATP1B1-mediated hepatic uptake appears to contribute to the significant increase in the blood concentration of statins after cyclosporine coadministration [22, 103, 104]. Because cyclosporine is an inhibitor of multiple transporters, including OATP1B1 and BCRP, inhibition of either BCRP or OATP1B1 may have contributed to the interaction between cyclosporine and rosuvastatin [105, 106]. Drugs such as ambrisentan are substrates for OATP1B1 and OATP1B3, and eltrombopag is an inhibitor of OATP1B1 (Table 13.2) [107].

Organic cation and organic anion transporters

A distinct family of proteins within the SLC superfamily is encoded by 22 genes of the human SLC22A family, and includes the electrogenic organic cation transporters (OCTs) (isoforms 1–3) and the organic anion transporters (OATs) (significant isoforms in humans include OAT1-4 and 7, and URAT1) [108–110]. Various compounds interact with human OCTs and OATs [110, 111]. OCTs transport relatively hydrophilic, low molecular mass organic cations including metformin (Table 13.3). Properties of inhibitors of OCT1 and OCT2 have been identified and include compounds with a net positive

TABLE 13.3 Association of transporter gene polymorphisms with drug pharmacokinetics, biomarkers, and/or clinical responses.[a]

Transporter	Model drugs or substrates	Outcome measures	Study results	Ref(s)
P-gp	Digoxin	Pharmacokinetics	TT homozygous C3435 associated with higher plasma concentrations	[112]
	Fexofenadine	Pharmacokinetics	TT homozygous C3435 associated with lower plasma concentrations	[113]
	Nelfinavir, efavirenz	Pharmacokinetics and immune recovery	TT homozygous C3435 associated with lower plasma concentrations, and greater rise in CD4 responses	[114]
	Antiepileptic drugs	Clinical response	CC homozygous C3435 associated with drug-resistant epilepsy	[115]
BCRP	Rosuvastatin, atorvastatin, sulfasalazine	Pharmacokinetics	AA homozygous c.421C>A associated with higher *AUC* and C_{max}	[56, 61, 105, 116]
	Rosuvastatin	Clinical response (GWAS)	rs1481012 (G allele) associated with reduction in LDL cholesterol. rs1481012 is in LD with rs2231142/c.421C>A ($r^2>0.8$)	[117, 118]
	Allopurinol	Clinical response (GWAS)	AA homozygous c.421C>A associated with poor response to allopurinol	[58, 60, 119]
MRP2	Methotrexate	Pharmacokinetics and clinical response	412A>G associated with impaired renal elimination and renal toxicity	[120]
	Platinum-based therapy	Pharmacokinetics	C-24T associated with increased platinum-based chemotherapy response in 113 advanced nonsmall cell lung cancer patients	[121]
OATP1B1	Pravastatin	Pharmacokinetics	*SLCO1B1*15* (Asp130Ala174) lower clearance	[122]
	Statins	Clinical response (GWAS)	rs4149056 (c.521T>C) associated with a higher incidence of myopathy	[98, 99]
	Pitavastatin	Clinical response	c.521T>C and c. 388A>G unrelated to lipid-lowering effect in Chinese patients	[123]
	Atorvastatin	Pharmacokinetics (GWAS)	c.521T>C associated with higher atorvastatin and its metabolite level	[124]
	Methotrexate	Pharmacokinetics (GWAS)	rs4149056 (c.521T>C) and rs4149080 are associated with lower methotrexate clearance. rs4149080 is in LD with rs4149056 ($r^2>0.7$)	[101, 102]
	Statins	Clinical response (GWAS)	rs2900478 (A allele) associated with a smaller LDL-lowering effect. rs2900478 is in LD with rs4149056/V174A ($r^2>0.8$)	[100, 125]

Continued

TABLE 13.3 Association of transporter gene polymorphisms with drug pharmacokinetics, biomarkers, and/or clinical responses.[a]—cont'd

Transporter	Model drugs or substrates	Outcome measures	Study results	Ref(s)
MATE2-K	Metformin	Clinical response	Homozygous for g.−130A associated with poorer response	[126, 127]
OCT1	Metformin	Pharmacokinetics and biomarkers	Reduced function alleles (i.e., R61C) associated with higher AUC levels and lower glucose tolerance test[b]	[128, 129]
		Clinical response	Reduced function alleles associated with increased risk of metformin-induced gastrointestinal side effects[b]	[130, 131]
	Tramadol	Pharmacokinetics and biomarkers	Reduced function alleles associated with higher plasma levels of *O*-desmethyltramadol (metabolite) and prolonged miosis[b]	[132]
		Clinical response	Reduced function alleles associated with lower consumption of tramadol dose in patients on patient-controlled analgesia (PCA)[b]	[133]
	Ondansetron, Tropisetron	Pharmacokinetics and clinical response	Reduced function alleles associated with increased drug levels and reduce episodes of vomiting[b]	[134]
	Morphine	Pharmacokinetics	Reduced function alleles associated with reduced morphine clearance[b]	[135]
		Clinical response	Reduced function alleles associated with morphine-related postoperative nausea and vomiting and a higher incidence of respiratory distress[b]	[136]
	Sumatriptan	Pharmacokinetics	Reduced function alleles associated with increased AUC[b]	[137]
	Fenoterol	Pharmacokinetics and Clinical response	Reduced function alleles associated with increased AUC, lower volume of distribution, and increase incidence of side effects (higher heart rate and blood glucose, lower potassium)[b]	[138]
OCT2	Metformin	Pharmacokinetics	Variant alleles (p.A270S, c.808G > T) associated with reduced renal clearance and net secretion in one study but opposite direction in another study	[139, 140]

[a]*Abbreviations:* ABCB1, *ATP-binding cassette family (ABC);* B1, *multidrug resistance (MDR1), a human gene that encodes P-glycoprotein (P-gp);* MRP, *multidrug resistance protein;* OATP-1B1, *organic anion transporting peptide 1B1.*

[b]*Reduced function alleles for OCT1 refer to nonsynonymous variants in SLC22A1 that have reduced transporter activity and altered substrates disposition, response, or adverse effects. In these studies, there is a significant correlation with the number of inactive OCT1 alleles with the studied drug disposition (pharmacokinetic effect, PK) and response and toxicity (pharmacodynamics effect, PD). These studies associated the phenotype with one or more of the most common functional amino acid substitutions found in Caucasians (Arg61Cys, Cys88Arg, Gly401Ser, Met420del, and Gly465Arg).*

charge and high lipophilicity [110]. OCT1 is mainly expressed in human liver (sinusoidal) while OCT2 is mainly expressed in human kidney (basolateral). OAT1, OAT3, and OAT4 mediate exchange of intracellular 2-oxoglutarate for extracellular substrates [141]. OAT1 and OAT3 mediate the basolateral cell-entry step in renal secretion of different structural classes of monovalent and selected divalent anions with a molecular weight of less than 500 Da (type I organic anions) [142]. In addition, OAT3 can also transport some basic drugs, such as cimetidine. OAT2, which is expressed in both kidney and liver, is a transporter with emerging clinical importance [89]. The ITC has highlighted the increasing number of clinical drugs that are substrates of OAT2 (e.g., antiviral nucleoside drugs, warfarin, tolbutamide), in addition to endogenous metabolites which are OAT2 substrates (e.g., creatinine, cyclic GMP) [89, 143–145].

Multidrug and toxin extrusion transporters

The multidrug and toxin extrusion transporter MATE1 (*SLC47A1*) is expressed in both kidney and liver cells at the apical side of the cell membrane, whereas MATE2-K (*SLC47A2*) is mainly expressed in the kidney (Fig. 13.2) [146–148]. In 2005 Otsuka et al. [148] identified and functionally characterized the human H^+/organic cation antiporter MATE1 and Masuda et al. [147] characterized a paralog (i.e., a gene copy created by a duplication event within the same genome locus), MATE2, the following year. Two isoforms of MATE2 have been identified, one of which, MATE2-K, has been characterized as a membrane transporter in the kidney [147]. Various drugs, including metformin, as well as endogenous substances such as guanidine, have been shown to be substrates of MATE1 [148]. MATE2-K, like MATE1, appears to transport an array of structurally diverse compounds, including many cationic drugs and endogenous compounds [149]. Komatsu et al. [150] characterized isoform 1 of MATE2 (NP_690872) and showed that both human MATE2 (isoform 1)

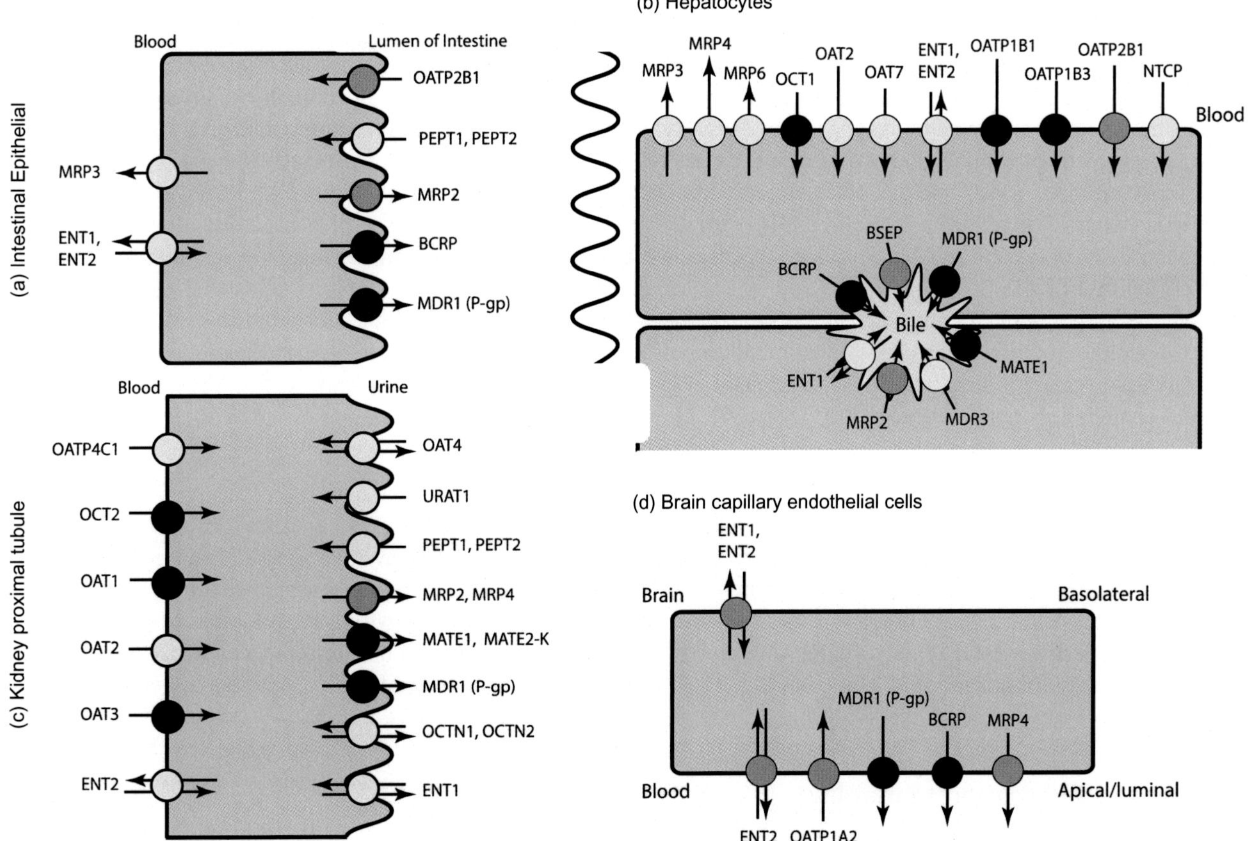

FIG. 13.2 Selected human transport proteins for drugs and endogenous substances. Transporters in plasma membrane domains of (A) intestinal epithelia, (B) hepatocytes, (C) kidney proximal tubules, and (D) blood-brain barrier. *Black circles* are transporters currently recommended for evaluation by the FDA and/or EMA. *Dark gray circles* are transporters recommended for retrospective mechanistic explanation of clinical observations. *Light gray circles* are other transporters discussed in this chapter. Refer to Ref. [89] for abbreviations of transporters listed in the figure. *(Reproduced with permission from the Nature Publishing Group and corresponding authors, Zamek-Gliszczynski MJ, Taub ME, Chothe PP, et al. Transporters in drug development: 2018 ITC recommendations for transporters of emerging clinical importance. Clin Pharmacol Ther 2018;104:890–899.)*

and MATE2-K (isoform 2): (1) operate in the kidney as electroneutral H^+/organic cation exchangers; (2) express and localize in the kidney, with MATE2-K being slightly more abundant than MATE2; (3) transport tetraethyl ammonium (TEA); and (4) have similar inhibitor specificities. Since some substrates (e.g., metformin) or inhibitors (e.g., cimetidine) recognized by OCT2 are also recognized by MATEs [149], MATEs may act in concert with OCT2 to mediate the excretion of some drugs [151–153]. On the other hand, many renal DDIs of basic drugs appear to be mediated by inhibition of MATE1 and MATE2, rather than by OCT2 [154, 155].

Role of transporters in pharmacokinetics and drug action

There is increasing recognition of the important roles played by membrane transporters in the processes of drug absorption, distribution, and elimination. This is particularly true with respect to the barrier and drug-eliminating functions of gastrointestinal epithelial cells (enterocytes), hepatocytes, and renal tubule cells. Fig. 13.2 indicates some of the known membrane transport systems that are expressed in various body tissues [49].

Role of membrane transport in the intestine

As discussed in Chapter 4, factors affecting the absorption of orally administered drugs include the physicochemical (e.g., lipophilicity, solubility, etc.) and pharmaceutical (e.g., dissolution and dosage form) properties of the drug, as well as physiological factors (e.g., gastric emptying rate and intestinal motility, metabolizing enzymes, and transporters). Transporters can either facilitate the absorption of a drug (e.g., absorptive transporters such as peptide transporters or OATP2B1) or limit its oral absorption (e.g., efflux transporters such as P-gp, BCRP, and MRP).

Absorptive (uptake) transporters

As described in Chapter 4, oligopeptide and monocarboxylic acid transporters facilitate the absorption of certain drugs, and these natural transport pathways have been exploited to enhance the bioavailability of some drugs. For example, the usefulness of acyclovir is limited by its poor bioavailability. However, valacyclovir is an amino acid ester of acyclovir (acyclovir conjugated with valine) and is a substrate for the PEPT1 transporter [156]. Consequently, the oral bioavailability of valacyclovir is three- to fivefold that of acyclovir in human subjects and, because it is readily hydrolyzed after absorption to release acyclovir, it functions as a useful prodrug for acyclovir [157]. This example represents a drug delivery strategy in which the absorption of an active drug can be significantly improved by coupling it with an amino acid that enables it to be transported by PEPT1.

Member of the OATP family, such as OATP2B1, have been identified as playing a role in the absorption of drugs such as fexofenadine. In vitro studies have shown that grapefruit juice inhibits OATP2B1-mediated fexofenadine uptake, presumably accounting for the clinical observation that grapefruit juice decreases fexofenadine exposure by three- to fourfold without changing its renal clearance [90, 158–160].

Efflux transporters

In contrast to absorptive transporters, efflux transporters such as P-gp and BCRP limit the intestinal absorption of drugs that are their substrates. These transporters are responsible for reducing the bioavailability of drugs such as digoxin, topotecan, and sulfasalazine (Table 13.1) and inhibitors of these transporters significantly increase their bioavailability. Consequently, the systemic exposure to these drugs is enhanced when they are coadministered with a P-gp inhibitor (e.g., quinidine's interaction with digoxin [161]) or a BCRP inhibitor (e.g., GF120918's interaction with topotecan [162], or curcumin's interaction with sulfasalazine [65], shown in Fig. 13.3). Because of their important role in limiting bioavailability, these two transporters are routinely studied during drug development.

Metabolism and transport interplay

Drugs that are substrates, inhibitors, or inducers of cytochrome P450 (CYP) or Phase II enzymes can also be substrates, inhibitors, or inducers of transporters. The effect on drug metabolism of interactions that modify transporter activity depends on the location of the transporters, and they may either enhance or reduce the access of drugs to the intracellular space where metabolism occurs [33, 163, 164]. The impact of this interplay between drug transporters and metabolizing enzymes has been demonstrated in both animal and human studies [163, 165]. As discussed in Chapters 4 and 14, both P-gp and CYP3A4 are colocalized in intestinal enterocytes and many of the substrates for CYP3A4 are also substrates for P-gp.

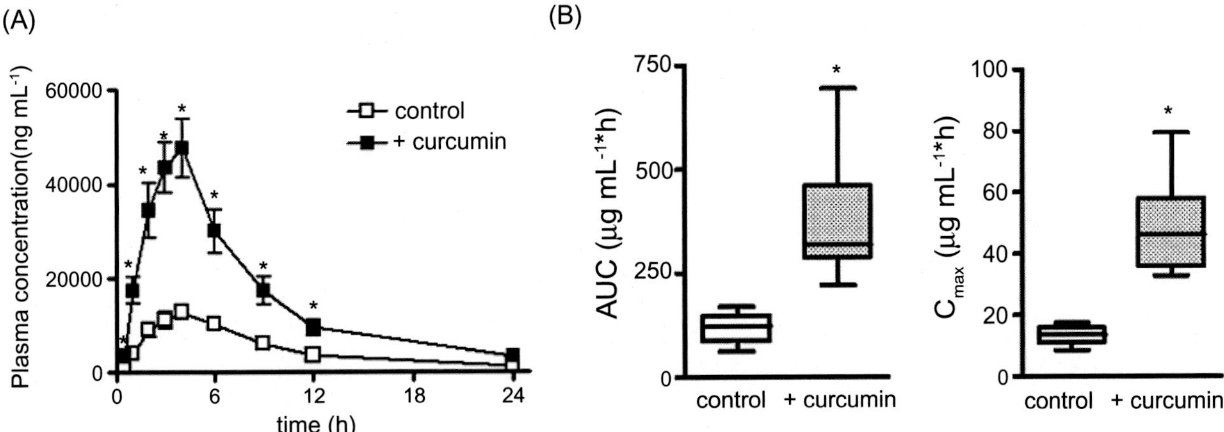

FIG. 13.3 The influence of breast cancer resistance protein (BCRP) on systemic exposure to sulfasalazine. (A) Plasma concentrations of sulfasalazine after an oral sulfasalazine dose of 2000 mg alone (□) and with a 2000mg oral dose of the BCRP inhibitor, curcumin (■) administered 30min before the sulfasalazine 2000mg oral dose. (B) Effect of curcumin on the AUC and C_{max} of sulfasalazine given orally. AUC and C_{max} were calculated from the data shown in (A). Values are expressed as box (lower and upper quartiles) and whisker plots (the furthest data points still within a distance of 1.5 interquartile ranges from the lower and upper quartiles) with medians shown as the *horizontal line*. *$P < .05$, significantly different from control; paired *t*-test. *(Based on data from Kusuhara H, Furuie H, Inano A, et al. Pharmacokinetic interaction study of sulphasalazine in healthy subjects and the impact of curcumin as an in vivo inhibitor of BCRP. Br J Pharmacol 2012;166:1794–1803.)*

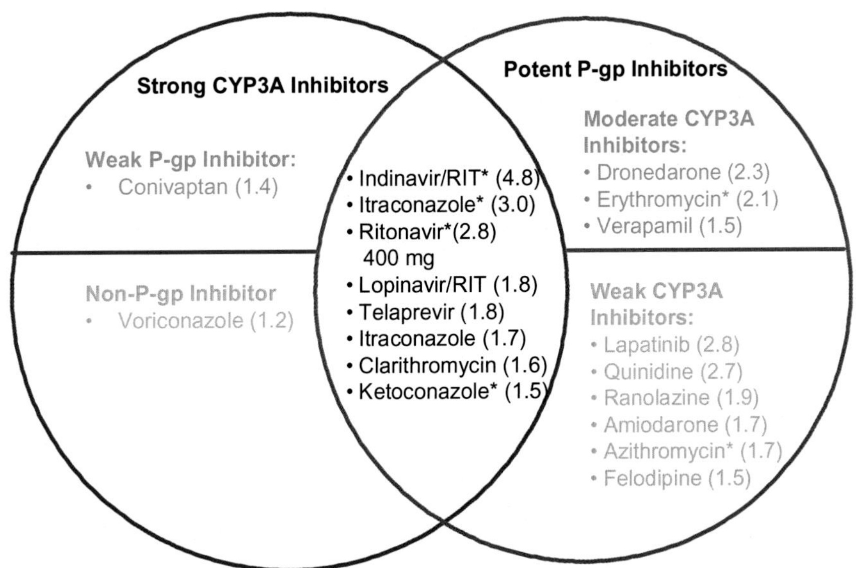

FIG. 13.4 Venn diagram illustrating the overlap between inhibitors of CYP3A and P-gp and their relative potency. The fold increases in the *AUC* of P-gp substrates are provided after the inhibitor drug names by the numbers in *parentheses*. Digoxin was the substrate drug, except when fexofenadine was used (indicated by an *asterisk*). *RIT*, ritonavir. *(Modified from Zhang L, Zhang YD, Huang SM. Scientific and regulatory perspectives on metabolizing enzyme-transporter interplay and its role in drug interactions: challenges in predicting drug interactions. Mol Pharm 2009;6:1766–1774 and US FDA. Drug development and drug interactions: Table of substrates, inhibitors and inducers; 2020. Available from: https://www.fda.gov/drugs/drug-interactions-labeling/drug-development-and-drug-interactions-table-substrates-inhibitors-and-inducers#major. [cited 2020].)*

Consequently, many CYP3A4 substrates may also be competing for transport by P-gp and bioavailability may be limited either by intestinal first-pass metabolism by CYP3A4 or by P-gp-mediated efflux.

Fig. 13.4 illustrates the overlap between CYP3A and P-gp inhibitors and indicates their relative potency [166]. Although many CYP3A inhibitors are also P-gp inhibitors, a strong CYP3A inhibitor does not necessarily cause a large increase in systemic exposure to a P-gp substrate, such as digoxin or fexofenadine. Thus the area under the plasma-level vs time curve (*AUC*) of digoxin, a P-gp substrate, was significantly increased when it was coadministered with some strong CYP3A inhibitors, such as itraconazole, clarithromycin, ketoconazole, but not when it was given with other strong CYP3A inhibitors, such as voriconazole. Similarly, some P-gp inhibitors, such as amiodarone and quinidine, increased digoxin *AUC* significantly and yet are weak CYP3A inhibitors. In many cases, known inhibitors of either CYP3A or P-gp have not been tested for their respective potency for the other entity, so it may be difficult to generalize interaction data generated from studies using these inhibitors to drugs that are substrates for both CYP3A and P-gp. For example, the net effect of tipranavir/ritonavir on the oral bioavailability and plasma concentrations of drugs that are dual substrates of CYP 3A and P-gp will vary depending on the relative affinity of the coadministered drugs for CYP3A and P-gp, and the extent of intestinal first-pass metabolism/efflux [166, 167].

Role of membrane transporters in drug distribution

Transporters are expressed in varying abundance in all tissues in the body where they govern the access of molecules to cells or their exit from cells, and thereby control the overall distribution of drugs to their intracellular site of action. For this reason, intracellular concentrations of drugs can in some cases change drastically enough to affect the efficacy or safety of a drug without this being reflected in the drug's *AUC*. Many tissues express the same drug export pumps that occur in the barrier epithelial tissues (e.g., P-gp, MRP, BCRP), and these may be important in normal tissues, as well as in drug-resistant cancers.

Transporters are also critical to target tissue uptake of drugs from the extravascular space. As discussed in Chapter 3, transport of drugs between the vascular and extravascular spaces, except in capillaries with tight junctions, generally occurs by nonmediated passive diffusion, and tissue specific uptake is mediated by plasma membrane transporters. For example, concentrations of metformin in the liver are highly determined by OCT1 as shown by studies in *Oct1* knockout mice, whereas this transporter has modest effects on systemic blood levels [128, 168]. Other transporters that play a role in drug distribution to tissues include the nucleoside transporter family that is responsible for antiviral and anticancer drug uptake [169, 170], and the reduced folate carrier which is essential for methotrexate uptake [171]. In capillaries with tight junctions such as the blood-brain, blood-germinal epithelium (blood-testis and blood-ovary), and blood-placental barriers, transporters play a critical role in the movement of substrates between intravascular space and interstitial space. Endothelial cells in each of these tissues express high levels of P-gp and BCRP as well as high levels of influx transporters in the SLC family.

A large body of research now focuses on the transcriptomic and proteomic levels of membrane transporters in tissues of drug absorption, distribution, and elimination, such as liver, intestine, and blood-brain barrier [172–174]. These data are increasingly important for understanding transporters' roles in drug distribution and establishing physiological parameters to predict in vivo outcomes [175].

Blood-brain barrier and blood-cerebrospinal fluid barrier

The blood-brain barrier largely results from the formation of tight junctions between brain endothelial cells and is enhanced by the action of a number of transporters (Fig. 13.2D) [49, 176, 177]. The blood-cerebrospinal fluid (CSF) barrier is formed by epithelial cells of the choroid plexus, and tight junctions limit drug transfer between blood and CSF [176, 177]. P-gp is the best studied transporter in the choroid plexus and is located on the apical surface analogous to its location in other tissues. Choroid plexus cells also have been shown to express MRP on their basolateral surface, consistent with a brain-protective role for this transport protein [178]. In addition, several other blood-brain barrier and choroid plexus transporters have been recognized, including BCRP, OATP1A2, OATP2B1, MRP4, and MRP5 [49, 179, 180]. OCTs on the apical surface of the choroid plexus appear to serve as efflux transporters, taking organic cations from the cerebrospinal fluid into epithelial cells. OCT3 is expressed at high levels in brain and has been shown to transport cimetidine, amphetamine, and methamphetamine, as well as serotonin and dopamine [110, 181].

The importance of P-gp in the blood-brain barrier was revealed by a laboratory incident in which ivermectin, routinely used in rodent facilities to control parasitic worms, was administered to *abcb1a/b* knockout mice. The day after one mouse colony was given standard ivermectin treatment, all of the homozygous *abcb1a/b* knockout mice were found dead, and ivermectin levels were 100-fold higher in their brains than in the brains of wild-type mice [182]. The clinical significance of P-gp in preventing the central nervous system (CNS) effects of loperamide was demonstrated in a study in which it was shown that coadministration of quinidine not only increased loperamide plasma concentrations but also resulted in a depressed respiratory response to carbon dioxide rebreathing that was not seen when loperamide was given by itself [183]. P-gp also may contribute to resistance to peptidomimetic HIV protease inhibitors (e.g., indinavir, saquinavir, and nelfinavir) in AIDS patients because it limits the access of these P-gp substrates to HIV within the CNS [184–187].

Placenta

The placenta, an organ of the fetus, serves to supply the fetus with essential nutrients, to eliminate fetal waste products, and to protect the fetus from potentially harmful chemicals that may be present in the maternal circulation. BCRP (*ABCG2*) was originally identified in human placenta [188], and may function in the human placenta to protect the fetus or to transport steroid hormones produced in the placenta. Specifically, estrogen sulfate (E_1S) and DHEAS are among the major estrogens produced and secreted by the placenta and are shown to be substrates for BCRP. Given its high expression in the syncytiotrophoblast near the apical surface at the chorionic villus, BCRP may help form the barrier between the maternal and fetal circulation systems and thus protect the fetus from endogenous and exogenous toxins.

Hepatocytes

Though transporters exist in all cells in the body, because of its major role in drug absorption and elimination, the liver and in particular, hepatocytes should be included in any discussion of drug distribution. From Fig. 13.2B [49], it is clear that many uptake transporters govern the entry and exit of drugs to and from the liver. OATP1B1, OATP1B3, OATP2B1, NTCP, OAT2, OAT7, and OCT1 are examples of uptake transporters, while MRP3, MRP4, and MRP6 are efflux transporters located in the basolateral (sinusoidal) membrane. On the apical (canalicular) side, P-gp, BSEP, BCRP, MRP2, and MATE1 are efflux transporters, which govern the secretion of drugs in the bile. Lapatinib is a substrate for efflux transporters P-gp and BCRP [189]. Rosuvastatin is a substrate for both BCRP and OATP1B1 [190], while pravastatin is a substrate for OATP1B1 and MRP2 [191] (Tables 13.1 and 13.2). As there are multiple pathways for clearance of these drugs, evaluation of a transporter's effect on a drug's plasma and tissue levels and its safety and efficacy needs to consider the multiple transport and enzymatic pathways involved in that drug's clearance.

Various recent clinical studies have evaluated the role of P-gp, OATP1B1, and BCRP in a drug's ADME and clinical effects. As mentioned earlier, a GWAS demonstrated that decreased OATP1B1 activity due to the presence of a genetic variant was associated with an increased incidence of myopathy in patients taking 40 or 80 mg of simvastatin (Table 13.4) [98]. Similarly, Maeda et al. [192] used a micro-dosing approach to demonstrate that OATP1B1 (and not CYP3A)

TABLE 13.4 Clinically relevant transporter variants and their allele frequencies in different populations.[a]

Protein name	AFR (%)	EUR (%)	EAS (%)	SAS (%)	AMR (%)
ABC transporters					
P-gp: p.I1145I, rs1045642, c.3435C>T	15	52	40	57	43
MRP2: 5′UTR, rs717620, c.-24C>T	3	21	22	10	17
BCRP: p.Q141K, rs2231142, c.421C>A	1	9	29	10	14
SLC transporters					
OCT1: p.R61C, rs12208357, c.181C>T	0	6	0	2	2
OCT1: p.G465R, rs34059508, c.1393G>A	0	2	0	0	2
OCT1: p.M420del, rs202220802, c.1258_1260ATG>deletion	5	18	0	15	29
OCT2: p.A270S, rs316019, c808G>T	19	11	14	13	9
OATP1B1: p.V174A, rs4149056, c.521T>C	1	16	12	4	13
OATP1B3: p.S112A, rs4149117, c.334T>G	36	86	70	91	84
OATP1B3: p.M233I, rs7311358, c.699G>A	36	86	70	91	84
OATP2B1: p.R312Q, rs12422149, c.935G>A	9	10	3	26	36
MATE1: 5′UTR, rs2252281, c.-66T>C	41	41	21	17	27
MATE2-K: 5′UTR, rs12943590, c.-130G>A	18	27	45	40	32

[a]*Abbreviations:* AFR, *African;* AMR, *Admixed Americans/Hispanics;* EUR, *European;* EAS, *East Asian,* SAS, *South Asian;* BCRP, *breast cancer resistance protein;* MATE, *multidrug and toxin extrusion;* MRP, *multidrug resistance-associated protein;* OATP, *organic anion transporting polypeptide;* OCT, *organic cation transporter;* P-gp, *P-glycoprotein.*
Modified from Yee SW, Brackman DJ, Ennis E, et al. Influence of transporter polymorphisms on drug disposition and response: a perspective from the International Transporter Consortium. Clin Pharmacol Ther 2018;104:803–817.

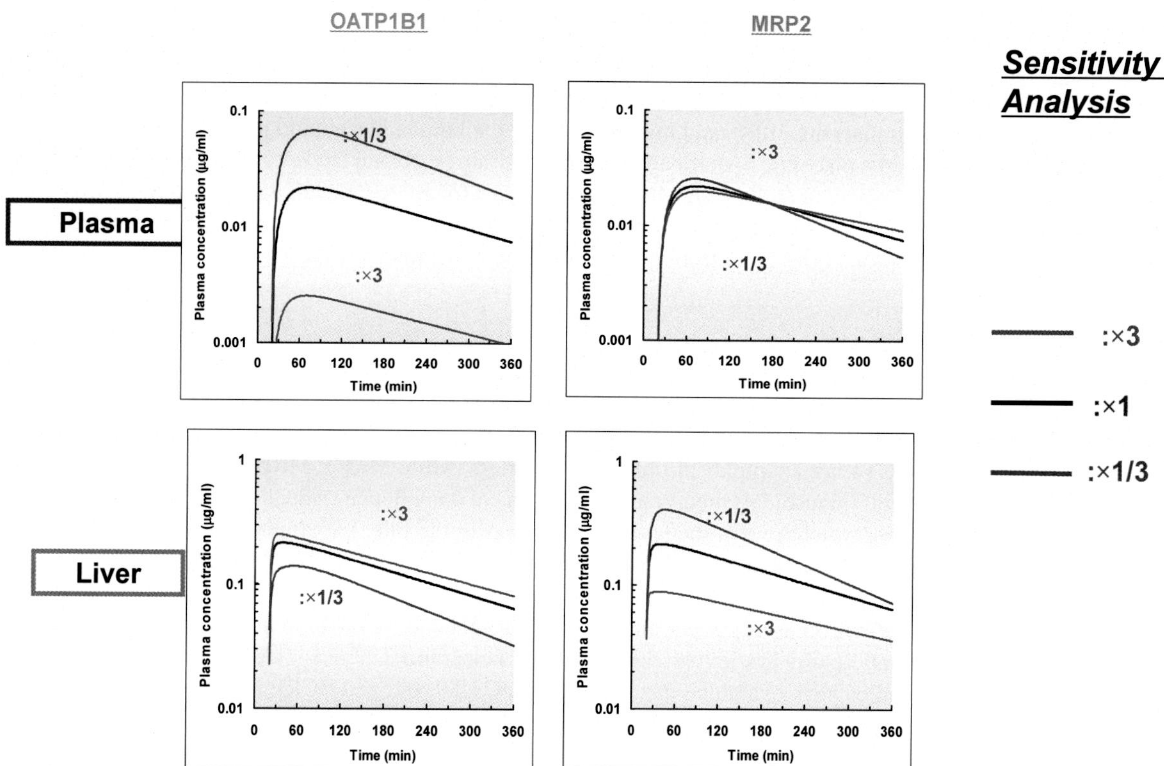

FIG. 13.5 Sensitivity analysis using physiologically based PK modeling to predict the effect of increases and decreases in the activity (1/3, 1, or 3 × normal activity) of OATP1B1-mediated hepatic uptake and MRP2-mediated biliary excretion on plasma and liver concentrations of pravastatin. *(Modified from Watanabe T, Kusuhara H, Maeda K, et al. Physiologically based pharmacokinetic modeling to predict transporter-mediated clearance and distribution of pravastatin in humans. J Pharmacol Exp Ther 2009;328:652–662.)*

determined the rate of hepatic clearance of another statin, atorvastatin. However, OATP1B1 appeared to have played only a small role in the LDL-cholesterol lowering effect of either rosuvastatin [193] or simvastatin [98].

Sugiyama's laboratory [191] has delineated how the activities of different transporters located in hepatocytes may have different effects on the plasma or tissue levels of a drug. As shown in Fig. 13.5, a sensitivity analysis showed that decreased activity of OATP1B1, which governs the entry of pravastatin to the liver, could result in an increased plasma level of pravastatin that could lead to increased adverse events. On the other hand, an increase in MRP2 activity, which is one of the pathways responsible for pravastatin's excretion into the bile, could result in decreased levels of pravastatin at its hepatic site of action, thereby diminishing its clinical efficacy while not affecting its plasma level. This sensitivity analysis used a systems approach based on physiologically based pharmacokinetic (PBPK) modeling, and is a useful approach for providing hypotheses for further evaluation or for interpreting laboratory or clinical observations related to the complex interplay of various elimination pathways, including those mediated by transporters [191, 194–196]. Further discussion on the utility of PBPK to study the interplay of metabolism and transport in DDI evaluation is provided in Chapter 16.

Role of membrane transporters in renal drug elimination

Many drugs are eliminated via the kidneys, either unchanged or after biotransformation into more polar metabolites. It is generally accepted that smaller and more hydrophilic (anionic or cationic) drugs are eliminated by the kidney, whereas bulkier and more hydrophobic drugs are eliminated by the liver [197, 198]. After filtration at the glomerulus, drugs pass through renal tubules that are the site of active drug secretion and reabsorption by various transporters. As discussed in Chapter 5, only the drug not bound to plasma proteins is filtered at the glomerulus, so an indicator of net tubular secretion or reabsorption can be obtained by comparing a drug's renal clearance (CL_R) with its glomerular filtration rate ($f_u \times$ GFR, where f_u is the fraction free in plasma and GFR is the glomerular filtration rate). If $CL_R \neq f_u \times$ GFR, then there is either net secretion or reabsorption and transporter involvement (CL_R could also equal $f_u \times$ GFR in the unlikely event that both the secretion and reabsorption processes cancel each other out).

Various transporters are responsible for the tubular secretion and reabsorption of drugs (Fig. 13.2C) [49, 197, 199]. P-gp expressed in the kidney is responsible for secreting digoxin and other large neutral compounds. In addition to P-gp, OCT2, MATE1, MATE2-K, OAT1, and OAT3 are the major drug transporters in human kidneys. Competitive inhibition of renal drug transporters can alter drug excretion and either enhanced or reduce systemic exposure. OCT2 is responsible for renal secretion of cytotoxic drugs (e.g., cisplatin and oxaliplatin) [200–202], antiretroviral agents [203], and adrenergic agonists and antagonists [204]. Both OCT2 inhibition and genetic polymorphisms have been shown to modulate the PK of these drugs [110, 132, 205]. Recent studies have shown that MATE, and not OCT2, is the rate-determining process in metformin renal elimination [126, 206].

Renal transporters and nephrotoxicity

OATs are involved in the development of organ-specific toxicity for some drugs and their metabolites [111, 197]. For example, as described in Chapter 16, OATs are responsible for the high renal tubular accumulation of antiviral drugs such as adefovir and cidofovir that is responsible for their nephrotoxicity [207, 208]. This nephrotoxicity can be reduced by coadministering OAT inhibitors, such as probenecid, that can inhibit the tubular accumulation of cidofovir and thus reduce its potential risk. For this reason, probenecid is now recommended in the cidofovir labeling as a nephroprotectant [209].

Transporter-mediated drug-drug interactions

For many years, important drug-drug interactions were thought to be mediated exclusively by drug-metabolizing enzymes; however, more recently, transporters in the intestine, liver, and kidney have been implicated as the target sites of many drug-drug interactions. Although animal models and whole cell systems, such as liver slices, have been used to evaluate transporter-mediated drug-drug interactions, a series of articles published by the ITC [8, 49, 89, 210] and the recently published FDA final drug-drug interaction guidances [3, 4] have recommended the use of in vitro models (e.g., membrane vesicles, oocytes, cell lines, single or double transfected cell lines, and hepatocytes) to determine a drug's potential as a substrate or inhibitor of several major transporters (P-gp, BCRP, OATP1B1, OATP1B3, OCT2, OAT1, OAT3, MATE1, and MATE2-K). These interactions are specifically discussed in Chapter 14.

Pharmacogenetics and pharmacogenomics of membrane transport

Genetic variants in many transporters have been identified and functionally characterized in a number of studies ([211] and references therein). Comparative studies in subjects with various transporter genotypes have helped to determine the relative contribution of the transporter to a drug's overall PK, even when a specific inhibitor drug was not available. Many techniques, including GWAS and candidate gene approaches, have been used to evaluate the associations of SNPs of transporter genes and clinical phenotypes which were related to drug concentrations in plasma and tissue, and to drug efficacy and safety. In 2013 the ITC highlighted the two clinically important polymorphisms in membrane transporters, BCRP and OATP1B1, missense variants, c.421C>A (p.Q141K) and c.521T>C (p.V174A), respectively [212]. These polymorphisms resulted in reduced protein levels on plasma membranes and hence reduced transporter function [102, 213]. Importantly, several GWAS and multiple candidate gene studies have consistently showed that these polymorphisms resulted in significant changes in drug PK and response (Table 13.3). These polymorphisms were found in populations across ancestral groups, with lower allele frequencies in individuals of sub-Saharan African ancestry (Table 13.4). In 2018 the ITC highlighted additional clinically important transporter polymorphisms including OCT1 [211]. The four OCT1 missense variants that were evaluated for their drug disposition or response phenotypes are OCT1 p.R61C, p.G401S, p.M420del, and p.G465R. These variants significantly reduced the transport of cationic drugs such as metformin, atenolol, and morphine in multiple candidate gene studies (Tables 13.3 and 13.4, and Fig. 13.6) [129, 134, 138, 214].

In addition to OATP1B1, BCRP, and OCT1, Table 13.3 presents the correlations that were made for selected substrates between genetic variants of P-gp, BSEP, MRP2, OATP1B3, MATE1, MATE2, OCT2, and other transporters and altered drug PK and/or clinical response [59, 98, 101, 105, 112–116, 120–122, 126, 128, 129, 132, 134, 137–139, 190, 214–218]. Many of these studies were exploratory and were conducted in a small number of healthy subjects (e.g., 10–30/arm), and some were case studies selected from cohorts of patients in large clinical trials or from electronic health records, such as the study on simvastatin and OATP1B1 for adverse events and response [98–100]. As discussed in Chapter 16, one of these studies showed the correlation of *SLCO1B1* variants with adverse events (e.g., myopathy) in patients taking 80 or 40 mg of simvastatin for up to 6 years and illustrated how GWAS could identify a clear contribution of transporter genetics to variability in clinical response [98].

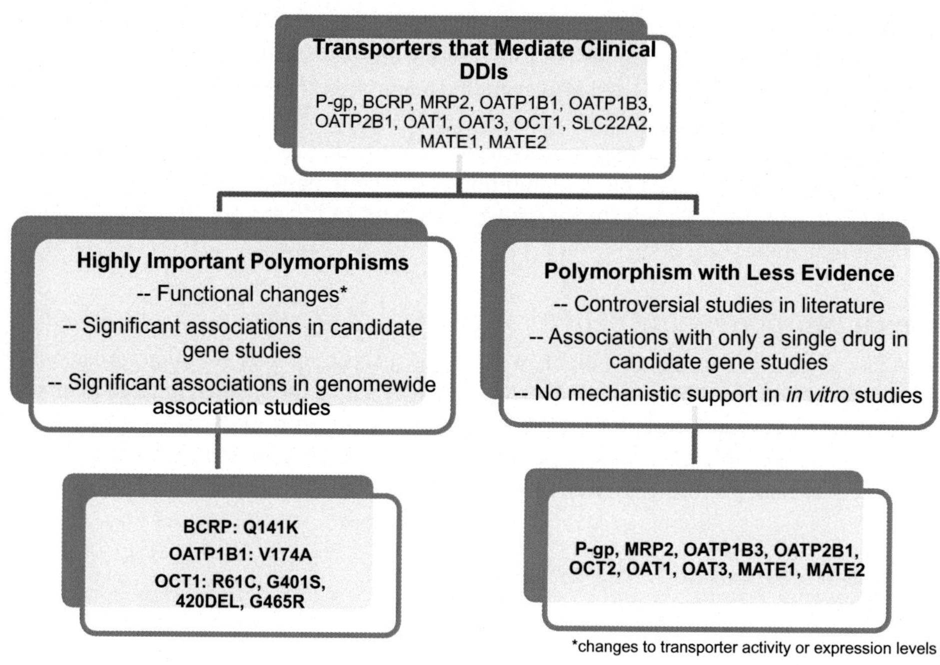

FIG. 13.6 Criteria used to select very important polymorphisms in transporters that mediate clinical drug-drug interactions. *(Reproduced with permission from Yee SW, Brackman DJ, Ennis EA, et al. Influence of transporter polymorphisms on drug disposition and response: a perspective from the International Transporter Consortium. Clin Pharmacol Ther 2018;104:803–817.)*

Because alterations in P-gp function can affect drug absorption and bioavailability, drug distribution to the brain and other tissues, and drug elimination, drugs are now routinely tested during their development to ascertain whether they are substrates, inhibitors, or inducers of P-gp. However, studies of genetic differences in P-gp expression have not provided consistent results [219, 220]. For example, although higher drug concentrations of one P-gp substrate, digoxin, were found in individuals with the TT homozygous C3435T variant of the *ABCB1* gene, lower concentrations of other P-gp substrates, fexofenadine, nelfinavir, and efavirenz, were found to be associated with this genotype (Table 13.4). This discrepancy possibly reflects different degrees of P-gp contribution to the overall PK of these drugs, as they are also substrates of other transporters and enzymes. In addition, other studies showed only a modest effect of *ABCB1* polymorphism on the PK of various P-gp substrate drugs. For the earlier reasons, *ABCB1* genetic testing has not been recommended in any drug label, and tests for its clinical use are not widely available.

Race/ethnic differences in allele frequencies of transporter polymorphisms

As discussed in Chapter 12, there are significant differences in the frequencies of some variant alleles in genes that encode metabolizing enzymes in different ancestral populations. Similarly, significant differences in frequencies of various alleles in genes encoding transporters exist in different ancestral groups. Such differences may contribute to apparent race or ethnic differences in drug disposition, response, and toxicity. Table 13.4 lists the distribution of various alleles in different populations for ABCB1, ABCG2, and SLCO1B1 [211, 221–223]. As shown in Fig. 13.7, statin plasma levels are variably affected by the genetics of P-gp, BCRP, and OATP1B1 [190].

The relative contributions of these transporters to each statin's PK and the ethnic distribution of the critical variant alleles may be one of the key factors determining the relative efficacy and safety profile of these statins in different race/ethnic groups. For example, Tomlinson et al. [116] studied 305 Chinese patients and found that the ABCG2 (C.421C>A) variant appeared to increase the LDL-cholesterol lowering effect of rosuvastatin. This drug had a 6.9% greater effect in reducing LDL-cholesterol in C.421AA variants than in C.421CC genotypes—an effect equivalent to doubling the dose in C.421CC patients (Table 13.4). Similarly, this variant has been shown to contribute to interindividual differences in LDL-cholesterol lowering response to rosuvastatin in large GWAS [117]. As shown in Chapter 16, Table 16.1, the FDA approved labeling for rosuvastatin recommends a lower starting and maximum daily dose in individuals of East Asian ancestry in comparison to individuals of European ancestry. Although controversial, this race-specific dosing recommendation for rosuvastatin, which is due to the higher bioavailability of the drug in East Asians, may ultimately be due to the higher allele frequency of the ABCG2 (C.421C>A) variant in these populations. On the other hand, based on evaluation of SLCO1B1 521T>C and 388A>G, OATP1B1 genetics appeared to be unrelated to the lipid-lowering effect of another statin drug, pitavastatin, in 140 Chinese patients (Table 13.3) [123].

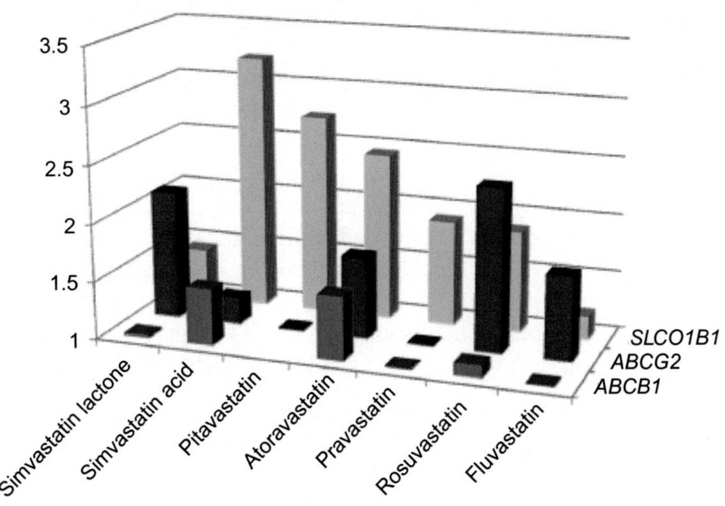

FIG. 13.7 Effects of *SLCO1B1*, *ABCG2*, and *ABCB1* genotypes on systemic exposure to various statins. Data are shown as multiples of *AUC* increase by *SLCO1B1* c.521CC, *ABCG2* c.421AA, and *ABCB1* c.1236TT-c.2677TT-c.3435TT genotype as compared with the reference genotype (c.521TT, c.421CC, and c.1236CC-c.2677GG-c.3435CC, respectively). Weighted mean values from various studies are shown for pitavastatin, rosuvastatin, and pravastatin. *(Reproduced with permission from Niemi M. Transporter pharmacogenetics and statin toxicity. Clin Pharmacol Ther 2010;87:130–133.)*

Conclusions and future perspectives

Drug-metabolizing enzymes and transporters work in concert, participating together in the absorption, distribution, metabolism, and excretion of many drugs. It is therefore important to understand how each of the processes alone and in combination contributes to individual variability in drug exposure and clinical response. Association studies linking genetics to drug exposure and clinical response have been increasingly conducted and are critical to elucidating the basis underlying variation in the response of individuals to drug treatments. Table 13.5 enumerates recommendations for improving the outcomes of association studies.

Based on cumulative evidence, genetic tests of enzyme polymorphisms are now available to help determine the initial dose of warfarin (*CYP2C9* and *VKORC1*), to suggest treatment alternatives to clopidogrel (*CYP2C19*), and to determine whether a high dose of tetrabenazine can be given (*CYP2D6*). The Clinical Pharmacogenetics Implementation Consortium (CPIC) has made enormous contributions to this effort by creating, curating, and publishing gene-based and evidence-supported clinical practice guidelines for various drugs (see https://cpicpgx.org/genes-drugs). However, for membrane transporters, only the *SLCO1B1* polymorphism, p.V174A, has sufficient evidence to warrant recommending specific prescribing actions for statin drugs, though the importance of the *ABCG2* (C.421C>A) variant as a guide to rosuvastatin dosing is being increasingly recognized [224]. In addition, the results of many of the studies of genetic polymorphisms in transporters summarized in Table 13.3 have helped to:

TABLE 13.5 Recommendations for conduct of future drug transporter association studies.

1. Conduct in vitro studies to evaluate if a drug is a substrate, inhibitor, and/or inducer of key drug transporters (e.g., P-gp, BCRP, OATP1B1, OATP1B3, OAT1, OAT3, OCT2, MATE1, MATE2-K). If positive, assess the relative contribution of these transporters to drug update and efflux; such studies are critical in providing basic data that will help the design and interpretation of in vivo human studies.
2. Develop needed technology platforms and tools to characterize the contribution of established and evolving allelic variations of drug transporter genes to better understand the genomic basis for individual variability in plasma levels and response to interacting drugs.
3. Conduct correlation studies with well-characterized in vivo phenotypes in order to enhance the interpretability of study results.
4. Design studies that consider multiple drug transporters and that have the potential to differentiate the impact of rate-limiting transporters for drugs that are substrates for multiple transporters that govern their uptake and efflux into and out of key eliminating organs (e.g., design studies to differentiate between the contributions of MATE2-K and OCT2 to metformin elimination).
5. Conduct studies that enroll a sufficient number of subjects with the major variant alleles of drug transporters that are representative of various race/ethnic groups.
6. Evaluate genetic association data along with drug-drug interaction data (i.e., the evaluation of comparative PK in subgroups genetically defined as high or low expressors) to provide crucial information on potential drug-drug interactions (e.g., rosuvastatin GWAS results revealed the impact of *ABCG2* variant alleles on response to rosuvastatin [117]).
7. Apply a systems biology approach that incorporates all data (in vitro and in vivo human studies) to improve understanding of the interplay between drug transporters, metabolizing enzymes (e.g., metabolism/transport, transporter/transporter, and/or metabolism/transport/orphan nuclear receptor interplay) and other patient factors (age, race, sex, organ impairment, disease, etc.).

1. Elucidate the role of specific transporters in a drug's absorption and elimination pathway (e.g., OATP1B1 and plasma levels of atorvastatin)
2. Explain variability in PK, PD, and drug response and clarify the role of one transporter vs another (e.g., OATP1B1 and simvastatin-induced myopathy; BCRP and the cholesterol lowering effect of rosuvastatin; the relative contribution of MATE2-K vs. OCT2 to metformin elimination)
3. Suggest a toxicity mechanism (e.g., BSEP and troglitazone liver toxicity) [70]
4. Provide data and input for a systems biology approach to analyzing complex pathways (e.g., differential roles of OATP1B1 and MRP2 in determining pravastatin's concentrations in plasma and in liver cells that may link to its adverse reactions and cholesterol-lowering effect [191]; OATP1B1 and increased levels of repaglinide in renal impairment [225]).
5. Provide data supporting the role of transporters as targets for drug-drug interactions (e.g., OCT1 polymorphisms leading to higher levels of morphine).

In its initial workshop in 2008, the ITC identified key transporters that warrant early evaluation in future clinical pharmacology studies, including P-gp, BCRP, OATP1B1/1B3, OAT1, OAT3, and OCT2 [10, 49]. In two subsequent workshops, the Consortium continued to evaluate the suitability of various in vitro, in vivo, and in silico methods for studying the above-mentioned key transporters and additional, emerging transporters (e.g., BSEP, MRPs, MATEs, OATP2B1, and OCT1) [89, 210]. Future research is needed that focuses on these emerging transporters as well as on changes in the expression levels of transporters in specific populations, such as pediatric populations and patients with renal and hepatic impairment.

Disclaimer

The views or opinions expressed in this chapter are those of the authors and should not be interpreted as the position of the U.S. Food and Drug Administration.

References

[1] Giacomini KM, Sugiyama Y. Membrane transporters and drug response. In: Brunton LL, editor. Goodman and Gilman's the pharmacological basis of therapeutics. USA: McGraw-Hill Education; 2018 [chapter 5].
[2] Morrissey KM, et al. The UCSF-FDA TransPortal: a public drug transporter database. Clin Pharmacol Ther 2012;92(5):545–546.
[3] U.S. Food and Drug Administration. In vitro drug interaction studies—cytochrome p450 enzyme- and transporter-mediated drug interactions. 2020.
[4] U.S. Food and Drug Administration. Clinical drug interaction studies—cytochrome P450 enzyme- and transporter-mediated drug interactions guidance for industry. 2020.
[5] European Medicines Agency. Guideline on the investigation of drug interactions. 2012.
[6] Ishiguro A, Sato R, Nagai N. Development of a new Japanese guideline on drug interaction for drug development and appropriate provision of information. Drug Metab Pharmacokinet 2020;35(1):12–17.
[7] Lai Y, Hsiao P. Beyond the ITC White Paper: emerging sciences in drug transporters and opportunities for drug development. Curr Pharm Des 2014;20(10):1577–1594.
[8] Tweedie D, et al. Transporter studies in drug development: experience to date and follow-up on decision trees from the International Transporter Consortium. Clin Pharmacol Ther 2013;94(1):113–125.
[9] Huang S-M, Woodcock J. Transporters in drug development: advancing on the critical path. Nat Rev Drug Discov 2010;9(3):175–176.
[10] Huang SM, Zhang L, Giacomini KM. The International Transporter Consortium: a collaborative group of scientists from academia, industry, and the FDA. Clin Pharmacol Ther 2010;87(1):32–36.
[11] Zamek-Gliszczynski MJ, et al. Highlights from the International Transporter Consortium second workshop. Clin Pharmacol Ther 2012;92 (5):553–556.
[12] Giacomini KM, Galetin A, Huang SM. The International Transporter Consortium: summarizing advances in the role of transporters in drug development. Clin Pharmacol Ther 2018;104(5):766–771.
[13] Povey S, et al. The HUGO Gene Nomenclature Committee (HGNC). Hum Genet 2001;109(6):678–680.
[14] Bai X, Moraes TF, Reithmeier RAF. Structural biology of solute carrier (SLC) membrane transport proteins. Mol Membr Biol 2017;34(1–2):1–32.
[15] Schlessinger A, et al. SLC classification: an update. Clin Pharmacol Ther 2013;94(1):19–23.
[16] Colas C, Ung PM, Schlessinger A. SLC transporters: structure, function, and drug discovery. MedChemComm 2016;7(6):1069–1081.
[17] Hediger MA, et al. The ABCs of solute carriers: physiological, pathological and therapeutic implications of human membrane transport proteins. Pflugers Arch Eur J Physiol 2004;447(5):465–468.
[18] Busti AJ, et al. Effects of atazanavir/ritonavir or fosamprenavir/ritonavir on the pharmacokinetics of rosuvastatin. J Cardiovasc Pharmacol 2008;51 (6):605–610.

[19] Kiser JJ, et al. Drug/drug interaction between lopinavir/ritonavir and rosuvastatin in healthy volunteers. J Acquir Immune Defic Syndr 2008;47 (5):570–578.

[20] Martin P, et al. Effects of fostamatinib on the pharmacokinetics of oral contraceptive, warfarin, and the statins rosuvastatin and simvastatin: results from phase I clinical studies. Drugs R D 2016;16(1):93–107.

[21] Shiveley L, et al. Pharmacokinetics of apricitabine, a novel nucleoside reverse transcriptase inhibitor, in healthy volunteers treated with trimethoprim-sulphamethoxazole. J Clin Pharm Ther 2008;33(1):45–54.

[22] Simonson SG, et al. Rosuvastatin pharmacokinetics in heart transplant recipients administered an antirejection regimen including cyclosporine. Clin Pharmacol Ther 2004;76(2):167–177.

[23] Allred AJ, et al. Eltrombopag increases plasma rosuvastatin exposure in healthy volunteers. Br J Clin Pharmacol 2011;72(2):321–329.

[24] Schinkel AH, Jonker JW. Mammalian drug efflux transporters of the ATP binding cassette (ABC) family: an overview. Adv Drug Deliv Rev 2003;55(1):3–29.

[25] Silva R, et al. Modulation of P-glycoprotein efflux pump: induction and activation as a therapeutic strategy. Pharmacol Ther 2015;149:1–123.

[26] Kishimoto W, et al. In vitro predictability of drug-drug interaction likelihood of P-glycoprotein-mediated efflux of dabigatran etexilate based on [I] 2/IC50 threshold. Drug Metab Dispos 2014;42(2):257–263.

[27] Chinn LW, Kroetz DL. ABCB1 pharmacogenetics: progress, pitfalls, and promise. Clin Pharmacol Ther 2007;81(2):265–269.

[28] Elmeliegy M, et al. Effect of P-glycoprotein (P-gp) inducers on exposure of P-gp substrates: review of clinical drug-drug interaction studies. Clin Pharmacokinet 2020.

[29] Wessler JD, et al. The P-glycoprotein transport system and cardiovascular drugs. J Am Coll Cardiol 2013;61(25):2495–2502.

[30] Takara K, Sakaeda T, Okumura K. An update on overcoming MDR1-mediated multidrug resistance in cancer chemotherapy. Curr Pharm Des 2006;12(3):273–286.

[31] Chu X, et al. Dabigatran etexilate and digoxin: comparison as clinical probe substrates for evaluation of P-gp inhibition. Clin Pharmacol Ther 2018;104(5):788–792.

[32] Fenner KS, et al. Drug–drug interactions mediated through P-glycoprotein: clinical relevance and in vitro–in vivo correlation using digoxin as a probe drug. Clin Pharmacol Ther 2008;85(2):173–181.

[33] Zhang L, et al. Predicting drug-drug interactions: an FDA perspective. AAPS J 2009;11(2):300–306.

[34] Agarwal S, Arya V, Zhang L. Review of P-gp inhibition data in recently approved new drug applications: utility of the proposed [I1]/IC50 and [I2]/IC50 criteria in the P-gp decision tree. J Clin Pharmacol 2013;53(2):228–233.

[35] Keppler D. Multidrug resistance proteins (MRPs, ABCCs): importance for pathophysiology and drug therapy. In: Handbook of experimental pharmacology. Berlin, Heidelberg: Springer; 2010. p. 299–323.

[36] Klaassen CD, Aleksunes LM. Xenobiotic, bile acid, and cholesterol transporters: function and regulation. Pharmacol Rev 2010;62(1):1–96.

[37] Kathawala RJ, et al. The modulation of ABC transporter-mediated multidrug resistance in cancer: a review of the past decade. Drug Resist Updat 2015;18:1–17.

[38] Cole S, et al. Overexpression of a transporter gene in a multidrug-resistant human lung cancer cell line. Science 1992;258(5088):1650–1654.

[39] Paulusma CC, et al. A mutation in the human canalicular multispecific organic anion transporter gene causes the Dubin-Johnson syndrome. Hepatology 1997;25(6):1539–1542.

[40] Zelcer N, et al. Mice lacking multidrug resistance protein 3 show altered morphine pharmacokinetics and morphine-6-glucuronide antinociception. Proc Natl Acad Sci U S A 2005;102(20):7274–7279.

[41] Zamek-Gliszczynski MJ, et al. Evaluation of the role of multidrug resistance-associated protein (Mrp) 3 and Mrp4 in hepatic basolateral excretion of sulfate and glucuronide metabolites of acetaminophen, 4-methylumbelliferone, and harmol in Abcc3-/- and Abcc4-/- mice. J Pharmacol Exp Ther 2006;319(3):1485–1491.

[42] Russel F, Koenderink J, Masereeuw R. Multidrug resistance protein 4 (MRP4/ABCC4): a versatile efflux transporter for drugs and signalling molecules. Trends Pharmacol Sci 2008;29(4):200–207.

[43] Schuetz JD, et al. MRP4: a previously unidentified factor in resistance to nucleoside-based antiviral drugs. Nat Med 1999;5(9):1048–1051.

[44] Wakabayashi K, et al. Human ABC transporter ABCG2 in xenobiotic protection and redox biology. Drug Metab Rev 2006;38(3):371–391.

[45] Doyle LA, et al. A multidrug resistance transporter from human MCF-7 breast cancer cells. Proc Natl Acad Sci U S A 1998;95(26):15665–15670.

[46] Robey RW, et al. ABCG2: a perspective. Adv Drug Deliv Rev 2009;61(1):3–13.

[47] van Herwaarden AE, Schinkel AH. The function of breast cancer resistance protein in epithelial barriers, stem cells and milk secretion of drugs and xenotoxins. Trends Pharmacol Sci 2006;27(1):10–16.

[48] Vlaming MLH, Lagas JS, Schinkel AH. Physiological and pharmacological roles of ABCG2 (BCRP): recent findings in Abcg2 knockout mice. Adv Drug Deliv Rev 2009;61(1):14–25.

[49] Giacomini KM, et al. Membrane transporters in drug development. Nat Rev Drug Discov 2010;9(3):215–236.

[50] Ishikawa T, et al. Emerging new technologies in pharamcogenomics: rapid SNP detection, molecular dynamic simulation, and QSAR analysis methods to validate clinically important genetic variants of human ABC Transporter ABCB1 (P-gp/MDR1). Pharmacol Ther 2010;126(1):69–81.

[51] Saito H, et al. A new strategy of high-speed screening and quantitative structure-activity relationship analysis to evaluate human ATP-binding cassette transporter ABCG2-drug interactions. J Pharmacol Exp Ther 2006;317(3):1114–1124.

[52] Cusatis G, et al. Pharmacogenetics of ABCG2 and adverse reactions to gefitinib. J Natl Cancer Inst 2006;98(23):1739–1742.

[53] Cusatis G, Sparreboom A. Pharmacogenomic importance of ABCG2. Pharmacogenomics 2008;9(8):1005–1009.

[54] Morisaki K, et al. Single nucleotide polymorphisms modify the transporter activity of ABCG2. Cancer Chemother Pharmacol 2005;56(2):161–172.

[55] Polgar O, Robey RW, Bates SE. ABCG2: structure, function and role in drug response. Expert Opin Drug Metab Toxicol 2007;4(1):1–15.

[56] Yamasaki Y, et al. Pharmacogenetic characterization of sulfasalazine disposition based on NAT2 and ABCG2 (BCRP) gene polymorphisms in humans. Clin Pharmacol Ther 2008;84(1):95–103.

[57] Zhang W, et al. Role of BCRP 421C > A polymorphism on rosuvastatin pharmacokinetics in healthy Chinese males. Clin Chim Acta 2006;373 (1–2):99–103.

[58] Brackman DJ, et al. Genome-wide association and functional studies reveal novel pharmacological mechanisms for allopurinol. Clin Pharmacol Ther 2019;106(3):623–631.

[59] Chu AY, et al. Genome-wide association study evaluating lipoprotein-associated phospholipase A2 mass and activity at baseline and after rosuvastatin therapy. Circ Cardiovasc Genet 2012;5(6):676–685.

[60] Wen CC, et al. Genome-wide association study identifies ABCG2 (BCRP) as an allopurinol transporter and a determinant of drug response. Clin Pharmacol Ther 2015;97(5):518–525.

[61] Urquhart BL, et al. Breast cancer resistance protein (ABCG2) and drug disposition: intestinal expression, polymorphisms and sulfasalazine as an in vivo probe. Pharmacogenet Genomics 2008;18(5):439–448.

[62] Zaher H, et al. Breast cancer resistance protein (Bcrp/abcg2) is a major determinant of sulfasalazine absorption and elimination in the mouse. Mol Pharm 2006;3(1):55–61.

[63] Miyata H, et al. Identification of febuxostat as a new strong ABCG2 inhibitor: potential applications and risks in clinical situations. Front Pharmacol 2016;7:518.

[64] Adkison KK, et al. Oral sulfasalazine as a clinical BCRP probe substrate: pharmacokinetic effects of genetic variation (C421A) and pantoprazole coadministration. J Pharm Sci 2010;99(2):1046–1062.

[65] Kusuhara H, et al. Pharmacokinetic interaction study of sulphasalazine in healthy subjects and the impact of curcumin as an in vivo inhibitor of BCRP. Br J Pharmacol 2012;166(6):1793–1803.

[66] Hirano M, et al. Bile salt export pump (BSEP/ABCB11) can transport a nonbile acid substrate, pravastatin. J Pharmacol Exp Ther 2005;314(2):876–882.

[67] Jansen PLM, et al. Hepatocanalicular bile salt export pump deficiency in patients with progressive familial intrahepatic cholestasis. Gastroenterology 1999;117(6):1370–1379.

[68] Strautnieks SS, et al. A gene encoding a liver-specific ABC transporter is mutated in progressive familial intrahepatic cholestasis. Nat Genet 1998;20(3):233–238.

[69] Noe J, et al. Impaired expression and function of the bile salt export pump due to three novel ABCB11 mutations in intrahepatic cholestasis. J Hepatol 2005;43(3):536–543.

[70] Ogimura E, Sekine S, Horie T. Bile salt export pump inhibitors are associated with bile acid-dependent drug-induced toxicity in sandwich-cultured hepatocytes. Biochem Biophys Res Commun 2011;416(3-4):313–317.

[71] Ali I, et al. Effect of a common genetic variant (p.V444A) in the bile salt export pump on the inhibition of bile acid transport by cholestatic medications. Mol Pharm 2019;16(3):1406–1411.

[72] Morgan RE, et al. Interference with bile salt export pump function is a susceptibility factor for human liver injury in drug development. Toxicol Sci 2010;118(2):485–500.

[73] Byrne JA, et al. The human bile salt export pump: characterization of substrate specificity and identification of inhibitors. Gastroenterology 2002;123(5):1649–1658.

[74] Stieger B. Role of the bile salt export pump, BSEP, in acquired forms of cholestasis. Drug Metab Rev 2010;42(3):437–445.

[75] Kis E, et al. Effect of membrane cholesterol on BSEP/Bsep activity: species specificity studies for substrates and inhibitors. Drug Metab Dispos 2009;37(9):1878–1886.

[76] Mano Y, Usui T, Kamimura H. Effects of bosentan, an endothelin receptor antagonist, on bile salt export pump and multidrug resistance-associated protein 2. Biopharm Drug Dispos 2007;28(1):13–18.

[77] Chan R, Benet LZ. Evaluation of the relevance of DILI predictive hypotheses in early drug development: review of in vitro methodologies vs BDDCS classification. Toxicol Res (Camb) 2018;7(3):358–370.

[78] Kenna JG, et al. Can bile salt export pump inhibition testing in drug discovery and development reduce liver injury risk? An International Transporter Consortium perspective. Clin Pharmacol Ther 2018;104(5):916–932.

[79] Garzel B, et al. The role of bile salt export pump gene repression in drug-induced cholestatic liver toxicity. Drug Metab Dispos 2014;42(3):318–322.

[80] Garzel B, et al. A change in bile flow: looking beyond transporter inhibition in the development of drug-induced cholestasis. Curr Drug Metab 2019;20(8):621–632.

[81] Kalliokoski A, Niemi M. Impact of OATP transporters on pharmacokinetics. Br J Pharmacol 2009;158(3):693–705.

[82] Stieger B, Hagenbuch B. Organic anion-transporting polypeptides. Curr Top Membr 2014;73:205–232.

[83] König J. Uptake transporters of the human OATP family. In: Handbook of experimental pharmacology. Berlin, Heidelberg: Springer; 2010. p. 1–28.

[84] Malagnino V, et al. OATP1B3-1B7 (LST-3TM12) is a drug transporter that affects endoplasmic reticulum access and the metabolism of ezetimibe. Mol Pharmacol 2019;96(2):128–137.

[85] Malagnino V, et al. LST-3TM12 is a member of the OATP1B family and a functional transporter. Biochem Pharmacol 2018;148:75–87.

[86] Drozdzik M, et al. Protein abundance of clinically relevant drug transporters in the human liver and intestine: a comparative analysis in paired tissue specimens. Clin Pharmacol Ther 2019;105(5):1204–1212.

[87] Gao B, et al. Differential cellular expression of organic anion transporting peptides OATP1A2 and OATP2B1 in the human retina and brain: implications for carrier-mediated transport of neuropeptides and neurosteriods in the CNS. Pflugers Arch 2015;467(7):1481–1493.

[88] Morita T, et al. pH-dependent transport kinetics of the human organic anion-transporting polypeptide 1A2. Drug Metab Pharmacokinet 2020;35 (2):220–227.
[89] Zamek-Gliszczynski MJ, et al. Transporters in drug development: 2018 ITC recommendations for transporters of emerging clinical importance. Clin Pharmacol Ther 2018;104(5):890–899.
[90] Yu J, et al. Intestinal drug interactions mediated by OATPs: a systematic review of preclinical and clinical findings. J Pharm Sci 2017;106 (9):2312–2325.
[91] Unger MS, et al. Clinically relevant OATP2B1 inhibitors in marketed drug space. Mol Pharm 2020;17(2):488–498.
[92] Khuri N, et al. Computational discovery and experimental validation of inhibitors of the human intestinal transporter OATP2B1. J Chem Inf Model 2017;57(6):1402–1413.
[93] Zou L, et al. Impact of pharmaceutical excipients on oral drug absorption: a focus on intestinal drug transporters. Clin Pharmacol Ther 2019;105 (2):323–325.
[94] Zou L, et al. Bacterial metabolism rescues the inhibition of intestinal drug absorption by food and drug additives. Proc Natl Acad Sci U S A 2020;117 (27):16009–16018.
[95] Mikkaichi T, et al. Isolation and characterization of a digoxin transporter and its rat homologue expressed in the kidney. Proc Natl Acad Sci U S A 2004;101(10):3569–3574.
[96] Chu XY, et al. Transport of the dipeptidyl peptidase-4 inhibitor sitagliptin by human organic anion transporter 3, organic anion transporting polypeptide 4C1, and multidrug resistance P-glycoprotein. J Pharmacol Exp Ther 2007;321(2):673–683.
[97] Scotcher D, et al. Delineating the role of various factors in renal disposition of digoxin through application of physiologically based kidney model to renal impairment populations. J Pharmacol Exp Ther 2017;360(3):484–495.
[98] SEARCH Collaborative Group, et al. SLCO1B1 variants and statin-induced myopathy—a genomewide study. N Engl J Med. 2008;359(8):789–99.
[99] Carr DF, et al. Genomewide association study of statin-induced myopathy in patients recruited using the UK clinical practice research datalink. Clin Pharmacol Ther 2019;106(6):1353–1361.
[100] Postmus I, et al. Pharmacogenetic meta-analysis of genome-wide association studies of LDL cholesterol response to statins. Nat Commun 2014;5:5068.
[101] Ramsey LB, et al. Genome-wide study of methotrexate clearance replicates SLCO1B1. Blood 2013;121(6):898–904.
[102] Trevino LR, et al. Germline genetic variation in an organic anion transporter polypeptide associated with methotrexate pharmacokinetics and clinical effects. J Clin Oncol 2009;27(35):5972–5978.
[103] Neuvonen P, Niemi M, Backman J. Drug interactions with lipid-lowering drugs: mechanisms and clinical relevance. Clin Pharmacol Ther 2006;80 (6):565–581.
[104] Shitara Y, et al. Inhibition of transporter-mediated hepatic uptake as a mechanism for drug-drug interaction between cerivastatin and cyclosporin A. J Pharmacol Exp Ther 2003;304(2):610–616.
[105] Keskitalo JE, et al. ABCG2 polymorphism markedly affects the pharmacokinetics of atorvastatin and rosuvastatin. Clin Pharmacol Ther 2009;86 (2):197–203.
[106] Xia CQ, et al. Interactions of cyclosporin A with breast cancer resistance protein. Drug Metab Dispos 2007;35(4):576–582.
[107] McFeely SJ, et al. Identification and evaluation of clinical substrates of organic anion transporting polypeptides 1B1 and 1B3. Clin Transl Sci 2019;12(4):379–387.
[108] Hediger MA, et al. The ABCs of membrane transporters in health and disease (SLC series): introduction. Mol Asp Med 2013;34(2–3):95–107.
[109] Koepsell H. The SLC22 family with transporters of organic cations, anions and zwitterions. Mol Asp Med 2013;34(2–3):413–435.
[110] Koepsell H. Organic cation transporters in health and disease. Pharmacol Rev 2020;72(1):253–319.
[111] Nigam SK. The SLC22 transporter family: a paradigm for the impact of drug transporters on metabolic pathways, signaling, and disease. Annu Rev Pharmacol Toxicol 2018;58:663–687.
[112] Hoffmeyer S, et al. Functional polymorphisms of the human multidrug-resistance gene: multiple sequence variations and correlation of one allele with P-glycoprotein expression and activity in vivo. Proc Natl Acad Sci U S A 2000;97(7):3473–3478.
[113] Kim RB, et al. Identification of functionally variant MDR1 alleles among European Americans and African Americans. Clin Pharmacol Ther 2001;70(2):189–199.
[114] Fellay J, et al. Response to antiretroviral treatment in HIV-1-infected individuals with allelic variants of the multidrug resistance transporter 1: a pharmacogenetics study. Lancet 2002;359(9300):30–36.
[115] Siddiqui A, et al. Association of multidrug resistance in epilepsy with a polymorphism in the drug-transporter gene ABCB1. N Engl J Med 2003;348 (15):1442–1448.
[116] Tomlinson B, et al. ABCG2 polymorphism is associated with the low-density lipoprotein cholesterol response to rosuvastatin. Clin Pharmacol Ther 2010;87(5):558–562.
[117] Chasman DI, et al. Genetic determinants of statin-induced low-density lipoprotein cholesterol reduction: the Justification for the Use of Statins in Prevention: an Intervention Trial Evaluating Rosuvastatin (JUPITER) trial. Circ Cardiovasc Genet 2012;5(2):257–264.
[118] Bailey KM, et al. Hepatic metabolism and transporter gene variants enhance response to rosuvastatin in patients with acute myocardial infarction: the GEOSTAT-1 study. Circ Cardiovasc Genet 2010;3(3):276–285.
[119] Wallace MC, et al. Association between ABCG2 rs2231142 and poor response to allopurinol: replication and meta-analysis. Rheumatology (Oxford) 2018;57(4):656–660.

[120] Hulot J-S, et al. A mutation in the drug transporter gene ABCC2 associated with impaired methotrexate elimination. Pharmacogenet Genomics 2005;15(5):277–285.
[121] Sun N, et al. MRP2 and GSTP1 polymorphisms and chemotherapy response in advanced non-small cell lung cancer. Cancer Chemother Pharmacol 2010;65(3):437–446.
[122] Nishizato Y, et al. Polymorphisms of OATP-C (SLC21A6) and OAT3 (SLC22A8) genes: consequences for pravastatin pharmacokinetics. Clin Pharmacol Ther 2003;73(6):554–565.
[123] Yang G-p, et al. Lack of effect of genetic polymorphisms of SLCO1B1 on the lipid-lowering response to pitavastatin in Chinese patients. Acta Pharmacol Sin 2010;31(3):382–386.
[124] Turner RM, et al. A genome-wide association study of circulating levels of atorvastatin and its major metabolites. Clin Pharmacol Ther 2020.
[125] Akao H, et al. Genetic variation at the SLCO1B1 gene locus and low density lipoprotein cholesterol lowering response to pravastatin in the elderly. Atherosclerosis 2012;220(2):413–417.
[126] Choi JH, et al. A common 5'-UTR variant in MATE2-K is associated with poor response to metformin. Clin Pharmacol Ther 2011;90(5):674–684.
[127] Stocker SL, et al. The effect of novel promoter variants in MATE1 and MATE2 on the pharmacokinetics and pharmacodynamics of metformin. Clin Pharmacol Ther 2013;93(2):186–194.
[128] Shu Y, et al. Effect of genetic variation in the organic cation transporter 1 (OCT1) on metformin action. J Clin Invest 2007;117(5):1422–1431.
[129] Shu Y, et al. Effect of genetic variation in the organic cation transporter 1, OCT1, on metformin pharmacokinetics. Clin Pharmacol Ther 2008;83 (2):273–280.
[130] Dujic T, et al. Organic cation transporter 1 variants and gastrointestinal side effects of metformin in patients with Type 2 diabetes. Diabet Med 2016;33(4):511–514.
[131] Dujic T, et al. Association of organic cation transporter 1 with intolerance to metformin in type 2 diabetes: a GoDARTS study. Diabetes 2015;64 (5):1786–1793.
[132] Tzvetkov MV, et al. The effects of genetic polymorphisms in the organic cation transporters OCT1, OCT2, and OCT3 on the renal clearance of metformin. Clin Pharmacol Ther 2009;86(3):299–306.
[133] Stamer UM, et al. Loss-of-function polymorphisms in the organic cation transporter OCT1 are associated with reduced postoperative tramadol consumption. Pain 2016;157(11):2467–2475.
[134] Tzvetkov MV, et al. Effects of OCT1 polymorphisms on the cellular uptake, plasma concentrations and efficacy of the 5-HT(3) antagonists tropisetron and ondansetron. Pharmacogenomics J 2012;12(1):22–29.
[135] Fukuda T, et al. OCT1 genetic variants influence the pharmacokinetics of morphine in children. Pharmacogenomics 2013;14(10):1141–1151.
[136] Balyan R, et al. OCT1 genetic variants are associated with postoperative morphine-related adverse effects in children. Pharmacogenomics 2017;18 (7):621–629.
[137] Matthaei J, et al. OCT1 mediates hepatic uptake of sumatriptan and loss-of-function OCT1 polymorphisms affect sumatriptan pharmacokinetics. Clin Pharmacol Ther 2016;99(6):633–641.
[138] Tzvetkov MV, et al. Increased systemic exposure and stronger cardiovascular and metabolic adverse reactions to fenoterol in individuals with heritable OCT1 deficiency. Clin Pharmacol Ther 2018;103(5):868–878.
[139] Chen Y, et al. Effect of genetic variation in the organic cation transporter 2 on the renal elimination of metformin. Pharmacogenet Genomics 2009;19(7):497–504.
[140] Wang ZJ, et al. OCT2 polymorphisms and in-vivo renal functional consequence: studies with metformin and cimetidine. Pharmacogenet Genomics 2008;18(7):637–645.
[141] Nigam SK, et al. The organic anion transporter (OAT) family: a systems biology perspective. Physiol Rev 2015;95(1):83–123.
[142] Wright SH. Role of organic cation transporters in the renal handling of therapeutic agents and xenobiotics. Toxicol Appl Pharmacol 2005;204 (3):309–319.
[143] Bi YA, et al. Role of hepatic organic anion transporter 2 in the pharmacokinetics of R- and S-warfarin: in vitro studies and mechanistic evaluation. Mol Pharm 2018;15(3):1284–1295.
[144] Lepist EI, et al. Contribution of the organic anion transporter OAT2 to the renal active tubular secretion of creatinine and mechanism for serum creatinine elevations caused by cobicistat. Kidney Int 2014;86(2):350–357.
[145] Cropp CD, et al. Organic anion transporter 2 (SLC22A7) is a facilitative transporter of cGMP. Mol Pharmacol 2008;73(4):1151–1158.
[146] Damme K, et al. Mammalian MATE (SLC47A) transport proteins: impact on efflux of endogenous substrates and xenobiotics. Drug Metab Rev 2011;43(4):499–523.
[147] Masuda S, et al. Identification and functional characterization of a new human kidney–specific H+/organic cation antiporter, kidney-specific multidrug and toxin extrusion 2. J Am Soc Nephrol 2006;17(8):2127–2135.
[148] Otsuka M, et al. A human transporter protein that mediates the final excretion step for toxic organic cations. Proc Natl Acad Sci U S A 2005;102 (50):17923–17928.
[149] Tanihara Y, et al. Substrate specificity of MATE1 and MATE2-K, human multidrug and toxin extrusions/H+-organic cation antiporters. Biochem Pharmacol 2007;74(2):359–371.
[150] Komatsu T, et al. Characterization of the human MATE2 proton-coupled polyspecific organic cation exporter. Int J Biochem Cell Biol 2011;43 (6):913–918.
[151] Burt HJ, et al. Metformin and cimetidine: physiologically based pharmacokinetic modelling to investigate transporter mediated drug-drug interactions. Eur J Pharm Sci 2016;88:70–82.

[152] Ito S, et al. Competitive inhibition of the luminal efflux by multidrug and toxin extrusions, but not basolateral uptake by organic cation transporter 2, is the likely mechanism underlying the pharmacokinetic drug-drug interactions caused by cimetidine in the kidney. J Pharmacol Exp Ther 2012;340(2):393–403.

[153] Kito T, et al. Investigation of non-linear Mate1-mediated efflux of trimethoprim in the mouse kidney as the mechanism underlying drug-drug interactions between trimethoprim and organic cations in the kidney. Drug Metab Pharmacokinet 2019;34(1):87–94.

[154] Elsby R, et al. Mechanistic in vitro studies confirm that inhibition of the renal apical efflux transporter multidrug and toxin extrusion (MATE) 1, and not altered absorption, underlies the increased metformin exposure observed in clinical interactions with cimetidine, trimethoprim or pyrimethamine. Pharmacol Res Perspect 2017;5(5).

[155] Muller F, et al. N(1)-methylnicotinamide as an endogenous probe for drug interactions by renal cation transporters: studies on the metformin-trimethoprim interaction. Eur J Clin Pharmacol 2015;71(1):85–94.

[156] Balimane PV, et al. Direct evidence for peptide transporter (PepT1)-mediated uptake of a nonpeptide prodrug, valacyclovir. Biochem Biophys Res Commun 1998;250(2):246–251.

[157] Li F, Maag H, Alfredson T. Prodrugs of nucleoside analogues for improved oral absorption and tissue targeting. J Pharm Sci 2008;97(3):1109–1134.

[158] Dresser GK, et al. Fruit juices inhibit organic anion transporting polypeptide-mediated drug uptake to decrease the oral availability of fexofenadine. Clin Pharmacol Ther 2002;71(1):11–20.

[159] Akamine Y, et al. Effects of one-time apple juice ingestion on the pharmacokinetics of fexofenadine enantiomers. Eur J Clin Pharmacol 2014;70(9):1087–1095.

[160] Akamine Y, et al. The change of pharmacokinetics of fexofenadine enantiomers through the single and simultaneous grapefruit juice ingestion. Drug Metab Pharmacokinet 2015;30(5):352–357.

[161] Fromm MF, et al. Inhibition of P-glycoprotein–mediated drug transport. Circulation 1999;99(4):552–557.

[162] Kruijtzer CMF, et al. Increased oral bioavailability of topotecan in combination with the breast cancer resistance protein and P-glycoprotein inhibitor GF120918. J Clin Oncol 2002;20(13):2943–2950.

[163] Benet LZ. The drug transporter-metabolism alliance: uncovering and defining the interplay. Mol Pharm 2009;6(6):1631–1643.

[164] Tachibana T, et al. Predicting drug – drug interactions involving the inhibition of intestinal CYP3A4 and P-glycoprotein. Curr Drug Metab 2010;11(9):762–777.

[165] Benet LZ, Cummins CL, Wu CY. Unmasking the dynamic interplay between efflux transporters and metabolic enzymes. Int J Pharm 2004;277(1–2):3–9.

[166] Zhang L, Zhang Y, Huang S-M. Scientific and regulatory perspectives on metabolizing enzyme – transporter interplay and its role in drug interactions: challenges in predicting drug interactions. Mol Pharm 2009;6(6):1766–1774.

[167] Dumond JB, et al. A phenotype-genotype approach to predicting CYP450 and P-glycoprotein drug interactions with the mixed inhibitor/inducer tipranavir/ritonavir. Clin Pharmacol Ther 2010;87(6):735–742.

[168] Wang DS, et al. Involvement of organic cation transporter 1 in hepatic and intestinal distribution of metformin. J Pharmacol Exp Ther 2002;302(2):510–515.

[169] Pastor-Anglada M, Perez-Torras S. Emerging roles of nucleoside transporters. Front Pharmacol 2018;9:606.

[170] Young JD. The SLC28 (CNT) and SLC29 (ENT) nucleoside transporter families: a 30-year collaborative odyssey. Biochem Soc Trans 2016;44(3):869–876.

[171] Rothem L, et al. Resistance to multiple novel antifolates is mediated via defective drug transport resulting from clustered mutations in the reduced folate carrier gene in human leukaemia cell lines. Biochem J 2002;367(Pt 3):741–750.

[172] Billington S, et al. Interindividual and regional variability in drug transporter abundance at the human blood-brain barrier measured by quantitative targeted proteomics. Clin Pharmacol Ther 2019;106(1):228–237.

[173] Drozdzik M, et al. Protein abundance of clinically relevant multidrug transporters along the entire length of the human intestine. Mol Pharm 2014;11(10):3547–3555.

[174] Prasad B, et al. Abundance of drug transporters in the human kidney cortex as quantified by quantitative targeted proteomics. Drug Metab Dispos 2016;44(12):1920–1924.

[175] Prasad B, et al. Toward a consensus on applying quantitative liquid chromatography-tandem mass spectrometry proteomics in translational pharmacology research: a white paper. Clin Pharmacol Ther 2019;106(3):525–543.

[176] Castro Dias M, et al. Structure and junctional complexes of endothelial, epithelial and glial brain barriers. Int J Mol Sci 2019;20(21).

[177] Liu L, Liu X. Contributions of drug transporters to blood-brain barriers. Adv Exp Med Biol 2019;1141:407–466.

[178] Rao VV, et al. Choroid plexus epithelial expression of MDR1 P glycoprotein and multidrug resistance-associated protein contribute to the blood-cerebrospinal-fluid drug-permeability barrier. Proc Natl Acad Sci U S A 1999;96(7):3900–3905.

[179] Gomez-Zepeda D, et al. ABC transporters at the blood-brain interfaces, their study models, and drug delivery implications in gliomas. Pharmaceutics 2019;**12**(1).

[180] Golden PL, Pollack GM. Blood–brain barrier efflux transport. J Pharm Sci 2003;92(9):1739–1753.

[181] Chen L, et al. Genetic and epigenetic regulation of the organic cation transporter 3, SLC22A3. Pharmacogenomics J 2013;13(2):110–120.

[182] Schinkel AH, et al. Disruption of the mouse mdr1a P-glycoprotein gene leads to a deficiency in the blood-brain barrier and to increased sensitivity to drugs. Cell 1994;77(4):491–502.

[183] Sadeque AJ, et al. Increased drug delivery to the brain by P-glycoprotein inhibition. Clin Pharmacol Ther 2000;68(3):231–237.

[184] Fromm MF. P-glycoprotein: a defense mechanism limiting oral bioavailability and CNS accumulation of drugs. Int J Clin Pharmacol Ther 2000;38 (02):69–74.
[185] Begley R, et al. Pharmacokinetics of tenofovir alafenamide when coadministered with other HIV antiretrovirals. J Acquir Immune Defic Syndr 2018;78(4):465–472.
[186] Gimenez F, Fernandez C, Mabondzo A. Transport of HIV protease inhibitors through the blood-brain barrier and interactions with the efflux proteins, P-glycoprotein and multidrug resistance proteins. J Acquir Immune Defic Syndr 2004;36(2):649–658.
[187] Owen A, Chandler B, Back DJ. The implications of P-glycoprotein in HIV: friend or foe? Fundam Clin Pharmacol 2005;19(3):283–296.
[188] Allikmets R, et al. A human placenta-specific ATP-binding cassette gene (ABCP) on chromosome 4q22 that is involved in multidrug resistance. Cancer Res 1998;58(23):5337–5339.
[189] Thomas-Schoemann A, et al. Drug interactions with solid tumour-targeted therapies. Crit Rev Oncol Hematol 2014;89(1):179–196.
[190] Niemi M. Transporter Pharmacogenetics and statin toxicity. Clin Pharmacol Ther 2009;87(1):130–133.
[191] Watanabe T, et al. Physiologically based pharmacokinetic modeling to predict transporter-mediated clearance and distribution of pravastatin in humans. J Pharmacol Exp Ther 2008;328(2):652–662.
[192] Maeda K, et al. Identification of the rate-determining process in the hepatic clearance of atorvastatin in a clinical cassette microdosing study. Clin Pharmacol Ther 2011;90(4):575–581.
[193] Bailey KM, et al. Hepatic metabolism and transporter gene variants enhance response to rosuvastatin in patients with acute myocardial infarction. Circ Cardiovasc Genet 2010;3(3):276–285.
[194] Guo Y, et al. Advancing predictions of tissue and intracellular drug concentrations using in vitro, imaging and physiologically based pharmacokinetic modeling approaches. Clin Pharmacol Ther 2018;104(5):865–889.
[195] Pan Y, et al. The application of physiologically based pharmacokinetic modeling to predict the role of drug transporters: scientific and regulatory perspectives. J Clin Pharmacol 2016;56(Suppl. 7):S122–S131.
[196] Huang SM, Rowland M. The role of physiologically based pharmacokinetic modeling in regulatory review. Clin Pharmacol Ther 2012;91 (3):542–549.
[197] Morrissey KM, et al. Renal transporters in drug development. Annu Rev Pharmacol Toxicol 2013;53:503–529.
[198] Meier PJ, et al. Substrate specificity of sinusoidal bile acid and organic anion uptake systems in rat and human liver. Hepatology 1997;26 (6):1667–1677.
[199] Li M, Anderson GD, Wang J. Drugdrug interactions involving membrane transporters in the human kidney. Expert Opin Drug Metab Toxicol 2006;2(4):505–532.
[200] Filipski KK, et al. Interaction of cisplatin with the human organic cation transporter 2. Clin Cancer Res 2008;14(12):3875–3880.
[201] Filipski KK, et al. Contribution of organic cation transporter 2 (OCT2) to cisplatin-induced nephrotoxicity. Clin Pharmacol Ther 2009;86 (4):396–402.
[202] Zhang S, et al. Organic cation transporters are determinants of oxaliplatin cytotoxicity. Cancer Res 2006;66(17):8847–8857.
[203] Jung N, et al. Relevance of the organic cation transporters 1 and 2 for antiretroviral drug therapy in human immunodeficiency virus infection. Drug Metab Dispos 2008;36(8):1616–1623.
[204] Jensen O, et al. Stereoselective cell uptake of adrenergic agonists and antagonists by organic cation transporters. Biochem Pharmacol 2020;171:113731.
[205] UCSF-FDA TransPortal. 2012. Available from: http://transportal.compbio.ucsf.edu/.
[206] Kusuhara H, et al. Effects of a MATE protein inhibitor, pyrimethamine, on the renal elimination of metformin at oral microdose and at therapeutic dose in healthy subjects. Clin Pharmacol Ther 2011;89(6):837–844.
[207] You G. Structure, function, and regulation of renal organic anion transporters. Med Res Rev 2002;22(6):602–616.
[208] Nieskens TT, et al. A human renal proximal tubule cell line with stable organic anion transporter 1 and 3 expression predictive for antiviral-induced toxicity. AAPS J 2016;18(2):465–475.
[209] U.S. Food and Drug Administration. Drugs@FDA: FDA-approved drugs, Available from: https://www.accessdata.fda.gov/scripts/cder/daf/; 2020. [cited 17 May 2020].
[210] Hillgren KM, et al. Emerging transporters of clinical importance: an update from the International Transporter Consortium. Clin Pharmacol Ther 2013;94(1):52–63.
[211] Yee SW, et al. Influence of transporter polymorphisms on drug disposition and response: a perspective from the International Transporter Consortium. Clin Pharmacol Ther 2018;104(5):803–817.
[212] Giacomini KM, et al. International Transporter Consortium commentary on clinically important transporter polymorphisms. Clin Pharmacol Ther 2013;94(1):23–26.
[213] Furukawa T, et al. Major SNP (Q141K) variant of human ABC transporter ABCG2 undergoes lysosomal and proteasomal degradations. Pharm Res 2009;26(2):469–479.
[214] Tzvetkov MV, et al. Morphine is a substrate of the organic cation transporter OCT1 and polymorphisms in OCT1 gene affect morphine pharmacokinetics after codeine administration. Biochem Pharmacol 2013;86(5):666–678.
[215] Eechoute K, et al. Environmental and genetic factors affecting transport of imatinib by OATP1A2. Clin Pharmacol Ther 2011;89(6):816–820.
[216] Lang C, et al. Mutations and polymorphisms in the bile salt export pump and the multidrug resistance protein 3 associated with drug-induced liver injury. Pharmacogenet Genomics 2007;17(1):47–60.
[217] Yamakawa Y, et al. Pharmacokinetic impact of SLCO1A2 polymorphisms on imatinib disposition in patients with chronic myeloid leukemia. Clin Pharmacol Ther 2011;90(1):157–163.

[218] Tzvetkov MV, et al. Genetically polymorphic OCT1: another piece in the puzzle of the variable pharmacokinetics and pharmacodynamics of the opioidergic drug tramadol. Clin Pharmacol Ther 2011;90(1):143–150.

[219] Hodges LM, et al. Very important pharmacogene summary: ABCB1 (MDR1, P-glycoprotein). Pharmacogenet Genomics 2011;21(3):152–161.

[220] Leschziner GD, et al. ABCB1 genotype and PGP expression, function and therapeutic drug response: a critical review and recommendations for future research. Pharmacogenomics J 2007;7(3):154–179.

[221] Cropp CD, Yee SW, Giacomini KM. Genetic variation in drug transporters in ethnic populations. Clin Pharmacol Ther 2008;84(3):412–416.

[222] Kroetz DL, Yee SW, Giacomini KM. The pharmacogenomics of membrane transporters project: research at the interface of genomics and transporter pharmacology. Clin Pharmacol Ther 2010;87(1):109–116.

[223] Yasuda SU, Zhang L, Huang SM. The role of ethnicity in variability in response to drugs: focus on clinical pharmacology studies. Clin Pharmacol Ther 2008;84(3):417–423.

[224] Ramsey LB, et al. The clinical pharmacogenetics implementation consortium guideline for SLCO1B1 and simvastatin-induced myopathy: 2014 update. Clin Pharmacol Ther 2014;96(4):423–428.

[225] Zhao P, et al. Evaluation of exposure change of nonrenally eliminated drugs in patients with chronic kidney disease using physiologically based pharmacokinetic modeling and simulation. J Clin Pharmacol 2012;52(S1):91S–108S.

Chapter 14

Drug-drug interactions

Aleksandra Galetin[a], Lei Zhang[b], A. David Rodrigues[c], and Shiew-Mei Huang[d]

[a]*Centre for Applied Pharmacokinetic Research, School of Health Sciences, The University of Manchester, Manchester, United Kingdom,* [b]*Office of Research and Standards, Office of Generic Drugs, Center for Drug Evaluation and Research, U.S. Food and Drug Administration, Silver Spring, MD, United States,* [c]*ADME Sciences, Medicine Design, Worldwide Research & Development, Pfizer Inc., Groton, CT, United States,* [d]*Office of Clinical Pharmacology, Office of Translational Sciences, Center for Drug Evaluation and Research, U.S. Food and Drug Administration, Silver Spring, MD, United States*

Introduction

A drug-drug interaction (DDI) can result from changes in the pharmacokinetics (PK) of a drug and/or its metabolites due to alteration in absorption, distribution, metabolism, and/or excretion. Although PK-based interactions are more prevalent, DDIs can also be a result of amplification or disruption of a pharmacodynamic (PD) effect of a drug. In either case, both the efficacy and safety implications of the DDI are important considerations. The risk of a DDI is particularly high when several medications are administered together to patients with multiple comorbidities. This chapter will focus primarily on PK interactions, although PD interactions are an important consideration for many classes of drugs.

Characterization of the potential for DDI is an integral part of drug development. Early characterization of a drug's route of elimination, including its specificity for drug-metabolizing enzymes and transporters, as well as its potential to either inhibit or induce enzymes and transporters, is critical for evaluating the need for subsequent clinical drug interaction studies. In this regard, the evaluation of DDI risk of a drug requires evaluation of the effect of other drugs on its PK (i.e., as a "victim" drug) and equally its ability to affect other drugs (i.e., as a "perpetrator"). A well-designed drug development program can often fully address the DDI potential of a new drug with a minimal number of clinical studies, if the studies are conceptualized and designed appropriately. Recent progress in incorporating physiologically based pharmacokinetic (PBPK) modeling in both drug development and regulatory submissions has added another approach for characterizing a drug's interaction potential without the need for extensive clinical studies and exemplifies application of the concept of model-informed drug development (MIDD).

This chapter will outline different mechanisms of PK-mediated DDIs, both enzyme- and transporter-based, and provide clinically relevant examples. In addition, in vitro techniques and modeling approaches used for the quantitative prediction of drug interactions will be described. Finally, this chapter will also address the implications of DDIs in product labeling with specific case examples.

PK interactions

PK-based drug-drug interactions usually occur as a result of either inhibition or induction of shared drug-metabolizing enzymes or transporter pathways. The most common in vivo metric used to assess the magnitude of a DDI is the fold change in maximal plasma concentration (C_{max}) or the area under the concentration-time curve (AUC) of the victim drug following multiple doses of a perpetrator (either inhibitor or inducer) relative to the control state [1, 2]. Inhibition of these pathways results in an increase in the exposure of victim or substrate drugs (measured by changes in C_{max} or AUC), whereas induction would reduce exposure (Fig. 14.1). Typically, clinical data are reported as AUC ($AUCR$) and C_{max} ratios (geometric means with 90% confidence interval). For example, the U.S. FDA guidance document for clinical drug interaction studies provides criteria for classifying an investigational drug that is a cytochrome P450 (CYP) inhibitor as a strong, moderate, or weak inhibitor, based on the fold increase in the AUC of an index substrate (e.g., midazolam in case of CYP3A4) [3]. For renally eliminated victim drugs, probes, or biomarkers, changes in renal clearance and renal secretory clearance are also reported [4, 5].

Transport-mediated interactions typically occur when a xenobiotic modulates the function of a particular transporter, thereby altering the absorption and elimination as well as the distribution and tissue-specific drug targeting of

Atkinson's Principles of Clinical Pharmacology. https://doi.org/10.1016/B978-0-12-819869-8.00013-6

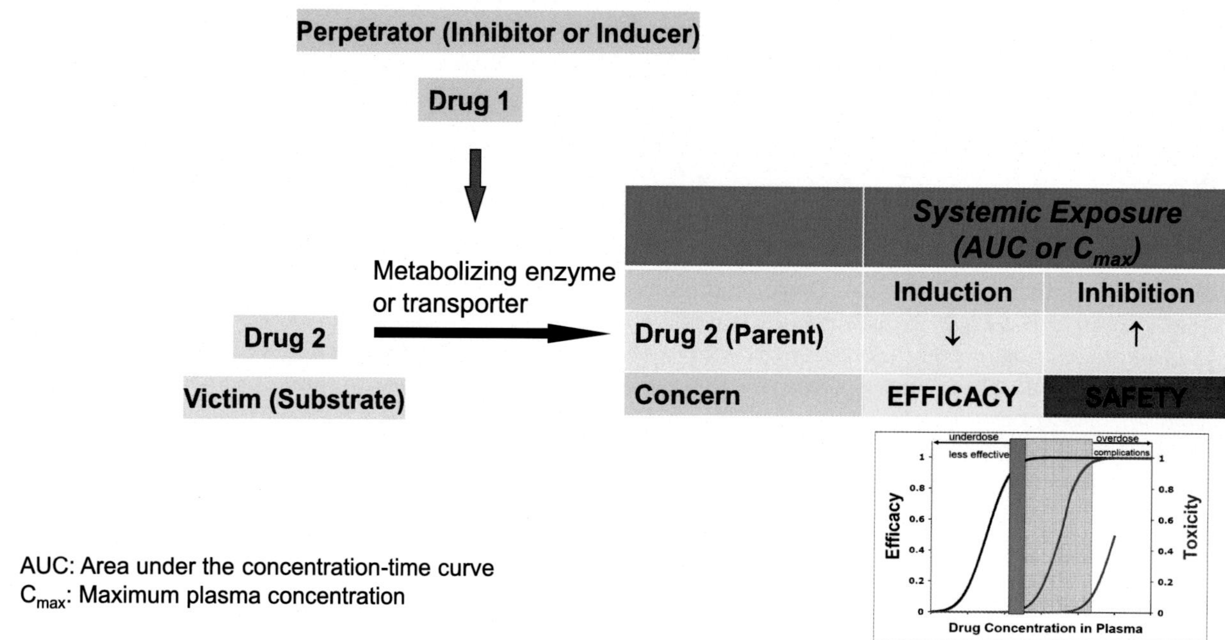

FIG. 14.1 Clinical implications of inhibition and induction of drug metabolizing enzymes or transporters.

coadministered drugs transported by these proteins. Out of more than 400 membrane transporters identified so far, a relatively small number (~30) have clinical relevance and compelling evidence for involvement in ADME processes and DDIs, although the list is continuously updated with the emerging data [6–8]. Transporter-mediated drug disposition and subsequently interactions mediated via these proteins often entail the complex interplay of multiple processes. As a result, significant DDIs can occur at the tissue level, which may not be differentiated in a typical clinical DDI study where only the systemic concentrations of the victim drug are measured in control and interaction phases. Some of these examples are highlighted in the following sections.

Interactions affecting drug elimination

Inhibition of metabolic enzymes

Enzyme inhibition decreases the rate of drug metabolism, thereby increasing the systemic exposure of a substrate drug, leading to an increased propensity for side effects and potential toxicity. Enzyme inhibition can be reversible and irreversible in its mechanism; interactions due to reversible metabolic inhibition can be further categorized into competitive and noncompetitive, the latter being more common [9, 10]. In the case of *reversible inhibition*, enzyme activity is regained by the systemic elimination of the inhibitor which decreases inhibitor concentration available for interaction with the drug-metabolizing enzyme. *Competitive inhibition* is characterized by competition between substrate and inhibitor for the enzyme's active site, i.e., binding of a substrate and competitive inhibitor is mutually exclusive. This reciprocity of inhibition means that competitive inhibition can be overcome by increasing the concentration of a substrate, thereby sustaining the velocity of the enzymatic reaction despite the presence of an inhibitor [9, 10]. In contrast, *noncompetitive inhibition* cannot be overcome by increasing the substrate concentration because the inhibitor binds to a separate binding site on the enzyme, rendering the enzyme-substrate complex nonfunctional. Ketoconazole is a classic example of a strong CYP3A4 inhibitor (it increases the *AUC* of a CYP3A substrate drug by more than 5-fold); but, due to hepatotoxicity concerns, this drug is no longer used for clinical evaluation of CYP3A4 DDIs and itraconazole is used instead [11].

Irreversible or *quasiirreversible inhibition* occurs when either the parent compound or a metabolic intermediate binds to the reduced ferrous heme portion of the P450 enzyme, thereby inactivating it [2]. In *irreversible inhibition*, or "suicide inhibition," the intermediate forms a covalent bond with the CYP protein or its heme component, causing permanent inactivation. In *quasiirreversible* inhibition, the intermediate is so tightly bound to the heme portion of the enzyme that it is practically irreversibly bound. Accordingly, quasiirreversible and irreversible mechanisms of inhibition are indistinguishable in vivo [12–15]. In this type of inhibition, also referred to as "mechanism-based inhibition" or "time-dependent inhibition," the recovery time is dependent upon the synthesis of a new enzyme, rather than the dissociation and elimination of the inhibitor, as in the case of reversible inhibition. The recovery time varies between CYP enzymes and shows large interindividual variability for some enzymes (e.g., for CYP3A4, it varies between 1 and 6 days) which also contributes to differences in the magnitude of interaction observed between individuals [13, 16]. Examples of irreversible inhibitors include the macrolide antibiotics (e.g., clarithromycin) and the HIV protease inhibitors (e.g., ritonavir). Interactions with grapefruit juice, one of the most characterized drug-food interactions, are also examples of this type of interaction, as furanocoumarins in grapefruit juice irreversibly inhibit CYP3A4 in the small intestine [17–19]. The maximal inhibitory effect of grapefruit juice on the activity of intestinal CYP3A4 is achieved when the juice is administered with, or up to four hours before, drug intake [20]; the extent of the interaction varies with the juice strength and the duration of administration [21]. Coadministration of grapefruit juice shows no effect on the clearance of substrates after IV administration, indicating that it has an exclusive presystemic effect in the small intestine [18, 19]. Intake of grapefruit juice causes increase in the bioavailability of a number of CYP3A4 substrates, including cyclosporine, calcium channel blockers, and certain HMG CoA-reductase inhibitors and this is reflected in the labeling for these drugs.

Inhibition of drug transporters

Mechanisms of drug transporter inhibition are less understood than enzyme inhibition mechanisms, but competitive inhibition is generally perceived as the most common mechanism. Both uptake and efflux transporters have displayed substrate-dependent inhibition, suggesting potential involvement of multiple transporter binding sites, thus highlighting the need to investigate transporter inhibition with relevant substrate comedications as well as prototypical probes [22–25]. In addition, a time-dependent increase in inhibitory potency of certain OATP1B1 inhibitors (e.g., cyclosporine and its main metabolite) toward OATP1B1/1B3 has been observed, although the mechanism is not fully understood [26–28]. The potential impact of pharmaceutical excipients on the potency of transporter inhibition has been highlighted for intestinal drug transporters such as BCRP and OATP2B1 [29, 30]. All of the earlier mentioned represent challenges in quantitatively predicting transporter-mediated DDI risk in drug development.

OATP1B1. Inhibition of OATP1B1 results in increased systemic exposure of a substrate drug, leading to an increased propensity for side effects and potential toxicity. For example, a single dose of rifampin causes strong inhibition of OATP1B1, as illustrated by increases of 125% for glyburide *AUC* and 520% for pitavastatin [31, 32]. In addition, the lopinavir-ritonavir combination has been reported to inhibit OATP1B1 (e.g., increased rosuvastatin *AUC* by 107%) [33]. Inhibition of hepatic OATP1B1 (and/or OATP1B3) by cyclosporine has resulted in large increases in the *AUC* and C_{max} of atorvastatin, rosuvastatin, pitavastatin, as well as other drugs [26] and endogenous biomarkers, such as coproporphyrin I (CP-I), tetradecanedioate, and glycochenodeoxycholic acid 3-sulfate [34]. Cyclosporine also inhibits a number of other transporters, including MPRs and intestinal P-gp and BCRP. Therefore, inhibition of OATP1B-mediated liver uptake is one of the mechanisms contributing to the DDI that is observed with drugs such as atorvastatin, lovastatin, simvastatin, rosuvastatin [26]. Some of these victim drugs (e.g., rosuvastatin) are substrates for a number of uptake and efflux transporters [35, 36] or interaction may involve inhibition of intestinal CYP3A4 metabolism and uptake via OATP1B1 (e.g., lovastatin and simvastatin). One of the factors confounding the interpretation of cyclosporine clinical DDI data is that majority of the studies report the magnitude of interaction in individuals receiving chronic dosing after organ transplantation in comparison to historic data obtained in healthy subjects [37]. Noteworthy exceptions to this are clinical studies with atorvastatin, repaglinide, and simvastatin in which the PK of the victim drug was assessed in the same individuals [38–40].

Significant increases in the plasma concentrations of many OATP1B victim drugs may lead to serious, potentially life-threatening toxicities, e.g., increased risk of myopathy and rhabdomyolysis in the case of statins. Despite these significant changes in systemic exposure of statins which result from OATP1B inhibition, most of these interactions do not substantially impact statin concentrations at their site of therapeutic action in the liver, hence the change in efficacy is minor. [41–43]. It is important to note that these concepts apply for statins that are predominantly eliminated via liver and where hepatic uptake is the rate-determining step in their hepatic disposition, as discussed in more detail elsewhere [44, 45].

OCTs/MATEs. Cimetidine is a well-known OCT2/MATEs inhibitor that is associated with reduced renal clearance of a number of concomitantly administered drugs, including metformin, pindolol, and dofetilide [6], but also endogenous biomarkers such as creatinine and N1-methylnicotinamide [4, 46, 47]. However, the magnitude of these interactions (both in terms of the effect on *AUC* and/or renal clearance of drugs) is quite low in comparison to the OATP1B inhibitory interactions described before. Many OCT/MATE DDIs are associated with metformin, but their interpretation can often be challenging due to its complex transporter-mediated disposition. Distribution of metformin to the liver, the primary site of its antihyperglycemic effect and rare toxicity (lactic acidosis), is mediated by the OCT1 transporter [48], whereas its renal elimination is via uptake (OCT2) and efflux (MATE1/2K) transport across proximal tubule cells [49, 50]. As a result, OCT/MATE-mediated DDIs may affect either metformin PK, efficacy, or safety when coadministered with drugs that inhibit these transporters [49]. For example, modulation of OCT/MATE may result in changes in metformin hepatic exposure that differ from changes in systemic drug concentrations, resulting in scenarios with minimal or no alterations in metformin systemic PK, yet potentially increased liver exposure and subsequent glucose lowering (PD) effect [51, 52]. Because these changes in metformin PD effect are occurring independently of changes in its systemic PK, any decision on metformin dose adjustment that is based solely on changes in systemic exposure may not be appropriate, as the DDI effect at the actual site of action (i.e., liver) may be neglected.

OATs. Probenecid is a prototypical inhibitor of OATs and increases plasma *AUC* of a number of clinical probe substrates, such as adefovir (OAT1 predominantly), furosemide (dual OAT1/3 substrate), and benzylpenicillin (more selective for OAT3) [4, 53–55]. In addition to clinical drugs, probenecid causes a decrease in renal clearance of endogenous molecules such as pyrodixic and homovanilic acid [56]. Probenecid protects against cidofovir-mediated nephrotoxicity by limiting its OAT1-mediated renal uptake [57]. In addition to probenecid, several other therapeutic agents have been associated with inhibition of the OATs in vitro, including pravastatin, cimetidine, thiazide and loop diuretics, and certain NSAIDs.

P-glycoprotein. P-glycoprotein (P-gp) encoded in the *ABCB1* gene is the most extensively studied transporter. Early studies in the 1980s established P-gp's association with drug resistance in cancer chemotherapy. Although P-gp is expressed in various tissues including intestine, liver, kidney, and brain where it provides protection against xenobiotics [6, 58, 59], inhibition of intestinal P-gp is the most relevant contributor to clinical DDIs. Digoxin is a drug with a narrow therapeutic index that is a well-known substrate for P-gp and DDIs with P-gp inhibitors such as itraconazole, verapamil, and clarithromycin have been reported [60]. Because of safety concerns, clinical DDI studies with digoxin are conducted for new drugs that are P-gp inhibitors. Although digoxin DDI studies are clinically relevant from the safety perspective, they do not capture the true "worst-case" scenario associated with intestinal P-gp inhibition. To that end, many recent studies have explored dabigatran etexilate as a clinical probe for studying intestinal P-gp inhibition [61, 62].

Inhibition or induction of P-gp function has physiological and pharmacological consequences. The pharmacologic effects of altering P-gp function could range from changes in drug absorption and bioavailability, to changes in drug distribution to the central nervous system and other organs, and to changes in drug elimination. For this reason, drugs are routinely tested during development to determine whether they are substrates or inhibitors of P-gp [50].

BCRP. Many drugs from various therapeutic areas have been identified as substrates or inhibitors of breast cancer resistance protein (BCRP) in vitro, including rosuvastatin, sulfasalazine, and topotecan [4, 36]. However, clinical DDIs attributed directly and specifically to BCRP inhibition are limited because probes used are also substrate drugs for other transporters, e.g., P-gp [36, 63]. Similarly, some perpetrator drugs are potent BCRP as well as OATP1B inhibitors and can cause elevated systemic exposure of dual substrates like rosuvastatin. Particularly challenging in the interpretation of rosuvastatin BCRP-mediated DDIs is the localization of this transporter in the intestine and liver as well as its polymorphic expression [36]. Inhibition of intestinal BCRP is expected to increase the bioavailability and systemic exposure of rosuvastatin, whereas inhibition of hepatic BCRP will affect rosuvastatin distribution in the liver and therefore its PD effect, with only a marginal effect on systemic exposure. Analogous to digoxin safety studies for P-gp inhibitor drugs, if a BCRP substrate drug has a narrow therapeutic range and/or identified safety concerns, then a DDI study will have direct clinical relevance by informing dose adjustment for the drug.

Induction of metabolic enzymes

Enzyme induction represents another DDI mechanism in which drug metabolism is increased, leading to decreased substrate concentrations or increased metabolite concentrations. Unlike CYP inhibition, which is an almost immediate response, the full impact of CYP induction is delayed because time is required to reach the steady-state enzyme levels that result from a new balance between the rate of enzyme biosynthesis and degradation [2, 9]. Similarly, it also takes time to return the enzyme to its basal level after discontinuing the treatment with the inducer. For example, exposure to the CYP3A probe substrate midazolam returned to baseline with a half-life of ~8 days after coadministration with rifampin (a CYP3A inducer) was discontinued [64]. Because of the time-dependent nature of the process, enzyme induction may complicate chronic drug therapy dosing regimens.

One of the intriguing aspects of CYPs is that some but not all of these enzymes are inducible [65, 66]. Major human CYP enzymes, CYP1A2, CYP2B6, CYP2C8, CYP2C9, CYP2C19, and CYP3A enzymes, are known to be inducible. In contrast, there is no evidence of CYP2D6 induction. Regulation of CYP enzymes involves an orphan nuclear receptor, pregnane X receptor (PXR), that transcriptionally activates the CYP3A genes by interacting with their PXR response elements. Studies have indicated that activation of this nuclear receptor actually results in the coinduction of both CYP3A and CYP2C. Thus a negative in vitro result for CYP3A induction may eliminate the need for additional induction studies for CYP2C enzymes. However, whether CYP2C and CYP3A are always coinduced may need further validation. CYP1A2 induction occurs mainly via the aryl hydrocarbon receptor (AhR), therefore, CYP1A2 is not likely to be coinduced with CYP3A. Although overlap exists between CYP2B6 and CYP3A inducers, there are data suggesting that certain CYP2B6 inducers selectively bind to the constitutive androstane receptor (CAR), and these inducers do not show significant CYP3A induction. Therefore the potential for induction of CYP1A2 and CYP2B6 should be evaluated separately regardless of the CYP3A induction result.

A new drug that induces a CYP enzyme can cause drug interactions with substrate drugs for that particular pathway leading to enhanced clearance. Therefore, understanding a new drug's potential to induce major CYP enzymes is recommended in regulatory guidance documents [3, 50, 67]. Human primary or cryopreserved hepatocytes are the preferred experimental system for the evaluation of P450 induction.

Induction of drug transporters

Akin to enzymes, transporters may be induced, also leading to decreased substrate concentrations. Induction of several transporters, including MRP2/3, and the organic solute transporters α/β, and P-gp has been reported as a result of either increased transporter mRNA and/or protein expression [58, 68–70]. Despite P-gp localization across multiple organs, only induction of intestinal P-gp causes clinically significant DDIs [64, 68]. In contrast to in vitro findings, clinical relevance is lacking for induction of P-gp expressed in the blood-brain barrier (directly demonstrated in clinical brain imaging studies), or in the liver and kidney (no evidence for decreased half-life of metabolically stable substrates) [71, 72]. Considerable overlap exists between CYP3A4 and P-gp inducers, including rifampin, dexamethasone, and St John's wort [64, 73–76]. This overlap is not surprising considering common regulatory mechanisms for CYP3A4 and *MDR1* genes and induction via PXR activation.

Induction of intestinal P-gp has been reported to increase P-gp protein expression in human intestinal biopsies by ~3–4-fold [73, 74]. Functionally, induction of intestinal P-gp following multiple doses of PXR activators (rifampin or St. John's wort) reduces the bioavailability of P-gp substrates (e.g., digoxin, talinolol) and results in a clinically relevant DDI [68, 75, 76]. Dabigatran etexilate, a prodrug considered a relatively specific intestinal P-gp substrate [61], exhibited up to a 67% decrease in total dabigatran exposure (parent plus glucuronide) after a 10-day treatment with 10–600 mg rifampin [76]. Similarly, following pretreatment with multiple doses of rifampin, the *AUC* of sofosbuvir and tenofovir alafenamide was decreased without the half-life being altered [72]. In addition to decreasing systemic exposure, intestinal P-gp induction is expected to attenuate both the fraction absorbed and absorption rate of substrate drugs [72].

The possibility of OATP1B induction has been suggested because the *AUC* of some OATP1B substrates (e.g., rosuvastatin) is reduced following multiple-dose rifampin administration (and relative to the DDI effect after single-dose rifampin). However, clinical and in vitro data supporting this concept are conflicting, as summarized recently [68, 72]. In interpreting such clinical findings, it is important to consider the effect of multiple-dose rifampin on other metabolizing enzymes (CYP3A4) or transporters (intestinal MRP2) that may contribute to drug elimination and DDI observed. Transcriptional regulation of OATP1B is complex, and involves the liver X receptor α, farnesoid X receptor (FXR), hepatic nuclear factor 1α and 4α, but not PXR and constitutive androstane receptor [68, 77, 78], highlighting the need to understand further the clinical relevance of other regulatory pathways beyond PXR. Any potential induction of hepatic OATP1B would have important implications for the efficacy and safety of many drugs, but clinical relevance of this type of DDI mechanism for OATP1B1 is still ambiguous.

Interactions affecting drug absorption

Absorption of an orally administered drug can be influenced by many factors, including drug release from a dosage unit, solubility and stability of the drug, gastric emptying, uptake and efflux transporters, and metabolic enzymes in the intestine. Coadministration with other drugs that affect these factors can alter absorption of the drug. For example, interactions affecting drug absorption could be caused by inhibition or induction of enzymes (e.g., CYP3A) or transporters in the intestine (e.g., P-gp and BCRP). Drugs that alter GI motility can affect drug absorption by changing the rate at which drugs are transported into and through the small intestine as described in Chapter 4. Another absorption-related DDI for drugs whose solubility is pH dependent can be caused by pH changes in the gastrointestinal tract that are induced by acid-reducing agents (e.g., proton pump inhibitors). Elevation of gastric pH by an acid-reducing agent may affect the absorption of these drugs, leading to altered systemic exposure. The solubility of some weak base drugs decreases with increases in pH, so their exposure can be decreased when coadministered with an acid-reducing agent. For example, exposure of atazanavir decreased 94% when atazanavir/ritonavir was coadministered with once daily 40mg omeprazole, leading to loss of therapeutic efficacy. pH-dependent DDI should be evaluated during drug development and a preliminary decision framework has been proposed to investigate this type of DDI [79], supported also by PBPK modeling efforts to predict pH-dependent DDI [80–82]. Drug absorption may also be limited by the formation of insoluble complexes that result when certain drugs are exposed to di- and trivalent cations in the GI tract. For example, exposure of raltegravir decreased 14%–76% in the presence of carbonate antacid or magnesium/aluminum hydroxide antacid [83]. Therefore coadministration of raltegravir and metal-containing antacids is not recommended.

Interactions affecting drug distribution

Displacement of a highly protein bound drug (>90%) by other drugs from its binding sites would increase the availability of the pharmacologically active free drug. However, very few clinically relevant DDIs result from disruption of protein binding. This mechanism of interaction is considered significant only for drugs that are highly protein bound, have a narrow therapeutic index, and a small volume of distribution. Warfarin, extensively bound to plasma albumin (>97%), is the most commonly reported victim drug associated with this DDI mechanism. Acidic highly albumin-bound drugs such as valproic acid may displace warfarin from albumin binding sites, resulting in increase in free warfarin plasma concentrations and rapid increases in International Normalized Ratio (INR) [84, 85]. However, increase in plasma concentrations of free warfarin leads to more rapid drug metabolic elimination and therefore the overall effect is often transient (see Fig. 7.2, Chapter 7). Thus, for restrictively metabolized drugs, the increased concentration of unbound drug due to the displacement interaction increases the elimination of unbound drug as to return unbound concentrations to their previous level, even though the fractional binding remains reduced.

Inhibition of certain drug transporters may limit the distribution of a drug to its site(s) of action. Examples include inhibition of P-gp that limits drug distribution across the blood-brain barrier, or inhibition of OATP1B1/1B3 that limits drug distribution into the liver. This is of particular relevance for drugs where liver is the pharmacological site of action, as in the case of HMG-CoA reductase inhibitors ("statins") or hepatitis C antivirals. As indicated earlier, concomitant administration of substrates with inhibitors of OATP1B1 (such as cyclosporine) results in increased statin plasma concentrations [26, 41] and risk of myopathy, with marginal effect on cholesterol-lowering efficacy (driven by liver drug exposure). However, another confounding factor for the disposition of statins is that inhibitors of OATP1B1 may often also inhibit BCRP, an important transporter for the oral absorption and biliary elimination of statins. The inhibition of hepatic BCRP may not cause significant changes in the plasma exposure of statins per se, but will affect drug accumulation in the hepatocytes and increase in liver exposure and, therefore, the cholesterol-lowering effect of drugs like rosuvastatin [36].

Other interactions

PD interactions

Antihypertensive drugs are a mainstay treating patients with arterial hypertension and PD interactions play a fundamental role in current therapeutic strategy. In the approach that was previously standard, treatment was begun with a single drug and other drugs were added stepwise if therapeutic response was suboptimal. However, in treating suboptimally responding patients, it has been shown that adding a second drug with a different mechanism of action is five times more effective than simply doubling the dose of the single drug that was initially prescribed [86]. The physiological basis for this is that the second drug not only has a different mechanism of pharmacological action, but also serves to block counterregulatory responses evoked by the first drug. Accordingly, current guidelines advocate beginning therapy with a diuretic together with an angiotensin-converting enzyme in patients with a systolic blood pressure ≥140mmHg or a diastolic pressure ≥90mmHg [87].

PD interactions may also exacerbate the toxic potential of drug combinations. As the COVID-19 (severe acute respiratory syndrome coronavirus 2 (SARS-CoV-2)) pandemic started in December 2019 and caused more than 1.32 million deaths globally as of November 2020, the search for effective new drugs was accelerated, but also focused on repurposed drugs [88–90]. One such drug is hydroxychloroquine, an antimalarial drug which, despite unproved efficacy in treating patients with COVID-19 [91, 92], has often been coadministered to these patients with a macrolide, such as azithromycin [93]. Both drugs prolong the electrocardiographic QT interval and their combination increased the incidence of cardiac arrest in one study of COVID-19 patients, although no increase was noted when either drug was given by itself [91].

Interaction of urine pH and renal urine flow with drug PK and toxicity

The PK of renally excreted drugs may be altered by changes in active tubular secretion mediated via renal transporters, as well as by changes in urinary pH and urine flow. Changes in pH of the luminal fluid in the renal tubule alter the extent of ionization of weakly acidic and basic drugs, thereby affecting their degree of passive diffusion and the magnitude of their passive reabsorption [94–97]. Examples include acidic drugs such as phenobarbital and aspirin, whose renal excretion increases with concurrent antacid or sodium bicarbonate administration [98]. For this reason, patients with phenobarbital and salicylate overdose have been treated with bicarbonate infusions to increase drug ionization, thus decreasing the renal tubular absorption and enhancing the renal excretion of these drugs. Urine flow and urine pH also can be important contributors to renal toxicity risk. Sulfamethoxazole and acyclovir are low solubility compounds, and crystalluria leading to acute kidney injury has been reported for these drugs and attributed to changes in urine flow and urine pH [95, 99].

Therapeutic protein-drug interactions

The increase in the clinical use and types of therapeutic proteins (e.g., monoclonal antibodies, replacement enzymes, cytokines, and growth factors) has drawn the attention to their propensity for DDIs [100–103]. Evaluation of therapeutic protein-drug interactions is still an evolving area. The 2020 FDA guidance for industry on clinical drug interaction studies did not include a section on DDIs for therapeutic proteins [3, 50], but a separate draft guidance document on DDI assessment for therapeutic proteins has now been published [104]. Although PBPK modeling may be applied to therapeutic protein-drug interactions to evaluate complex mechanisms and explore the potential for clinically significant interactions, this approach is currently not comprehensive enough to substitute for in vivo studies.

As therapeutic proteins do not typically depend on mechanisms of metabolism or transport for clearance, there is less potential for concomitantly administered drugs to affect their disposition and/or elimination. However, evolving data indicate that therapeutic proteins may affect the disposition of coadministered small molecule drugs by causing downregulation or suppression of drug-metabolizing enzymes or transporters. For example, administration of immunological proteins, such as interferons and interleukins, may alter the metabolic capacity of the liver, similar to what has been observed during acute infection or inflammation. Systemic pro-inflammatory cytokines released during infection, inflammation, or cancer suppress gene transcription, resulting in downregulation of CYP enzymes [105]. Treatment of rheumatoid arthritis patients with tocilizumab, a monoclonal anti-IL-6 receptor antibody, reversed the enzyme suppression caused by IL-6 and normalized CYP3A4-mediated clearance of simvastatin [106]. Therapeutic peptides such as native glucagon and fibroblast growth factor-21 have also been reported to cause downregulation of CYP3A4 [107]. However, any potential regulatory effect of these peptides on clinically relevant drug transporters (e.g., OATP1B1) is currently unknown [104]. An overview of clinically reported therapeutic protein-drug interactions and the information included in product package inserts has recently been summarized elsewhere [100].

Integrated investigation of DDI risk in drug development

This section illustrates how current drug development employs an integrated approach for evaluating potential DDI risk, i.e., from in vitro data via in silico modeling to clinical evaluation (Fig. 14.2). The most common in vivo metric used to assess the magnitude of either metabolic enzyme- or transporter-mediated DDIs is the fold change in *AUC* of the victim drug following multiple dosing with a perpetrator (inhibitor or inducer) relative to the control state [1, 2]. Although multiple dosing of a perpetrator drug is a more standard practice, in certain instances a single dose of a perpetrator is used in clinical studies to assess inhibition (e.g., inhibition of OAT1B1 by rifampin) [3, 32, 50]. Single-dose rifampin is a potent inhibitor of this hepatic transporter, whereas multiple-dose rifampin is used extensively to investigate induction effects mediated by PXR (e.g., CYP3A4 with midazolam as a clinical probe). Regulatory guidance for clinical DDIs classifies them based on the effect of the investigational drug when given at the highest clinical dose and the shortest dosing interval within its therapeutic dose range/dosing regimen [3]. Drugs classified as strong inhibitors cause ≥5-fold increase in the *AUC*, moderate inhibitors increase the *AUC* by ≥2-fold but <5-fold, and weak inhibitors increase the *AUC* of a sensitive substrate by ≥1.25-fold but <2-fold [3] (Table 14.1). Assignment to the latter two classes needs to be based on evaluations with sensitive index substrates. Many advanced tools have been introduced in recent years to evaluate DDI risks during drug development. Examples include the increasing use of PBPK modeling for evaluating DDI risk in different patient populations and/or ethnic groups and for informing the drug labeling (e.g., simeprevir, letermovir) [44, 108], the use of positron emission tomography (PET) imaging [109], and the consideration of using endogenous biomarkers (e.g., coproporphyrin I) to evaluate transporter-mediated perpetrator DDIs during early drug development [110–113].

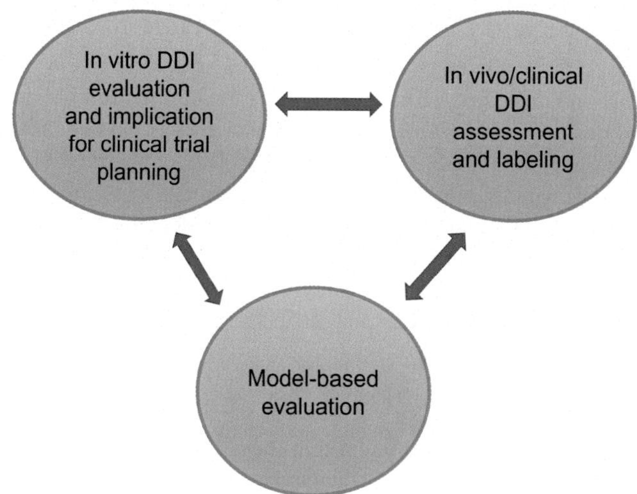

FIG. 14.2 Integrated DDI evaluation approach in drug development.

TABLE 14.1 Classification of strong and moderate perpetrators for CYP enzymes.

Variable	Strong inhibitor[a]	Moderate inhibitor	Weak inhibitor
Change in AUC of a sensitive index substrate	↑ ≥5-fold	↑ ≥2- to <5-fold	↑ ≥1.25- to <2-fold
Variable	**Strong inducer[a]**	**Moderate inducer**	**Weak inducer**
Change in AUC of a sensitive index substrate	↓ ≥80%	↓ ≥50% to <80%	↓ ≥20% to <50%

AUC, area under the concentration-time curve.
[a]*For strong inhibitors or inducers, data may be from nonsensitive index substrates.*

In vitro evaluation of DDIs and in silico prediction of DDI risk

The identification of metabolic pathways relevant for drug elimination during early drug development [114] allows the prediction of in vivo DDIs and can indicate what clinical DDI studies may be warranted during subsequent clinical development. In vitro enzyme/transporter inhibition data (i.e., enzyme-inhibitor dissociation constant (K_i)), together with the maximum unbound plasma concentration of inhibitor achieved in vivo, anticipated gut concentrations of the drug (e.g., estimated as dose/250mL for CYP3A or P-gp) or maximum unbound inlet concentrations (e.g., for OATP1B1), are used to predict the likelihood and magnitude (i.e., fold change in *AUC*) of a clinical interaction. The assessment is usually done in a stepwise manner, applying models that differ in their complexity, starting with basic models [15, 115], progressing to static mechanistic models [16, 116–118], and then to dynamic PBPK models [119–122].

Application of basic models

The simplest approach is to evaluate the potential for an investigational drug to be an enzyme or transporter inhibitor by using a basic model such as the I/K_i approach [1, 2, 15, 123–125]. This approach often overestimates the magnitude of the in vivo DDI, as it assumes that metabolism or transport of the victim drug occurs exclusively via a particular enzyme or transporter that can be inhibited (e.g., OATP1B1) and that any potential contributing effects of passive diffusion or inhibition of other processes (efflux/metabolism) are negligible. Although this model provides a conservative initial estimate (the "worst-case" scenario), it may eliminate the need for later clinical investigations of DDIs if it indicates a low potential for interactions. When the I/K_i value is above proposed cut-off values and suggests that an interaction potential exists, then more complex modeling approaches need to be considered to further investigate the DDI potential and determine the need to conduct a clinical study [50].

Application of mechanistic static models

Mechanistic static models incorporate more detailed drug disposition and drug interaction mechanisms for both drugs in an interaction combination [126]. For example, parameters such as the fraction metabolized by specific CYP enzymes or the intestinal availability of victim drugs are incorporated along with K_i values for inhibitors [118, 126]. Although these models allow multiple interaction mechanisms to be incorporated (e.g., simultaneous time-dependent inhibition and induction of metabolic enzymes), their scope is to some extent limited [15, 16, 124, 126]. For example, assessment of complex interactions via multiple transporters and/or transporter-enzyme interplay in different tissues is difficult to investigate by the static approach. One reason that contributes to this is that static models assume that there is no change in the concentration of an inhibitor during the dosing interval, so that the level of inhibition remains constant. In some instances, the plasma concentrations considered in assessing the DDIs are not reflective of the intracellular concentration of an inhibitor interacting, for example, with biliary efflux transporters. If the predicted AUC ratio is ≥ 1.25 based on static mechanistic models or dynamic mechanistic models (e.g., PBPK models), then a clinical DDI study using a sensitive index substrate or a drug that is likely to be coadministered may need to be conducted.

Application of PBPK models

PBPK modeling is the most advanced modeling approach and is now commonly used in drug development and regulatory submissions [108, 120, 122, 127–130] (Fig. 14.3). This translational tool provides a dynamic framework for integrating physiological or system data (e.g., organ blood flows, tissue volumes, enzyme/transporter abundance) with drug-dependent

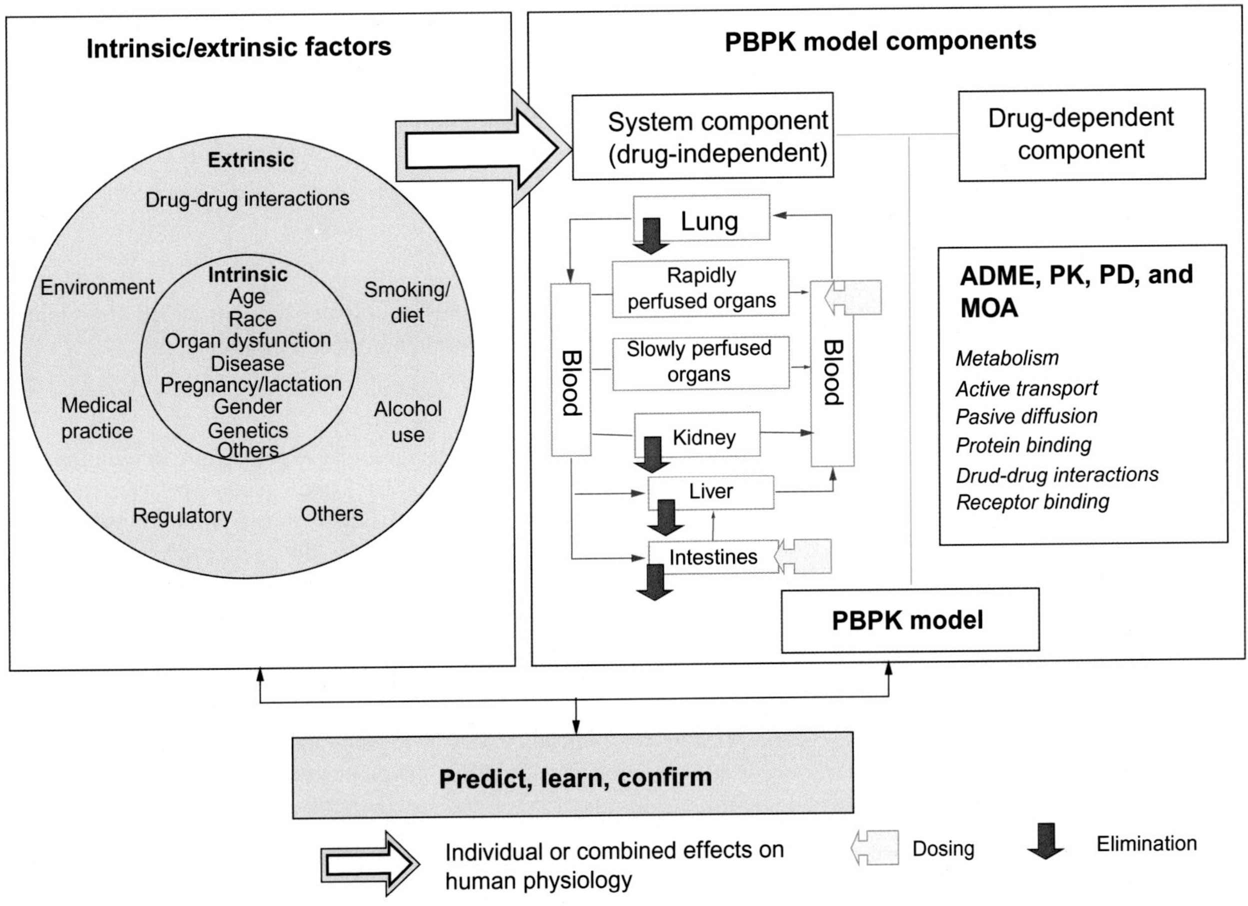

FIG. 14.3 (A) Intrinsic and extrinsic patient factors that can affect drug exposure and response (B) Drug-dependent components and drug-independent (system) components of the PBPK model that can act individually or in combination to affect drug exposure. *ADME*, absorption, distribution, metabolism, and excretion; *MOA*, mechanism of action; *PD*, pharmacodynamics; *PK*, pharmacokinetics. *(Reproduced with permission from Zhao P, Zhang L, Grillo JA, Liu Q, Bullock JM, Moon YJ, et al. Applications of physiologically based pharmacokinetic (PBPK) modeling and simulation during regulatory review. Clin Pharmacol Ther 2011;89:259–267.)*

parameters (e.g., in vitro metabolic clearance, permeability, or transporter kinetic data) [26, 44, 45, 120, 121, 131, 132]. By integrating these parameters in a whole body PBPK model in a "bottom-up" manner, both systemic and tissue exposure resulting from changes in enzyme and/or transporter activity can be simulated [22, 41, 42, 44, 133].

The increased use of PBPK modeling in drug development is reflected in the number and diversity of examples reported in the literature and in recent regulatory submissions, together with DDI and PBPK guidance documents from regulatory agencies [44, 50, 122, 129, 130, 134–136].

Verified PBPK models offer the following advantages over static models:

1. Investigation of the effect of an interacting drug on the entire PK profile of the victim drug.
2. Incorporation of multiple DDI mechanisms, such as simultaneous induction and inhibition, the effect of inhibitory metabolites, etc.
3. Investigation of dynamic changes in transporter activity at multiple membranes/organs (e.g., intestine and liver) and transporter-metabolism interplay using relevant (e.g., enterocytic) inhibitor concentrations for the evaluation of interaction risk
4. Investigation of DDIs in the presence of multiple intrinsic and/or extrinsic factors and provision of a link to drug effect through PBPK-PD models.
5. Simulation of various scenarios in order to elucidate potential causes of uncertainty and variability

Verified victim drug PBPK models, in combination with corresponding perpetrator PBPK model(s), are crucial to inform and guide the design of prospective clinical DDI and/or pharmacogenetic studies and to support decision-making in drug development and regulatory submissions [41, 108, 129, 130, 136, 137]. In addition, there is an increasing use of PBPK models to predict PK in specific populations (e.g., pediatric, pregnant women) or DDI magnitude in various clinical situations, including those with multiple concurrent patient factors such as renal or hepatic impairment [44, 45, 133, 138–145]. Integrating various patient-intrinsic and patient-extrinsic factors in these mechanistic models can provide an understanding of the potentially complex changes in exposure-response relationships in patients in whom multiple covariates are present. These models provide the ability to design precision dosing regiments for patients with multiple comorbidities and coadministered medications [146–148].

Clinical DDI evaluation

Clinical DDI studies are conducted using appropriate index substrates/perpetrators or likely coadministered drugs that are expected to satisfy criteria of selectivity and specificity for a particular enzyme/transporter of interest [4].

Probe selection

Clinical probe needs to show appropriate sensitivity, i.e., that the extent of change in its exposure due to inhibition correlates with the potency of coadministered inhibitor. In addition, probes for clinical DDI studies should be selected that can be measured with robust and validated bioanalytical methods. For CYP enzymes, DDI results from index substrates or perpetrators can generally be extrapolated to other substrates or perpetrators that share the same pathway with similar DDI sensitivity or potency (Tables 14.1 and 14.2). However, there is a general lack of index substrates or perpetrators for most transporters, so such extrapolation generally is not possible. The doses of probe and perpetrator drugs should be clinically relevant for appropriate characterization of a DDI risk. For certain probes (e.g., dabigatran etexilate), potential saturation of drug transporters (e.g., intestinal P-gp) needs to be considered, as it may reduce the sensitivity of the measurements [61].

Lists of recommended clinical probes and perpetrators for clinically relevant enzymes and transporters are available on the FDA website https://www.fda.gov/drugs/drug-interactions-labeling/drug-development-and-drug-interactions-table-substrates-inhibitors-and-inducers (Tables 14.3–14.5). The majority of the listed transporter substrates, inducers, or

TABLE 14.2 Classification of sensitive and moderate sensitive substrate for CYP enzymes.

Variable	Sensitive substrate[a]	Moderate sensitive substrate
Change in AUC with a strong index inhibitor	↑ ≥5-fold	↑ ≥2- to <5-fold

AUC, area under the concentration-time curve.
[a]*For sensitive substrates, data may be from any known index inhibitors for a particular pathway or whose AUC ratio in poor metabolizers for a specific enzyme is greater than or equal to 5-fold compared with extensive metabolizers.*

TABLE 14.3 Examples of strong clinical inhibitors and inducers for CYP-mediated metabolisms (for concomitant use clinical DDI studies and/or drug labeling).

	Strong inhibitors	Moderate inhibitors	Strong inducers	Moderate inducers
CYP1A2	Ciprofloxacin, enoxacin, fluvoxamine[a]	Methoxsalen, mexiletine, oral contraceptives		Phenytoin,[b] rifampin,[c] ritonavir,[d,e] smoking, teriflunomide
CYP2B6	–	–	Carbamazepine[f]	Efavirenz[f], rifampin[b]
CYP2C8	Gemfibrozil[g]	Clopidogrel,[h] deferasirox, teriflunomide	–	Rifampin[b]
CYP2C9	–	Amiodarone, fluconazole,[i] miconazole, piperine	–	Enzalutamide,[j] rifampin[b]
CYP2C19	Fluconazole,[i] fluoxetine,[k] fluvoxamine,[a] ticlopidine	Felbamate	Rifampin[c]	Apalutamide, efavirenz,[f,l] enzalutamide,[j] phenytoin[c]
CYP2D6	Bupropion, fluoxetine,[k] paroxetine, quinidine,[m] terbinafine	Abiraterone, cinacalcet, duloxetine, lorcaserin, mirabegron	–	–
CYP3A4	Boceprevir, cobicistat,[m] danoprevir and ritonavir,[n] elvitegravir and ritonavir,[n] grapefruit juice,[o] indinavir and ritonavir,[n] itraconazole,[m] ketoconazole, lopinavir and ritonavir,[m,n] paritaprevir and ritonavir and (ombitasvir and/or dasabuvir),[n] posaconazole, ritonavir,[m,n] saquinavir and ritonavir,[m,n] telaprevir,[m] tipranavir and ritonavir,[m,n] telithromycin, troleandomycin, voriconazole **≥10-fold increase:** Clarithromycin,[m] idelalisib, nefazodone, nelfinavir[m]	Aprepitant, ciprofloxacin, conivaptan,[p] crizotinib, cyclosporine, diltiazem,[q] dronedarone,[m] erythromycin, fluconazole,[i] fluvoxamine,[a] imatinib, tofisopam, verapamil[m]	Apalutamide, carbamazepine,[f] enzalutamide,[j] mitotane, phenytoin,[b] rifampin,[c] St. John's wort[r]	Bosentan, efavirenz,[l] etravirine, phenobarbital, primidone

Note:

- Strong, moderate, and weak inhibitors are drugs that increase the AUC of sensitive index substrates of a given metabolic pathway ≥5-fold, ≥2 to <5-fold, and ≥1.25 to <2-fold, respectively (Table 14.1). For strong inhibitors, data may be from nonsensitive index substrates.
- Strong, moderate, and weak inducers are drugs that decreases the AUC of sensitive index substrates of a given metabolic pathway by ≥80%, ≥50% to <80%, and ≥20% to <50%, respectively (Table 14.1). For strong inducers, data may be from nonsensitive index substrates.
- Index substrates have a well-understood contribution of a specific cytochrome P-450 (CYP) pathway to their elimination and a well-defined interaction effect with index inhibitors and inducers, and are safe for use in healthy subjects.
- Index perpetrators (inhibitors or inducers) have predictable effect size, are known to alter the function of a given metabolic pathway, and are safe for use in healthy subjects.

This table is prepared to provide examples of clinical inhibitors and is not intended to be an exhaustive list. Lists of recommended clinical probes and perpetrators for clinically relevant enzymes and transporters are available on the FDA website https://www.fda.gov/drugs/drug-interactions-labeling/drug-development-and-drug-interactions-table-substrates-inhibitors-and-inducers.
DDI data were collected based on a search of the University of Washington Drug Interaction Solutions (also known as "UW Metabolism and Transport Drug Interaction Database," https://www.druginteractionsolutions.org/).
Abbreviations: *AUC*, area under the concentration-time curve; *CYP*, cytochrome P450; *DDI*, drug-drug interaction; *HIV*, human immunodeficiency virus; *HCV*, hepatitis C virus; *OATP1B1*, organic anion transporting polypeptide 1B1; *OAT3*, organic anion transporter 3; *P-gp*, P-glycoprotein.
[a]*Strong inhibitor of CYP1A2 and CYP2C19. Moderate inhibitor of CYP3A and weak inhibitor of CYP2D6.*
[b]*Strong inducer of CYP3A and moderate inducer of CYP1A2, CYP2C19.*
[c]*Strong inducer of CYP2C19, CYP3A, and moderate inducer of CYP1A2, CYP2B6, CYP2C8, CYP2C9.*
[d]*Moderate inducer of CYP1A2 with dose of 800 mg/day ritonavir (not with other anti-HIV drugs). Effect on CYP1A2 at lower doses of ritonavir is unknown.*
[e]*Weak inducer of CYP2B6, CYP2C9, and CYP2C19. Classification is based on studies conducted with ritonavir itself (not with other anti-HIV drugs) at doses of 100–200 mg/day, although larger effects have been reported in literature for high doses of ritonavir.*
[f]*Strong inducer of CYP2B6, CYP3A, and weak inducer of CYP2C9.*
[g]*Strong inhibitor of CYP2C8 and inhibitor of OATP1B1 and OAT3.*
[h]*Moderate inhibitor of CYP2C8 and weak inhibitor of CYP2B6.*
[i]*Strong inhibitor of CYP2C19 and moderate inhibitor of CYP2C9 and CYP3A.*
[j]*Strong inducer of CYP3A and moderate inducer of CYP2C9, and CYP2C19.*
[k]*Strong inhibitors of CYP2C19 and CYP2D6.*
[l]*Moderate inducer of CYP2B6, CYP2C19, and CYP3A.*
[m]*Inhibitor of P-gp (defined as those increasing AUC of digoxin to ≥1.25-fold).*
[n]*Ritonavir is usually given in combination with other anti-HIV or anti-HCV drugs in clinical practice. Caution should be used when extrapolating the observed effect of ritonavir alone to the effect of combination regimens on CYP3A activities.*
[o]*The effect of grapefruit juice varies widely among brands and is concentration-, dose-, and preparation-dependent. Studies have shown that it can be classified as a "strong CYP3A inhibitor" when a certain preparation was used (e.g., high dose, double strength) or as a "moderate CYP3A inhibitor" when another preparation was used (e.g., low dose, single strength).*
[p]*The classification is based on studies conducted with intravenously administered conivaptan.*
[q]*Diltiazem increased AUC of certain sensitive CYP3A substrates (e.g., buspirone) more than 5-fold.*
[r]*The effect of St. John's wort varies widely and is preparation dependent.*

TABLE 14.4 Examples of clinical substrates for CYP-mediated metabolism (for concomitant use clinical DDI studies and/or drug labeling).

	Sensitive substrates	Moderate sensitive substrates
CYP1A2	Alosetron, caffeine, duloxetine, melatonin, ramelteon, tasimelteon, tizanidine	Clozapine, pirfenidone, ramosetron, theophylline
CYP2B6	Bupropion[a]	Efavirenz[a]
CYP2C8	Repaglinide[b]	Montelukast, pioglitazone, rosiglitazone
CYP2C9	Celecoxib[c]	Glimepiride, phenytoin, tolbutamide, warfarin
CYP2C19	*S*-Mephenytoin, omeprazole	Diazepam, lansoprazole,[d] rabeprazole, voriconazole
CYP2D6	Atomoxetine, desipramine, dextromethorphan, eliglustat,[e] nebivolol, nortriptyline, perphenazine, tolterodine, *R*-venlafaxine	Encainide, imipramine, metoprolol, propafenone, propranolol, tramadol, trimipramine, *S*-venlafaxine
CYP3A	Alfentanil, avanafil, buspirone, conivaptan, darifenacin, darunavir,[f] ebastine, everolimus, ibrutinib, lomitapide, lovastatin,[g] midazolam, naloxegol, nisoldipine, saquinavir,[f] simvastatin,[g] sirolimus, tacrolimus, tipranavir,[f] triazolam, vardenafil **Sensitive substrates of CYP3A with ≥10-fold increase in AUC by coadministration of strong index inhibitors:** Budesonide, dasatinib, dronedarone, eletriptan, eplerenone, felodipine, indinavir,[f] lurasidone, maraviroc, quetiapine, sildenafil, ticagrelor, tolvaptan	Alprazolam, aprepitant, atorvastatin,[c] colchicine, eliglustat,[e] pimozide, rilpivirine, rivaroxaban, tadalafil

Lists of recommended clinical probes and perpetrators for clinically relevant enzymes and transporters are available on the FDA website https://www.fda.gov/drugs/drug-interactions-labeling/drug-development-and-drug-interactions-table-substrates-inhibitors-and-inducers.
Note:

- Sensitive substrates are drugs that demonstrate an increase in AUC of ≥5-fold with strong index inhibitors of a given metabolic pathway in clinical DDI studies (Table 14.2). For sensitive substrates, data may be from any known index inhibitors for a particular pathway or whose AUC ratio in poor metabolizers for a specific enzyme is greater than or equal to 5-fold compared to extensive metabolizers.
- Moderate sensitive substrates are drugs that demonstrate an increase in AUC of ≥2 to <5-fold with strong index inhibitors of a given metabolic pathway in clinical DDI studies (Table 14.2).
- Other elimination pathways may also contribute to the elimination of the substrates listed in the table above and should be considered when assessing the drug interaction potential.

This table is prepared to provide examples of clinical substrates and not intended to be an exhaustive list. DDI data were collected based on a search of the University of Washington Drug Interaction Solutions (also known as "UW Metabolism and Transport Drug Interaction Database," https://www.druginteractionsolutions.org/).
Abbreviations: *AUC*, area under the concentration-time curve; *CYP*, cytochrome P450; *DDI*, drug-drug interaction; *EM*, extensive metabolizer; *OATP1B1*, organic anion transporting polypeptide 1B1.
[a]*Listed based on an in vivo induction study and the observed effect might be partly attributable to induction of other pathway(s).*
[b]*OATP1B1 substrate.*
[c]*Listed based on pharmacogenetic studies.*
[d]*S-Lansoprazole is a sensitive substrate in CYP2C19 EM subjects.*
[e]*Sensitive substrate of CYP2D6 and moderate sensitive substrate of CYP3A.*
[f]*Usually administered to patients in combination with ritonavir, a strong CYP3A inhibitor.*
[g]*Acid form is an OATP1B1 substrate.*

inhibitors cannot be considered as index drugs for prospective DDI studies because they lack specificity for one transporter and are often substrates of multiple transporters and/or enzymes. However, clinical interaction studies conducted with these drugs can provide useful information about potential DDIs with coadministered drugs (Fig. 14.4). For example, pitavastatin, rosuvastatin, and atorvastatin are clinical probes that are widely used to evaluate OATP1B-mediated DDIs, either following standard oral dose or as a microdose in transporter cocktail studies [50, 61]. Among these probes, pitavastatin is considered the most sensitive based on the contribution of OATP1B1, estimated from in vitro, *SLCO1B1* (OATP1B1) c.521T > C pharmacogenomic data, and DDI studies [62]. Although widely used, rosuvastatin is also a substrate of BCRP and several other transporters (e.g., OATP1B3, OATP2B1, NTCP, and OAT3) [61]. In the case of atorvastatin, the potential effect of inhibiting intestinal CYP3A4 and BCRP/P-gp efflux needs to be considered when interpreting the observed changes in its systemic exposure [149, 150].

One promising approach to address the issue of overlapping selectivity of transporters and enzymes is to use a transporter and enzyme probe drug cocktail [53, 151, 152] or to consider a specific study with design/end point measurements

TABLE 14.5 Examples of clinical substrates and inhibitors for transporters (for use in clinical DDI studies and drug labeling).

Transporter	Gene	Substrates	Inhibitors
P-gp	*ABCB1*	Dabigatran etexilate, digoxin, fexofenadine[c]	Amiodarone, carvedilol, clarithromycin, dronedarone, itraconazole, lapatinib, lopinavir and ritonavir, propafenone, quinidine, ranolazine, ritonavir, saquinavir and ritonavir, telaprevir, tipranavir and ritonavir, verapamil
BCRP	*ABCG2*	Rosuvastatin, sulfasalazine	Curcumin, cyclosporine A, eltrombopag
OATP1B1, OATP1B3	*SLCO1B1, SLCO1B3*	Asunaprevir, atorvastatin, bosentan, danoprevir, docetaxel,[b] fexofenadine,[c] glyburide, nateglinide, paclitaxel, pitavastatin,[d] pravastatin, repaglinide, rosuvastatin,[d] simvastatin acid	Atazanavir and ritonavir, clarithromycin, cyclosporine, erythromycin, gemfibrozil, lopinavir and ritonavir, rifampin (single dose), simeprevir
OAT1, OAT3	*SLC22A6, SLC22A8*	Adefovir,[e] cefaclor, ceftizoxime, famotidine,[a] furosemide, ganciclovir,[e] methotrexate, oseltamivir carboxylate,[a] penicillin G[a]	*p*-Aminohippuric acid (PAH),[f] probenecid, teriflunomide
MATE1, MATE2-K	*SLC47A1, SLC47A2*	Metformin	Cimetidine, dolutegravir, isavuconazole, ranolazine, trimethoprim, vandetanib

This table is prepared to provide examples of clinical substrates for various transporters and not intended to be an exhaustive list. Lists of recommended clinical probes and perpetrators for clinically relevant enzymes and transporters are available on the FDA website https://www.fda.gov/drugs/drug-interactions-labeling/drug-development-and-drug-interactions-table-substrates-inhibitors-and-inducers.
DDI data were collected based on a search of the University of Washington Drug Interaction Solutions (also known as "UW Metabolism and Transport Drug Interaction Database," https://www.druginteractionsolutions.org/).
Note:
Criteria for selecting clinical substrates are as follows:

- P-gp: (1) AUC fold-increase ≥2 with verapamil or quinidine coadministration and (2) in vitro transport by P-gp expression systems, but not extensively metabolized.
- BCRP: (1) AUC fold-increase ≥2 with pharmacogenetic alteration of ABCG2 (421C>A) and (2) in vitro transport by BCRP expression systems.
- OATP1B1/OATP1B3: (1) AUC fold-increase ≥2 with rifampin (single dose) or cyclosporine A coadministration, or pharmacogenetic alteration of SLCO1B1 (521T>C) and (2) in vitro transport by OATP1B1 or OATP1B3 expression systems.
- OAT1/OAT3: (1) AUC fold-increase ≥1.5 with probenecid coadministration, (2) fraction excreted unchanged into urine as an unchanged drug ≥0.5, and (3) in vitro transport by OAT1 or OAT3 expression systems.
- OCT2/MATE: Well-established substrate of cationic transport system (metformin).

Criteria for selecting in vivo inhibitors are as follows:

- P-gp: (1) AUC fold-increase of digoxin ≥2 with co-administration and (2) in vitro inhibitor.
- BCRP: (1) AUC fold-increase of sulfasalazine ≥1.5 with co-administration and (2) in vitro inhibitor. Cyclosporine A and eltrombopag were also included, although the available DDI information was with rosuvastatin, where inhibition of both BCRP and OATPs may have contributed to the observed interaction.
- OATP1B1/OATP1B3: (1) AUC fold-increase ≥2 for at least one of clinical substrates in this table with co-administration and (2) in vitro inhibitor.
- OAT1/OAT3: (1) AUC fold-increase ≥1.5 for at least one of clinical substrates in this table with co-administration and (2) in vitro inhibitor.
- OCT2/MATE: (1) AUC fold-increase of metformin ≥ 1.5 with co-administration and (2) in vitro inhibitor.

Abbreviations: *AUC*, area under the concentration-time curve.
[a] *In vitro data suggested higher contribution of OAT3 than OAT1.*
[b] *In vitro data suggested higher contribution of OATP1B3 than OATP1B1.*
[c] *Fexofenadine is a substrate for both P-gp and OATP1B.*
[d] *In vitro and pharmacogenetic data suggested higher contribution of OATP1B1 than OATP1B3.*
[e] *In vitro data suggested higher contribution of OAT1 than OAT3.*
[f] *In vivo data suggested specific inhibition of OAT1.*

that would allow differentiation of interaction mechanisms [36, 49]. Probe drug cocktails have been successfully applied in drug development and recognized by regulatory agencies for evaluation of metabolic DDI [153], but their use to investigate transporter-mediated DDIs is still relatively limited [53, 62, 151, 152]. Use of a cocktail approach at either the microdose or therapeutic dose level requires confirmation that there is no interaction between different transporter probes and validation of the method to allow translation of the data to clinical DDIs. The extent of DDI with a microdose can be higher compared with the therapeutic dose due to the saturation of transporters at therapeutic doses. In such cases, microdose DDI data can be considered as the "worst-case" scenario for evaluating the impact of a particular DDI [4].

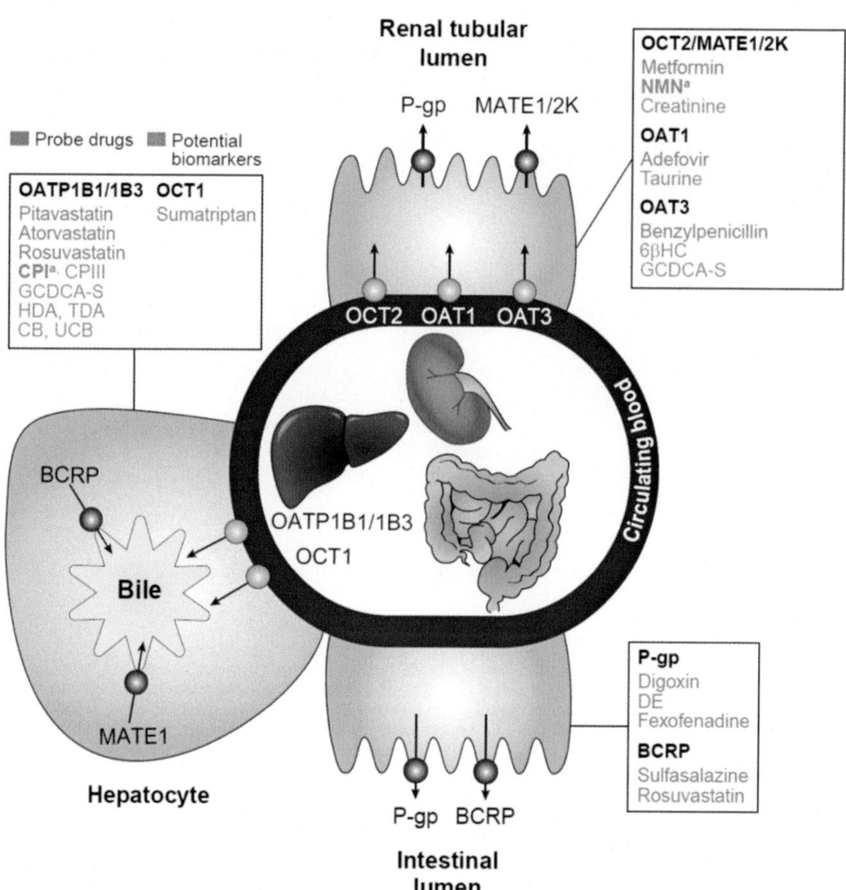

FIG. 14.4 Transporters and recommended probe drugs for clinical DDI studies to evaluate inhibitory effects of an investigational drug on major drug transporters expressed in gut, liver, and kidney.[a] *(Reproduced with permission from Chu X, Liao M, Shen H, Yoshida K, Zur AA, Arya V, et al. Clinical probes and endogenous biomarkers as substrates for transporter drug-drug interaction evaluation: perspectives from the International Transporter Consortium. Clin Pharmacol Ther 2018;104:836–864.)*
[a]Potential endogenous biomarkers with relatively higher selectivity and/or sensitivity for clinical evaluation based on current literature data. Green colored circles: uptake transporters; and purple colored circles: efflux transporters.

In the case of BCRP, selective clinical substrate probes and inhibitors are lacking and consensus has not been reached on the optimal way to evaluate clinical BCRP victim and perpetrator DDI potential [36]. Following a comprehensive review of in vitro, clinical DDI, and pharmacogenomic data, sulfasalazine has been proposed as the best available probe for intestinal BCRP and oral rosuvastatin as the best available probe for both intestinal and hepatic BCRP, either as a standard dose or microdose [36, 151, 152]. The analysis also identified oral curcumin (2000 mg) and lapatinib (subefficacious 250 mg dose) as the best available BCRP inhibitors. To evaluate individual contribution of intestinal and hepatic BCRP, i.v. rosuvastatin is proposed to evaluate contribution of hepatic BCRP inhibition, whereas oral administration of the probe reflects the effect on both intestinal and hepatic BCRP [4, 36].

OCT/MATE DDI evaluation represents an additional example where alternative study design/end point measurements are beneficial. Metformin is a well-known and routinely used clinical probe to study drugs that inhibit the renal uptake transporter OCT2 and efflux transporters (MATE1/-2K) [49, 50]. In addition to renal elimination, OCT/MATE modulators may affect metformin distribution in the liver (via OCT1) and therefore its glucose lowering PD effect. Considering these complexities, recent recommendations proposed that metformin DDI studies in drug development investigate both PK and PD endpoints to enable rational dose adjustment, i.e., changes in metformin renal clearance as well as its antihyperglycemic effects, with an oral glucose tolerance test for example [49].

Endogenous biomarkers

Theoretically, endogenous substances that are enzyme or transporter substrates could be used to determine the activity of enzymes and transporters in vivo, and their concentrations could be altered when enzyme/transporter activity is modulated by an interacting drug. Therefore, these endogenous substances have the potential to serve as biomarkers to study enzyme/transporter function in vivo and could be used in early clinical studies to determine whether new drugs are enzyme/transporter inhibitors. With appropriate validation, these results could obviate the need for dedicated clinical DDI studies. For example, plasma 4β-hydroxycholesterol (4β-OHC), which is the metabolite of CYP3A4/5-mediated cholesterol metabolism, has been advocated as an endogenous biomarker for CYP3A. Further, 4β-OHC and 4β-OHC:cholesterol and

6β-hydroxycortisol:cortisol ratios and have been suggested as a probe for CYP3A activity in the drug development process [154]. Due to its long half-life, 4β-OHC:cholesterol marker is more suitable to study CYP3A induction and is not sensitive to CYP3A inhibition. However, endogenous biomarkers are generally not recommended for the index studies because it is not possible to consistently extrapolate the effect on an endogenous substrate to other substrates of the same enzyme. Beyond CYP3A, no selective and validated biomarkers have identified for other CYPs such as CYP2D6, CYP2B6, CYP2C9, CYP2C19, CYP2C8 [154].

Compared with CYPs and other drug-metabolizing enzymes, there has been considerable recent progress to identify, characterize, and qualify endogenous biomarkers as selective substrates of transporters in early phase clinical studies [4, 56, 110, 111, 155–157]. These biomarkers can provide an early indication of potential transporter-mediated DDIs and inform the need for subsequent studies with clinical transporter probes. However, a number of factors, including selectivity, sensitivity, and kinetic determinants of their exposure, need to be verified before these endogenous compounds can be used to evaluate transporter function in vivo.

So far, characterization of endogenous compounds as substrates and potential biomarkers of drug transporters is most advanced for the hepatic transporter OATP1B1. Many endogenous molecules have been identified as substrates of this transporter including coproporphyrins (CP), bile acids, sulfated and glucuronidated bile acids, fatty acid dicarboxylates, conjugated and unconjugated bilirubin, among others. Among them, CP-I, a by-product of heme synthesis, shows the most promising potential as endogenous biomarker for clinical evaluation of OATP1B1-mediated DDIs in early drug development [61, 110–113, 155, 158–160]. Metabolic stability, minimal interindividual variability in its baseline plasma concentrations, and sensitivity in its response to a range of perpetrators are the key advantages of CP-I as a biomarker, in comparison to glycochenodeoxycholate-3-*O*-sulfate (GCDCA-S), tetradecanedioate (TDA), glycodeoxycholate 3-*O*-glucuronide (GDCA-3G) that may be monitored along with CP-I to determine if OATP1B activities change in the presence of an inhibitor or transporter polymorphism [34, 111, 157, 161]. The benefit of monitoring combined biomarkers (e.g., CP-I, bile acid conjugate, and/or one fatty acid) needs to be confirmed with larger data sets and against multiple OATP1B clinical probes and perpetrators.

Recent studies have also reported that CP-I is sensitive to the genetic polymorphism of OATP1B1. Subjects with the *SLCO1B1* 521 CC allelic variant associated with reduced transporter activity have increased exposure to OATP1B1 substrates, including CP-I [34, 162–164]. In addition, multiple studies have used mechanistic modeling approaches to understand CP-I formation and elimination mechanisms in order to optimize design of clinical studies with this biomarker [112, 165]. Clinical studies are also emerging in which CP-I has been used to assess OATP1B1 function and transporter-mediated interaction risk in specific patient populations, e.g., in renal impairment [166].

Additional factors impacting drug interactions

Impact of enzyme/transporter genetic polymorphisms on DDI magnitude

As discussed in Chapters 10 and 13, genetic polymorphisms occur in many CYP enzymes and transporters and significantly affect drug metabolism and transport. This genotypic variation also may affect the magnitude of the DDIs associated with these proteins. For example, rifampin, a potent inducer of multiple CYP enzymes, has been found to have a differential effect on exposure to the antiretroviral drug efavirenz, which is metabolized primarily by CYP2B6, that depends on a patient's CYP2B6 genotype. Efavirenz exposure would be expected to decrease dramatically during coadministration with rifampin. However, in patients carrying the *CYP2B6* single nucleotide polymorphism (SNP) 516G>T, which confers reduced CYP2B6 enzyme activity, efavirenz clearance is significantly lower in the presence of rifampin, relative to intermediate or normal metabolizer genotypes [167].

Over recent years, the clinical implications of drug-gene interactions on DDIs with respect to recommended codeine dosage regimens have been discussed extensively [168, 169]. Approximately 5%–10% of codeine is metabolized via CYP2D6 O-demethylation to the pharmacologically active metabolite morphine. Quinidine, a potent CYP2D6 inhibitor, significantly alters codeine's conversion to morphine in CYP2D6 extensive metabolizers. However, the rate of codeine's metabolism is already substantially diminished in genetically poor CYP2D6 metabolizers, so coadministration of quinidine has only a minimal additive effect on codeine PK and PD in these patients [170].

In some cases, differences in drug PK among genetically diverse groups of subjects can be used to predict potentially significant DDIs. For example, clopidogrel is metabolized by CYP2C19 to form an active metabolite. Subjects who are poor metabolizers of CYP2C19 due to genetic polymorphism have a decreased active metabolite formation and diminished inhibition of platelet aggregation. A similar decrease in metabolite formation and anticoagulant response occurs when clopidogrel is coadministered with omeprazole, a CYP2C19 inhibitor [171]. Thus, a clinically significant effect in a genetically poor metabolizer population may predict the likelihood for a clinically significant effect in patients that are coadministered an inhibitor of the same pathway. Similarly, the risk of statin myopathy that is increased in association with the *SLCO1B1* 521T > C allelic variant, in which OATP1B1 activity and hepatic uptake are reduced, is also apparent when statins are coadministered with potent inhibitors of this transporter [37, 41, 172]. Recent studies have reported differential cyclosporine DDI effects in SLCO1B1 c.521T > C genotype groups that are evident not just for the clinical drug probe, pravastatin, but also for the endogenous biomarker CP-I that has been proposed for evaluation of OATP1B1 function in vivo [34].

Particularly careful consideration is required in evaluating DDI risk when multiple polymorphic transporters/enzymes are involved in the metabolism and transport of a drug. In the case of rosuvastatin, genetic polymorphisms of both *SLCO1B1* c.521 T > C and *ABCG2* c.421C.A affect its PK. To avoid any potential confounding effect of OATP1B1 polymorphism, evaluation of rosuvastatin BCRP DDI risk should exclude any subjects with *SLCO1B1* 521 TC or CC polymorphic variants and enroll subjects that are homozygous for the *ABCG2* reference allele c.421C/C (most prevalent in non-Asian ethnicities) [36]. Otherwise, the impact of multiple genetic covariates (e.g., coexistence of *SLCO1B1* and *ABCG2* polymorphisms in the same subject) would need to be considered together with ethnicity, and these studies would need to be adequately powered to identify high-risk combination patterns that could cause an increase in rosuvastatin exposure, as it has been done for simvastatin [173]. PBPK modeling is particularly useful for exploring the consequences of these complex clinical scenarios [41, 133, 174]. For example, PBPK modeling was applied to explore the impact of coexisting *CYP2C8*3* and *SLCO1B1* polymorphisms on repaglinide PK and DDI [137]. PBPK modeling can also be applied to explore DDI risk in *CYP2C19* poor metabolizers in the case in which a parallel nonpolymorphic pathway (e.g., via CYP3A4) is completely inhibited (e.g., by ketoconazole) [175].

Contribution of metabolites to DDIs

Current regulatory guidance recommends that the DDI potential of a major metabolite (e.g., $\geq$25% of parent exposure for metabolites that are less polar than the parent) as perpetrators of drug-metabolizing enzymes and major drug transporters should be assessed along with that of the parent drug [50]. In general, metabolites are less likely to cause clinical CYP-mediated DDIs because of their increased polarity and metabolic stability. But they can be important contributor to the magnitude of DDIs observed with some inhibitors (e.g., itraconazole, diltiazem) and are considered in conjunction with a parent drug in PBPK-based evaluation of CY3A4 DDI risk [45, 176, 177]. In addition, a review of available drug interaction data for 129 clinical CYP-inhibitor drugs reported 2% of inhibitors would not even have been predicted as perpetrators without considering the inhibitory contribution of their metabolites (e.g., amiodarone, bupropion, and sertraline) [178]. Pharmacologically active metabolites require particular attention with respect to their DDI potential, as in the case of abemaciclib and evaluation of its DDI risk with multiple CYP3A4 modulators [179].

Following reports of severe interactions when gemfibrozil was coadministered with cerivastatin or repaglinide, there has been an increased interest on the effect of glucuronide metabolites on either metabolic enzymes or transporters [180, 181]. Subsequent in vitro studies identified that gemfibrozil acyl-glucuronide is an irreversible inhibitor of CYP2C8 following hydroxylation at a site distal to the glucuronide moiety, whereas the parent molecule was only a weak reversible inhibitor of this enzyme. In addition, both gemfibrozil and its glucuronide are inhibitors of hepatic uptake transporter OATP1B1 [182]. Thus, the apparent DDI potential of gemfibrozil toward either CYP2C8 or OATP1B1 cannot be understood without considering its glucuronide, as well as the systemic and intracellular exposure of both drug and metabolite [183]. Other glucuronides (e.g., clopidogrel glucuronide) have also shown inhibitory effects against metabolic enzymes, although in most cases the most pronounced inhibition is observed against CYP2C8 [184]. The complexity of these DDIs highlights the importance of prospective characterization of the inhibitory potential of glucuronide metabolites [185]; the current regulatory recommendation being that these should be investigated on a case-by-case basis [50]. PBPK modeling can facilitate evaluation of the interaction potential of metabolites, as illustrated by the case of the cyclosporine monohydroxylated metabolite AM1 which is a potent inhibitor of OATP1B1 [26]. However, wider use of this approach is restricted by the general lack of either exposure or potency data for metabolites in the early stages of drug development.

Labeling and DDI management

Drug interactions in product labeling

Drug interaction information is generally included in the DRUG INTERACTIONS (Section 7) and CLINICAL PHARMACOLOGY (Section 12) sections of the US prescribing information. When DDI information has important implications for the safe and effective use of the drug, it is also often included in varying levels of detail in other sections of the labeling, such as DOSAGE AND ADMINISTRATION (Section 2), CONTRAINDICATIONS (Section 4), WARNINGS AND PRECAUTIONS (Section 5), or HIGHLIGHTS. The labeling should include clinically relevant information about metabolic and transport pathways, metabolites, PK and/or PD interactions, and clinical implications of PK and/or PD interactions or genetic polymorphisms of drug-metabolizing enzymes and transporters, if applicable. When relevant, the description of clinical implications should include monitoring and dose adjustment recommendations [3, 186].

Drug interaction information in labeling may not always result from a clinical DDI study. In some cases, in vitro studies can rule out a specific type of drug interaction. In other cases, information can be extrapolated from a study conducted with one drug to another drug, when similar results are expected. Additionally, modeling approaches (such as PBPK) have been used to informed labeling recommendations. The following cases illustrate recent labeling examples.

Case 1

Rivaroxaban was approved for the prophylaxis of deep vein thrombosis. It is a substrate for CYP3A4, CYP2J2, P-gp, and BCRP, and also is eliminated renally as unchanged drug [187]. Coadministration of rivaroxaban with ketoconazole or ritonavir, both strong CYP3A and P-gp inhibitors, resulted in a clinically significant, ~2.5-fold increase in rivaroxaban *AUC* and anticoagulation effect (factor Xa inhibition and prothrombin time prolongation). However, studies with other inhibitors such as erythromycin and clarithromycin caused only 1.3- and 1.5-fold increases in rivaroxaban *AUC*, respectively, that were not deemed clinically relevant. Further, when rivaroxaban was evaluated in subjects with renal impairment and with CL_{CR} values down to 15 mL/min, the *AUC* was increased 1.4- to 1.6-fold compared with subjects with normal renal function. Thus, it was considered important to address the question of whether a combination of mild-to-moderate renal impairment plus concomitant administration of a mild-to-moderate CYP3A4 inhibitor, each of which by itself would be deemed insignificant, could result in a clinically significant increase in rivaroxaban exposure. This question was answered by PBPK analysis, which indicated that this combination of factors could increase rivaroxaban *AUC* by twofold or more [128, 188]. Therefore, there was a postmarketing requirement (PMR 1797-2) to "perform a clinical trial to evaluate the effect of renal impairment (i.e., mild, moderate, severe) plus the concurrent use of P-gp inhibitors and moderate inhibitors of CYP3A4 on the PK, PD, and safety of rivaroxaban in volunteers so that appropriate dosing recommendations could be developed in these populations" [189]. In the meantime, the labeling indicates:

> *"Based on simulated pharmacokinetic data, patients with renal impairment receiving XARELTO with drugs that are combined P-gp and weak or moderate CYP3A4 inhibitors (e.g., erythromycin, azithromycin, diltiazem, verapamil, quinidine, ranolazine, dronedarone, amiodarone, and felodipine) may have significant increases in exposure compared with patients with normal renal function and no inhibitor use, since both pathways of rivaroxaban elimination are affected. Since these increases may increase bleeding risk, use XARELTO in this situation only if the potential benefit justifies the potential risk."*

Following the completion of the PMR study, the labeling was updated with the DDI study results and updated recommendations. The current XARELTO labeling states [190]:

> ***"7 DRUG INTERACTIONS***
>
> ***7.2 Drugs that Inhibit Cytochrome P450 3A Enzymes and Drug Transport Systems***
>
> *Interaction with Combined P-gp and Moderate CYP3A Inhibitors in Patients with Renal Impairment*
>
> *XARELTO should not be used in patients with creatinine clearance (CrCL) 15 to <80 mL/min who are receiving concomitant combined P-gp and moderate CYP3A inhibitors (e.g., erythromycin) unless the potential benefit justifies the potential risk [see Warnings and Precautions (5.4) and Clinical Pharmacology (12.3)].*
>
> ***12 CLINICAL PHARMACOLOGY***
>
> ***12.3 Pharmacokinetics***
>
> *Drug-Disease Interactions with Drugs that Inhibit Cytochrome P450 3A Enzymes and Drug Transport Systems*
>
> *In a pharmacokinetic trial, XARELTO was administered as a single dose in subjects with mild (CrCl = 50 to 79 mL/min) or moderate renal impairment (CrCl = 30 to 49 mL/min) receiving multiple doses of erythromycin (a combined P-gp and moderate CYP3A inhibitor). Compared with XARELTO administered alone in subjects with normal renal function (CrCl >80 mL/min), subjects with mild and moderate renal impairment concomitantly receiving erythromycin reported a 76% and 99% increase in AUCinf and a 56% and 64% increase in Cmax, respectively. Similar trends in pharmacodynamic effects were also observed."*

Case 2

Simeprevir, a hepatitis C virus NS3/4A protease inhibitor, is actively taken up into liver by OATP1B1/OATP1B3 transporters, followed by metabolism via CYP3A4, and biliary elimination of the parent drug and its metabolites [108]. Information on the DDI risk in the drug labeling is supported extensively by PBPK modeling which was used to simulate simeprevir exposure in different patient populations and for a number of untested clinical scenarios [191]. Higher simeprevir plasma exposure was predicted when moderate/strong CYP3A inhibitors were coadministered with multiple doses of simeprevir compared with a single dose due to the saturation of CYP3A4/OATP1B. Concomitant administration of moderate/strong CYP3A inhibitors is not recommended per simeprevir US labeling. Simeprevir PBPK modeling was also used to evaluate changes in liver concentrations, as the target organ [44, 191]. Simulations of 100mg daily administration to Chinese and Japanese patients and 150mg daily to Caucasian patients resulted in comparable predicted liver exposure in all these populations. Although no dose adjustment was initially recommended based on ethnicity, the FDA issued a postmarketing requirement (PMR 2105-4) for simeprevir to evaluate safety signals in patients with East Asian ancestry. The labeling states [192]:

> *"**8 USE IN SPECIFIC POPULATIONS***
> ***8.6 Race***
> *Patients of East Asian ancestry exhibit higher simeprevir plasma exposures, but no dosage adjustment is required based on race [see Adverse Reactions (6.1), Clinical Pharmacology (12.3) and Clinical Studies (14.3)]."*

Postmarketing surveillance and real-world data for DDI

Drug interaction evaluation is an integral part of drug development, and DDIs, if not managed, can cause adverse drug events (ADEs). Although some drug interactions can be predicted through analysis of ADME pathways and be evaluated prior to approval to mitigate DDI risk, others become apparent only with clinical observations after the drugs are on the market. Postmarketing surveillance of potential drug interactions may utilize a "big data" approach that involves the identification of drug-ADE associations by data mining various electronic sources, including adverse event reports, the medical literature, electronic health records (EHRs), and social media. This approach has been useful in assisting the US FDA and other regulatory agencies in monitoring and decision-making regarding drug safety. Data mining can also assist pharmaceutical companies in drug safety surveillance efforts, in adhering to risk management plans, and in gathering real-world evidence to supplement clinical trial data [193, 194]. For example, potential drug interactions between the lipid-lowering agent pravastatin and the antidepressant paroxetine, two widely prescribed drugs, were studied through mining the US FDA's adverse event reporting system (AERS) for side-effect profiles involving glucose homeostasis [195]. There was a surprisingly strong signal for comedication with pravastatin and paroxetine, and they had a synergistic effect on increasing blood glucose when these two drugs were administered together. Further confirmation of this DDI was provided by a retrospective observational study of patients on combined paroxetine and pravastatin therapy which showed that the average increase in blood glucose was 19mg/dL (1.0mmol/L) overall and 48mg/dL (2.7mmol/L) in patients with diabetes. In contrast, neither drug administered individually was associated with a significant increase in glucose levels. This DDI was unexpected because an increase in glucose levels is not a general effect of combined therapy with selective serotonin reuptake inhibitors and statins. Thus, unpredictable or unidentified DDIs may be detected through postmarketing surveillance that utilizes real-world data. Other examples of uncovering PK- or PD-based drug interactions via the AERS system include DDIs involving St John's wort and oral contraceptives, that resulted in unexpected pregnancies, and with St John's wort and cyclosporine [196].

Conclusions

- Concomitant use of drugs is common, especially in elderly patients. Understanding drug metabolism, transport, and DDIs is critical to the benefit/risk assessment of a drug for personalized dosing in the era of polypharmacy. However, most clinical DDI studies are conducted with single perpetrator-victim combinations employing normal healthy volunteers and careful translation to the elderly population is needed
- An integrated approach that incorporates in vitro, in vivo, and in silico metabolism and transport studies to elucidate underlying DDI mechanisms and to evaluate the potential for drug interactions can optimize our knowledge and reduce the number of clinical studies that are needed

- Endogenous biomarkers can support de-risking of DDIs in early stages of drug development and guide the design of subsequent clinical studies with relevant drug substrates
- PBPK models can be used to predict multiple drug interactions and can help guide further clinical studies
- The clinical significance of DDIs should be interpreted based on well-defined exposure–response data and analyses
- Classification of CYP inhibitors and substrates can aid in DDI study design and cross-labeling of drugs
- DDI information should be appropriately placed in the labeling
- With improved understanding of the molecular basis of DDIs and the interplay of various intrinsic and extrinsic factors affecting these interactions, risks associated with DDIs can be assessed and managed to minimize untoward effects

Disclaimer

The views or opinions expressed in this chapter are those of the authors and should not be interpreted as the position of the U.S. Food and Drug Administration.

References

[1] Huang SM, Temple R, Throckmorton DC, Lesko LJ. Drug interaction studies: study design, data analysis, and implications for dosing and labeling. Clin Pharmacol Ther 2007;81(2):298–304.

[2] Houston J, Galetin A. In vitro techniques to study drug-drug interactions of drug metabolism: cytochrome P450. In: Pang KS, Rodrigues AD, Peter RM, editors. Enzymatic- and transporter-based drug-drug interactions: progress and future challenge. New York: Springer; 2010. p. 169–217.

[3] FDA. Clinical drug interaction studies—study design, data analysis, and clinical implications. Guidance for industry, https://www.fda.gov/media/134581/download; 2020.

[4] Chu X, Liao M, Shen H, Yoshida K, Zur AA, Arya V, et al. Clinical probes and endogenous biomarkers as substrates for transporter drug-drug interaction evaluation: perspectives from the International Transporter Consortium. Clin Pharmacol Ther 2018;104(5):836–864.

[5] Gessner A, Konig J, Fromm MF. Clinical aspects of transporter-mediated drug-drug interactions. Clin Pharmacol Ther 2019;105(6):1386–1394.

[6] Giacomini KM, Huang SM, Tweedie DJ, Benet LZ, Brouwer KL, Chu X, et al. Membrane transporters in drug development. Nat Rev Drug Discov 2010;9(3):215–236.

[7] Zamek-Gliszczynski MJ, Taub ME, Chothe PP, Chu X, Giacomini KM, Kim RB, et al. Transporters in drug development: 2018 ITC recommendations for transporters of emerging clinical importance. Clin Pharmacol Ther 2018;104(5):890–899.

[8] Yee SW, Brackman DJ, Ennis EA, Sugiyama Y, Kamdem LK, Blanchard R, et al. Influence of transporter polymorphisms on drug disposition and response: a perspective from the International Transporter Consortium. Clin Pharmacol Ther 2018;104(5):803–817.

[9] Thummel K, Kunze K, Shen DD. Metabolically-based drug–drug interactions: principles and mechanisms. In: Levy RH, Thummel KE, Trager WF, editors. Metabolic drug interactions. Philadelphia: Lippincott Williams & Williams; 2000. p. 3–47.

[10] Houston JB, Kenworthy KE, Galetin A. Typical and atypical enzyme kinetics. In: Fisher M, Lee J, Obach S, editors. Drug metabolizing enzymes: cytochrome P450 and other enzymes in drug discovery and development. Lausanne: Fontis Media; 2003. p. 211–254.

[11] Liu L, Bello A, Dresser MJ, Heald D, Komjathy SF, O'Mara E, et al. Best practices for the use of itraconazole as a replacement for ketoconazole in drug-drug interaction studies. J Clin Pharmacol 2016;56(2):143–151.

[12] Obach RS, Walsky RL, Venkatakrishnan K. Mechanism-based inactivation of human cytochrome p450 enzymes and the prediction of drug-drug interactions. Drug Metab Dispos 2007;35(2):246–255.

[13] Rowland Yeo K, Walsky RL, Jamei M, Rostami-Hodjegan A, Tucker GT. Prediction of time-dependent CYP3A4 drug-drug interactions by physiologically based pharmacokinetic modelling: impact of inactivation parameters and enzyme turnover. Eur J Pharm Sci 2011;43(3):160–173.

[14] Venkatakrishnan K, Obach RS. Drug-drug interactions via mechanism-based cytochrome P450 inactivation: points to consider for risk assessment from in vitro data and clinical pharmacologic evaluation. Curr Drug Metab 2007;8(5):449–462.

[15] Vieira ML, Kirby B, Ragueneau-Majlessi I, Galetin A, Chien JY, Einolf HJ, et al. Evaluation of various static in vitro-in vivo extrapolation models for risk assessment of the CYP3A inhibition potential of an investigational drug. Clin Pharmacol Ther 2014;95(2):189–198.

[16] Galetin A, Burt H, Gibbons L, Houston JB. Prediction of time-dependent CYP3A4 drug-drug interactions: impact of enzyme degradation, parallel elimination pathways, and intestinal inhibition. Drug Metab Dispos 2006;34(1):166–175.

[17] Kupferschmidt HH, Fattinger KE, Ha HR, Follath F, Krahenbuhl S. Grapefruit juice enhances the bioavailability of the HIV protease inhibitor saquinavir in man. Br J Clin Pharmacol 1998;45(4):355–359.

[18] Bailey DG, Malcolm J, Arnold O, Spence JD. Grapefruit juice-drug interactions. Br J Clin Pharmacol 1998;46(2):101–110.

[19] Gertz M, Davis JD, Harrison A, Houston JB, Galetin A. Grapefruit juice-drug interaction studies as a method to assess the extent of intestinal availability: utility and limitations. Curr Drug Metab 2008;9(8):785–795.

[20] Lundahl J, Regardh CG, Edgar B, Johnsson G. Relationship between time of intake of grapefruit juice and its effect on pharmacokinetics and pharmacodynamics of felodipine in healthy subjects. Eur J Clin Pharmacol 1995;49(1–2):61–67.

[21] Edgar B, Bailey D, Bergstrand R, Johnsson G, Regardh CG. Acute effects of drinking grapefruit juice on the pharmacokinetics and dynamics of felodipine–and its potential clinical relevance. Eur J Clin Pharmacol 1992;42(3):313–317.

[22] Zamek-Gliszczynski MJ, Lee CA, Poirier A, Bentz J, Chu X, Ishikawa T, et al. ITC recommendations on transporter kinetic parameter estimation and translational modeling of transport-mediated PK and DDIs in humans. Clin Pharmacol Ther 2013;94(1):64–79.

[23] Lee CA, Kalvass JC, Galetin A, Zamek-Gliszczynski MJ. ITC commentary on the prediction of digoxin clinical drug-drug interactions from in vitro transporter assays. Clin Pharmacol Ther 2014;96(3):298–301.

[24] Izumi S, Nozaki Y, Komori T, Maeda K, Takenaka O, Kusano K, et al. Substrate-dependent inhibition of organic anion transporting polypeptide 1B1: comparative analysis with prototypical probe substrates estradiol-17beta-glucuronide, estrone-3-sulfate, and sulfobromophthalein. Drug Metab Dispos 2013;41(10):1859–1866.

[25] Mathialagan S, Rodrigues AD, Feng B. Evaluation of renal transporter inhibition using creatinine as a substrate in vitro to assess the clinical risk of elevated serum creatinine. J Pharm Sci 2017;106(9):2535–2541.

[26] Gertz M, Cartwright CM, Hobbs MJ, Kenworthy KE, Rowland M, Houston JB, et al. Cyclosporine inhibition of hepatic and intestinal CYP3A4, uptake and efflux transporters: application of PBPK modeling in the assessment of drug-drug interaction potential. Pharm Res 2013;30(3):761–780.

[27] Shitara Y, Sugiyama Y. Preincubation-dependent and long-lasting inhibition of organic anion transporting polypeptide (OATP) and its impact on drug-drug interactions. Pharmacol Ther 2017;177:67–80.

[28] Park JE, Shitara Y, Lee W, Morita S, Sahi J, Toshimoto K, et al. Improved prediction of the drug-drug interactions of pemafibrate caused by cyclosporine A and rifampicin via PBPK modeling: consideration of the albumin-mediated hepatic uptake of pemafibrate and inhibition constants with preincubation against OATP1B. J Pharm Sci 2021;110(1):517–528.

[29] Zou L, Pottel J, Khuri N, Ngo HX, Ni Z, Tsakalozou E, et al. Interactions of oral molecular excipients with breast cancer resistance protein. BCRP Mol Pharm 2020;17(3):748–756.

[30] Zou L, Spanogiannopoulos P, Pieper LM, Chien HC, Cai W, Khuri N, et al. Bacterial metabolism rescues the inhibition of intestinal drug absorption by food and drug additives. Proc Natl Acad Sci U S A 2020;117(27):16009–16018.

[31] Zheng HX, Huang Y, Frassetto LA, Benet LZ. Elucidating rifampin's inducing and inhibiting effects on glyburide pharmacokinetics and blood glucose in healthy volunteers: unmasking the differential effects of enzyme induction and transporter inhibition for a drug and its primary metabolite. Clin Pharmacol Ther 2009;85(1):78–85.

[32] Prueksaritanont T, Chu X, Evers R, Klopfer SO, Caro L, Kothare PA, et al. Pitavastatin is a more sensitive and selective organic anion-transporting polypeptide 1B clinical probe than rosuvastatin. Br J Clin Pharmacol 2014;78(3):587–598.

[33] Kiser JJ, Gerber JG, Predhomme JA, Wolfe P, Flynn DM, Hoody DW. Drug/drug interaction between lopinavir/ritonavir and rosuvastatin in healthy volunteers. J Acquir Immune Defic Syndr 2008;47(5):570–578.

[34] Yee SW, Giacomini MM, Shen H, Humphreys WG, Horng H, Brian W, et al. Organic anion transporter polypeptide 1B1 polymorphism modulates the extent of drug-drug interaction and associated biomarker levels in healthy volunteers. Clin Transl Sci 2019;12(4):388–399.

[35] Ho RH, Tirona RG, Leake BF, Glaeser H, Lee W, Lemke CJ, et al. Drug and bile acid transporters in rosuvastatin hepatic uptake: function, expression, and pharmacogenetics. Gastroenterology 2006;130(6):1793–1806.

[36] Lee CA, O'Connor MA, Ritchie TK, Galetin A, Cook JA, Ragueneau-Majlessi I, et al. Breast cancer resistance protein (ABCG2) in clinical pharmacokinetics and drug interactions: practical recommendations for clinical victim and perpetrator drug-drug interaction study design. Drug Metab Dispos 2015;43(4):490–509.

[37] Simonson SG, Raza A, Martin PD, Mitchell PD, Jarcho JA, Brown CD, et al. Rosuvastatin pharmacokinetics in heart transplant recipients administered an antirejection regimen including cyclosporine. Clin Pharmacol Ther 2004;76(2):167–177.

[38] Lemahieu WP, Hermann M, Asberg A, Verbeke K, Holdaas H, Vanrenterghem Y, et al. Combined therapy with atorvastatin and calcineurin inhibitors: no interactions with tacrolimus. Am J Transplant 2005;5(9):2236–2243.

[39] Ichimaru N, Takahara S, Kokado Y, Wang JD, Hatori M, Kameoka H, et al. Changes in lipid metabolism and effect of simvastatin in renal transplant recipients induced by cyclosporine or tacrolimus. Atherosclerosis 2001;158(2):417–423.

[40] Kajosaari LI, Niemi M, Neuvonen M, Laitila J, Neuvonen PJ, Backman JT. Cyclosporine markedly raises the plasma concentrations of repaglinide. Clin Pharmacol Ther 2005;78(4):388–399.

[41] Galetin A, Zhao P, Huang SM. Physiologically based pharmacokinetic modeling of drug transporters to facilitate individualized dose prediction. J Pharm Sci 2017;106(9):2204–2208.

[42] Chu X, Korzekwa KR, Elsby R, Fenner KS, Galetin A, Lai Y, et al. Intracellular drug concentrations and transporters: measurement, modeling and implications in the liver. Clin Pharmacol Ther 2013;94(1):126–141.

[43] Link E, Parish S, Armitage J, Bowman L, Heath S, Matsuda F, et al. SLCO1B1 variants and statin-induced myopathy–a genomewide study. N Engl J Med 2008;359(8):789–799.

[44] Guo Y, Chu X, Parrott NJ, Brouwer KLR, Hsu V, Nagar S, et al. Advancing predictions of tissue and intracellular drug concentrations using in vitro, imaging and physiologically based pharmacokinetic modeling approaches. Clin Pharmacol Ther 2018;104(5):865–889.

[45] Tsamandouras N, Dickinson G, Guo Y, Hall S, Rostami-Hodjegan A, Galetin A, et al. Development and application of a mechanistic pharmacokinetic model for simvastatin and its active metabolite simvastatin acid using an integrated population PBPK approach. Pharm Res 2015;32 (6):1864–1883.

[46] Chu X, Bleasby K, Chan GH, Nunes I, Evers R. The complexities of interpreting reversible elevated serum creatinine levels in drug development: does a correlation with inhibition of renal transporters exist? Drug Metab Dispos 2016;44(9):1498–1509.

[47] Dutt MK, Moody P, Northfield TC. Effect of cimetidine on renal function in man. Br J Clin Pharmacol 1981;12(1):47–50.

[48] Gong L, Goswami S, Giacomini KM, Altman RB, Klein TE. Metformin pathways: pharmacokinetics and pharmacodynamics. Pharmacogenet Genomics 2012;22(11):820–827.

[49] Zamek-Gliszczynski MJ, Chu X, Cook JA, Custodio JM, Galetin A, Giacomini KM, et al. ITC commentary on metformin clinical drug-drug interaction study design that enables an efficacy- and safety-based dose adjustment decision. Clin Pharmacol Ther 2018;104(5):781–784.
[50] FDA. In vitro metabolism- and transporter-mediated drug-drug interaction studies. Guidance for industry, https://www.fda.gov/media/134582/download; 2020.
[51] Hibma JE, Zur AA, Castro RA, Wittwer MB, Keizer RJ, Yee SW, et al. The effect of famotidine, a MATE1-selective inhibitor, on the pharmacokinetics and pharmacodynamics of metformin. Clin Pharmacokinet 2016;55(6):711–721.
[52] Cho SK, Kim CO, Park ES, Chung JY. Verapamil decreases the glucose-lowering effect of metformin in healthy volunteers. Br J Clin Pharmacol 2014;78(6):1426–1432.
[53] Trueck C, Hsin CH, Scherf-Clavel O, Schaeffeler E, Lenssen R, Gazzaz M, et al. A clinical drug-drug interaction study assessing a novel drug transporter phenotyping cocktail with adefovir, sitagliptin, metformin, pitavastatin, and digoxin. Clin Pharmacol Ther 2019;106(6):1398–1407.
[54] Maeda K, Tian Y, Fujita T, Ikeda Y, Kumagai Y, Kondo T, et al. Inhibitory effects of p-aminohippurate and probenecid on the renal clearance of adefovir and benzylpenicillin as probe drugs for organic anion transporter (OAT) 1 and OAT3 in humans. Eur J Pharm Sci 2014;59:94–103.
[55] Mathialagan S, Piotrowski MA, Tess DA, Feng B, Litchfield J, Varma MV. Quantitative prediction of human renal clearance and drug-drug interactions of organic anion transporter substrates using in vitro transport data: a relative activity factor approach. Drug Metab Dispos 2017;45(4):409–417.
[56] Shen H, Nelson DM, Oliveira RV, Zhang Y, McNaney CA, Gu X, et al. Discovery and validation of pyridoxic acid and homovanillic acid as novel endogenous plasma biomarkers of organic anion transporter (OAT) 1 and OAT3 in cynomolgus monkeys. Drug Metab Dispos 2018;46(2):178–188.
[57] Lacy SA, Hitchcock MJ, Lee WA, Tellier P, Cundy KC. Effect of oral probenecid coadministration on the chronic toxicity and pharmacokinetics of intravenous cidofovir in cynomolgus monkeys. Toxicol Sci 1998;44(2):97–106.
[58] Lin JH. Drug-drug interaction mediated by inhibition and induction of P-glycoprotein. Adv Drug Deliv Rev 2003;55(1):53–81.
[59] Schinkel AH, Jonker JW. Mammalian drug efflux transporters of the ATP binding cassette (ABC) family: an overview. Adv Drug Deliv Rev 2003;55(1):3–29.
[60] Fenner KS, Troutman MD, Kempshall S, Cook JA, Ware JA, Smith DA, et al. Drug-drug interactions mediated through P-glycoprotein: clinical relevance and in vitro-in vivo correlation using digoxin as a probe drug. Clin Pharmacol Ther 2009;85(2):173–181.
[61] Chu X, Galetin A, Zamek-Gliszczynski MJ, Zhang L, Tweedie DJ, International Transporter Consortium. Dabigatran etexilate and digoxin: comparison as clinical probe substrates for evaluation of P-gp inhibition. Clin Pharmacol Ther 2018;104(5):788–792.
[62] Prueksaritanont T, Tatosian DA, Chu X, Railkar R, Evers R, Chavez-Eng C, et al. Validation of a microdose probe drug cocktail for clinical drug interaction assessments for drug transporters and CYP3A. Clin Pharmacol Ther 2017;101(4):519–530.
[63] Poirier A, Portmann R, Cascais AC, Bader U, Walter I, Ullah M, et al. The need for human breast cancer resistance protein substrate and inhibition evaluation in drug discovery and development: why, when, and how? Drug Metab Dispos 2014;42(9):1466–1477.
[64] Reitman ML, Chu X, Cai X, Yabut J, Venkatasubramanian R, Zajic S, et al. Rifampin's acute inhibitory and chronic inductive drug interactions: experimental and model-based approaches to drug-drug interaction trial design. Clin Pharmacol Ther 2011;89(2):234–242.
[65] Lin JH. CYP induction-mediated drug interactions: in vitro assessment and clinical implications. Pharm Res 2006;23(6):1089–1116.
[66] Hakkola J, Hukkanen J, Turpeinen M, Pelkonen O. Inhibition and induction of CYP enzymes in humans: an update. Arch Toxicol 2020;94(11):3671–3722.
[67] European Medicines Agency (EMA). Guideline on the investigation of drug interactions, EMA website [online] http://www.ema.europa.eu; 2012.
[68] Rodrigues AD, Lai Y, Shen H, Varma MVS, Rowland A, Oswald S. Induction of human intestinal and hepatic organic anion transporting polypeptides: where is the evidence for its relevance in drug-drug interactions? Drug Metab Dispos 2020;48(3):205–216.
[69] Marschall HU, Wagner M, Zollner G, Fickert P, Diczfalusy U, Gumhold J, et al. Complementary stimulation of hepatobiliary transport and detoxification systems by rifampicin and ursodeoxycholic acid in humans. Gastroenterology 2005;129(2):476–485.
[70] Williamson B, Dooley KE, Zhang Y, Back DJ, Owen A. Induction of influx and efflux transporters and cytochrome P450 3A4 in primary human hepatocytes by rifampin, rifabutin, and rifapentine. Antimicrob Agents Chemother 2013;57(12):6366–6369.
[71] Kalvass JC, Polli JW, Bourdet DL, Feng B, Huang SM, Liu X, et al. Why clinical modulation of efflux transport at the human blood-brain barrier is unlikely: the ITC evidence-based position. Clin Pharmacol Ther 2013;94(1):80–94.
[72] Zamek-Gliszczynski MJ, Patel M, Yang X, Lutz JD, Chu X, Brouwer KLR, et al. Intestinal P-gp and putative hepatic OATP1B induction: ITC perspective on drug development implications. Clin Pharmacol Ther 2021;109(1):55–64.
[73] Westphal K, Weinbrenner A, Zschiesche M, Franke G, Knoke M, Oertel R, et al. Induction of P-glycoprotein by rifampin increases intestinal secretion of talinolol in human beings: a new type of drug/drug interaction. Clin Pharmacol Ther 2000;68(4):345–355.
[74] Greiner B, Eichelbaum M, Fritz P, Kreichgauer HP, von Richter O, Zundler J, et al. The role of intestinal P-glycoprotein in the interaction of digoxin and rifampin. J Clin Invest 1999;104(2):147–153.
[75] Lutz JD, Kirby BJ, Wang L, Song Q, Ling J, Massetto B, et al. Cytochrome P450 3A induction predicts P-glycoprotein induction; part 2: prediction of decreased substrate exposure after rifabutin or carbamazepine. Clin Pharmacol Ther 2018;104(6):1191–1198.
[76] Lutz JD, Kirby BJ, Wang L, Song Q, Ling J, Massetto B, et al. Cytochrome P450 3A induction predicts P-glycoprotein induction; part 1: establishing induction relationships using ascending dose rifampin. Clin Pharmacol Ther 2018;104(6):1182–1190.
[77] Alam K, Crowe A, Wang X, Zhang P, Ding K, Li L, et al. Regulation of organic anion transporting polypeptides (OATP) 1B1- and OATP1B3-mediated transport: an updated review in the context of OATP-mediated drug-drug interactions. Int J Mol Sci 2018;19(3).
[78] Niu C, Wang Y, Zhao X, Tep S, Murakami E, Subramanian R, et al. Organic anion-transporting polypeptide genes are not induced by the pregnane X receptor activator rifampin: studies in hepatocytes in vitro and in monkeys in vivo. Drug Metab Dispos 2019;47(12):1433–1442.

[79] FDA. Framework for assessing pH-dependent drug-drug interactions, https://www.govinfo.gov/content/pkg/FR-2018-05-22/pdf/2018-10927.pdf; 2018.

[80] Zhang L, Wu F, Lee SC, Zhao H, Zhang L. pH-dependent drug-drug interactions for weak base drugs: potential implications for new drug development. Clin Pharmacol Ther 2014;96(2):266–277.

[81] Mitra A, Parrott N, Miller N, Lloyd R, Tistaert C, Heimbach T, et al. Prediction of pH-dependent drug-drug interactions for basic drugs using physiologically based biopharmaceutics modeling: industry case studies. J Pharm Sci 2020;109(3):1380–1394.

[82] Dong Z, Li J, Wu F, Zhao P, Lee SC, Zhang L, et al. Application of physiologically-based pharmacokinetic modeling to predict gastric pH-dependent drug-drug interactions for weak base drugs. CPT Pharmacometrics Syst Pharmacol 2020;9(8):456–465.

[83] Krishna R, East L, Larson P, Valiathan C, Butterfield K, Teng Y, et al. Effect of metal-cation antacids on the pharmacokinetics of 1200 mg raltegravir. J Pharm Pharmacol 2016;68(11):1359–1365.

[84] Panjehshahin MR, Bowmer CJ, Yates MS. Effect of valproic acid, its unsaturated metabolites and some structurally related fatty acids on the binding of warfarin and dansylsarcosine to human albumin. Biochem Pharmacol 1991;41(8):1227–1233.

[85] Yoon HW, Giraldo EA, Wijdicks EF. Valproic acid and warfarin: an underrecognized drug interaction. Neurocrit Care 2011;15(1):182–185.

[86] Wald DS, Law M, Morris JK, Bestwick JP, Wald NJ. Combination therapy versus monotherapy in reducing blood pressure: meta-analysis on 11,000 participants from 42 trials. Am J Med 2009;122(3):290–300.

[87] Whelton PK, Carey RM, Aronow WS, Casey DE Jr, Collins KJ, Dennison Himmelfarb C, et al. 2017 ACC/AHA/AAPA/ABC/ACPM/AGS/APhA/ASH/ASPC/NMA/PCNA guideline for the prevention, detection, evaluation, and management of high blood pressure in adults: executive summary: a report of the American College of Cardiology/American Heart Association Task Force on Clinical Practice Guidelines. Circulation 2018;138(17):e426–e483.

[88] Arshad U, Pertinez H, Box H, Tatham L, Rajoli RKR, Curley P, et al. Prioritization of anti-SARS-Cov-2 drug repurposing opportunities based on plasma and target site concentrations derived from their established human pharmacokinetics. Clin Pharmacol Ther 2020;108(4):775–790.

[89] van der Graaf PH, Giacomini KM. COVID-19: a defining moment for clinical pharmacology? Clin Pharmacol Ther 2020;108(1):11–15.

[90] Peck RW, Weiner D, Cook J, Robert Powell J. A real-world evidence framework for optimizing dosing in all patients with COVID-19. Clin Pharmacol Ther 2020;108(5):921–923.

[91] Rosenberg ES, Dufort EM, Udo T, Wilberschied LA, Kumar J, Tesoriero J, et al. Association of treatment with hydroxychloroquine or azithromycin with in-hospital mortality in patients with COVID-19 in New York state. JAMA 2020;323(24):2493–2502.

[92] Geleris J, Sun Y, Platt J, Zucker J, Baldwin M, Hripcsak G, et al. Observational study of hydroxychloroquine in hospitalized patients with Covid-19. N Engl J Med 2020;382(25):2411–2418.

[93] Gautret P, Lagier JC, Parola P, Hoang VT, Meddeb L, Mailhe M, et al. Hydroxychloroquine and azithromycin as a treatment of COVID-19: results of an open-label non-randomized clinical trial. Int J Antimicrob Agents 2020;56(1):105949.

[94] Scotcher D, Jones C, Rostami-Hodjegan A, Galetin A. Novel minimal physiologically-based model for the prediction of passive tubular reabsorption and renal excretion clearance. Eur J Pharm Sci 2016;94:59–71.

[95] Matsuzaki T, Scotcher D, Darwich AS, Galetin A, Rostami-Hodjegan A. Towards further verification of physiologically-based kidney models: predictability of the effects of urine-flow and urine-ph on renal clearance. J Pharmacol Exp Ther 2019;368(2):157–168.

[96] Blanchard J, Sawers SJ. Relationship between urine flow rate and renal clearance of caffeine in man. J Clin Pharmacol 1983;23(4):134–138.

[97] Birkett DJ, Miners JO. Caffeine renal clearance and urine caffeine concentrations during steady state dosing. Implications for monitoring caffeine intake during sports events. Br J Clin Pharmacol 1991;31(4):405–408.

[98] Proudfoot AT, Krenzelok EP, Vale JA. Position paper on urine alkalinization. J Toxicol Clin Toxicol 2004;42(1):1–26.

[99] Perazella MA. Crystal-induced acute renal failure. Am J Med 1999;106(4):459–465.

[100] Jing X, Ji P, Schrieber SJ, Fletcher EP, Sahajwalla C. Update on therapeutic protein-drug interaction: information in labeling. Clin Pharmacokinet 2020;59(1):25–36.

[101] Kenny JR, Liu MM, Chow AT, Earp JC, Evers R, Slatter JG, et al. Therapeutic protein drug-drug interactions: navigating the knowledge gaps-highlights from the 2012 AAPS NBC roundtable and IQ Consortium/FDA workshop. AAPS J 2013;15(4):933–940.

[102] Evers R, Dallas S, Dickmann LJ, Fahmi OA, Kenny JR, Kraynov E, et al. Critical review of preclinical approaches to investigate cytochrome p450-mediated therapeutic protein drug-drug interactions and recommendations for best practices: a white paper. Drug Metab Dispos 2013;41(9):1598–1609.

[103] Huang SM, Zhao H, Lee JI, Reynolds K, Zhang L, Temple R, et al. Therapeutic protein-drug interactions and implications for drug development. Clin Pharmacol Ther 2010;87(4):497–503.

[104] FDA. Drug-drug interaction assessment for therapeutic proteins. Guidance for industry, https://www.fda.gov/media/140909/download; 2020.

[105] Morgan ET, Goralski KB, Piquette-Miller M, Renton KW, Robertson GR, Chaluvadi MR, et al. Regulation of drug-metabolizing enzymes and transporters in infection, inflammation, and cancer. Drug Metab Dispos 2008;36(2):205–216.

[106] Schmitt C, Kuhn B, Zhang X, Kivitz AJ, Grange S. Disease-drug-drug interaction involving tocilizumab and simvastatin in patients with rheumatoid arthritis. Clin Pharmacol Ther 2011;89(5):735–740.

[107] Woolsey SJ, Beaton MD, Mansell SE, Leon-Ponte M, Yu J, Pin CL, et al. A fibroblast growth factor 21-pregnane X receptor pathway downregulates hepatic CYP3A4 in nonalcoholic fatty liver disease. Mol Pharmacol 2016;90(4):437–446.

[108] Snoeys J, Beumont M, Monshouwer M, Ouwerkerk-Mahadevan S. Mechanistic understanding of the nonlinear pharmacokinetics and intersubject variability of simeprevir: A PBPK-guided drug development approach. Clin Pharmacol Ther 2016;99(2):224–234.

[109] Billington S, Shoner S, Lee S, Clark-Snustad K, Pennington M, Lewis D, et al. Positron emission tomography imaging of [(11) C]rosuvastatin hepatic concentrations and hepatobiliary transport in humans in the absence and presence of cyclosporin A. Clin Pharmacol Ther 2019;106(5):1056–1066.

[110] Jones NS, Yoshida K, Salphati L, Kenny JR, Durk MR, Chinn LW. Complex DDI by fenebrutinib and the use of transporter endogenous biomarkers to elucidate the mechanism of DDI. Clin Pharmacol Ther 2020;107(1):269–277.

[111] Barnett S, Ogungbenro K, Menochet K, Shen H, Humphreys WG, Galetin A. Comprehensive evaluation of the utility of 20 endogenous molecules as biomarkers of OATP1B inhibition compared with rosuvastatin and coproporphyrin I. J Pharmacol Exp Ther 2019;368(1):125–135.

[112] Barnett S, Ogungbenro K, Menochet K, Shen H, Lai Y, Humphreys WG, et al. Gaining mechanistic insight into coproporphyrin I as endogenous biomarker for OATP1B-mediated drug-drug interactions using population pharmacokinetic modeling and simulation. Clin Pharmacol Ther 2018;104(3):564–574.

[113] Kunze A, Ediage EN, Dillen L, Monshouwer M, Snoeys J. Clinical investigation of coproporphyrins as sensitive biomarkers to predict mild to strong OATP1B-mediated drug-drug interactions. Clin Pharmacokinet 2018;57(12):1559–1570.

[114] Zientek MA, Youdim K. Reaction phenotyping: advances in the experimental strategies used to characterize the contribution of drug-metabolizing enzymes. Drug Metab Dispos 2015;43(1):163–181.

[115] Ito K, Brown HS, Houston JB. Database analyses for the prediction of in vivo drug-drug interactions from in vitro data. Br J Clin Pharmacol 2004;57 (4):473–486.

[116] Brown HS, Galetin A, Hallifax D, Houston JB. Prediction of in vivo drug-drug interactions from in vitro data : factors affecting prototypic drug-drug interactions involving CYP2C9, CYP2D6 and CYP3A4. Clin Pharmacokinet 2006;45(10):1035–1050.

[117] Fahmi OA, Hurst S, Plowchalk D, Cook J, Guo F, Youdim K, et al. Investigation of different algorithms for predicting clinical drug-drug interactions, based on the use of CYP3A4 in vitro data; predictions of compounds as precipitants of interaction. Drug Metab Dispos 2009;37 (8):1658–1666.

[118] Galetin A, Gertz M, Houston JB. Contribution of intestinal cytochrome P450-mediated metabolism to drug-drug inhibition and induction interactions. Drug Metab Pharmacokinet 2010;25(1):28–47.

[119] Rowland M, Peck C, Tucker G. Physiologically-based pharmacokinetics in drug development and regulatory science. Annu Rev Pharmacol Toxicol 2011;51:45–73.

[120] Zhao P, Zhang L, Grillo JA, Liu Q, Bullock JM, Moon YJ, et al. Applications of physiologically based pharmacokinetic (PBPK) modeling and simulation during regulatory review. Clin Pharmacol Ther 2011;89(2):259–267.

[121] Jones HM, Chen Y, Gibson C, Heimbach T, Parrott N, Peters SA, et al. Physiologically based pharmacokinetic modeling in drug discovery and development: a pharmaceutical industry perspective. Clin Pharmacol Ther 2015;97(3):247–262.

[122] Wagner C, Zhao P, Pan Y, Hsu V, Grillo J, Huang SM, et al. Application of physiologically based pharmacokinetic (PBPK) modeling to support dose selection: report of an FDA public workshop on PBPK. CPT Pharmacometrics Syst Pharmacol 2015;4(4):226–230.

[123] Bjornsson TD, Callaghan JT, Einolf HJ, Fischer V, Gan L, Grimm S, et al. The conduct of in vitro and in vivo drug-drug interaction studies: a Pharmaceutical Research and Manufacturers of America (PhRMA) perspective. Drug Metab Dispos 2003;31(7):815–832.

[124] Yoshida K, Zhao P, Zhang L, Abernethy DR, Rekic D, Reynolds KS, et al. In vitro-in vivo extrapolation of metabolism- and transporter-mediated drug-drug interactions-overview of basic prediction methods. J Pharm Sci 2017;106(9):2209–2213.

[125] Tucker GT, Houston JB, Huang SM. Optimizing drug development: strategies to assess drug metabolism/transporter interaction potential-toward a consensus. Clin Pharmacol Ther 2001;70(2):103–114.

[126] Fahmi OA, Maurer TS, Kish M, Cardenas E, Boldt S, Nettleton D. A combined model for predicting CYP3A4 clinical net drug-drug interaction based on CYP3A4 inhibition, inactivation, and induction determined in vitro. Drug Metab Dispos 2008;36(8):1698–1708.

[127] Rostami-Hodjegan A. Physiologically based pharmacokinetics joined with in vitro-in vivo extrapolation of ADME: a marriage under the arch of systems pharmacology. Clin Pharmacol Ther 2012;92(1):50–61.

[128] Huang SM, Rowland M. The role of physiologically based pharmacokinetic modeling in regulatory review. Clin Pharmacol Ther 2012;91 (3):542–549.

[129] Grimstein M, Yang Y, Zhang X, Grillo J, Huang SM, Zineh I, et al. Physiologically based pharmacokinetic modeling in regulatory science: an update from the U.S. Food and Drug Administration's Office of Clinical Pharmacology. J Pharm Sci 2019;108(1):21–25.

[130] Shebley M, Sandhu P, Emami Riedmaier A, Jamei M, Narayanan R, Patel A, et al. Physiologically based pharmacokinetic model qualification and reporting procedures for regulatory submissions: a consortium perspective. Clin Pharmacol Ther 2018;104(1):88–110.

[131] Gertz M, Houston JB, Galetin A. Physiologically based pharmacokinetic modeling of intestinal first-pass metabolism of CYP3A substrates with high intestinal extraction. Drug Metab Dispos 2011;39(9):1633–1642.

[132] Watanabe T, Kusuhara H, Maeda K, Shitara Y, Sugiyama Y. Physiologically based pharmacokinetic modeling to predict transporter-mediated clearance and distribution of pravastatin in humans. J Pharmacol Exp Ther 2009;328(2):652–662.

[133] Rostami-Hodjegan A. Reverse translation in PBPK and QSP: going backwards in order to go forward with confidence. Clin Pharmacol Ther 2018;103(2):224–232.

[134] FDA. Physiologically based pharmacokinetic analyses—format and content. Guidance for industry, https://www.fda.gov/media/101469/download; 2018.

[135] European Medicines Agency (EMA). EMA/CHMP/458101/2016—Guideline on the qualification and reporting of physiologically based pharmacokinetic (PBPK) modelling and simulation, https://www.ema.europa.eu/en/documents/scientific-guideline/guideline-reporting-physiologically-based-pharmacokinetic-pbpk-modelling-simulation_en.pdf; 2018.

[136] Taskar KS, Pilla Reddy V, Burt H, Posada MM, Varma M, Zheng M, et al. Physiologically-based pharmacokinetic models for evaluating membrane transporter mediated drug-drug interactions: current capabilities, case studies, future opportunities, and recommendations. Clin Pharmacol Ther 2020;107(5):1082–1115.

[137] Gertz M, Tsamandouras N, Sall C, Houston JB, Galetin A. Reduced physiologically-based pharmacokinetic model of repaglinide: impact of OATP1B1 and CYP2C8 genotype and source of in vitro data on the prediction of drug-drug interaction risk. Pharm Res 2014;31(9):2367–2382.

[138] Zhao P, Vieira Mde L, Grillo JA, Song P, Wu TC, Zheng JH, et al. Evaluation of exposure change of nonrenally eliminated drugs in patients with chronic kidney disease using physiologically based pharmacokinetic modeling and simulation. J Clin Pharmacol 2012;52(1 Suppl):91S–108S.

[139] Scotcher D, Jones CR, Galetin A, Rostami-Hodjegan A. Delineating the role of various factors in renal disposition of digoxin through application of physiologically based kidney model to renal impairment populations. J Pharmacol Exp Ther 2017;360(3):484–495.

[140] Hsueh CH, Hsu V, Zhao P, Zhang L, Giacomini KM, Huang SM. PBPK modeling of the effect of reduced kidney function on the pharmacokinetics of drugs excreted renally by organic anion transporters. Clin Pharmacol Ther 2018;103(3):485–492.

[141] Abduljalil K, Jamei M, Rostami-Hodjegan A, Johnson TN. Changes in individual drug-independent system parameters during virtual paediatric pharmacokinetic trials: introducing time-varying physiology into a paediatric PBPK model. AAPS J 2014;16(3):568–576.

[142] Ke AB, Greupink R, Abduljalil K. Drug dosing in pregnant women: challenges and opportunities in using physiologically based pharmacokinetic modeling and simulations. CPT Pharmacometrics Syst Pharmacol 2018;7(2):103–110.

[143] Salerno SN, Burckart GJ, Huang SM, Gonzalez D. Pediatric drug-drug interaction studies: barriers and opportunities. Clin Pharmacol Ther 2019;105 (5):1067–1070.

[144] El-Khateeb E, Achour B, Scotcher D, Al-Majdoub ZM, Athwal V, Barber J, et al. Scaling factors for clearance in adult liver cirrhosis. Drug Metab Dispos 2020;48(12):1271–1282.

[145] Takita H, Scotcher D, Chinnadurai R, Kalra PA, Galetin A. Physiologically-based pharmacokinetic modelling of creatinine-drug interactions in the chronic kidney disease population. CPT Pharmacometrics Syst Pharmacol 2020;9(12):695–706.

[146] Polasek TM, Rostami-Hodjegan A. Virtual twins: understanding the data required for model-informed precision dosing. Clin Pharmacol Ther 2020;107(4):742–745.

[147] Sorich MJ, Mutlib F, van Dyk M, Hopkins AM, Polasek TM, Marshall JC, et al. Use of physiologically based pharmacokinetic modeling to identify physiological and molecular characteristics driving variability in axitinib exposure: a fresh approach to precision dosing in oncology. J Clin Pharmacol 2019;59(6):872–879.

[148] Darwich AS, Polasek TM, Aronson JK, Ogungbenro K, Wright DFB, Achour B, et al. Model-informed precision dosing: background, requirements, validation, implementation, and forward trajectory of individualizing drug therapy. Annu Rev Pharmacol Toxicol 2021;61:225–245.

[149] Maeda K, Ikeda Y, Fujita T, Yoshida K, Azuma Y, Haruyama Y, et al. Identification of the rate-determining process in the hepatic clearance of atorvastatin in a clinical cassette microdosing study. Clin Pharmacol Ther 2011;90(4):575–581.

[150] Kashihara Y, Ieiri I, Yoshikado T, Maeda K, Fukae M, Kimura M, et al. Small-dosing clinical study: pharmacokinetic, pharmacogenomic (SLCO2B1 and ABCG2), and interaction (atorvastatin and grapefruit juice) profiles of 5 probes for OATP2B1 and BCRP. J Pharm Sci 2017;106(9):2688–2694.

[151] Stopfer P, Giessmann T, Hohl K, Hutzel S, Schmidt S, Gansser D, et al. Optimization of a drug transporter probe cocktail: potential screening tool for transporter-mediated drug-drug interactions. Br J Clin Pharmacol 2018;84(9):1941–1949.

[152] Stopfer P, Giessmann T, Hohl K, Sharma A, Ishiguro N, Taub ME, et al. Pharmacokinetic evaluation of a drug transporter cocktail consisting of digoxin, furosemide, metformin, and rosuvastatin. Clin Pharmacol Ther 2016;100(3):259–267.

[153] Zhou H, Tong Z, McLeod JF. "Cocktail" approaches and strategies in drug development: valuable tool or flawed science? J Clin Pharmacol 2004;44 (2):120–134.

[154] Magliocco G, Thomas A, Desmeules J, Daali Y. Phenotyping of human CYP450 enzymes by endobiotics: current knowledge and methodological approaches. Clin Pharmacokinet 2019;58(11):1373–1391.

[155] Rodrigues AD, Taskar KS, Kusuhara H, Sugiyama Y. Endogenous probes for drug transporters: balancing vision with reality. Clin Pharmacol Ther 2018;103(3):434–448.

[156] Rodrigues AD, Rowland A. Profiling of drug-metabolizing enzymes and transporters in human tissue biopsy samples: a review of the literature. J Pharmacol Exp Ther 2020;372(3):308–319.

[157] Neuvonen M, Hirvensalo P, Tornio A, Rago B, West M, Lazzaro S, et al. Identification of glycochenodeoxycholate 3-O-glucuronide and glycodeoxycholate 3-O-glucuronide as highly sensitive and specific OATP1B1 biomarkers. Clin Pharmacol Ther 2021;109(3):646–657.

[158] Lai Y, Mandlekar S, Shen H, Holenarsipur VK, Langish R, Rajanna P, et al. Coproporphyrins in plasma and urine can be appropriate clinical biomarkers to recapitulate drug-drug interactions mediated by organic anion transporting polypeptide inhibition. J Pharmacol Exp Ther 2016;358 (3):397–404.

[159] Cheung KWK, Yoshida K, Cheeti S, Chen B, Morley R, Chan IT, et al. GDC-0810 pharmacokinetics and transporter-mediated drug interaction evaluation with an endogenous biomarker in the first-in-human, dose escalation study. Drug Metab Dispos 2019;47(9):966–973.

[160] Mori D, Kimoto E, Rago B, Kondo Y, King-Ahmad A, Ramanathan R, et al. Dose-dependent inhibition of OATP1B by rifampicin in healthy volunteers: comprehensive evaluation of candidate biomarkers and OATP1B probe drugs. Clin Pharmacol Ther 2020;107(4):1004–1013.

[161] Takehara I, Yoshikado T, Ishigame K, Mori D, Furihata KI, Watanabe N, et al. Comparative study of the dose-dependence of OATP1B inhibition by rifampicin using probe drugs and endogenous substrates in healthy volunteers. Pharm Res 2018;35(7):138.

[162] Yee SW, Giacomini MM, Hsueh CH, Weitz D, Liang X, Goswami S, et al. Metabolomic and genome-wide association studies reveal potential endogenous biomarkers for OATP1B1. Clin Pharmacol Ther 2016;100(5):524–536.

[163] Mori D, Kashihara Y, Yoshikado T, Kimura M, Hirota T, Matsuki S, et al. Effect of OATP1B1 genotypes on plasma concentrations of endogenous OATP1B1 substrates and drugs, and their association in healthy volunteers. Drug Metab Pharmacokinet 2019;34(1):78–86.

[164] Suzuki Y, Sasamoto Y, Koyama T, Yoshijima C, Nakatochi M, Kubo M, et al. Substantially increased plasma coproporphyrin-I concentrations associated with OATP1B1*15 allele in Japanese general population. Clin Transl Sci 2021;14(1):382–388.

[165] Yoshida K, Guo C, Sane R. Quantitative prediction of OATP-mediated drug-drug interactions with model-based analysis of endogenous biomarker kinetics. CPT Pharmacometrics Syst Pharmacol 2018;7(8):517–524.

[166] Tatosian DA, Yee KL, Zhang Z, Mostoller K, Paul E, Sutradhar S, et al. A microdose cocktail to evaluate drug interactions in patients with renal impairment. Clin Pharmacol Ther 2021;109(2):403–415.

[167] Kwara A, Lartey M, Sagoe KW, Xexemeku F, Kenu E, Oliver-Commey J, et al. Pharmacokinetics of efavirenz when co-administered with rifampin in TB/HIV co-infected patients: pharmacogenetic effect of CYP2B6 variation. J Clin Pharmacol 2008;48(9):1032–1040.

[168] Crews KR, Gaedigk A, Dunnenberger HM, Leeder JS, Klein TE, Caudle KE, et al. Clinical Pharmacogenetics Implementation Consortium guidelines for cytochrome P450 2D6 genotype and codeine therapy: 2014 update. Clin Pharmacol Ther 2014;95(4):376–382.

[169] Fulton CR, Zang Y, Desta Z, Rosenman MB, Holmes AM, Decker BS, et al. Drug-gene and drug-drug interactions associated with tramadol and codeine therapy in the INGENIOUS trial. Pharmacogenomics 2019;20(6):397–408.

[170] Samer CF, Daali Y, Wagner M, Hopfgartner G, Eap CB, Rebsamen MC, et al. Genetic polymorphisms and drug interactions modulating CYP2D6 and CYP3A activities have a major effect on oxycodone analgesic efficacy and safety. Br J Pharmacol 2010;160(4):919–930.

[171] Ma TK, Lam YY, Tan VP, Kiernan TJ, Yan BP. Impact of genetic and acquired alteration in cytochrome P450 system on pharmacologic and clinical response to clopidogrel. Pharmacol Ther 2010;125(2):249–259.

[172] Ramsey LB, Johnson SG, Caudle KE, Haidar CE, Voora D, Wilke RA, et al. The clinical pharmacogenetics implementation consortium guideline for SLCO1B1 and simvastatin-induced myopathy: 2014 update. Clin Pharmacol Ther 2014;96(4):423–428.

[173] Tsamandouras N, Dickinson G, Guo Y, Hall S, Rostami-Hodjegan A, Galetin A, et al. Identification of the effect of multiple polymorphisms on the pharmacokinetics of simvastatin and simvastatin acid using a population-modeling approach. Clin Pharmacol Ther 2014;96(1):90–100.

[174] Zhao P, Rowland M, Huang SM. Best practice in the use of physiologically based pharmacokinetic modeling and simulation to address clinical pharmacology regulatory questions. Clin Pharmacol Ther 2012;92(1):17–20.

[175] Collins C, Levy R, Ragueneau-Majlessi I, Hachad H. Prediction of maximum exposure in poor metabolizers following inhibition of nonpolymorphic pathways. Curr Drug Metab 2006;7(3):295–299.

[176] Chen Y, Cabalu TD, Callegari E, Einolf H, Liu L, Parrott N, et al. Recommendations for the design of clinical drug-drug interaction studies with itraconazole using a mechanistic physiologically-based pharmacokinetic model. CPT Pharmacometrics Syst Pharmacol 2019;8(9):685–695.

[177] Lang J, Vincent L, Chenel M, Ogungbenro K, Galetin A. Simultaneous ivabradine parent-metabolite PBPK/PD modelling using a Bayesian estimation method. AAPS J 2020;22(6):129.

[178] Yeung CK, Fujioka Y, Hachad H, Levy RH, Isoherranen N. Are circulating metabolites important in drug-drug interactions?: Quantitative analysis of risk prediction and inhibitory potency. Clin Pharmacol Ther 2011;89(1):105–113.

[179] Posada MM, Morse BL, Turner PK, Kulanthaivel P, Hall SD, Dickinson GL. Predicting clinical effects of CYP3A4 modulators on abemaciclib and active metabolites exposure using physiologically based pharmacokinetic modeling. J Clin Pharmacol 2020;60(7):915–930.

[180] Backman JT, Kyrklund C, Neuvonen M, Neuvonen PJ. Gemfibrozil greatly increases plasma concentrations of cerivastatin. Clin Pharmacol Ther 2002;72(6):685–691.

[181] Niemi M, Backman JT, Neuvonen M, Neuvonen PJ. Effects of gemfibrozil, itraconazole, and their combination on the pharmacokinetics and pharmacodynamics of repaglinide: potentially hazardous interaction between gemfibrozil and repaglinide. Diabetologia 2003;46(3):347–351.

[182] Hinton LK, Galetin A, Houston JB. Multiple inhibition mechanisms and prediction of drug-drug interactions: status of metabolism and transporter models as exemplified by gemfibrozil-drug interactions. Pharm Res 2008;25(5):1063–1074.

[183] Varma MV, Lin J, Bi YA, Kimoto E, Rodrigues AD. Quantitative rationalization of gemfibrozil drug interactions: consideration of transporters-enzyme interplay and the role of circulating metabolite gemfibrozil 1-O-beta-glucuronide. Drug Metab Dispos 2015;43(7):1108–1118.

[184] Ma Y, Fu Y, Khojasteh SC, Dalvie D, Zhang D. Glucuronides as potential anionic substrates of human cytochrome P450 2C8 (CYP2C8). J Med Chem 2017;60(21):8691–8705.

[185] Zamek-Gliszczynski MJ, Chu X, Polli JW, Paine MF, Galetin A. Understanding the transport properties of metabolites: case studies and considerations for drug development. Drug Metab Dispos 2014;42(4):650–664.

[186] Tran MT, Grillo JA. Translation of drug interaction knowledge to actionable labeling. Clin Pharmacol Ther 2019;105(6):1292–1295.

[187] Xarelto® rpi. Xarelto®, rivaroxaban [package insert]. Ttusville, NJ: Janssen Pharmaceuticals, Inc; 2011 [package insert approved 7/2011].

[188] Grillo JA, Zhao P, Bullock J, Booth BP, Lu M, Robie-Suh K, et al. Utility of a physiologically-based pharmacokinetic (PBPK) modeling approach to quantitatively predict a complex drug-drug-disease interaction scenario for rivaroxaban during the drug review process: implications for clinical practice. Biopharm Drug Dispos 2012;33(2):99–110.

[189] Fan Y, Sun B, Agarwal S, Zhang L. Review of transporter-related postmarketing requirement or postmarketing commitment studies. J Clin Pharmacol 2016;56(Suppl. 7):S193–S204.

[190] XARELTO® label. https://wwwaccessdatafdagov/drugsatfda_docs/label/2020/202439s031,022406s035lblpdf.

[191] Snoeys J, Beumont M, Monshouwer M, Ouwerkerk-Mahadevan S. Elucidating the plasma and liver pharmacokinetics of simeprevir in special populations using physiologically based pharmacokinetic modelling. Clin Pharmacokinet 2017;56(7):781–792.

[192] OLYSIO® label. https://wwwaccessdatafdagov/drugsatfda_docs/label/2017/205123s014lblpdf.

[193] Ventola CL. Big data and pharmacovigilance: data mining for adverse drug events and interactions. PT 2018;43(6):340–351.

[194] Antonazzo IC, Poluzzi E, Forcesi E, Salvo F, Pariente A, Marchesini G, et al. Myopathy with DPP-4 inhibitors and statins in the real world: investigating the likelihood of drug-drug interactions through the FDA adverse event reporting system. Acta Diabetol 2020;57(1):71–80.

[195] Tatonetti NP, Denny JC, Murphy SN, Fernald GH, Krishnan G, Castro V, et al. Detecting drug interactions from adverse-event reports: interaction between paroxetine and pravastatin increases blood glucose levels. Clin Pharmacol Ther 2011;90(1):133–142.

[196] Liu Q, Ramamoorthy A, Huang SM. Real-world data and clinical pharmacology: a regulatory science perspective. Clin Pharmacol Ther 2019;106(1):67–71.

Chapter 15

Biochemical mechanisms of drug toxicity

Jack Uetrecht[a], Denis M. Grant[b], and Peter G. Wells[a]

[a]*Faculty of Pharmaceutical Sciences, University of Toronto, Toronto, ON, Canada,* [b]*Department of Pharmacology and Toxicology, University of Toronto, Toronto, ON, Canada*

Introduction

Adverse reactions (ADRs) are so diverse in nature and mechanism that is difficult to fit them all into a simple classification. One general classification was proposed by Rawlins and Thomas [1]. Specifically, a Type A reaction refers to an "augmented, but qualitatively normal pharmacologic response," whereas a Type B reaction represents a "qualitatively bizarre pharmacological effect." This classification is used less often today, and a Type B reaction is usually translated to mean an idiosyncratic, allergic, or hypersensitivity reaction. Idiosyncratic means specific to an individual. This includes ADRs such as malignant hyperthermia, whereas allergic or hypersensitivity refers to an immune-mediated ADR. Different people can use the same term to mean different things. For example, the term idiosyncratic is usually used to refer to an ADR that does not occur in most patients and does not involve the therapeutic mechanism of the drug. Many such ADRs are immune mediated. However, when a clinical immunologist uses the term idiosyncratic, it usually specifically excludes any ADR that is immune mediated. When an ADR has clear evidence of an immune mechanism it is usually referred to as an allergic or hypersensitivity reaction, but to many, the term allergic reaction is associated with ADRs characterized by fever and rash, which would exclude many immune-mediated ADRs. Therefore the best way to avoid confusion when describing a specific ADR is to describe its characteristics rather than to depend on a label. Ultimately, we need a better mechanistic understanding of ADRs.

Type B reactions or idiosyncratic ADRs are commonly referred to as dose independent [2]; in fact, nothing is dose independent! By definition, most patients will not have an idiosyncratic ADR (IDR) at any dose of a drug. In general, the mechanism of a Type B or IDR is different from that of the therapeutic effect. Therefore there is no reason that the dose-response curve for the idiosyncratic effect should be in the same dose range as the therapeutic effect. The dose-response curve for susceptible patients may be shifted well to the left relative to that of the therapeutic effect such that there will not be a change in the incidence of an IDR within the therapeutic range, which in general is quite narrow. These characteristics may give an IDR the appearance of being dose independent; however, in many cases there is an increase in the risk of an IDR at higher doses within the therapeutic range. It is important to realize that the typical dose of a drug is about 10^{20} molecules, and it is axiomatic that a dose can always be found below which no one will have an IDR. For example, if penicillin is essential for the treatment of a serious infection in a patient who is highly allergic to penicillin, it is usually possible to administer 1/10,000 the usual dose and escalate to the therapeutic dose. Even 1/10,000 the usual dose is a very large number of molecules. Furthermore, drugs given at a high daily dose are more likely to cause IDRs, and drugs given at a dose of 10 mg/day or less are unlikely to cause IDRs [3]. Therefore it is important to know that Type B or IDRs are not dose independent.

Approximately 70%–80% of ADRs can be classified as Type A. Although diverse, the mechanisms of type A ADRs, which involve an extension of the therapeutic effects or general off-target effects of a drug, are relatively straightforward. This chapter will have an emphasis on Type B reactions or IDRs. Although IDRs are less common than Type A reactions, they can be quite serious, and their idiosyncratic or unpredictable nature makes them very difficult to study and to prevent. In addition, IDRs are a major source of risk for the process of drug development because they are usually only discovered late in phase III trials or after the drug has been approved. In addition, the related issues of drug-induced carcinogenicity and teratogenicity will be discussed because some of the same issues and mechanisms are involved.

Given the idiosyncratic nature of IDRs, they are virtually impossible to study prospectively in humans, and they are also idiosyncratic in animals. Therefore mechanistic studies are difficult, and little is known with certainty about their mechanisms. Most animal models represent acute toxicity with high doses of drug, and the mechanism is almost surely different than the mechanism in humans. There are many in vitro models, but again, the concentrations used are routinely 100-fold

Atkinson's Principles of Clinical Pharmacology. https://doi.org/10.1016/B978-0-12-819869-8.00015-X

higher than the therapeutic C_{max} [4], and it is unlikely that they represent events that occur in humans. It is essential that any mechanistic hypothesis be consistent with observations in humans.

Role of reactive metabolites and covalent binding in adverse drug reactions

Many years ago the Millers discovered that reactive metabolites play an important role in the mechanism of carcinogenesis [5]. This husband and wife team found that many of the chemicals that cause cancer are metabolized to chemically reactive species that covalently bind to DNA and cause mutations as discussed later in the chapter. It was largely through the work in B.B. Brodie's Chemical Pharmacology lab at the US National Institutes of Health (NIH) that it was discovered that many of the toxic effects of drugs are also due to their metabolites. This is chronicled in the book "Apprentice to Genius" [6]. They also found that the metabolism of a drug was usually similar in rodents and humans, which facilitated the study of drug metabolism. A classic study involved acetanilide- and phenacetin-induced methemoglobinemia. Methemoglobin is formed by the oxidation of the usual ferrous form of iron in hemoglobin to the ferric form, which does not readily release oxygen to tissues [7]. Both acetanilide and phenacetin can be converted to acetaminophen: acetanilide by para-hydroxylation and phenacetin by *O*-dealkylation (Fig. 15.1). However, acetaminophen does not cause methemoglobinemia. Both acetanilide

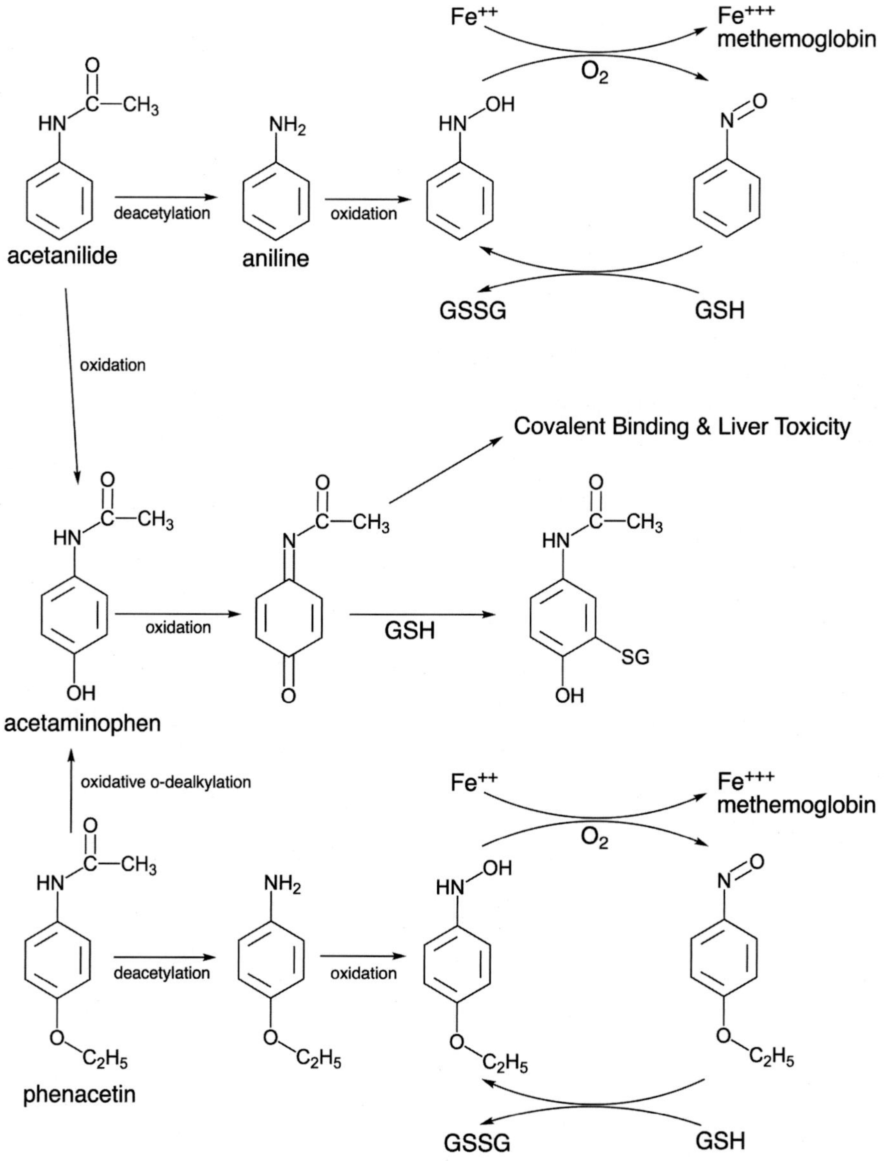

FIG. 15.1 Drug-induced methemoglobinemia. Methemoglobinemia is produced when aromatic amines are oxidized and redox cycle between hydroxylamine and nitroso metabolites. This leads to the oxidation of the heme iron of hemoglobin from the ferrous form, which carries oxygen, and the ferric form, which also binds to oxygen, but the affinity is higher such that insufficient oxygen is released in tissues. Even under normal circumstances, methemoglobin is constantly being formed, but it is reduced back to the ferrous form by NADH methemoglobin reductase. This pathway can be overwhelmed by the redox cycling of aromatic amines and other oxidants.

and phenacetin are deacetylated to primary aromatic amines, and it is the hydroxylamine metabolites of these two agents that are responsible for production of methemoglobinemia by undergoing redox cycling (Fig. 15.1). Acetaminophen can also be deacetylated, but when the product, *p*-aminophenol, is oxidized, the product is an iminoquinone rather than a hydroxylamine, and although this metabolite can also redox cycle, it has less potential to cause methemoglobinemia. Phenacetin was withdrawn from the market because it not only causes methemoglobinemia, but it is also associated with renal toxicity and an increase in renal tumors.

The NIH Chemical Pharmacology lab also made several other seminal discoveries. Although acetaminophen is safer than acetanilide or phenacetin, it is the leading cause of acute liver failure in the United States [8]. They discovered that reactive metabolites are responsible for the liver toxicity caused by acetaminophen and several other chemicals [9]. Acetaminophen causes a similar liver injury in mice as in humans, although rats are relatively resistance. The availability of the mouse animal model has allowed detailed mechanistic studies of acetaminophen-induced liver injury. The liver injury only occurs when the glutathione levels are depleted by 80%–90% [10]. Paradoxically, a deficiency in glutathione transferase in the mouse model was protective, presumably because this deficiency decreased glutathione depletion [11]. Many other drugs that cause liver injury can deplete glutathione in vitro, and it has been proposed that this is involved in the mechanism of liver injury. However, it is unlikely that this occurs with other drugs given at therapeutic doses, and it only occurs with acetaminophen with large overdoses. With the exception of some anticancer drugs, few drugs today are cytotoxic, hence the focus on IDRs.

Other drugs that cause liver injury were studied at the NIH Chemical Pharmacology laboratory, including isoniazid and halothane. However, unlike the injury caused by acetaminophen, the injury caused by these drugs is idiosyncratic, i.e., it does not occur in most patients, and the time to onset is delayed. They found that isoniazid causes acute liver injury in rats. In this model, the injury appears to be caused by oxidation of acetylhydrazine, a metabolite of isoniazid; this will be discussed again later. The major metabolic pathway of halothane involves oxidative dehalogenation to form trifluoroacetyl chloride, which is very reactive.

Most reactive metabolites are formed by P450-mediated oxidation in the liver. In general, reactive metabolites are electrophiles, i.e., they are relatively electron deficient and react with biological nucleophiles, usually thiols or amino groups. A classic class of drugs that is associated with IDRs is the β-lactam. β-Lactams are intrinsically reactive because of the ring strain of the β-lactam ring. These reactive species, i.e., the trifluoroacetyl chloride metabolite of halothane, the reactive iminoquinone of acetaminophen, and β-lactams, represent the three major types of reactive metabolites (Fig. 15.2). Specifically, the trifluoroacetyl chloride metabolite of halothane is very electrophilic because of the electronegative fluorine atoms and it has a good leaving group, i.e., chloride. Chloride is a good leaving group because it readily accepts a negative charge. The oxidized acetylhydrazine also has a good leaving group, i.e., nitrogen gas. The iminoquinone metabolite of acetaminophen is electrophilic (electron deficient) and has a carbon-carbon bond that is polarized by a carbonyl group analogous to a Michael acceptor. A Michael acceptor does not require a good leaving group because the nucleophile can add across the double bond. Finally, the β-lactams are reactive because of ring strain, i.e., the normal bond angle of a carbonyl group is 120 degrees, but it is forced to be 90 degrees because it is part of a 4-membered ring. This ring strain is relieved when the ring is attacked by a nucleophile leading to ring opening. One other class of reactive metabolite that is relatively unique is the carbene (Fig. 15.2). A carbene is a divalent carbon formed by the oxidation of a methylenedioxy aromatic compound. This is important because carbenes bind to the heme iron of cytochromes P450 leading to inhibition of the enzyme. This pathway is involved in the mechanism by which piperonyl butoxide works synergistically with insecticides to slow down their clearance by insects. When present in drugs, the methylenedioxy group leads to a longer half-life of the drug and drug-drug interactions. Examples include paroxetine and tadalafil.

In addition to electrophilic reactive metabolites, free radicals are another class of reactive metabolite. It is convenient to include reactive oxygen species in this class. Free radical chemistry can be quite complex. In general, free radicals abstract hydrogen atoms from other molecules rather than covalently binding to proteins. However, they do add across the double bonds of unsaturated lipids, and the hydroxy radical is extremely reactive and can react with DNA as discussed in a later section of this chapter. The balance of formation and detoxication of reactive metabolites and their potential adverse effects are summarized in Fig. 15.3.

There is a large amount of circumstantial evidence that most IDRs are caused by chemically reactive drugs or reactive metabolites. However, this is very difficult to prove, and it is always dangerous to assume that association represents causation. The liver is the major site of drug metabolism, and that is presumably a major reason that it is the target of many IDRs; however, another factor is that many drugs are concentrated in the liver. Most reactive metabolites are too reactive to get far from where they are formed. In fact, many reactive metabolites are so reactive that they bind to the enzyme that formed them, often leading to inactivation of the enzyme. This is referred to as mechanism-based inhibition.

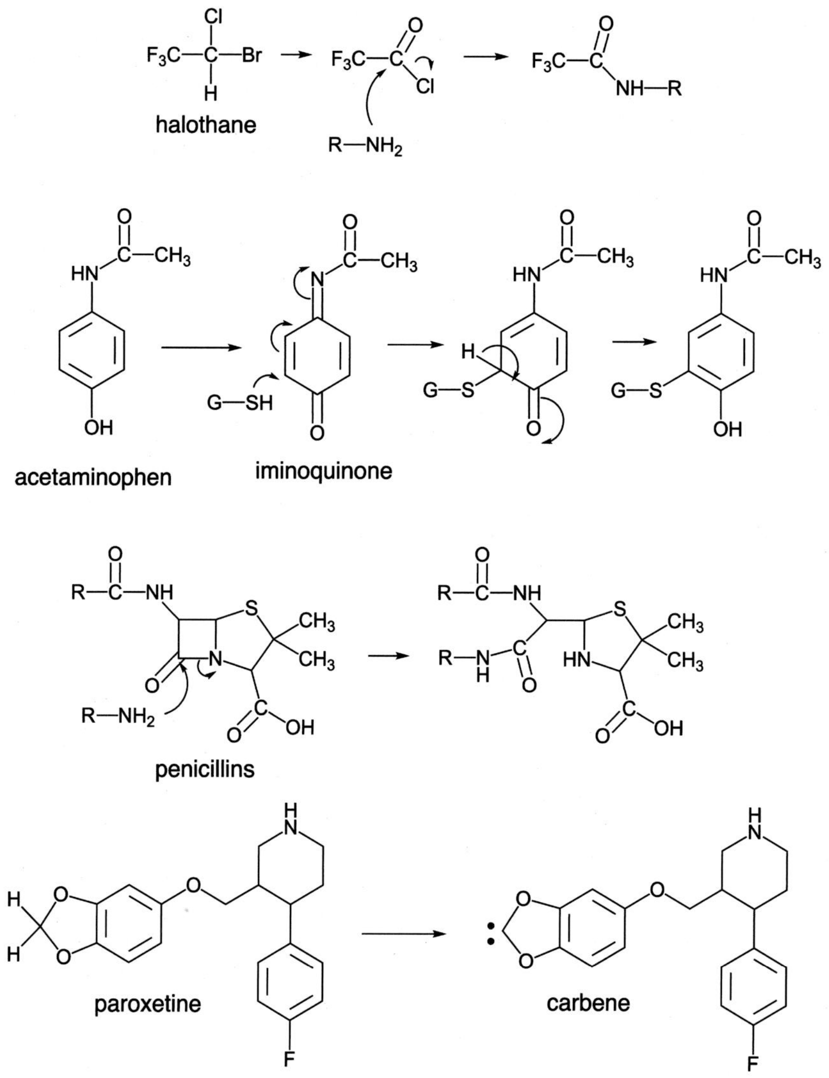

FIG. 15.2 Types of reactive metabolites. In general, reactive metabolites are electrophiles that react with tissue nucleophiles such as amino groups on proteins ($R\text{-}NH_2$) or thiols such as glutathione (G-SH). One type of reactive metabolite has a good leaving group that can be displaced by the attacking nucleophile as illustrated by halothane. Halothane is oxidized to trifluoroacetyl chloride. The fluorine atoms make it very electron deficient, and the chloride is a good leaving group because it can readily accept a negative charge. Another type of reactive metabolite is analogous to a Michael acceptor. It is also electron deficient because of the carbonyl group, but in this case no leaving group is required because the tissue nucleophile adds across the carbon-carbon double bond. This is illustrated by the iminoquinone of acetaminophen. This type of reactive metabolite predominantly reacts with tissue thiols such as glutathione. The final type of reactive metabolite is reactive because of ring strain. In the case of penicillins, the carbonyl group normally has a bond angle of 120 degrees, but it is forced to be 90 degrees because it is part of a 4-membered ring. Reaction with a nucleophile opens up the ring and relieves the ring strain. A special type of reactive metabolite is the carbene: a divalent carbon with only two bonds. During its formation by cytochromes P450 it immediately binds to the heme iron leading to inhibition of the enzyme. It is formed by the oxidation of methylenedioxy compounds such as paroxetine.

Even though the liver is a frequent target for IDRs, many other organs such as the skin and bone marrow are often the targets of IDRs. Nevirapine can cause both serious liver injury and skin rashes. There are several possible reactive metabolites of nevirapine. The major pathway involves oxidation of the methyl group to a transient free radical (Fig. 15.4). This free radical can lose another hydrogen atom to form a very reactive quinone methide, which covalently binds to proteins in the liver and also leads to mechanism-based P450 inhibition [12]. This reactive metabolite is presumably responsible for nevirapine-induced liver injury. The P450-generated nevirapine free radical can also undergo oxygen rebound to produce a benzylic alcohol, 12-hydroxynevirapine. This is the major observed metabolite of nevirapine in the serum. This benzylic alcohol undergoes sulfation in the skin to form a weakly reactive benzylic sulfate that is responsible for the skin rash [13]. The evidence for involvement of this sulfate in the mechanism of the skin rash is very strong. Nevirapine causes an immune-mediated skin rash in female Brown Norway rats with characteristics very similar to those of the skin rash in humans. Application of a topical sulfotransferase inhibitor to the rats prevents covalent binding of nevirapine where it is applied, and it also prevents the skin rash where it is applied. This is one of the few animal models of an IDR with characteristics similar to the IDR in humans [14], and one of the few cases where it was possible to test the involvement of a specific reactive metabolite in the mechanism of an IDR. In general, the skin has low activity of enzymes that can metabolize drugs, but sulfotransferase is an exception [15]. Most sulfate conjugates are not chemically reactive; the sulfate conjugate of 12-hydroxynevirapine is an exception. However, it is likely that there are other drugs that cause skin rashes that involve bioactivation by sulfotransferase. In other cases, a skin rash may involve chemically reactive drugs such as penicillin or reactive metabolites with low reactivity that are formed in the liver but have a sufficient half-life to reach the skin.

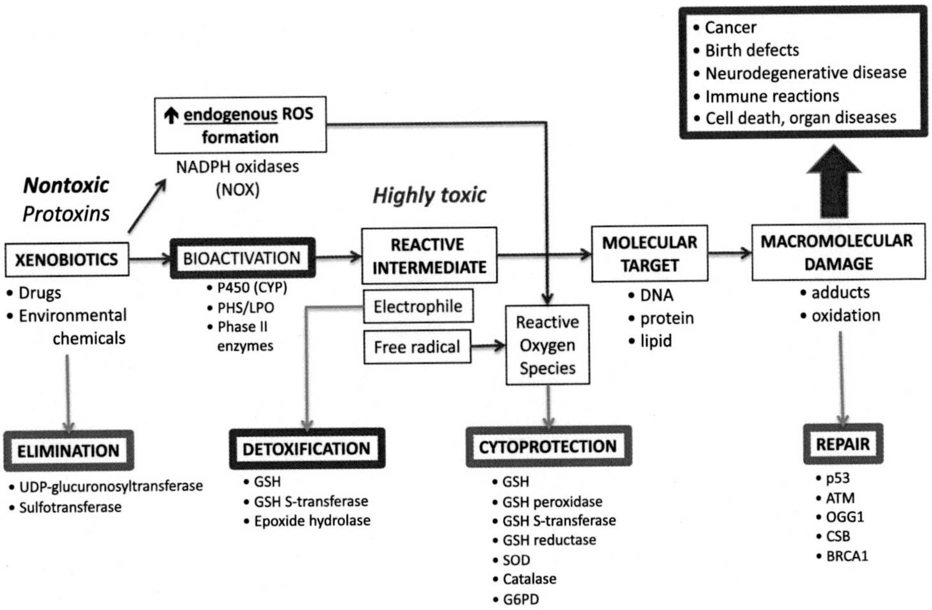

FIG. 15.3 Balance of biochemical pathways involved in the mechanism and determinants of risk for xenobiotic toxicity mediated by bioactivation to electrophilic or free radical reactive intermediates and formation of reactive oxygen species (ROS). If not eliminated via phase II pathways of drug metabolism, relatively nontoxic xenobiotics can be bioactivated to highly toxic reactive intermediates. Common enzymes that catalyze xenobiotic bioactivation include cytochromes P450 (CYPs), prostaglandin H synthases, and lipoxygenases. Some xenobiotics also can enhance endogenous pathways for ROS formation, such as NADPH oxidases. For a limited number of xenobiotics, phase II pathways catalyzed by UDP-glucuronosyltransferases, sulfotransferases, or glutathione *S*-transferases can result in the formation of electrophilic reactive intermediates. The pathways for the detoxification of electrophilic and free radical reactive intermediates and ROS are mostly different except for the shared role of glutathione and GSH S-transferase. Risk is determined by the balance between xenobiotic bioactivation or ROS formation vs. phase II pathways for xenobiotic elimination, reactive intermediate detoxification, ROS cytoprotection, and repair of macromolecular damage. An unfavorable imbalance in these pathways can result in toxicity even at a therapeutic drug concentration or reportedly safe exposure level for an environmental chemical. Abbreviations: ATM, ataxia telangiectasia mutated protein; BRCA1, breast cancer 1 protein; CSB, Cockayne syndrome B protein; G6PD, glucose-6-phosphate dehydrogenase; GSH, glutathione; LPO, lipoxygenase; OGG1, oxoguanine glycosylase 1; PHS, prostaglandin H synthase; P450, cytochrome P450 (CYP); SOD, superoxide dismutase. *(Modified from Wells PG, Bhuller Y, Chen CS, et al. Molecular and biochemical mechanisms in teratogenesis involving reactive oxygen species. Toxicol Appl Pharmacol 2005;207(2 Suppl):354–366.)*

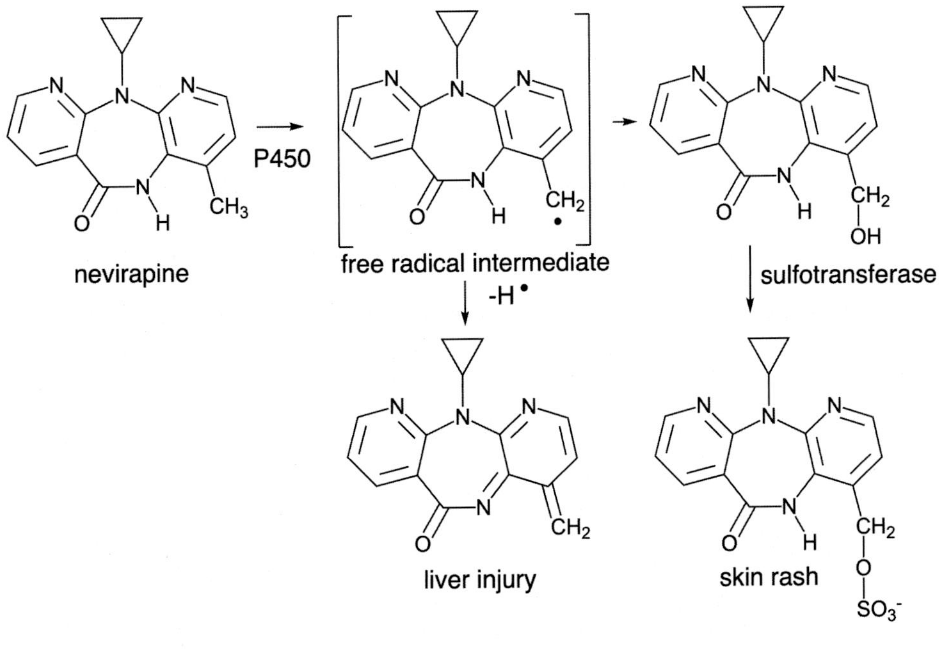

FIG. 15.4 Nevirapine forms two reactive metabolites. Nevirapine is oxidized by cytochromes P450 to a free radical intermediate. (It is shown in brackets because it has a very transient existence.) The most common fate of this free radical is oxygen rebound to form an alcohol, and this is the major metabolite of nevirapine in the blood. However, the free radical can also lose a hydrogen atom to form a very reactive quinone methide. This metabolite is responsible for most of the covalent binding in the liver, and it is presumably responsible for the liver injury that nevirapine can cause. It also leads to mechanism-based inhibition of cytochromes P450. In contrast, the alcohol is not reactive, but it can reach the skin where it forms a reactive sulfate metabolite that is responsible for the skin rash.

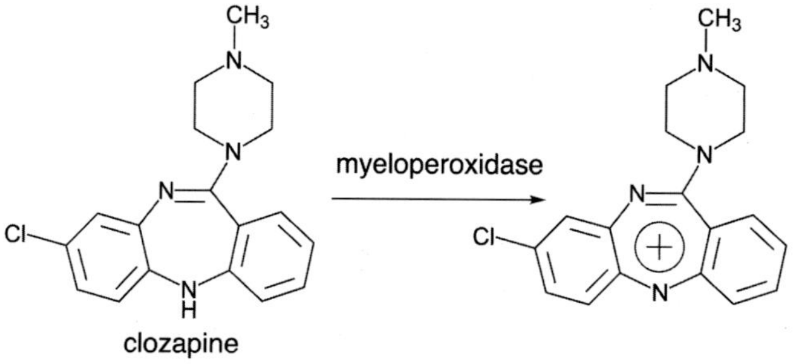

FIG. 15.5 Clozapine is oxidized to a reactive nitrenium ion by myeloperoxidase, which is present in neutrophils, neutrophil precursors, and monocytes. This nitrenium ion binds to neutrophils and their precursors in most patients who take the drug; however, most patients do not develop agranulocytosis.

The bone marrow is also a frequent target of IDRs such as agranulocytosis and aplastic anemia. Like the skin, bone marrow cells also have low P450 activity; however, neutrophils, monocytes, and some of their precursors contain high levels of myeloperoxidase and also NADPH oxidase, which generates superoxide [16]. The superoxide is converted to hydrogen peroxide by superoxide dismutase, and the hydrogen peroxide converts myeloperoxidase to compound I. Compound I is a strong oxidant that can oxidize drugs. Compound I also reacts with chloride to form hypochlorite, which is also a strong oxidant. Compound I and hypochlorite are not sufficiently strong oxidants to oxidize a C—H bond analogous to P450, but they can oxidize many nitrogen- and sulfur-containing drugs. A good example is clozapine, a drug that is associated with a relatively high incidence of agranulocytosis (Fig. 15.5). Clozapine is very rapidly oxidized to a reactive nitrenium ion by hypochlorite, and there is covalent binding of clozapine to the neutrophils of patients treated with the drug [17].

There are certain functional groups that readily form reactive metabolites such as primary aromatic amines, nitro groups, and thiono sulfur groups, and these are known as structural alerts [18]. Medicinal chemists try to avoid such functional groups, but it is almost impossible to completely avoid the possibility that a drug will form a reactive metabolite. For example, aromatic rings have the potential to form reactive epoxides (otherwise known as arene oxides), and most drugs possess an aromatic ring, although whether arene oxides are commonly involved in the mechanism of IDRs is controversial. Another controversial structural alert is the carboxylic acid. Carboxylic acids have the potential to form weakly reactive acyl glucuronides and also reactive Co-A esters, but the relevance of these metabolites to the mechanism of IDRs is also controversial [19].

Although there is a significant correlation between the ability of a drug to form reactive metabolites and the risk that it will cause IDRs, the correlation is far from perfect even when taking into account total daily dose [20]. For example, ethacrynic acid is chemically reactive and binds to proteins that have a thiol group, and yet it is not associated with a significant risk of IDRs. It appears that not all reactive metabolites have the same potential to cause IDRs. On the other side of the coin, ximelagatran, allopurinol, and pyrazinamide do not appear to form reactive metabolites and yet are associated with a relatively high risk of serious drug-induced liver injury.

Role of the immune system in the mechanism of IDRs

There is little question that penicillin-induced anaphylaxis is immune mediated. Penicillin covalently binds to proteins, and it is IgE antibodies that recognize penicillin-modified proteins that lead to the manifestations of anaphylaxis. In fact most IDRs appear to be immune mediated; the major question has been with idiosyncratic drug-induced liver injury (IDILI). It has been characterized as either metabolic or immune idiosyncrasy [21].

The characteristics of halothane-induced liver injury suggest that it is immune mediated, and it has been classed as immune idiosyncrasy [21]. Specifically, the onset of jaundice is usually preceded by fever and sometimes eosinophilia. Unlike other drugs, halothane is administered briefly during a procedure rather than over a period of weeks or months. Liver injury rarely occurs after the first exposure to halothane; it almost always occurs after a previous exposure, especially if the prior exposure was within the previous 3 months. Often the previous exposure was accompanied by a delayed fever. The time to onset is shorter than most idiosyncratic drug-induced liver injury with a peak at 3–7 days, but in the unusual cases in which liver injury occurs with the first exposure the delay in onset is longer. These characteristics strongly suggest that patients are sensitized during the first exposure, which is too short to produce a full adaptive immune response, but on subsequent exposure the immune system is primed to respond. Consistent with this hypothesis, patients with halothane-induced liver injury usually have antibodies against trifluoroacetylated proteins as well as autoantibodies [22].

In contrast to halothane-induced liver injury, the injury associated with isoniazid is not usually associated with typical signs of an immune response such as fever. Isoniazid-induced liver injury has been characterized as metabolic idiosyncrasy rather than immune idiosyncrasy [21]. In part this is due to the rat model in which it was shown that a high dose of isoniazid caused liver injury, and evidence suggested that the injury was caused by bioactivation of *N*-acetylhydrazine, a metabolite of isoniazid [23]. This led to the idea that the idiosyncratic nature of isoniazid was due to differences in metabolism of isoniazid, i.e., metabolic idiosyncrasy. However, although patients with a slow acetylator phenotype appear to be at increased risk, this does not explain the idiosyncratic nature of isoniazid-induced liver injury because the difference in risk is very small. In fact, it has been difficult to clearly demonstrate that polymorphisms in any drug-metabolizing enzyme are relevant to the risk of idiosyncratic drug-induced liver injury [24]. In addition, the liver injury in the rat model is very different from the injury in humans; in particular, it occurs almost immediately rather than having a delay in onset. This suggests that the mechanism in the rat model is different from the IDR in humans. In addition, the metabolism of isoniazid in rats is different from that in humans, and most of the bioactivation of isoniazid in mice and humans involves direct oxidation of isoniazid [25]. There are also antidrug and anticytochrome P450 antibodies in patients with isoniazid-induced liver failure [26]. Another reason to believe that isoniazid-induced liver injury was not immune mediated is that it often did not occur immediately on rechallenge. Patients who experience an increase in ALT (alanine transaminase) can often be rechallenged with a lower dose, and the dose increased to a therapeutic dose without liver injury. This is similar to the adaptation discussed later. However, when patients with more significant isoniazid-induced liver injury are rechallenged, the onset of injury is usually rapid and serious [27].

In fact, there are multiple lines of evidence that most IDILI is immune mediated. This includes the histology of the lesions. In the case of hepatocellular injury, which is the type most commonly associated with liver failure, the histology is very similar to that of viral hepatitis with a mononuclear infiltrate including CD8 T cells [28]. In some cases, there is an association between a specific HLA genotype and the risk of IDILI caused by a specific drug [29]. Although this has not been demonstrated for most drugs that cause IDILI, there are two likely reasons for this: there are insufficient cases available to study, and if the immune response is directed against drug-modified peptides, it is likely that there are many drug-modified peptides that could induce an immune response. For example, the reactive metabolite of isoniazid reacts with amino groups, and most proteins contain one or more lysines [25]; therefore there are multiple drug-modified peptides that could bind to different HLA molecules. Another study found that patients with a polymorphism in PTPN22, which is a risk factor for various autoimmune diseases, also had an increase in the risk of IDILI, which was independent of the drug [30]. This provides additional evidence that most IDILI is immune mediated.

Given that the existing evidence suggests that most IDRs are immune mediated, it is logical that it might be possible to produce animal models by stimulation of the immune system. There is such a model in which cotreatment with lipopolysaccharide, which stimulates immune cells through toll-like receptor 4, caused liver injury with some drugs that cause idiosyncratic drug-induced liver injury [31]. However, this model is different from IDILI in humans. Specifically, it occurs within hours, and the liver histology is characterized by an infiltration of neutrophils rather than the mononuclear infiltrate that is characteristic of IDILI in humans. We have tried to develop animal models by stimulation of the immune system, and it was never successful. This is consistent with the clinical observation that patients with inflammatory conditions such as ulcerative colitis and whose livers are exposed to many inflammatory molecules such as lipopolysaccharide are not at significantly increased risk of IDILI when treated with drugs that can cause such IDRs. We also tried to increase the immune-mediated liver injury caused by amodiaquine by immunization with amodiaquine-modified hepatic proteins. However, the immunization actually prevented mild injury, and this was associated with an increase in T regulatory cells [32]. Any drug that can cause a serious IDR always causes a higher incidence of mild IDRs affecting the same target organ, and the mild IDR often resolves despite continued treatment with the drug. If the IDR is immune mediated and resolves despite continued treatment with the drug, the resolution must involve immune tolerance. In the case of liver injury this is referred to as adaptation, and this is the basis of Temple's corollary, i.e., drugs that cause serious IDILI always cause a higher incidence of mild liver injury [33]. The dominant immune response in the liver is immune tolerance. This is presumably because it is exposed to many "foreign" molecules and bacterial products that come from the intestine. A strong immune response to these molecules would be very damaging, and yet the liver still needs to be able to respond to pathogens such as the viruses that cause hepatitis.

If the dominant immune response to drugs that can cause IDRs is immune tolerance it might be possible to develop animal models by impairing immune tolerance. A major advance in the treatment of cancer has been the development of immune checkpoint inhibitors that block immune tolerance, and this discovery led to the 2018 Nobel Prize in physiology or medicine. Two major immune checkpoints are programmed cell death protein-1 (PD-1) and cytotoxic T-lymphocyte-associated protein-4 (CTLA-4). Amodiaquine is an antimalarial drug that is readily oxidized to a reactive iminoquinone by both cytochromes P450 and myeloperoxidase [34]. Its use is associated with a relatively high risk of liver injury and/or agranulocytosis, and this has limited its use [35]. When mice or rats are treated with amodiaquine it leads to a very mild delayed onset liver injury that resolves despite continued with the drug [36]. When PD-1$^{-/-}$ mice are treated with a combination of anti-CTLA-4 antibodies and amodiaquine it results in delayed onset liver injury, which does not resolve with continued treatment, and the histology is characterized by piecemeal necrosis very similar to idiosyncratic drug-induced liver injury in humans [37]. This injury is prevented by treatment with antibodies that deplete CD8 T cells [38]. This impaired immune tolerance model unmasks the liver injury of other drugs that cause idiosyncratic liver injury, but with other drugs the injury is mild and resolves despite continued treatment [39]. Immune checkpoint inhibitors also increase the risk of liver injury caused by coadministered drugs in patients being treated for cancer [40].

Involvement of the immune system in the mechanism of other types of IDRs is less controversial. Certainly, various types of autoimmune reactions, whether specific to one cell type such as antibody-mediated thrombocytopenia or generalized autoimmunity that is similar to lupus, must be immune mediated. There is also little controversy about the involvement of the immune system in the mechanism of most skin rashes, although the type of immune response is different for different types of rashes. In several cases there is an HLA association with a specific type of IDR [41]. This is also true for idiosyncratic drug-induced agranulocytosis [42, 43]. However, even if a patient has the required HLA genotype and is treated with the associated drug, it is unlikely that they will have a significant IDR. For example, carbamazepine-induced Stevens-Johnson Syndrome and toxic epidermal necrolysis are associated with HLA-B*1502, but if a patient with that genotype is treated with carbamazepine it is unlikely that they will develop a serious skin rash [44]. There must be other factors; this will be discussed later.

Hapten hypothesis

If reactive drugs or reactive metabolites are responsible for most IDRs it begs the question: how do reactive metabolites induce an immune response? The prevailing theory in immunology for many years was that the immune system ignored "self" and only responded to "foreign" molecules. Almost a century ago, Landsteiner found that small molecules were not immunogenic unless they were covalently bound to proteins [45]. A small molecule that is covalently linked to a macromolecule and induces an immune response is referred to as a hapten. In general, the molecules presented by APCs are peptides produced by processing proteins, and the modification of proteins by reactive drugs or metabolites would make them foreign, which is consistent with the hapten hypothesis.

Danger hypothesis

Even though the immune system appears to respond to "foreign" molecules, it was observed that, in general, foreign proteins do not provoke a significant immune response in the absence of an adjuvant. Janeway referred to adjuvants as the "immunologist's dirty little secret." In addition to being foreign, pathogens release pathogen-associated molecule pattern molecules (PAMPs) that act as adjuvants to activate APCs. Polly Matzinger proposed that foreign molecules are ignored unless they are associated with some type of cell damage [46]. This is referred to as the danger hypothesis. The cell damage causes a release of damage-associated molecular pattern molecules (DAMPs) that activate APCs similar to PAMPs. Activation of APCs is referred to as signal 2 where T cell recognition of peptides presented by APCs is referred to as signal 1. Both signals are required for an immune response; signal 1 in the absence of signal 2 results in immune tolerance. Thus the hapten and danger hypotheses are complementary. The hapten and danger hypotheses are summarized in Fig. 15.6.

P-I hypothesis

Pichler found that lymphocytes from patients who had sustained an IDR would proliferate on exposure to drug in the absence of reactive metabolite formation. He proposed that reversible binding of a drug to the MHC-II/T cell receptor combination could lead to an immune response [47]. However, there is an unstated assumption: the agent that the T cells respond to is what invoked the immune response. This is not always true. For example, we have shown that a reactive benzylic sulfate of nevirapine is responsible for the skin rash that it can cause, and yet both in the animal model and in humans, the parent drug is able to stimulate T cells from affected patients [14]. Therefore the assumption is false, but in some cases the hypothesis could still be true. This could explain how some drugs such as ximelagatran and pyrazinamide that do not appear to form reactive metabolites are associated with a relatively high risk of IDRs.

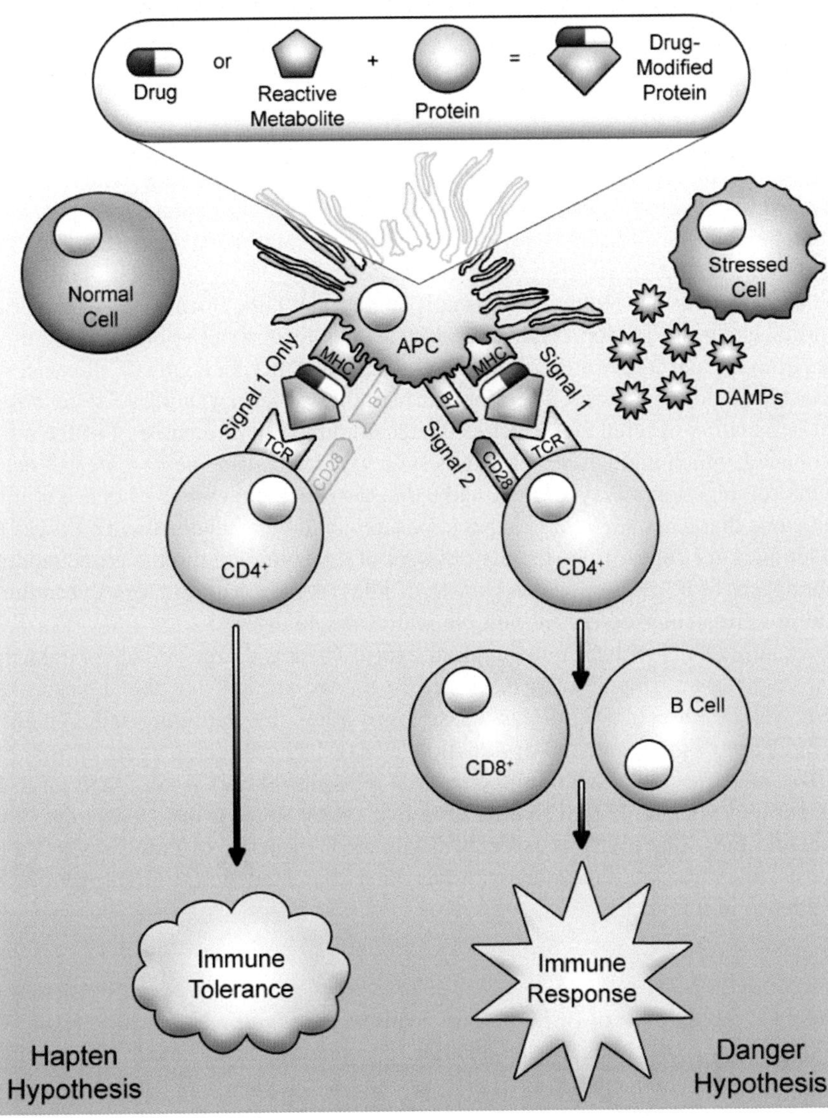

FIG. 15.6 A graphic depiction of the hapten and danger hypotheses. The generation of an immune response requires two signals: signal 1 is produced by the recognition of an antigen presented in the context of MHC by a T cell, and signal 2 is produced by the upregulation of costimulatory molecules such as B7 on APCs. Signal 1 without signal 2 results in immune tolerance. Generation of drug-modified peptides that can result in signal 1, and this is the basis of the hapten hypothesis. The upregulation of costimulatory molecules by DAMPs is the basis of the danger hypothesis. *(Modified from Cho T, Uetrecht J. How reactive metabolites induce an immune response that sometimes leads to an idiosyncratic drug reaction. Chem Res Toxicol 2017;30:295.)*

Altered peptide repertoire hypothesis

Abacavir is associated with a relatively high incidence of severe hypersensitivity reactions. This is associated with the HLA-B*5701 genotype [48]. Unlike other HLA associations, if a patient who carries the B*5701 gene and is treated with abacavir there is a high probability that they will have a hypersensitivity reaction. It has been demonstrated that abacavir binds noncovalently to B*5701 and alters the endogenous peptides that bind to it [49, 50]. Because the immune system has not "seen" these peptides previously there is no immune tolerance, and this can lead to an immune response. This is similar, but distinct, from the p-i hypothesis. It is interesting that abacavir also forms a reactive metabolite [51]. The reactive metabolite is not believed to be involved in the mechanism of abacavir-induced hypersensitivity reactions; however, it could be involved in the production of DAMPs. Although it has been proposed that other drugs cause IDRs by binding to MHC-II and altering the endogenous peptides presented to T cells, at the present time, this does not appear to be common.

Mechanistic hypotheses for IDRs other than immune activation

As discussed, there is ample evidence that most IDRs are immune mediated. The only significant debate has been whether there are other mechanisms of IDILI. In particular, it has been proposed that mitochondrial injury and/or bile acid-mediated liver injury caused by inhibition of bile salt export protein (BSEP) could be responsible for IDILI [52]. Even if these mechanisms are not solely responsible for some cases of IDILI, they could cause the release of DAMPs and contribute to immune-mediated liver injury.

Mitochondrial injury

Mitochondria are the powerhouses of the cell, and when damaged, can release DAMPs. It has been proposed that mitochondrial injury is a major cause of IDILI. The two major assays used to screen drugs for their ability to cause mitochondrial injury involve oxygen uptake and effects of a drug on hepatocytes cultured in galactose [53]. Oxygen uptake by hepatocytes is decreased by drugs that inhibit the mitochondrial electron transport chain, and it is increased by drugs that uncouple oxidative phosphorylation. Inhibition of the mitochondrial electron transport chain leads to lactic acidosis. Many drugs decrease the rate of oxygen uptake, but the concentrations required are usually higher that the clinical C_{max} of the drug. However, drugs that inhibit the mitochondrial electron transport chain at or near therapeutic concentrations, and therefore can cause serious lactic acidosis, e.g., phenformin and metformin, seldom if ever cause IDILI. In contrast, idiosyncratic drug-induced liver injury is seldom associated with lactic acidosis. Therefore the hypothesis does not fit with clinical observations. In addition, it was reported that combination of rotenone, which is the classic inhibitor of complex I of the mitochondrial electron transport chain, and isoniazid, which inhibits complex II, is synergistic in causing hepatocyte cell death in vitro [54]. However, in vivo, although the combination was synergistic and lethal to mice, there was no evidence of liver injury [55]. At slightly lower doses of rotenone that were not lethal so that exposure could be extended there still was no evidence of liver injury. Therefore the liver does not appear to be the major target of drugs that inhibit the mitochondrial electron transport chain, and this does not appear to be a common mechanism of idiosyncratic drug-induced liver injury. This is a good example where theory and in vitro studies do not fit with clinical observations.

However, there are drugs that cause liver injury that involves mitochondrial injury. There is a large amount of evidence that acetaminophen-induced liver injury involves mitochondria as discussed in a later section, but the injury is not idiosyncratic. Several nucleoside reverse transcriptase inhibitors can cause liver injury by inhibiting mitochondrial DNA synthesis, but it is associated with evidence of mitochondrial dysfunction such as lactic acidosis, and it is not idiosyncratic [56]. Chronic linezolid causes liver injury by inhibition of mitochondrial protein synthesis similar to its antibacterial mechanism, but again the injury is not idiosyncratic [57]. The only drug that causes idiosyncratic liver injury that clearly involves mitochondria is valproic acid [58]. The injury is associated with clear evidence of mitochondrial dysfunction such as lactic acidosis and steatosis, and although idiosyncratic, it has other characteristics different from those of most IDILI such as a much higher incidence in infants [59].

BSEP inhibition

Bile acids are toxic. A genetic defect leading to the absence of BSEP activity leads to liver failure early in life [60]. The injury is characterized by a cholestatic pattern, and although the alkaline phosphatase is elevated, the gamma-glutamyltransferase is usually normal [61]. The formation and transport of bile acids is complex [62]. There are several compensatory mechanisms for decreased BSEP activity [63], and milder forms of BSEP deficiency are not associated with serious liver injury. The composition of bile acids in rodents is different from that in humans; therefore, development of a valid animal model is a challenge. The hypothesis that BSEP inhibition plays a role in the mechanism of IDILI is quite plausible, and screening drug candidates for their ability to inhibit BSEP is quite common [64]. If BSEP inhibition were the cause of IDILI it would be expected that the IDILI would have a cholestatic pattern, but many of the drugs that have been proposed to cause IDILI through this mechanism cause hepatocellular IDILI. Therefore it is more plausible that BSEP inhibition plays a role in the mechanism of IDILI by leading to the production of DAMPs, and the IDILI is immune mediated. Although the role of BSEP inhibition in the mechanism of IDILI is widely accepted, most of the data are in vitro with high concentrations of drug, and there is little clinical data to support the hypothesis that BSEP inhibition causes or contributes to the mechanism of IDILI. Specifically, there are few examples where drugs that inhibit BSEP have even been shown to increase the concentrations of bile acids in the blood. There is one exception: it has been shown that bosentan inhibits BSEP in vitro, causes an increase in serum bile acids in patients, and is associated with IDILI. Furthermore, coadministration of glyburide, which inhibits BSEP but is not associated with a significant incidence of IDILI, causes a further increase in serum bile acids and increases the incidence of bosentan-induced ALT elevations [65].

Types of IDRs

IDRs can affect any organ, but liver, skin, and blood cells are the most common. Some IDRs affect several organs, sometimes simultaneously. Some drugs can cause autoimmune reactions, which either target a specific organ, or cause a generalized autoimmune syndrome that resembles idiopathic lupus. As mentioned previously, the reason that the liver is a common target is presumably because that is where most reactive metabolites are formed. However, the dominant immune response in the liver is immune tolerance. In contrast, the skin has much lower drug-metabolizing activity, but it is immunologically very active. The bone marrow has little cytochrome P450 activity, but it does have myeloperoxidase, which can oxidize some drugs to reactive metabolites.

Liver injury

Acetaminophen

As mentioned previously, acetaminophen is a major cause of liver injury, and it is responsible for the greatest number of cases of acute liver failure in North America [8]. Although acetaminophen-induced liver injury is not idiosyncratic, i.e., it occurs acutely and in virtually everyone who takes a high dose, the individual sensitivity varies significantly. Most of the cases of severe injury occur only with an overdose of more than 10g of acetaminophen. However, many of the cases of acetaminophen-induced liver failure occur by accident. An interesting study found that when the maximal therapeutic dose of acetaminophen was given to normal subjects, approximately 1/3 of them developed a significant increase in ALT [66]. This has led to a decrease in the recommended upper therapeutic dose in some countries. Alcohol intake has been claimed to increase the risk of acetaminophen-induced liver injury, but the interaction is complex. One aspect of the interaction is that while chronic use of alcohol induces CYP 2E1, a significant enzyme in the bioactivation of acetaminophen, alcohol acutely inhibits CYP 2E1 leading to a decrease in bioactivation [67]. The liver injury caused by acetaminophen clearly involves mitochondria [68]. This increases reactive oxygen and reactive nitrogen species, which eventually leads to mitochondrial permeability transition. This, in turn, leads to a depletion of ATP and cell death. It is interesting that the isomer of acetaminophen in which the hydroxy group is meta to the nitrogen covalently binds to hepatic proteins to approximately the same degree as acetaminophen, and yet it does not cause liver injury under comparable conditions. A significant difference is that more of the covalent binding of acetaminophen is to mitochondrial proteins compared to the covalent binding of the meta isomer [69]. Given its clinical importance and the availability of an animal model, acetaminophen-induced liver injury has been the subject of more than 1000 publications. The general mechanism of acetaminophen-induced liver injury has been defined: formation of the reactive imidoquinone metabolite, covalent binding, glutathione depletion, and mitochondrial injury [70]. Yet several controversies remain, especially with respect to the involvement of the innate immune system in the mechanism of the injury [71, 72].

Other than drug-induced cardiac arrhythmias, the type of IDR leading to drug-candidate failure or withdrawal from the market is IDILI. It has been proposed that liver injury caused by other drugs involves a similar mechanism as that of acetaminophen. However, other drugs are not directly toxic at therapeutic doses, and the injury is idiosyncratic; therefore, this seems unlikely. The three major types of IDILI are hepatocellular, cholestatic, and autoimmune. The type most responsible for liver failure is hepatocellular; however, cholestatic liver injury is far from benign and usually resolves very slowly [73]. The distinction is based on the ratio of ratios of ALT relative to the upper limit of normal divided by alkaline phosphatase relative to its upper limit of normal. If the ratio is >5 it is considered hepatocellular, if <2 it is considered cholestatic, and between 2 and 5 is considered mixed hepatocellular cholestatic injury. Drug-induced autoimmune hepatitis is diagnosed on the same basis as idiopathic autoimmune hepatitis. It usually responds to corticosteroids, but unlike idiopathic autoimmune hepatitis, it does not usually recur when the steroid treatment is stopped. Most IDILI occurs after 1–3 months of exposure to a drug, but the delay in onset of autoimmune IDILI is often more than a year. With some drugs such as telithromycin [74] and fluoroquinolones the onset can be much shorter, which is difficult to explain if the injury is mediated by the adaptive immune system.

Skin rash

Skin rashes are said to be the most common type of IDR; however, a mild skin rash is easily detected because the skin is visible. In contrast, other mild IDRs such as a small increase in ALT because of liver injury are not usually detected if they are asymptomatic.

Maculopapular rash

The most common type of skin rash is a maculopapular rash. It appears that this type of skin rash is mediated by CD4 T cells [75]. In general, these rashes are not serious, and it is often possible to treat through the rash, i.e., despite continuation of the responsible drug, the rash goes away. This is similar to the "adaptation" that occurs with drugs that can cause IDILI.

However, the early phase of a serious rash may be difficult to differentiate from a minor maculopapular rash. One important feature is fever; if a rash is associated with a fever, which is an indication of the release of significant amounts of cytokines, it is likely to be the harbinger of a serious IDR.

Anaphylaxis

Anaphylactic reactions are more serious, not because of the rash, which is characterized as urticaria, but because they can be accompanied by airway obstruction and shock. The classic example is penicillin-induced anaphylaxis, which is mediated by IgE antibodies that recognize penicillin-modified proteins. As mentioned previously, penicillin is chemically reactive because of ring strain; therefore, it covalently binds to endogenous proteins. This leads to an immune response; however, in most cases the immune response leads to production of IgG antibodies, and this does not usually lead to an IDR. Anaphylaxis only occurs if the immune response leads to a significant production of IgE antibodies. These antibodies bind to mast cells and basophils leading to degranulation and the release of mediators such as histamine, leukotrienes, etc. This is one of the few examples where it is possible to actually prove that covalent binding of a drug is responsible for an IDR. Approximately 10% of patients have a history of penicillin "allergy"; however, more than 90% of these patients are not allergic to penicillin, either because they were falsely labeled, or the allergy resolved over time. This leads to the use of inappropriate and more expensive alternative antibiotics. A recent study demonstrated that skin testing with a combination of penicilloyl polylysine (referred to as the major determinant), a minor determinant mixture of penicillin breakdown products, and amoxicillin had a negative predictive value of >97% [76]. Skin testing is not available in many locations, and a two-step oral challenge with amoxicillin for low-risk patients (patients with a reaction to penicillin restricted to the skin that occurred more than 1 year ago) in the absence of skin testing is a relatively safe alternative [77].

Although the IDRs caused by nonsteroidal antiinflammatory drugs can look very similar to a true IgE-mediated anaphylactic reaction, most are not true immune-mediated reactions. They are caused by inhibition of prostaglandin production leading to a diversion of the arachidonic acid precursor to the production of leukotrienes. It is the leukotrienes that produce the manifestations of the reaction [78].

Skin rashes mediated by CD8 T cells

Other serious skin rashes include fixed drug eruptions, drug hypersensitivity reactions/drug reaction with eosinophilia and systemic symptoms (DRESS), and Stevens-Johnson Syndrome/toxic epidermal necrolysis (SJS/TEN). These reactions involve CD8 T cells. Fixed drug eruptions involve memory T cells and recur in the same fixed location with rechallenge. When localized, fixed drug reactions are not life threatening, although when extensive they are serious and associated with systemic symptoms. Drug hypersensitivity reactions, a term that is used mostly for systemic adverse reactions to aromatic anticonvulsants, overlap with DRESS. As the name implies, DRESS usually involves eosinophils as well at CD8 T cells. It is a serious IDR that usually involves the liver and other organs as well as the skin. SJS and TEN are believed to be the same entity, the difference being the extent of skin involvement in which TEN involves more than 30% of the skin [79]. TEN is associated with a >30% mortality rate, and those patients who survive usually have permanent sequelae such scaring and even blindness. TEN is mediated by cytotoxic T cells that release granulysin resulting in the death of keratinocytes and epidermal detachment [80].

Given that the skin has few enzymes that can metabolize drugs, it is not clear what chemical entity is responsible for skin rashes. In the case of penicillin and other β-lactams the drug itself is intrinsically reactive. Some reactive metabolites such as acyl glucuronides have a sufficiently long half-life that they can be formed in the liver and reach the skin in significant concentrations. As mentioned, one of the few drug-metabolizing enzymes that has significant activity in the skin is sulfotransferase. Most sulfate conjugates are not chemically reactive, but sulfate is a good "leaving group," and some sulfate conjugates are chemically reactive. It was found in an animal model of nevirapine-induced skin rash that a benzylic metabolite of nevirapine is further metabolized in the skin to a reactive benzylic sulfate [13]. This sulfate covalently binds in the skin, and this covalent binding is responsible for the rash as discussed earlier. There are other drugs that have the potential to form chemically reactive sulfate conjugates, but most drugs that cause skin rashes do not have this potential. It is possible that some skin rashes involve the p-i mechanism discussed earlier, but conclusive evidence is lacking.

IDRs involving blood cells

Bone marrow toxicity is usually the dose-limiting toxicity of cytotoxic agents that target dividing cells and used to treat cancer because bone marrow cells also have a very high rate of proliferation. However, blood cells can also be the target of IDRs in the absence of overt cytotoxicity, and these IDRs also appear to be immune mediated as discussed later.

Agranulocytosis

Agranulocytosis is usually defined as a peripheral neutrophil count of <500 neutrophils/μL of blood. A classic example is the agranulocytosis caused by aminopyrine. In order to determine the mechanism, an investigator injected himself with serum from a patient with aminopyrine-induced agranulocytosis [81]. His neutrophil count immediately plummeted. This provided conclusive evidence that aminopyrine-induced agranulocytosis is caused by drug-dependent antiaminopyrine antibodies that deplete mature neutrophils. Aminopyrine is oxidized by myeloperoxidase-generated hypochlorite to a very reactive dication [82].

In contrast to aminopyrine, clozapine-induced agranulocytosis affects neutrophil precursors in the bone marrow [83]. Although <1% of patients treated with clozapine develop agranulocytosis, most patients have a transient innate immune response with an increase in serum IL-6 and TNFα levels and a paradoxical neutrophilia [84]. Clozapine-induced agranulocytosis is associated with specific HLA genotypes [42], and leukocytes from patients with a history of clozapine-induced agranulocytosis are activated by clozapine [85]. This is very strong evidence that clozapine-induced agranulocytosis is immune mediated. In this case it may be a cell-mediated immune response directed against neutrophil precursors. Clozapine is also oxidized by hypochlorite produced by neutrophils, and patients treated with clozapine have clozapine irreversibly bound to their neutrophils [17].

Drug-induced thrombocytopenia

Several drugs have the potential to cause thrombocytopenia. In most cases this appears to be mediated by drug-dependent antiplatelet antibodies. The most common example is heparin-induced thrombocytopenia. The mechanism involves IgG antibodies that recognize the molecular complex of platelet factor-4 and heparin [86]. Another interesting example is thrombocytopenia caused by quinidine and its diastereomer, quinine. The mechanism involves an antibody that recognizes the complex between drug and a platelet membrane glycoprotein [87]. Covalent binding of the drug to the glycoprotein is not required for binding of the antibody. However, these drugs have the potential to form reactive metabolites, and it is possible that induction of antibody production does involve covalent binding of a reactive metabolite. Some drugs can also cause the production of antiplatelet autoantibodies [88].

Drug-induced hemolytic anemia

Several drugs can induce the formation of antibodies that result in hemolytic anemia [89]. In some cases, the antibodies only bind to red cells in the presence of drug as in the case of hemolytic anemia associated with penicillin. However, in other cases such as α-methyldopa, the antibodies are true autoantibodies. Most patients treated with α-methyldopa develop antired cell antibodies, but only a few patients actually develop anemia. α-methyldopa is a catechol and has the potential to form a reactive ortho-quinone metabolite, but it is not clear what chemical species is responsible for this IDR.

Aplastic anemia

Aplastic anemia is the absence of all blood-forming elements in the bone marrow. The diagnosis is made with a bone marrow biopsy, which shows fat replacing the blood-forming cells. It is presumably immune mediated because it is associated with γ-interferon-producing T cells, and it usually responds to immunosuppression independent of whether it is drug induced or idiopathic [90]. The classic drug that is associated with aplastic anemia is chloramphenicol [91]. It has an aromatic nitro group, which has the potential to form reactive metabolites, and this is presumably involved in the mechanism.

Drug-induced autoimmunity

There are many drugs that can induce an autoimmune reaction. In some cases, this is directed against a specific target such as autoimmune hepatitis or autoimmune hemolytic anemia as mentioned. In other cases, the autoimmune syndrome is more generalized and resembles idiopathic lupus. The drug associated with the highest incidence of drug-induced lupus is procainamide; however, it is no longer commonly used. Most patients treated with procainamide develop antinuclear antibodies, but only about 20% develop clinical autoimmunity [92]. In general, drug-induced lupus is less severe than idiopathic lupus, and involvement of kidneys and central nervous system is uncommon. Patients with a history of procainamide-induced lupus can be treated with *N*-acetylprocainamide without recurrence even though a small amount of the *N*-acetylprocainamide is converted back to procainamide [93]. This implies that the aromatic amine functional group is required for the induction of autoimmunity.

The aromatic amine functional group is oxidized by hypochlorite and myeloperoxidase to reactive metabolites [94]. Procainamide is also associated with a significant incidence of agranulocytosis. Therefore it is likely that reactive metabolites formed by the myeloperoxidase of monocytes/macrophages are responsible for the lupus-like syndrome, while oxidation by the myeloperoxidase in neutrophils and their precursors is likely responsible for agranulocytosis. However, there is no direct evidence for this hypothesis. Another drug associated with autoimmunity is minocycline. It can cause either autoimmune hepatitis or a generalized lupus-like syndrome. It is also oxidized by myeloperoxidase to a reactive metabolite [95].

The use of biological drugs that modify the immune response has dramatically increased in recent years. As mentioned, the development of immune checkpoint inhibitors has been a major advance in the treatment of cancer. Although these agents are free from many of the adverse effects associated with the older cancer treatments, they can cause autoimmunity affecting many organs, especially the intestine, liver, skin, and pituitary gland [96]. It is not surprising that agents designed to impair immune tolerance could cause autoimmune reactions; what is surprising is that agents used to decrease inflammation can also provoke autoimmune reactions. For example, anti-TNFα antibodies such as infliximab, used to treat inflammatory bowel disease and rheumatoid arthritis, can cause a lupus-like syndrome and autoimmune hepatitis [97]. Another example is daclizumab, an anti-CD25 antibody used to treat multiple sclerosis, which can cause autoimmune hepatitis or DRESS [98].

IDR risk factors

There are genetic risk factors for IDRs as evidenced by strong HLA associations with specific IDRs. However, with the exception of abacavir-induced hypersensitivity, if a patient with the genotype associated with an increased risk of a specific IDR is treated with the drug associated with an increased risk of that IDR, it is unlikely that the IDR will occur. For example, patients who carry the HLA-B*5710 gene are at a much higher risk of developing flucloxacillin-induced liver injury; however, even if a patient has that genotype and is treated with flucloxacillin there is less than a 1 in 500 chance that they will develop liver injury [99]. Therefore, even in cases where an HLA genotype is a significant risk factor for a specific IDR, it is often not practical to screen patients to prevent the IDR. Gene-wide association studies have not yet revealed many strong non-HLA genetic risk factors for IDRs, even those involved in drug metabolism [100].

If IDRs are immune mediated then it would be expected that an inflammatory stimulus would increase risk; however, as mentioned earlier, even inflammatory bowel disease does not significantly increase the risk of IDILI. In general, Zimmerman stated that preexisting liver disease does not increase the risk of IDIDI [21], although there are probably exceptions. In addition, patients with liver disease have a lower hepatic reserve; therefore, they are more likely to develop liver failure. The incidence of many IDRs is higher in females than males, and the elderly are at increased risk of IDRs caused by some drugs such as isoniazid [101], but as mentioned earlier, infants are at increased risk of valproate-induced liver injury [59]. However, these risk factors are relatively minor and do not permit prediction of IDR risk.

Overall, the known non-HLA risk factors are quite small and do not explain the idiosyncratic nature of IDRs. Since even when there is a strong HLA association, patients with that genotype are unlikely to have an IDR when treated with the associated drug, there must be another major risk factor or factors. Probably the most important factor is the T cell receptor repertoire [102]. The T cell receptor repertoire is produced by random gene recombination, and it is different even in "identical" twins. It even changes over time in the same individual in response to various pathogens and other immunogens. Because of this random recombination of the genes that code for the T cell receptor, the number of antigens that can be recognized is virtually limitless; however, the number of lymphocytes is not. It has been found that the same T cell receptor can recognize several different antigens even if they have very different structures. This is possible because there are multiple ways by which an antigen can interact with the T cell receptor. This is referred to as heterologous immunity [103]. This makes it possible for the immune system to respond to a larger number of antigens, but it also means that if a T cell that was primed by response to a pathogen also recognizes a drug-modified protein it can lead to an inappropriate immune response. Fortunately, the immune system usually gets it right. The incidence of serious IDRs is low; in most cases the response is immune tolerance. Even though most patients do not have the HLA/T cell repertoire required to develop a serious IDR, most patients do form the reactive metabolite involved in the induction of an immune response. Therefore most patients probably have a subclinical innate immune response to drugs that cause IDRs. This is summarized in Fig. 15.7. Overall, in most cases, it is presently impossible to predict who is likely to develop an IDR.

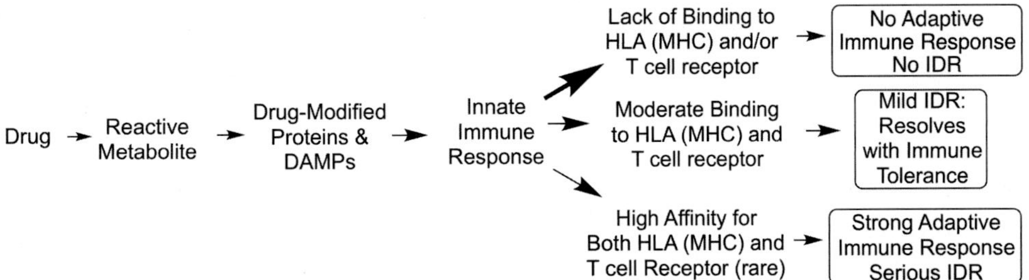

FIG. 15.7 Reactive metabolites can lead to drug-modified proteins and also cause the release of DAMPs. This can lead to activation of the innate immune system. This probably occurs in most patients and even many animals treated with the drug, and it is therefore not idiosyncratic. It is only if this innate immune response leads to an adaptive immune response that an IDR occurs. An adaptive immune response depends on binding of the drug-modified peptides to specific HLA molecules (the human form of the major histocompatibility molecule) and T cell receptors. Even if the drug-modified peptides do bind to both HLA and the T cell receptor, it does not usually result in a serious IDR, and the response resolves with immune tolerance. It is only if the affinity is very high that it is likely to lead to a serious IDR. Although this provides a simple explanation for the idiosyncratic nature of IDRs, this hypothesis has yet to be rigorously tested, and certainly the details are unknown.

IDR treatment

The major treatment of an IDR is to stop the responsible drug, but serious IDRs progress even after the drug is discontinued. Given that most IDRs are immune mediated, corticosteroids are often used to treat serious IDRs such as toxic epidermal necrolysis, but there is little evidence that they decrease mortality. Other immunosuppressive therapies have been tried such as cyclosporine and intravenous immunoglobulins for toxic epidermal necrolysis [104] and mycophenolate for serious liver injury, but again there is a lack of evidence that these treatments decrease mortality [105]. The one exception is that cyclosporine and antithymocyte globulins are effective in the treatment of aplastic anemia, whether it is drug induced or idiopathic [106].

Carcinogenic effects of drugs

It is now almost 250 years since Percival Pott's first epidemiological observations (reviewed in [107]) of a high incidence of scrotal cancer in British chimney sweeps who were occupationally exposed to coal tars that are now known to contain polycyclic aromatic hydrocarbon (PAH) procarcinogens. The first association between a therapeutic agent and cancer risk occurred in the 19th century during the use of arsenic for the treatment of syphilis [108]. Today, of the approximately 250 chemicals that are currently recognized by the International Agency for Research on Cancer (IARC) or the US National Toxicology Program (NTP) as being carcinogenic to humans [109–111], fewer than 30 are either past or present pharmaceutical agents [109, 112]. This relatively small number is not surprising, given that carcinogenicity screening during early preclinical stages of drug development is presumably designed to effectively eliminate cancer-causing chemicals from further development and use in humans. On the other hand, although earlier reviews on the topic had suggested that the vast majority of currently available pharmacotherapy agents have no evidence of carcinogenic associations [113, 114], more recent compilations suggest that as much as 65% of chronically administered drugs have no data on carcinogenicity in humans [115]. Furthermore, drugs for which both animal and human data are available show only 30% concordance in carcinogenicity predictions between species.

Of the identified potentially cancer-causing drugs that do remain in use, these fall under three general classes (Table 15.1), which will be further discussed in this section: (i) traditional cancer chemotherapeutic agents utilized specifically for genotoxic effects that are intended to result in the death or arrested proliferation of cancer cells, but which may also lead to the subsequent occurrence of secondary cancers arising from mutations in surviving healthy cells; (ii) immunosuppressive agents that target proliferating immune cells using similar genotoxic mechanisms as cancer chemotherapies, or suppress the immune surveillance response that may clear precancerous lesions; and (iii) hormonal therapies that target receptor-mediated cellular signaling mechanisms, many of which are now known to be key pathways in enabling cancer progression. Due to space limitations, this section will focus on key selected examples from Table 15.1 that illustrate each of the three classes of cancer-causing drugs.

As our understanding of cancer cells and their complex pathway interactions within the cancer microenvironment evolves, it is now clear that genotoxicity is but one enabling feature of cancer-producing processes, and that exposures to nongenotoxic agents that may impact those processes also have the potential to contribute to cancer development

TABLE 15.1 Known or probably carcinogenic drugs [109, 110, 112, 116].

		Mechanism(s)			
Agent	**Cancer site**	**Genotoxic**	**Immune**	**Signaling**	**Other**
In current use					
Aristolochic acid	Renal pelvis, ureter	Yes			
Azacitidine	Multiple sites	Yes			DNA hypomethylation
Azathioprine	Lymphoma, skin	Yes	Yes		
BCNU (carmustine)	Leukemia	Yes			
Busulfan	Leukemia	Yes			
Chlorambucil	Leukemia	Yes	Yes		
Chloramphenicol	Leukemia	Yes			Mitochondrial protein synthesis inhibition
Chlorozotocin	Leukemia	Yes			
Cisplatin	Leukemia	Yes	Yes		
Cyclophosphamide	Bladder, leukemia	Yes			
Cyclosporine	Lymphoma, skin		Yes		
Diethylstilbestrol	Vagina, cervix	Yes		Estrogen receptor	Epigenetic programming
Estrogen	Uterus, breast	Yes		Estrogen receptor	
Doxorubicin	Leukemia, bone				Topo II inhibitor
Etoposide	Leukemia	Yes			Topo II inhibitor
Melphalan	Leukemia	Yes			
Methoxypsoralen/ UVA	Skin	Yes			
Methyl-CCNU	Leukemia	Yes			
MOPP combined therapy	Leukemia	Yes			
Nitrogen mustard	Skin, leukemia	Yes			
N-Nitroso-*N*-methylurea	Leukemia	Yes			
Oxymetholone	Liver			Androgen receptor	
Procarbazine	Leukemia	Yes			
Tamoxifen	Uterus	Yes		Estrogen receptor	
Thiotepa	Leukemia	Yes			
Treosulfan	Leukemia	Yes			

TABLE 15.1 Known or probably carcinogenic drugs [109, 110, 112, 116]—cont'd

Agent	Cancer site	Mechanism(s)			
		Genotoxic	Immune	Signaling	Other
No longer used					
Arsenic trioxide	Multiple sites	Yes			
Chlornaphazine	Bladder	Yes			
Phenacetin	Renal pelvis, ureter	Yes			

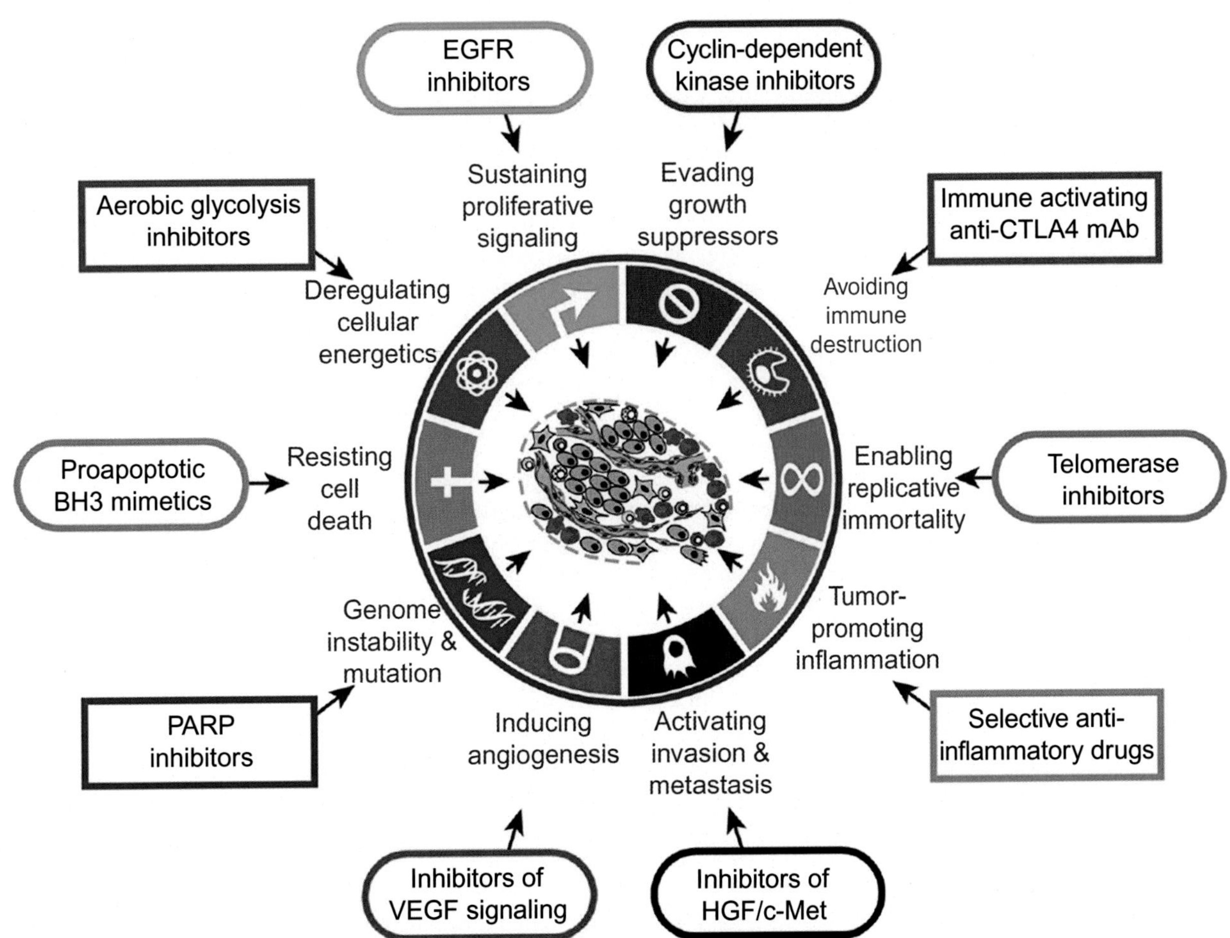

FIG. 15.8 The hallmarks of cancer. *(Modified from Hanahan D, Weinberg RA. Hallmarks of cancer: the next generation. Cell 2011;144:646–674.)*

[115, 117–119]. This suggests that methods for preclinical testing of agents for potential carcinogenicity should also continue to move beyond simple screening for DNA damaging potential or conventional hormone signaling effects. In 2011 Hanahan and Weinberg published an updated version [120] of their seminal 2001 paper [121]] describing the so-called hallmarks of cancer, which provides a useful mechanistic framework to explain some of the key phenotypic and enabling features of cancer cells and tissues, and of the underlying processes of cancer cell growth (Fig. 15.8). The hallmark features of cancerous cells and tissues are sustained proliferative signaling, evasion of growth suppressors, avoidance of immune destruction, replicative immortality, activated invasion and metastasis, induction of angiogenesis, resistance to cell death, and deregulation of cellular energetics. The model also recognizes genotoxicity (genome instability and mutation) and chronic inflammation (a pathological consequence of innate immune system activation) as two key enabling processes that can initiate or sustain the other 8 phenotypic hallmarks.

Since chemicals used in conventional cancer chemotherapy or immunotherapy often kill cells by genotoxic mechanisms, it is clear that such DNA damage may also enable the cancerous phenotypes of cells that happen to survive chemotherapeutic regimens, by producing mutations and consequent dysfunction in the products of genes that control any of these hallmark processes. Genotoxic drugs, therefore, comprise the majority of Table 15.1 and are a main focus of the subsequent discussions in this section. However, it should be appreciated that much effort is understandably being undertaken to develop novel drugs as potential anticancer therapies that more selectively target mechanistic processes underlying each of the hallmark features outlined in Fig. 15.8 [120]. Drug makers will need to ensure that new drugs in development, either for cancer or for unrelated pathologies, do not have the potential to interact with any of these processes in such a manner as to further enable rather than reduce the survival and proliferation of genotoxicant-initiated cells, and thus to cause cancer.

Genotoxic agents leading to myelodysplastic syndrome and secondary leukemia

Although solid tumor chemotherapy with alkylating agents or topoisomerase inhibitors is only rarely followed by the development of therapy-induced myelodysplastic syndrome (tMDS) leading to secondary acute myeloid leukemia (tAML) [122], mortality from tAML is high (78%, with median survival of 7 months) and about 75% of tMDS/tAML cases that occur within 5 years after chemotherapy can be attributed to the therapy [123, 124]. tMDS is characterized by impaired cellular maturation of myeloid stem cells and impaired hematopoiesis, and in some patients, it progresses to tAML with a risk timeline that peaks between 5 and 10 years after chemotherapy. Although the pathogenesis of tMDS/tAML is likely to be heterogeneous among the individuals in chemotherapy-exposed populations, animal studies suggest that an underlying initial feature of the disease caused by DNA alkylating agents is likely to be the alkylation of DNA in hematopoietic stem cells, followed by a loss of stem cell reserve and restoration of hematopoiesis by successive stem cell clones [125]. Subsequent development of a chromosomal abnormality in one of these clones then provides it with a selective growth advantage. Several different genetic alterations have been observed in human patients with tMDS/tAML, the majority of which involve the loss of part or all of chromosomes 5 and 7 [126, 127]. It is not yet known how the observed chromosomal changes produce both increased hematopoietic stem cell proliferation and increased apoptosis that results in the paradoxical combination of normal or increased bone marrow cellularity and pancytopenia seen in patients with tMDS. Subsequent progression from tMDS to tAML, which occurs in about two-thirds of cases, can be mediated in part by progressive loss of function of genes that encode hematopoietic transcription factors such as Runx1 (AML1), activation of genes that regulate cytokine signaling pathways, loss of function of the cell cycle checkpoint regulator p53, epigenetic silencing of the cyclin-dependent kinase p15, and mutations in receptor tyrosine kinases [126].

The tAML that occurs following topoisomerase II-inhibitory drugs differs from that produced by alkylating agents in several respects. Firstly, the onset is more rapid, with appearance within only 2–3 years of chemotherapy. Secondly, it is rarely preceded by tMDS. Thirdly, it is associated with balanced chromosomal translocations that are relatively unique to separate members of this class of chemotherapeutic agents [128], and which produce fusion proteins that cause dysregulation of cell growth and leukemic transformation [129]. For example, the epipodophyllotoxin etoposide causes a balanced translocation at chromosome 11q23 that combines the leukemic proto-oncogene *MLL* with one of a number of partner genes [130]. The resultant fusion proteins bind to the *MEN1* tumor suppressor gene product menin and inappropriately maintain *HOX* homeobox gene function [131]. This hyperexpression of *HOX* function results in leukemogenic transformation. On the other hand, exposure to anthracyclines such as doxorubicin is often associated with balanced translocations at chromosomes 21q22 or 16q22 that lead to chimeric proteins arising from the core binding factor genes *AML1* and *CBFβ* [132], which normally heterodimerize and transcriptionally activate hematopoietic genes [133]. Loss of this function presumably contributes to the development of tAML.

The risk factors for development of tMDS/tAML in only a small subset of chemotherapy-treated patients have not been extensively investigated. Among the possible contributions to risk are the dose, duration, and schedule of the original chemotherapy; interindividual differences in the biotransformation (both detoxication and bioactivation) of the drugs; and genetic factors related to target susceptibility and DNA repair capacity [134, 135]. For example, etoposide is metabolized largely by the cytochrome P450 isoform CYP3A4 to potentially genotoxic catechol and quinone metabolites, and individuals with a variant allele of CYP3A4 have decreased etoposide metabolism and reduced susceptibility to tAML [130]. On the other hand, patients with inactivating mutations in the quinone detoxifying enzyme NAD(P)H:quinone oxidoreductase (NQO1) have increased susceptibility to tAML [136]. DNA repair capacity is also genetically determined, and patients who are deficient in DNA mismatch repair have an increased incidence of tAML [135].

Immunosuppressive agents and cancer risk

As indicated in Table 15.1, azathioprine, chlorambucil, and cisplatin are agents that possess both genotoxic and immunosuppressive actions. Indeed, many agents that act to kill proliferating cells will be effective at killing both malignant cells and activated cells of the immune system, with the key distinguishing feature being the dosing schedules employed. As such, any of the carcinogenic mechanisms that operate for genotoxic/cytotoxic drugs will be similar between those used primarily for immunosuppression and those used primarily for cancer chemotherapy. Azathioprine is a case in point, since it is used primarily as an immunosuppressant, but it is in fact a prodrug of 6-mercaptopurine, which is used primarily as a cancer chemotherapeutic agent.

Cyclosporine is an example of a carcinogenic drug with purely immunosuppressant activity. It impairs the function of T cells of the innate immune system by binding to T cell cyclophilin, thus inhibiting calcineurin activity and inhibiting the transcription of genes encoding immune system activating cytokines such as interleukin-2, interleukin-3, and interferon gamma [137]. Patients given cyclosporine for the prevention of organ transplant rejection or for the treatment of psoriasis or rheumatoid arthritis have higher incidences of lymphoma, Kaposi sarcoma, and skin cancer [110]. Although animal and in vitro studies have provided no evidence for direct DNA damage after cyclosporine exposure, it is able to promote the development of lymphoid, liver, intestinal, and cervical cancers in rodents that were initially exposed to nitrosamine, nitrosourea, or polycyclic aromatic hydrocarbon genotoxicants. Although the exact mechanism by which cyclosporine promotes tumor growth is not known, the most likely explanation is that it suppresses the immune surveillance function that would normally act to recognize and destroy carcinogen-initiated cells.

Hormonal therapies and cancer risk: Diethylstilbestrol and vaginal cancer

Diethylstilbestrol (DES) is a nonsteroidal estrogen mimic that was formerly used therapeutically to prevent spontaneous abortion and premature delivery, until it was found to be associated with an increased incidence of clear cell vaginal carcinoma in the female offspring of mothers to whom it was administered [138, 139]. As presented in Table 15.1, DES is likely to have both nongenotoxic and genotoxic modes of action in producing this malignancy. Firstly, during fetal development DES crosses the placenta, binds to intracellular estrogen receptors of the ER-α subtype in the fetal genital tract, and this binding results in persistent proliferation of Muellerian-derived columnar epithelial cells rather than their normal replacement with squamous epithelium from the vaginal plate [140]. At the same time, DES may be genotoxic by virtue of the fact that it can be bioactivated by cytochrome P450 enzymes to a chemically reactive semiquinone and then further oxidized to a quinone [141, 142]. The quinone and semiquinone metabolites can then undergo redox cycling catalyzed by cytochrome b_5 reductase and cytochrome P450 to yield reactive oxygen species (ROS) that oxidatively damage DNA, while the semiquinone and minor epoxide metabolites can also covalently bind to DNA as either stable or depurinating adducts [143]. Depurinating adducts are thought to be the primary initiators of carcinogenesis, and that mutations occur from misrepair or misreplication of the apurinic sites [143]. Although specific gene mutations have not been identified in DES-induced clear cell adenomas in humans, upregulation of p53 gene expression has been observed [144], and this has been attributed to the cellular response to persistent DNA damage. Another study provided evidence of microsatellite instability in DES-induced clear cell adenoma tissue samples, supporting the idea that defective DNA repair is a key molecular feature of this tumor type [145].

On the other hand, strong evidence that DES-triggered ER-α activation itself is a requisite event in DES-induced tumor development comes from observations that DES-induced uterine hyperplasia and cancer in mice is enhanced by ER-α overexpression and absent in ER-α knockout mice [146, 147]. DES treatment of wild-type, but not ER-α knockout mice, also downregulated the uterine expression of Wnt7a, which controls tissue patterning during critical periods of embryogenesis [146]. Taken together, the earlier studies suggest a model whereby DES genotoxicity may initiate tumorigenesis while DES-mediated ER-α signaling promotes the proliferation of initiated cells.

Teratogenic effects of drugs

This section reviews general concepts of mechanisms of chemical teratogenesis, followed by a more focused discussion of two important and well-investigated human teratogens: ethanol (fetal alcohol spectrum disorders) and the sedative/hypnotic drug thalidomide (in utero death, limb defects, and other malformations).

General concepts of mechanisms of chemical teratogenesis

Teratological effects following in utero exposure of an embryo or fetus to harmful agents include both morphological and functional abnormalities. The former are exemplified by fetal death and shortened or missing limbs caused by thalidomide [148] and the latter by cognitive deficits and behavioral disorders caused by alcohol (ethanol) [149]. Each teratogen causes a characteristic abnormality, or pattern of abnormalities, in the fetus, such as shortened limbs or phocomelia resulting from maternal therapy with thalidomide [148]. However, even known teratogens will not exert a teratogenic effect unless they are given during the relevant embryonic or fetal periods of pregnancy when a tissue or organ is developing morphologically or functionally. The morphological formation of organs, or organogenesis, occurs mostly within the embryonic period, or first trimester of pregnancy, and exposure to teratogens during this period can result in morphological birth defects. In contrast, functional development occurs primarily during the later fetal period, or second and third trimesters, and in the brain continuing postnatally up to around 25 years of age. Exposure to teratogens during the fetal period can cause postnatal functional disorders like alterations in brain function leading to cognitive and motor disorders. In addition, embryonic and fetal xenobiotic exposure must also exceed a critical threshold for teratogenesis to occur.

The level of embryonic and fetal drug exposure is determined by: (a) maternal metabolism and elimination, which reduces the amount of drug available for placental transfer; (b) the rate of drug transfer across the placenta, which depends upon the balance of influx/efflux placental drug transport activities; and (c) embryonic and fetal clearance mechanisms. Some examples of these determinants, virtually all of which have been examined only in animal models with respect to teratogenicity, are discussed later.

Maternal metabolism and elimination

Maternal drug metabolism and elimination can reduce the amount of drug available for transfer to the embryo/fetus. Most drugs are converted in phase 1 reactions catalyzed by cytochromes P450 (CYPs) enzymes to stable metabolites, which in turn are metabolized by phase 2 enzymes like UDP-glucuronosyltransferases (UGTs) to form water-soluble products that are excreted via the kidney (Fig. 15.3). For example, pretreatment of pregnant mice with the CYP inducer, phenobarbital, reduced the teratogenicity of phenytoin in the progeny, presumably due to enhanced maternal CYP-catalyzed metabolism of phenytoin, which reduced maternal plasma phenytoin concentrations and fetal exposure [150]. Conversely, pretreatment with the CYP inhibitors, SKF 525A or fluconazole, enhanced teratogenicity, presumably due to reduced maternal phenytoin metabolism resulting in increased maternal plasma phenytoin concentrations and fetal exposure.

UGT-catalyzed glucuronidation is a major phase 2 pathway of elimination for most xenobiotics, and hence a likely maternal metabolic pathway for reducing the amount of drug entering the embryo or fetus, thereby reducing its teratogenic effect. In pregnant rats with a genetic UGT deficiency, maternal administration of a single, normally nontoxic dose (25 mg/kg i.p.) of the teratogen/carcinogen benzo[a]pyrene on gestational day (GD) 10 increased embryonic in utero death, or resorptions, compared both to untreated UGT-deficient controls and to benzo[a]pyrene-treated wild-type UGT-normal dams [151]. Among wild-type UGT-normal dams, embryonic death was not enhanced by this low dose of benzo[a]pyrene compared to vehicle controls, corroborating the protective role of maternal glucuronidation.

Placental drug transporters

Placental drug transporters, and particularly the efflux transporters phospho-glycoprotein (P-gp) and breast cancer resistance protein (BCRP), extrude a wide range of drugs from the embryo and fetus back into the maternal circulation [152]. This potentially protective effect is highly gestationally variable, as the expression of both transporters is high early in pregnancy but declines dramatically near term [152]. The magnitude of this protective effect, which varies for each drug substrate, can be substantial, as shown in pregnant double knockout mice lacking both multidrug resistance (*Mdr1*) genes coding for the two P-gp isoforms MDR1A and MDR1B [153]. Importantly, both placental isoforms of P-gp, while facing the maternal circulation, are derived from embryonic rather than maternal tissue, so the embryonic genotype is the key determinant. Following maternal treatment with the anticancer drug paclitaxel on GD 15, the ratio of the fetal-to-maternal plasma concentrations of paclitaxel was 16-fold higher in the *null* double knockout fetuses compared to the ratio in their wild-type P-gp-normal littermates.

Embryonic and fetal drug clearance

In human embryonic and fetal liver, activities of phase 1 and phase 2 drug-metabolizing enzymes, and particularly CYPs are not detectable until around the last week of the embryonic period (8th week of pregnancy), and during the first trimester typically reach only about 1%–10% of adult activities, depending upon the enzyme [154]. Although the activities for some enzymes increase somewhat during the second and third trimesters (the fetal period), most, and particularly most CYP isoforms, still do not exceed 10% of adult levels until after birth. One notable exception is CYP3A7, a "fetal" CYP that is highly expressed in fetal liver, but it declines after birth and is generally undetectable after 1 year of age. Retinoic acid is a CYP3A7 substrate, so this CYP isoform may provide protection against highly teratogenic retinoid drugs used topically or orally by young mothers during pregnancy to treat a variety of skin disorders [155]. However, CYP3A7 has a limited repertoire of drug substrates, and its catalytic efficacy for most, albeit not all, of these substrates is considerably lower than that for other CYP3A enzymes (primarily CYP3A4, CYP3A5), which are minimally expressed in fetal liver [154–156]. In general, the metabolism of most drugs by the fetal liver is highly limited, and fetal drug clearance does not provide substantial protection against most potential teratogens.

Xenobiotic bioactivation and oxidative stress in the embryo and fetus

Xenobiotics typically cause their pharmacological effects via the reversible binding of the xenobiotic and/or one or more of its stable metabolites to a specific receptor [157]. This is particularly true for the therapeutic effect of most drugs, including retinoid drugs that cause both their therapeutic and teratogenic affects by reversibly binding to retinoic acid receptors.

However, many of the more severe adverse effects of xenobiotics, including teratogenesis, often result from a relatively nontoxic xenobiotic, or "proteratogen," being enzymatically metabolized, or "bioactivated," within the embryo or fetus to a highly toxic and short-lived reactive intermediate (Fig. 15.3) [150, 151]. These include electrophilic reactive intermediates, which covalently or irreversibly bind to cellular macromolecules such as proteins and DNA, permanently altering their function. Toxicity is dependent upon the balance between the enzymatic pathway for formation of the electrophilic reactive intermediate, such as an epoxide, vs. one or both of two detoxifying pathways: (a) insertion of water at the electrophilic site to form a nontoxic diol metabolite, catalyzed by epoxide hydrolase; and, (b) conjugation with the peptide glutathione (GSH) to form a usually nontoxic GSH conjugate, catalyzed by GSH *S*-transferases.

Alternatively, xenobiotics can be bioactivated to free radical reactive intermediates and/or enhance the formation of reactive oxygen species (ROS), including hydrogen peroxide (H_2O_2), superoxide anion ($O_2^{\bullet -}$), and hydroxyl radicals ($HO^{\bullet}$) (Fig. 15.9). H_2O_2 can reversibly oxidize sulfhydryl (thiol) groups on specific signal transduction proteins, while $HO^{\bullet}$ can cause irreversible oxidative damage to all cellular macromolecules, in either case altering their function [157–159]. ROS-mediated oxidative damage to DNA, in particular, can be enzymatically repaired, providing one last level of protection, as discussed later. The oxidation of protein thiols by H_2O_2 is readily reversed by reaction with soluble cellular reducing agents like GSH, and this process plays a major role in regulating signal transduction in many physiologically processes. Drug free radical intermediates also can covalently bind to cellular protein and DNA, exemplified by the covalent binding of the phenytoin free radical intermediate to DNA, although a causal role for such drug-DNA adducts in developmental disorders remains uncertain. As with electrophilic reactive intermediates, toxicity is dependent upon the balance of free radical intermediate/ROS formation vs ROS detoxification and DNA repair. ROS are detoxified via an array of antioxidants and antioxidative enzymes (Fig. 15.9) that are mostly different from the enzymes that detoxify electrophilic reactive intermediates, with the exception of GSH discussed as follows and later under ROS detoxification (Fig. 15.3) [151].

GSH is the one major protective component shared by both the electrophilic and the free radical/ROS pathways. However, in the former pathway GSH serves as a cosubstrate that reacts with the drug electrophilic reactive intermediate and is eliminated as a GSH-drug conjugate, while in the latter pathway GSH serves as a cofactor and is oxidized to form glutathione disulfide (GSSG) during the reduction of the free radical or H_2O_2 to stable nontoxic products (Fig. 15.9). Thus electrophilic reactive intermediates deplete GSH, and protective homeostasis is maintained by the synthesis of new GSH, while GSSG produced during the detoxification of free radicals and H_2O_2 is maintained by the reduction of GSSG to two molecules of GSH, catalyzed by glutathione reductase. This difference is important in distinguishing the teratological mechanism and for developing therapeutic approaches for mitigating developmental disorders, as discussed later for specific teratogens.

Due to their chemical instability, both electrophilic and free radical reactive intermediates typically must be both formed and detoxified within the embryo or fetus, rather than in maternal tissues. There may be exceptions for intermediates of lesser reactivity that might cross the placenta intact. However, this has not been observed for teratogens that have been investigated to date, particularly in embryo culture lacking any maternal bioactivating source, and in genetically modified mouse models where developmental disorders are dependent upon the fetal rather than the maternal genotype, as discussed later. Therefore maternal biochemical measurements usually do not predict embryonic or fetal risk, aside from determining the maternal plasma concentration of a proteratogen that can cross the placenta, as discussed later.

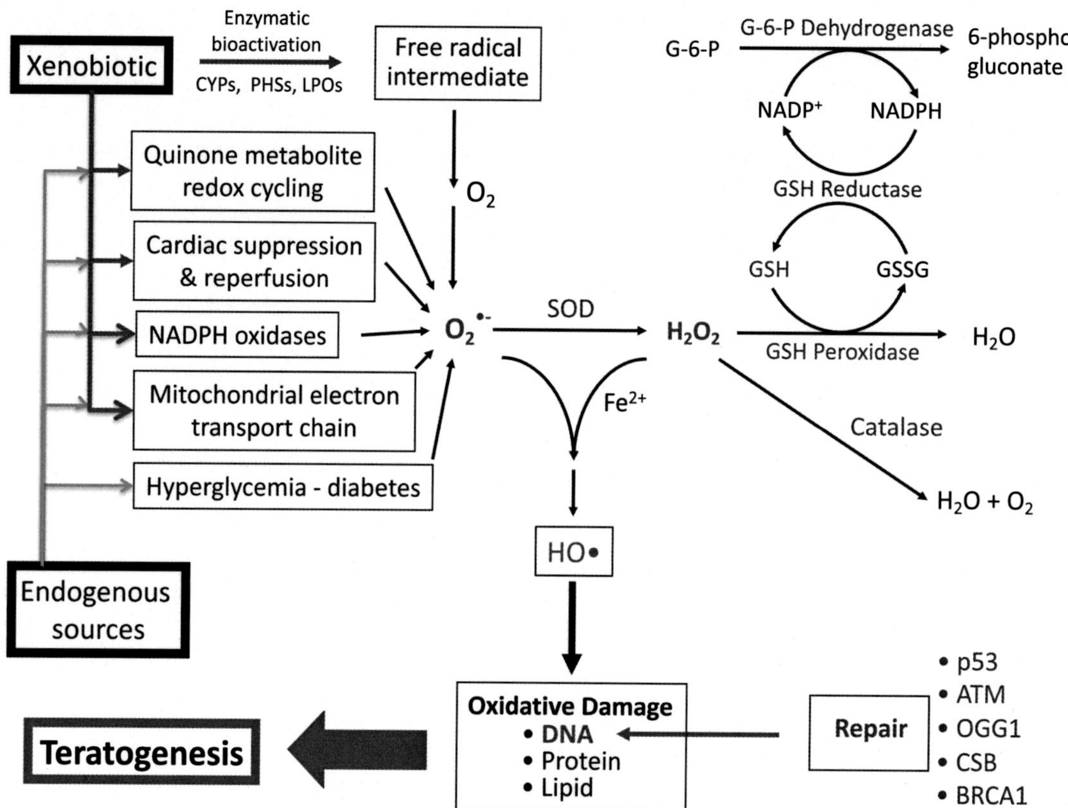

FIG. 15.9 Biochemical pathways for physiological and ethanol (EtOH)-enhanced formation and detoxification of reactive oxygen species (ROS). ROS include superoxide anions ($O_2^{\bullet -}$), hydrogen peroxide (H_2O_2), and hydroxyl radicals ($HO^{\bullet}$). Teratogenesis is postulated to result from H_2O_2-mediated reversible alterations in embryonic/fetal signal transduction in target tissues, and/or irreversible macromolecular damage caused primarily by $HO^{\bullet}$, and in some circumstances by H_2O_2. If embryonic or fetal ROS formation exceeds the proximal capacity for ROS detoxification and/or repair of cellular macromolecules, this imbalance can result in enhanced teratogenesis, even at a therapeutic drug concentration or generally "safe" exposure level for an environmental chemical. Many of the same ROS-forming pathways that are enhanced by xenobiotics are also responsible for physiological ROS formation, and imbalances between conceptal ROS formation versus detoxification and the repair of oxidatively damaged DNA can have pathogenic consequences even under normal conditions in the absence of xenobiotic exposures. Abbreviations: ATM, ataxia telangiectasia mutated protein; BRCA1, breast cancer 1 protein; CSB, Cockayne syndrome B protein; CYPs, cytochromes P450; Fe, iron; G-6-P, glucose-6-phosphate; GSH, glutathione; GSSG, glutathione disulfide; LPOs, lipoxygenases; NADP+, nicotinamide adenine dinucleotide phosphate; OGG1, oxoguanine glycosylase 1; PHSs, prostaglandin H synthases; SOD, superoxide dismutase. *(Modified from Wells PG, McCallum GP, Chen CS, et al. Oxidative stress in developmental origins of disease: teratogenesis, neurodevelopmental deficits and cancer. Toxicol Sci 2009;108:4–18.)*

Multiple contributing mechanisms of teratogenesis

The earlier mentioned mechanisms of teratogenesis are not mutually exclusive, and xenobiotics may cause developmental disorders by one or a combination of mechanisms mediated via reversible reactions with receptors, and irreversible reactions of an electrophilic reactive intermediate or a drug free radical intermediate or ROS. Moreover, the relative contributions of these mechanisms may vary with the xenobiotic, time of gestational exposure, the embryonic/fetal target tissue or cell type, and environmental factors. This variability arises in part because the earlier teratological mechanisms are enzymatically or protein dependent, and the ontogeny of gene expression and levels of their functional protein products can change dramatically throughout gestation. Further variation can result from environmental influences such as exposure to exogenous chemicals, as well as from inherent differences in gene expression by race and, in animal models, by species and strain.

Enzymes such as CYPs, which commonly bioactivate xenobiotics to electrophilic reactive intermediates, are negligible in the human embryo and low in the fetus, and even lower in the fetuses of rodents. For this and other reasons, the importance of this mechanism in teratogenesis is somewhat controversial. For example, the antiepileptic drug phenytoin causes morphological and neurodevelopmental disorders in humans, characterized as the fetal hydantoin syndrome (FHS), and early studies in humans and rodents implicated an electrophilic epoxide reactive intermediate in the mechanism [150]. However, results from subsequent studies of phenytoin and structurally related antiepileptic drugs in rodent models are not consistent with the involvement of an epoxide intermediate, and suggest a role for a free radical intermediate and ROS formation, among other mechanisms. Studies relating to electrophilic reactive intermediates in teratogenesis, including the FHS, are reviewed elsewhere [150, 157].

ROS formation

In contrast to limited embryonic/fetal CYP-catalyzed formation of an electrophilic reactive intermediate, several pathways for ROS formation are highly active in both the rodent and human embryo and fetus (Fig. 15.9) [150, 158]. There are two particularly important embryonic/fetal pathways for enzymatic ROS formation. The first is bioactivation of xenobiotics by peroxidases such as prostaglandin H synthases (PHSs) and lipoxygenases (LPOs), which are highly expressed in the embryo, to free radical intermediates that enhance ROS formation, exemplified by benzo[a]pyrene, phenytoin and structurally related antiepileptic drugs, thalidomide and methamphetamine. The second pathway is xenobiotic-induced activation of NADPH oxidases (NOXs) that produce ROS directly, exemplified by ethanol, methanol, and possibly methamphetamine [149, 150, 159]. A third and less well examined pathway involves the formation of ROS and related reactive nitrogen species (RNS) by nitric oxide synthases (NOS), which has been implicated to some extent in the teratogenicity of phenytoin and benzo[a]pyrene [150]. Due to their highly unstable nature, ROS, and particularly $HO^{\bullet}$, need to be formed within the embryo and fetus, and even within target tissues/cells and subcellular organelles (e.g., nucleus), rather than via maternal production and transport to the embryo or fetus. This localized embryonic/fetal enzymatic dependence is corroborated by rodent embryo culture studies, which in the absence of maternal tissues demonstrate enzyme-catalyzed ROS formation, as well as ROS detoxification and DNA repair, all within the embryo. A corollary of this embryonic/fetal dependence is that measurements in the mother (or dam, for rodents) do not necessarily provide relevant information about genetic or environmental determinants of teratological risk for their embryo or fetus.

ROS detoxification

ROS are essential regulators of numerous signaling pathways required for normal development and life, but they can have pathogenic effects even at normal levels in a biochemically predisposed embryo or fetus [149, 158–160]. The embryo and fetus are particularly susceptible to the pathogenic potential of ROS because the activity of several protective embryonic antioxidative enzymes is only about 5% of maternal hepatic levels, including superoxide dismutase (SOD), which converts $O_2^{\bullet-}$ to H_2O_2; and, catalase and glutathione peroxidase, both of which detoxify H_2O_2 (Fig. 15.9). These pathways, while quantitatively minor, provide important protection against both physiological and drug-enhanced levels of fetal ROS formation, as progeny genetically deficient in antioxidative enzymes such as catalase are more susceptible to even physiological levels of ROS formation, and more so to drug-enhanced ROS formation. The pathogenic role of ROS and the embryoprotective importance of catalase were confirmed by pretreatment with a stabilized form of catalase that is conjugated with polyethylene glycol (PEG). Maternal pretreatment with PEG-catalase increases embryonic and fetal catalase activity and blocks the developmental toxicity of drugs such as phenytoin in vivo and in embryo culture. In contrast, other enzymes important for antioxidative protection may equal or exceed maternal levels, exemplified by glucose-6-phosphate dehydrogenase (G6PD), which generates the cofactor NADPH necessary for the regeneration of GSH from GSSG (glutathione disulfide), the latter reaction being catalyzed by glutathione reductase. In the detoxification of free radicals and H_2O_2, as discussed earlier, GSH either nonenzymatically reduces free radicals or serves as a cofactor for antioxidative enzymes such as glutathione peroxidase that detoxify hydroperoxides including H_2O_2, in either case being oxidized to GSSG, which can be enzymatically converted back to two molecules of GSH. The central role of embryonic/fetal GSH in protecting against ROS-initiating teratogens has been supported by several lines of evidence, exemplified by phenytoin teratogenicity, which was enhanced by the following approaches: (a) pretreatment with GSH-depleting agents like diethyl maleate and acetaminophen, or an inhibitor of GSH synthesis, buthionine sulfoximine; (b) pretreatment with a low, non-teratogenic dose of the glutathione reductase inhibitor *bis*-choroethyl-nitrosourea (BCNU); and (c) maternal dietary depletion of selenium, the essential cofactor for glutathione peroxidase, sufficient to reduce fetal enzyme activity [150]. In the latter case, selenium repletion restored fetal glutathione peroxidase activity and abolished the enhanced teratogenicity in progeny exposed to a selenium-deficient diet.

ROS-initiated transient effects and irreversible macromolecular damage

If not detoxified: (a) H_2O_2 can transiently and reversibly oxidize protein sulfhydryl groups on regulatory proteins, either increasing or decreasing signal transduction pathways during critical periods of development [158, 159]; (b) H_2O_2 at higher levels can irreversibly oxidize protein sulfhydryl groups; and/or (c) H_2O_2 reacts with $O_2^{\bullet-}$ to form highly reactive $HO^{\bullet}$, which irreversibly oxidizes cellular macromolecules such as lipids, proteins, RNA, and DNA thereby permanently altering their function (Fig. 15.9) [150, 158, 159]. Mutant or knockout mouse progeny deficient in one of several antioxidative enzymes (e.g., catalase, G6PD), when exposed in embryo culture or in utero to a ROS-initiating teratogen, exhibit enhanced oxidative DNA damage and developmental disorders compared to their normal wild-type littermates. Embryonic/fetal cellular macromolecules other than DNA, including RNA, proteins and lipids, are also oxidatively damaged by ROS, and may contribute to teratological mechanisms, but models have not been developed to evaluate their selective pathogenic contribution.

Oxidative DNA damage and repair

ROS cause over 20 different DNA lesions, the most prevalent of which is 8-oxoguanine (**8-oxoG**) [161]. These molecular lesions are rapidly repaired by an array of DNA repair enzymes/proteins including oxoguanine glycosylase 1 (OGG1), which initiates repair by cleaving the 8-oxoG lesion from DNA, thereby releasing free 8-oxoG (Fig. 15.10). The formation of 8-oxoG is not random, being concentrated in guanine-rich regulatory elements of the promoters and 5′-untranslated regions of selective genes [162]. Knockout mouse progeny deficient in key proteins involved in the cellular recognition and response to DNA damage (e.g., p53, ataxia telangiectasia mutated (ATM)) or the repair of DNA damage (e.g., oxoguanine glycosylase 1 (OGG1), Cockayne syndrome B (CSB)), when exposed to ROS-initiating agents, such as ionizing

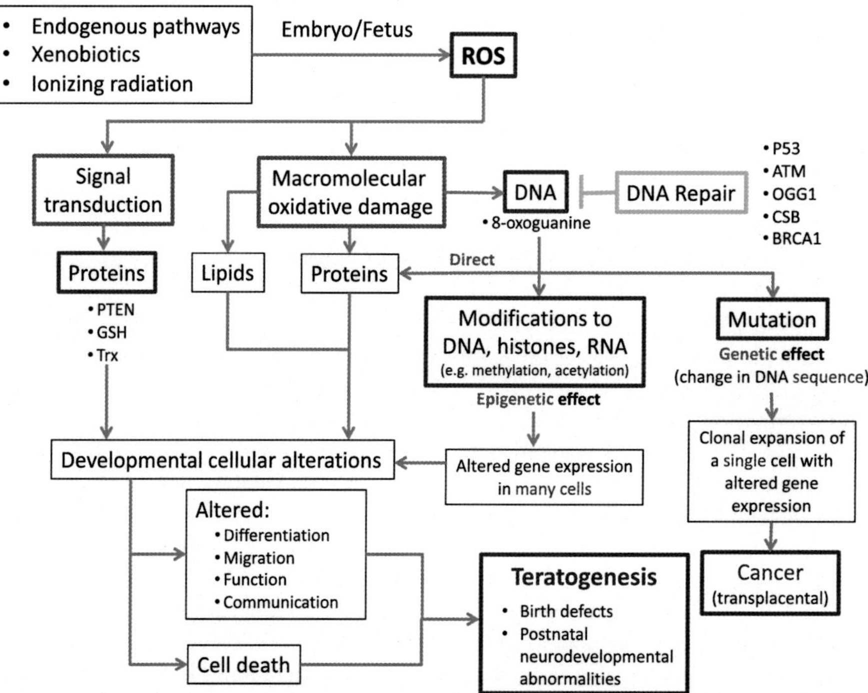

FIG. 15.10 Alternative biochemical mechanisms by which xenobiotic-enhanced formation of reactive oxygen species (ROS) can cause developmental disorders. Physiological or xenobiotic-enhanced levels of embryonic and fetal ROS can adversely affect development via one or both of the following two general mechanisms: (1) Irreversible oxidative damage to cellular macromolecules including DNA, proteins, peptides, and lipids. 8-Oxoguanine is the most prevalent of over 20 DNA lesions initiated by ROS, and this lesion is repaired by oxoguanine glycosylase 1 (OGG1), one of several DNA repair proteins regulated by breast cancer protein 1 (BRCA1) and known to protect the developing embryo and fetus from ROS-initiated DNA damage. DNA lesions like 8-oxoguanine (8-oxoG) can result in: (a) genetic mutations involving a change in DNA sequence in a single cell resulting in cellular immortalization, clonal expansion leading to postnatal cancer. Alternatively, 8-oxoG lesions can result in (b) direct or indirect epigenetic modifications to DNA, histones, or RNA that do not involve a change in DNA sequence, but alter gene expression in many cells, contributing to teratogenesis in the form of birth defects and postnatal neurodevelopmental abnormalities. (2) Reversible oxidative modification of signaling molecules, exemplified by phosphatase and tensin homolog (PTEN), glutathione (GSH), and thioredoxin (Trx). The degree to which either or both of these two alternative pathways contribute to the pathogenic mechanism may vary with the particular nature and timing of ROS initiation and the conceptal target tissue, among other factors. These biochemical changes can lead to nonapoptotic alterations in cellular function, including differentiation, migration, function, and communication, or may result in cell death. If these cellular alterations occur during critical windows of development, they may cause gross morphological birth defects or postnatal neurodevelopmental abnormalities. *(Modified from Bhatia S, Drake DM, Miller L, Wells PG. Oxidative stress and DNA damage in the mechanism of fetal alcohol spectrum disorders. Birth Defects Res 2019;111:714–748.)*

radiation and xenobiotics (e.g., benzo[a]pyrene, phenytoin, methamphetamine, ethanol), exhibit enhanced oxidative DNA damage and developmental disorders compared to their wild-type littermates with normal DNA repair [149, 150, 158, 159, 161]. The enhanced developmental disorders exhibited in DNA repair-deficient knockout progeny compared to their wild-type littermates implicate oxidative damage to DNA, as distinct from damage to other macromolecules, in the teratological mechanism, and embryonic/fetal DNA repair as an important determinant of risk.

Oxidative DNA damage, and particularly the 8-oxoG lesion, are well known to cause gene mutations in a single cell that result in the unregulated clonal expansion of a cell line, typically due to permanently activated oncogenes and/or down-regulated tumor suppressor genes, which ultimately can lead to cancer. This mutational mechanism can occur in the embryo or fetus following enhanced ROS exposure, leading to transplacental carcinogenesis arising postnatally (Fig. 15.10). For example, in utero exposure to the synthetic estrogen diethylstilbestrol can lead to vaginal and testicular tumors developing in female and male children, respectively, as discussed in the previous section. At the molecular level, carcinogenic mutations involve a "genetic" change, or a change in the sequence of nucleotides in DNA.

In contrast to carcinogenesis, developmental disorders, or teratogenesis, require changes in a critical mass of cells in the target tissue within the time window for the morphological and/or functional development of a tissue, organ, or system to be adversely affected (Fig. 15.10). At the molecular level, oxidative DNA damage initiates teratogenesis (aside from transplacental carcinogenesis) via nonmutational mechanisms including, but not limited to: (a) direct effects on developmental signal transduction proteins; and, (b) altered gene expression due to an "epigenetic" change, which involves the modification of a target gene or its surrounding histone proteins without changing the nucleotide sequence of the gene (Fig. 15.11). A direct effect of 8-oxoG on signal transduction proteins is exemplified by the complexing of cytosolic OGG1 with its excised repair product, the free base 8-oxoG, resulting in altered OGG1 binding activity [163]. This free OGG1-8-oxoG complex can serve as a guanine nucleotide exchange factor (GEF), binding to and activating small GTPases, which in turn bind to downstream signaling pathway proteins that regulate signal transduction. Small GTPases subject to OGG1-8-oxoG regulation include the RAS protein family, which plays a role in carcinogenesis and possibly in phenytoin-initiated developmental disorders [150].

Alternatively, the 8-oxoG lesion in DNA can serve as a nonrandom epigenetic modification, typically enriched in regulatory regions of the promoter regions of selective genes (Fig. 15.11). The 8-oxoG modification, either alone or by recruiting OGG1, alters the local three-dimensional conformation of DNA and binding of transcription factors and regulatory proteins, which can switch gene expression either on or off depending on numerous local molecular factors including the specific guanine residues oxidized to 8-oxoG [163–165]. For example, the OGG1-8-oxoG complex in DNA enhances binding of the transcription factor NF-κB to the promoter regions of multiple target genes [166], and 8-oxoG alone in DNA facilitates recruitment of regulatory proteins to the promoter region of the *Kras* gene [167]. Both NF-κB and RAS proteins are involved in developmental signal transduction pathways, as noted before for phenytoin teratogenesis. Also, ROS-initiated 8-oxoG formation, with or without recruitment of OGG1, may alter epigenetic marks on DNA (methylation) or histone proteins (methylation, acetylation, etc.) via various mechanisms, thereby dysregulating gene expression [168, 169]. For example, in addition to direct effects on gene-transcription factor binding, 8-oxoG formation can alter the binding of repressor regulatory proteins such as methyl-CpG-binding proteins (MBPs), facilitating gene transcription [165]. These epigenetic modifications, which in some cases may be sustained over the lifespan of the exposed progeny and into subsequent generations (i.e., heritable), could result either from the altered binding of epigenetic modifiers (DNA demethylases and methyltransferases, histone deacetylases and acetyltransferases, etc.), or an alteration in their activity. In one example of ROS-initiated alterations in epigenetic DNA marks, the OGG1-8-oxoG complex in DNA recruits ten-eleven translocation methylcytosine dioxygenase 1 (TET1) [169], which oxidizes adjacent 5-methylcytosines (5-mC) to 5-hydroxymethylcytosine (5-hmC) in the first step of a 5-mC demethylation process that restores cytosine and gene activation. Another potential epigenetic mechanism potentially initiated by 8-oxoG alone or in combination with OGG1 is an alteration in the levels of noncoding RNAs (ncRNAs) including long noncoding RNAs (lncRNAs), which interact with transcriptional machinery and initiate chromatin compaction at commonly imprinted genes, and microRNAs (miRNAs) and small inhibiting RNAs (siRNAs), which bind to messenger RNAs (mRNAs), initiating their degradation and altering translation [170]. Altered levels of miRNAs, which can bind to many related mRNA transcripts and regulate entire gene networks, have been implicated in the mechanism of ethanol teratogenicity, discussed later [170], although the role of ROS-initiated 8-oxoG formation and repair by OGG1 in this mechanism has yet to be determined. RNAs also are highly susceptible to guanine oxidation [165], but the developmental implications this reaction have not been investigated.

There is a growing appreciation that the earlier direct and epigenetic roles for OGG1 and 8-oxoG are important for physiologically essential processes involving gene expression and signal transduction, as well as for potential pathogenic mechanisms arising from altered levels of ROS or DNA repair (Fig. 15.11) [163–165]. 8-OxoG formation can accordingly be considered either a molecular lesion or a physiological epigenetic modification, depending upon the context.

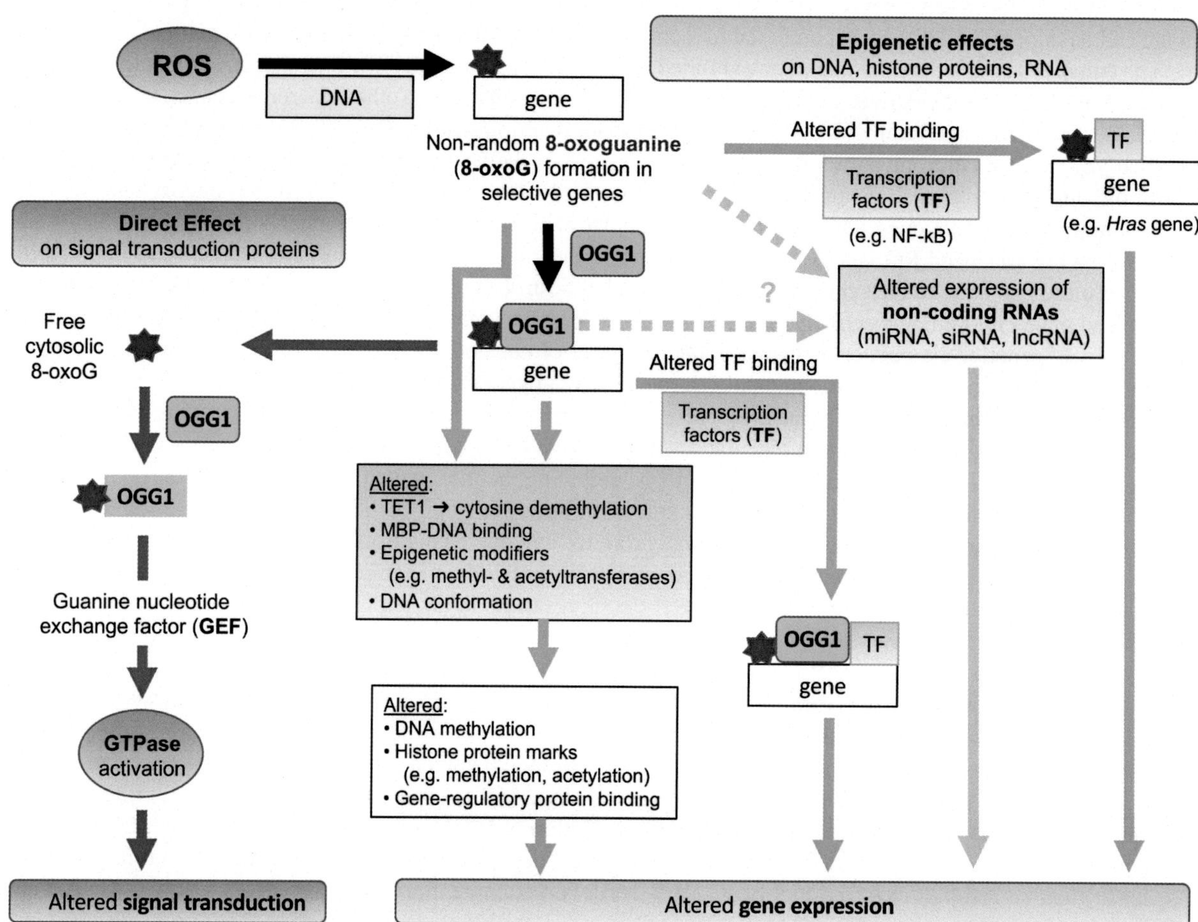

FIG. 15.11 Nonmutational mechanisms of teratogenesis initiated by the DNA lesion 8-oxoguanine (8-oxoG). Physiological or xenobiotic-enhanced levels of reactive oxygen species (ROS) in embryonic and fetal tissues oxidize guanine residues in DNA to form 8-oxoG, which is repaired by the enzyme oxoguanine glycosylase 1 (OGG1). 8-OxoG formation is nonrandom, and is particularly enriched in promoter regions of selective genes, leading to localized effects. 8-OxoG alone or bound to OGG1 can initiate changes in signal transduction or gene expression by a variety of nonmutational mechanisms including direct or epigenetic effects, for which some examples are illustrated (see text for details). (1) Direct effect: Cytosolic free 8-oxoG excised by OGG1 from oxidized DNA binds to OGG1 causing a conformation change in OGG1 that allows it to bind to cytosolic GTPases, thereby serving as a guanine nucleotide exchange factor (GEF) that activates the GTPase, altering signal transduction. (2) Epigenetic effects: (a) 8-OxoG alone or the 8-oxoG-OGG1complex can bind to selective genes, altering the binding of transcription factors and gene expression. Alternatively, 8-oxoG alone or the 8-oxoG-OGG1complex can: (b) alter TET binding and cytosine demethylation; alter the binding of methyl binding proteins (MBPs); alter the level and/or activity of epigenetic modifiers like DNA/histone protein methyltransferases or demethylases and histone/nonhistone protein acetyltransferases or deacetylases; and cause discrete conformation changes in selective DNA regions, all of which can alter gene expression. (c) 8-OxoG alone or the 8-oxoG-OGG1complex may directly affect RNAs, which are highly susceptible to oxidation by ROS, or alter their expression. Changes particularly in micro RNAs (miRNAs) have been associated with xenobiotic-initiated developmental disorders, but the role of ROS in these processes has yet to be determined.

With respect to the pathogenic consequences of oxidative DNA damage, DNA repair appears to have evolved primarily to protect the developing embryo and fetus from ROS-initiated developmental disorders, as opposed to its more widely appreciated role in tumor suppression. For example, in the case of BRCA1, which regulates multiple DNA repair pathways, the loss of even one *Brca1* allele renders BRCA1-deficient fetuses more susceptible to DNA damage and developmental disorders, in contrast to increased carcinogenesis, which requires the loss of both *Brca1* alleles [149]. Similarly, *Ogg1 null* mice are more susceptible to neurodevelopmental disorders caused by ROS-initiating drugs, but do not get cancer. These two DNA repair proteins accordingly appear to be more important in protecting the embryo and fetus from ROS-initiated developmental disorders than from cancer, which is consistent with the levels of both proteins being about twofold higher in fetal than maternal brains [149, 150].

Balance of embryonic/fetal pathways determines risk

As noted earlier for both electrophilic and free radical reactive intermediates, the risk of ROS-initiated developmental disorders accordingly depends upon the balance within each embryo or fetus among the pathways for ROS formation vs. ROS detoxification and DNA repair. This means that exposure to the embryo or fetus to even a therapeutic drug dose, or a generally accepted safe level of an environmental chemical, can be teratogenic in a biochemically predisposed embryo or fetus, which has, for either genetic or environmental reasons, an enhanced pathway for ROS formation, or an inadequate level of a key protein/enzyme for ROS detoxification or DNA damage repair. Because these pathways all lie within the embryo or fetus, an increased risk will not necessarily be detected by maternal biochemical measurements. One reason for this discrepancy is evident in studies of knockout mice lacking a particular protein, where heterozygous (+/−) parents with a deficiency in a particular protein are bred to produce progeny with all three genotypes (+/+, +/−, and −/−) in the same litter. Although the +/− littermates may have the same level of the protein as the (+/−) dam, the +/+ progeny typically have a higher level than the dam, and the −/− littermates a lower level. Another reason for fetal/maternal discrepancy is that embryonic and fetal protein/enzyme levels are often very different from maternal levels even with the same genotype. For example, embryonic/fetal levels of the antioxidative enzymes SOD and catalase are <5% of maternal levels, whereas levels of the DNA repair proteins OGG1 and BRCA1 are both about twofold higher in fetal than maternal brains.

The ROS sensor nuclear factor-erythroid 2-related factor 2 (NRF2), which is actively expressed in the embryo and fetus, regulates the expression of an array of proteins that contribute to the protective component of this balance, including enzymes that catalyze xenobiotic metabolism, ROS detoxification, and repair of oxidative DNA damage [159]. For example, NRF2 protects the embryo and fetus from ethanol-initiated embryonic ROS formation and apoptosis in vivo, and from oxidative DNA damage in fetal brain and postnatal neurodevelopmental disorders caused by in utero exposure to methamphetamine.

Pathogenic potential of normal levels of ROS formation

Even in the absence of exposure to an environmental teratogen, the embryos or fetuses with genetically reduced levels of either an important antioxidative enzyme (e.g., catalase or G6PD) or proteins involved in DNA repair (e.g., p53, ATM, BRCA1) (Figs. 15.9 and 15.10) exhibit increased oxidative DNA damage and developmental disorders [149, 150, 159]. This enhanced intrinsic risk reveals the pathogenic potential of even normal levels of ROS formation in a biochemically predisposed embryo or fetus, which may be relevant to developmental disorders like autism.

Multiple contributing mechanisms of teratogenesis

As noted earlier, the various mechanisms involving receptor- and reactive intermediate/ROS-mediated reactions are not mutually exclusive, and more than one mechanism may variably contribute to a teratological outcome. However, at least in animal models, the developmental disorders in embryo culture or in vivo caused by some xenobiotics (e.g., phenytoin, ethanol, thalidomide, methamphetamine, benzo[a]pyrene) can be definitively modified by genetic or pharmacological manipulation of pathways for ROS formation, ROS detoxification, and repair of oxidative DNA damage. This suggests that ROS-initiated effects, including oxidative DNA damage, play a central role in their mechanism of teratogenicity (Fig. 15.10).

The fetal alcohol syndrome and fetal alcohol spectrum disorders

In 1973 Kenneth Jones, David Smith, and colleagues characterized a combination of morphological and functional abnormalities in children exposed in utero to alcohol (ethanol) as the fetal alcohol syndrome (FAS) [171, 172]. Over the ensuing four decades, many studies have expanded our understanding of the human developmental consequences of in utero ethanol exposure. This includes a broader and variable array of teratological outcomes, including complex abnormalities in brain function [173], collectively termed fetal alcohol spectrum disorders (FASDs), with similar outcomes in animal models, reviewed elsewhere [149]. A recent well-controlled study of over 13,000 children found the prevalence of FASDs to be at least 1%–5%, and possibly as high as 3%–10% [174, 175], making ethanol one of the leading causes of preventable neurodevelopmental disorders [173].

Extensive studies have indicated multiple and complex potential mechanisms of FASDs and related risk factors involving genetic [176, 177] and epigenetic [170, 178, 179] mechanisms, and direct effects on proteins [149]. The cited studies and reviews here and later are only representative of a much broader body of evidence, much of which is included in the cited reviews. One complexity arises in the variable dose and duration of ethanol exposure in different studies and the extensive array of potential developmental effects of ethanol. Even within a particular gestational period, a limited number of mechanisms and resulting developmental disorders, and particularly some neurodevelopmental abnormalities, occur at lower ethanol doses and with briefer exposure periods than the majority of potential morphological and functional components of FASD. As the dose is increased, an increasing number of additional teratological molecular mechanisms are recruited along with an increasing range and severity of disorders. Increasing the duration of exposure within and beyond a particular gestational window further increases the number of teratological mechanisms and range and severity of resulting disorders to ultimately include the full spectrum and maximal severity of FASD. This section will focus on representative studies in animal models relating primarily to limited ethanol exposures that involve a more constrained number of teratological mechanisms, and particularly the role of ROS and oxidative DNA damage. More detailed reviews can be found elsewhere [159, 180], including genetic [176, 177] and epigenetic [170, 178] mechanisms that may or may not involve ROS.

Maternal metabolism

Maternal metabolism and elimination of ethanol by alcohol dehydrogenase (ADH) and acetaldehyde dehydrogenase appear to be developmentally protective in reducing maternal plasma concentrations and fetal exposure to ethanol and acetaldehyde. In three strains of maternal mice with differing levels of ADH, increasing maternal ADH activities correlated with decreasing maternal plasma ethanol concentrations and decreased fetal abnormalities [181].

ROS formation

Within the embryo and fetus, as well as in the adult brain, ethanol can induce/activate multiple NOX isoforms [182, 183], and ethanol increased ROS formation, oxidative DNA damage, embryonic caspase-3 activation, and apoptosis in mouse embryos in vivo, all of which were blocked by the NOX inhibitor diphenyleneiodonium chloride (DPI) [182]. Although apoptosis typically leads to developmental disorders, this study did not assess morphological or postnatal functional abnormalities, and definitive proof remains to be demonstrated. However, another alcohol, methanol, similarly upregulated in vivo embryonic NOX mRNA and protein levels, and enhanced oxidative protein damage, the latter of which was blocked by pretreatment with either DPI or the free radical spin trapping agent PBN [184]. Both DPI and PBN also blocked methanol-enhanced NOX mRNA and protein expression, although the apparent reduction in methanol-enhanced NOX protein expression by PBN was not significant. In mouse embryo culture, methanol-enhanced oxidative protein damage and embryopathies were both blocked by either DPI or PBN, corroborating NOX-catalyzed ROS formation in the pathogenic mechanism. Methanol embryopathies were not blocked by the dual PHS/LPO inhibitor ETYA, indicating that methanol, and perhaps ethanol, are not substrates for peroxidase-catalyzed bioactivation to a free radical intermediate, unlike phenytoin and some other xenobiotics. Ethanol also can form ROS during its metabolism by ADHs, acetaldehyde dehydrogenases and CYP2E1 [149], but the ability of DPI to block ethanol-initiated caspase-3 activation and apoptosis, and the relatively low levels of these enzymes in rodent embryos, suggest that embryonic NOXs constitute an important, if not the predominant, mechanism of proximate ROS formation by ethanol and methanol.

The pathogenic role of ROS in ethanol embryopathies in culture and teratogenicity in vivo has been corroborated by multiple approaches including: (a) direct measure of ethanol-enhanced ROS formation in embryo culture using fluorescent probes or nitroblue tetrazolium; (b) increased oxidative damage to embryonic/fetal DNA, proteins and lipids; (c) protection against oxidative damage to cellular macromolecules and embryopathies in culture or teratogenicity in vivo provided by pretreatment with PBN, antioxidants such as vitamin E, and exogenous antioxidative enzymes such as SOD and polyethylene glycol (PEG)-conjugated catalase; and, (d) genetically modified mice with progeny exhibiting either elevated or deficient embryonic levels of catalase compared to catalase-normal progeny were, respectively, resistant or more susceptible to ethanol-initiated DNA oxidation and embryopathies in culture or in utero death (resorptions) and morphological birth defects (Fig. 15.10) [149, 159]. This protective effect of endogenous catalase is remarkable given that embryonic catalase activity is only about 5% of maternal levels.

Pathogenic role of DNA damage in DNA repair-deficient progeny

DNA repair-deficient OGG1 knockout mouse progeny, compared to their wild-type littermates, exhibit enhanced ethanol-initiated oxidative DNA damage in embryos in culture [185] and in fetal brain in vivo [186], congruent with enhanced embryopathies in culture and neurodevelopmental deficits in vivo (Figs. 15.9 and 15.10). The development of fetal brain function is particularly sensitive to ROS, as neurodevelopmental abnormalities occur at lower ethanol doses than are necessary to cause the majority of morphological components of FASD. These results indicate that oxidative DNA damage, and particularly the 8-oxoguanine (8-oxoG) lesion, is a central component of the mechanism of ethanol teratogenicity, and that embryonic/fetal DNA repair activity is an important determinant of FASD risk. Preliminary studies in *Ogg1* knockout mice suggest that the 8-oxoG lesion alone and/or together with OGG1 epigenetically alter DNA methylation [168], and other nonmutational mechanisms discussed previously will likely be found. A developmentally pathogenic role for oxidative DNA damage nevertheless does not exclude potential pathogenic contributions from other ROS-mediated mechanisms yet to be determined, such as oxidative damage to other cellular macromolecules (proteins, lipids) and reversible oxidation of protein sulfhydryl groups.

NRF2 and the balance of embryonic pathways in determining risk

The risk of FASD is determined, at least in part, by the balance of embryonic/fetal pathways for ethanol-initiated ROS formation vs. ROS detoxification and repair of oxidative DNA damage [149], and nuclear factor-E2-related factor 2 (NRF2) is a ROS sensor and regulator of many of these pathways [159]. Maternal ethanol administration induced embryonic *Nrf2* mRNA and protein, NRF2 binding to the antioxidant response element of target genes, and expression of mRNA and protein for several antioxidative enzymes, all of which were enhanced by pretreatment with the NRF2 inducer 3*H*-1,2-dithiole-3-thione (D3T) [187]. D3T pretreatment also inhibited ethanol-initiated embryonic ROS formation and apoptosis, consistent with a ROS-dependent mechanism of ethanol teratogenicity. Although morphological or functional disorders were not evaluated in this study, apoptosis is typically associated with developmental disorders, and NRF2 was protective against postnatal neurodevelopmental deficits caused by in utero exposure to another ROS-initiating teratogen, methamphetamine [188].

Thalidomide teratogenicity

The history and potential mechanisms of thalidomide teratogenicity have been extensively reviewed elsewhere [148], and this section will focus upon two more recently investigated mechanisms that are not mutually exclusive: (a) thalidomide-enhanced embryonic ROS initiation and oxidative DNA damage; and, (b) thalidomide binding to the adaptor protein cereblon (CRBN). Maternal use of the sedative/hypnotic drug thalidomide during pregnancy in the early 1960s caused severe limb abnormalities and other malformations in over 10,000 children exposed in utero, and many others died before birth [148]. There is a remarkable species specificity among animal models, with rats, mice and hamsters being virtually resistant, particularly to limb malformations, while rabbits, zebrafish, chickens and several other species are susceptible [148, 189]. Although the mechanisms of thalidomide teratogenicity remain to be definitively established, particularly in humans, there is compelling evidence for the involvement of ROS, altered expression or inhibition of transcription factors including NF-κB, bone morphogenetic proteins (BMPs), fibroblast growth factor 9 (FGF8) and sonic hedgehog (SHH), and inhibition of angiogenesis [148]. Most recently, thalidomide binding to the Cullin 4 (CUL4)-cereblon (CRBN) E3 ubiquitin ligase complex, which ubiquitinates developmentally important transcription factors and targets them for degradation, has also been shown to play an important role in the mechanism of thalidomide teratogenesis (Fig. 15.12) [190–192]. However, whether or how, and to what extent and in what sequence this mechanism interacts with those earlier remains to be established [189].

Embryonic PHS/LPO-catalyzed bioactivation of thalidomide and hydrolysis products and ROS formation

In pregnant rabbits, thalidomide enhanced embryonic oxidative DNA damage (8-oxoG) and teratogenicity, both of which were blocked by pretreatment with the free radical spin trapping agent PBN [193], as was teratogenicity by pretreatment with the PHS inhibitor acetylsalicylic acid (ASA) [194]. Remarkably, thalidomide did not cause oxidative DNA damage in mouse embryos, which are completely resistant to thalidomide teratogenicity, providing a basis for the species specificity in susceptibility to thalidomide teratogenesis. Fibroblast studies suggest the resistance of mice to thalidomide-initiated, ROS-mediated teratogenesis may be due at least in part to higher GSH levels [195]. In rabbit embryo culture, similar to in vivo studies, oxidative DNA damage and embryopathies, including limb bud abnormalities, were initiated by thalidomide and by two of its many hydrolysis products, and both DNA damage and embryopathies were blocked by pretreatment with either ASA, the dual PHS/LPO inhibitor ETYA or PBN [196]. These studies in vivo and in embryo culture showed that thalidomide as well as two of its more stable hydrolysis products are bioactivated by embryonic PHSs and possibly by LPOs to reactive intermediates that initiate ROS formation and pathogenic oxidative DNA damage.

Thalidomide binding to the adaptor protein cereblon (CRBN)

In this pathway (Fig. 15.12) [189], a series of comprehensive in vivo and in vitro studies have shown that thalidomide binds to the embryonic CRBN component of the CUL4-CRBN E3 ubiquitin ligase complex [191], resulting in the recruitment

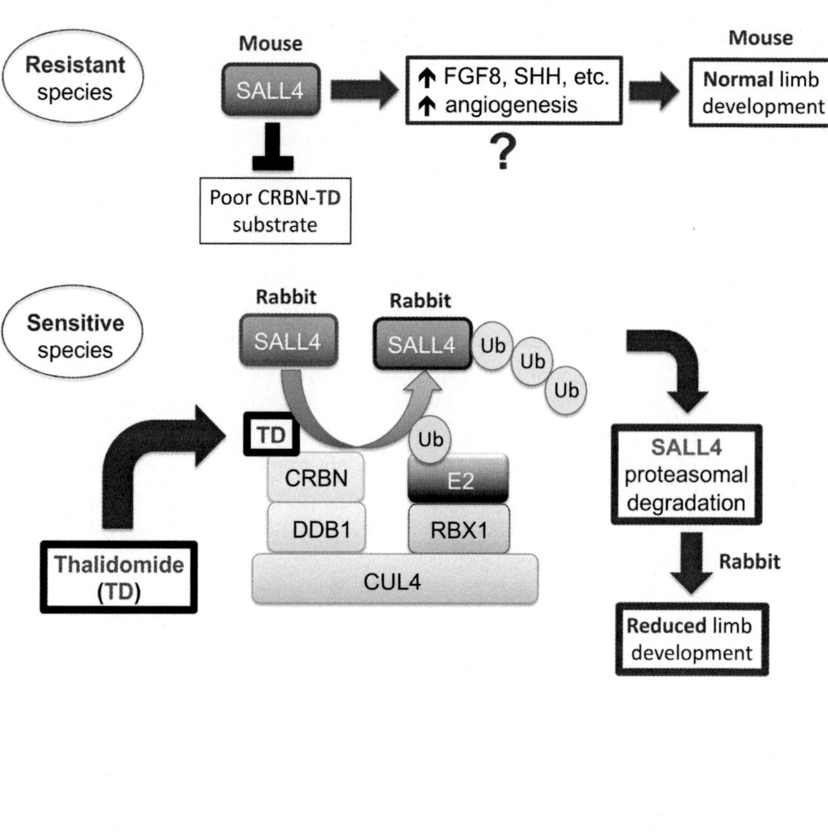

FIG. 15.12 Thalidomide binding to the adaptor protein cereblon (CRBN). Variants of spalt-like transcription factor 4 (SALL4) are a determinant of the species-specific nature of susceptibility to thalidomide (TD) teratogenicity. In sensitive species (rabbits, zebrafish, and chicks), TD binds to the CBRN component of the CUL4-CRBN E3 ubiquitin ligase complex, resulting in the recruitment and ubiquitination of SALL4, which targets SALL4 for proteasomal degradation. In contrast, resistant species (mice, rats) express a SALL4 variant that binds minimally to the TD-CRBN complex and are protected from SALL4 degradation and TD teratogenicity. SALL4 expression in mice may lead directly or indirectly to altered expression of fibroblast growth factor 8 (FGF8), Sonic hedgehog (SHH), and other transcription factors, as well as to increased angiogenesis in embryonic limb buds, which results in normal limb formation. The sequence of the latter two processes (transcription factor expression and angiogenesis) may differ among species, and it is not known if these processes are SALL4/CRBN-dependent, nor whether or how these processes relate to TD teratogenesis mediated by reactive oxygen species (see text). Additional potential CRBN-dependent and possibly independent mechanisms are discussed in the text. Components of the CUL4-CRBN E3 ubiquitin (Ub) ligase complex include Cullin 4 (CUL4), cereblon (CRBN), DNA damage binding protein 1 (DDB1), ring box protein (RBX1) and an E2 ubiquitin-conjugating enzyme. *(Modified from Wells PG. A new target for thalidomide. Nat Chem Biol 2018;14:904–905.)*

and ubiquitination of the developmental transcription factor spalt-like transcription factor 4 (SALL4), which targets SALL4 for rapid degradation by the 26S proteasome [190, 192]. Thalidomide binds with similar efficacy to CRBN in both mice and rabbits, which are respectively resistant and susceptible to thalidomide teratogenicity, so while thalidomide binding to CRBN is necessary for teratogenesis, it is not sufficient to explain the critical difference in species-specific susceptibility. The latter is explained by the binding of SALL4 to the thalidomide-CRBN-Cul4 complex, which occurs in humans and rabbits, resulting in the degradation of SALL4, failed signal transduction and teratogenesis in these species. In contrast, mice, which are resistant to thalidomide teratogenesis, express a SALL4 variant that does not substantially bind to the thalidomide-CRBN-Cul4 complex, leaving SALL4 intact to fulfill its normal role in signal transduction and development.

Multiple mechanisms of thalidomide teratogenesis

It remains to be determined: (a) if the earlier two mechanisms (ROS and CBRN) constitute alternative pathways of teratogenesis, sequential pathways or interacting pathways; (b) if the CRBN/SALL4 pathway is relevant to the two embryopathic hydrolysis products of thalidomide; (c) how either the ROS or CRBN/SALL4 pathways relate to the inhibition of angiogenesis, as well as the other transcription factors already associated with thalidomide teratogenesis in animal models; and, (d) whether among thalidomide-sensitive species the relative contributions of the ROS and CBRN/SALL4 pathways vary with species, strain, gestational stage of thalidomide exposure, thalidomide dose, and genetic or environmental factors that alter the component genes and proteins constituting each pathway [189]. Similar questions remain for the other mechanisms implicated in thalidomide teratogenesis, including alterations in transcription factors (NF-κB, BMPs, FGF8, SHH) and impaired angiogenesis.

References

[1] Rawlins MD, Thomas SHL. Mechanisms of adverse drug reactions. In: Davies DM, Ferner RE, de Glanville H, editors. Davies's textbook of adverse drug reactions. 5th ed. London: Chapman & Hall Medical; 1998. p. 40–64.

[2] Edwards IR, Aronson JK. Adverse drug reactions: definitions, diagnosis, and management. Lancet 2000;356:1255–1259.

[3] Uetrecht JP. New concepts in immunology relevant to idiosyncratic drug reactions: the "danger hypothesis" and innate immune system. Chem Res Toxicol 1999;12:387–395.

[4] Xu JJ, Henstock PV, Dunn MC, Smith AR, Chabot JR, de Graaf D. Cellular imaging predictions of clinical drug-induced liver injury. Toxicol Sci 2008;105:97–105.

[5] Miller EC, Miller JA. Mechanisms of chemical carcinogenesis: nature of proximate carcinogens and interactions with macromolecules. Pharmacol Rev 1966;18:805–838.

[6] Kanigel R. Apprentice to genius. New York: MacMillan; 1986.

[7] Brodie BB, Axelrod J. The fate of acetanilide in man. J Pharmacol Exp Ther 1948;94:29–38.

[8] Ostapowicz G, Fontana RJ, Schiodt FV, et al. Results of a prospective study of acute liver failure at 17 tertiary care centers in the United States. Ann Intern Med 2002;137:947–954.

[9] Mitchell JR, Snodgrass WR, Gillette JR. The role of biotransformation in chemical-induced liver injury. Environ Health Perspect 1976;15:27–38.

[10] Mitchell JR, Thorgeirsson SS, Potter WZ, Jollow DJ, Keiser H. Acetaminophen-induced hepatic injury: protective role of glutathione in man and rationale for therapy. Clin Pharmacol Ther 1974;16:676–684.

[11] Henderson CJ, Wolf CR, Kitteringham N, Powell H, Otto D, Park BK. Increased resistance to acetaminophen hepatotoxicity in mice lacking glutathione S-transferase Pi. Proc Natl Acad Sci U S A 2000;97:12741–12745.

[12] Sharma AM, Li Y, Novalen M, Hayes MA, Uetrecht J. Bioactivation of nevirapine to a reactive quinone methide: implications for liver injury. Chem Res Toxicol 2012;25:1708–1719.

[13] Sharma AM, Novalen M, Tanino T, Uetrecht JP. 12-OH-nevirapine sulfate, formed in the skin, is responsible for nevirapine-induced skin rash. Chem Res Toxicol 2013;26:817–827.

[14] Chen X, Tharmanathan T, Mannargudi B, Gou H, Uetrecht JP. A study of the specificity of lymphocytes in nevirapine-induced skin rash. J Pharmacol Exp Ther 2009;331:836–841.

[15] Sharma AM, Uetrecht J. Bioactivation of drugs in the skin: relationship to cutaneous adverse drug reactions. Drug Metab Rev 2014;46:1–18.

[16] Klebanoff SJ, Kettle AJ, Rosen H, Winterbourn CC, Nauseef WM. Myeloperoxidase: a front-line defender against phagocytosed microorganisms. J Leukoc Biol 2013;93:185–198.

[17] Gardner I, Leeder JS, Chin T, Zahid N, Uetrecht JP. A comparison of the covalent binding of clozapine and olanzapine to human neutrophils in vitro and in vivo. Mol Pharmacol 1998;53:999–1008.

[18] Kalgutkar AS, Gardner I, Obach RS, et al. A comprehensive listing of bioactivation pathways of organic functional groups. Curr Drug Metab 2005;6:161–225.

[19] Stachulski AV, Baillie TA, Park BK, et al. The generation, detection, and effects of reactive drug metabolites. Med Res Rev 2013;33:985–1080.

[20] Kalgutkar AS, Dalvie D. Predicting toxicities of reactive metabolite-positive drug candidates. Annu Rev Pharmacol Toxicol 2015;55:35–54.

[21] Zimmerman H. Hepatotoxicity: the adverse effects of drugs and other chemicals on the liver. Philadelphia, PA: Lippincott Williams & Wilkins; 1999.

[22] Satoh H, Martin BM, Schulick AH, Christ DD, Kenna JG, Pohl LR. Human anti-endoplasmic reticulum antibodies in sera of patients with halothane-induced hepatitis are directed against a trifluoroacetylated carboxylesterase. Proc Natl Acad Sci U S A 1989;86:322–326.

[23] Timbrell JA, Mitchell JR, Snodgrass WR, Nelson SD. Isoniazid hepatotoxicity: the relationship between covalent binding and metabolism *in vivo*. J Pharmacol Exp Ther 1980;213:364–369.

[24] Daly AK. Are polymorphisms in genes relevant to drug disposition predictors of susceptibility to drug-induced liver injury. Pharm Res 2017;34:1564–1569.

[25] Metushi IG, Nakagawa T, Uetrecht J. Direct oxidation and covalent binding of isoniazid to rodent liver and human hepatic microsomes: humans are more like mice than rats. Chem Res Toxicol 2012;25:2567–2576.

[26] Metushi IG, Sanders C, Lee WM, Uetrecht J. Detection of anti-isoniazid and anti-cytochrome P450 antibodies in patients with isoniazid-induced liver failure. Hepatology 2014;59:1084–1093.

[27] Maddrey WC, Boitnott JK. Isoniazid hepatitis. Ann Intern Med 1973;79:1–12.

[28] Foureau DM, Walling TL, Maddukuri V, et al. Comparative analysis of portal hepatic infiltrating leucocytes in acute drug-induced liver injury, idiopathic autoimmune and viral hepatitis. Clin Exp Immunol 2015;180:40–51.

[29] Daly AK, Day CP. Genetic association studies in drug-induced liver injury. Drug Metab Rev 2012;44:116–126.

[30] Cirulli ET, Nicoletti P, Abramson K, et al. A missense variant in PTPN22 is a risk factor for drug-induced liver injury. Gastroenterology 2019;156:1707–1716.e2.

[31] Luyendyk JP, Maddox JF, Cosma GN, Ganey PE, Cockerell GL, Roth RA. Ranitidine treatment during a modest inflammatory response precipitates idiosyncrasy-like liver injury in rats. J Pharmacol Exp Ther 2003;307:9–16.

[32] Mak A, Uetrecht J. Immunization with amodiaquine-modified hepatic proteins prevents amodiaquine-induced liver injury. J Immunotoxicol 2015;12:361–367.

[33] Watkins PB, Desai M, Berkowitz SD, et al. Evaluation of drug-induced serious hepatotoxicity (eDISH): application of this data organization approach to phase III clinical trials of rivaroxaban after total hip or knee replacement surgery. Drug Saf 2011;34:243–252.

[34] Harrison AC, Kitteringham NR, Clarke JB, Park BK. The mechanism of bioactivation and antigen formation of amodiaquine in the rat. Biochem Pharmacol 1992;43:1421–1430.
[35] Neftel KA, Woodtly W, Schmid M, Frick PG, Fehr J. Amodiaquine induced agranulocytosis and liver damage. Br Med J (Clin Res Ed) 1986;292:721–723.
[36] Metushi IG, Cai P, Dervovic D, et al. Development of a novel mouse model of amodiaquine-induced liver injury with a delayed onset. J Immunotoxicol 2015;12:247–260.
[37] Metushi IG, Hayes MA, Uetrecht J. Treatment of PD-1(-/-) mice with amodiaquine and anti-CTLA4 leads to liver injury similar to idiosyncratic liver injury in patients. Hepatology 2015;61:1332–1342.
[38] Mak A, Uetrecht J. The role of CD8 T cells in amodiaquine-induced liver injury in PD1-/- mice cotreated with anti-CTLA-4. Chem Res Toxicol 2015;28:1567–1573.
[39] Mak A, Uetrecht J. The combination of anti-CTLA-4 and PD1-/- mice unmasks the potential of isoniazid and nevirapine to cause liver injury. Chem Res Toxicol 2015;28:2287–2291.
[40] Suzman DL, Pelosof L, Rosenberg A, Avigan MI. Hepatotoxicity of immune checkpoint inhibitors: an evolving picture of risk associated with a vital class of immunotherapy agents. Liver Int 2018;38:976–987.
[41] Osanlou O, Pirmohamed M, Daly AK. Pharmacogenetics of adverse drug reactions. Adv Pharmacol 2018;83:155–190.
[42] Chowdhury NI, Remington G, Kennedy JL. Genetics of antipsychotic-induced side effects and agranulocytosis. Curr Psychiatry Rep 2011;13:156–165.
[43] Hallberg P, Eriksson N, Ibañez L, et al. Genetic variants associated with antithyroid drug-induced agranulocytosis: a genome-wide association study in a European population. Lancet Diabetes Endocrinol 2016;4:507–516.
[44] Chung WH, Hung SI, Hong HS, et al. Medical genetics: a marker for Stevens-Johnson syndrome. Nature 2004;428:486.
[45] Landsteiner K, Jacobs J. Studies on the sensitization of animals with simple chemical compounds. J Exp Med 1935;61:643–656.
[46] Matzinger P. Tolerance, danger and the extended family. Annu Rev Immunol 1994;12:991–1045.
[47] Pichler WJ. Pharmacological interaction of drugs with antigen-specific immune receptors: the p-i concept. Curr Opin Allergy Clin Immunol 2002;2:301–305.
[48] Mallal S, Nolan D, Witt C, et al. Association between presence of HLA-B*5701, HLA-DR7, and HLA-DQ3 and hypersensitivity to HIV-1 reverse-transcriptase inhibitor abacavir. Lancet 2002;359:727–732.
[49] Norcross MA, Luo S, Lu L, et al. Abacavir induces loading of novel self-peptides into HLA-B*57: 01: an autoimmune model for HLA-associated drug hypersensitivity. AIDS 2012;26:F21–F29.
[50] Ostrov DA, Grant BJ, Pompeu YA, et al. Drug hypersensitivity caused by alteration of the MHC-presented self-peptide repertoire. Proc Natl Acad Sci U S A 2012;109:9959–9964.
[51] Walsh JS, Reese MJ, Thurmond LM. The metabolic activation of abacavir by human liver cytosol and expressed human alcohol dehydrogenase isozymes. Chem Biol Interact 2002;142:135–154.
[52] Aleo MD, Luo Y, Swiss R, Bonin PD, Potter DM, Will Y. Human drug-induced liver injury severity is highly associated with dual inhibition of liver mitochondrial function and bile salt export pump. Hepatology 2014;60:1015–1022.
[53] Will Y, Dykens J. Mitochondrial toxicity assessment in industry—a decade of technology development and insight. Expert Opin Drug Metab Toxicol 2014;10:1061–1067.
[54] Lee KK, Fujimoto K, Zhang C, et al. Isoniazid-induced cell death is precipitated by underlying mitochondrial complex I dysfunction in mouse hepatocytes. Free Radic Biol Med 2013;65:584–594.
[55] Cho T, Wang X, Uetrecht J. Rotenone increases isoniazid toxicity but does not cause significant liver injury: implications for the hypothesis that inhibition of the mitochondrial electron transport chain is a common mechanism of idiosyncratic drug-induced liver injury. Chem Res Toxicol 2019;32:1423–1431.
[56] Montessori V, Harris M, Montaner JS. Hepatotoxicity of nucleoside reverse transcriptase inhibitors. Semin Liver Dis 2003;23:167–172.
[57] De Bus L, Depuydt P, Libbrecht L, et al. Severe drug-induced liver injury associated with prolonged use of linezolid. J Med Toxicol 2010;6:322–326.
[58] Zimmerman HJ, Ishak KG. Valproate-induced hepatic injury: analyses of 23 fatal cases. Hepatology 1982;2:591–597.
[59] Bryant AE, Dreifuss FE. Valproic acid hepatic fatalities. III. U.S. experience since 1986. Neurology 1996;46:465–469.
[60] Strautnieks SS, Bull LN, Knisely AS, et al. A gene encoding a liver-specific ABC transporter is mutated in progressive familial intrahepatic cholestasis. Nat Genet 1998;20:233–238.
[61] Jacquemin E. Progressive familial intrahepatic cholestasis. Clin Res Hepatol Gastroenterol 2012;36(Suppl 1):S26–S35.
[62] Rodrigues AD, Lai Y, Cvijic ME, Elkin LL, Zvyaga T, Soars MG. Drug-induced perturbations of the bile acid pool, cholestasis, and hepatotoxicity: mechanistic considerations beyond the direct inhibition of the bile salt export pump. Drug Metab Dispos 2014;42:566–574.
[63] Köck K, Ferslew BC, Netterberg I, et al. Risk factors for development of cholestatic drug-induced liver injury: inhibition of hepatic basolateral bile acid transporters multidrug resistance-associated proteins 3 and 4. Drug Metab Dispos 2014;42:665–674.
[64] Kenna JG, Uetrecht J. Do in vitro assays predict drug candidate idiosyncratic drug-induced liver injury risk. Drug Metab Dispos 2018;46:1658–1669.
[65] Fattinger K, Funk C, Pantze M, et al. The endothelin antagonist bosentan inhibits the canalicular bile salt export pump: a potential mechanism for hepatic adverse reactions. Clin Pharmacol Ther 2001;69:223–231.
[66] Watkins PB, Kaplowitz N, Slattery JT, et al. Aminotransferase elevations in healthy adults receiving 4 grams of acetaminophen daily: a randomized controlled trial. JAMA 2006;296:87–93.
[67] Prescott LF. Paracetamol, alcohol and the liver. Br J Clin Pharmacol 2000;49:291–301.

[68] Hinson JA, Roberts DW, James LP. Mechanisms of acetaminophen-induced liver necrosis. Handb Exp Pharmacol 2010;369–405.

[69] Myers TG, Dietz EC, Anderson NL, Khairallah EA, Cohen SD, Nelson SD. A comparative study of mouse liver proteins arylated by reactive metabolites of acetaminophen and its nonhepatotoxic regioisomer, 3'-hydroxyacetanilide. Chem Res Toxicol 1995;8:403–413.

[70] Ramachandran A, Jaeschke H. Mechanisms of acetaminophen hepatotoxicity and their translation to the human pathophysiology. J Clin Transl Res 2017;3:157–169.

[71] Fannin RD, Gerrish K, Sieber SO, Bushel PR, Watkins PB, Paules RS. Blood transcript immune signatures distinguish a subset of people with elevated serum ALT from others given acetaminophen. Clin Pharmacol Ther 2016;99:432–441.

[72] Ju C, Reilly T. Role of immune reactions in drug-induced liver injury (DILI). Drug Metab Rev 2012;44:107–115.

[73] Chalasani N, Bonkovsky HL, Fontana R, et al. Features and outcomes of 899 patients with drug-induced liver injury: the DILIN prospective study. Gastroenterology 2015;148: 1340-52.e7.

[74] Clay KD, Hanson JS, Pope SD, Rissmiller RW, Purdum III PP, Banks PM. Brief communication: severe hepatotoxicity of telithromycin: three case reports and literature review. Ann Intern Med 2006;144:415–420.

[75] Hoetzenecker W, Nägeli M, Mehra ET, et al. Adverse cutaneous drug eruptions: current understanding. Semin Immunopathol 2016;38:75–86.

[76] Solensky R, Jacobs J, Lester M, et al. Penicillin allergy evaluation: a prospective, multicenter, open-label evaluation of a comprehensive penicillin skin test kit. J Allergy Clin Immunol Pract 2019;7:1876–1885.e3.

[77] Mustafa SS, Conn K, Ramsey A. Comparing direct challenge to penicillin skin testing for the outpatient evaluation of penicillin allergy: a randomized controlled trial. J Allergy Clin Immunol Pract 2019;7:2163–2170.

[78] Kowalski ML, Asero R, Bavbek S, et al. Classification and practical approach to the diagnosis and management of hypersensitivity to nonsteroidal anti-inflammatory drugs. Allergy 2013;68:1219–1232.

[79] Roujeau JC, Chosidow O, Saiag P, Guillaume JC. Toxic epidermal necrolysis (Lyell syndrome). J Am Acad Dermatol 1990;23:1039–1058.

[80] Suda G, Yamamoto Y, Nagasaka A, et al. Serum granulysin levels as a predictor of serious telaprevir-induced dermatological reactions. Hepatol Res 2015;45:837–845.

[81] Moeschlin S, Wagner K. Agranulocytosis due to the occurrence of leukocyte-agglutinins. Acta Haematol 1952;8:29–41.

[82] Uetrecht JP, Ma HM, MacKnight E, McClelland R. Oxidation of aminopyrine by hypochlorite to a reactive dication: possible implications for aminopyrine-induced agranulocytosis. Chem Res Toxicol 1995;8:226–233.

[83] Pisciotta AV. Drug-induced agranulocytosis. Peripheral destruction of polymorphonuclear leukocytes and their marrow precursors. Blood Rev 1990;4:226–237.

[84] Pollmacher T, Hinze-Selch D, Mullington J. Effects of clozapine on plasma cytokine and soluble cytokine receptor levels. J Clin Psychopharmacol 1996;16:403–409.

[85] Regen F, Herzog I, Hahn E, et al. Clozapine-induced agranulocytosis: Evidence for an immune-mediated mechanism from a patient-specific in-vitro approach. Toxicol Appl Pharmacol 2017;316:10–16.

[86] Warkentin TE. Heparin-induced thrombocytopenia: pathogenesis and management. Br J Haematol 2003;121:535–555.

[87] Visentin GP, Newman PJ, Aster RH. Characteristics of quinine- and quinidine-induced antibodies specific for platelet glycoproteins IIb and IIIa. Blood 1991;77:2668–2676.

[88] Arnold DM, Nazi I, Warkentin TE, et al. Approach to the diagnosis and management of drug-induced immune thrombocytopenia. Transfus Med Rev 2013;27:137–145.

[89] Garratty G. Immune hemolytic anemia caused by drugs. Expert Opin Drug Saf 2012;11:635–642.

[90] Sloand E, Kim S, Maciejewski JP, Tisdale J, Follmann D, Young NS. Intracellular interferon-gamma in circulating and marrow T cells detected by flow cytometry and the response to immunosuppressive therapy in patients with aplastic anemia. Blood 2002;100:1185–1191.

[91] Polak BCP, Wesseling H, Schut D, Herxheimer A, Meyler L. Blood dyscrasias attributed to chloramphenicol: a review of 576 published and unpublished cases. Acta Med Scand 1972;192:409–414.

[92] Woosley RL, Drayer DE, Reidenberg MM, Nies AS, Carr K, Oates JA. Effect of acetylator phenotype on the rate at which procainamide induces antinuclear antibodies and the lupus syndrome. N Engl J Med 1978;298:1157–1159.

[93] Kluger J, Drayer DE, Reidenberg MM, Lahita R. Acetylprocainamide therapy in patients with previous procainamide-induced lupus syndrome. Ann Intern Med 1981;95:18–23.

[94] Uetrecht JP, Zahid N. N-Chlorination and oxidation of procainamide by myeloperoxidase:toxicological implications. Chem Res Toxicol 1991;4:218–222.

[95] Mannargudi B, McNally D, Reynolds W, Uetrecht J. Bioactivation of minocycline to reactive intermediates by myeloperoxidase, horseradish peroxidase, and hepatic microsomes: implications for minocycline-induced lupus and hepatitis. Drug Metab Dispos 2009;37:1806–1818.

[96] Khan S, Gerber DE. Autoimmunity, checkpoint inhibitor therapy and immune-related adverse events: A review. Semin Cancer Biol 2019;64:93–101.

[97] Shovman O, Tamar S, Amital H, Watad A, Shoenfeld Y. Diverse patterns of anti-TNF-α-induced lupus: case series and review of the literature. Clin Rheumatol 2018;37:563–568.

[98] Cohan SL, Lucassen EB, Romba MC, Linch SN. Daclizumab: mechanisms of action, therapeutic efficacy, adverse events and its uncovering the potential role of innate immune system recruitment as a treatment strategy for relapsing multiple sclerosis. Biomedicine 2019;7:18.

[99] Daly AK, Donaldson PT, Bhatnagar P, et al. HLA-B*5701 genotype is a major determinant of drug-induced liver injury due to flucloxacillin. Nat Genet 2009;41:816–819.

[100] Daly AK. Using genome-wide association studies to identify genes important in serious adverse drug reactions. Annu Rev Pharmacol Toxicol 2012;52:21–35.

[101] Dossing M, Wilcke JT, Askgaard DS, Nybo B. Liver injury during antituberculosis treatment: an 11-year study. Tuber Lung Dis 1996;77:335–340.

[102] Ko TM, Chung WH, Wei CY, et al. Shared and restricted T-cell receptor use is crucial for carbamazepine-induced Stevens-Johnson syndrome. J Allergy Clin Immunol 2011;128:1266–1276.e11.

[103] Welsh RM, Selin LK. No one is naive: the significance of heterologous T-cell immunity. Nat Rev Immunol 2002;2:417–426.

[104] Sassolas B, Haddad C, Mockenhaupt M, et al. ALDEN, an algorithm for assessment of drug causality in Stevens-Johnson syndrome and toxic epidermal necrolysis: comparison with case-control analysis. Clin Pharmacol Ther 2010;88:60–68.

[105] Andrade RJ, Chalasani N, Björnsson ES, et al. Drug-induced liver injury. Nat Rev Dis Primers 2019;5:58.

[106] Young NS, Calado RT, Scheinberg P. Current concepts in the pathophysiology and treatment of aplastic anemia. Blood 2006;108:2509–2519.

[107] Waldron HA. A brief history of scrotal cancer. Br J Ind Med 1983;40:390–401.

[108] Hutchinson J. Salvarsan ("606") and arsenic cancer. Br Med J 1911;1:976–977.

[109] IARC. Pharmaceuticals. *IARC monographs on the evaluation of carcinogenic risks to humans* **100A**:1-403 (2012).110;2014. 13th Report on Carcinogens.

[110] 13th Report on Carcinogens. National toxicology program, http://ntp.niehs.nih.gov/pubhealth/roc/roc13/index.html; 2014.

[111] Known and Probable Human Carcinogens. American cancer society, www.cancer.org/cancer/cancer-causes/general-info/known-and-probable-human-carcinogens.html; 2020.

[112] Grosse Y, Baan R, Straif K, et al. A review of human carcinogens—part A: pharmaceuticals. Lancet Oncol 2009;10:13–14.

[113] Anon. Harvard report on cancer prevention. Causes of human cancer. Prescription drugs. Cancer Causes Control 1996;7(Suppl 1). S45-7.

[114] Smith PG, Jick H. Regular drug use and cancer. J Natl Cancer Inst 1977;59:1387–1391.

[115] Brambilla G, Mattioli F, Robbiano L, Martelli A. Update of carcinogenicity studies in animals and humans of 535 marketed pharmaceuticals. Mutat Res 2012;750:1–51.

[116] Marselos M, Vainio H. Carcinogenic properties of pharmaceutical agents evaluated in the IARC monographs programme. Carcinogenesis 1991;12:1751–1766.

[117] Kobets T, Iatropoulos MJ, Williams GM. Mechanisms of DNA-reactive and epigenetic chemical carcinogens: applications to carcinogenicity testing and risk assessment. Toxicol Res (Camb) 2019;8:123–145.

[118] Luijten M, Olthof ED, Hakkert BC, et al. An integrative test strategy for cancer hazard identification. Crit Rev Toxicol 2016;46:615–639.

[119] Moggs JG, MacLachlan T, Martus HJ, Bentley P. Derisking drug-induced carcinogenicity for novel therapeutics. Trends Cancer 2016;2:398–408.

[120] Hanahan D, Weinberg RA. Hallmarks of cancer: the next generation. Cell 2011;144:646–674.

[121] Hanahan D, Weinberg RA. The hallmarks of cancer. Cell 2000;100:57–70.

[122] Shenolikar R, Durden E, Meyer N, Lenhart G, Moore K. Incidence of secondary myelodysplastic syndrome (MDS) and acute myeloid leukemia (AML) in patients with ovarian or breast cancer in a real-world setting in the United States. Gynecol Oncol 2018;151:190–195.

[123] Guru Murthy GS, Abedin S. Myeloid malignancies after treatment for solid tumours. Best Pract Res Clin Haematol 2019;32:40–46.

[124] Morton LM, Dores GM, Schonfeld SJ, et al. Association of chemotherapy for solid tumors with development of therapy-related myelodysplastic syndrome or acute myeloid leukemia in the modern era. JAMA Oncol 2019;5:318–325.

[125] List AF, Jacobs A. Biology and pathogenesis of the myelodysplastic syndromes. Semin Oncol 1992;19:14–24.

[126] Pedersen-Bjergaard J, Andersen MK, Andersen MT, Christiansen DH. Genetics of therapy-related myelodysplasia and acute myeloid leukemia. Leukemia 2008;22:240–248.

[127] Qian Z, Joslin JM, Tennant TR, et al. Cytogenetic and genetic pathways in therapy-related acute myeloid leukemia. Chem Biol Interact 2010;184:50–57.

[128] Leone G, Mele L, Pulsoni A, Equitani F, Pagano L. The incidence of secondary leukemias. Haematologica 1999;84:937–945.

[129] Smith MA, McCaffrey RP, Karp JE. The secondary leukemias: challenges and research directions. J Natl Cancer Inst 1996;88:407–418.

[130] Felix CA, Kolaris CP, Osheroff N. Topoisomerase II and the etiology of chromosomal translocations. DNA Repair (Amst) 2006;5:1093–1108.

[131] Yokoyama A, Somervaille TC, Smith KS, Rozenblatt-Rosen O, Meyerson M, Cleary ML. The menin tumor suppressor protein is an essential oncogenic cofactor for MLL-associated leukemogenesis. Cell 2005;123:207–218.

[132] Pedersen-Bjergaard J, Christiansen DH, Desta F, Andersen MK. Alternative genetic pathways and cooperating genetic abnormalities in the pathogenesis of therapy-related myelodysplasia and acute myeloid leukemia. Leukemia 2006;20:1943–1949.

[133] Kurokawa M, Hirai H. Role of AML1/Runx1 in the pathogenesis of hematological malignancies. Cancer Sci 2003;94:841–846.

[134] Godley LA, Larson RA. Therapy-related myeloid leukemia. Semin Oncol 2008;35:418–429.

[135] Seedhouse C, Russell N. Advances in the understanding of susceptibility to treatment-related acute myeloid leukaemia. Br J Haematol 2007;137:513–529.

[136] Larson RA, Wang Y, Banerjee M, et al. Prevalence of the inactivating 609C–>T polymorphism in the NAD(P)H:quinone oxidoreductase (NQO1) gene in patients with primary and therapy-related myeloid leukemia. Blood 1999;94:803–807.

[137] Beyaert R, Beaugerie L, Van Assche G, et al. Cancer risk in immune-mediated inflammatory diseases (IMID). Mol Cancer 2013;12:98.

[138] Hatch EE, Palmer JR, Titus-Ernstoff L, et al. Cancer risk in women exposed to diethylstilbestrol in utero. JAMA 1998;280:630–634.

[139] Herbst AL, Ulfelder H, Poskanzer DC. Adenocarcinoma of the vagina. Association of maternal stilbestrol therapy with tumor appearance in young women. N Engl J Med 1971;284:878–881.

[140] Herbst AL. Behavior of estrogen-associated female genital tract cancer and its relation to neoplasia following intrauterine exposure to diethylstilbestrol (DES). Gynecol Oncol 2000;76:147–156.

[141] Haaf H, Metzler M. In vitro metabolism of diethylstilbestrol by hepatic, renal and uterine microsomes of rats and hamsters. Effects of different inducers. Biochem Pharmacol 1985;34:3107–3115.

[142] Roy D, Palangat M, Chen CW, et al. Biochemical and molecular changes at the cellular level in response to exposure to environmental estrogen-like chemicals. J Toxicol Environ Health 1997;50:1–29.

[143] Cavalieri E, Frenkel K, Liehr JG, Rogan E, Roy D. Estrogens as endogenous genotoxic agents—DNA adducts and mutations. J Natl Cancer Inst Monogr 2000;75–93.

[144] Waggoner SE, Baunoch DA, Anderson SA, Leigh F, Zagaja VG. Bcl-2 protein expression associated with resistance to apoptosis in clear cell adenocarcinomas of the vagina and cervix expressing wild-type p53. Ann Surg Oncol 1998;5:544–547.

[145] Boyd J, Takahashi H, Waggoner SE, et al. Molecular genetic analysis of clear cell adenocarcinomas of the vagina and cervix associated and unassociated with diethylstilbestrol exposure in utero. Cancer 1996;77:507–513.

[146] Couse JF, Dixon D, Yates M, et al. Estrogen receptor-alpha knockout mice exhibit resistance to the developmental effects of neonatal diethylstilbestrol exposure on the female reproductive tract. Dev Biol 2001;238:224–238.

[147] Dickson RB, Stancel GM. Estrogen receptor-mediated processes in normal and cancer cells. J Natl Cancer Inst Monogr 2000;135–145.

[148] Vargesson N. Thalidomide-induced teratogenesis: history and mechanisms. Birth Defects Res C Embryo Today 2015;105:140–156.

[149] Bhatia S, Drake DM, Miller L, Wells PG. Oxidative stress and DNA damage in the mechanism of fetal alcohol spectrum disorders. Birth Defects Res 2019;111:714–748.

[150] Wells PG, McCallum GP, Chen CS, et al. Oxidative stress in developmental origins of disease: teratogenesis, neurodevelopmental deficits and cancer. Toxicol Sci 2009;108:4–18.

[151] Wells PG, Bhuller Y, Chen CS, et al. Molecular and biochemical mechanisms in teratogenesis involving reactive oxygen species. Toxicol Appl Pharmacol 2005;207:354–366.

[152] Iqbal M, Audette MC, Petropoulos S, Gibb W, Matthews SG. Placental drug transporters and their role in fetal protection. Placenta 2012;33:137–142.

[153] Smit JW, Huisman MT, van Tellingen O, Wiltshire HR, Schinkel AH. Absence or pharmacological blocking of placental P-glycoprotein profoundly increases fetal drug exposure. J Clin Investig 1999;204:1441–1447.

[154] Hines RN. The ontogeny of drug metabolism enzymes and implications for adverse drug events. Pharmacol Ther 2008;118:250–267.

[155] Leeder JS, Gaedigk R, Marcucci KA, et al. Variability of CYP3A7 expression in human fetal liver. J Pharmacol Exp Ther 2005;314:626–635.

[156] Williams JA, Ring BJ, Cantrell VE, et al. Comparative metabolic capabilities of CYP3A4, CYP3A5 and CYP3A7. Drug Metab Dispos 2002;30:883–891.

[157] Wells PG, Lee CJJ, McCallum GP, Perstin J, Harper PA. Receptor- and reactive intermediate-mediated mechanisms of teratogenesis. In: Uetrecht JP, editor. Handbook of experimental pharmacology. Mechanisms of adverse drug reactions, vol. 196. Heidelberg: Springer; 2009. p. 131–162 [chapter 6].

[158] Wells PG, Miller-Pinsler L, Shapiro AM. Impact of oxidative stress on development. In: Dennery PA, Buonocore G, Saugstad O, editors. Perinatal and prenatal disorders. Berlin: Humana Press, Springer Science; 2014. p. 1–37.

[159] Wells PG, Bhatia S, Drake DM, Miller-Pinsler L. Fetal oxidative stress mechanisms of neurodevelopmental deficits and exacerbation by methamphetamine and ethanol. Birth Defects Res C Embryo Today 2016;108:108–130.

[160] Hansen J, Jones DP, Harris C. The redox theory of development. Antioxid Redox Signal 2020;32:715–740.

[161] Wells PG, McCallum GP, Lam KCH, Henderson JT, Ondovcik SL. Oxidative DNA damage and repair in teratogenesis and neurodevelopmental deficits. Birth Defects Res C Embryo Today 2010;90:103–109.

[162] Ding Y, Fleming AM, Burrows CJ. Sequencing the mouse genome for the oxidatively modified base 8-oxo-7,8-dihydroguanine by OG-seq. J Am Chem Soc 2017;139:2569–2572.

[163] Ba X, Boldogh I. 8-Oxoguanine DNA glycosylase 1: beyond repair of the oxidatively modified base lesions. Redox Biol 2018;14:669–678.

[164] Fleming AM, Burrows CJ. Interplay of guanine oxidation and G-quadruplex folding in gene promoters. J Am Chem Soc 2020;142:1115–1136.

[165] Giorgio M, Dellino IG, Gambino V, Roda N, Pelicci PG. On the epigenetic role of guanosine oxidation. Redox Biol 2020;29:101398.

[166] Pan L, Hao W, Zheng X, et al. OGG1-DNA interactions facilitate NF-κB binding to DNA targets. Sci Rep 2017;7:43297.

[167] Cogoi S, Ferino A, Miglietta G, Pedersen EB, Xodo LE. The regulatory G4 motif of the Kirsten ras (KRAS) gene is sensitive to guanine oxidation: implications on transcription. Nucleic Acids Res 2018;46:661–676.

[168] Bhatia S, Arslan E, Wells PG. Loss of the DNA repair enzyme oxoguanine glycosylase 1 (OGG1) increases DNA strand breaks and decreases DNA methylation in the brain, possibly contributing to a sex-dependent increase in postnatal behavioural disorders, In: Society for neuroscience 2019 neuroscience online meeting planner session 718—Autism: molecular & cellular mechanisms (nanosymposium). Abstract No. 718.08; 2019.

[169] Zhou X, Zhuang Z, Wang W, et al. OGG1 is essential in oxidative stress induced DNA demethylation. Cell Signal 2016;28:1163–1171.

[170] Mahnke AH, Miranda RC, Homanics GE. Epigenetic mediators and consequences of excessive alcohol consumption. Alcohol 2017;60:1–6.

[171] Jones KL, Smith DW, Ulleland CN, Streissguth AP. Pattern of malformation in offspring of chronic alcoholic mothers. Lancet 1973;301:1267–1271.

[172] Jones KL, Smith DW. Recognition of the fetal alcohol syndrome in early infancy. Lancet 1973;302:999–1001.

[173] Mattson SN, Crocker N, Nguyen TT. Fetal alcohol spectrum disorders: neuropsychological and behavioral features. Neuropsychol Rev 2011;21:81–101.

[174] Lange S, Rehm J, Popova S. Implications of higher than expected prevalence of fetal alcohol spectrum disorders. JAMA 2018;319:448–449.

[175] May PA, Chambers CD, Kalberg WO, et al. Prevalence of fetal alcohol spectrum disorders in 4 US communities. JAMA 2018;319:474–482.

[176] Lovely CB. Animal models of gene–alcohol interactions. Birth Defects Res 2019. https://doi.org/10.1002/bdr2.1623 [Epub date Nov. 2019].

[177] Zarrei M, Hicks GG, Reynolds JN, et al. Copy number variation in fetal alcohol spectrum disorder. Biochem Cell Biol 2018;96:161–166.

[178] Mahnke AH, Salem NA, Tseng AM, Chung DD, Miranda RC. Nonprotein-coding RNAs in fetal alcohol spectrum disorders. Prog Mol Biol Transl Sci 2018;157:299–342.

[179] Xu W, Liyanage VRB, MacAulay A, et al. Genome-wide transcriptome landscape of embryonic brain-derived neural stem cells exposed to alcohol with strain-specific cross-examination in BL6 and CD1 mice. Sci Rep 2019;9:206.

[180] Drake DM, Tran J, Wells PG. Ethanol-enhanced fetal proteasomal degradation of BRCA1 protein and macromolecular damage in the brains of Brca1 knockout mice, In: Proceedings of the annual meeting of the society of toxicology of Canada. 37 (Abstract No. 7); 2018.

[181] Chernoff GF. The fetal alcohol syndrome in mice: maternal variables. Teratology 1980;22:71–75.

[182] Dong J, Sulik KK, Chen S-Y. The role of NOX enzymes in ethanol-induced oxidative stress and apoptosis in mouse embryos. Toxicol Lett 2010;193:94–100.

[183] Wang X, Chen G, Xu M, et al. Cdc42-dependent activation of NADPH oxidase is involved in ethanol-induced neuronal oxidative stress. PLoS One 2012;7:e38075.

[184] Miller-Pinsler L, Sharma A, Wells PG. Enhanced NADPH oxidases and reactive oxygen species in the mechanism of methanol-initiated protein oxidation and embryopathies in vivo and in embryo culture. Arch Toxicol 2016;90:717–730.

[185] Miller-Pinsler L, Wells PG. Deficient DNA repair exacerbates ethanol-initiated DNA oxidation and embryopathies in ogg1 knockout mice: gender risk and protection by a free radical spin trapping agent. Arch Toxicol 2016;90:415–425.

[186] Miller-Pinsler L, Pinto D, Wells PG. Oxidative DNA damage in the in utero initiation of postnatal neurodevelopmental deficits by normal fetal and ethanol-enhanced oxidative stress in oxoguanine glycosylase 1 (ogg1) knockout mice. Free Radic Biol Med 2015;78:23–29.

[187] Dong J, Sulik KK, Chen S-Y. Nrf2-mediated transcriptional induction of antioxidant response in mouse embryos exposed to ethanol in vivo: implications for the prevention of fetal alcohol spectrum disorders. Antioxid Redox Signal 2008;10:2023–2033.

[188] Ramkissoon A, Wells PG. Developmental role of nuclear factor-E2-related factor 2 (Nrf2) in protecting against methamphetamine fetal toxicity and postnatal neurodevelopmental deficits. Free Radic Biol Med 2013;65:620–631.

[189] Wells PG. A new target for thalidomide. Nat Chem Biol 2018;14:904–905.

[190] Donovan KA, An J, Nowak R, et al. Thalidomide promotes degradation of SALL4, a transcription factor implicated in Duane Radial Ray Syndrome, eLife 2018;7. https://doi.org/10.7554/eLife.38430. e38430 https://elifesciences.org/articles/38430.

[191] Ito T, Ando H, Suzuki T, et al. Identification of a primary target of thalidomide teratogenicity. Science 2010;327:1345–1350.

[192] Matyskiela ME, Couto S, Zheng X, et al. SALL4 mediates teratogenicity as a thalidomide-dependent cereblon substrate. Nat Chem Biol 2018;14:981–987.

[193] Parman T, Wiley MJ, Wells PG. Free radical-mediated oxidative DNA damage in the mechanism of thalidomide teratogenicity. Nat Med 1999;5:582–585.

[194] Arlen RR, Wells PG. Inhibition of thalidomide teratogenicity by acetylsalicylic acid: evidence for prostaglandin H synthase-catalysed bioactivation of thalidomide to a teratogenic reactive intermediate. J Pharmacol Exp Ther 1996;277:1649–1658.

[195] Knobloch J, Reimann K, Klotz LO, Ruther U. Thalidomide resistance is based on the capacity of the glutathione-dependent antioxidant defense. Mol Pharm 2008;5:1138–1144.

[196] Lee CJJ, Goncalves LL, Wells PG. Embryopathic effects of thalidomide and its hydrolysis products in rabbit embryo culture: evidence for a prostaglandin H synthase (PHS)-dependent, reactive oxygen species (ROS)-mediated mechanism. FASEB J 2011;25:2468–2483.

Chapter 16

Pharmacogenomic mechanisms of drug toxicity

Shiew-Mei Huang[a], Ligong Chen[b], and Kathleen M. Giacomini[b]

[a]*Office of Clinical Pharmacology, Office of Translational Sciences, Center for Drug Evaluation and Research, U.S. Food and Drug Administration, Silver Spring, MD, United States,* [b]*Department of Bioengineering and Therapeutic Sciences, University of California, San Francisco, CA, United States*

Many drugs have been discontinued in development or withdrawn from the market after approval because of serious adverse drug reactions (ADRs), including fatalities due to acute liver failure, *torsades de pointes*, rhabdomyolysis, and Stevens-Johnson syndrome [1–3]. For drugs on the market, the spontaneous adverse event reporting, continual monitoring of patient responses, and additional studies conducted postmarketing also can lead to changes in safety information in the labeling [4, 5]. These labeling changes resulted in either restricted distribution or use with increased or decreased warnings and precautions in the drug labeling, especially in the first 10 years after their initial approval [6].

Many ADRs may go unrecognized prior to drug approval due to the limited size and subgroups of patients who have been exposed to the drug during Phase 1–3 clinical trials. However, with increased understanding of molecular mechanisms, risks for ADRs can be assessed prior to market approval and managed via labeling, education, and/or postmarketing risk evaluation and mitigation strategies established at the time of regulatory approval. The need to collect and store DNA samples in clinical trials to facilitate the identification of genetic basis of ADRs has been emphasized [7–9]. Tetrabenazine is an example of a drug for which a premarket evaluation of genetic effects on drug toxicity resulted in labeling that described the relation between a patient's CYP2D6 activity and the potential of this drug to prolong the QT interval [10–12]. Multiple factors, including both patient-specific factors (such as genetics, race, age) and environmental factors (such as drug-drug interactions), can influence adverse drug response [13]. Understanding the pharmacologic mechanisms of ADRs is therefore critical to provide appropriate treatment decisions for individual patients and to develop safer medications. This chapter will focus on the pharmacogenomic mechanisms that are responsible for a variety of ADRs.

ADRS with a pharmacogenomic basis

ADRs may be related to increased systemic exposure in some patients receiving the same dosage regimens as others. This high exposure can be due to variations in genes that encode metabolizing enzymes, transporters, or environmental factors such as diet and concomitantly administered drugs that affect drug metabolism and/or transport. In other cases, factors other than those affecting the patient's systemic exposure have contributed to ADRs.

For some drugs, the prevalence of certain genotypes in a specific population can explain the different dosing regimens being used in the patient population in certain regions or race and ethnic groups [14, 15]. For example, data showing a higher frequency of warfarin-sensitive genotype (s) of *VKORC1* in Asians compared to Caucasians are consistent with the past FDA labeling of warfarin, and practices in some Asian countries based on evidence that Asians need a lower starting dose than Caucasians. Similarly, although Stevens-Johnson syndrome due to the antiepileptic drug carbamazepine is not completely explained by the presence of HLA-B * 1502, allele frequency differences among various ancestral groups could explain why the adverse event may be more prevalent in some but not in other populations (Table 16.1).

Drug metabolizing enzyme-mediated pharmacogenomic mechanisms of drug toxicity

Genetic variants in drug-metabolizing enzymes were among the first to be recognized as increasing an individual's susceptibility to drug toxicity, and truly ushered in the area of pharmacogenetics. A few additional examples in which genetic variants in metabolizing enzymes play a critical role in drug toxicity are described later.

Atkinson's Principles of Clinical Pharmacology. https://doi.org/10.1016/B978-0-12-819869-8.00002-1

TABLE 16.1 Recent FDA drug product labeling examples that included ethnicity or genetic information[a] [12].

Therapeutic area	Drug products' generic (brand) names	Ethnicity information	Genetic information[b]
Cardio-renal	Angiotensin II antagonists and ACE inhibitor	Smaller effects in Blacks[c]	Angiotensin II antagonists and ACE inhibitor
	Clopidogrel (Plavix)		Boxed warning for CYP2C19 PM
	Isosorbide dinitrate/ hydralazine (Bidil)	Indicated for self-identified Blacks	
	Prasugrel		No relevant effect of genetic variation in CYP2B6, CYP2C9, CYP2C19, or CYP3A5
Metabolic	Rosuvastatin (Crestor)	Lower dose for Asians	Clinical pharmacology and SLCO1B1
	Simvastatin (Zocor)	Chinese (on lipid-modifying doses of niacin-containing drugs) not to take 80 mg	
Transplant or Rheumatology	Azathiopurine (Imuran)		Dose adjustments for TPMT or NUDT15 deficiency
	Tacrolimus (Protopic)	Higher dose for Blacks	
Oncology	Afatinib		Indicated for EGFR
	Alectinib		Indicated for ALK
	Atezolizumab		Indicated for CD274 (PD-L1), EGFR, ALK
	Cetuximab		Boxed warning for K-Ras and EGFR
	Crizotinib		Indicated for ALK and ROS1
	Dasatinib		Indicated for Philadelphia chromosome
	Erlotinib (Tarceva)		Different survival and tumor response in EGFR-positive and EGFR-negative patients reported
	Imatinib		Indicated for C-kit
	Irinotecan (Camptosar)		Dose reduction for UGT1A1*28
	Lapatinib		Indicated for HER2 overexpression
	6-Mercaptopurine (Purinethol)		Dose adjustments for TPMT variants
	Nicotinib		Indicated for Philadelphia chromosome
	Panitumumab		Boxed warning for KRAS variants
	Pembrolizumab		Indicated for BRAF, CD274 (PD-L1), microsatellite instability, mismatch repair, EGFR, ALK
	Tamoxifen (Nolvadex)		Estrogen receptor positive more likely to benefit
	Trastuzumab (Herceptin)		Indicated for HER2 overexpression
	Vemurafenib (Zelboraf)		Indicated for BRAF ^{v600E} mutation
	Crizotinib (Xalkori)		Indicated for AKL-positive

TABLE 16.1 Recent FDA drug product labeling examples that included ethnicity or genetic information—cont'd

Therapeutic area	Drug products' generic (brand) names	Ethnicity information	Genetic information
Antiviral	Abacavir		Boxed warning for HLA-B*5701
	Maraviroc (Selzentry)		Indicated for CCR5-positive
	Oseltamivir (Tamiflu)	Neuropsychiatric events mostly reported in Japan	
Pain	Codeine		Warnings for nursing mothers that CYP2D6 UM metabolized codeine to morphine more rapidly and completely
Hematology	Warfarin (Coumadin)	Lower dose for Asians	Lower initial dose for CYP2C9 and VKORC1 sensitive variants
	Avatrombopag		Warnings F2, F5, PROC, PROS1, SERPINCI, CYP2C9
Psychopharm	Atomoxetine (Strattera)		Dosage adjustments for CYP2D6 PM; no drug interactions with strong CYP2D6 inhibitors expected for PM
	Citalopram		Limit dose based on CYP2C29 (QT prolongation)
	Thioridazine (Mellaril)		Contraindication for CYP2D6 PM
Neuropharm	Amifampridine		Dose and NAT2
	Carbamazepine (Tegretol)	Boxed warning in Asians with variant alleles of HLA-B*1502	Boxed warning in Asians with variant alleles of HLA-B*1502
	Tetrabenazine (Xenazine)		Dose limitation for CYP2D6 PM
Rare Diseases (Inborn Errors of Metabolism)	Eliglustat		Dosing based on CYP2D6

[a]*PM, poor metabolizer; UM, ultra-rapid metabolizer; TPMT, thiopurine methyl transferase; UGT, uridine diphosphate glucuronosyl transferase; HER2, human epidermal growth factor receptor 2; EGFR, epidermal growth factor receptor; CCR5, chemokine (C—C motif) receptor 5; VKORC, vitamin K reductase complex; HLA, human leukocyte antigen; BRAF, B-type Raf kinase; ALK, anaplastic lymphoma kinase.*
[b]*Genetic information may include information about polymorphisms in germline DNA or mutations and/or expression levels of genes in tumors.*
[c]*A general statement in the candesartan (Atacand) labeling.*
Modified from Huang SM, Temple R. Clin Pharmacol Ther 2008;84:287–294.

Thiopurine methyltransferase and thiopurine myelotoxicity

Thiopurines are used to treat nonmalignant immune disorders as well as various lymphomas and leukemias. There are three thiopurines approved for clinical use: azathioprine, 6-mercaptopurine (6-MP), and thioguanine [16]. Azathioprine is a prodrug of 6-MP and is used as adjunctive therapy to prevent rejection in renal homotransplantations and to reduce signs and symptoms in patients with active rheumatoid arthritis. 6-MP is used as part of a combination regimen for maintenance therapy of patients with acute lymphatic (lymphocytic, lymphoblastic) leukemia [17]. Thioguanine is used in the treatment of myeloid leukemias.

Both thioguanine and 6-MP are direct substrates of thiopurine methyltransferase (TPMT), a polymorphic enzyme that is responsible for converting 6-MP into the inactive metabolite methyl-6-MP (meMP) (Fig. 16.1) and thioguanine into the inactive, methylthioguanine [16, 17]. About 10% of Caucasians and African Americans have intermediate TPMT activity and 0.3% of them have low or absent activity. There are several major reduced-function polymorphisms of TPMT. *TPMT*2* (rs1800462) has an alanine to proline mutation at position 80 and is associated with reduced function. *TPMT*3A* has two base pair changes leading to the amino acid changes, p.A154T (rs1800460) and p.Y240C (rs1142345), and is the most

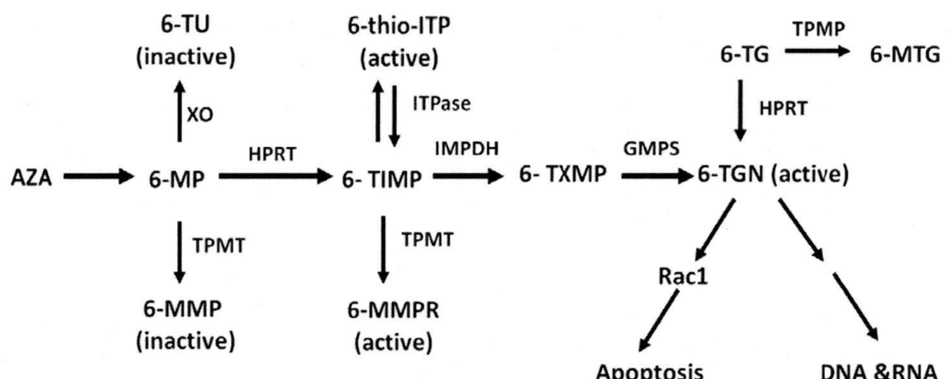

FIG. 16.1 Metabolism of thiopurines. The prodrug azathioprine (AZA) is converted through a nonenzymatic reaction to 6-mercaptopurine (6-MP). 6-MP then undergoes extensive metabolism through three competing pathways mediated by the following: xanthine oxidase (XO), thiopurine *S*-methyltransferase (TPMT), and hypoxanthine guanine phosphoribosyl transferase (HPRT). The XO-mediated pathway produces an inactive metabolite, 6-thiouric acid (6-TU). The TPMT-mediated pathway produces a second inactive metabolite, 6-methymercaptopurine (6-MMP). The HPRT-mediated pathway produces 6-thioinosine monophosphate (6-TIMP). 6-TIMP can then undergo one of the following: (1) transformation into thioguanine nucleotides (6-TGN) by inosine-5-monophosphate dehydrogenase (IMPDH) and guanine monophosphate synthetase (GMPS); (2) methylation by TPMT into 6-methylmercaptopurine ribonucleotides (6-MMPR); (3) phosphorylation to 6-thio-inosine triphosphate (6-thio-ITP). In healthy cells, inosine triphosphatase (ITPase) converts 6-thio-ITP back to 6-TIMP to prevent the accumulation of 6-thio-ITP to toxic levels. AZA can act as an immunosuppressant if 2′-deoxy-6-TGTP is randomly incorporated into DNA and RNA, or, as recent studies suggest, by inhibiting the guanosine triphosphatase Rac1 in T lymphocytes [17–19]. NUDT15 (shown in Fig. 16.3) is involved in the inactivation of TGNs via conversion to TXMPs.

common reduced-function polymorphism of *TPMT* in Caucasians. *TPMT*3B* has only the p.A154T change and is associated with reduced function. Finally, *TPMT*3C* is the most common reduced-function polymorphism in African Americans and has a single amino acid change, p.Y240C. Though other reduced-function alleles of TPMT have been identified, these alleles, *TPMT*2, TPMT*3A, TPMT*3B, and TPMT*3C*, have been most commonly associated with reduced TPMT activity in various populations [20]. The mechanism for reduced function appears to be enhanced protein instability and increased degradation. A recent genomewide association study and meta-analysis examining whether other genes may potentially influence TPMT activity identified genetic polymorphisms in TPMT as the primary determinant of TPMT activity (Fig. 16.2) in blood samples from 884 individuals in which activity of the enzyme was quantified [21]. The enhanced toxicity of 6-MP in patients with TPMT reduced-function polymorphisms is related to accumulation of bioactive thioguanine nucleotides that cause myelosuppression. Thus these patients are at increased risk of myelotoxicity if a conventional dose of azathioprine, 6-thioguanine, or 6-MP is administered [22, 23]. Paradoxically, a number of studies have suggested that individuals with these same reduced-function variants of TPMT have a lower rate of relapse, particularly heterozygotes who are at reduced risk for myelotoxicity. Ultimately, clinicians must select doses for patients with various TPMT genotypes that maximize efficacy and minimize toxicity.

In July 2003, the FDA Pediatric Subcommittee of the Oncology Drug Advisory Committee (ODAC) discussed TPMT pharmacogenetics and debated whether relabeling 6-MP with genetic information was warranted [24]. Based on the evidence presented, the Subcommittee recommended that the label of 6-MP should be updated with TPMT genetic information. According to the ODAC recommendation, the labels for both 6-MP and subsequently, azathioprine were revised to include TPMT genetic information [11]. Current FDA recommendations for 6-MP include recommendations for genetic testing of the **2*, **3A*, and **3C* alleles of TPMT, and FDA updated tables include recommendations for genetic testing to inform dosing of azathioprine as well as thioguanine (see https: //www.fda.gov/medical-devices/precision-medicine/table-pharmacogenetic-associations). The current view is that TPMT testing, when combined with other tests, e.g., phenotypic testing of TPMT activity and clinical observations, can lead to informed decisions about drug selection and drug dosing that will further decrease the risk of severe and preventable bone marrow toxicity, yet provide the desired benefit from therapy with these drugs. In addition, a survey of TPMT genotyping in patients with acute lymphoblastic leukemia in four European countries (Germany, Ireland, The Netherlands, and the UK) suggested its cost-effectiveness in clinical practice [25].

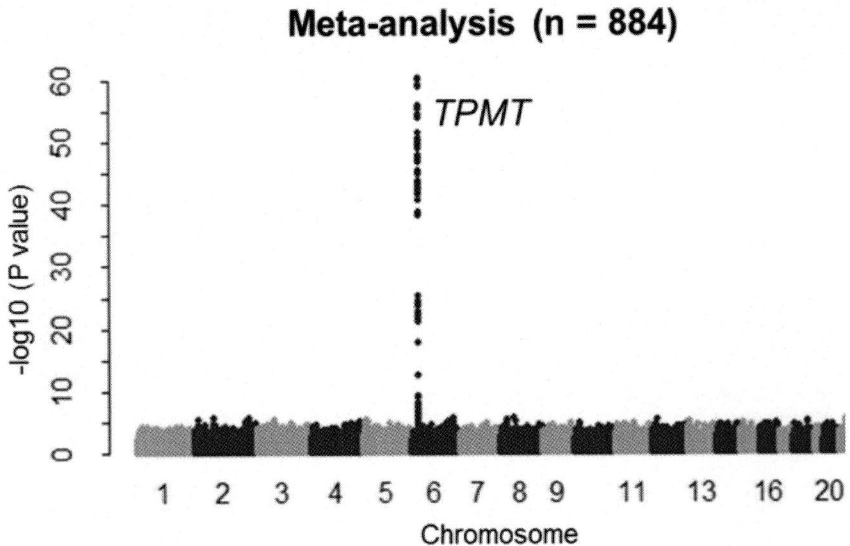

FIG. 16.2 Thiopurine methyltransferase activity in red blood cells is largely a monogenic trait. Figure represents a Manhattan plot of the -log*P* value for the association of SNPs across the human genome (by chromosome) with methyl transferase enzymatic activity in blood samples from 884 individuals. SNPs in only one gene, *TPMT*, are associated with methyl transferase enzymatic activity at genomewide levels of significance ($p < 10^{-8}$). *Reproduced with permission from Tamm R, Mägi R, Tremmel R, et al. Polymorphic variation in TPMT is the principal determinant of TPMT phenotype: A meta-analysis of three genome-wide association studies. Clin Pharmacol Ther 2017;101(5):684–695.*

NUDT15 and thiopurine myelotoxicity

Myelotoxicity to thiopurines has also been associated with genetic polymorphisms in nudix (nucleoside diphosphate linked moiety X)-type motif 15 (NUDT15) [16, 26]. NUDT15 is a nucleoside diphosphatase that catalyzes the conversion of thioguanine triphosphate metabolites (TGTP) to less toxic monophosphate metabolites (Fig. 16.3). A nonsynonymous genetic variant in NUDT15, p.R139C (rs116855232), has been associated with loss of catalytic activity and protein stability in in vitro studies. Clinically, children homozygous for p.R139C are at risk for severe myelosuppression and tolerate only 8% of the standard dose of 6-MP. Presumably, in these children highly active and toxic TGTP accumulate to extremely high levels that result in myelosuppression. Alleles that include the risk allele, p.R139C, are termed *NUDT15*2* and *NUDT15*3*. The reference allele is conventionally termed *NUDT15*1*. *NUDT15*2* has a population frequency of about 4% in East Asians and Latinos, and *NUDT15*3* has an allele frequency of 7% in South Asians and 6% in East Asians. Both the **2* and **3* alleles are found at much lower frequencies in other populations. Though other alleles of NUDT15 have been identified, these are even rarer. Most clinical studies have focused on 6-MP, but cellular studies indicate that the variant allele, p.R139C, has similar effects on the cytotoxicities of both azathioprine and thioguanine. In various populations, variant alleles of TPMT are the primary genetic basis for thiopurine intolerance and myelosuppression in populations of African and European ancestries, whereas NUDT15 alleles are the major cause of thiopurine-related myelosuppression in Asians and Hispanic populations. More details are available in dosing guidelines from the Clinical Pharmacogenetics Implementation Consortium [16].

UGT1A1 and irinotecan neutropenia

Irinotecan is an antineoplastic agent of the topoisomerase I inhibitor class that, in combination with 5-fluorouracil and leucovorin, is used for first-line therapy of patients with metastatic carcinoma of the colon or rectum. It is also indicated for patients with metastatic carcinoma of the colon or rectum whose disease has recurred or progressed following initial fluorouracil-based therapy [11]. Although irinotecan increases survival, it causes severe diarrhea and neutropenia.

Irinotecan is hydrolyzed by carboxylesterase enzymes to its active metabolite, SN-38 (Fig. 16.4). UDP-glucuronosyl transferase 1A1 (UGT1A1) is primarily responsible for inactivating SN-38 [30] by forming a glucuronide metabolite. *UGT1A1*28*, a variant allele, is associated with decreased enzyme activity. The variant occurs in the promoter region of the gene and is a variant of TA tandem repeats, which range between five and eight copies. The most common is six TA repeats and the allele, *UGT1A1*28*, contains seven TA repeats. Reporter assays suggest that the *UGT1A1*28* allele results in reduced transcription rates of UGTIA1, and therefore a reduced level of the enzyme and consequently reduced

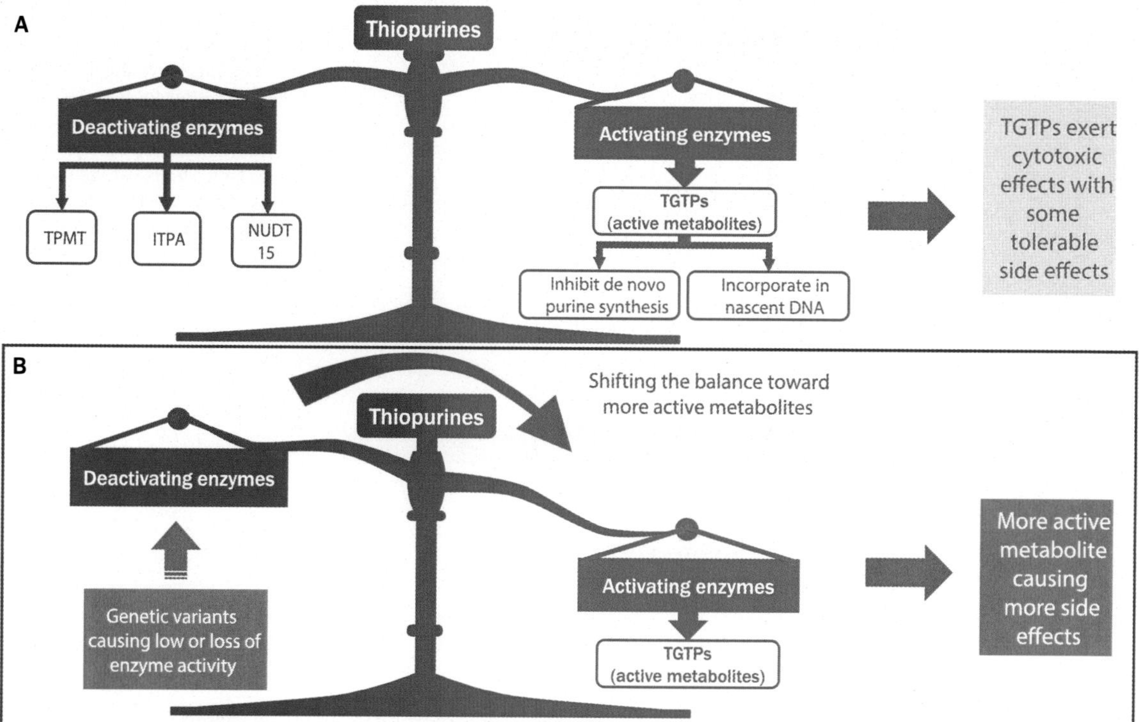

FIG. 16.3 The significant pathways of thiopurine activation and deactivation in pediatric acute lymphocytic leukemia, and the effects of some genetic variants. ITPA, inosine triphosphate pyrophosphatase; NUDT15, nucleoside diphosphate-linked moiety X motif 15; TGTP, thioguanine triphosphate nucleotide; TPMT, thiopurine methyltransferase. *Modified from Zeina N Al-Mahayri, George P Patrinos, and Bassam R Ali, Pharmacogenomics in pediatric acute lymphoblastic leukemia: promises and limitations. Pharmacogenomics 2017 18:7, 687–699. Figure kindly prepared by Giang Ho.*

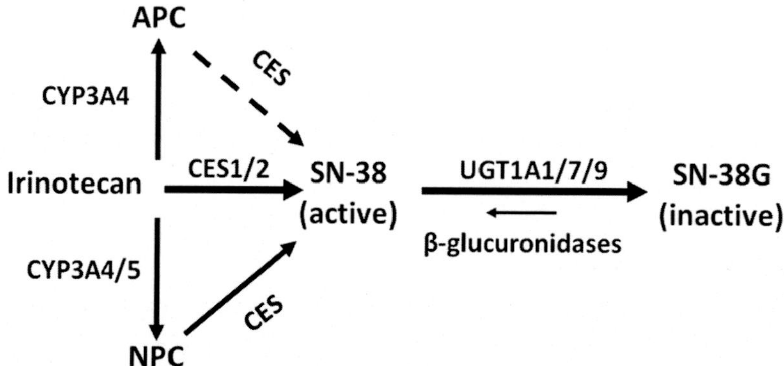

FIG. 16.4 Metabolism of irinotecan. Irinotecan is metabolized into its active metabolite SN-38 (7-ethyl-10-hydroxycamptothecin) via carboxylesterases (CES). SN-38 is then metabolized to its inactive glucuronide conjugate, SN-38G, by one of the following uridine diphosphate glucuronosyltransferases (UGTs), listed from most to least significant: UGT1A1, 1A7, and 1A9. Hepatobiliary excretion occurs, then SN-38G is reconverted into active SN-38 by β-glucuronidase containing intestinal bacteria. A second irinotecan detoxification pathway is via CYP3A (cytochrome P450 isoforms 3A4 and 3A5)-mediated oxidation of irinotecan to APC (7-ethyl-10-[4-*N*-(5-aminopentanoic acid)-1-piperidino]-carbonyloxy-camptothecin) and NPC (7-ethyl-10-[4-amino-1-piperidino]-carbonyloxy-camptothecin). CES facilitates conversion of NPC, and possibly APC, into SN-38 [27–29].

function. Because they inactivate SN-38 at a slower rate, patients with *UGT1A1*28* are at increased risk of neutropenia from irinotecan treatment [31]. Approximately 10% of the North American population is homozygous for the *UGT1A1*28* allele.

In a study of 66 patients who received irinotecan as a single agent (350 mg/m^2 once every 3 weeks), the incidence of grade 4 neutropenia in patients homozygous for the *UGT1A1*28* allele was 50%, and in patients heterozygous for this allele the incidence was 12.5%. No grade 4 neutropenia was observed in patients homozygous for the wild-type allele (*UGT1A1* *1 genotype). In a prospective study to investigate the role of *UGT1A1*28* polymorphism in the development of toxicity in 250 patients treated with irinotecan (180 mg/m^2) in combination with infusional 5-FU/LV, the incidence of grade 4 neutropenia in patients homozygous for the *UGT1A1*28* allele was 4.5%, compared to an incidence of 5.3% in patients heterozygous for this allele [11]. Grade 4 neutropenia was observed in 1.8% of patients homozygous for the wild-type allele [11]. In another study in which 109 patients were treated with irinotecan (100–125 mg/m^2) in combination with bolus 5-FU/LV, the incidence of grade 4 neutropenia in patients homozygous for the *UGT1A1*28* allele was 18.2%, and in patients heterozygous for this allele the incidence was 11.1%. Grade 4 neutropenia was observed in 6.8% of patients homozygous for the wild-type allele [11]. In November 2004, the FDA Advisory Committee for Pharmaceutical Science—Clinical Pharmacology Subcommittee (CPSC) discussed these findings [32]. Based on their recommendation, the label of irinotecan was updated to include *UGT1A1* genetic information and the recommendation that patients who are homozygous for *UGT1A1*28* alleles start irinotecan therapy with a reduced dose because of an increased risk of neutropenia [11].

Additional *UGT1A* polymorphisms have been evaluated, and Cecchin et al. [33] suggested that *UGT1A1* variants in addition to *UGT1A1*28* or haplotypes of *UGT1A1*, *UGT1A7*, and *UGT1A9* may describe the status of SN-38 glucuronidation more completely and thus contribute to a better characterization of individual variation in the clinical response to irinotecan. Another recent study has explored the association of a haplotype of ABCC2, which encodes MRP2 (an efflux transporter), with irinotecan-related diarrhea, and suggested that patients with this haplotype may have less diarrhea because their hepatobiliary secretion of irinotecan is reduced [34]. The significance of this association in modifying patient treatment awaits further evaluation. As *UGT1A1*28* is rare in Asians, recent studies had focused on *UGT1A1*6* which is more common in Asian populations. A meta-analysis of 11 studies showed that this polymorphism is associated with an increased risk of severe neutropenia [35]. In addition, while the risk of severe diarrhea was not significantly increased in the group heterozygous for *UGT1A1*6*, the homozygous group showed an increased risk (OR = 3.51; 95%CI 1.41–8.73, $p = 0.007$).

N-acetyltransferases and drug-induced toxicity

Acetylation of drugs in which an acetyl group is introduced into a drug molecule occurs via a Phase II reaction that is catalyzed by *N*-acetyltransferases, NAT1 and NAT2, that are both expressed at high levels in the liver and at lower levels in other tissues. Acetylation plays a major role in the metabolism of a number of drugs, including isoniazid, hydralazine, procainamide, and several sulfonamides, such as sulfamethoxazole, sulfanilamide, and sulfapyridine. Both enzymes have been found to be polymorphic, with over 25 alleles of NAT1 and 80 alleles of NAT2 that have been assigned official gene symbols [36]. *NAT1*4* and *NAT2*4* have been designated the reference alleles for each of the two genes. Of the two genes, NAT2 has many variants that are functionally significant and result in different enzyme activities. In general, NAT2 enzyme activity is associated with three phenotypes: slow acetylator (two slow alleles), intermediate acetylator (one slow and one rapid allele), and rapid acetylator (two rapid alleles). Rapid alleles are largely *NAT2*4*, and commonly observed slow alleles include *NAT2*5*, *NAT2*6*, and *NAT2*7*.

Drugs in which metabolism by NAT1 or NAT2 is a major route of elimination may have drug concentrations and adverse effects that are dependent on the level of *N*-acetyltransferase activity and thus, pharmacogenetic factors. As discussed in Chapter 14, there are reports of associations between drug-induced liver injury and NAT2 slow acetylator phenotypes or alleles [36]. Sulfamethoxazole pharmacokinetics also depend on NAT2 genotypes and phenotypes, and adverse effects such as skin rash and liver injury have also been associated with slow acetylator alleles of NAT2. Sulfasalazine, used in the treatment of Crohn's disease, is converted to sulfapyridine by gut bacteria. Sulfapyridine is subsequently metabolized by *N*-acetylation. NAT2 slow acetylator alleles (**5*, **6* or **7*) have been associated with higher levels of sulfapyridine and increased risk of sulfasalazine-associated toxicities [36]. Finally, slow acetylators of hydralazine are at an increased risk of developing antinuclear antibodies and a systemic lupus erythematosus-like adverse reaction [37]. The higher levels of hydralazine in the slow acetylators are presumably the mechanism for the increased risk for this reaction, though this needs further investigation. Collectively, the data support a role of NAT2 genetic polymorphisms in adverse effects of drugs that undergo acetylation; however, there is currently insufficient evidence available to warrant official recommendations, such as those of CPIC, regarding genotype-guided dosing or drug selection of NAT2 substrate drugs.

Transporter-mediated pharmacogenomic mechanisms of drug toxicity

In addition to drug-metabolizing enzymes, genes associated with exposure-related drug toxicity include those coding for drug transporters, which play a role in both influx and efflux of drugs into all cells in the body [38, 39]. Polymorphisms in transporter genes may enhance drug accumulation into target tissues responsible for toxicity, either directly or indirectly through pharmacokinetic mechanisms, and thereby increase susceptibility to ADRs. For example, a polymorphism in a hepatic transporter may result in reduced hepatic uptake and metabolism of a drug, and therefore higher systemic drug levels (Fig. 16.5) [39, 40]. The resulting higher systemic drug concentrations may in turn cause toxicity in various body organs. Other mechanisms by which transporter polymorphisms may be associated with drug toxicity include modulation of endogenous substrate accumulation. For example, polymorphisms in bile acid transporters in the liver may be associated with changes in bile salt disposition that result in drug-induced cholestasis [39, 41].

The organic anion transporter 1B1 (OATP1B1) and statin-induced myopathy

Statins (HMG-CoA reductase inhibitors) are among the most widely prescribed drugs and are used as lipid-lowering medications. The major side effect of statins is muscle toxicity or myopathy. Symptoms of statin-induced myopathy include fatigue, muscle pain, tenderness, weakness, and cramping, which can occur with or without an increase in blood creatine kinase concentration. In general, statin-induced myopathy is mild and reversible, but at times a more severe myopathy may result from statin therapy [41, 42]. The incidence of statin-induced myopathy ranges from a mild and relatively common myalgia in 5%–10% of statin users/year to a life-threatening and rare rhabdomyolysis in 0.001%–0.005% of statin users/year [36, 38]. Known risk factors for statin-induced myopathy and rhabdomyolysis include a high statin dose, drug-drug interactions (especially those that raise statin plasma concentrations), old age, existence of multiple concomitant diseases, hypothyroidism, and certain inherited muscle disorders [43, 44]. The mechanism by which statins cause myopathy remains unknown, but appears to be related to statin concentrations in blood and muscle [45]. As described in Chapter 13, polymorphisms in the hepatic uptake transporter, OATP1B1 (SLCO1B1), have been associated with statin-induced myopathy [46]. Accordingly, CPIC guidelines for drug and dose selection based on genotype have been published and provide information on use of genetic information to inform drug selection and dosing for simvastatin and other statins [47]. In

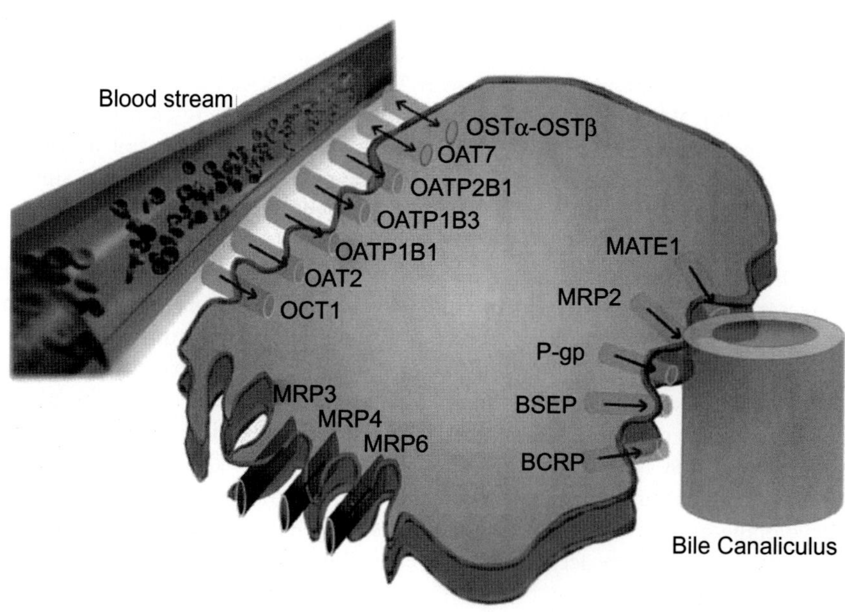

FIG. 16.5 Selected transporters for endogenous compounds and xenobiotics, expressed on the sinusoidal and canalicular membranes of human hepatocytes [59, 117]. Not shown is the heteromeric organic solute transporter (NTCP) which is expressed on the sinusoidal membrane and contributes to the uptake of bile salts from the portal circulation. BSEP, bile salt export pump; MATE1, multidrug and toxin extrusion protein 1; MRP, multiple drug resistance protein; OAT, organic anion transporter; OCT, organic cation transporter; OSTα-OSTβ.

particular, dosing recommendations are made on the basis of the increased risk of developing statin-induced myopathy that has been associated with the genotype of the reduced-function variant, rs4149056T > C (p.V174A) in *SLCO1B1*, which is present in several haplotypes.

Transporters in drug-induced liver injury (DILI)

DILI is the primary cause of drug attrition due to safety issues. Indeed, over 1000 approved drugs have been linked to DILI [48]. DILI takes multiple forms including highly predictable DILI, which is dependent on drug dose and hepatic accumulation and idiosyncratic DILI, a much more difficult form of the injury. Of the five major classes of DILI including necrosis, cholestasis, steatosis, vascular injury, and cytoplasmic alterations [48], cholestatic liver injury accounts for the greatest number of cases of DILI and represents the most severe form. Cholestatic liver injury is characterized by impaired bile flow, which is mediated by transporters on both canalicular and sinusoidal membranes of hepatocytes. The primary transporter involved in bile acid flow on the sinusoidal membrane is the sodium-taurocholate cotransporter polypeptide (NTCP, SLC10A1), whereas the major efflux pump on the canalicular membrane is the bile salt export protein (BSEP, ABCB11). Other transporters that contribute to bile acid disposition in the liver include multidrug resistance associated proteins 2 (MRP2, ABCC2) on the apical membrane, and 3 (MRP3, ABCC3) and 4 (MRP4, ABCC4) on the sinusoidal membranes. Several lines of evidence support the notion that polymorphisms in bile acid transporters may play a role in drug-induced cholestasis. First, small molecule inhibitors of bile acid transporters can cause cholestatic liver injury [49–51]. Second, familial forms of cholestatic liver injury such as Dubin-Johnson syndrome and pregnancy-induced cholestasis are associated with rare missense variants ABCC2 [52]. However, there have been few studies to date that associate polymorphisms in hepatic bile acid transporters with DILI [53], and most are underpowered. For example, a recent study suggests that patients heterozygous for reduced-function alleles of BSEP may be at elevated risk for DILI [48] and that individuals with genetic variants of ABCC2 are at elevated risk for liver injury from the nonsteroidal antiinflammatory drug, diclofenac [53]. With the evidence that hepatic bile acid transporters appear to be involved in DILI, more studies with larger sample sizes are needed to understand the role that common and rare variants in these transporters play in the occurrence of DILI.

Transporters and tenofovir renal toxicity

Tenofovir disoproxil fumarate (TDF) is an orally bioavailable prodrug of tenofovir (TFV), an acyclic nucleotide analog reverse transcriptase inhibitor [54]. Cases of renal failure and kidney tubular dysfunction, including development of Fanconi syndrome, have been reported, leading to concerns regarding long-term TDF use [55]. Owing to the high interindividual variability in the presentation of kidney function abnormalities, researchers have recently focused on host genetic factors predisposing to TFV-associated renal dysfunction [56]. Transporter proteins involved in the renal elimination of TFV, such as organic anion transporters (OATs) or MRP 2, 4, or 10, have been the focus of these studies (Fig. 16.6). Notably, several genetic polymorphisms in these transporters have been associated with an increased risk of kidney tubulopathy in TDF-treated patients [56, 58–61]. Relevant pharmacogenetic factors that may play a role in the risk of renal toxicity associated with the use of tenofovir are summarized in Table 16.2.

MRP2, encoded by the *ABCC2* gene, is localized apically in cellular membranes. Associations between polymorphisms in this gene and TFV-associated tubulopathy have been reported in two studies. [56, 61, 67]. Polymorphisms in ABCB1 and OAT1, the main transporter taking tenofovir into the proximal tubular cell, also have been investigated but the overall results suggest that these polymorphisms have no effect on TFV-associated renal dysfunction [56, 61]. In addition to genetic factors, nongenetic factors such as age, body weight, and gender have to some extent been related to the incidence of renal dysfunction in TFV-treated patients. For example, it has been reported that renal toxicity occurs more frequently in males than females [59]. Other variables that may increase risk of renal toxicity from TFV include preexisting renal impairment and DDI resulting from concomitant use of nephrotoxic drugs such as didanosine, protease inhibitors, and, in particular, ritonavir [68].

Genetic mechanisms for drug-induced hypersensitivity reactions

As discussed in Chapter 15, ADRs have traditionally been classified into two major subtypes: A and B. Type A reactions are dose dependent, based on pharmacological mechanism of action, and generally predictable, whereas type B reactions are idiosyncratic, allergic, or hypersensitivity reactions that are not predictable. Among type B reactions, hypersensitivity reactions have been the most thoroughly studied and are responsible for substantial morbidity and mortality. Drug allergies are a class of hypersensitivity reactions that can range from mild skin rashes to more severe, less common syndromes. In particular, toxic epidermal necrolysis (TEN) and Stevens-Johnson syndrome (SJS) are two life-threatening hypersensitivity

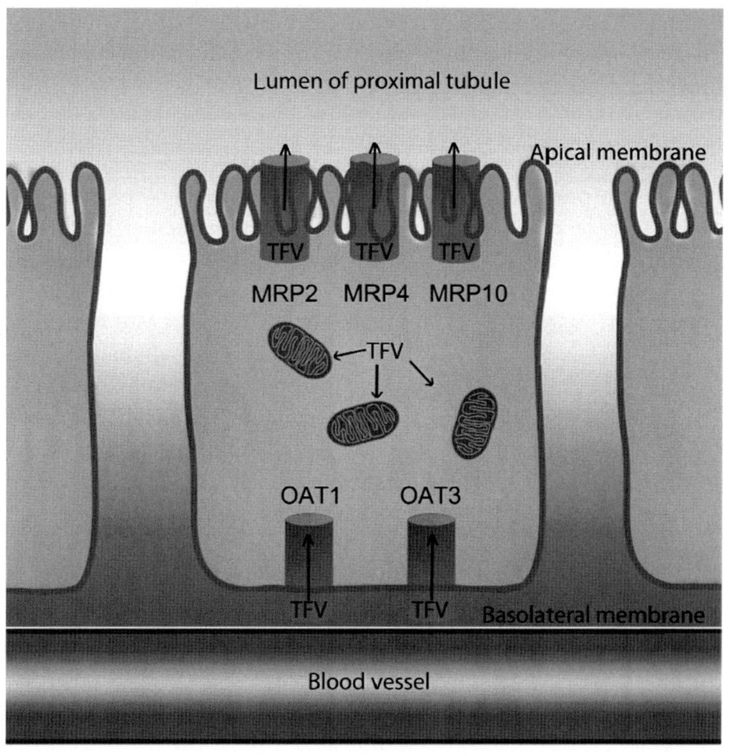

FIG. 16.6 Between 20% and 30% of an administered tenofovir dose is excreted unchanged in the urine through active secretion by proximal tubular cells and several transporter proteins are involved in this process. OAT1 is the main transporter taking tenofovir from blood into the proximal tubular cell, although OAT3 also contributes. Once in the proximal tubular cells, tenofovir is extruded into the tubular lumen by MRP2 and MRP4. Recently, MRP10 has also been implicated in TFV transport (not shown in figure). Proximal tubular cells are uniquely susceptible to tenofovir toxicity because they express transporters that increase intracellular concentrations of the drug and are rich in mitochondria [57]. MRP, multidrug resistant protein; OAT, organic anion transporter protein; TFV, tenofovir.

reactions in which several drugs or their metabolites are implicated. Particular drugs and classes of drugs that are associated with SJS and TEN include nonsteroidal antiinflammatory drugs (NSAIDS), sulfonamides, antiretroviral drugs, antibiotics, corticosteroids, antiepileptic agents, methotrexate, and allopurinol.

For years, hypersensitivity reactions have been known to vary in prevalence among human populations. For example, East Asians are particularly sensitivity to carbamazepine-induced hypersensitivity reactions. More recently, genetic polymorphisms in the human leukocyte antigen (HLA) system, the major histocompatibility complex (MHC), have been implicated in drug-induced hypersensitivity reactions. Though the mechanisms by which HLA polymorphisms may lead to risk for drug hypersensitivity reactions are not well understood, recent studies have shed some light on the genetic mechanisms of abacavir-induced hypersensitivity reactions.

Haptens interact with HLA molecules in a polymorphic-specific manner

To produce a robust T-cell or immunologic response, the neoself peptides, formed by the drug or its metabolite reacting with proteins and the proteins being digested into smaller peptides, must bind to the HLA molecule (Fig. 16.7). HLA-B polymorphisms have been associated with a variety of drug-induced hypersensitivity reactions. HLA genes are found on chromosome 6 in the region of the MHC. MHC class 1, including HLA-A, HLA—B, and HLA—C, are primarily involved in the presentation of peptides on the cell surface, which, if foreign, will attract CD8-positive T-cells. The HLA-B gene, located on chromosome 6 p21.3, is involved in hypersensitivity reactions to various drugs, including allopurinol, carbamazepine, and abacavir [68–70], and in flucloxacillin hepatotoxicity [71]. Hundreds of HLA-B polymorphisms have been described. These are numbered, and many have been associated with human disease, including infectious disease such as AIDS and reactive arthritis [72–74]. Though the exact drug-modified peptide for abacavir sensitivity has not been discovered, the reaction appears to be dependent on key residues in HLA-B*5701, which are not present in other HLA-B polymorphisms. This mechanism explains how an HLA polymorphism may lead to a drug-induced hypersensitivity reaction.

Though patients with particular HLA-B polymorphisms are at increased risk for SJS and TEN, most do not get these hypersensitivity reactions when exposed to the drugs that have the potential to cause these ADRs. Thus HLA-B polymorphisms seem to be necessary, but not sufficient, to elicit these drug hypersensitivity reactions. The mechanisms for this phenomenon are not clear. However, it is possible that patients with certain T-cell receptor polymorphisms may be at risk

TABLE 16.2 Transporter polymorphisms and their association with renal damage.

Gene (protein)	rs Number	SNPs/haplotypes	Amino acid change	Functional alteration	Association with renal damage
ABCC2 (MRP2)	rs717620	−24C>T	5′-UTR	No clear influence on DNA-protein binding and the mRNA stability did not differ significantly. In transfected HEK293T/17 cells; significantly lower protein expression [62]	The carriers of the −24T allele excreted 19% more TFV than carriers of the common allele; CC genotype is more frequent in patients with tubular damage [59, 61]
ABCC2 (MRP2)	rs7080681	1058G>A	Arg353His	N.A.	No association with renal damage
ABCC2 (MRP2)	rs2273697	1249G>A	Val417Ile	Vmax ↓; Km ↓(for certain substrates in sf9 cell [63]; significantly increased protein expression (HEK293T/17 cell) [62]	AA genotype is more frequent in patients with proximal tubular damage; no association with renal damage [56, 61]
	rs8187694	3563T>A	Val1188Glu	N.A.	TT genotype is more frequent in patients with proximal tubular damage; no association with renal damage [56, 61]
	rs3740066	3972C>T	Ile1324Ile	Significantly increased protein expression (HEK293T/17 cell) [62]	No association with renal damage [56, 61]
	rs8187710	4544G>A	Cys1515Tyr	N.A.	A allele is not present in patients with proximal tubular damage; no association with renal damage [56, 61]
ABCC2 (MRP2)	–	Haplotype CATC	–	Significantly increased protein expression (HEK293T/17 cell) [62]	Risk of proximal tubular damage [56]
ABCC4 (MRP4)	rs11568685	559G>T	Gly187Trp	Reduced function and Decreased expression (HEK 293T) [64]	No association with renal damage [56]
	rs899494	669C>T	Ile223Ile	N.A.	T allele is more frequent in patients with proximal tubular damage; no association with renal damage [56, 61]
	rs2274407	912G>T	Lys304Asn	No functional alternation (HEK 293T) [64]	No association with renal damage [56]
	rs2274406)	951G>A	Arg317Arg	N.A.	
	rs2274405)	969G>A	Ser323Ser	N.A.	
	rs1557070	1497C>T	Tyr499Tyr	N.A.	
	rs11568655	3310T>C	Leu1104Leu	N.A.	
	rs1751034	3348A>G	Lys1116Lys	N.A.	
	rs11568695	3609G>A	Ala1203Ala	N.A.	

Continued

TABLE 16.2 Transporter polymorphisms and their association with renal damage—cont'd

Gene (protein)	rs Number	SNPs/haplotypes	Amino acid change	Functional alteration	Association with renal damage
ABCC4 (MRP4)	rs3742106	4135T>G	3′UTR	N.A.	No association with TFV clearance and no association with renal damage [59, 61]
ABCC10 (MRP7)	rs9349256	2137G>A	Intron	N.A.	Significantly associated with kidney tubular dysfunction (KTD); urine phosphorus wasting and β2 microglobulinuria [60]
ABCC10 (MRP7)	rs2125739	2843T>C	Ile948Thr	N.A.	
ABCC10 (MRP7)	–	HaplotypeGGC	–	N.A.	
ABCC10 (MRP7)–*ABCC1* (MRP2)	–	HaplotypeGGC-CGTC	–	N.A.	Significantly higher in the KTD group than in the controls [60]
ABCB1 (P-gp)	rs1128503	1236C>T	Gly412Gly	N.A.	No association with renal damage [56, 61]
	rs2032582	2677G>A/T	Ala893Ser/Thr	Enhanced efflux of digoxin [65]	
	rs1045642	3435C>T	Ile1145Ile	N.A.	
SLC22A6 (OAT1)	rs11568634	1361G>A	Arg454Gln	Nonfunctional with respect to adenovir assayed in *X. laevis* oocytes [66]	No difference in renal clearance and secretory clearance of adefovir in family-based studies [59, 61]
SLC22A11 (OAT4)	rs11231809	g.64302950T>A	–	N.A.	No association with renal damage [61]

N.A., not available.

for drug-induced hypersensitivity reactions [75]. Additional studies are clearly needed to explain why many individuals with polymorphic HLA-B risk alleles do not get these hypersensitivity reactions. Further, in addition to hapten-specific binding to HLA-B polymorphisms, other mechanisms should be studied which may lead to HLA-B polymorphism-specific drug hypersensitivity reactions [75].

Abacavir-induced hypersensitivity reactions

Abacavir hypersensitivity reactions have been associated in many studies with the HLA polymorphism HLA-B*5701 [70, 76]. These reactions are known to vary in frequency among racial and ethnic groups, paralleling the allele frequencies of HLA-B*5701 in these populations [77]. Abacavir is a prodrug that is activated to carbovir triphosphate, a reactive drug which may be responsible for the formation of immunogenic peptides in the body. The mechanism of the HLA-B*5701-dependent abacavir hypersensitivity reaction was studied by Chessman and coworkers [78], who conducted in vitro experiments suggesting that abacavir-induced hypersensitivity reactions are mediated by the activation of cytotoxic $CD8^+$ T-cells, which corresponded to the known increased abundance of $CD8^+$ T-cells in the skin of patients with abacavir hypersensitivity reactions. Abacavir stimulation of $CD8^+$ T-cells in vitro occurred with lymphoblastoid cell lines expressing HLA-B*5701, but not HLA-B*5702 or HLA-B*5801. By comparing the amino acid substitutions in the antigen-binding pocket among the three HLA-B polymorphisms, the investigators speculated that HLA-B*5702 and *5801 may not bind abacavir neoself peptide (s) (which was not identified) because of differences in the antigen-binding cleft. Alternatively, they speculated that these HLA-B polymorphisms may bind abacavir neoself peptides, but present them in an altered configuration that is not recognized by $CD8^+$ T-cells. Further site-directed mutagenesis studies demonstrated that the amino acid substitution of a polar serine at position 116 of HLA-B*5701 to a tyrosine residue of HLA-B*5702 resulted in lack of

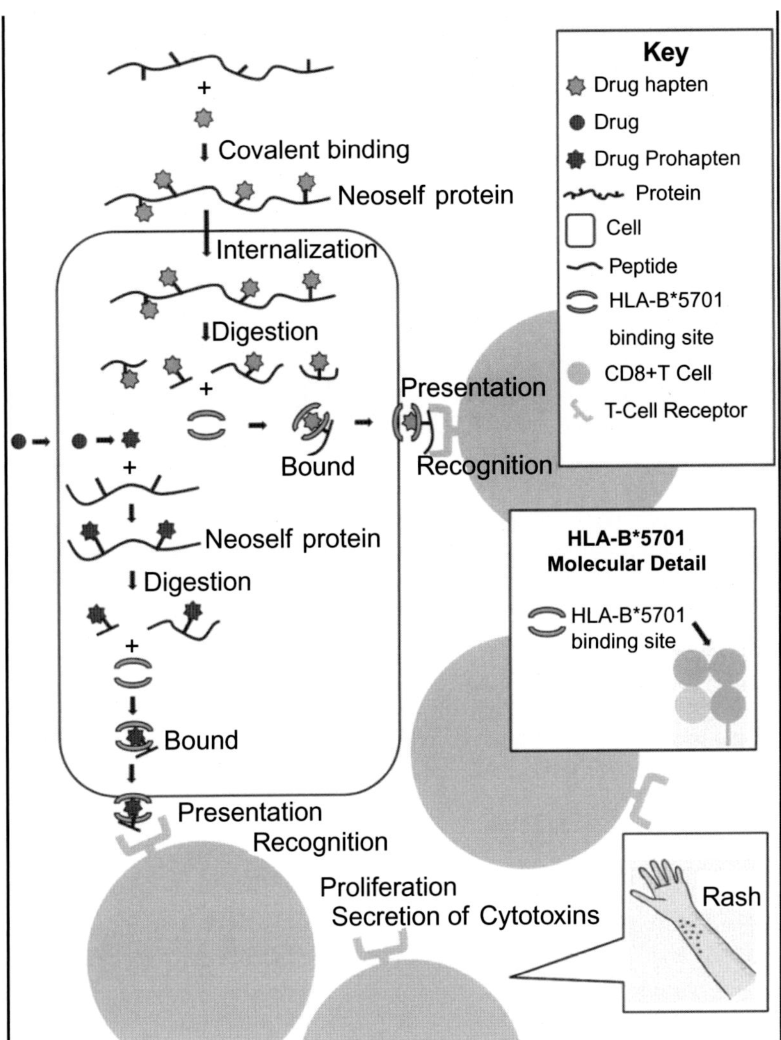

FIG. 16.7 Mechanisms by which HLA-B*5701 mediates hypersensitivity reactions of drugs including abacavir. The key describes the symbols, and the details of the mechanisms are described in the text.

recognition by abacavir-specific $CD8^+$ T-cells. Though residue 116 is clearly critical in the hypersensitivity reaction of abacavir, the study did not identify the abacavir hapten. Collectively, the data suggest that a unique ligand(s) or neoself peptide(s) is created with abacavir and an endogenous protein(s). Importantly, there is selective binding and presentation of the abacavir neoself peptide(s) by cells expressing the HLA-B*5701, due to amino acid differences in the antigen-binding cleft.

Drug-induced liver injury (DILI) mediated by the HLA system

Studies of polymorphisms in the HLA system and ADRs related to this have primarily centered on drug-induced skin rashes, SJS, and TEN. However, it has become increasingly clear that hypersensitivity reactions mediated by this system may lead to other adverse drug reactions, in particular in the liver [79]. Daly et al. [71] conducted a genomewide association study (GWAS) that showed a strong association with DILI caused by treatment with flucloxacillin. In 51 cases of flucloxacillin-mediated DILI and 282 controls, a highly significant association ($P < 8.7 \times 10^{-33}$) was identified with a genetic polymorphism (rs2395029) in complete linkage disequilibrium with HLA-B*5701 (Fig. 16.8). The genetic association of this rare adverse drug reaction was replicated in a second, smaller cohort in which HLA-B*5701 was present in 64% of the cases of flucloxacillin-mediated DILI. This striking association raised awareness in the field of pharmacogenomics that HLA polymorphisms may also contribute to DILI in addition to TEN and SJS.

DILI due to ximelagatran, an anticoagulant, has also been associated with an HLA polymorphism, in particular, HLA-DRB1*0701 [80]. HLA polymorphisms also have been found to be associated with DILI due to administration

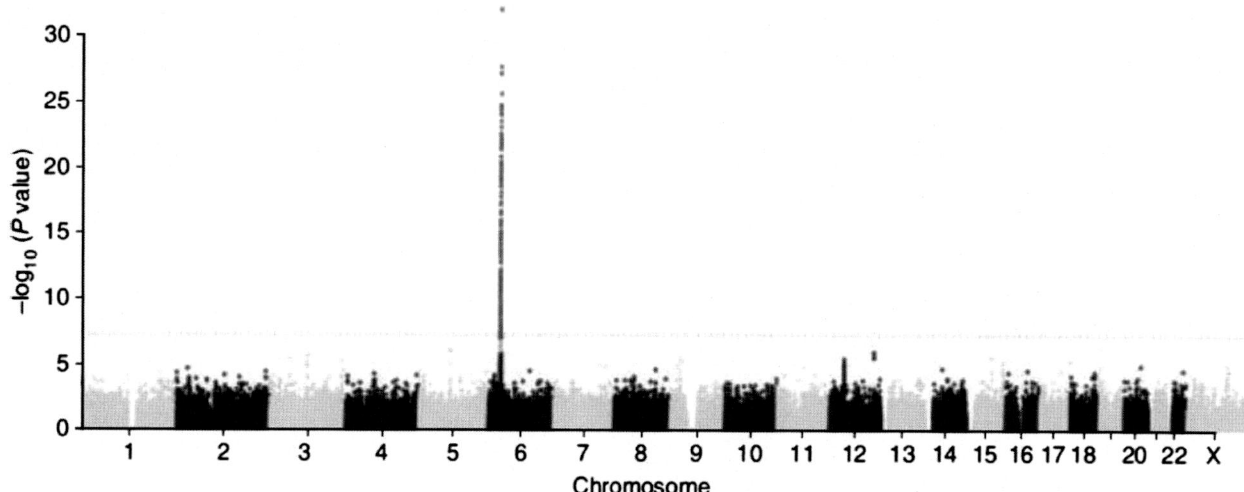

FIG. 16.8 Flucloxacillin DILI GWAS result. Each dot represents a SNP. The *x*-axis represents the chromosomal position of the SNP. The *y*-axis represents the −log10 of the Cochran–Armitage trend P value of the SNP in the case–control association study. The strong signal in chromosome 6 lies in the MHC region. A total of 51 DILI cases and 282 population controls were included in the study. *Reproduced with permission for Daly AK, Donaldson PT, Bhatnagar P, Shen Y, Pe'er I, Floratos A, et al. HLA-B*5701 genotype is a major determinant of drug-induced liver injury due to flucloxacillin. Nat Genet 2009;41:816–819.*

of several drugs used in the treatment of tuberculosis, including isoniazid, rifampin, and ethambutol [81]. Since most of these reports have been published only recently, the mechanisms responsible for their polymorphism-based risk for DILI have not been elucidated, but this is likely to be the subject of considerable future research.

FDA labeling of drugs for pharmacogenomic information

After the draft of the human genome was published more than two decades ago [82, 83], there was high hope that this information could be utilized to develop personalized medical therapy. Subsequently, there has been exponential growth in research exploring the utility of this genomic information, and rapid advancement in understanding the mechanisms that underlie interindividual differences in drug response, resulting in greater appreciation of the role that genetic factors play in such response. One result has been that many drugs have been relabeled to describe these new findings when they have critical implications for patient treatment. The timing of relabeling varies depending on the availability of new information, and may occur within a few years after the drugs have been on the market, as shown for abacavir in Fig. 16.9, or decades after their initial approvals, as with warfarin and codeine, which have been relabeled to include critical pharmacogenomic information more than 50 years after their initial approvals (Table 16.1).

Considerable controversy exists about the clinical utility of genomic tests and how to translate pharmacogenomic findings into useful tools in clinical practice [84–86]. Although randomized clinical trials (RCTs) have been considered as the gold standard for providing evidential basis for many interventions of medicine, there are other complementary sources of evidence (mechanistic, pharmacological, and observational studies) that can contribute to establishing clinical utility [87, 88]. For example, the recommendation and high utility of a test for patients' HLA genotype prior to treatment with abacavir [89, 90] were based on a prospective RCT that showed associations between hypersensitivity and HLA-B*5701 [91]. On the other hand, case-control or cohort studies have identified the genetic basis of other ADRs, including those in patients taking carbamazepine [92].

To transition from the discovery of a diagnostic test, such as the genetic tests related to ADRs discussed in this chapter, to their routine clinical use, key questions related to their clinical utility must be addressed, and can include the following [87]:

1. Is there an informative marker that correlates with a clinical state?
2. Does the test measure the biomarker reliably?
3. Does the test predict the clinical state?
4. Does the test provide reliable information?
5. Is the test worth doing?

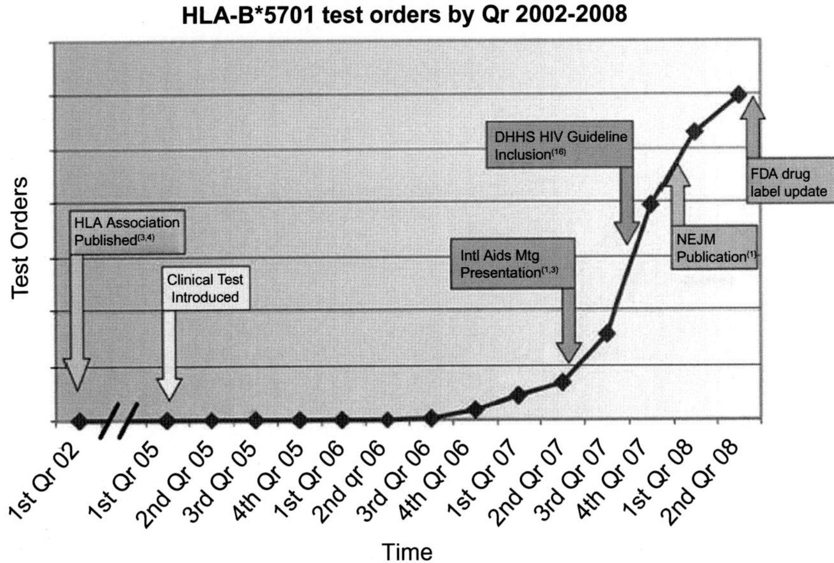

FIG. 16.9 HLA-B*5701 test orders received by quarter at a US-based National Reference Laboratory showing rapid adoption of the HLA-B*5701 genetic test. *Adapted with permission from Lai-Goldman M, Faruki H. Abacavir hypersensitivity: a model system for pharmacogenetic test adoption. Genet Med 2008;10(12):874–878.*

6. For biomarkers used in drug development, does the test predict the desired clinical outcome?
7. Is the test worth paying for?

Some of the earlier mentioned questions have been addressed via RCTs, others via case-control, cohort studies, or clinical studies in naturalistic settings [93].

A drug's labeling may be changed after an association has been established between a gene and a drug response. This often follows intensive review of the available association data and their clinical implication at various FDA internal interdisciplinary team meetings, open public meetings such as the FDA advisory committee meetings, other public scientific debates and publications, and FDA meetings with the NDA/BLA holders of the affected drug products and with other regulatory agencies such as EMA.

After the drug labeling has been revised, many factors affect the clinical uptake and implementation of the genetic tests. These may include the knowledge of the healthcare providers, the test's availability when the drug is initially prescribed, the peer-reviewed guidelines, and the availability of alternate dosages or drugs for patients with high-risk genotypes [94]. For example, the management of hypersensitivity reactions to abacavir, by requiring HLA-B*5701 genotyping prior to prescription of this drug was adopted by the HIV community as soon as strong clinical association data became available [89], even before the FDA labeling was changed to include a blackbox warning about this association (Fig. 16.9). On the other hand, widespread implementation of genetic testing to guide warfarin dosing has not occurred, and reimbursement for this testing remains uncertain or restricted [95, 96], even after FDA relabeling to describe how patients' CYP2C9 and VKORC1 genotypes can affect warfarin dosing requirements. As discussed in Chapter 17, the FDA has published both procedural guidance on biomarker qualifications and recommendations related to the evaluation of pharmacogenomic associations prior to marketing approval [97, 98]. The European Medicinal Agency has also provided guidelines in these areas [99].

The role of modeling and simulation in elucidating pharmacogenomic ADR mechanisms

As most ADRs cannot be attributed to a single patient factor, it is important to understand the risks associated with multiple factors—both genetic and nongenetic. Mathematical simulations using population-based, physiological models (e.g., physiologically based pharmacokinetic (PBPK) models) that simultaneously integrate various patient intrinsic and extrinsic factors can provide an understanding of the potential complex changes in exposure-response relationships in patients in whom multiple covariates affect drug response. Some applications of these physiologically based models including the design of clinical trials to evaluate the effects of drug-metabolizing enzyme polymorphisms on pharmacokinetics and pharmacodynamics are described in Chapter 31 and have been summarized in a recent review [100]. For example, simulations have been used to evaluate the impact of drug interactions on patients with CYP2C9 polymorphisms. Simulations indicated that coadministration of a CYP2C9 inhibitor to warfarin-treated patients who are extensive metabolizers of CYP2C9

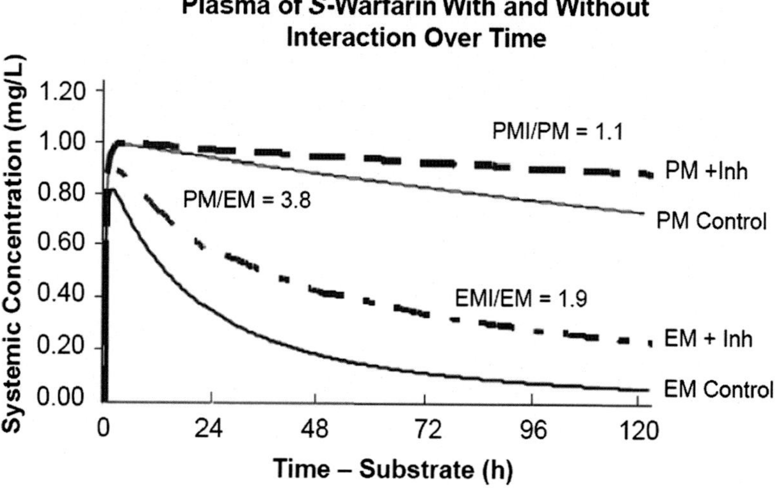

FIG. 16.10 Simulated inhibition of *S*-warfarin metabolism by a CYP2C9 inhibitor in subjects who are extensive vs. poor metabolizers of CYP2C9 (simulation, simcyp v8.20; PM, poor metabolizer of CYP2C9; EM, extensive metabolizer of CYP2C9; male/female ratio = 1; age 20–40 years. *S*-warfarin single dose, 10 mg on Day 1, sulfaphenazole (CYP2C9 inhibitor) once a day 2000 mg for 5 days). The intrinsic clearance values for 7-hydroxy warfarin (μL/min/pmol of CYP) were assigned to be 0.034 and 0.005, for EM (*1/*1) and PM (*3/*3) of CYP2C9, respectively.

substrates could result in a twofold increase in the plasma levels of *S*-warfarin, the active isomer of warfarin (Fig. 16.10) [101]. On the other hand, if a patient has two copies of variant alleles of CYP2C9 *3 and has been on a stable warfarin dosing regimen, coadministration of drugs that are strong CYP2C9 inhibitors would not be expected to lead to any significant increase in plasma *S*-warfarin levels.

PBPK models also can be developed to simulate tissue levels at the sites of adverse or therapeutic drug action and to evaluate their relationships (or lack thereof) to systemic exposure levels [102–104]. In addition, simulations can be used to provide hypotheses on observed clinical effects not predicted by systemic drug levels or to provide optimal study designs to address further questions. Finally, PBPK modeling and simulation can play an important role in regulatory review, and their utility and limitations in this context have been discussed in both FDA publications [105–107] and in guidance documents [18].

Acknowledgment

The authors would like to acknowledge support from GM115370, a grant from the National Institute of General Medical Sciences, NIH.

References

[1] Giacomini KM, Krauss RM, Roden DM, Eichelbaum M, Hayden MR, Nakamura Y. When good drugs go bad. Nature 2007;446:975–977.
[2] Friedman MA, Woodcock J, Lumpkin MM, Shuren JE, Hass AE, Thompson LJ. The safety of newly approved medicines: do recent market removals mean there is a problem? JAMA 1999;281:1728–1734.
[3] Berndt ER, Gottschalk AH, Philipson TJ, Strobeck MW. Industry funding of the FDA: effects of PDUFA on approval times and withdrawal rates. Nat Rev Drug Discov 2005;4(7):545–554.
[4] CDER, CBER. Safety labeling changes—implementation of section 505(o)(4) of the Federal Food, Drug, and Cosmetic Act. Guidance for Industry. Rockville, MD: FDA; 1988, (Internet atwww.fda.gov/downloads/Drugs/GuidanceComplianceRegulatoryInformation/Guid, cited April 15, 2011).
[5] FDA Drug Safety-related Labeling Changes (SrLC): n.d., https://www.accessdata.fda.gov/scripts/cder/safetylabelingchanges/ accessed June 21, 2020
[6] Liu Q, Ramamoorthy A, Huang S. Real-world data and clinical pharmacology: a regulatory science perspective. Clin Pharmacol Ther 2019;106:67–71.
[7] CDER, CBER CDRH. Clinical pharmacogenomics: Premarketing evaluation in early phase clinical studies. Guidance for Industry. Rockville, MD: FDA; 2011, (Internet at http://www.fda.gov/downloads/Drugs/GuidanceComplianceRegulatoryInformation/Guidances/UCM243702.pdfcited April 7, 2011.).
[8] Amur S, Frueh FW, Lesko LJ, Huang SM. Integration and use of biomarkers in drug development, regulation and clinical practice: a US regulatory perspective. Biomark Med 2008;2(3):305–311.
[9] Woodcock J, Lesko LJ. Pharmacogenetics—tailoring treatment for the outliers. N Engl J Med 2009;360(8):811–813.
[10] Xenazine. n.d. Xenazine® (Tetrabenazine) [package insert issued 5/2008]. Washington, DC: Prestwick Pharmaceuticals, Inc. (Internet at, www.accessdata.fda.gov/drugsatfda_docs/label/2008/021894lbl.pdf.).
[11] FDA general labeling. n.d. Drugs@FDA; Internet at https://www.accessdata.fda.gov/scripts/cder/daf/index.cfm; Accessed July 26, 2020

[12] CDER. n.d. Table of pharmacogenomic biomarkers in drug labeling (Internet at, https://www.fda.gov/drugs/science-and-research-drugs/table-pharmacogenomic-biomarkers-drug-labeling) Accessed 26 July 2020
[13] Huang SM, Temple R. Is this the drug or dose for you? Impact and consideration of ethnic factors in global drug development, regulatory review, and clinical practice. Clin Pharmacol Ther 2008;84(3):287–294.
[14] Yasuda SU, Zhang L, Huang SM. The role of ethnicity in variability in response to drugs: focus on clinical pharmacology studies. Clin Pharmacol Ther 2008;84(3):417–423.
[15] Green D, Brooks MM, Burckart GJ, Figg II WD, Troutman SM, Ferrell R, Chinnock R, Canter C, Addonizio L, Bernstein D, Kirklin JK, Naftel D, Price DK, Sissung TM, Girnita DM, Zeevi A, Webber SA. The influence of race and genetics on outcomes after pediatric heart transplantation. Am J Transplant 2017. https://doi.org/10.1111/ajt.14153.
[16] Relling MV, Schwab M, Whirl-Carrillo M, et al. Clinical pharmacogenetics implementation consortium guideline for Thiopurine dosing based on TPMT and NUDT15 genotypes: 2018 update. Clin Pharmacol Ther 2019;105(5):1095–1105.
[17] Zaza G, Cheok M, Krynetskaia N, Thorn C, Stocco G, Hebert JM, et al. Thiopurine pathway. Pharmacogenet Genomics 2010;20(9):573–574.
[18] FDA guidance: Physiologically Based Pharmacokinetic Analyses—Format and Content Guidance for Industry September 2018 (Internet site: https://www.fda.gov/media/101469/download)
[19] Roberts RL, Gearry RB, Barclay ML, Kennedy MA. IMPDH1 promoter mutations in a patient exhibiting azathioprine resistance. Pharmacogenomics J 2007;7(5):312–317.
[20] Murugesan R, Vahab SA, Patra S, et al. Thiopurine S-methyltransferase alleles, TPMT(*)2, (*)3B and (*)3C, and genotype frequencies in an Indian population. Exp Ther Med 2010;1(1):121–127.
[21] Tamm R, Mägi R, Tremmel R, et al. Polymorphic variation in TPMT is the principal determinant of TPMT phenotype: a meta-analysis of three genome-wide association studies. Clin Pharmacol Ther 2017;101(5):684–695.
[22] Otterness D, Szumlanski C, Lennard L, Klemetsdal B, Aarbakke J, Park-Hah JO, et al. Human thiopurine methyltransferase pharmacogenetics: gene sequence polymorphisms. Clin Pharmacol Ther 1997;62(1):60–73.
[23] McLeod HL, Krynetski EY, Relling MV, Evans WE. Genetic polymorphism of thiopurine methyltransferase and its clinical relevance for childhood acute lymphoblastic leukemia. Leukemia 2000;14(4):567–572.
[24] CDER. Pediatric Subcommittee of the Oncology Drug Advisory Committee meeting transcript. Rockville, MD: FDA; 2003, (Internet atwww.fda.gov/OHRMS/DOCKETS/AC/03/transcripts/3971T1.pdf).
[25] van den Akker-van Marle ME, Gurwitz D, Detmar SB, Enzing CM, Hopkins MM, Gutierrez de Mesa E, et al. Cost-effectiveness of pharmacogenomics in clinical practice: a case study of thiopurine methyltransferase genotyping in acute lymphoblastic leukemia in Europe. Pharmacogenomics 2006;7(5):783–792.
[26] Lee SHR, Yang JJ. Pharmacogenomics in acute lymphoblastic leukemia. Best Pract Res Clin Haematol 2017;30(3):229–236.
[27] Klein TE, Chang JT, Cho MK, Easton KL, Fergerson R, Hewett M, et al. Integrating genotype and phenotype information: an overview of the PharmGKB project. Pharmacogenomics J 2001;1:167–170.
[28] de Jong FA, van der Bol JM, Mathijssen RH, van Gelder T, Wiemer EA, Sparreboom A, et al. Renal function as a predictor of irinotecan-induced neutropenia. Clin Pharmacol Ther 2008;84(2):254–262.
[29] van der Bol JM, Mathijssen RH, Loos WJ, Friberg LE, van Schaik RH, de Jonge MJ, et al. Cigarette smoking and irinotecan treatment: pharmacokinetic interaction and effects on neutropenia. J Clin Oncol 2007;25(19):2719–2726.
[30] Hanioka N, Ozawa S, Jinno H, Ando M, Saito Y, Sawada J. Human liver UDP-glucuronosyltransferase isoforms involved in the glucuronidation of 7-ethyl-10-hydroxycamptothecin. Xenobiotica 2001;31(10):687–699.
[31] Innocenti F, Undevia SD, Iyer L, Chen PX, Das S, Kocherginsky M, et al. Genetic variants in the UDP–glucuronosyltransferase 1A1 gene predict the risk of severe neutropenia of irinotecan. J Clin Oncol 2004;22(8):1382–1388.
[32] CDER. Clinical Pharmacology Subcommittee of the Advisory Committee for Pharmaceutical Science. Briefing information Gaithersburg, MD: FDA; 2004, (Internet at www.fda.gov/ohrms/dockets/ac/04/briefing/2004-4079b1.htm).
[33] Cecchin E, Innocenti F, D'Andrea M, Corona G, De Mattia E, Biason P, et al. Predictive role of the UGT1A1, UGT1A7, and UGT1A9 genetic variants and their haplotypes on the outcome of metastatic colorectal cancer patients treated with fluorouracil, leucovorin, and irinotecan. J Clin Oncol 2009;27(15):2457–2465.
[34] de Jong FA, Scott-Horton TJ, Kroetz DL, McLeod HL, Friberg LE, Mathijssen RH, et al. Irinotecan-induced diarrhea: functional significance of the polymorphic ABCC2 transporter protein. Clin Pharmacol Ther 2007;81(1):42–49.
[35] Cheng L, et al. Cancer Chemother Pharmacol 2014;73:551–560.
[36] McDonagh EM, Boukouvala S, Aklillu E, Hein DW, Altman RB, Klein TE. PharmGKB summary: very important pharmacogene information for N-acetyltransferase 2. Pharmacogenet Genomics 2014;24(8):409–425.
[37] Russell GI, Bing RF, Jones JA, Thurston H, Swales JD. Hydralazine sensitivity: clinical features, autoantibody changes and HLA-DR phenotype. Q J Med 1987;65(246):845–852.
[38] Ho RH, Leake BF, Kilkenny DM, Meyer Zu Schwabedissen HE, Glaeser H, Kroetz DL, et al. Polymorphic variants in the human bile salt export pump (BSEP; ABCB11): functional characterization and interindividual variability. Pharmacogenet Genomics 2010;20(1):45–57.
[39] Wilke RA, Lin DW, Roden DM, Watkins PB, Flockhart D, Zineh I, et al. Identifying genetic risk factors for serious adverse drug reactions: current progress and challenges. Nat Rev Drug Discov 2007;6(11):904–916.
[40] Nakamura Y. Pharmacogenomics and drug toxicity. N Engl J Med 2008;359(8):856–858.

[41] Niemi M, Pasanen MK, Neuvonen PJ. SLCO1B1 polymorphism and sex affect the pharmacokinetics of pravastatin but not fluvastatin. Clin Pharmacol Ther 2006;80(4):356–366.

[42] Ghatak A, Faheem O, Thompson PD. The genetics of statin-induced myopathy. Atherosclerosis 2010;210(2):337–343.

[43] Staffa JA, Chang J, Green L. Cerivastatin and reports of fatal rhabdomyolysis. N Engl J Med 2002;346(7):539–540.

[44] Graham DJ, Staffa JA, Shatin D, Andrade SE, Schech SD, La Grenade L, et al. Incidence of hospitalized rhabdomyolysis in patients treated with lipid-lowering drugs. JAMA 2004;292(21):2585–2590.

[45] Thompson PD, Clarkson P, Karas RH. Statin-associated myopathy. JAMA 2003;289(13):1681–1690.

[46] Yee SW, Brackman DJ, Ennis EA, et al. Influence of transporter polymorphisms on drug disposition and response: a perspective from the international transporter consortium. Clin Pharmacol Ther 2018;104(5):803–817.

[47] Ramsey LB, Johnson SG, Caudle KE, et al. The clinical pharmacogenetics implementation consortium guideline for SLCO1B1 and simvastatin-induced myopathy: 2014 update. Clin Pharmacol Ther 2014;96(4):423–428.

[48] Garzel B, Zhang L, Huang SM, Wang H. A change in bile flow: looking beyond transporter inhibition in the development of drug-induced cholestasis. Curr Drug Metab 2019;20(8):621–632.

[49] Qiu X, Zhang Y, Liu T, et al. Disruption of BSEP function in HepaRG cells alters bile acid disposition and is a susceptive factor to drug-induced Cholestatic injury. Mol Pharm 2016;13(4):1206–1216.

[50] Woodhead JL, Yang K, Siler SQ, et al. Exploring BSEP inhibition-mediated toxicity with a mechanistic model of drug-induced liver injury. Front Pharmacol 2014;5:240.

[51] Sanoh S, Tamura Y, Fujino C, et al. Changes in bile acid concentrations after Administration of Ketoconazole or rifampicin to chimeric mice with humanized liver. Biol Pharm Bull 2019;42(8):1366–1375.

[52] Kularatnam GAM, Warawitage HD, Vidanapathirana DM, et al. Correction to: Dubin-Johnson syndrome and intrahepatic cholestasis of pregnancy in a Sri Lankan family: a case report. BMC Res Notes 2017;10(1):492.

[53] Daly AK. Are polymorphisms in genes relevant to drug disposition predictors of susceptibility to drug-induced liver injury? Pharm Res 2017;34(8):1564–1569.

[54] Rodriguez-Novoa S, Labarga P, Soriano V. Pharmacogenetics of tenofovir treatment. Pharmacogenomics 2009;10(10):1675–1685.

[55] Cooper RD, Wiebe N, Smith N, Keiser P, Naicker S, Tonelli M. Systematic review and meta-analysis: renal safety of tenofovir disoproxil fumarate in HIV-infected patients. Clin Infect Dis 2010;51(5):496–505.

[56] Izzedine H, Hulot JS, Villard E, Goyenvalle C, Dominguez S, Ghosn J, et al. Association between ABCC2 gene haplotypes and tenofovir-induced proximal tubulopathy. J Infect Dis 2006;194(11):1481–1491.

[57] Klaassen CD, Aleksunes LM. Xenobiotic, bile acid, and cholesterol transporters: function and regulation. Pharmacol Rev 2010;62(1):1–96.

[58] Labarga P, Barreiro P, Martin-Carbonero L, Rodriguez-Novoa S, Solera C, Medrano J, et al. Kidney tubular abnormalities in the absence of impaired glomerular function in HIV patients treated with tenofovir. AIDS 2009;23(6):689–696.

[59] Kiser JJ, Carten ML, Aquilante CL, Anderson PL, Wolfe P, King TM, et al. The effect of lopinavir/ritonavir on the renal clearance of tenofovir in HIV-infected patients. Clin Pharmacol Ther 2008;83(2):265–272.

[60] Pushpakom SP, Liptrott NJ, Rodriguez-Novoa S, Labarga P, Soriano V, Albalater M, et al. Genetic variants of ABCC10, a novel tenofovir transporter, are associated with kidney tubular dysfunction. J Infect Dis 2011;204(1):145–153.

[61] Rodriguez-Novoa S, Labarga P, Soriano V, Egan D, Albalater M, Morello J, et al. Predictors of kidney tubular dysfunction in HIV-infected patients treated with tenofovir: a pharmacogenetic study. Clin Infect Dis 2009;48(11):e18–e116.

[62] Laechelt S, Turrini E, Ruehmkorf A, Siegmund W, Cascorbi I, Haenisch S. Impact of ABCC2 haplotypes on transcriptional and posttranscriptional gene regulation and function. Pharmacogenomics J 2011;11(1):25–34.

[63] Megaraj V, Zhao T, Paumi CM, Gerk PM, Kim RB, Vore M. Functional analysis of nonsynonymous single nucleotide polymorphisms of multidrug resistance-associated protein 2 (ABCC2). Pharmacogenet Genomics 2011;21(8):506–515.

[64] Abla N, Chinn LW, Nakamura T, Liu L, Huang CC, Johns SJ, et al. The human multidrug resistance protein 4 (MRP4, ABCC4): functional analysis of a highly polymorphic gene. J Pharmacol Exp Ther 2008;325(3):859–868.

[65] Kim RB, Leake BF, Choo EF, Dresser GK, Kubba SV, Schwarz UI, et al. Identification of functionally variant MDR1 alleles among European Americans and African Americans. Clin Pharmacol Ther 2001;70(2):189–199.

[66] Fujita T, Brown C, Carlson EJ, Taylor T, de la Cruz M, Johns SJ, et al. Functional analysis of polymorphisms in the organic anion transporter, SLC22A6 (OAT1). Pharmacogenet Genomics 2005;15(4):201–209.

[67] Kiser JJ, Aquilante CL, Anderson PL, King TM, Carten ML, Fletcher CV. Clinical and genetic determinants of intracellular tenofovir diphosphate concentrations in HIV-infected patients. J Acquir Immune Defic Syndr 2008;47(3):298–303.

[68] Zimmermann AE, Pizzoferrato T, Bedford J, Morris A, Hoffman R, Braden G. Tenofovir-associated acute and chronic kidney disease: a case of multiple drug interactions. Clin Infect Dis 2006;42(2):283–290.

[69] Chung WH, Hung SI, Hong HS, Hsih MS, Yang LC, Ho HC, et al. Medical genetics: a marker for Stevens-Johnson syndrome. Nature 2004;428:486.

[70] Hetherington S, Hughes AR, Mosteller M, Shortino D, Baker KL, Spreen W, et al. Genetic variations in HLA-B region and hypersensitivity reactions to abacavir. Lancet 2002;359(9312):1121–1122.

[71] Daly AK, Donaldson PT, Bhatnagar P, Shen Y, Pe'er I, Floratos A, et al. HLA-B*5701 genotype is a major determinant of drug-induced liver injury due to flucloxacillin. Nat Genet 2009;41:816–819.

[72] Brown MA, Crane AM, Wordsworth BP. Genetic aspects of susceptibility, severity, and clinical expression in ankylosing spondylitis. Curr Opin Rheumatol 2002;14(4):354–360.

[73] Colmegna I, Cuchacovich R, Espinoza LR. HLA-B27-associated reactive arthritis: Pathogenetic and clinical considerations. Clin Microbiol Rev 2004;17(2):348–369.

[74] Carrington M, O'Brien SJ. The influence of HLA genotype on AIDS. Annu Rev Med 2003;54:535–551.

[75] Pichler WJ, Naisbitt DJ, Park BK. Immune pathomechanism of drug hypersensitivity reactions. J Allergy Clin Immunol 2011;127(Suppl 3): S74–S81.

[76] Martin AM, Nolan D, Gaudieri S, Almeida CA, Nolan R, James I, et al. Predisposition to abacavir hypersensitivity conferred by HLA-B*5701 and a haplotypic Hsp70-hom variant. Proc Natl Acad Sci U S A 2004;101:4180–4185.

[77] Hughes AR, Mosteller M, Bansal AT, Davies K, Haneline SA, Lai EH, et al. Association of genetic variations in HLA-B region with hypersensitivity to abacavir in some, but not all, populations. Pharmacogenomics 2004;5(2):203–211.

[78] Chessman D, Kostenko L, Lethborg T, Purcell AW, Williamson NA, Chen Z, et al. Human leukocyte antigen class I-restricted activation of $CD8^+$ TCells provides the immunogenetic basis of a systemic drug hypersensitivity. Immunity 2008;28:822–832.

[79] Posadas SJ, Pichler WJ. Delayed drug hypersensitivity reactions – new concepts. Clin Exp Allergy 2007;37:989–999.

[80] Kindmark A, Jawaid A, Harbron CG, Barratt BJ, Bengtsson OF, Andersson TB, et al. Genome-wide pharmacogenetic investigation of a hepatic adverse event without clinical signs of immunopathology suggests an underlying immune pathogenesis. Pharmacogenomics J 2008;8:186–195.

[81] Sharma SK, Balamurugan A, Saha PK, Pandey RM, Mehra NK. Evaluation of clinical and immunogenetic risk factors for the development of hepatotoxicity during antituberculosis treatment. Am J Respir Crit Care Med 2002;166:916–919.

[82] Venter JC, Adams MD, Myers EW, Li PW, Mural RJ, Sutton GG, et al. The sequence of the human genome. Science 2001;291(5507):1304–1351.

[83] Lander ES, Linton LM, Birren B, Nusbaum C, Zody MC, Baldwin J, et al. Initial sequencing and analysis of the human genome. Nature 2001;409 (6822):860–921.

[84] Lesko LJ, Zineh I, Huang SM. What is clinical utility and why should we care? Clin Pharmacol Ther 2010;88(6):729–733.

[85] O'Kane D. An outsider's viewpoint: The FDA should regulate clinical pharmacogenetic/genomic tests, but. Clin Pharmacol Ther 2010;88 (6):746–748.

[86] Epstein RS. Pharmacy benefit managers: evaluating clinical utility in the real world. Clin Pharmacol Ther 2010;88(6):880–882.

[87] Woodcock J. Assessing the clinical utility of diagnostics used in drug therapy. Clin Pharmacol Ther 2010;88(6):765–773.

[88] Temple R. Enrichment of clinical study populations. Clin Pharmacol Ther 2010;88(6):774–778.

[89] Lai-Goldman M, Faruki H. Abacavir hypersensitivity: a model system for pharmacogenetic test adoption. Genet Med 2008;10(12):874–878.

[90] ZIAGEN®, n.d. Abacavir sulfate [package insert, issued 2008]. Research Triangle Park, NC: GlaxoSmithKline. Internet at, www.accessdata.fda.gov/drugsatfda_docs/label/2008/020977s019, 020978s022lbl.pdf; Accessed 15 April 2011.

[91] Mallal S, Nolan D, Witt C, Masel G, Martin AM, Moore C, et al. Association between presence of HLA-B*5701, HLA-DR7, and HLA-DQ3 and hypersensitivity to HIV-1 reverse-transcriptase inhibitor abacavir. Lancet 2002;359:727–732.

[92] Hung S, Chung W, Chen Y. HLA-B genotyping to detect carbamazepine-induced Stevens-Johnson syndrome: implications for personalizing medicine. Pers Med 2005;2(3):225–237.

[93] Epstein RS, Moyer TP, Aubert RE, Kane DJ, Xia F, et al. Warfarin genotyping reduces hospitalization rates results from the MM-WES (Medco-Mayo warfarin effectiveness study). J Am Coll Cardiol 2010;55(25):2804–2812.

[94] Relling MV, Klein TE. CPIC: clinical pharmacogenetics implementation consortium of the pharmacogenomics research network. Clin Pharmacol Ther 2011;89(3):464–467.

[95] CMS. Pharmacogenomic testing for warfarin response. Medicare Learning Network Matters 2010; Internet at www.cms.gov/MLNMattersArticles/downloads/MM6715.pdf; Accessed 15 April 2011.

[96] Ansell J, Hirsh J, Hylek E, Jacobson A, Crowther M, Palareti G, et al. Pharmacology and management of the vitamin K antagonists: American College of Chest Physicians evidence-based clinical practice guidelines (8th edition). Chest 2008;133(Suppl 6):160S–198S.

[97] CDER. Qualification process for drug development tools. Guidance for Industry. Rockville, MD: FDA; 2010, (Internet atwww.fda.gov/downloads/Drugs/GuidanceComplianceRegulatoryInformation/Guidances/UCM230597.pdf.2010).

[98] CDER, CBER, CDRH. Clinical Pharmacogenomics: Premarketing evaluation in early phase clinical studies. Guidance for Industry. Rockville, MD: FDA; 2011, (Internet atwww.fda.gov/downloads/Drugs/GuidanceComplianceRegulatoryInformation/Guidances/UCM243702.pdf, cited April 15, 2011).

[99] European Medicines Agency (EMA). Guideline on the use of pharmacogenetic methodologies in the pharmacokinetic evaluation of medicinal products. London: EMA; 2010, (Internet atwww.ema.europa.eu/docs/en_GB/document_library/Scientific_guideline/2010/05/WC500090323.pdf.).

[100] Rowland M, Peck C, Tucker G. Physiologically-based pharmacokinetics in drug development and regulatory science. Annu Rev Pharmacol Toxicol 2011;51:45–73.

[101] Zhao P, Zhang L, Lesko L, Huang SM. Evaluating complex drug–drug interactions using modeling and simulations: application and challenges in regulatory review. In: Presentation at the Land o' Lakes Conference on Drug Metabolism/Applied Pharmacokinetics, Merrimac, WI: September 17; 2009.

[102] Watanabe T, Kusuhara H, Maeda K, Shitara Y, Sugiyama Y. Physiologically based pharmacokinetic modeling to predict transporter-mediated clearance and distribution of pravastatin in humans. J Pharmacol Exp Ther 2009;328(2):652–662.

[103] Galetin A, Zhao P, Huang SM. Physiologically based pharmacokinetic modeling of drug transporters to facilitate individualized dose prediction. J Pharm Sci 2017;106(9):2204–2208.

[104] Guo Y, Chu X, Parrott NJ, et al. Advancing predictions of tissue and intracellular drug concentrations using in vitro, imaging and physiologically based pharmacokinetic modeling approaches. Clin Pharmacol Ther 2018;104(5):865–889.

[105] Zhao P, Zhang L, Grillo JA, Liu Q, Bullock JM, Moon YJ, et al. Applications of physiologically based pharmacokinetic (PBPK) modeling and simulation during regulatory review. Clin Pharmacol Ther 2011;89(2):259–267.
[106] Huang SM, Abernethy DR, Wang Y, Zhao P, Zineh I. The utility of modeling and simulation in drug development and regulatory review. J Pharm Sci 2013;102(9):2912–2923.
[107] Grimstein M, Yang Y, Zhang X, et al. Physiologically based pharmacokinetic modeling in regulatory science: an update from the U.S. Food and Drug Administration's Office of Clinical Pharmacology. J Pharm Sci 2019;108(1):21–25.

Chapter 17

Biomarkers in drug development

Robert N. Schuck[a], Jana G. Delfino[b], Christopher Leptak[b], and John A. Wagner[c]

[a]*Office of Clinical Pharmacology, Center for Drug Evaluation and Research, U.S. Food and Drug Administration, Silver Spring, MD, United States,* [b]*Office of New Drugs, Center for Drug Evaluation and Research, U.S. Food and Drug Administration, Silver Spring, MD, United States,* [c]*Cygnal Therapeutics, Cambridge, MA, United States*

Introduction

A *biomarker* (biological marker) is a characteristic that is objectively measured and evaluated as an indicator of normal biological processes, pathogenic processes, or pharmacologic response to a therapeutic intervention [1, 2]. In the practice of medicine, biomarkers are commonly used to aid in diagnosis, monitor disease status, assess the effectiveness and safety of a therapeutic intervention, and provide information about a patient's prognosis or risk of developing a disease. In drug development, biomarkers have many additional uses, such as providing information on target engagement and efficacy, as well as drug safety.

Biomarkers have been historically used as an integral component of both medicine and drug development. Arguably, biomarker use and the practice of medicine—as well as drug development—go hand-in-hand. The practice of medicine and treatment of patients have been enabled by biomarker discovery and development, from the invention of the thermometer allowing more precise understanding of fever to next generation DNA sequencing (NGS) driving precision definition of cancers and other diseases. In drug development, use of biomarkers increases the probability of success of therapeutic programs [3]. In addition, use of clinically validated surrogate endpoints—biomarkers that are used in clinical trials as a substitute for a direct measure of how a patient feels, functions, or survives—has been shown to enable effective development and more rapid availability of new therapies [4].

Despite the obvious utility of biomarkers, there are a number of pitfalls to their use in drug development. For instance, there may not be enough evidence to clinically validate a biomarker or new evidence may arise questioning its clinical validation. This was most dramatically illustrated by the Cardiac Arrhythmia Suppression Trial (CAST), in which therapy with antiarrhythmic drugs was demonstrated to increase mortality risk despite suppression of ventricular ectopy [5]. The completely unexpected results of this study led to an outpouring of negative commentary regarding the reliability of biomarker responses—particularly when used as the basis for new drug approval—that obscured their actual utility for a time [6]. To help overcome this roadblock, the U.S. Food and Drug Administration (FDA) and National Institutes of Health (NIH) Biomarkers Definitions Working Group adopted the broad definition of a *surrogate endpoint* as "a biomarker that is intended to substitute for a clinical endpoint and is expected to predict clinical benefit (or harm or lack of benefit or harm) based on epidemiologic, therapeutic, pathophysiologic, or other scientific evidence"; this, and other efforts, helped accelerated biomarker discovery, development, and utilization to the rapid pace seen today [1]. In addition to issues with clinical validation of surrogate endpoints, there are a number of other pitfalls of biomarker use that should be avoided, including not adjusting for multiplicity and failure to predefine acceptance criteria for biomarker data.

When biomarkers are appropriately clinically validated, one of their most beneficial uses in drug development is as surrogate endpoints, substituting for clinical endpoints in regulatory approval of new therapeutics. From a historical perspective, the acquired immunodeficiency syndrome (AIDS) epidemic was likely the single biggest factor increasing interest and use of biomarkers as surrogate endpoints to accelerate the evaluation and approval of antiretroviral drugs. Although a number of potentially useful biomarkers were considered, only suppression in the level of human immunodeficiency virus (HIV) RNA emerged as sufficiently reliable to serve as the basis for accelerated antiretroviral drug approval [7]. In addition, the success of combination antiretroviral therapy made it increasingly impractical to require traditional clinical criteria for the approval of new antiretroviral drugs. As a result, the FDA, after deliberation with academic and industry colleagues, issued guidance for using plasma HIV RNA measurements for antiretroviral drug approval [8].

Recognizing both the potential benefits and pitfalls of biomarker use in drug development, the FDA proactively highlighted the role of appropriate biomarker use in drug development more than 15 years ago in the 2004 white paper

Atkinson's Principles of Clinical Pharmacology. https://doi.org/10.1016/B978-0-12-819869-8.00029-X

"Innovation or Stagnation: Challenge and Opportunity on the Critical Path to New Medical Products" [9]. As detailed in the white paper, effective drug development relies on the considered use of a reliable toolkit of scientific and technical methods, including biomarkers for prediction of safety and effectiveness. In addition, a formal process, designated the Biomarker Qualification Program (see "FDA/CDER Biomarker Qualification Program" section), was implemented, which allows individuals and groups developing biomarkers to interact with the FDA in both initial consultative and advisory stages as well as a subsequent review stage. This initiative launched a broad effort to form public-private partnerships, working precompetitively to develop evidence supporting use of biomarkers and other drug development tools for medical product development. As a result of these efforts, coupled with scientific and technological advancements in biomarker discovery and development, biomarkers now have a crucial role in drug development and medical practice, and have played a foundational role in medical advancements such as precision medicine.

Definitions and concepts

Definitions

Biomarkers have been an integral component of medicine and drug development for many years; however, consensus definitions were established only recently. Efforts to reduce ambiguity and harmonize terminology related to biomarkers began with an expert working group convened by the National Institutes of Health to develop preferred definitions for biomarkers and a conceptual framework for use of biomarkers as surrogate endpoints in clinical trials more than 20 years ago [1]. More recently, the FDA-NIH Joint Leadership Council identified the harmonization of terms used in translational science and medical product development as a priority need and developed the Biomarkers EndpointS and other Tools (BEST) Resource, which further develops terminology related to biomarkers [2]. BEST is a glossary that clarifies important definitions and describes hierarchical relationships, connections, and dependencies among terms (Table 17.1). It is intended to be a "living" resource that is updated periodically with new terms and clarifying information based on input from stakeholders.

Biomarker modalities

Among the most common biomarkers used in medicine and drug development are physiologic measures and biochemical analytes measured in blood. Blood pressure, for example, is a physiologic biomarker that is used clinically to diagnose and monitor hypertension, and also has multiple uses in drug development including as a clinical trial endpoint to demonstrate efficacy for hypertension treatments and as a safety biomarker for all drug classes. Biochemical analytes include white blood cell counts, which are measured to diagnose and monitor infections; blood glucose concentrations and hemoglobin A1c (HbA1c), which are quantified to diagnose and monitor type 1 and type 2 diabetes; and alanine aminotransferase (ALT) and aspartate aminotransferase (AST), which are biomarkers of liver damage that are used to diagnose and monitor liver diseases and are also used as safety biomarkers to monitor drug-induced liver injury. Physiologic measures and blood analytes are commonly used in medicine and drug development because they provide valuable information about the patient's status for many conditions and can usually be easily obtained in the clinical setting with low risk of harm to the patient.

While many well-known biomarkers are physiologic measures or blood analytes, there are many other types of biomarkers that also have important uses in medicine and drug development. Biomarkers may be measured in other biological matrices such as urine (e.g., urine protein), feces (e.g., fecal calprotectin), and sweat (e.g., sweat chloride), or may be measured within the organ or tissue of interest by obtaining a sample via a biopsy procedure (e.g., hepatic biopsy). Biomarkers measured in tissue or organ samples may provide more direct information about disease status compared to other types of samples because they are more proximal to the physiologic process of interest; however, depending on the organ being biopsied, the biopsy procedure may be complex and may pose risk to the patient. Therefore biopsy samples are typically collected only when the test is expected to provide information that cannot be obtained by other tests, and the samples are typically collected less frequently (e.g., at baseline and at the end of a clinical study rather than at every study visit).

Imaging biomarkers are integral in diagnosing and monitoring many diseases and are also frequently used in drug development (see Chapter 18). In cancer, the Response Evaluation Criteria in Solid Tumors (RECIST) is a set of rules developed by an international working group to assess the change in tumor burden in clinical trials of cancer therapeutics [10]. The images required to assess a tumor using RECIST criteria may be obtained using X-ray, computerized tomography (CT) scan, magnetic resonance imaging (MRI), and other technologies. The RECIST criteria provide standardized instructions on how to measure tumor lesions and lymph nodes and assess patient response. Imaging biomarkers are obtained using

TABLE 17.1 BEST biomarker categories and definitions.

Term	Definition
Biomarker	A defined characteristic that is measured as an indicator of normal biological processes, pathogenic processes, or responses to an exposure or intervention, including therapeutic interventions. Molecular, histologic, radiographic, or physiologic characteristics are types of biomarkers. A biomarker is not an assessment of how an individual feels, functions, or survives
Diagnostic biomarker	A biomarker used to detect or confirm presence of a disease or condition of interest or to identify individuals with a subtype of the disease
Monitoring biomarker	A biomarker measured serially for assessing status of a disease or medical condition or for evidence of exposure to (or effect of) a medical product or an environmental agent
Pharmacodynamic/response biomarker	A biomarker used to show that a biological response has occurred in an individual who has been exposed to a medical product or an environmental agent
Predictive biomarker	A biomarker used to identify individuals who are more likely than similar individuals without the biomarker to experience a favorable or unfavorable effect from exposure to a medical product or an environmental agent
Prognostic biomarker	A biomarker used to identify likelihood of a clinical event, disease recurrence or progression in patients who have the disease or medical condition of interest
Reasonably likely surrogate endpoint	An endpoint supported by strong mechanistic and/or epidemiologic rationale such that an effect on the surrogate endpoint is expected to be correlated with an endpoint intended to assess clinical benefit in clinical trials, but without sufficient clinical data to show that it is a validated surrogate endpoint
Safety biomarker	A biomarker measured before or after an exposure to a medical product or an environmental agent to indicate the likelihood, presence, or extent of toxicity as an adverse effect
Surrogate endpoint	An endpoint that is used in clinical trials as a substitute for a direct measure of how a patient feels, functions, or survives. A surrogate endpoint does not measure the clinical benefit of primary interest in and of itself, but rather is expected to predict that clinical benefit or harm based on epidemiologic, therapeutic, pathophysiologic, or other scientific evidence
Susceptibility/risk biomarker	A biomarker that indicates the potential for developing a disease or medical condition in an individual who does not currently have clinically apparent disease or the medical condition
Validated surrogate endpoint	An endpoint supported by a clear mechanistic rationale and clinical data providing strong evidence that an effect on the surrogate endpoint predicts a specific clinical benefit

noninvasive procedures and provide quantifiable information that can be used to guide patient care or assess patient response to a therapeutic intervention. However, use of imaging biomarkers is often limited because the test is time consuming, imaging technologies are often expensive, and quantification often depends on subjective interpretation by a human operator, which can lead to interoperator variability. Newer approaches including machine learning image analyses are being developed.

Discovery and validation

Biomarker discovery is generally divided into two approaches. In one approach, the mechanism of a disease or drug action is elucidated, and biomarkers to assess the drug or disease are proposed based on that mechanism. For example, dipeptidyl peptidase-4 (DPP-4) inhibitors are a class of oral antihyperglycemic agents for treatment of patients with type 2 diabetes, for which the mechanism of action involves incretin hormones such as glucagon-like peptide-1 (GLP-1) related to regulation of blood glucose levels. In this approach biomarker discovery moves hand-in-hand with drug discovery. Another approach begins with hypothesis-free quantification and screening of a large number of candidate analytes in samples from human or animal studies, and assessing the association between the candidate biomarkers and a biological process, disease state, response to a drug, or other phenotype of interest [11]. For instance, a microarray technique was used to assess expression of approximately 25,000 genes in breast cancer tissue to develop a 70 gene signature that provides prognostic information on breast cancer patients. [12, 13] In this approach, a large number of potential biomarkers are screened without considering prior knowledge of how they are related to the phenotype. Because of the large number of candidate biomarkers screened, appropriate statistical methods and replication of findings are important when using this approach.

When promising biomarker candidates are identified, additional biomarker development studies are conducted to begin the process of biomarker validation. Validation is the process to establish that the performance of a test, tool, or instrument is acceptable for its intended purpose, and includes both analytical and clinical validation [2]. Analytical validation is the process that assesses the acceptability of the test in terms of its ability to measure the analyte(s) it claims to measure, and clinical validation is the evidentiary process that establishes that the test acceptably identifies, measures, or predicts the clinical phenotype of interest [2]. Additional studies may also be necessary to optimize the performance of the test (e.g., refine cutoffs for a continuous biomarker or number of inputs for a multiplex test). For biomarkers that show promise for a specific context of use in drug development, biomarker developers may also begin the process of having the biomarker formally accepted for use as a drug development tool by the FDA through the Center for Drug Evaluation and Research (CDER) Biomarker Qualification Program, and similar programs at other global regulatory agencies. It should be noted that during biomarker development the processes of analytical validation, clinical validation, and qualification do not need to take place sequentially or independently; there is significant interplay between these processes (Fig. 17.1).

Analytical method validation

Analytical validity depends on important assay characteristics such as accuracy, precision, sensitivity, specificity, and reproducibility [11]. Validated analytical methods for the quantitative evaluation of biomarkers in a given biological matrix (e.g., blood, plasma, serum, or urine) are critical for the successful conduct of nonclinical and clinical studies that rely on biomarkers to make decisions about the efficacy or safety of a therapeutic intervention [14].

Analytical method validation of biomarkers is challenging for a number of reasons. First, results from biomarker assays will only be valid if sample integrity is maintained from sample collection through analysis [15]. As such, it is important to understand the impact of preanalytical factors such as sample collection and handling, and the analyte's short-term and long-term stability [15]. Furthermore, biomarkers present unique challenges in analytical validation because they are endogenous analytes, and thus there is inherent biological variability that is not always fully understood (e.g., diurnal variation, changes induced by therapy, differences between healthy individuals and the patient population of interest) [16]. Because of the complexity of analytical method validation for biomarkers, a fit-for-purpose approach to address the extent to which a biomarker assay should be validated has been proposed [15]. Using this approach, the intended purpose for which the data are being generated guides the extent of validation that is necessary. Assays that quantify biomarkers used for less critical decisions (e.g., a pharmacodynamic biomarker used in nonclinical models) undergo less rigorous analytical validation than biomarkers used for more critical decisions (e.g., a surrogate endpoint used to support drug approval). The same biomarker may need to undergo iteratively more rigorous analytical validation as it progresses through drug development or is used for more critical decisions. The FDA recommends that when biomarker data will be used to support regulatory decision-making, such as the pivotal determination of safety and/or effectiveness or to support dosing instructions in product labeling, the assay should be fully validated, whereas for assays intended to support early drug development

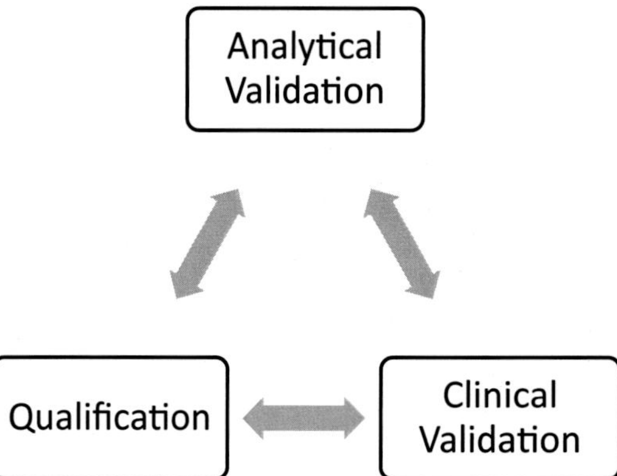

FIG. 17.1 Biomarker development. The biomarker development processes of analytical validation, clinical validation, and qualification do not necessarily need to take place sequentially or independently; there is significant interplay between these processes. In general, biomarkers used for internal decision-making early in the development process need lesser degrees of validation than those used for regulatory purposes, and no biomarker requires formal qualification through the CDER Biomarker Qualification Program to be used in a specific drug development program.

BOX 17.1 Key considerations for analytical method validation

- Does the method measure the intended analyte?
  - Does anything interfere with the measurement?
  - Is the method specific or selective for the analyte?
- What is the variability associated with these measurements?
  - What are the accuracy and precision of the method?
- What is the range in measurements that provide reliable data?
  - What is the sensitivity of the method (e.g., what is the lower limit of quantitation (LLOQ) of the method)?
  - What is the upper limit of quantitation the method (ULOQ)?)
- How do sample collection, handling, and storage affect the reliability of the data from the bioanalytical method?
  - What steps need to be followed while collecting samples?
  - Do the samples need to be frozen during shipping?
  - What temperatures are required to store the samples?
  - How long can the samples be stored?

Key considerations for analytical method validation for biomarker assays

- What are the physiochemical properties of the biomarker (e.g., isoforms and protein families)?
- How much precision, sensitivity, range, and stability are needed?
- How large of a difference is there between the healthy and patient values?
- What is the range of intra- and interpatient variability?
- What are the expected changes with therapy?

(Based on Arnold ME, Booth B, King L, Ray C. Workshop report: crystal city VI-bioanalytical method validation for biomarkers. AAPS J 2016;18:1366–1372; U. S. Food and Drug Administration. Guidance for industry and FDA staff—biomarker qualification: evidentiary framework. Accessed from: https://www.fda.gov/media/122319/download.)

the drug developer should validate the method to the extent they deem appropriate [14]. Some key questions to consider for bioanalytical method validation of a biomarker are provided in Box 17.1.

Clinical validation

Clinical validation of a biomarker is the evidentiary and statistical process of linking a biomarker to biologic and/or clinical endpoints [15]. Often, the novel biomarker is compared to a "gold standard" biomarker or diagnostic test to assess its sensitivity and specificity for its intended use; however, there may not be a well-accepted gold standard to compare the novel biomarker to, and many gold standard tests have their own limitations. As such, the process for clinical validation is dependent on the intended use of the biomarker. Similar to the fit-for-purpose approach for analytical validation of a biomarker, a novel biomarker intended for less critical purposes in drug development, such as to aid in prognostic enrichment of a clinical trial, may require different methods and less extensive clinical validation than a biomarker that is used for more critical purposes, such as a surrogate endpoint in a clinical trial. Again, the same biomarker may need to undergo iteratively more rigorous clinical validation as it progresses through drug development or is used for more critical decisions.

Clinical validation of biomarkers may take into consideration the biological plausibility of the relationship between the biomarker and the outcome of interest (e.g., based on known biology and experimental models), as well as the body of clinical evidence supporting the specific association. The clinical evidence supporting clinical validation of a biomarker may come from a number of different sources, including case reports, observational registry information, retrospective clinical studies, and prospective randomized controlled clinical trials. Similar to evidence to support the safety and efficacy of a therapeutic intervention, the strongest level of evidence to support the association of a biomarker with an outcome of interest comes from prospective studies that are specifically designed and powered to assess the association [17]. However, data supporting the clinical validation of biomarkers is often obtained from studies that were designed for other purposes, such as clinical trials of therapeutic products or observational studies. The paucity of well-designed studies intended to clinically validate biomarkers has resulted in lack of a strong evidentiary base for many biomarkers and a historical hesitancy of regulators to accept use of novel biomarkers in clinical trials. However, more recently the FDA has sought to facilitate the process of biomarker development through programs such as the CDER Biomarker Qualification Program (see "FDA/CDER Biomarker Qualification Program" section) [18].

Biomarkers in drug development

Biomarkers play a critical role in all phases of drug development (Fig. 17.2). In general, biomarkers are utilized throughout drug development to provide information about safety and efficacy of a compound being evaluated as a new therapy. Drug discovery and development is commonly schematized as a "pipeline" or "chevron" diagram as in Fig. 17.2. In reality this conception is a useful oversimplification; this is particularly true for biomarker discovery and development, which can iteratively occur across the usual depiction of the development pipeline and medical practice [19].

The biomarker categories defined by the BEST glossary are overlapping and not mutually exclusive, and all types of biomarkers are utilized for various purposes in drug development. Monitoring biomarkers are frequently used as pharmacodynamic biomarkers or safety biomarkers in drug development. Depending on the information desired, one type of biomarker may be more useful for certain assessments than other types of biomarkers. For example, in early clinical studies where one important goal of a biomarker assessment is to demonstrate target engagement, a biomarker that occurs early in the pathophysiologic cascade and closer in proximity to the drug's site of action may be ideal; these biomarkers are often referred to as target engagement or proximal biomarkers [20]. In contrast, in mid-stage or later phase clinical studies, where the goal is to generate evidence of efficacy or determine the dose (or dose range) to be assessed in confirmatory efficacy studies, a biomarker that occurs later in the physiologic pathway may be appropriate; these biomarkers are often referred to as disease-related or distal biomarkers (Fig. 17.3) [20]. In some cases, a biomarker may be utilized as a surrogate endpoint; in these cases, the drug's approval is based on its impact on a biomarker rather than a direct assessment of how a patient feels, functions, or survives. The utility of some of the most common types of biomarkers used in drug development is discussed in the following sections.

Pharmacodynamic biomarkers

A pharmacodynamic biomarker (pharmacodynamic/response biomarker in BEST) is defined as a biomarker used to show that a biological response has occurred in an individual who has been exposed to a medical product or an environmental agent. Pharmacodynamic biomarkers are used throughout all phases of drug development, from nonclinical studies through late phase clinical trials and beyond. Biomarker assessments can be used in conjunction with data from other studies such as transgenic or knockout mouse models and pharmacological challenge models (e.g., euglycemic clamp) to help understand mechanism or the effects of pharmacological modulation of the drug target. Although not defined in BEST, there are generally three types of pharmacodynamic biomarkers: target engagement biomarkers, pathway modulation or "intermediate" biomarkers, and disease-related biomarkers (Table 17.2). In early nonclinical studies, pharmacodynamic biomarkers may be used to generate preliminary efficacy information, such as pharmacodynamic effects related to target engagement. As the drug development program progresses into first-in-human and other early phase 1 studies, pharmacodynamic biomarkers are used to assess target engagement, to begin characterization of the pharmacokinetic/pharmacodynamic relationship, and to identify a range of doses to evaluate more thoroughly in larger phase 2 studies. Since phase 2 studies are designed to establish proof-of-concept and make decisions as to whether or not larger phase 3 clinical trials are warranted, these studies often evaluate pathway modulation or disease-related pharmacodynamic biomarkers that are more closely related to the clinical outcome of interest. To illustrate, early clinical studies of an antihyperglycemic agent

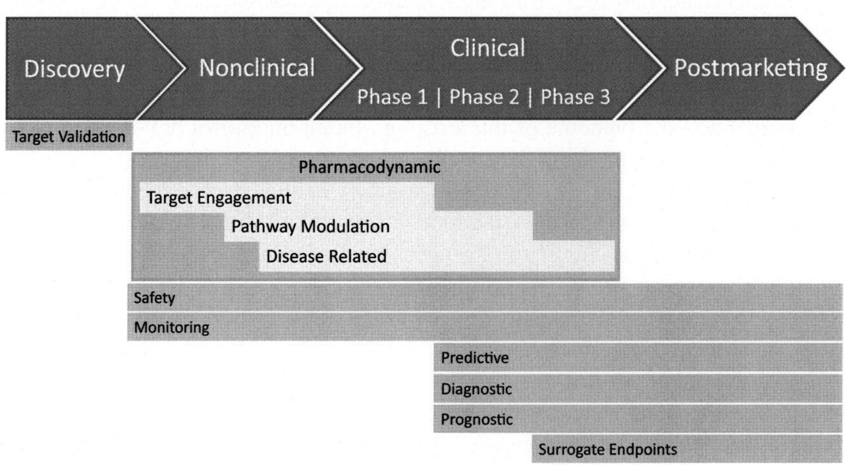

FIG. 17.2 Biomarkers in drug discovery and development. The purpose of biomarkers and the types of biomarkers used often change as drug development progresses from discovery through nonclinical and clinical trials and postmarketing studies. Some biomarkers such as target validation biomarkers are typically used in earlier phases, while others such as predictive biomarkers and surrogate endpoints are used in later phases. Pharmacodynamic biomarkers can be categorized as target engagement, pathway modulation, and disease related; these different types of pharmacodynamic biomarkers are important for assessing different aspects of drug response as drug development progresses.

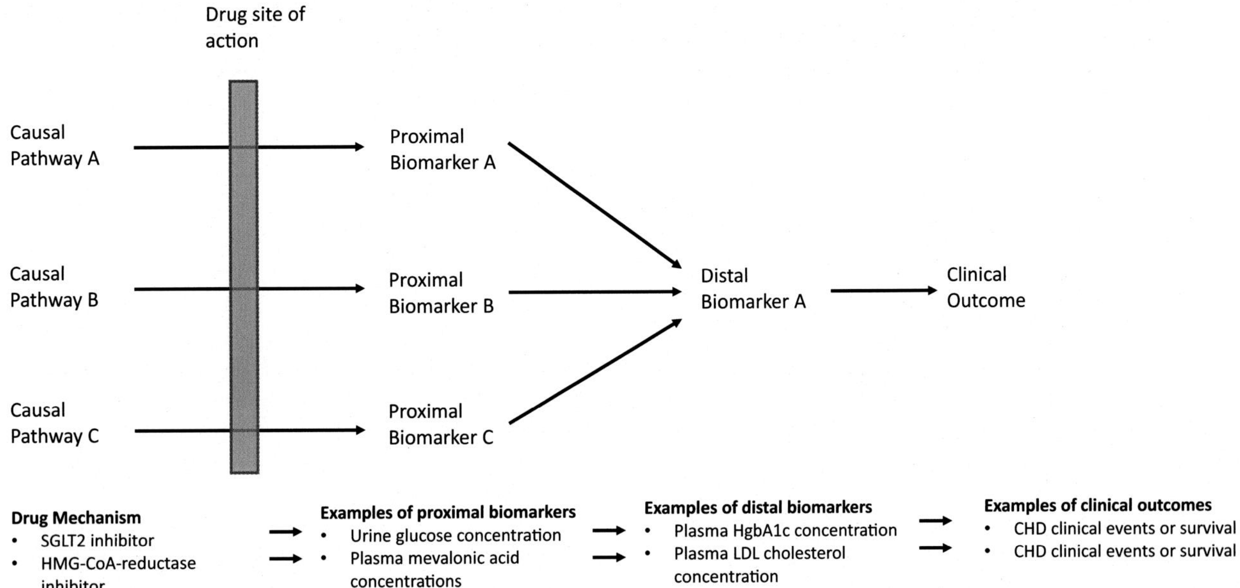

FIG. 17.3 Proximal and distal biomarkers. There may be multiple biomarkers along a causal pathway of disease. Proximal biomarkers are earlier in the pathway and are proximal to the drug site of action, making them useful as pharmacodynamic biomarkers of drug activity, but less likely to be useful as surrogate endpoints. Distal or disease-related biomarkers are later in the causal pathway, making them more likely to be correlated with clinical outcomes, and thus potential surrogate endpoints, but less useful as a biomarker of drug activity because factors other than activity of the drug are likely to impact biomarkers later in the pathway.

TABLE 17.2 Pharmacodynamic biomarker types.

Term	Definition
Target engagement	A pharmacodynamic biomarker that occurs early in the pathophysiologic cascade and proximal to the mechanism of action is known as target engagement or proximal biomarker. Target engagement biomarkers inform on physical or biological interactions with the molecular target of the drug, and estimate how "hard" the drug is "hitting" the target
Pathway modulation (intermediate)	A pharmacodynamic biomarker that occurs in the middle of pathophysiologic cascade is known as pathway modulation or intermediate biomarker. Pathway modulation biomarkers inform on physical or biological manifestations of activating (or antagonizing) the molecular pathway targeted by the drug. A change in a pathway modulation biomarker is thought to be meaningful within the context of the disease, but not necessarily expected to predict clinical benefit
Disease related	A pharmacodynamic biomarker that occurs late in the pathophysiologic cascade is known as disease-related or distal biomarker. Clinically validated disease-related biomarkers are intended to predict clinical benefit

may utilize proximal biomarkers of target engagement, such as inhibition of plasma DPP-4 activity using an ex vivo assay assessing DPP-4 inhibition, proof-of-concept studies may use pathway modulation and disease-related biomarkers such as GLP-1 modulation and glucose excursion after a glucose load, respectively, and phase 3 clinical trials may use HbA1c percentage as a surrogate endpoint [20].

Safety biomarkers

A safety biomarker is measured before or after an exposure to a medical product or an environmental agent to indicate the likelihood, presence, or extent of toxicity as an adverse effect. Some drug-related adverse events are rare; therefore, extensive safety assessments are taken throughout all phases of drug development from nonclinical studies through postmarketing studies, and biomarkers are a key component of these safety assessments. In nonclinical toxicology studies, biomarkers are used to gain insight into the drug's potential for hepatotoxicity, nephrotoxicity, phospholipidosis, cardiotoxicity, gonadotoxicity, and other potential safety issues [21]. Findings from these studies are subsequently used to inform potential adverse events that may occur in humans, and implement appropriate measures to avoid harm to patients and monitor for potential toxicity. For example, safety biomarker panels can be used in drug development programs, and range from the traditional use of ALT and AST as safety biomarkers to monitor drug-induced liver injury, to more recently identified kidney tubular injury biomarkers in phase 1 trials in healthy volunteers, which have been qualified through CDER's Biomarker Qualification program for this Context of sUe (Table 17.3) [22]. Safety biomarkers continue to be assessed throughout all phases of drug development to allow a thorough evaluation of a drug's safety profile prior to marketing.

Predictive biomarkers

Predictive biomarkers are used to identify individuals who are more likely than similar individuals without the biomarker to experience a favorable or unfavorable effect from exposure to a medical product or an environmental agent. Predictive biomarkers are used in some drug development programs for predictive enrichment strategies, which may include choosing patients who are more likely to respond to the drug treatment than other patients with the condition being treated, thus resulting in a larger effect size (both absolute and relative), and can permit use of a smaller study population [23]. In some cases, predictive biomarkers and/or predictive enrichment strategies may be used to develop targeted therapies, which are drugs that, based on their mechanism of action, are designed to target subsets of patients with specific molecular alterations among the larger population of patients with a clinically defined disease [24]. An example being nonsmall cell lung cancer (NSCLC) patients, who have certain somatic mutations in the epidermal growth factor receptor (*EGFR*) gene are likely to respond to EGFR tyrosine kinase inhibitors, but patients without these "sensitizing" mutations do not respond to this drug class. Therefore EGFR tyrosine kinase inhibitors are approved as targeted therapies for NSCLC patients who have sensitizing *EGFR* mutations, and these *EGFR* mutations are considered a predictive biomarker of EGFR tyrosine kinase inhibitor response [25].

TABLE 17.3 Select examples of biomarkers used as surrogate endpoints for drug approval or licensure.

Biomarker	Type of biomarker	Applicable drug mechanism(s)	Disease or use	Type of approval
Blood pressure	Physiologic	Alpha and beta adrenergic agonist; vasopressin analog	Distributive shock	Traditional
Blood pressure	Physiologic	Multiple antihypertensive agents	Hypertension	Traditional
Durable objective overall response rate (ORR)	Imaging	Mechanism agnostic[a]	Cancer (multiple solid tumor types)	Accelerated or traditional[b]
Forced expiratory volume in 1 second (FEV1)	Physiologic	Corticosteroid; beta-2 adrenergic agonist	Asthma	Traditional
Minimal residual disease (MRD) response rate	Laboratory (bone marrow and/or blood)	Mechanism agnostic[a]	Hematological malignancies	Accelerated
Alpha-1 proteinase inhibitor	Laboratory (plasma)	Alpha-1 protease inhibitor augmentation	Alpha-1-antitrypsin deficiency	Traditional
Potassium	Laboratory (serum)	Potassium binder	Hyperkalemia	Traditional
Uric acid	Laboratory (serum)	Xanthine oxidase inhibitor; URAT1 inhibitor	Gout	Traditional
Sustained viral response (HCV-RNA)	Laboratory (plasma)	Antiviral	Hepatitis C virus	Traditional

[a]*Mechanism agnostic refers to cases where there are many mechanisms of action associated with a surrogate endpoint, so it is not directly related to a particular causal pathway.*
[b]*Endpoints based on changes in tumor burden may be used for both traditional and accelerated approval depending on context of use, including factors such as disease, effect size, effect duration, residual uncertainty, and benefits of other available therapy.*
Based on U.S. Food and Drug Administration. Table of surrogate endpoints that were the basis of drug approval or licensure; 2019. https://www.fda.gov/drugs/development-resources/table-surrogate-endpoints-were-basis-drug-approval-or-licensure [Accessed November 2019], not a comprehensive list.

Diagnostic biomarkers

A biomarker used to detect or confirm presence of a disease or condition of interest or to identify individuals with a subtype of the disease. Diagnostic biomarkers are increasingly common in drug development and used for patient segmentation in precision medicine strategies. For example, certain genetic variants in the cystic fibrosis transmembrane conductance regulator (*CFTR*) may be used as diagnostic biomarkers in clinical trials evaluating potential therapeutic interventions for cystic fibrosis, to select patients with a disease subtype that is more likely to respond to a particular treatment (i.e., as a predictive biomarker for clinical trial enrichment).

Prognostic biomarkers

Prognostic biomarkers are used to identify the likelihood of a clinical event, disease recurrence or progression in patients who have the disease or medical condition of interest. Although prognostic biomarkers are not used universally across drug development programs, they may be used in some clinical trials for prognostic enrichment. Prognostic enrichment strategies make detection of a drug effect (if one is in fact present) more likely by enrolling patients with a greater likelihood of having a disease-related endpoint event (for event-driven studies) or a substantial worsening in condition (for continuous measurement endpoints) [23].

Monitoring biomarkers

A monitoring biomarker is defined as a biomarker measured serially for assessing status of a disease or medical condition or for evidence of exposure to (or effect of) a medical product or an environmental agent. The serial nature of the measurements increases the importance of change in the biomarker value as an indicator of current or future condition, beneficial or adverse effect of a drug or other intervention, or effect of an exposure over time. The BEST monitoring biomarker category therefore includes other biomarkers defined in the glossary, when they are measured serially. In the drug development context, monitoring biomarkers are usually used as pharmacodynamic or safety biomarkers to gain insight into a drug's potential efficacy and toxicity.

Surrogate endpoints

From a regulatory standpoint, surrogate endpoints and potential surrogate endpoints are biomarkers characterized by the level of clinical validation they have undergone (Table 17.4). A validated surrogate endpoint is an endpoint supported by a clear mechanistic rationale and clinical data providing strong evidence that an effect on the surrogate endpoint predicts a specific clinical benefit. A reasonably likely surrogate endpoint is an endpoint supported by strong mechanistic and/or epidemiologic rationale such that an effect on the surrogate endpoint is expected to be correlated with an endpoint intended to assess clinical benefit in clinical trials, but without sufficient clinical data to show that it is a validated surrogate endpoint. A candidate surrogate endpoint has the least robust evidence associated and is generally considered an endpoint still under evaluation for its ability to predict clinical benefit.

In some cases, biomarkers may be used as surrogate endpoints for the basis for approval of a drug, rather than a direct measure of a clinical endpoint. A reasonably likely surrogate may support accelerated approval under subpart H of the Code of Federal Regulations [26]. Drugs approved under the accelerated approval pathway may be required to confirm clinical

TABLE 17.4 Types of surrogate endpoints characterized by the level of clinical validation.

Term	Definition
Candidate surrogate endpoint	An endpoint still under evaluation for its ability to predict clinical benefit
Reasonably likely surrogate endpoint	An endpoint supported by strong mechanistic and/or epidemiologic rationale such that an effect on the surrogate endpoint is expected to be correlated with an endpoint intended to assess clinical benefit in clinical trials, but without sufficient clinical data to show that it is a validated surrogate endpoint
Validated surrogate endpoint	An endpoint supported by a clear mechanistic rationale and clinical data providing strong evidence that an effect on the surrogate endpoint predicts a specific clinical benefit

benefit in postmarketing studies evaluating clinical endpoints. Alternatively, a validated surrogate endpoint can support full approval of a drug, without requirements for postmarketing studies to confirm clinical benefit. The critical role of biomarkers as surrogate endpoints is discussed in detail in the following section.

Common pitfalls of biomarkers in drug development

Despite the obvious utility of biomarkers, there are a number of pitfalls to their use in drug development. Three of the most common pitfalls for use of biomarkers in drug development are a lack of prespecified criteria for biomarker performance, selection of a biomarker lacking fit-for-purpose analytical and clinical validation for the specific decision, and false positive findings secondary to biomarker multiplicity. It is critical to prospectively determine criteria for biomarker performance. Often the performance criteria should be related to a clinically or scientifically important change. Without appropriate prespecified performance criteria, preclinical or clinical studies cannot be properly powered statistically and drug development decisions can be misinformed. Another related issue includes selection of performance criteria that are insufficient (e.g., too low) or incorrect. Selection of a biomarker lacking fit-for-purpose clinical validation for the specific decision may also misinform critical decisions. Often this issue is encountered in transitions between Phase 2 and 3, in which exciting biomarker evidence in Phase 2 is used to justify progression to Phase 3; however, the clinical link between the biomarker evidence and the registration clinical endpoint is not strong enough, leading to divergent results [27]. Finally, biomarker multiplicity, using too many biomarkers, can lead to false discovery if not adequately controlled for statistically. For example, selecting one endpoint for Phase 3 out of a number of mixed-result biomarker endpoints in Phase 1 or 2, with no definitive Phase 2 data is problematic.

Surrogate endpoints

Using surrogate endpoints in clinical trials, rather than directly assessing the clinical outcome of interest using a clinical endpoint, may be advantageous for a number of reasons. The surrogate endpoint may be measured sooner during a clinical trial than the clinical outcome, may be easier or safer to measure, or may be less expensive to measure, speeding new therapies to patients. One of the most appealing reasons for the use of surrogate endpoints is that they may be more sensitive in identifying the effect of an intervention, thus allowing a clinical trial to demonstrate drug effects faster and more efficiently, often using smaller numbers of patients, compared to clinical endpoints [28]. However, there are significant potential adverse consequences of using surrogate endpoints [6]. These include the risk of not identifying major safety issues because of the smaller clinical trials, risk of patients suffering drug-related adverse events that are not offset by clinical benefit, risk of forgoing alternative therapies that are indeed effective, and financial costs of the health care system paying for ineffective therapies.

Clinical and analytical validation of surrogate endpoints

Clinical validation of a surrogate endpoint is the evidentiary process of linking a biomarker to a clinical endpoint, which includes assessing the causal association between the biomarker and the disease process, and the accuracy and reproducibility of the biomarker in predicting the effect of a treatment on the clinical outcome [1]. Ideally, a biomarker used as a surrogate endpoint would be on the only causal pathway for the disease process and would fully capture the net effect of treatment on the clinical outcome [6, 29]. However, the pathophysiology of most diseases is highly complex with multiple causal pathways and a biomarker will rarely, if ever, capture the full net effect of a treatment on a clinical outcome (Fig. 17.4). In fact, HbA1c reduction, a well-accepted surrogate endpoint for reduction of microvascular complications associated with diabetes, is not directly in the causal pathway for the disease, but a wealth of clinical trial data has established this biomarker as a surrogate endpoint [30, 31]. Therefore establishing a biomarker as a surrogate endpoint often involves multiple types and sources of scientific and clinical evidence to convincingly demonstrate the association between the surrogate endpoint the clinical endpoint. In addition, rigorous analytical validation of the assay used to measure the surrogate endpoint in clinical trials is critical to ensure appropriate interpretation of trial results.

Clinical trial data demonstrating that an effect on a surrogate endpoint predicts the clinical outcome for several different classes of drugs generally provides the most convincing evidence of a surrogate endpoint's clinical validity [28, 32]. However, other types of evidence supporting the biological plausibility of the surrogate endpoint may also be supportive. Such evidence may include epidemiologic studies that demonstrate a consistent relationship between the surrogate endpoint and clinical endpoint, animal studies that contribute to understanding of drug mechanism or disease pathology,

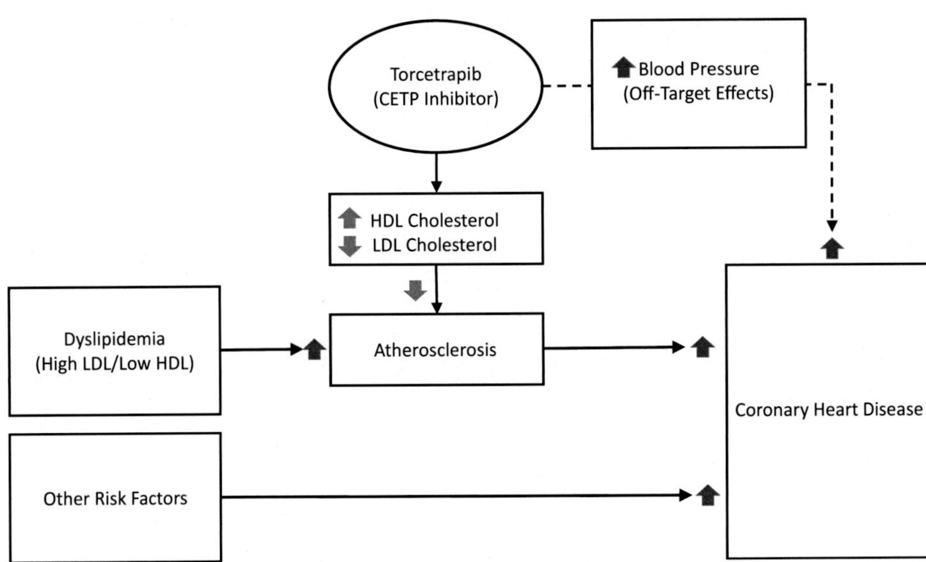

FIG. 17.4 Multiple causal pathways may influence a clinical outcome. Low HDL and high LDL cholesterol levels are associated with CHD risk; however, other factors also contribute to CHD risk. Torcetrapib is a CETP inhibitor that was hypothesized to reduce CHD risk by increasing HDL cholesterol concentrations and decreasing LDL cholesterol concentrations. However, in clinical trials torcetrapib was found to increase risk of cardiovascular events and death, likely because it had an off-target effect of increasing blood pressure, which is another causal pathway for CHD. Blue arrows indicate positive effects and red arrows represent negative effects on the disease process.

and inherent properties of the surrogate such as being late or distal on the biological pathway and closely related to the clinical outcome (disease-related biomarkers) [28].

Potential problems with the use of surrogates

Although a strong correlation may exist between a biomarker and a clinical outcome, this does not mean that the biomarker can be used as a surrogate endpoint. The effect of the intervention on the biomarker must predict the effect of the intervention on the clinical outcome, and in many circumstances a biomarker that is strongly correlated with a clinical endpoint may nevertheless fail to adequately predict the impact of an intervention on a clinical outcome [6, 32].

There are several reasons why a biomarker that is correlated with a clinical outcome may fail to predict clinical outcomes in response to an intervention (Fig. 17.5). The biomarker may not be in the causal pathway of the disease process, there may be many causal pathways while the intervention only impacts the pathway mediated through the biomarker, the intervention may have important off-target effects that are not captured by the biomarker (thus negating the positive effect mediated through the pathway captured by the biomarker), or the intervention may impact one causal pathway of the disease process while the biomarker is in another causal pathway (thus resulting in a false negative conclusion) [32]. Moreover, when the biomarker does capture effects on the principal causal pathway of the disease process, it may remain

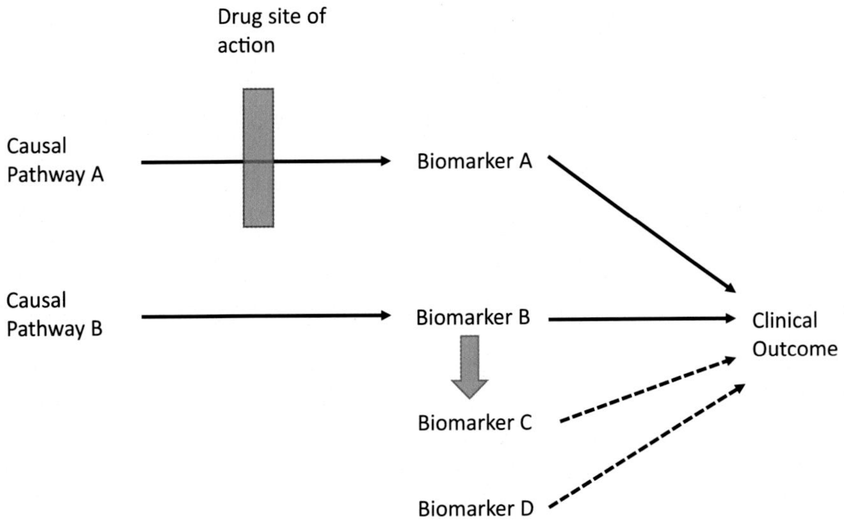

FIG. 17.5 Potential complications in use of biomarkers as surrogate endpoints. A biomarker may occur on a causal pathway of the disease where the drug exerts its effect (Biomarker A) but other causal pathways may exist that impact clinical outcomes. A biomarker may also occur on a causal pathway other than the one where the drug exerts its effect (Biomarker B), may be correlated with a biomarker on the causal pathway but not actually be on the causal pathway (Biomarker C), or may correlate with a clinical outcome but not be on the causal pathway of disease (Biomarker D). In any of these cases, the biomarker may not be a valid surrogate endpoint in spite of being correlated with the clinical outcome of interest.

unclear what magnitude and duration of effect on the biomarker is necessary to improve clinical outcomes [32]. Since there are significant potential adverse consequences of using surrogate endpoints that do not in fact predict clinical benefit, it is important to understand the potential reasons for failure of surrogate endpoints and have appropriate standards for analytical and clinical validation of surrogate endpoints before using them as substitutes for clinical endpoints.

Surrogate endpoint examples

Many biomarkers have been evaluated as potential surrogate endpoints, but relatively few are considered robust predictors of clinical outcomes such that they can be used to demonstrate efficacy of a therapeutic product for regulatory decision-making. FDA now maintains a list of surrogate endpoints that have been used to support either accelerated or traditional approval or licensure of a therapeutic product, or that could be used as surrogate endpoints to support approval or licensure (see Table 17.4) [33]. This list includes surrogate endpoints that are considered validated only for a specific mechanism of action, as well as surrogate endpoints that are considered validated irrespective of drug mechanism.

The process for regulatory acceptance of a surrogate endpoint to demonstrate efficacy of a therapeutic product requires convincing evidence of clinical validity, and the acceptance of the validity of a surrogate endpoint as a predictor of clinical outcomes may change over time. This process is exemplified by the use of low-density lipoprotein (LDL) cholesterol and high-density lipoprotein (HDL) cholesterol as surrogate endpoints for cardiovascular disease clinical outcomes.

LDL cholesterol

Atherosclerosis is the accumulation of lipids and atheromatous plaques in the arterial wall [34]. Over time, coronary heart disease (CHD) develops as fibrous plaques form in the coronary arteries; these growing plaques may cause clinical manifestations such as ischemic heart disease or may rupture and cause formation of a thrombus resulting in myocardial infarction or stroke. The primary event initiating atherosclerosis is accumulation of LDL cholesterol in the subendothelial matrix of arteries, and this accumulation is greater when circulating levels of LDL cholesterol are higher [35].

There is a strong mechanistic basis for the role of LDL cholesterol in atherosclerotic lesion formation. The integral role of LDL cholesterol in atherosclerosis has been demonstrated in numerous nonclinical models of disease, including apolipoprotein E (apoE) and LDL receptor knockout mouse models, and high-fat/high-cholesterol diet models, which result in high levels of LDL cholesterol and the development of atherosclerotic plaques [34, 35]. In addition, epidemiologic data from multiple studies demonstrates higher LDL correlates with occurrence of CHD clinical events [36, 37]. Genetic data in humans also support a causal relationship between LDL cholesterol and atherosclerosis. Familial hypercholesterolemia is caused by genetic variants in the LDL receptor and results in very high plasma LDL cholesterol levels [38]. Patients with homozygous familial hypercholesterolemia begin to develop atherosclerosis in childhood, with the severity related to the extent and duration of elevated LDL cholesterol levels [38]. Moreover, genetic association studies have demonstrated gain-of-function variants in proprotein convertase subtilisin/kexin type 9 (*PCSK9*) are associated with hypercholesterolemia and higher risk of CHD [37, 38]. Conversely, individuals with loss-of-function *PCSK9* variants demonstrate lower plasma LDL levels and lower risk of CHD [39]. Genetic variants in many other genes that have a relatively small impact on LDL cholesterol levels have also been associated with risk of CHD [39]. Collectively, the experimental, epidemiological, and genetic data make a convincing case for a causal relationship between LDL cholesterol and CHD clinical events.

Randomized clinical trials have demonstrated that multiple therapeutic products that lower LDL cholesterol by different physiological mechanisms also reduce the occurrence of CHD clinical events. 3-hydroxy-3-methylglutaryl coenzyme A reductase (HMG CoA reductase) inhibitors (statins) are LDL cholesterol-lowering agents, and clinical trial evidence convincingly supports the efficacy of multiple statins to improve clinical outcomes [40]. In addition, a Niemann-Pick C1-Like 1 (NPC1L1) inhibitor (ezetimibe) and PCSK9 inhibitors (evolocumab and alirocumab) represent diverse classes of LDL-lowering agents and have both been shown to improve clinical outcomes [41–43]. More recently, inclisiran was submitted for FDA review and approval based on the LDL surrogate endpoint and outcomes studies remain to be completed [44]. Moreover, older classes of LDL-lowering agents such as niacin, fibrates, and bile acid sequestrants have at least some evidence of benefit on clinical outcomes in CHD [45].

Collectively, these diverse lines of data suggest that lowering LDL cholesterol is a valid surrogate endpoint for CHD clinical events. However, there are important limitations of LDL cholesterol as a surrogate endpoint. It should be noted that LDL cholesterol does not reflect the entire disease burden of CHD; even in patients treated with highly effective LDL cholesterol-lowering agents, considerable risk of CHD clinical events remains [34]. This is anticipated, since CHD is a complex multifactorial disease, and other pathways not captured by LDL cholesterol contribute to the occurrence of CHD clinical events. Moreover, LDL cholesterol will not capture off-target effects caused by LDL-lowering agents.

For example, use of statins may be associated with new onset diabetes; however, statins were initially thought to reduce risk of diabetes, and the risk was not discovered until after several statins had been approved and used for many years [46]. Finally, LDL cholesterol may not fully capture the extent of CHD reduction, particularly across classes of LDL cholesterol-lowering agents. One example being the cholesterol ester transfer protein (CETP) inhibitor anacetrapib markedly reduced LDL cholesterol, but had only a modest impact on CHD clinical events [47]. Because of these limitations, the use of LDL cholesterol levels for regulatory approval of therapies that lower LDL cholesterol is not universally accepted.

HDL cholesterol

HDL cholesterol removes excess cholesterol from peripheral tissues and transports it to the liver for excretion, a process known as reverse cholesterol transport [34]. Since HDL cholesterol promotes cholesterol efflux, it has been hypothesized to be protective against atherosclerosis and the resulting manifestations of CHD [48]. Consistent with this hypothesis, multiple nonclinical studies demonstrate that HDL cholesterol can promote regression of atherosclerosis and numerous epidemiological studies have demonstrated a strong inverse correlation between HDL cholesterol levels and risk of CHD [48, 49]. However, human genetic studies have demonstrated that genetic variants that are associated with lower HDL cholesterol are not associated with increased risk of CHD clinical events [50]. Similarly, genetic variants that are associated with higher HDL cholesterol do not lower the risk of CHD clinical events [51]. Thus, despite the mechanistic and epidemiological evidence supporting an inverse relationship between HDL cholesterol and development of atherosclerosis, the evidence from human genetic studies suggests that HDL cholesterol levels may not be causally related to risk of CHD clinical events.

Several drugs that raise HDL cholesterol levels have been evaluated in randomized controlled clinical trials to assess their impact on CHD clinical events. Niacin (nicotinic acid) raises HDL cholesterol, and in initial clinical trials demonstrated a reduction in CHD clinical events [52]. However, niacin also lowers LDL cholesterol, making it difficult to isolate the impact of the HDL cholesterol-raising effect. Moreover, recent clinical trials of niacin have failed to demonstrate an effect on CHD clinical events, in spite of increasing HDL cholesterol [53]. Similarly, fibrates raise HDL cholesterol, but also impact triglycerides and LDL cholesterol, and have not consistently demonstrated positive effects on CHD clinical events [53]. Recently, cholesterol ester transfer protein (CETP) inhibitors have been developed; despite potent HDL cholesterol-raising effects, these agents have not consistently produced positive effects on CHD clinical events [54]. Anacetrapib modestly reduced the number of CHD clinical events; however, this agent both raises HDL cholesterol and lowers LDL cholesterol [47]. In contrast, torcetrapib caused excess deaths and CHD, which may have been caused by its off-target effect on blood pressure (Fig. 17.4) [55].

The experimental, epidemiological, genetic, and clinical trial data do not provide sufficient evidence to support a strong causal relationship between HDL cholesterol and CHD clinical events. As such, raising HDL cholesterol is not considered a valid surrogate endpoint for reducing CHD clinical events, and it is not accepted in regulatory submissions to support drug approval.

FDA/CDER biomarker qualification program

Historically, biomarkers have gained acceptance for use in drug development after evidence from scientific and medical communities led to recognition and consensus regarding the role and value of the biomarker. Biomarkers have been incorporated into many drug-specific development efforts based on data sufficient to justify use of the biomarker in specific settings. This focused development of biomarkers has demonstrated the utility of individual biomarkers in individual drug development programs but has not fostered generalized applicability of biomarkers across varied drug development programs. Until the CDER Biomarker Qualification Program was first proposed, a formal FDA regulatory process had not existed to recognize the broader utility of a biomarker independent from a specific drug development program. Similar approaches to the formal acceptance of biomarkers for use in drug development are used outside the U.S., such as the European Medicines Agency's biomarker qualification program which provides qualification opinions on biomarkers and other drug development tools [56].

Recognizing that biomarkers have the potential to advance public health by increasing the availability of more effective drugs, providing earlier access to medical therapies, and enhancing knowledge of the drug or disease process under development, CDER initially established the Biomarker Qualification Program in 2007 to provide a pathway for biomarker development outside of a specific drug development program. The goals of FDA's Biomarker Qualification program were to support outreach to stakeholders for the identification and development of new biomarkers, to provide a framework for the review of biomarkers for use in regulatory decision-making, and to publicly qualify biomarkers for specific contexts of use that address specified drug development needs. However, it is important to note that a biomarker does not need to be formally qualified to be accepted by the FDA for use within a specific drug development program or regulatory submission.

Qualification is a formal conclusion by FDA that, within a stated Context of Use (COU), the biomarker can be relied upon to have a specific interpretation and application in drug development and regulatory review. The COU is a concise description of the biomarker's specified use in drug development that includes two components: (1) the BEST biomarker category and (2) the biomarker's intended use in drug development. The drug development use may include defining inclusion/exclusion criteria, defining treatment arms, establishing a drug's proof of concept in a patient population, supporting clinical dose selection, enriching clinical trials for an event or population of interest, or evaluating treatment response, and other uses.

Qualified biomarkers are publicly available and can be used in any drug development program for their qualified COU. That is, a qualified biomarker can be included in IND, NDA, or BLA submissions without the need for FDA to reconsider and reaffirm its suitability; this holds true provided the biomarker is used within its qualified COU and no new or conflicting scientific facts have emerged since qualification.

The current FDA drug development tools qualification process

The Biomarker Qualification program was officially enacted into law as part of the 21st Century Cures Act, added to the Federal Food, Drug, and Cosmetic Act [57]. The 21st Century Cures Act outlines a formal, transparent process for the Qualification of Drug Development Tools (DDT), which may include biomarkers, clinical outcome assessments, and animal models. The legislation outlines a three-step process for formal qualification of a DDT. This three-step process consists of (1) a Letter of Intent (LOI) that provides initial information about the biomarker and drug development need; (2) a Qualification Plan (QP) that describes the detailed proposal for providing the information necessary to qualify the biomarker for the proposed COU (e.g., the study designs); and (3) a Full Qualification Package (FQP), which is a comprehensive compilation of all the evidence supporting the biomarker's proposed COU (Fig. 17.6).

Qualified biomarkers

As stated previously, qualification of a biomarker is a formal conclusion by FDA that within the stated COU, the biomarker can be relied upon to have a specific interpretation and application across development programs in drug development and regulatory review. Information about a qualified biomarker is publicly available and the biomarker may be used within its qualified COU in any applicable drug development program. The public FDA website [58] maintains a current list of qualified biomarkers. The list of qualified biomarkers at the time of printing is provided in Table 17.5.

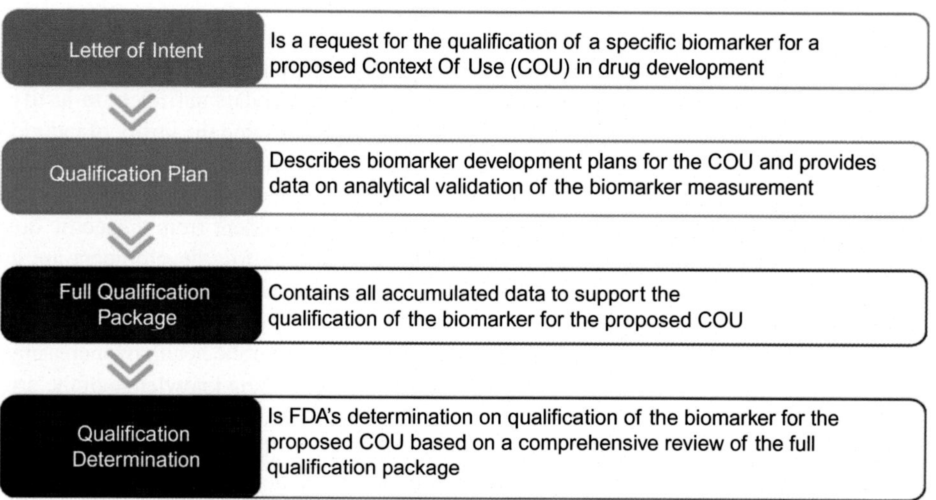

FIG. 17.6 The steps of the FDA biomarker qualification process. The Biomarker Qualification process starts with a Letter of Intent then proceeds to the Qualification Plan and the Full Qualification Package before FDA makes a qualification determination based on comprehensive review of the submission.

TABLE 17.5 Examples of qualified biomarkers.

Biomarker	Abbreviated COU[a]
Albumin, β2-microglobulin, clusterin, cystatin C, KIM-1, total protein, and trefoil factor-3	Safety biomarker to be used with traditional indicators to indicate renal injury in rat
Clusterin, renal papillary antigen (RPA-1)	Safety biomarker to be used with traditional indicators to indicate renal injury in rat
Cardiac troponins T (cTnT) and I (cTnI)	Safety biomarker to indicate cardiotoxicity in rats, dogs, or monkeys when testing known cardiotoxic drugs and may be used to help estimate nontoxic human dose
Galactomannan	Diagnostic biomarker used with other clinical and host factors to identify patients with invasive aspergillosis
Fibrinogen	Prognostic biomarker used with other characteristics to enrich for COPD exacerbations
Total kidney volume (TKV)	Prognostic biomarker with patient age and baseline glomerular filtration rate for autosomal dominant polycystic kidney disease
Clusterin (CLU), cystatin-C (CysC), Kidney injury molecule-1 (KIM-1), *N*-acetyl-beta-D-glucosaminidase (NAG), neutrophil gelatinase-associated lipocalin (NGAL), and osteopontin (OPN)	Safety biomarker panel to aid in the detection of kidney tubular injury in phase 1 trials in healthy volunteers
Plasmodium 18S rRNA/rDNA	Monitoring biomarker informs initiation of treatment with antimalarial drug following controlled human malaria infection (CHMI) with *Plasmodium falciparum* sporozoites in healthy subjects in clinical studies for vaccine and/or drug development

[a]Please refer to the FDA website (https://www.fda.gov/drugs/cder-biomarker-qualification-program/list-qualified-biomarkers) for complete information regarding the biomarker's qualified context of use (COU).

Contemporary approaches to biomarker development

Until recently, most assays used to measure candidate biomarkers for evaluation as tools in medical practice and drug development were only able to detect one or a few analytes at a time. This made screening large quantities of potential biomarkers both laborious and costly. As such, biomarker discovery and development for use in medical practice largely took place in academic labs, and the pharmaceutical industry developed fit-for-purpose biomarkers to assess individual therapeutic products during drug development. However, recent technological advancements in instrumentation, which now allows researchers to capture enormous numbers of data points, coupled with advanced computational approaches such as machine learning and artificial intelligence, have transformed biomarker development into a more high-throughput process [59]. Current approaches often use large amounts of data, collected both in academic studies and clinical trials from drug development programs, to screen and validate candidate biomarkers using a hypothesis-free approach. Advances in health care such as use of electronic health records and other technologies such as mobile devices have allowed collection of new forms of data that can be utilized in both medical practice and drug development. In addition, use of these technologies to advance our understanding of the molecular underpinnings of disease has led to the development of targeted therapies and precision medicine approaches to treatment of diseases, where biomarkers play a critical role in identifying disease subtypes that are more likely to respond to certain treatments.

Omics technologies

Current biomarker discovery and development strategies often incorporate genomic, transcriptomic, proteomic, and metabolomic technologies and data. Advancements in these "omics" sciences have made collection, processing, and analysis of large amounts of data more practical and cost effective. In the oncology setting, testing instruments are now able to use blood samples to perform liquid biopsies to help detect cancer at an early stage, identify genomic aberrations that may help guide the choice of therapy, [60] or assess minimal residual disease in order to monitor treatment response or for recurrence [61].

Moreover, the creation of biobanks, which store large numbers of biological samples (often coupled with clinical data) for research purposes, has provided researchers with vast datasets to conduct omics studies [62].

Omics data have many applications in drug development. Genomic technologies such as NGS now allow sequencing of the entire genome or exome in a short amount of time at increasingly lower costs. These technologies are rapidly advancing and new techniques such as single-cell RNA sequencing are constantly improving our ability to understand disease pathology and drug effects [63]. Genomic studies are now frequently used in drug development to inform target identification and genomic biomarkers are also incorporated into clinical trials for analysis, stratification, or enrichment [64]. Transcriptomics is the study of mRNA transcripts in a cell or tissue of interest; transcriptomic studies have been made possible by RNA microarrays and more recently transcriptome sequencing (RNA-Seq) platforms [65]. Technologies such as mass spectrometry (MS), protein arrays, and immune-based platforms have allowed for proteomics studies, which measure the expressed proteins in a system [65]. Similarly, metabolomics studies measure small molecule metabolites or chemicals, including lipids, nucleotides, dipeptides, and hormones using MS and nuclear magnetic resonance spectroscopy (NMR)-based methods [65]. Genomic, transcriptomic, metabolomic, and proteomic data are utilized in many areas of drug development, including identification and validation of drug targets, informing assay development for screening of leads, and generating potential biomarkers to inform efficacy and safety assessments [66].

Multimodal biomarkers

Omics technologies and other high-throughput assays now allow fast detection of multiple biomarkers simultaneously. Since a test for a single biomarker may not have sufficient performance characteristics (e.g., sensitivity, specificity, positive-predictive value, negative predictive value), there is now interest in developing tests that simultaneously detect multiple biomarkers and use them individually to provide distinct pieces of information about a patient (i.e., multiplex tests) or integrating the biomarkers to provide a single output (i.e., integrative tests). In fact, there are now multiplex NGS tests for tumor profiling that detect variants in hundreds of genes that are considered clinically significant or potentially clinically significant [67]. Similarly, there are many tests that integrate multiple biomarkers into a single output for purposes including cancer screening or prognostic assessments [68]. Although omics technologies are enabling, multimodal biomarkers are not a new concept in medical practice or drug development. Integrative multimodal biomarkers derive a single calculated value from a defined set of biomarkers and a known algorithm. A rudimentary example of an integrative multimodal biomarker is the HDL/LDL cholesterol ratio, a simple algorithm supported by epidemiological data [69]. Multiplex multimodal biomarkers are multiple single biomarkers used individually in a panel or for pattern recognition. A rudimentary example of a multiplex multimodal biomarker is a traditional vital sign panel used for clinical pattern recognition by clinicians. Both types have been used extensively as multimodal biomarkers in drug development and medical practice.

Electronic health records

The widespread use of electronic health records (EHR) and other technologies in the practice of medicine has resulted in new sources of data for health care research. As discussed in Chapter 36, these real-world data (RWD) sources and the translation of RWD into real-world evidence (RWE) allow insights into the patient experience that otherwise would not be apparent. Moreover, data from the EHR such as patient diagnosis codes and prescription records can be combined with other data such as genomic biomarkers for observational studies, or even collected prospectively as a component of a pragmatic clinical trial [70]. There are many potential uses of these data in drug development, including optimization of clinical trial design, assessment of rare safety events, or to provide supportive evidence of effectiveness of a therapeutic intervention [70, 71].

Digital monitoring technologies

Data can now be collected from myriad electronic devices including passive sensors (e.g., smartphones) and active sensors (e.g., wearables such as patches and ingestible sensors, or motion sensors placed in the home) [72]. These electronic devices may be used as RWD sources when worn for patient care or personal reasons. Sensors may also be integrated into clinical trials to provide more detailed data on a patient than is feasible in a typical short study visit that takes place a few times throughout the duration of a clinical trial [73]. Data collected from these devices may be processed to develop biomarkers that have many potential uses in medical practice as well as drug development, including monitoring adherence to a study drug, monitoring health status (e.g., in a Parkinson's disease trial), and detecting safety events such as a fall [74].

Precision medicine

Precision medicine is an approach to disease treatment and prevention that takes into account individual variability in genes, environment, and lifestyle for each person. Biomarkers often play a critical role in precision medicine by identifying patient subsets who are more likely to respond to a therapeutic intervention, less likely to experience an adverse event, or who require altered dosages, thus improving the probability of therapeutic success for each individual patient. Targeted therapies may offer improvements in efficacy over standard-of-care therapies, but only in a biomarker-defined subset of patients (e.g., *EGFR* mutation-positive NSCLC, as discussed previously). Similarly, a safety biomarker such as the *HLA-B*5701* allele can identify individuals with risk of serious and potentially fatal skin reactions when treated with abacavir, thus, *HLA-B*5701* screening may be used as a precision medicine strategy to improve the risk profile of abacavir. Biomarkers may also identify patients who require different dosages of therapeutic products than the general population in which the drug is used. For instance, warfarin dose requirements and bleeding risk are impacted by genetic variants in *CYP2C9* (a drug-metabolizing enzyme that contributes to warfarin metabolism) and *VKORC1* (the warfarin drug target). As such, the drug labeling for warfarin provides recommendations for starting dosages that incorporate these genetic variants. Precision medicine approaches such as these may also be incorporated prospectively into drug development programs, thus maximizing the benefit-risk profile of the drug and improving the likelihood of approval. As discussed in Chapter 12, where measuring the biomarker is essential to the safe and effective use of the drug (e.g., for identifying the population for which the drug is indicated), an in vitro companion diagnostic device is developed and authorized contemporaneously with the drug to ensure the biomarker is accurately measured prior to prescribing the drug.

Trial design and enrichment

Biomarker use has fostered novel clinical trial designs in drug development that now allow more rapid assessments of drugs in multiple patient populations. As discussed before, predictive and prognostic biomarkers are both frequently used for clinical trial enrichment and can help improve clinical trial efficiency. There are several ways to incorporate biomarkers into a clinical trial: only "biomarker-positive" patients may be enrolled in the study, patients may be stratified into biomarker-positive and biomarker-negative groups and analyzed separately, or a biomarker-based treatment strategy may be compared to a standard-of-care treatment strategy [75]. Clinical trials may also incorporate multiple biomarkers and/or multiple drugs and simultaneously assess different treatment strategies in master protocols such as basket trials, umbrella trials, and platform trial designs, which have become common in oncology clinical trials [76]. Umbrella designs screen multiple biomarkers within a single disease and match patients to a therapy they are hypothesized to respond to; in contrast, basket designs enroll patients with different tumor types who have a biomarker that is hypothesized to make them sensitive to the drug. In addition, platform trials may study multiple drugs within a disease in a perpetual manner by incorporating an adaptive element where ineffective therapies are dropped from the study and other therapies may enter. The I-SPY 2 TRIAL (Investigation of Serial Studies to Predict Your Therapeutic Response with Imaging and Molecular Analysis) was an adaptive breast cancer trial in the setting of neoadjuvant chemotherapy, which improved biomarker use for breast cancer, helped establish a new clinical endpoint (pathological complete response as a potential predictor of breast cancer survival), and to date has aided the development of multiple therapies in breast cancer [77].

Role of consortia

In recent years, the potential utility of biomarkers in drug development has been recognized by both drug developers and regulatory authorities. However, there is often a lack of robust data to support reliance on a biomarker for decisional purposes in drug development. The resources needed to develop and validate a biomarker for generalized use in drug development are often beyond the capabilities of a single entity. Therefore collaborative groups such as public-private partnerships or consortia have been formed increasingly in recent years to foster biomarker development [78, 79]. Such collaborative efforts allow multiple interested parties to pool resources and data, thus decreasing cost, expediting drug development, and facilitating regulatory review. The role of consortia and other collaborative approaches is becoming increasingly important as new technologies allow screening of large numbers of analytes and large studies are needed to adequately clinically validate candidate biomarkers. An example is the Biomarkers Consortium, which is a public-private biomedical research partnership that operates under the Foundation for the National Institutes of Health as a neutral convener. Over its history, the Biomarkers Consortium has worked with multiple diverse stakeholders to develop and clinically validate biomarkers that have facilitated many areas of drug development [80].

Summary

Biomarkers play an important role in all phases of drug development by providing information about the safety and efficacy of drug candidates. Some critical uses of biomarkers in drug development include the use of safety biomarkers for detecting adverse events in response to the drug, pharmacodynamic biomarkers for characterizing drug activity, and surrogate endpoints used in clinical trials as a substitute for a direct measure of how a patient feels, functions, or survives. While biomarkers have many uses in drug development, it is critical that they are appropriately validated for the purpose for which they are being used; biomarkers used for more critical decisions require more extensive validation than biomarkers used for less critical decisions throughout the drug development process. Recognizing the importance of biomarkers in facilitating drug development, stakeholders from academia, pharmaceutical industry, regulatory agencies, and consortia have worked together in recent years in an effort to standardize biomarker nomenclature and conduct studies to appropriately analytically and clinically validate biomarkers for use in drug development and in the practice of medicine. In the future, efforts to more rigorously evaluate biomarkers, as well as advancements in instrumentation and data analysis, will facilitate more effective use of biomarkers in drug development, ultimately improving our ability to develop safe and effective therapies for patients, and advance medical care more broadly.

References

[1] Biomarkers Definitions Working Group. Biomarkers and surrogate endpoints: preferred definitions and conceptual framework. Clin Pharmacol Ther 2001;69:89–95.

[2] FDA-NIH Biomarker Working Group. BEST (biomarkers, endpoints, and other tools) resource [internet]. Silver Spring, MD: Food and Drug Administration (US); 2016. Glossary. 2016 Jan 28 [Updated 2016 Apr 28]. Available from: https://www.ncbi.nlm.nih.gov/books/NBK338448/Co-published by National Institutes of Health (US), Bethesda (MD).

[3] Wong CH, Siah KW, Lo AW. Estimation of clinical trial success rates and related parameters. Biostatistics 2019;20:273–286.

[4] Lathia CD, Amakye D, Dai W, Girman C, Madani S, Mayne J, et al. The value, qualification, and regulatory use of surrogate end points in drug development. Clin Pharmacol Ther 2009;86:32–43.

[5] Echt DS, Liebson PR, Mitchell LB, Peters RW, Obias-Manno D, Barker AH, et al. Mortality and morbidity in patients receiving encainide, flecainide, or placebo. The cardiac arrhythmia suppression trial. N Engl J Med 1991;324:781–788.

[6] Fleming TR, DeMets DL. Surrogate end points in clinical trials: are we being misled? Ann Intern Med 1996;125:605–613.

[7] Chuang-Stein C, Demasi R. Surrogate endpoints in AIDS drug development: current status. Drug Inf J 1998;32:439–448.

[8] U.S. Food and Drug Administration. Human immunodeficiency virus-1 infection: developing antiretroviral drugs for treatment—guidance for industry. Accessed from: https://www.fda.gov/media/86284/download.

[9] U.S. Food and Drug Administration. Innovation or stagnation: challenge and opportunity on the critical path to new medical products. Washington DC. Available from: https://www.fda.gov/oc/initiatives/criticalpath/whitepaper.html; 2004.

[10] Eisenhauer EA, Therasse P, Bogaerts J, Schwartz LH, Sargent D, Ford R, et al. New response evaluation criteria in solid tumours: revised RECIST guideline (version 1.1). Eur J Cancer 2009;45:228–247.

[11] Kraus VB. Biomarkers as drug development tools: discovery, validation, qualification and use. Nat Rev Rheumatol 2018;14:354–362.

[12] van de Vijver MJ, He YD, van't Veer LJ, Dai H, AAM H, Voskuil DW, et al. A gene-expression signature as a predictor of survival in breast cancer. N Engl J Med 2002;347:1999–2009.

[13] van't Veer LJ, Dai H, van de Vijver MJ, He YD, AAM H, Mao M, et al. Gene expression profiling predicts clinical outcome of breast cancer. Nature 2002;415:530–536.

[14] U.S. Food and Drug Administration. Guidance for industry—bioanalytical method validation. Accessed from: https://www.fda.gov/media/70858/download; 2018.

[15] Lee JW, Devanarayan V, Barrett YC, Weiner R, Allinson J, Fountain S, et al. Fit-for-purpose method development and validation for successful biomarker measurement. Pharm Res 2006;23:312–328.

[16] Arnold ME, Booth B, King L, Ray C. Workshop report: crystal city VI-bioanalytical method validation for biomarkers. AAPS J 2016;18:1366–1372.

[17] U.S. Food and Drug Administration. Guidance for industry and FDA staff—biomarker qualification: evidentiary framework. Accessed from: https://www.fda.gov/media/122319/download.

[18] Woodcock J. Assessing the clinical utility of diagnostics used in drug therapy. Clin Pharmacol Ther 2010;88:765–773.

[19] Wagner JA, Dahlem AM, Hudson LD, Terry SF, Altman RB, Gilliland CT, et al. Application of a dynamic map for learning, communicating, navigating, and improving therapeutic development. Clin Transl Sci 2018;11:166–174.

[20] Wagner JA. Strategic approach to fit-for-purpose biomarkers in drug development. Annu Rev Pharmacol Toxicol 2008;48:631–651.

[21] Muller PY, Dieterle F. Tissue-specific, non-invasive toxicity biomarkers: translation from preclinical safety assessment to clinical safety monitoring. Expert Opin Drug Metab Toxicol 2009;5:1023–1038.

[22] U.S. Food and Drug Administration. Qualification decision and executive summary on qualification of biomarker: clusterin (CLU), cystatin-C (CysC), kidney injury molecule-1 (KIM-1), N-acetyl-beta-D-glucosaminidase (NAG), neutrophil gelatinase-associated lipocalin (NGAL), and osteopontin (OPN). Available from: https://www.fda.gov/media/115713/download; 2018.

[23] U.S. Food and Drug Administration. Draft guidance for industry and food and drug administration staff—enrichment strategies for clinical trials to support approval of human drugs and biological products. Accessed from: http://www.fda.gov/downloads/drugs/guidancecomplianceregulatoryinformation/guidances/ucm332181.pdf; 2012.

[24] Schuck RN, Woodcock J, Zineh I, Stein P, Jarow J, Temple R, et al. Considerations for developing targeted therapies in low-frequency molecular subsets of a disease. Clin Pharmacol Ther 2018;104:282–289.

[25] Schuck RN, Charlab R, Blumenthal GM. Leveraging genomic factors to improve benefit-risk. Clin Transl Sci 2017;10:78–83.

[26] 21 CFR, Secs. 314.500–314.560.

[27] U.S. Food and Drug Administration. 22 Case studies where phase 2 and phase 3 trials had divergent results. Available from: https://www.fda.gov/media/102332/download. Accessed December 2019.

[28] Temple R. Are surrogate markers adequate to assess cardiovascular disease drugs? JAMA 1999;282:790–795.

[29] Prentice RL. Surrogate endpoints in clinical trials: definition and operational criteria. Stat Med 1989;8:431–440.

[30] Holman RR, Paul SK, Bethel MA, Matthews DR, Neil HAW. 10-Year follow-up of intensive glucose control in type 2 diabetes. N Engl J Med 2008;359:1577–1589.

[31] Nathan DM, Cleary PA, Backlund J-YC, et al. Intensive diabetes treatment and cardiovascular disease in patients with type 1 diabetes. N Engl J Med 2005;353:2643–2653.

[32] Fleming TR, Powers JH. Biomarkers and surrogate endpoints in clinical trials. Stat Med 2012;31:2973–2984.

[33] U.S. Food and Drug Administration. Table of surrogate endpoints that were the basis of drug approval or licensure, https://www.fda.gov/drugs/development-resources/table-surrogate-endpoints-were-basis-drug-approval-or-licensure; 2019. Accessed November 2019.

[34] Libby P, Ridker PM, Hansson GK. Progress and challenges in translating the biology of atherosclerosis. Nature 2011;473:317–325.

[35] Lusis AJ. Atherosclerosis. Nature 2000;407:233–241.

[36] Prospective Studies C, Lewington S, Whitlock G, Clarke R, Sherliker P, Emberson J, et al. Blood cholesterol and vascular mortality by age, sex, and blood pressure: a meta-analysis of individual data from 61 prospective studies with 55,000 vascular deaths. Lancet 2007;370:1829–1839.

[37] Pekkanen J, Linn S, Heiss G, Suchindran CM, Leon A, Rifkind BM, et al. Ten-year mortality from cardiovascular disease in relation to cholesterol level among men with and without preexisting cardiovascular disease. N Engl J Med 1990;322:1700–1707.

[38] Rader DJ, Cohen J, Hobbs HH. Monogenic hypercholesterolemia: new insights in pathogenesis and treatment. J Clin Invest 2003;111:1795–1803.

[39] Holmes MV, Asselbergs FW, Palmer TM, Drenos F, Lanktree MB, Nelson CP, et al. Mendelian randomization of blood lipids for coronary heart disease. Eur Heart J 2015;36:539–550.

[40] Baigent C, Keech A, Kearney PM, Blackwell L, Buck G, Pollicino C, et al. Efficacy and safety of cholesterol-lowering treatment: prospective meta-analysis of data from 90,056 participants in 14 randomised trials of statins. Lancet 2005;366:1267–1278.

[41] Cannon CP, Blazing MA, Giugliano RP, McCagg A, White JA, Theroux P, et al. Ezetimibe added to statin therapy after acute coronary syndromes. N Engl J Med 2015;372:2387–2397.

[42] Sabatine MS, Giugliano RP, Wiviott SD, Raal FJ, Blom DJ, Robinson J, et al. Efficacy and safety of evolocumab in reducing lipids and cardiovascular events. N Engl J Med 2015;372:1500–1509.

[43] Schwartz GG, Steg PG, Szarek M, Bhatt DL, Bittner VA, Diaz R, et al. Alirocumab and cardiovascular outcomes after acute coronary syndrome. N Engl J Med 2018;379:2097–2107.

[44] Ray KK, Landmesser U, Leiter LA, Kallend D, Dufour R, Karakas M, et al. Inclisiran in patients at high cardiovascular risk with elevated LDL cholesterol. N Engl J Med 2017;376:1430–1440.

[45] Schuck RN, Mendys PM, Simpson RJ Jr. Beyond statins: lipid management to reduce cardiovascular risk. Pharmacotherapy 2013;33:754–764.

[46] Kamran H, Kupferstein E, Sharma N, Karam JG, Myers AK, Youssef I, et al. Statins and new-onset diabetes in cardiovascular and kidney disease cohorts: a meta-analysis. Cardiorenal Med 2018;8:105–112.

[47] Bowman L, Hopewell JC, Chen F, et al. Effects of anacetrapib in patients with atherosclerotic vascular disease. N Engl J Med 2017;377:1217–1227.

[48] Feig JE, Hewing B, Smith JD, Hazen SL, Fisher EA. High-density lipoprotein and atherosclerosis regression: Evidence from preclinical and clinical studies. Circ Res 2014;114:205–213.

[49] Gordon DJ, Rifkind BM. High-density lipoprotein—the clinical implications of recent studies. N Engl J Med 1989;321:1311–1316.

[50] Haase CL, Tybjaerg-Hansen A, Qayyum AA, Schou J, Nordestgaard BG, Frikke-Schmidt R. LCAT, HDL cholesterol and ischemic cardiovascular disease: a mendelian randomization study of HDL cholesterol in 54,500 individuals. J Clin Endocrinol Metab 2012;97:E248–E256.

[51] Voight BF, Peloso GM, Orho-Melander M, Frikke-Schmidt R, Barbalic M, Jensen MK, et al. Plasma HDL cholesterol and risk of myocardial infarction: a mendelian randomisation study. Lancet 2012;380:572–580.

[52] Bruckert E, Labreuche J, Amarenco P. Meta-analysis of the effect of nicotinic acid alone or in combination on cardiovascular events and atherosclerosis. Atherosclerosis 2010;210:353–361.

[53] Kingwell BA, Chapman MJ, Kontush A, Miller NE. Hdl-targeted therapies: progress, failures and future. Nat Rev Drug Discov 2014;13:445–464.

[54] Tall AR, Rader DJ. Trials and tribulations of CETP inhibitors. Circ Res 2018;122:106–112.

[55] Barter PJ, Caulfield M, Eriksson M. Effects of torcetrapib in patients at high risk for coronary events. J Vasc Surg 2008;47:893.

[56] Manolis E, Koch A, Deforce D, Vamvakas S. The european medicines agency experience with biomarker qualification. In: Vlahou A, Makridakis M, editors. Clinical proteomics: methods and protocols. New York, NY: Springer New York; 2015. p. 255–272.

[57] 21st Century Cures Act. Public law 114-255, section 507-qualification of drug development tools; December 2016.

[58] U.S. Food and Drug Administration. List of qualified biomarkers. Available from: https://www.fda.gov/drugs/cder-biomarker-qualification-program/list-qualified-biomarkers; 2019. Accessed December 2019.

[59] Koromina M, Pandi MT, Patrinos GP. Rethinking drug repositioning and development with artificial intelligence, machine learning, and omics. OMICS 2019;23:539–548.
[60] Lianidou E, Pantel K. Liquid biopsies. Genes Chromosom Cancer 2019;58:219–232.
[61] Berry DA, Zhou S, Higley H, Mukundan L, Fu S, Reaman GH, et al. Association of minimal residual disease with clinical outcome in pediatric and adult acute lymphoblastic leukemia: a meta-analysis. JAMA Oncol 2017;3:e170580.
[62] De Souza YG, Greenspan JS. Biobanking past, present and future: responsibilities and benefits. AIDS 2013;27:303–312.
[63] Hwang B, Lee JH, Bang D. Single-cell RNA sequencing technologies and bioinformatics pipelines. Exp Mol Med 2018;50:96.
[64] Stuart T, Butler A, Hoffman P, Hafemeister C, Papalexi E, Mauck III WM, et al. Comprehensive integration of single-cell data. Cell 2019;177:1888–1902. e21.
[65] Berg EL. Systems biology in drug discovery and development. Drug Discov Today 2014;19:113–125.
[66] Matthews H, Hanison J, Nirmalan N. "Omics"-informed drug and biomarker discovery: opportunities, challenges and future perspectives. Proteome 2016;4:28.
[67] U.S. Food and Drug Administration. CDRH's approach to tumor profiling next generation sequencing tests. Accessed from: https://www.fda.gov/media/109050/download.
[68] Beaver JA, Tzou A, Blumenthal GM, McKee AE, Kim G, Pazdur R, et al. An fda perspective on the regulatory implications of complex signatures to predict response to targeted therapies. Clin Cancer Res 2017;23:1368–1372.
[69] Kannel WB, Castelli WP, Gordon T. Cholesterol in the prediction of atherosclerotic disease. new perspectives based on the Framingham study. Ann Intern Med 1979;90:85–91.
[70] Miksad RA, Abernethy AP. Harnessing the power of real-world evidence (RWE): a checklist to ensure regulatory-grade data quality. Clin Pharmacol Ther 2018;103:202–205.
[71] Corrigan-Curay J, Sacks L, Woodcock J. Real-world evidence and real-world data for evaluating drug safety and effectiveness. JAMA 2018;320:867–868.
[72] Sim I. Mobile devices and health. N Engl J Med 2019;381:956–968.
[73] Goldsack JC, Izmailova ES, Menetski JP, Hoffmann SC, Groenen PMA, Wagner JA. Remote digital monitoring in clinical trials in the time of COVID-19. Nat Rev Drug Discov 2020;19:378–379.
[74] Coravos A, Goldsack JC, Karlin DR, Nebeker C, Perakslis E, Zimmerman N, et al. Digital medicine: a primer on measurement. Digit Biomark 2019;3:31–71.
[75] Lin JA, He P. Reinventing clinical trials: a review of innovative biomarker trial designs in cancer therapies. Br Med Bull 2015;114:17–27.
[76] Woodcock J, LaVange LM. Master protocols to study multiple therapies, multiple diseases, or both. New Engl J Med 2017;377:62–70.
[77] Das S, Lo AW. Re-inventing drug development: a case study of the I-SPY 2 breast cancer clinical trials program. Contemp Clin Trials 2017;62:168–174.
[78] Zhao X, Modur V, Carayannopoulos LN, Laterza OF. Biomarkers in pharmaceutical research. Clin Chem 2015;61:1343–1353.
[79] Anderson DC, Kodukula K. Biomarkers in pharmacology and drug discovery. Biochem Pharmacol 2014;87:172–188.
[80] Menetski JP, Hoffmann SC, Cush SS, Kamphaus TN, Austin CP, Herrling PL, et al. The foundation for the national institutes of health biomarkers consortium: past accomplishments and new strategic direction. Clin Pharmacol Ther 2019;105:829–843.

Chapter 18

Imaging in drug development

Owen Carmichael
Pennington Biomedical Research Center, Baton Rouge, LA, United States

Introduction

Novel drug discovery is becoming progressively more difficult. Many diseases are today well served by existing agents, making the hurdle increasingly high for the differentiation of novel therapeutics that clearly demonstrate increased therapeutic benefits. Additionally, diseases with the greatest impact on quality of life and health economics are both chronic, developing over years to decades, and multifactorial, with a variety of contributing factors that often include diet and exercise. Examples include Alzheimer's disease, diabetes, and heart failure. There is still, however, room for improvement in the treatment of many disorders. Increased scientific understanding has recognized that what appears as one disease can in fact be deconstructed into constellations of disease subtypes and "symptom clusters" that are only partly treated by current therapeutics, giving opportunity for new therapies to improve patient care.

New drug candidates need to demonstrate a clear advantage over currently available drugs, and novel unprecedented mechanisms are often the means to reach this goal. Drugs with a novel mechanism of action carry greater inherent risk of failure. As discussed in Chapter 28, strategies for early decision-making are therefore critical to cost-effective drug development, as deferring *proof of concept* on poorly validated targets to late clinical trials is financially unsustainable. New, more efficient drug discovery paradigms could fundamentally allow evaluation of a greater number of targets, many of which today have only preclinical face validity, and prevent late-stage testing and extensive human exposure to molecules that have no chance of clinical success. Stopping work on targets and mechanisms that show little early evidence of significant biological benefit allows clinical development resources and energy to be focused on the best candidates and the best-validated hypotheses. As discussed in Chapter 17, the use of biomarkers has the promise to reinvigorate the drug discovery process through improved success rates that help bring useful medicines to patients sooner [1].

Advances in imaging methods are playing an increasingly important role in our ability to use imaging as a translational endpoint in assessing molecules, mechanisms, and therapeutic hypotheses [2, 3]. In early phase studies, imaging can help validate drug targets in models of disease and symptomatology and focus research on those drug candidates that achieve the highest target engagement with the lowest exposure, thereby maximizing the therapeutic index. Linking the degree of target engagement and the time-on-target to preclinical measures of efficacy is critical to molecule selection and hypothesis generation. In early clinical development, imaging can be used to link target engagement to drug-induced biological changes that are expected to produce clinical benefit—so-called *proof-of-mechanism* or activity testing.

Proof of concept can be declared when target engagement can be linked to a change in a clinically meaningful imaging endpoint. If a drug has adequate target engagement but does not produce the expected biological or clinical effects, the therapeutic concept is flawed and development can be stopped. In later phase studies (Phases 2 and 3), imaging measures are more likely to be used to demonstrate normalization of a disease-related imaging signal, at one or very few dose levels. Imaging can also be used in this setting to identify individuals most likely to demonstrate a therapeutic response for trial recruitment. Such studies may be submitted to regulators as part of an application for new drug approval.

Molecular imaging technologies

A variety of imaging technologies are used to visualize, characterize, and quantify anatomical structures and biological processes with high spatial and biochemical resolution at the cellular and subcellular levels in a physiologically relevant tissue context [4]. Each technology generates images in different ways, and each has its strengths and weaknesses in terms of spatial resolution, sensitivity, and imaging probe characteristics (Table 18.1). X-ray computed tomography (CT) is a mainstay for anatomical (structural) and perfusion imaging. Magnetic resonance imaging (MRI), on the other hand, yields rich information on structure, metabolites, and functional physiology. Molecular imaging modalities enable the spatial,

Atkinson's Principles of Clinical Pharmacology. https://doi.org/10.1016/B978-0-12-819869-8.00022-7

TABLE 18.1 The molecular imaging toolbox.

Modality	Parameter	Probe dosing characteristics	Spatial resolution	Molecular sensitivity	Applications
CT	X-rays	High mass contrast	~20–50 μm	*	**Tissue anatomy/density** Tumors Bone
MRI/MRS	Radiowaves	High mass contrast (nanoparticles)	~100 μm	**	**Tissue anatomy/blood flow/and content** Tumors Atherosclerotic plaque Vascular edema Brain structure, function and biochemistry
US	High frequency acoustic	High mass microbubbles (targeted)	~100 μm	***	**Anatomy/blood flow/tissue structure** Atherosclerotic plaque
SPECT/PET	Low/high energy gamma radiation	Low mass high specific activity (targeted)	PET: 1–2 mm	****	**Blood flow/metabolism receptor density/molecular markers of health and disease** Brain receptors/pathology Tumor physiology
Optical	Fluorescence Bioluminescence Near-IR	Gene reporters and activatable probes	μm to mm	*****	Enzyme activity/metabolism/receptors/genes **Tumors** **Atherosclerosis**

Note: * represents low molecular sensitivity, ***** represents high molecular sensitivity, and ** through **** are intermediate levels of molecular sensitivity.

temporal, and in vivo characterization of biological processes at the molecular level by employing various types of exogenously applied imaging probes. Application of each of these imaging technologies for drug development purposes requires integration of many disciplines, including medicine, biology, chemistry, pharmacology, medical imaging physics, applied computer sciences and mathematics, and bioinformatics.

The most commonly used imaging technique in the early phases of drug development is nuclear imaging, which visualizes radiolabeled probes or radiotracers interacting with protein targets within or on the surface of cells. The two key radionuclide imaging modalities are PET, which uses tracers labeled with positron-emitting radioisotopes (^{11}C and ^{18}F), and single photon emission computed tomography (SPECT), which detects tracers labeled with gamma-emitting radioactive isotopes (e.g., ^{123}I). Both can be used to track small molecule and biologic therapeutics. Radiotracers are versatile and sensitive, and can be designed to track the drug itself, image the drug target, or monitor key biochemical and physiological processes. Novel molecular tracer probes are usually needed as they are the only way to quantitatively measure receptor populations and pharmacology at picomolar to nanomolar concentrations in vivo in both animals and humans. The use of structural imaging modalities such as CT and MRI in combination with PET or SPECT enables precise spatial and anatomical localization of molecular activity.

Advances in the development of small animal tomographic cameras (microPET or microSPECT with CT) have facilitated translational bridging between preclinical and clinical research. Radionuclide imaging modalities, especially PET, have become powerful tools for drug discovery and development, particularly in oncology, where [^{18}F] FDG PET imaging of glucose metabolism is part of routine clinical care, and in the neurosciences, due to the inaccessibility of the brain and the paucity of specific CNS-specific markers to drive accurate drug dosing.

The other widely used imaging technique used in drug development, especially for CNS applications, is MRI which provides predominantly dynamic data either by blood oxygenation level dependent (BOLD) [5, 6] or arterial spin labeling (ASL) perfusion MRI [7] sequences. There are three experimental settings within which fMRI data is collected. First, *task-based fMRI* uses sensory or cognitive stimuli to provoke responses from brain regions or circuits involved in responding to the stimuli. These provoked responses include changes in fMRI signal amplitudes (i.e., activations or deactivations) as well as changes in functional connectivity (low-frequency temporal correlations in fMRI signals between brain regions).

Second, *resting state fMRI* (rsfMRI) is used to examine functional connectivity during ostensible rest times [8]. Third, *pharmacological MRI* (phMRI) records fMRI signals following the administration of pharmacological agents [9]. Static MRI imagery, representing the structure of healthy or lesioned bodily tissues, are also collected in drug development studies.

Uses for imaging in drug development

Participant stratification/selection

There is a growing interest in patient-specific, disease-specific, and outcome-specific imaging biomarkers that are independent of specific therapeutic mechanisms and molecules. Imaging approaches that can be used to stratify patients for clinical trials will enable enrichment of clinical proof-of-concept studies, potentially leading to shorter, smaller, and more definitive clinical trials. Stratification using imaging may not only improve the drug development process but ultimately could also drive personalized medicine approaches to therapy, delivering the right drug at the right dose to the right patient. In addition, there is increasing interest in disease- and outcome-specific imaging biomarkers that can be used to study disease progression and remission, potentially serving as surrogate endpoints that could support and speed marketing approval of new disease-modifying drug therapies.

The development of disease-modifying agents for Alzheimer's disease provides an example in which a range of imaging biomarkers have been used to select and stratify patients in clinical trials designed to test the amyloid cascade hypothesis [10]. PET imaging with radiotracers that visualize amyloid and tau protein is being used to select patients with high amyloid and tau burden [11], while structural MRI is used to select individuals with early brain atrophy in the entorhinal cortex and hippocampus—regions that are markedly affected during the progression of the disease [12]. Sequential imaging during therapy can also be used to monitor treatment response by providing objective measures of the preservation, slowing, or reversal of pathological, anatomical, or fluid-based biomarkers. Future efforts will be aimed toward the development of molecular tracers for other hallmark pathological processes in Alzheimer's disease, such as neuroinflammation [13].

The validation and qualification of selection and stratification biomarkers that are independent of drug target and mechanism require long-term studies, so they are increasingly being conducted through public-private consortia that share the risk and considerable cost. Large consortia are developing and standardizing CNS imaging biomarker measurements in Alzheimer's disease (ADNI: Alzheimer's Disease Neuroimaging Initiative; www.nia.nih.gov/Alzheimers/ResearchInformation/ClinicalTrials/ADNI.htm) and Parkinson's disease (www.michaeljfox.org/living_PPMI.cfm Parkinson's Progression Markers Initiative) that characterize disease progression in patient populations to provide robust baselines for therapeutic trials. Data collected from these initiatives could lead to the development of objective standard assessment tools to define the most appropriate patients to treat, and so could become an important part of personalized medicine and the drug application, review, and approval process. In the United States, the foundation for the National Institutes of Health (fNIH) set up the Biomarker Consortium (www.fnih.org) as a direct response to the FDA Critical Path Initiative that called for a greater emphasis on biomarkers to speed drug discovery and development. Other groups, such as the Innovative Medicines Initiative (IMI: www.imi.europa.eu/ a partnership between the EU and pharmaceutical companies) and the European Medicines Agency (www.ema.europa.eu), have also championed these approaches.

Imaging target engagement

The goal of any early development program is always to test the mechanism and not the molecule in order to support additional research investments in late-phase clinical trials. Confirmation that drugs reach their targets using imaging markers of engagement and pharmacodynamics constitutes a valuable proof of mechanism and is therefore central to successful clinical proof-of-concept testing, particularly in CNS drug development. All too often, suboptimal molecules that fail to test hypotheses have been advanced to the clinic and so confuse and complicate paths for future development of new drug entities, especially in neuropsychiatric disease. Indeed, the lack of an appropriate imaging "biomarker tool box" probably explains why so many neuroscience targets from the 1990s are still being pursued and have not yet been shown to work. It is a sobering thought that many different companies continue to base drug development on these same targets and keep failing because they still lack the appropriate CNS biomarkers needed to guide Go/No Go decision-making and dose selection.

In nuclear medicine, medicinal chemists together with radiochemists now play an increasingly important role in developing PET tracers to establish brain penetration and target engagement of candidate drugs that can guide interpretation of preclinical experiments and help select doses for clinical trial. Accordingly, an important feature of most CNS drug discovery programs is now the design, in parallel with drug candidate synthesis, of precursor molecules suitable for rapid labeling at high specific activity with ^{11}C and ^{18}F radionuclides to produce imaging radioligands that have high receptor affinity, target selectivity, fast brain penetration, and physicochemical properties that minimize nonspecific binding and maximize signal-to-noise sensitivity.

There are many examples of drug development go/no-go decisions that have been influenced significantly by PET radionucleotides in this way. NPY5 receptor agonists [14], cannabinoid-1 receptor inverse agonists (CB1R) [15, 16], H_3-receptor inverse agonists [17, 18], $GABA_A$ agonists [19], μ-opioid antagonists [20–23], striatal D2 dopamine receptor agonists [24], and neurokinin 1 (NK1) antagonists [25] are all examples.

Dose ranging using PET data can facilitate the registration of new therapies. For example, PET imaging (Fig. 18.1) was used to support final dose selection for aprepitant, a selective neurokinin-1-(NK1) receptor antagonist [26] that prevents acute and delayed chemotherapy-induced nausea and vomiting [26]. In this application, PET studies were used to pick the lowest doses that demonstrated full CNS target engagement, thereby maximizing efficacy while optimizing the therapeutic window [1, 27]. This was especially important as aprepitant is used in conjunction with complex oncologic drug therapy regimes where the potential for drug interactions is high. NK-1R PET imaging also was used in a novel study to show receptor occupancy over 5 days of dosing with a single daily IV dose of 150 mg fosaprepitant (the water-soluble phosphate prodrug of aprepitant) that was equivalent to that provided by a single oral dose of 165 mg aprepitant [28]. This study provided critical support for registration of new single-dose options for the drug. Finally, imaging was also used to select doses of aprepitant or the investigational NK-1R antagonist L-759,274 needed to block central NK1 receptors "around the clock" in a series of unsuccessful Phase 2/3 trials of this mechanism in patients with depression [29] and anxiety [30].

Imaging biology

Beyond assessing target engagement, imaging procedures are also useful for measuring a variety of biological processes associated with the disease of interest, and in turn can be used to assess the effects of novel treatments on those processes.

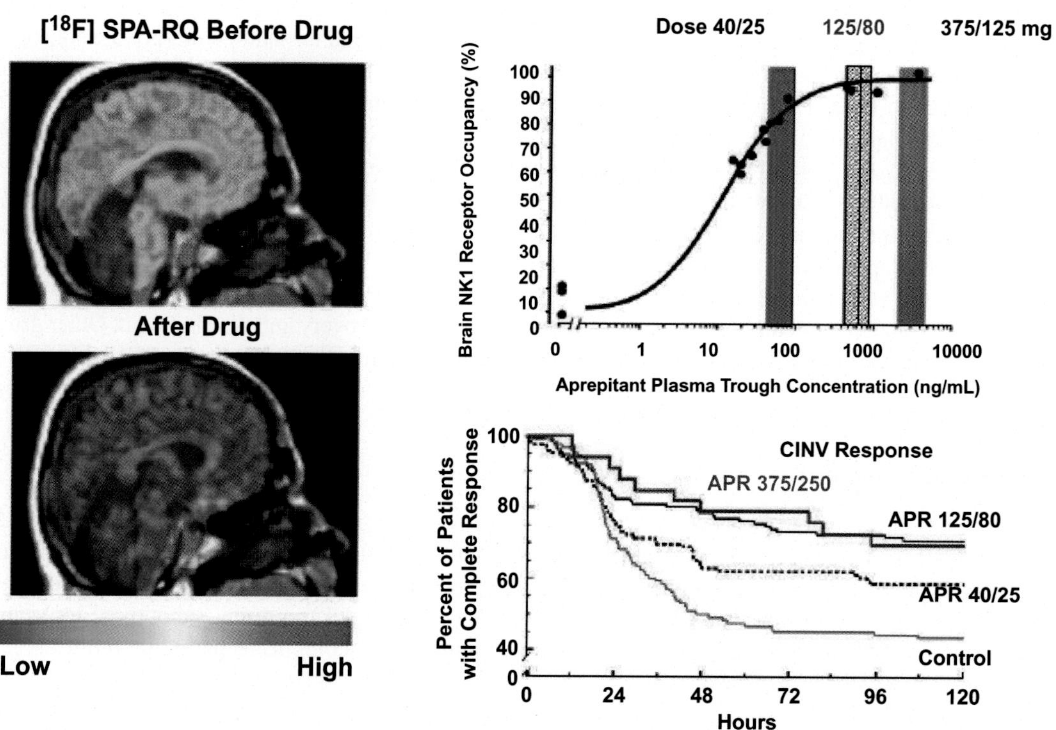

FIG. 18.1 Substance P NK1-receptor imaging with [^{18}F] SPA-RQ. The *left panels* show [^{18}F] SPA-RQ imaging of NK1 receptors in the brain *(top)* in the absence of aprepitant (EMEND) and *(bottom)* after a fully blocking dose of aprepitant. The *right lower panel* shows dose-response curves for aprepitant in preventing emesis caused by a highly emetogenic chemotherapy such as cisplatin. Note that the response is submaximal at 40/25 mg and then is complete at doses of 125/80 mg, with no further effect at the higher dose of 375/250 mg. The *right upper panel* shows that this is the case because receptor occupancy is ~75% at the lowest dose and then >90% saturated at the higher doses. The 125/80-mg dose was chosen for registration because it optimized the therapeutic window for aprepitant.

Applications of imaging in this regard have been observed in a variety of disease settings, including oncology, pulmonology, bone diseases, heart conditions, and the brain. Examples from these domains are described as follows.

Cancer

Molecular imaging has the potential to aid the development of oncology therapeutics since it fits into the existing framework of medical care, where PET/CT is a mainstay of diagnostic evaluation and response monitoring [31, 32]. PET radiotracers are being developed as early response markers to assess the impact of novel therapeutics on various universal molecular characteristics of tumor physiology (Fig. 18.2). The most widely used molecular imaging marker in oncology is [^{18}F]-fluorodeoxyglucose ([^{18}F] FDG), which can monitor glucose uptake and metabolism by glycolysis and thereby can be applied as a diagnostic to identify and track tumors and metastases that have increased glucose demands. Decreases in [^{18}F] FDG uptake, resulting from downregulation of glucose transporters, decreased glucose metabolism by cells, or fewer cells, have been proposed as an early signal that an experimental treatment may show promise in affecting tumor physiology [33, 34].

Imaging also has an important role to play in assessing changes in tumor burden, which are useful endpoints in clinical trials. Guidelines for these tumor assessments, called RECIST (Response Evaluation Criteria in Solid Tumors), were published in 2000 and revised in 2009, and have been widely used to evaluate treatment outcomes. These guidelines cover imaging recommendations on the optimal anatomical assessment of lesions, which and how many lesions to measure, and clear definitions of progression. Interestingly, detection of new lesions, including the interpretation of [^{18}F] FDG scan assessment, is now a consideration in denoting disease progression [35].

In comparison to [^{18}F] FDG PET, other applications of nuclear imaging for oncologic drug development include tracers that can monitor cell proliferation ([^{18}F] FLT and [^{18}F] FMAU), angiogenesis (integrin $\alpha v\beta 3$ directed tracers), hypoxia ([^{18}F] MISO and [^{64}Cu] ATSM), apoptosis (Annexin-V based tracers and caspase-3 and -9 directed tracers) [36], and skeletal metastasis ([^{18}F]-NaF) [37]. Optical and MR-based tracers that monitor cell physiology are also under development [38, 39].

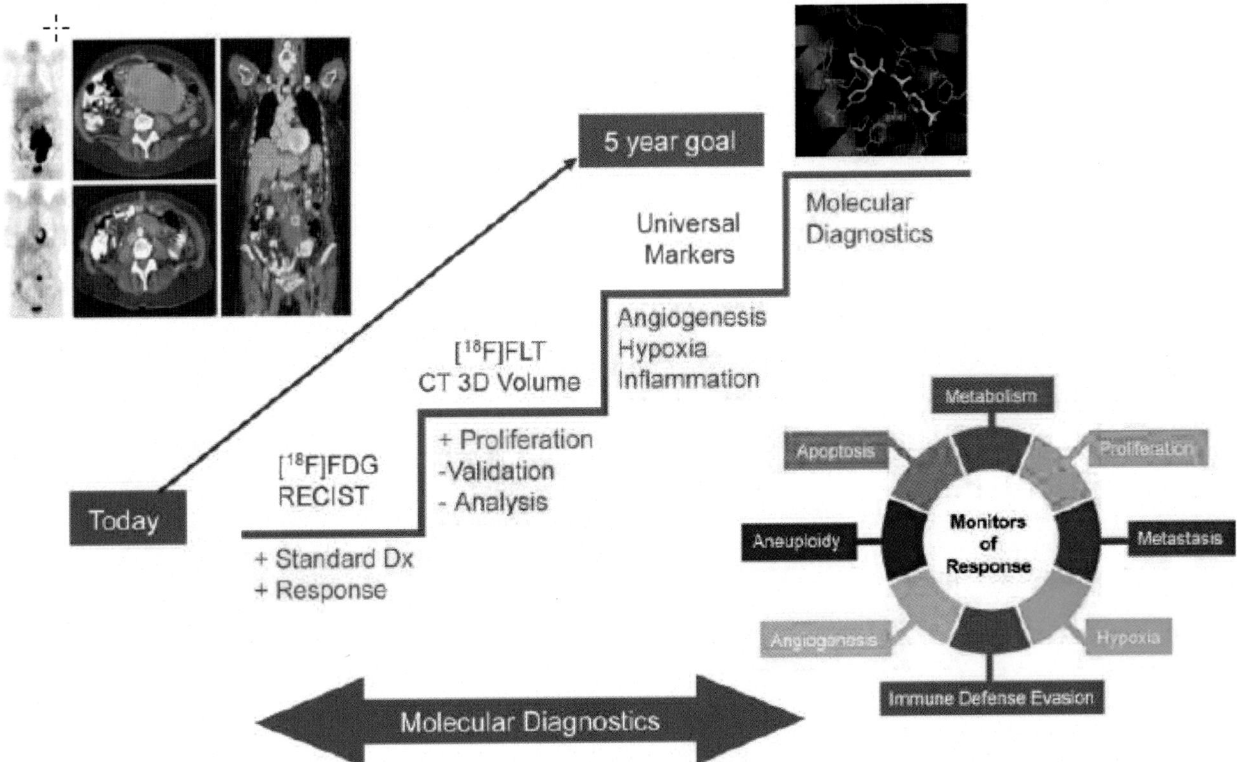

FIG. 18.2 An oncology imaging roadmap in which steps of increasing value are shown as we move from today's imaging metrics to the development of universal markers of tumor physiology and molecular diagnostics for cancer pathways. *(Based on Hargreaves RJ. The role of molecular imaging in drug discovery and development. Clin Pharmacol Ther 2008;83:349–353, with thanks to Dr S. Stroobants for use of the PET/CT images.)*

Finally, MRI techniques also play an important role in imaging cancer biology. One technique of particular note is dynamic contrast-enhanced magnetic resonance imaging (T_1-weighted DCE-MRI), which is now frequently used to assess dose-dependent biological responses in early clinical trial assessment of many antiangiogenic drug candidates [40]. Combined PET-MRI markers collected simultaneously on integrated PET-MRI systems are also in development [41, 42]. Whether such MRI changes are predictive of drug efficacy or could be used as a tumor progression marker are still subjects of debate. As with many imaging modalities, critical issues for the future development and application of DCE-MRI are standardization of data acquisition, analysis, and modeling.

Lung

With the advent of novel imaging modalities (Fig. 18.3), it is now possible to evaluate COPD and asthma phenotypes in clinical studies using noninvasive or minimally invasive imaging methods such as CT and MRI to complement traditional physiological measurements such as forced expiratory volumes (FEV_1) [43, 44]. CT is the imaging modality of choice for the lung, enabling the extent of emphysema to be estimated objectively in patients with COPD. It is now possible to obtain high-resolution images of the lung with less than a 10-s breath-hold. The volume of the lung and its individual lobes can be measured and lung mass, tissue volume, and airspace volumes can be calculated by using the apparent X-ray attenuation values of the lung to estimate lung density.

MRI with the hyperpolarized noble gases ^{129}Xe and ^{3}He can help in developing drugs for respiratory diseases such as asthma and COPD. These imaging agents provide excellent MRI contrast and, within a single breath-hold, enable quantitative images of the airways and airspaces of the entire lung to be captured that distinguish areas involved in normal ventilation from those that are impaired by disease. Diffusion-weighted MR methods are used to detect signals that reflect the random Brownian motion of the hyperpolarized gas. During inhalation, gas diffusion is restricted by the dimension of the airways and airspaces, so the average displacement of the gas is similar to alveolar diameters (a few hundred micrometers) and thus reflects alveolar integrity. An apparent diffusion coefficient (ADC) can be derived from the MRI and mapped quantitatively to examine lung integrity in pulmonary disease. In healthy young adults the ADC signal is homogeneous, whereas "focal" defects are observed in COPD and, as shown in Fig. 18.4, the ADC can be used to map disease progress and severity [45]. Fluorine-based MRI imaging of sulfur hexafluoride (SF6) has also been investigated in this setting, eliminating the need for hyperpolarization and its associated technical challenges [46].

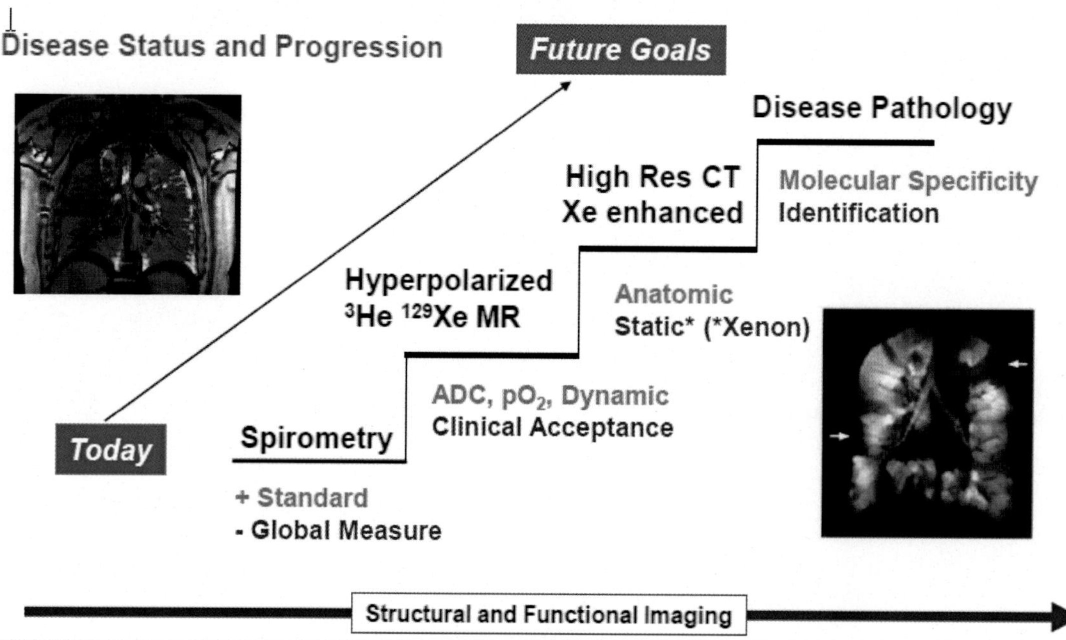

FIG. 18.3 A respiratory imaging roadmap in which steps of increasing value are shown as we move from today's respiratory physiology measurements to imaging lung structure and function with a goal of discovering molecular diagnostics for respiratory disease pathology. *(Lung images kindly provided by Dr G. Parraga.)*

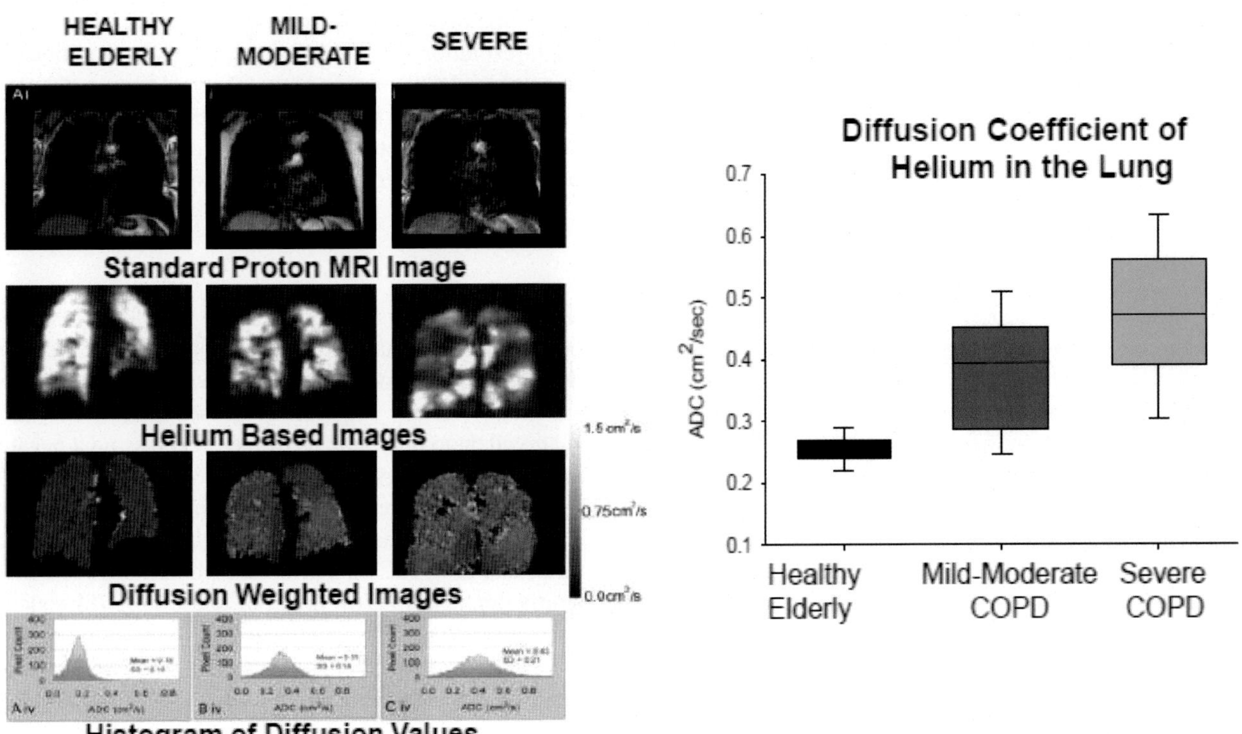

FIG. 18.4 Imaging studies in patients with chronic obstructive pulmonary disease (COPD) in which the *left panels* show representative standard proton MRI images, ^{3}He images, and calculated diffusion-weighted images for healthy elderly, mild-moderate and severe COPD patients. The histograms of diffusion values show the increasing spread with disease indicative of loss of alveolar integrity and increased diffusional characteristics (ADC) of the hyperpolarized gas. The *right panel* shows the mean data for each group, and indicates that ADC derived from ^{3}He MR imaging could be a sensitive marker for disease progression and therapeutic outcome. *(Preliminary data from studies with Drs G. Santyr, G. Parraga, and R. Fogel.)*

Heart

Cardiovascular medicine is another area in which imaging has become a routine part of medical practice. The chronic and progressive nature of atherosclerosis requires the registration of new therapies for this condition to be based on long-term clinical outcome trials. As with any disease-modifying therapy, there is a critical need to select and prioritize drug targets and to personalize therapy by identifying atherosclerotic plaque subtypes (e.g., high-risk vulnerable plaques) that can be used to select the most appropriate therapeutic interventions (www.hrpinitiative.com/hrpinit). Molecular imaging agents directed against plaque-specific targets could be used to identify patients for clinical trials and in the future could form the basis of diagnostic molecular imaging alongside conventional CT- and MRI-based structural and intravascular imaging approaches [47, 48]. However, despite considerable effort to use genetic and proteomic analysis of atherosclerotic plaque to identify targets, no molecular imaging agents have yet progressed into routine experimental use or been incorporated into clinical trials.

Studies have attempted to use [^{18}F] FDG to highlight active plaque by imaging increased glucose metabolic rates due to macrophage infiltration [49], and these have had varying degrees of success [50]. In the field of vascular imaging, important advances have been made in three-dimensional carotid ultrasound techniques to quantitatively capture plaque volumes. Developments in optical coherence tomography (OCT) may allow intravascular coronary imaging to advance beyond the intravascular ultrasound (IVUS) techniques used today to image the vessel wall at the ultrastructural (macrophage) level [51], and all intravascular techniques now permit combined measurements (ultrasound, OCT, near IR spectroscopy) to be made with a single catheter [52].

Bone

The development of bone imaging biomarkers [53] was spurred by the development of effective drug therapies such as the bisphosphonates, drug registrations such as the RANK ligand denosumab [54], and investigational drugs such as the cathepsin K inhibitor odanacatib [55]. Biomarkers have advanced from fluid markers of bone formation and resorption to include dual energy X-ray imaging (DEXA) of bone density (allowing bone to be distinguished from soft tissue due to differential absorption at the two energies) and, most recently, high-resolution CT and MR imaging of bone architecture (Fig. 18.5). These high-resolution structural measurements can be combined with ex vivo biomechanical testing of bone to form the basis for computational algorithms, such as finite element analysis (FEA), that can estimate bone strength, thereby complementing bone density estimates and potentially differentiating between treatment effects [56]. Hopefully these estimates of bone strength ultimately will displace the current need to use bone fracture development as a metric in clinical drug development trials (Fig. 18.6).

Brain

Functional MRI of the brain has been shown to be sensitive to brain functional changes following both acute (i.e., after a single dose) or chronic (i.e., multiple dose) administration of drugs and food products [57]. The vast majority of these studies have been academic investigations using marketed drugs whose efficacy and effective doses have already been established. One prominent example is the fMRI response of the amygdala to photographs of faces expressing a negative affect, which can be normalized in depressed individuals by antidepressant drugs at clinically effective doses [58, 59]. Intravenous ketamine (an NMDA receptor antagonist) elicits a widespread fMRI response [60–66] that is blocked by antiglutamatergic compounds [61, 62], and reverses the phMRI signal evoked by some (but not all) antipsychotic agents and compounds designed to attenuate glutamate release [67, 68]. Additional drug classes that induce phMRI signals include antiepileptics [69], analgesics [70–74], antipsychotics [75], cognitive enhancers [76], drugs of abuse [77, 78], calcium channel blockers [79, 80], cyclooxygenase-2 (COX-2) inhibitors [81], muscarinic acetylcholine receptor modulators [82–84], monoamine stabilizers [85], and therapies traditionally thought to impact solely immune system activity [86]. In addition to traditional phMRI studies, pharmacological modulation of resting state functional connectivity has also been reported in animal models and humans [87–92].

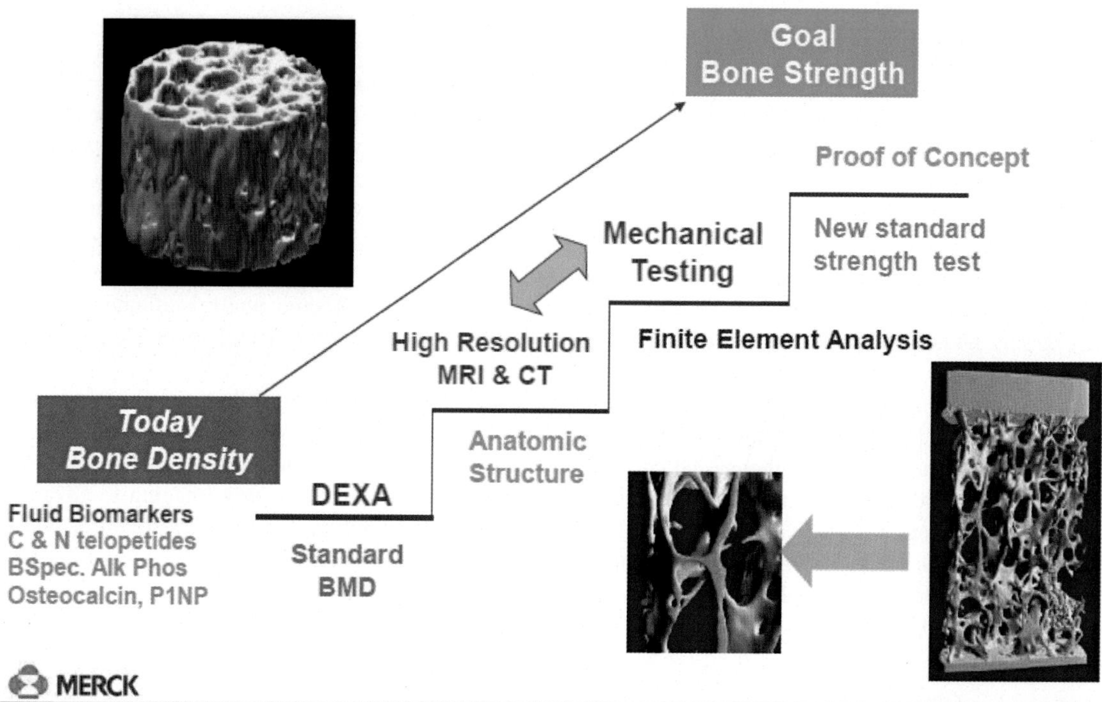

FIG. 18.5 A bone imaging roadmap in which steps of increasing value are shown as we move from today's fluid biomarkers of bone formation and resorption, to measurements of bone density (DEXA), to imaging of bone architecture accompanied by functional analysis of bone strength through mechanical testing and finite element analysis.

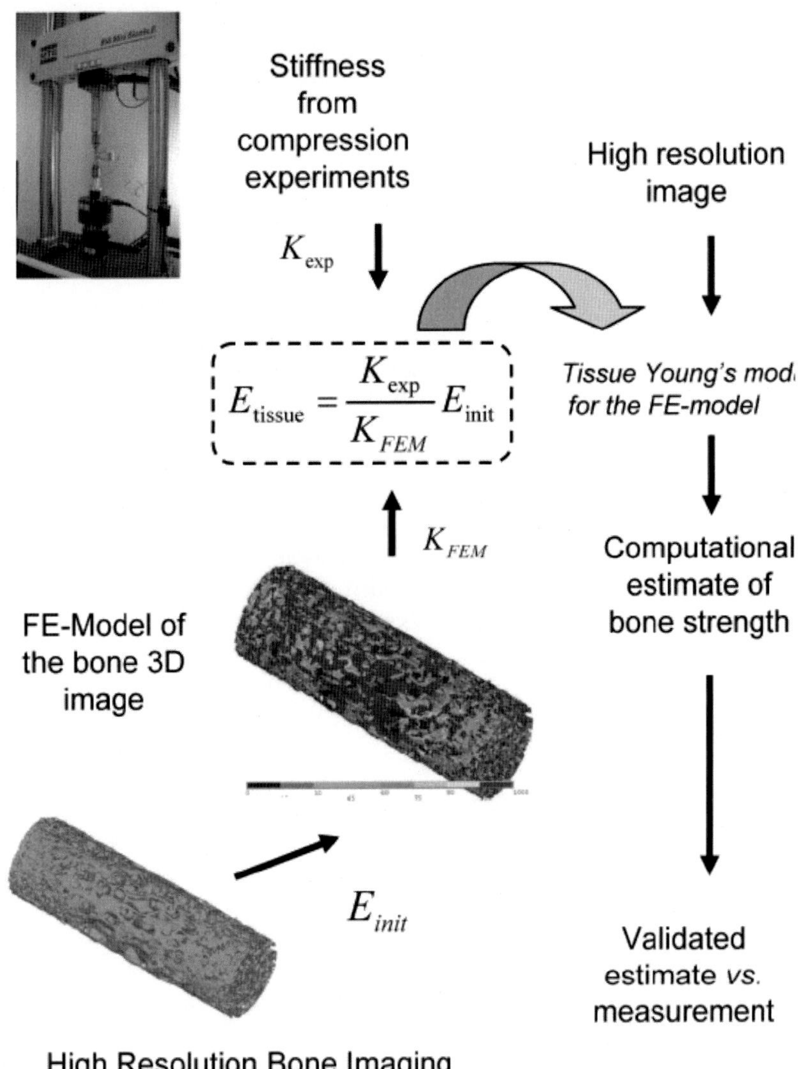

FIG. 18.6 Steps in the finite element analysis calculation of bone strength, starting with the acquisition of the in vivo bone trabecular images, leading to a mathematical model derived from mechanical testing of bone samples that allows virtual testing and calculation of an index of bone strength from the images. *(Images kindly provided by Drs D. Williams and A. Cabal.)*

Challenges to using imaging in drug development

Optimal acquisition and quantification of imaging data

Each imaging acquisition experiment includes a large number of design parameters, both at the acquisition and postprocessing stages. For example, for fMRI, Ben Inglis [93] provides a listing of dozens of parameters that must be set and breaks those down into those that should be required to be reported in publications. Postprocessing steps for imaging exams can include coregistration, normalization to a template space, segmentation into tissues, and smoothing [94]. Additional steps for dynamic acquisitions can include regressing out motion and physiological artifacts. Each postprocessing step is implemented differently in different software packages, each with its own set of operating parameters. Exact guidance on how to set these operating parameters is sparse and incomplete, with some noteworthy exceptions. Poldrack et al. [95], for example, provide guidelines for task-related fMRI experimental design, preprocessing, and statistical modeling, including how many experimental sessions and volumes per session should be acquired. Van Dijk et al. [96] evaluated a variety of acquisition and postprocessing parameters for resting state fMRI, to determine if settings of these parameters made any appreciable difference in detecting default mode and attention networks, against a reference network. Carp [97] evaluated 6912 unique analysis pipelines for a single event-related fMRI experiment, and reported substantial variability across pipelines in terms of BOLD signal strength, localization, and spatial extent. These types of studies necessarily only provide partial guidance about the large design spaces involved in imaging data analysis and suggest that greater knowledge of optimal methods for acquisition and processing of fMRI remains a major research need.

A related challenge involves reducing a high-dimensional medical image to a small number of predefined numeric summary values that can be used as biomarkers in drug development studies. There are several motivations for summary values. (1) The drastically lower dimensionality allows results of imaging experiments to be imported into standard databases, combined with other data such as pharmacokinetics, and analyzed by accredited statisticians. These databases are auditable and operate under strict revision and access control, safeguards that assure a high level of data integrity. (2) Defining summary readouts as primary endpoints before conducting a study requires the practitioner to formulate specific and simple a priori hypotheses, an exercise that can highlight uncertainty in the anticipated outcome and prevent false positive rate inflation [98]. (3) Summary values can reduce the multiple comparison burden, and thus avoid ill-defined choices among correction schemes. Unfortunately, there is no widespread agreement on optimal approaches for this type of imaging data summary. Graph-theoretical summaries [99, 100] and factor analytic methods such as independent components analysis (ICA) [101, 102] are used extensively in exploratory research studies, but these methods have many variants and operating parameters. The more traditional approach of selecting a region of interest (ROI) in an image and reducing all signals in a region to a single summary score [103] requires a choice of summary score (for example, the mean, median, or mode). More recent machine learning-based techniques use complex computational machinery to perform data reduction in a supervised or unsupervised setting [104]. The optimal summary measure for any given clinical trial is unclear and may depend on the hypothesized action of the drug. One reason for the lack of broad agreement on standardized summary measures for imaging exams is that the range of acquisition protocols, pharmacological mechanisms, and imaging sites involved is large, and few standardization studies have been published.

Need for significant resources

As with all biomarkers, imaging markers undergo the fit-for-purpose scientific validation and clinical qualification process that is described in Chapter 17 and elsewhere [2, 105]. However, there are diverse practical challenges that are specific to using imaging markers to characterize patients, identify responders, monitor drug actions, and define therapeutic outcomes. Imaging requires specialized equipment and trained individuals, but its successful routine use most importantly depends on assay validation through assessment of the true magnitude of effect and purposeful harmonization of data acquisition techniques, together with the development of "turn-key" applications using standardized tools for data collection and analysis. These requirements add complexity, especially in multicenter clinical imaging trials, in as much as detailed imaging manuals, standardized acquisition protocols (across different instruments from different manufacturers), data transfer, image reconstruction, and data processing algorithms (to annotate images with patient-specific information to permit confidential independent data review) are also required. Clinical qualification is a graded evidentiary process that is needed to link the biomarker to biology and clinical endpoints, and is dependent upon the intended use of the biomarker (Chapter 17). The intended use may be for internal, regulatory, or clinical trial design and decision-making. But qualifying imaging biomarkers for use in regulatory approval processes is especially difficult, even when a biomarker is scientifically validated and well defined, ultimately requiring assessment in the context of clinical care or through integration into trials with proven active agents. This is clearly an issue when novel mechanisms and novel markers are developed together. Indeed, most biomarkers continue to be used at risk for decision-making during drug discovery and development, and few ever reach the level of surrogacy where they can substitute for a clinical outcome.

Specificity of molecular imaging targets

Proprietary molecular imaging biomarkers rarely have applicability across different targets even within the same disease area, and the cost of developing them has to be justified and accounted for in the context of specific drug discovery programs. In contrast, disease imaging biomarkers can generally be considered platform technologies that can characterize patient populations, disease state, and therapeutic response, so they have a potentially broad cross-target utility with value to diverse therapeutic approaches within a common disease area. In this case, the barrier is that there is little incentive for any one company to bear the considerable cost of clinical qualifying of the biomarker, so a different shared solution is required, in some cases entailing creation of public-private consortia.

Molecular drivers of other imaging signals not fully understood

Outside of PET imaging, the molecular events that drive the emergence of observed imaging signals are more indirectly tied to the administered drug and more complex. In classical BOLD fMRI, for example, signals are determined by at least three physiological effects—changes to cerebral blood volume (CBV), cerebral blood flow (CBF), and the cerebral metabolic rate of oxygen metabolism (CMRO2)—as well as glucose metabolism [106, 107]. Past research shows an association between cerebral hemodynamics and activity of neuronal populations, although exact relationships are still a matter of debate [108–113]. There is a consensus that graded increases in neuronal metabolism result in graded increases in the BOLD response, while corresponding decreases in neuronal metabolism result in reduced BOLD responses [114–117]. However, a precise understanding of the relative contributions of metabolic, vascular, and neural processes to the BOLD signal is still being elucidated. For some pharmacological treatments, such a lack of physiological specificity may be a major limitation to the ability to make development decisions based on phMRI results. Emerging approaches could help to identify distinct physiological changes induced by the treatment, including calibrated BOLD [118–121], quantitative BOLD, "qBOLD" [122], TRUST [123], and QUIXOTIC [124, 125]. Simultaneous BOLD and FDG PET could also help disentangle the multiple physiological effects of treatments [126].

Compounds with slow pharmacokinetics

In studies that use imaging techniques to interrogate the acute effects of novel compounds, the test agent is typically administered partway through the imaging exam, allowing the temporal response to the agent to be quantified [61, 127–131]. This approach works well for compounds whose route of administration (e.g., intravenous) and pharmacokinetics lead to a rapid, easily detectable signal change. But compounds entering clinical drug development are often formulated for oral administration and/or have extended pharmacokinetic profiles. For such compounds, the time required for the imaging exam would be impractically long. A proposed solution to this problem has been to rely on imaging techniques that provide absolute, rather than relative, readouts [132]. Perfusion MRI, for example, yields quantified maps of cerebral blood flow in absolute physiological units, thus allowing CBF measures to be compared between scans taken on different hours or days [133]. Agonist-antagonist fMRI designs are yet another approach. In these designs, a "probe" compound (e.g., ketamine) is administered intravenously and elicits a strong phMRI response [62, 127]. The compounds of interest are administered beforehand, such that the imaging exam coincides with the time of high exposure to the test compound, allowing any modulatory effect on the probe signal (e.g., reversal) to be examined.

Conclusion

Imaging has the potential to play an important role in the clinical evaluation and development of new molecules and mechanisms across diverse therapeutic areas. The value proposition in drug discovery is to use imaging biomarkers to focus research activities on the patients and molecules most likely to test therapeutic hypotheses and achieve beneficial clinical outcomes. The hope is that the use of imaging biomarkers in early discovery and development, despite adding cost to early trials, will increase return on research investments by leading to fewer expensive late-stage failures by quickly eliminating the approaches that are most likely to fail. Perhaps most valuable are imaging biomarkers that could be used to drive new medical practice paradigms for patients in the latent phase of progressive disorders. This would enable prediction, prevention, and tracking of disease in a paradigm shift from today's approaches that have to see clinically overt disease before beginning treatment.

References

[1] Frank R, Hargreaves R. Clinical biomarkers in drug discovery and development. Nat Rev Drug Discov 2003;2:566–580.

[2] Hargreaves R, Wagner J. Imaging as a biomarker for decision making in drug development. In: Beckmann N, editor. In vivo MRI techniques in drug discovery and development. New York, NY: Taylor & Francis; 2006. p. 31–46.

[3] Hargreaves RJ. The role of molecular imaging in drug discovery and development. Clin Pharmacol Ther 2008;83:349–353.

[4] Rudin M, Weissleder R. Molecular imaging in drug discovery and development. Nat Rev Drug Discov 2003;2:123–131.

[5] Logothetis NK, Pfeuffer J. On the nature of the BOLD fMRI contrast mechanism. Magn Reson Imaging 2004;22:1517–1531.

[6] Logothetis NK, Wandell BA. Interpreting the BOLD signal. Annu Rev Physiol 2004;66:735–769.

[7] Petersen ET, Zimine I, Ho YC, Golay X. Non-invasive measurement of perfusion: a critical review of arterial spin labelling techniques. Br J Radiol 2006;79:688–701.

[8] van den Heuvel MP, Hulshoff Pol HE. Exploring the brain network: a review on resting-state fMRI functional connectivity. Eur Neuropsychopharmacol 2010;20:519–534.

[9] Wandschneider B, Koepp MJ. Pharmaco fMRI: determining the functional anatomy of the effects of medication. Neuroimage Clin 2016;12:691–697.

[10] Tolar M, Abushakra S, Sabbagh M. The path forward in Alzheimer's disease therapeutics: reevaluating the amyloid cascade hypothesis. Alzheimers Dement 2020. https://doi.org/10.1016/j.jalz.2019.09.075.

[11] Barthel H, Seibyl J, Lammertsma AA, Villemagne VL, Sabri O. Exploiting the full potential of β-amyloid and tau PET imaging for drug efficacy testing. J Nucl Med 2020;61:1105–1106.

[12] Fujishima M, Kawaguchi A, Maikusa N, Kuwano R, Iwatsubo T, Matsuda H. Sample size estimation for Alzheimer's disease trials from Japanese ADNI serial magnetic resonance imaging. J Alzheimers Dis 2017;56:75–88.

[13] Lagarde J, Sarazin M, Bottlaender M. In vivo PET imaging of neuroinflammation in Alzheimer's disease. J Neural Transm 2018;125:847–867.

[14] Erondu N, Gantz I, Musser B, et al. Neuropeptide Y5 receptor antagonism does not induce clinically meaningful weight loss in overweight and obese adults. Cell Metab 2006;4:275–282.

[15] Burns HD, Van Laere K, Sanabria-Bohorquez S, et al. [18F]MK-9470, a positron emission tomography (PET) tracer for in vivo human PET brain imaging of the cannabinoid-1 receptor. Proc Natl Acad Sci U S A 2007;104:9800–9805.

[16] Van Laere K, Casteels C, Dhollander I, Goffin K, Grachev J, Bormans G, et al. Widespread decrease of type 1 cannabinoid receptor availability in Huntington disease in vivo. J Nucl Med 2010;51:1413–1417.

[17] Iannone R, Palcza J, Renger JJ, Calder NA, Cerechio KA, Gotesdiener KM, et al. Acute alertness-promoting effects of a novel histamine subtype-3 receptor inverse agonist in healthy sleep-deprived male volunteers. Clin Pharmacol Ther 2010;88:831–839.

[18] Iannone R, Renger J, Potter W, Dijk D, Boyle J, Palcza J, et al. The relationship between brain receptor occupancy (RO) and alerting effects in humans support MK-0249 and MK-3134 as inverse agonists at the histamine subtype-3 pre-synaptic receptor (H3R). (Poster), In: American College of neuropsychopharmacology (ANCP) 48th annual conference. Hollywood, Florida; December; 2009.

[19] Atack JR, Wafford KA, Street LJ, Dawson GR, Tye S, Van Laere K, et al. MRK-409 (MK-0343), a GABAA receptor subtype-selective partial agonist, is a non-sedating anxiolytic in preclinical species but causes sedation in humans. J Psychopharmacol 2011;25:314–328.

[20] Nathan PJ, O'Neill BV, Bush MA, Koch A, Tao WX, Maltby K, et al. Opioid receptor modulation of hedonic taste preference and foodiIntake: a single-dose safety, pharmacokinetic, and pharmacodynamic investigation with GSK1521498, a novel μ-opioid receptor inverse agonist. J Clin Pharmacol 2012;52:464–474.

[21] Rabiner EA, Beaver J, Makwana A, Searle G, Long C, Nathan PJ, et al. Pharmacological differentiation of opioid receptor antagonists by molecular and functional imaging of target occupancy and food reward-related brain activation in humans. Mol Psychiatry 2011;16:826–835.

[22] Yeomans MR, Gray RW. Opioid peptides and the control of human ingestive behaviour. Neurosci Biobehav Rev 2002;26:713–728.

[23] Yeomans MR, Wright P. Lower pleasantness of palatable foods in nalmefene-treated human volunteers. Appetite 1991;16:249–259.

[24] Wong DF, Tauscher J, Gründer G. The role of imaging in proof of concept for CNS drug discovery and development. Neuropsychopharmacology 2009;34:187–203.

[25] Borsook D, Upadhyay J, Klimas M, Schwarz AJ, Coimbra A, Baumgartner R, et al. Decision-making using fMRI in clinical drug development: revisiting NK-1 receptor antagonists for pain. Drug Discov Today 2012;17:964–973.

[26] Hargreaves R, Ferreira JC, Hughes D, Brands J, Hale J, Mattson B, et al. Development of aprepitant, the first neurokinin-1 receptor antagonist for the prevention of chemotherapy-induced nausea and vomiting. Ann N Y Acad Sci 2011;1222:40–48.

[27] Bergstrom M, Hargreaves RJ, Burns HD, Goldberg MR, Sciberras D, Reines SA, et al. Human positron emission tomography studies of brain neurokinin 1 receptor occupancy by aprepitant. Biol Psychiatry 2004;55:1007–1012.

[28] Van Laere K, De Hoon J, Bormans G, Koole M, Derdelinckx I, De Lepeleire I, et al. Equivalent dynamic human brain NK1-receptor occupancy following single-dose i.v. fosaprepitant vs. oral aprepitant as assessed by PET imaging. Clin Pharmacol Ther 2012;92:243–250.

[29] Keller M, Montgomery S, Ball W, Morrison M, Snavely D, Liu G, et al. Lack of efficacy of the substance p (neurokinin1 receptor) antagonist aprepitant in the treatment of major depressive disorder. Biol Psychiatry 2006;59:216–223.

[30] Michelson D, Hargreaves R, Alexander R, Ceesay P, Hietala J, Lines C, et al. Lack of efficacy of L-759274, a novel neurokinin 1 (substance P) receptor antagonist, for the treatment of generalized anxiety disorder. Int J Neuropsychopharmacol 2013;16:1–11.

[31] Shields AF. Positron emission tomography measurement of tumor metabolism and growth: its expanding role in oncology. Mol Imaging Biol 2006;8:141–150.

[32] Weissleder R. Molecular imaging in cancer. Science 2006;312:1168–1171.

[33] MacManus MP, Seymour JF, Hicks RJ. Overview of early response assessment in lymphoma with FDG-PET. Cancer Imaging 2007;7:10–18.

[34] Stroobants S, Goeminne J, Seegers M, Dimitrijevic S, Dupont P, Nuyts J, et al. 18FDG-Positron emission tomography for the early prediction of response in advanced soft tissue sarcoma treated with imatinib mesylate (Glivec). Eur J Cancer 2003;39:2012–2020.

[35] Eisenhauer EA, Therasse P, Bogaerts J, Schwartz LH, Sargent D, Ford R, et al. New response evaluation criteria in solid tumours: revised RECIST guideline (version 1.1). Eur J Cancer 2009;45:228–247.

[36] Shields AF, Grierson JR, Dohmen BM, Machulla HJ, Stayanoff JC, Lawhorn-Crews JM, et al. Imaging proliferation in vivo with [F-18]FLT and positron emission tomography. Nat Med 1998;4:1334–1336.

[37] Velez EM, Desai B, Jadvar H. Treatment response assessment of skeletal metastases in prostate cancer with 18 F-NaF PET/CT. Nucl Med Mol Imaging 2019;53:247–252.

[38] Pysz MA, Gambhir SS, Willmann JK. Molecular imaging: current status and emerging strategies. Clin Radiol 2010;65:500–516.

[39] Weissleder R, Pittet MJ. Imaging in the era of molecular oncology. Nature 2008;452:580–589.

[40] O'Connor JP, Jackson A, Parker GJ, Jayson GC. DCE-MRI biomarkers in the clinical evaluation of antiangiogenic and vascular disrupting agents. Br J Cancer 2007;96:189–195.

[41] Gao S, Du S, Lu Z, Xin J, Gao S, Sun H. Multiparametric PET/MR (PET and MR-IVIM) for the evaluation of early treatment response and prediction of tumor recurrence in patients with locally advanced cervical cancer. Eur Radiol 2020;30:1191–1201.

[42] Xu C, Sun H, Du S, Xin J. Early treatment response of patients undergoing concurrent chemoradiotherapy for cervical cancer: an evaluation of integrated multi-parameter PET-IVIM MR. Eur J Radiol 2019;117:1–8.

[43] Coxson HO, Mayo J, Lam S, Santyr G, Parraga G, Sin DD. New and current clinical imaging techniques to study chronic obstructive pulmonary disease. Am J Respir Crit Care Med 2009;180:588–597.

[44] Schuster DP. The opportunities and challenges of developing imaging biomarkers to study lung function and disease. Am J Respir Crit Care Med 2007;176:224–230.

[45] Kirby M, Mathew L, Heydarian M, Etemad-Rezai R, McCormack DG, Parraga G. Chronic obstructive pulmonary disease: quantification of bronchodilator effects by using hyperpolarized (3)He MR imaging. Radiology 2011;261:283–292.

[46] Ruiz-Cabello J, Barnett BP, Bottomley PA, Bulte JW. Fluorine (19F) MRS and MRI in biomedicine. NMR Biomed 2011;24:114–129.

[47] Jaffer FA, Libby P, Weissleder R. Molecular imaging of cardiovascular disease. Circulation 2007;116:1052–1061.

[48] Sanz J, Fayad ZA. Imaging of atherosclerotic cardiovascular disease. Nature 2008;451:953–957.

[49] Rudd JH, Myers KS, Bansilal S, Machac J, Pinto CA, Tong C, et al. Atherosclerosis inflammation imaging with 18F-FDG PET: carotid, iliac, and femoral uptake reproducibility, quantification methods, and recommendations. J Nucl Med 2008;49:871–878.

[50] Myers KS, Rudd JH, Hailman EP, Bolognese JA, Burke J, Pinto CA, et al. Correlation between arterial FDG uptake and biomarkers in peripheral artery disease. JACC Cardiovasc Imaging 2012;5:38–45.

[51] Liu L, Gardecki JA, Nadkarni SK, Toussaint JD, Yagi Y, Bouma BE, et al. Imaging the subcellular structure of human coronary atherosclerosis using micro-optical coherence tomography. Nat Med 2011;17:1010–1014.

[52] Yoo H, Kim JW, Shishkov M, Namati E, Morse T, Shubochkin R, et al. Intra-arterial catheter for simultaneous microstructural and molecular imaging in vivo. Nat Med 2011;17:1680–1684.

[53] Guglielmi G, Muscarella S, Bazzocchi A. Integrated imaging approach to osteoporosis: state-of-the-art review and update. Radiographics 2011;31:1343–1364.

[54] Kendler DL, Roux C, Benhamou CL, Brown JP, Lillestol M, Siddhanti S, et al. Effects of denosumab on bone mineral density and bone turnover in postmenopausal women transitioning from alendronate therapy. J Bone Miner Res 2010;25:72–81.

[55] Eisman JA, Bone HG, Hosking DJ, McClung MR, Reid IR, Rizzoli R, et al. Odanacatib in the treatment of postmenopausal women with low bone mineral density: three-year continued therapy and resolution of effect. J Bone Miner Res 2011;26:242–251.

[56] Jayakar RY, Cabal A, Szumiloski J, Sardesai S, Phillips EA, Laib A, et al. Evaluation of high-resolution peripheral quantitative computed tomography, finite element analysis and biomechanical testing in a pre-clinical model of osteoporosis: a study with odanacatib treatment in the ovariectomized adult rhesus monkey. Bone 2012;50:1379–1388.

[57] Carmichael OT, Pillai S, Shankapal P, McLellan A, Kay DG, Gold BT, et al. A combination of essential fatty acids, Panax ginseng extract, and green tea catechins modifies brain fMRI signals in healthy older adults. J Nutr Health Aging 2018;22:837–846.

[58] Delaveau P, Jabourian M, Lemogne C, Guionnet S, Bergouignan L, Fossati P. Brain effects of antidepressants in major depression: a meta-analysis of emotional processing studies. J Affect Disord 2011;130:66–74.

[59] van Wingen GA, Tendolkar I, Urner M, van Marle HJ, Denys D, Verkes RJ, et al. Short-term antidepressant administration reduces default mode and task-positive network connectivity in healthy individuals during rest. NeuroImage 2014;88:47–53.

[60] Corlett PR, Honey GD, Krystal JH, Fletcher PC. Glutamatergic model psychoses: prediction error, learning, and inference. Neuropsychopharmacology 2011;36:294–315.

[61] Deakin JF, Lees J, McKie S, Hallak JE, Williams SR, Dursun SM. Glutamate and the neural basis of the subjective effects of ketamine: a pharmaco-magnetic resonance imaging study. Arch Gen Psychiatry 2008;65:154–164.

[62] Doyle OM, De Simoni S, Schwarz AJ, Brittain C, O'Daly OG, Williams SC, et al. Quantifying the attenuation of the ketamine pharmacological magnetic resonance imaging response in humans: a validation using antipsychotic and glutamatergic agents. J Pharmacol Exp Ther 2013;345:151–160.

[63] Joules R, Doyle OM, Schwarz AJ, O'Daly OG, Brammer M, Williams SC, et al. Ketamine induces a robust whole-brain connectivity pattern that can be differentially modulated by drugs of different mechanism and clinical profile. Psychopharmacology 2015;232:4205–4218.

[64] Krystal JH, Abi-Saab W, Perry E, D'Souza DC, Liu N, Gueorguieva R, et al. Preliminary evidence of attenuation of the disruptive effects of the NMDA glutamate receptor antagonist, ketamine, on working memory by pretreatment with the group II metabotropic glutamate receptor agonist, LY354740, in healthy human subjects. Psychopharmacology 2005;179:303–309.

[65] Large CH. Do NMDA receptor antagonist models of schizophrenia predict the clinical efficacy of antipsychotic drugs? J Psychopharmacol 2007;21:283–301.

[66] Yu H, Li Q, Wang D, Shi L, Lu G, Sun L, et al. Mapping the central effects of chronic ketamine administration in an adolescent primate model by functional magnetic resonance imaging (fMRI). Neurotoxicology 2012;33:70–77.

[67] Chin CL, Upadhyay J, Marek GJ, Baker SJ, Zhang M, Mezler M, et al. Awake rat pharmacological magnetic resonance imaging as a translational pharmacodynamic biomarker: metabotropic glutamate 2/3 agonist modulation of ketamine-induced blood oxygenation level dependence signals. J Pharmacol Exp Ther 2011;336:709–715.

[68] Gozzi A, Large CH, Schwarz A, Bertani S, Crestan V, Bifone A. Differential effects of antipsychotic and glutamatergic agents on the phMRI response to phencyclidine. Neuropsychopharmacology 2008;33:1690–1703.

[69] Xiao F, Koepp MJ, Zhou D. Pharmaco-fMRI: A tool to predict the response to antiepileptic drugs in epilepsy. Front Neurol 2019;10:1203. https://doi.org/10.3389/fneur.2019.01203.

[70] Duff EP, Vennart W, Wise RG, Howard MA, Harris RE, Lee M, et al. Learning to identify CNS drug action and efficacy using multistudy fMRI data. Sci Transl Med 2015;7. https://doi.org/10.1126/scitranslmed.3008438. 274ra216.

[71] Gear R, Becerra L, Upadhyay J, Bishop J, Wallin D, Pendse G, et al. Pain facilitation brain regions activated by nalbuphine are revealed by pharmacological fMRI. PLoS One 2013;8. https://doi.org/10.1371/journal.pone.0050169.

[72] Liu CH, Greve DN, Dai G, Marota JJ, Mandeville JB. Remifentanil administration reveals biphasic phMRI temporal responses in rat consistent with dynamic receptor regulation. NeuroImage 2007;34:1042–1053.

[73] Upadhyay J, Anderson J, Schwarz AJ, Coimbra A, Baumgartner R, Pendse G, et al. Imaging drugs with and without clinical analgesic efficacy. Neuropsychopharmacology 2011;36:2659–2673.

[74] Wager TD, Atlas LY, Lindquist MA, Roy M, Woo CW, Kross E. An fMRI-based neurologic signature of physical pain. N Engl J Med 2013;368:1388–1397.

[75] Sarpal DK, Robinson DG, Lencz T, Argyelan M, Ikuta T, Karlsgodt K, et al. Antipsychotic treatment and functional connectivity of the striatum in first-episode schizophrenia. JAMA Psychiatry 2015;72:5–13.

[76] Risacher SL, Wang Y, Wishart HA, Rabin LA, Flashman LA, McDonald BC, et al. Cholinergic enhancement of brain activation in mild cognitive impairment during episodic memory encoding. Front Psychiatry 2013;4:105. https://doi.org/10.3389/fpsyt.2013.00105.

[77] Breiter HC, Gollub RL, Weisskoff RM, Kennedy DN, Makris N, Berke JD, et al. Acute effects of cocaine on human brain activity and emotion. Neuron 1997;19:591–611.

[78] Stein EA, Pankiewicz J, Harsch HH, Cho JK, Fuller SA, Hoffmann RG, et al. Nicotine-induced limbic cortical activation in the human brain: a functional MRI study. Am J Psychiatry 1998;155:1009–1015.

[79] Governo RJ, Morris PG, Marsden CA, Chapman V. Gabapentin evoked changes in functional activity in nociceptive regions in the brain of the anaesthetized rat: an fMRI study. Br J Pharmacol 2008;153:1558–1567.

[80] Hooker BA, Tobon G, Baker SJ, Zhu C, Hesterman J, Schmidt K, et al. Gabapentin-induced pharmacodynamic effects in the spinal nerve ligation model of neuropathic pain. Eur J Pain 2014;18:223–237.

[81] Upadhyay J, Baker SJ, Rajagovindan R, Hart M, Chandran P, Hooker BA, et al. Pharmacological modulation of brain activity in a preclinical model of osteoarthritis. NeuroImage 2013;64:341–355.

[82] Baker S, Chin CL, Basso AM, Fox GB, Marek GJ, Day M. Xanomeline modulation of the blood oxygenation level-dependent signal in awake rats: development of pharmacological magnetic resonance imaging as a translatable pharmacodynamic biomarker for central activity and dose selection. J Pharmacol Exp Ther 2012;341:263–273.

[83] Byun NE, Grannan M, Bubser M, Barry RL, Thompson A, Rosanelli J, et al. Antipsychotic drug-like effects of the selective M4 muscarinic acetylcholine receptor positive allosteric modulator VU0152100. Neuropsychopharmacology 2014;39:1578–1593.

[84] Kocsis P, Gyertyán I, Éles J, Laszy J, Hegedűs N, Gajári D, et al. Vascular action as the primary mechanism of cognitive effects of cholinergic, CNS-acting drugs, a rat phMRI BOLD study. J Cereb Blood Flow Metab 2014;34:995–1000.

[85] Berginström N, Nordström P, Ekman U, Eriksson J, Nyberg L, Nordström A. Pharmaco-fMRI in patients with traumatic brain injury: a randomized controlled trial with the monoaminergic stabilizer (–)-OSU6162. J Head Trauma Rehabil 2019;34:189–198.

[86] Rech J, Hess A, Finzel S, Kreitz S, Sergeeva M, Englbrecht M, et al. Association of brain functional magnetic resonance activity with response to tumor necrosis factor inhibition in rheumatoid arthritis. Arthritis Rheum 2013;65:325–333.

[87] Cole DM, Beckmann CF, Oei NY, Both S, van Gerven JM, Rombouts SA. Differential and distributed effects of dopamine neuromodulations on resting-state network connectivity. NeuroImage 2013;78:59–67.

[88] Gass N, Schwarz AJ, Sartorius A, Cleppien D, Zheng L, Schenker E, et al. Haloperidol modulates midbrain-prefrontal functional connectivity in the rat brain. Eur Neuropsychopharmacol 2013;23:1310–1319.

[89] Gass N, Schwarz AJ, Sartorius A, Schenker E, Risterucci C, Spedding M, et al. Sub-anesthetic ketamine modulates intrinsic BOLD connectivity within the hippocampal-prefrontal circuit in the rat. Neuropsychopharmacology 2014;39:895–906.

[90] Grimm O, Gass N, Weber-Fahr W, Sartorius A, Schenker E, Spedding M, et al. Acute ketamine challenge increases resting state prefrontal-hippocampal connectivity in both humans and rats. Psychopharmacology 2015;232:4231–4241.

[91] Kelly C, de Zubicaray G, Di Martino A, Copland DA, Reiss PT, Klein DF, et al. L-dopa modulates functional connectivity in striatal cognitive and motor networks: a double-blind placebo-controlled study. J Neurosci 2009;29:7364–7378.

[92] Khalili-Mahani N, Zoethout RM, Beckmann CF, Baerends E, de Kam ML, Soeter RP, et al. Effects of morphine and alcohol on functional brain connectivity during "resting state": a placebo-controlled crossover study in healthy young men. Hum Brain Mapp 2012;33:1003–1018.

[93] Inglis B. A checklist for fMRI acquisition methods reporting in the literature, Winnower 2015;3. https://doi.org/10.15200/winn.143191.17127. e143191.17127. Published May 17, 2015. Internet at https://pdfs.semanticscholar.org/43f8/c3d86b93c0caad26b1b876cf6832fc43a75c.pdf?_ga=2.262343372.1385639421.1602425936-466399296.1602425936.

[94] Glasser MF, Sotiropoulos SN, Wilson JA, Coalson TS, Fischl B, Andersson JL, et al. The minimal preprocessing pipelines for the human connectome project. NeuroImage 2013;80:105–124.

[95] Poldrack RA, Fletcher PC, Henson RN, Worsley KJ, Brett M, Nichols TE. Guidelines for reporting an fMRI study. NeuroImage 2008;40:409–414.

[96] Van Dijk KR, Hedden T, Venkataraman A, Evans KC, Lazar SW, Buckner RL. Intrinsic functional connectivity as a tool for human connectomics: theory, properties, and optimization. J Neurophysiol 2010;103:297–321.
[97] Carp J. On the plurality of (methodological) worlds: estimating the analytic flexibility of fMRI experiments. Front Neurosci 2012;6:149. https://doi.org/10.3389/fnins.2012.00149.
[98] Gelman A, Loken E. The garden of forking paths: why multiple comparisons can be a problem, even when there is no "fishing expedition" or "p-hacking" and the research hypothesis was posited ahead of time. Department of Statistics, Columbia University; 2013.
[99] Bullmore E, Sporns O. Complex brain networks: graph theoretical analysis of structural and functional systems. Nat Rev Neurosci 2009;10:186–198.
[100] Karwowski W, Vasheghani Farahani F, Lighthall N. Application of graph theory for identifying connectivity patterns in human brain networks: a systematic review. Front Neurosci 2019;13:585. https://doi.org/10.3389/fnins.2019.00585.
[101] Calhoun VD, Liu J, Adalı T. A review of group ICA for fMRI data and ICA for joint inference of imaging, genetic, and ERP data. NeuroImage 2009;45:S163–S172.
[102] Morioka H, Calhoun V, Hyvärinen A. Nonlinear ICA of fMRI reveals primitive temporal structures linked to rest, task, and behavioral traits. NeuroImage 2020. https://doi.org/10.1016/j.neuroimage.2020.116989. 116989.
[103] Poldrack RA. Region of interest analysis for fMRI. Soc Cog Affect Neurosci 2007;2:67–70.
[104] Bhagwat N, Pipitone J, Voineskos AN. Chakravarty MM; Alzheimer's disease neuroimaging initiative. An artificial neural network model for clinical score prediction in Alzheimer disease using structural neuroimaging measures. J Psychiatry Neurosci 2019;44:246–260.
[105] Borsook D, Hargreaves RJ, Becerra L. Can functional magnetic resonance imaging improve success rates in central nervous system drug discovery? Expert Opin Drug Discovery 2011;6:597–617.
[106] Sheth SA, Nemoto M, Guiou M, Walker M, Pouratian N, Toga AW. Linear and nonlinear relationships between neuronal activity, oxygen metabolism, and hemodynamic responses. Neuron 2004;42:347–355.
[107] Gauthier CJ, Fan AP. BOLD signal physiology: models and applications. NeuroImage 2019;187:116–127.
[108] Amunts K, Zilles K. Advances in cytoarchitectonic mapping of the human cerebral cortex. Neuroimaging Clin N Am 2001;11:151–169 vii.
[109] Ogawa S, Menon R, Tank D, Kim SG, Merkle H, Ellermann JM, et al. Functional brain mapping by blood oxygenation level-dependent contrast magnetic resonance imaging. A comparison of signal characteristics with a biophysical model. Biophys J 1993;64:803–812.
[110] Toga AW, editor. Brain mapping: an encyclopedic reference. 1st ed. London: Academic Press; 2015.
[111] Wohlschläger AM, Specht K, Lie C, Wohlschläger A, Bente K, Pietrzyk U, et al. Linking retinotopic fMRI mapping and anatomical probability maps of human occipital areas V1 and V2. NeuroImage 2005;26:73–82.
[112] Zilles K, Palomero-Gallagher N, Amunts K. Cytoarchitecture and maps of the human cerebral cortex. In: Brain mapping. San Diego, CA: Elsevier; 2015. p. 115–135.
[113] Lu H, Jaime S, Yang Y. Origins of the resting-state functional MRI signal: potential limitations of the "neurocentric" model. Front Neurosci 2019;13. https://doi.org/10.3389/fnins.2019.01136.
[114] Mathiesen C, Caesar K, Akgoren N, Lauritzen M. Modification of activity-dependent increases of cerebral blood flow by excitatory synaptic activity and spikes in rat cerebellar cortex. J Physiol 1998;512(Pt 2):555–566.
[115] Shmuel A, Grinvald A. Functional organization for direction of motion and its relationship to orientation maps in cat area 18. J Neurosci 1996;16:6945–6964.
[116] Shulman RG, Rothman DL, Behar KL, Hyder F. Energetic basis of brain activity: implications for neuroimaging. Trends Neurosci 2004;27:489–495.
[117] Smith AJ, Blumenfeld H, Behar KL, Rothman DL, Shulman RG, Hyder F. Cerebral energetics and spiking frequency: the neurophysiological basis of fMRI. Proc Natl Acad Sci U S A 2002;99:10765–10770.
[118] Ances B, Vaida F, Ellis R, Buxton R. Test–retest stability of calibrated BOLD-fMRI in HIV– and HIV+ subjects. NeuroImage 2011;54:215662.
[119] Goodwin JA, Vidyasagar R, Balanos GM, Bulte D, Parkes LM. Quantitative fMRI using hyperoxia calibration: reproducibility during a cognitive Stroop task. NeuroImage 2009;47:573–580.
[120] Leontiev O, Buxton RB. Reproducibility of BOLD, perfusion, and CMRO 2 measurements with calibrated-BOLD fMRI. NeuroImage 2007;35:175–184.
[121] Wey H-Y, Wang DJ, Duong TQ. Baseline CBF, and BOLD, CBF, and CMRO2 fMRI of visual and vibrotactile stimulations in baboons. J Cereb Blood Flow Metab 2011;31:715–724.
[122] He X, Yablonskiy DA. Quantitative BOLD: mapping of human cerebral deoxygenated blood volume and oxygen extraction fraction: default state. Magn Reson Med 2007;57(1):115–126.
[123] Lu H, Ge Y. Quantitative evaluation of oxygenation in venous vessels using T2-relaxation-under-spin-tagging MRI. Magn Reson Med 2008;60:357–363.
[124] Bolar DS, Rosen BR, Sorensen A, Adalsteinsson E. Quantitative imaging of extraction of oxygen and tissue consumption (QUIXOTIC) using venular-targeted velocity-selective spin labeling. Magn Reson Med 2011;66:1550–1562.
[125] Yablonskiy DA, Sukstanskii AL, He X. Blood oxygenation level-dependent (BOLD)-based techniques for the quantification of brain hemodynamic and metabolic properties–theoretical models and experimental approaches. NMR Biomed 2013;26:963–986.
[126] Wehrl HF, Hossain M, Lankes K, Liu CC, Bezrukov I, Martirosian P, et al. Simultaneous PET-MRI reveals brain function in activated and resting state on metabolic, hemodynamic and multiple temporal scales. Nat Med 2013;19:1184–1189.
[127] De Simoni S, Schwarz AJ, O'Daly OG, Marquand AF, Brittain C, Gonzales C, et al. Test–retest reliability of the BOLD pharmacological MRI response to ketamine in healthy volunteers. NeuroImage 2013;64:75–90.

[128] Leppä M, Korvenoja A, Carlson S, Timonen P, Martinkauppi S, Ahonen J, et al. Acute opioid effects on human brain as revealed by functional magnetic resonance imaging. NeuroImage 2006;31:661–669.

[129] McKie S, Richardson P, Elliott R, Völlm BA, Dolan MC, Williams SR, et al. Mirtazapine antagonises the subjective, hormonal and neuronal effects of m-chlorophenylpiperazine (mCPP) infusion: a pharmacological-challenge fMRI (phMRI) study. NeuroImage 2011;58:497–507.

[130] Völlm BA, de Araujo IE, Cowen PJ, Rolls ET, Kringelbach ML, Smith KA, et al. Methamphetamine activates reward circuitry in drug naive human subjects. Neuropsychopharmacology 2004;29:1715–1722.

[131] Wise RG, Williams P, Tracey I. Using fMRI to quantify the time dependence of remifentanil analgesia in the human brain. Neuropsychopharmacology 2004;29:626–635.

[132] Chen Y, Wan HI, O'Reardon JP, Wang DJ, Wang Z, Korczykowski M, et al. Quantification of cerebral blood flow as biomarker of drug effect: arterial spin labeling phMRI after a single dose of oral citalopram. Clin Pharmacol Ther 2011;89:251–258.

[133] Bruns A, Kunnecke B, Risterucci C, Moreau JL, von Kienlin M. Validation of cerebral blood perfusion imaging as a modality for quantitative pharmacological MRI in rats. Magn Reson Med 2009;61:1451–1458.

Chapter 19

Dose-effect and concentration-effect analysis

Jiang Liu[a], Justin C. Earp[a], Juan J.L. Lertora[b,c], and Yaning Wang[a]

[a]*Office of Clinical Pharmacology, Office of Translational Sciences, Center for Drug Evaluation and Research, US Food and Drug Administration, Silver Spring, MD, United States,* [b]*Adjunct Professor, Division of Clinical Research, Pennington Biomedical Research Center, Louisiana State University, Baton Rouge, LA, United States,* [c]*Adjunct Professor, Department of Medicine, Duke University School of Medicine, Durham, NC, United States*

Background

The intensity and duration of a drug's pharmacological effect are proportional to the dose of the drug administered and the concentration of the drug at its site of action. This simple fundamental principle of pharmacology has a pervasive influence on our approach to the study and use of drugs, from the basic research laboratory to the management of patients receiving drug therapy in the clinic. *Pharmacodynamics* is the discipline that quantifies the relationship between drug concentration at the site of drug action and the drug's pharmacological effect. A drug's pharmacological effect can be monitored and quantified at several levels, including at a molecular or cellular level in vitro, in a tissue or organ in vitro or in vivo, or in the whole organism (Table 19.1). The endpoint that is used to measure effect may differ at each level even for the same drug, and at the organism level the overall pharmacological effect may be the sum of multiple drug effects and the physiologic response of the organism to these drug effects.

When the drug-effect endpoint, such as change in blood pressure, is measured on a continuous scale, the dose-effect relationship is termed *graded*, whereas an all-or-none endpoint, such as alive or dead, results in a dose-effect relationship that is *quantal*. Graded dose-effect relationships can be measured in a single biological unit that is exposed to a range of doses, and dose or drug concentration is related to the *intensity* of the effect. Quantal dose-effect relationships are measured in a population of subjects that are treated with a range of doses, and the dose is related to the *frequency* of the all-or-none effect at each dose level.

Fig. 19.1 illustrates a graded dose-effect relationship for recombinant human erythropoietin (rhEPO) in patients with end-stage renal disease [1]. Erythropoietin, which is produced by the kidney in response to hypoxia, is a naturally occurring hematopoietic growth factor that stimulates bone marrow production of erythrocytes. Patients with end-stage renal disease are deficient in erythropoietin, and, as a result, they are usually severely anemic and transfusion dependent. Fig. 19.1 is based on the results of a dose-finding study in which 18 patients with end-stage renal disease and baseline hematocrit <20% were treated with rhEPO at doses ranging from 1.5 to 500 units/kg in cohorts of 3–5 patients per dose level [1]. The effect of the rhEPO is measured as the peak absolute increment in the hematocrit. At the lowest dose levels (1.5 and 5 units/kg) there was no effect on hematocrit, but starting at a dose of 15 units/kg the hematocrit increased by 4%–22% as the rhEPO dose increased. The shape of the dose-effect curve is a rectangular hyperbola, which asymptotically approaches a maximum effect. This means that there is a "diminishing return" at higher doses because the incremental increase in hematocrit is smaller with each incremental increase in rhEPO dose.

Drug-receptor interactions

The pharmacological effects of rhEPO and most drugs result from their noncovalent interaction with *receptors* (Fig. 19.2). A receptor can be any cellular macromolecule to which a drug selectively binds to initiate its pharmacological effect. Cellular proteins are the most important class of drug receptors, especially cellular proteins that are receptors for endogenous regulatory ligands, such as hormones, growth factors, and neurotransmitters. The drug's chemical structure is the primary determinant of the class of receptors with which it will interact. Receptors on the cell surface have two functional domains—a *ligand-binding domain*, which is the drug-binding site, and an *effector domain*, which propagates a

Atkinson's Principles of Clinical Pharmacology. https://doi.org/10.1016/B978-0-12-819869-8.00039-2

TABLE 19.1 Endpoints for measuring drug effect at different levels for the new class of molecularly targeted anticancer drugs that inhibit farnesyl protein transferase.

Level	Endpoint
Molecular	Inhibition of farnesyl protein transferase, farnesylation of target substrate proteins such as HDJ2
Cellular	Inhibition of cellular proliferation in vitro induction of apoptosis
Tissue	Change in the size of measurable tumors
Organism	Prolonged survival reduction in tumor-related symptoms enhanced quality of life

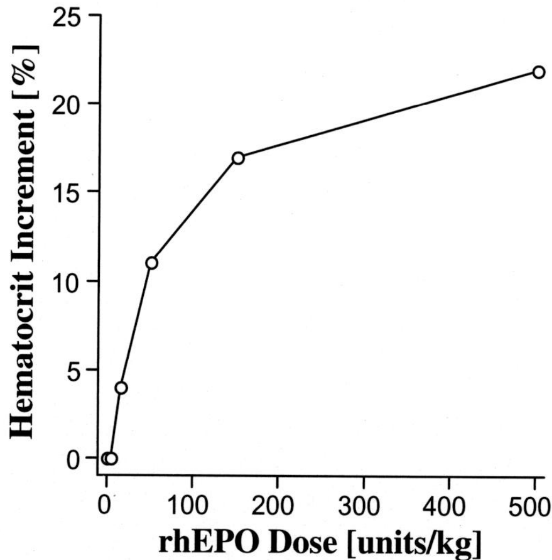

FIG. 19.1 Dose-effect curve for recombinant human erythropoietin in patients with end-stage renal disease. Each point represents the mean absolute increase in hematocrit in a cohort of three to five patients. *(Adapted from data published by Eschbach JW, Egrie JC, Downing MR, Browne JK, Adamson JW. Correction of the anemia of end-stage renal disease with recombinant human erythropoietin: results of a combined phase I and II clinical trial. N Engl J Med 1987;316:73–78.)*

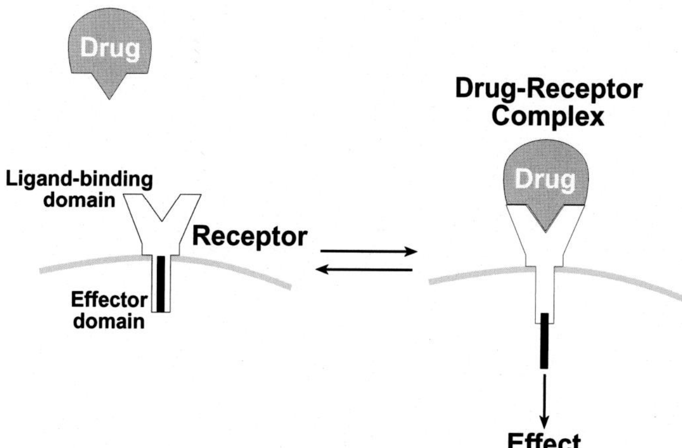

FIG. 19.2 Drug-receptor interaction. A drug molecule binds reversibly to the ligand-binding domain of a receptor on the cell surface and the receptor propagates the signal into the cell via its effector domain, resulting in a pharmacological effect.

signal and results in an effect (Fig. 19.2). The interaction of a drug and its receptor is reversible and conforms to the *law of mass action*:

$$C + R \underset{k_2}{\overset{k_1}{\rightleftharpoons}} C - R \tag{19.1}$$

where C is the free drug concentration at the site of action, R is the concentration of unoccupied receptor in tissue, $C - R$ is the concentration of receptors occupied by drug, and k_1 and k_2 are the proportionality constants for the formation and dissociation of the drug-receptor complex.

Receptor occupation theory

The receptor *occupation theory* of drug action equates drug effect to receptor occupancy. The *intensity* of drug effect is proportional to the number of receptors that are occupied by drug and the *maximum* effect occurs when all receptors are occupied by drug. The relationship between drug effect and the concentration of free drug at the site of action (C) can be described at equilibrium by the following equation:

$$\text{Effect} = \frac{\text{Maximum Effect} \cdot C}{K_D + C} \tag{19.2}$$

where Maximum Effect is the intensity of the pharmacological effect that occurs when all of the receptors are occupied, and K_D, which equals k_2/k_1 (see Eq. 19.1), is the equilibrium dissociation constant of the drug-receptor complex. The dissociation constant (K_D) is also a measure of the *affinity* of a drug for its receptor, analogous to the Michaelis-Menten constant (K_m), which is a measure of the affinity of a substrate for its enzyme. The expression C/K_D+C in Eq. 19.2 represents the fraction of receptors that are occupied with drug. When $C \gg K_D$, the expression equals 1 (i.e., all of the receptors are occupied with drug), and the Effect = Maximum Effect.

In relating a drug's pharmacological effect to its concentration, Eq. 19.2 describes a hyperbolic function that is shown graphically in Fig. 19.3A. As free drug concentration increases, the drug effect asymptotically approaches the maximum effect. When the free drug concentration on the *x*-axis is transformed to a logarithmic scale, the dose-effect curve becomes sigmoidal, with a central segment that is nearly log-linear (Fig. 19.3B). Semilogarithmic dose-effect curves allow for a better assessment of the dose-effect relationship at low doses and of a wide range of higher doses on the same plot. The EC_{50} is the dose at which 50% of the maximum effect is produced or the concentration of drug at which the drug is half-maximally effective. On a semilogarithmic plot, the EC_{50} is located at the midpoint or inflection point of the curve. When the relationship between receptor occupancy and effect is linear, $K_D = EC_{50}$. If there is amplification between receptor occupancy and effect, such as if the receptor has catalytic activity when the ligand is bound to the receptor, then the EC_{50} lies to the left of the K_D.

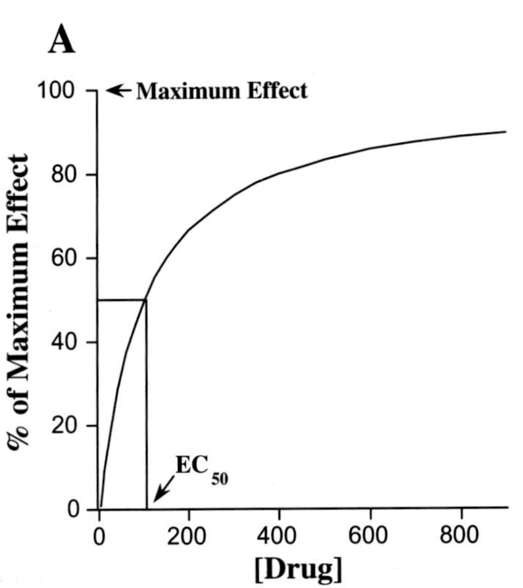

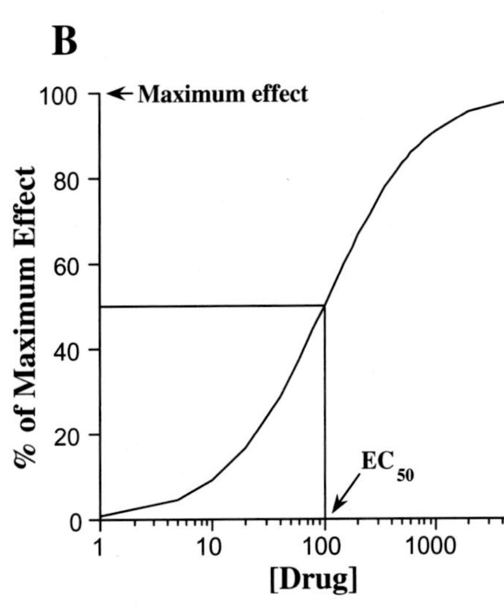

FIG. 19.3 Dose-effect curves plotted using a (A) linear or (B) logarithmic scale for drug dose/concentration on the *x*-axis. The function relating effect to dose/concentration is based on the receptor occupation theory described in the text. The relationship is nonlinear, and with each increment in dose/concentration there is diminishing increment in effect. EC_{50} is the dose/concentration producing half of the maximum effect.

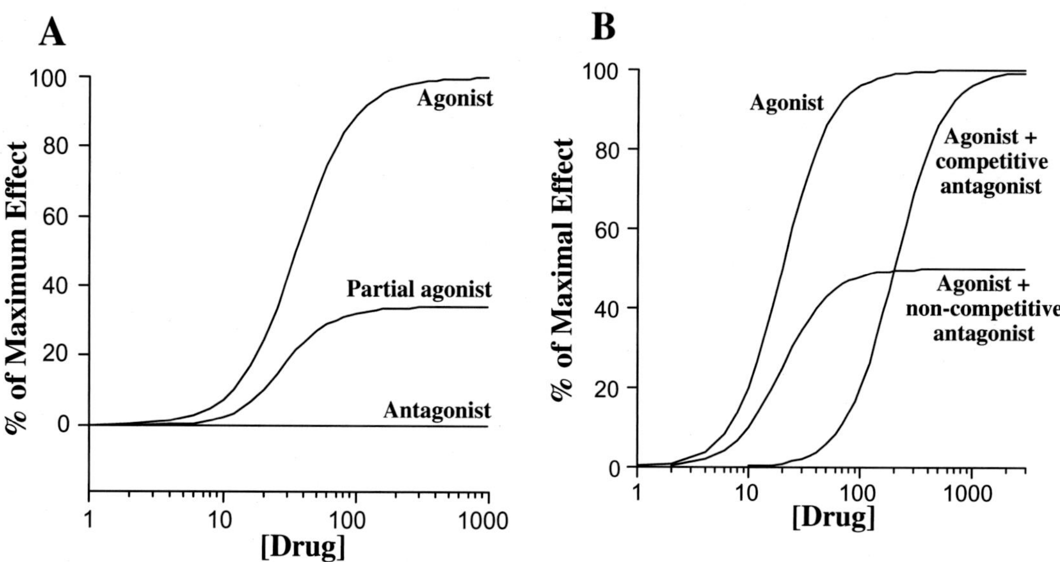

FIG. 19.4 (A) Dose-effect curves describing the types of pharmacological effects produced when a drug interacts with its receptor. An *agonist* produces the maximum stimulatory effect, a *partial agonist* produces less than the maximum stimulatory effect, and an *antagonist* elicits no effect but inhibits the effect of an agonist. (B) Dose-effect curves for the combination of an agonist and antagonist. A competitive antagonist reduces the potency of the agonist but not the maximum effect. A noncompetitive antagonist reduces the efficacy (maximum effect) but does not alter the potency of the agonist.

Receptor-mediated effects

Fig. 19.4A shows dose-effect curves for the types of pharmacological effects that can be elicited when a drug interacts with its receptor. Drugs that interact with a receptor and elicit the same stimulatory effect as the receptor's endogenous ligand are called *agonists*. An agonist that produces less than the maximum effect at doses or concentrations that saturate the receptor is a *partial agonist*. An *antagonist* binds to a receptor but produces no effect. Antagonists produce their pharmacological effects by inhibiting the action of an agonist that binds to the same receptor.

Dose-effect curves are also useful for studying pharmacodynamic drug interactions (Fig. 19.4B). A *competitive antagonist* binds to the same binding site as does the agonist, and the competitive antagonist can be displaced from the binding site by an excess of the agonist. Therefore the maximum effect of an agonist can still be achieved in the presence of a competitive antagonist, if a sufficient dose or concentration of the agonist is used. The competitive antagonist lowers the potency of the agonist but does not alter its efficacy. A *noncompetitive antagonist* binds irreversibly to the same binding site as does the agonist, or it interacts with other components of the receptor to diminish or eliminate the effect of the drug binding to the receptor. A noncompetitive antagonist prevents the agonist, at any concentration, from producing its maximum effect. Typically, a dose-effect curve with this type of interaction will reveal a reduced apparent efficacy, but the potency of the drug is unchanged.

The graded dose-effect relationship

The drug-receptor concept of drug action and the receptor occupation theory describe a graded dose-effect relationship as one in which the responding system is capable of showing progressively increasing effect with increasing dose or drug concentration. Graded dose-effect relationships are measured by exposing a single subject or a specific organ or tissue to increasing amounts of drug and quantifying the resulting effect on a continuous scale. Although the dose-effect curve can take on a variety of shapes, the classical graded dose-effect curve is the rectangular hyperbola that was described previously (Fig. 19.3A).

Fig. 19.5 demonstrates a graded concentration-effect study of an intravenous infusion of lidocaine at a rate of 8.35 mg/min in patients with neuropathic pain [2]. The severity of pain was measured at 10-min intervals using a visual analog pain scale, and blood levels of lidocaine were also measured at 10-min intervals. Patients had a median pain score of 7 prior to the initiation of therapy, and the maximal effect, no pain, had a score of 0. The concentration-effect curve for

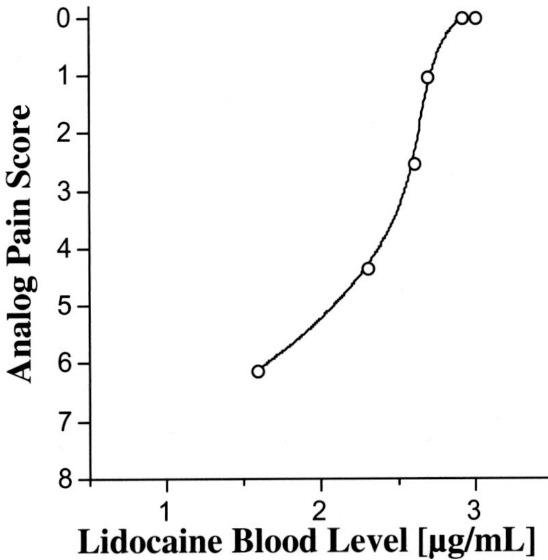

FIG. 19.5 Graded concentration-effect curve for intravenous lidocaine in patients with neuropathic pain. Pain was scored from 0 to 10 with an analog pain scale. The median pretreatment pain score was 7 and a score of 0 meant no pain. Blood levels of lidocaine were measured every 10 min, and pain was scored at the same time points. The graph relates the blood level of lidocaine to the severity of pain. *(Adapted from data published by Ferrante FM, Paggioli J, Cherukuri S, Arthur GR. The analgesic response to intravenous lidocaine in the treatment of neuropathic pain. Anesth Analg 1996;82:91–97.)*

lidocaine is very steep. The pain decreased over a concentration range of 0.62 μg/mL. This steep concentration-effect curve indicates that the response to intravenous lidocaine is characterized by a precipitous break in pain over a narrow range in lidocaine concentrations.

Fig. 19.6 demonstrates a typical example of a graded dose-effect curve from a study that evaluated the dose-effect relationship for the antihyperglycemic agent metformin. Metformin lowers blood glucose concentrations by increasing insulin sensitivity in peripheral tissues and inhibiting hepatic glucose production. Patients with a fasting plasma glucose (FPG) exceeding 180 mg/dL were randomized to receive either a placebo or metformin at 1 of 5 escalating doses ranging from 500 to 2500 mg/day [3]. The monitored endpoints of the study included FPG and levels of glycosylated hemoglobin (HbA_{1c}), a biomarker for chronic hyperglycemia. At the end of the study, FPG had declined by 19–84 mg/dL and HbA_{1c}

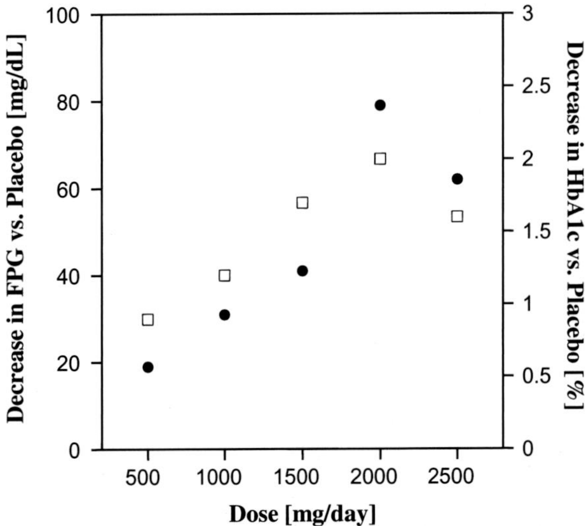

FIG. 19.6 Graded dose-effect curves for the oral antihyperglycemic agent, metformin, relative to a placebo in patients with a fasting plasma glucose (FPG) exceeding 180 mg/dL. Reductions in FPG (●) and HbA_{1c} (□) occurred in a dose-dependent manner. *(Adapted from data published by Garber AJ, Duncan TG, Goodman AM, Mills DJ, Rohlf JL. Efficacy of metformin in type II diabetes: results of a double-blind, placebo-controlled, dose-response trial. Am J Med 1997;102:491–497.)*

had declined by 0.6%–2.0% in patients receiving metformin compared to placebo. Predictably, the decreases in FPG and HbA_{1c} were disproportionate due to the slow turnover of hemoglobin. Metformin reduced both FPG and HbA_{1c} in a dose-related fashion, with the maximum effect on both endpoints occurring at the upper limits of the dose range (2000 mg). The minimum effective dose was found to be 500 mg/day rather than 1500 mg/day, as was previously thought. This allowed metformin therapy in subsequent clinical practice to be started at 500 mg/day with an upward dose titration above this minimum only if needed to achieve the target effect.

Dose-effect parameters

Potency and *efficacy* are parameters that are derived from graded dose-effect curves and that can be used to compare drugs that elicit the same pharmacological effect. Potency, which is a measure of the sensitivity of a target organ or tissue to a drug, is a relative term that relates the amount of one drug required to produce a desired level of effect to the amount of a different drug required to produce the same effect. On a semilogarithmic graded dose-effect plot, the curve of the more potent agent is to the left, and the EC_{50} is lower. A drug's potency is influenced by its affinity for its receptor. In Fig. 19.7, Drug A is more potent than Drug B.

Fig. 19.8 shows the in vitro dose-effect curves for two thiopurine analogs, thioguanine (TG) and mercaptopurine (MP). The thiopurines are antimetabolites that are used in the treatment of acute leukemia. Both drugs have multiple sites of action, but their primary mechanism of action is felt to be the result of their incorporation into DNA strands. Effect is measured in vitro as the percentage of leukemic cells killed in the presence of drug compared to untreated controls for three different leukemic cell lines [4]. The dose-effect curves show that TG is approximately 10-fold more potent than MP, despite the fact that they both have very similar chemical structures and are converted to the same active intracellular metabolite (deoxy-thioguanosine triphosphate) prior to their incorporation into DNA. The two drugs appear to have similar efficacy in this in vitro study. Considerable weight is placed on these in vitro concentration-effect studies for anticancer drugs because it has not been possible to define therapeutic concentrations in vivo in either animal models or patients.

Efficacy is the drug property that allows the receptor-bound drug to produce its pharmacological effect. The relative efficacy of two drugs that elicit the same effect can be measured by comparing the maximum effects of the drugs. In Fig. 19.7, Drugs A and B are more efficacious than is Drug C. *Intrinsic activity* (α), which is a proportionality factor that relates drug effect in a specific tissue to receptor occupancy, has become a standard parameter for quantifying the ability of a drug to produce a response:

$$\text{Effect} = \alpha \cdot \left(\frac{\text{Maximum Effect} \cdot \text{Dose}}{K_D + \text{Dose}}\right) \tag{19.3}$$

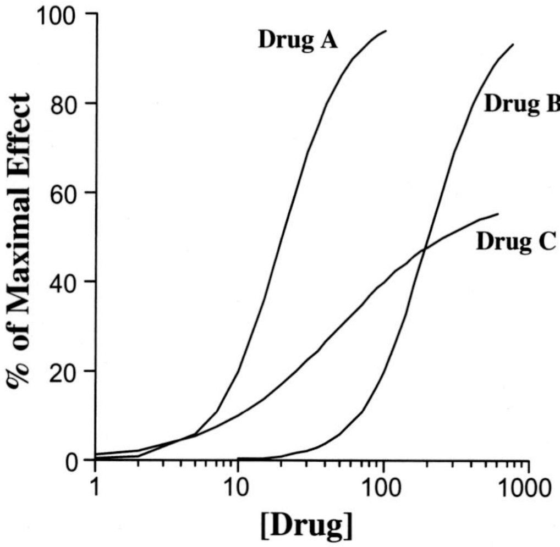

FIG. 19.7 Evaluation of the relative potency and efficacy of drugs that produce the same pharmacological effect. Drug A is more potent than Drug B although both have a similar maximum effect. On the other hand, drugs A and B are more efficacious than Drug C which has a lower maximum effect.

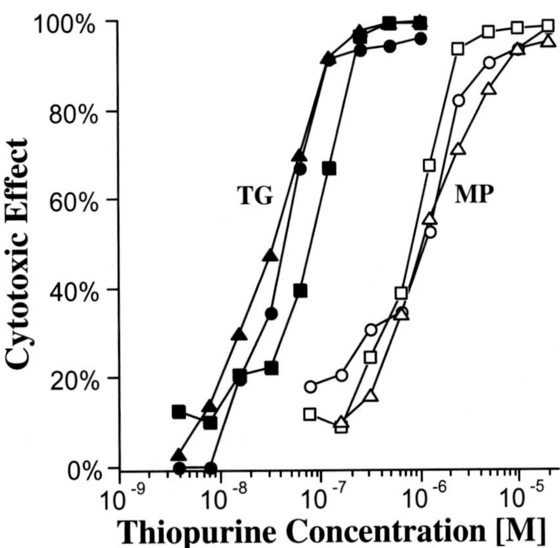

FIG. 19.8 Concentration-effect curves for the thiopurine analogs, mercaptopurine (MP, *open symbols*) and thioguanine (TG, *closed symbols*). Effect is the percentage of cells killed in vitro relative to an untreated control in MOLT 4 (*squares*), CCRF-CEM (*triangles*), and Wilson (*circles*) leukemia cell lines. TG is 10-fold more potent than is MP. *(Reproduced with permission from Adamson PC, Poplack DG, Balis FM. The cytotoxicity of thioguanine vs mercaptopurine in acute lymphoblastic leukemia. Leuk Res 1994;18:805–810.)*

The value for intrinsic activity ranges from 1 for a full agonist to 0 for an antagonist, and the fractional values between these extremes represent partial agonists. Intrinsic activity is a property of both the drug and the tissue in which drug effect is measured.

Comparing the dose-effect curves of drugs that produce the same pharmacological effect can also provide information about the site of action of the drugs. Drugs A and B in Fig. 19.7 have parallel dose-effect curves with identical shapes and the same level of maximal response. This suggests, but does not prove, that these two drugs act through the same receptor. Conversely, Drugs A and C have nonparallel dose-response curves, suggesting that they have different sites of action.

Dose effect and site of drug action

Graded concentration-effect studies may be useful for establishing the mechanism of action of a drug at a molecular or biochemical level by assessing the drug-receptor interaction. The xanthine analog, theophylline, which is a potent relaxant of bronchial smooth muscle, is used for the treatment of asthma. However, theophylline has a narrow therapeutic range, and at concentrations above this therapeutic range patients can experience vomiting, tremor, seizures, and cardiac arrhythmias. Theophylline interacts with multiple receptors that could account for its antiasthmatic effect and its toxicity. Theophylline is an adenosine receptor antagonist and it inhibits phosphodiesterase (PDE). These two mechanisms have been proposed as the basis for the antiasthmatic effects of theophylline and other xanthines.

In Fig. 19.9, the concentration of theophylline and a series of xanthine analogs that is required to elicit in vitro relaxation of tracheal smooth muscle in isolated guinea pig tracheal segments is related to the drug concentrations required to antagonize the A_1-adenosine receptor (Fig. 19.9A) or to inhibit brain-soluble PDE (Fig. 19.9B) [5]. The relative potency of these xanthine analogs as adenosine receptor antagonists does not correlate with their potencies as tracheal relaxants. However, there is an association between PDE inhibition and tracheal relaxant activity, suggesting that PDE inhibition is the primary mechanism of drug action. This type of graded concentration-effect analysis can lead to the development of more selective agents. This case demonstrates the possibility that xanthine analogs that are more potent PDE inhibitors and weaker adenosine receptor antagonists may be more effective and less toxic antiasthmatics.

The quantal dose-effect relationship

Whereas a graded dose-effect relationship relates drug dose and concentration to the intensity of a drug's effect that is measured on a continuous scale in a single biological unit, the *quantal* dose-effect relationship relates dose to the frequency of an all-or-none effect in a population of individuals. The minimally effective dose, or *threshold dose*, of the drug that evokes the all-or-none effect is identified by gradually increasing the dose in each subject. When displayed graphically

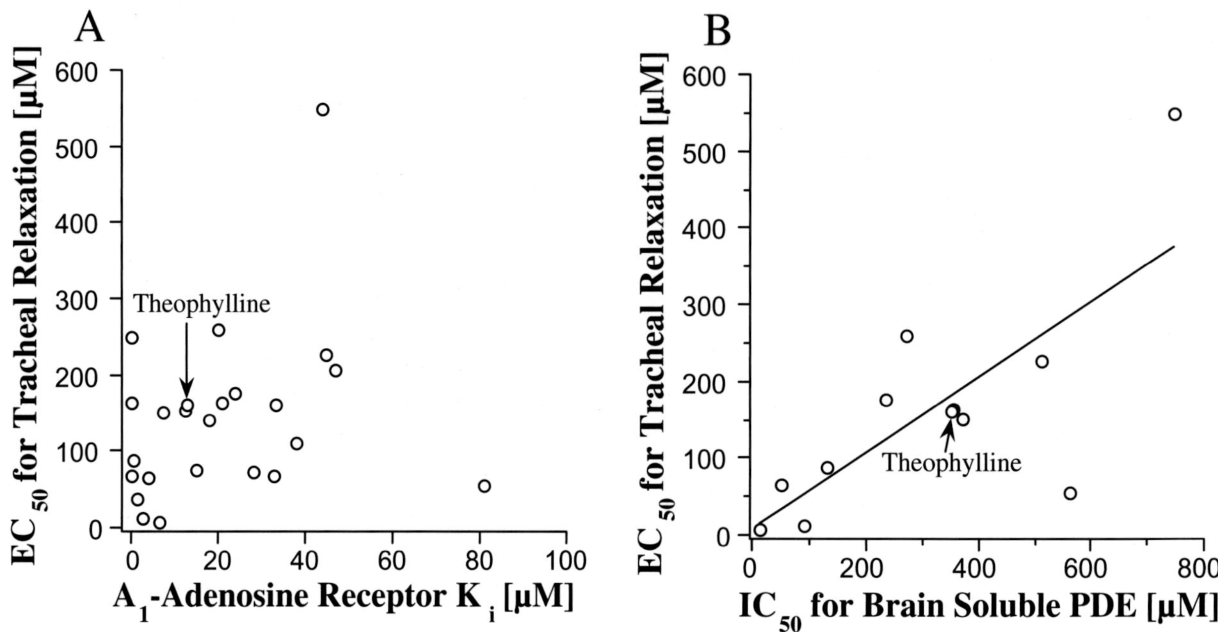

FIG. 19.9 Correlation between concentration-effect at the tissue level measured by EC_{50} for relaxation of guinea pig trachea and concentration-effect at the receptor level for (A) antagonism of the A_1-adenosine receptor and (B) inhibition of phosphodiesterase for a series of xanthine analogs, including theophylline. The correlation between EC_{50} for tracheal relaxation and IC_{50} for phosphodiesterase inhibition suggests that phosphodiesterase inhibition is the primary site of action for the antiasthmatic effects of these drugs. *(Reproduced with permission from Brackett LE, Shamim MT, Daley JW. Activities of caffeine, theophylline, and enprofylline analogs as tracheal relaxants. Biochem Pharmacol 1990;39:1897–1904.)*

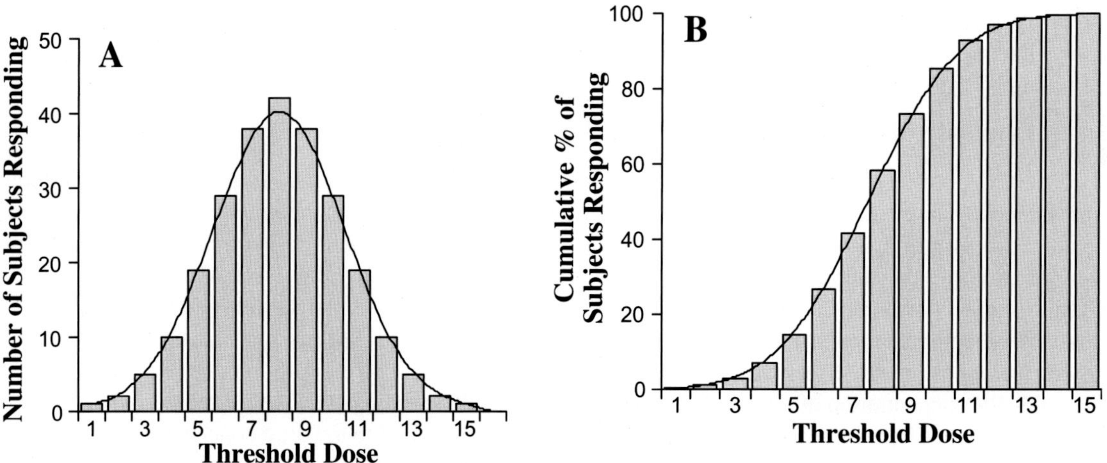

FIG. 19.10 Population-based, quantal dose-effect curves plotted in (A) as a frequency distribution histogram relating the threshold dose that is required to produce an all-or-none effect to the number of patients responding at each threshold dose; and in (B) as a cumulative distribution, in which the cumulative fraction of patients responding at each dose is plotted as a function of the dose.

as a frequency distribution histogram with threshold dose levels as the independent variable (x-axis) and the number of subjects who respond at each threshold dose level on the y-axis, the quantal dose-effect curve assumes a normal frequency distribution or bell-shaped curve (Fig. 19.10A). The threshold dose level at which the effect occurs with maximum frequency is in the middle portion of the dose range. For most drugs, a wide range of threshold doses is required to produce the all-or-none effect in a population of individuals. This variability results from differences in pharmacokinetics and in end-organ or tissue sensitivity to the drug (pharmacodynamics) within the population.

A quantal dose-effect relationship can also be graphically displayed as a cumulative dose-effect curve, in which the cumulative percentage of individuals experiencing an effect is plotted as a function of the threshold dose. The normal frequency distribution in Fig. 19.10A takes on a sigmoidal shape when the same data are plotted as a cumulative dose-effect curve (Fig. 19.10B). The median effective dose (ED_{50}) for the quantal dose-effect relationship is the dose at which 50% of the population on the cumulative dose-effect curve responds to the drug. The cumulative dose-effect curve reflects the manner in which most quantal dose-effect studies are performed in a population of individuals. It is usually not practical in human or animal trials to define the threshold dose for each subject by gradually increasing the dose in each individual. Therefore, in most studies, groups of individuals are treated at each different dose level, and the fraction of individuals who respond at each dose level represents the cumulative proportion of those whose threshold dose is at or below the administered dose. This is equivalent to the cumulative distribution.

Quantal dose-effect curves are best suited to analyzing situations in which drug concentration is related to a pharmacological effect that is either present or absent, such as sleep, or is a defined cutoff for a continuous effect, such as diastolic blood pressure <90 mmHg in a patient with hypertension. The specific pharmacological effect is present when the drug concentration is greater that a threshold level required to produce the effect, and the effect is absent when the drug concentration is below the threshold. This type of dose-response relationship is analyzed using what is technically described as a fixed-effect pharmacodynamic model. The effective threshold concentration varies among individuals, and the fixed-effect model quantifies the likelihood or probability that a given concentration will produce an all-or-none effect based on the population distribution of threshold concentrations. This model is used primarily in the clinical setting.

When administered to an organism, a drug that produces a desired therapeutic effect is also likely to produce at least one toxic effect. As a result, a single dose-effect curve does not adequately characterize the full spectrum of effects from the drug. The toxic effects of a drug can also be described by separate quantal dose-effect curves and analyzed with a fixed-effect model. The safety of a drug depends on the degree of separation between the dose that produces the therapeutic effect and the dose that produces unacceptable toxic effects. For example, in a study correlating digoxin levels with toxicity, the probability of toxicity was found to be 48% at a digoxin level of ≥3 ng/mL [6].

Cardiotoxicity, which can lead to congestive heart failure and death, is a toxic effect of the anticancer drug—doxorubicin. A cumulative dose-effect analysis demonstrated that doxorubicin cardiotoxicity is related to the lifetime dose of the drug (Fig. 19.11) and provided the basis for the definition of safe lifetime dose levels [7]. The lifetime dose of doxorubicin is now limited to less than 400–450 mg/m^2, which is associated with a <5% risk of developing congestive heart failure.

Therapeutic indices

Therapeutic indices quantify the relative safety of a drug and can be estimated from the cumulative quantal dose-effect curves of a drug's therapeutic and toxic effects. Fig. 19.12 shows the doses that are used in the calculation of these indices.

The *therapeutic ratio* is a ratio [TD_{50}/ED_{50}] of the dose at which 50% of subjects experience the toxic effect (TD_{50}) to the dose at which 50% of patients experience the therapeutic effect. A therapeutic ratio of 2.5 means that approximately 2.5 times as much drug is required to cause toxicity in half of the patients than is needed to produce a therapeutic effect in the

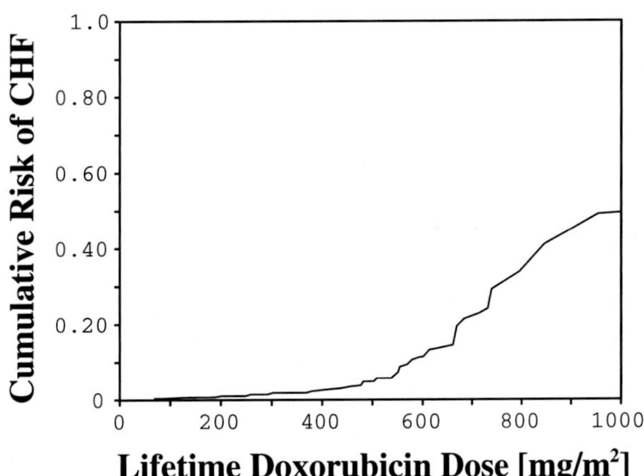

FIG. 19.11 Cumulative risk of developing congestive heart failure (CHF) as a function of the lifetime dose of doxorubicin. *(Reproduced with permission from Von Hoff DD, Layard MW, Basa P, Davis HL, Von Hoff AL, Rozencweig M, et al. Risk factors for doxorubicin-induced congestive heart failure. Ann Intern Med 1979;91:710–717.)*

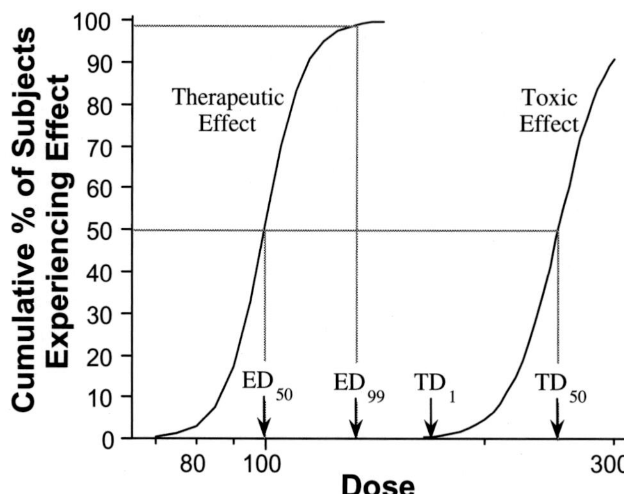

FIG. 19.12 Cumulative quantal dose-effect curves for a drug's therapeutic and toxic effects. The ED_{50} and ED_{99} are the doses required to produce the drug's therapeutic effect in 50% and 99% of the population, respectively. The TD_1 and TD_{50} are the doses that cause the toxic effect in 1% and 50% of the population, respectively.

same proportion of patients. However, this ratio of toxic to therapeutic dose may not be consistent across the entire dose range if the dose-effect curves for the therapeutic and toxic effects are not parallel.

The goal of drug therapy is to achieve the desired therapeutic effect in all patients without producing toxic effects in any patients. Therefore an index that uses the lowest toxic and highest therapeutic doses is more consistent with this goal than the therapeutic ratio. The *certainty safety factor* (CSF) is the ratio of $[TD_1/ED_{99}]$. A CSF > 1 indicates that the dose effective in 99% of the population is less than the dose that would be toxic in 1% of the population. If the CSF < 1, there is overlap between the maximally effective (ED_{99}) and minimally toxic (TD_1) doses. Unlike the therapeutic ratio, this measure is independent of the shapes of the cumulative quantal dose-effect curves for the therapeutic and toxic effects. The *standard safety margin* $\{[(TD_1 - ED_{99})/ED_{99}] \times 100\}$ also uses TD_1 and ED_{99} but is expressed as the percentage by which the ED_{99} must be increased before the TD_1 is reached.

Dose-effect and defining optimal dose

Characterization of the dose-effect relationship is an important component of clinical trials performed during the initial stages of clinical drug development. These early trials frequently follow a dose-escalation design, in which increasing dose levels of drug are administered to cohorts of patients until the maximal effect is achieved or dose-limiting toxicity is encountered. The optimal dose is identified from these dose-effect relationships for the therapeutic and toxic effects.

Johnston [8] reviewed the dose-finding studies of a variety of antihypertensive agents and compared the initial recommended dosage range from these dose-finding studies with the lowest effective dose identified in subsequent randomized clinical trials and the currently recommended dose (Table 19.2). Based on this dose-effect meta-analysis, he concluded that many antihypertensive agents were introduced into clinical practice at excessively high doses. He attributed this to reliance on a dose-escalation trial design in which the dose was escalated too rapidly, resulting in a failure to define the lower part of the dose-effect relationship. In many of the cases the initial dose produced the maximum therapeutic effect, but the dose continued to be escalated without any clear evidence of increased efficacy. The initial recommended doses often appeared to be on the plateau of the dose-effect curve, considerably higher than the range of doses adequate to achieve the desired therapeutic response. At these higher doses, there was very little added benefit but a significantly greater risk for toxicity. A current trend is to avoid this pitfall by identifying the minimum dose required for satisfactory effect (MDSE) [9].

For anticancer drugs, tumor response is often related to *dose intensity*, and this dose-effect relationship is the basis for treating cancer patients with the maximum tolerated dose of these drugs, administered at the shortest possible dosing interval. Dose intensity, or dose rate, is the amount of drug administered within a defined period of time (e.g., mg/week). The strong relationship between doxorubicin dose intensity and the percentage of patients with osteogenic sarcoma who

TABLE 19.2 Comparison of recommended doses for antihypertensive agents based on initial dose-finding clinical trials and subsequent experience in randomized clinical trials and clinical practice.

	Dose range (mg)		
Drug	Early studies	Present dose	Lowest effective dose (mg)
Propranolol	160–5000	160–320	80
Atenolol	100–2000	50–100	25
Hydrochlorothiazide	50–400	25–50	12.5
Captopril	75–1000	50–150	37.5
Methyldopa	500–6000	500–3000	750

Data from Johnston GD. Dose-response relationships with antihypertensive drugs. Pharmacol Ther 1992;55:53–93; CDER, CBER. Exposure–response relationships—study design, data analysis, and regulatory applications. Guidance for industry. Rockville, MD: FDA; 2003, (Internet at www.fda.gov/downloads/Drugs/GuidanceComplianceRegulatoryInformation/Guidances/UCM072109.pdf).)

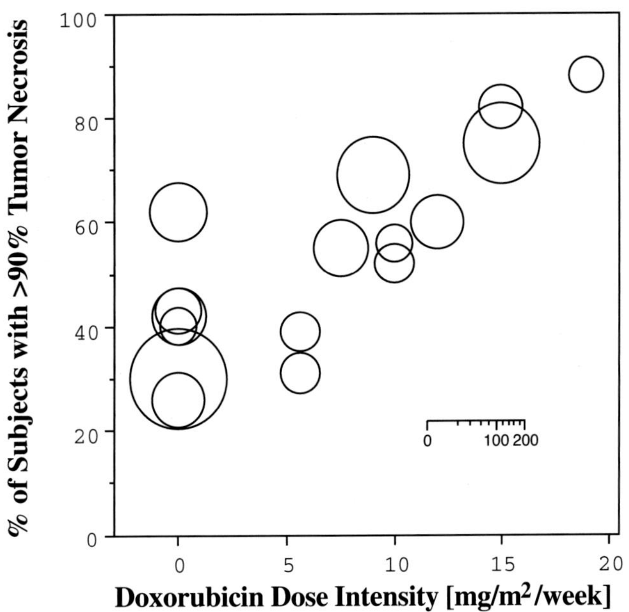

FIG. 19.13 Dose intensity meta-analysis for doxorubicin in patients with osteosarcoma. Each bubble represents a separate clinical trial, and the size of the bubble is proportional to the number of patients treated during the trial. Doxorubicin was administered prior to definitive surgical resection and effect is >90% necrosis of tumor in the resected specimen. Dose intensity or dose rate is measured in mg/m^2/week. *(Reproduced with permission from Smith MA, Ungerleider RS, Horowitz ME, Simon R. Influence of doxorubicin dose intensity on response and outcome for patients with osteogenic sarcoma and Ewing's sarcoma. J Natl Cancer Inst 1991;83:1460–1470.)*

achieved greater than 90% tumor necrosis is shown in Fig. 19.13 [10]. A dose-intensity analysis such as this one is useful in defining the optimal dose of an anticancer drug if a relationship between dose and therapeutic effect is observed.

FDA guidance on exposure-response relationships

In 2003 the United States Food and Drug Administration (FDA) produced a guidance document with nonbinding recommendations for sponsors of investigational new drugs (INDs) and applicants submitting new drug applications (NDAs) or biologics license applications (BLAs) on the use of exposure-response information in the development of these therapeutic agents [11]. This guidance recognizes that exposure-response information is integral to determining the safety and effectiveness of drugs. However, like all FDA guidance documents, it does not establish legally enforceable responsibilities but presents only recommendations that are consistent with the FDA's current thinking on a topic.

Pharmacodynamic models

Pharmacodynamic models mathematically relate a drug's pharmacological effect to its concentration at the effect site. Unlike pharmacokinetic models, pharmacodynamic models are in themselves time independent but, as described in Chapter 20, can be linked to models of a drug's pharmacokinetics. Examples of the types of pharmacodynamic models that have been employed include the fixed-effect model, maximum-effect models (E_{max} and sigmoid E_{max}), and linear and log-linear models [12]. However, simpler linear models are necessary when effects are linear over narrow concentration ranges. Semilogarithmic plots should not be used to linearize curvilinear dose-effect relationships and maximum effect models are often required when concentration-response relationships are modeled over a broad drug concentration range.

Evaluating dose/exposure-response relationships in drug development

Dose/exposure-response (D/E-R) analyses can be conducted at various phases of clinical trials as well as from nonclinical studies for integrated understanding of the drug effects and simulations for untested scenarios to inform better clinical trial design in the subsequent program or provide justifications for drug development or regulatory decisions. It is generally advisable to use a fit-for-purpose approach for evaluating dose/exposure-response relationships in drug development. The rigor of the D/E-R analysis and the methodology being applied depend on the intent of use of the D/E-R analyses and the identified relationships [13]. For this reason, it is important to examine the entire drug development program for potential applications of D/E-R relationships.

Application during drug discovery and early development

During drug discovery and early development, the D/E-R analyses would be more descriptive and exploratory, because their intent of use is typically for integrating information for improving understanding and generating hypothesis for future trial designs. The analyses generally are based on inadequately controlled data where associations between exposure and outcomes are evaluated. Therefore the degree of methodological rigor in checking assumptions and model performance is likely to be less intensive. Physiologically based modeling approaches and statistical Bayesian approaches are well suited for integrating previous understanding of disease, patient factors, therapeutics, and trials conducting into the dose/exposure-response analyses. The physiological plausibility and predictability of the analyses will be further assessed in the future confirmatory setting.

Application during clinical development

Fundamentally, the goal of a D/E-R analysis is to provide essential information for the health care provider to safely and effectively use the drug [14]. Appropriate dose/exposure-response analyses that can establish causality or provide a mechanistic understanding of a drug's effect are well suited for this purpose. Adequate and well-controlled clinical trials that investigate several fixed doses and/or measure systemic exposure levels, when analyzed using scientifically reasonable causal models, can provide substantial clinical evidence of effectiveness and providing an ability to incorporate the benefits and risks when selecting doses. A comparison across doses/exposures and the control with a consistent ordering of responses, or an established slope for the dose/exposure-response relationship can represent internal consistency and within-trial replication as convincing evidence of drug effect. The established exposure-response relationships for safety and/or efficacy may provide plausible hypotheses about the effects of alternative doses and dosage regimens not clinically tested. This can suggest ways to optimize dosage regimens and to individualize treatment in specific patient subsets for which there are limited data. Creating a theory or rationale to explain exposure-response relationships through modeling and simulation allows interpolation and reasonable extrapolation to better doses and responses in the general population and to subpopulations defined by certain intrinsic and extrinsic factors. For these decision-making purposes, the highest standard in methodology for data quality, assumption validation, model qualification, and physiological plausibility and predictability of its use will be required.

It is preferable that exposure-response analyses strategy be carefully planned while planning clinical trials in which decisions based on dose/exposure-response analyses are likely to be critical [15]. In the plan, the following good practices for the D/E-R analyses are generally expected:

- *Objectives*: The dose/exposure-response analyses should be an issue-driven process. Thus the objectives of the analyses with respect to the intended use should be explicitly described.

- *Data*: Justification for selecting and pooling data from the studies should be provided. The adequacy of data with regard to the number of subjects and samples and sampling at informative time points should also be discussed. Any potential impact from data handling, including transformation of exposure or response variables, simulation of exposure variables, imputation for missing covariates, or determination of outliers, on the capability to address the research questions should be considered.
- *Analysis tools*: Statistical software, such as R and SAS, and population PK/PD software, such as NONMEM, Phoenix, and Monolix, are commonly used for evaluating the D/E-R relationships. For answering regulatory questions, any novel platform should be verified to ensure validity of the D/E-R results.
- *Selection of exposure matrix*: The most appropriate exposure variable will depend on the trial objectives, the trial design, and the nature of the relationship between exposure and response. If response varies substantially with time within a dosage interval, then the maximum information on exposure-response will normally be retrieved by relating response to concentration at various time points within the group and individual subjects. When a single clinical outcome is evaluated, it may be more appropriate to represent the exposure by more simplified metrics such as dose or C_{max}, C_{trough}, or AUC at steady state. Rationales for specific exposure and response (e.g., biomarkers or clinical outcomes; continuous, categorical, or time to event) should also be documented. Inclusion of active metabolites and their contribution to response should also be justified.
- *Assumptions*: Modeling analyses are always associated with assumptions. Examples of those assumptions include mechanism of the drug actions for efficacy and adverse effects, immediate or cumulative clinical effects, response in a placebo group, disease state progression, absence or presence of an effect compartment or a latent variable, development of tolerance or absence of tolerance, drug-induced inhibition or induction of PK processes, circadian variations in basal conditions, influential covariates, distributions of intra- and interindividual variability in parameters, etc. Careful consideration of those assumptions before collecting data, conducting analyses, or interpreting the results is needed. Justifications of the appropriateness of model assumptions can be supported by preliminary data assessments.
- *Model selection, evaluation, and qualification*: The strategy for model selection for the determination of model structure and inclusion of covariate and random effect should be carefully planned. In general, model selection will be based on the mechanism of action of a drug, assumptions made and supported by data, the goodness that the model can describe the data, and its intended use. The simplest model structure that serves the analysis objective is usually preferable. The model selection process could be a series of trial and evaluation steps. Statistical comparison and visual inspection of goodness of fit are commonly used. The predictability of the model can then be validated based on internal and external data. Qualifying a model for its intended use depends on the data adequacy, the predication capability, and the potential risks of a decision based on the D/E-R analyses.
- *Simulations*: To inform the trial design for drug development or the safe and effective use of the drug in an individual patient based on the established D/E-R relationships, simulations can be conducted for predictions for various scenarios that may not be adequately studied. Depending on the purpose of simulation, various levels of uncertainty (for model parameters) and variability (for between subjects and for within subjects) could be included to answer a specific "what-if" question for trial design or drug use.

Methodology for dose/exposure-response analysis

The methodology for evaluating dose/exposure-response relationships ranges from physiologically based approaches to more empirical statistical approaches of comparison and regression for data dependence relationship analyses. In addition, novel methodologies such as machine learning approaches may also be applied [16–18].

Physiologically based bottom-up approaches are based on the current understanding of the underlying pharmacological processes, including drug site of action distribution, target occupancy, signal transduction or up/down regulation of a pathway, systemic network interaction, etc., which can be complicated and rely on assumptions that may lack the direct support of high-quality in vivo data. The systemic model may range in complexity from a simple reaction process to a large network of drug and virtual patient interaction. Commonly, most model parameters are derived from alternative sources, such as in vitro studies, and may not be estimable using the available clinical trial data [19].

The statistical approaches are generally data-driven top-down methods. Statistical comparisons of responses among different dose/exposure groups are relatively straightforward and make fewer assumptions regarding the underlying relationship between dose/exposure and response. However, this kind of analyses generally has less prediction power for responses at unstudied dose/exposure levels, dosing regimens, treatment durations, or various other unstudied scenarios.

Statistical regression analyses evaluating the relationship between dose/exposure and responses are often called dose/exposure-response modeling. The purpose of the modeling is to predict responses at different dose/exposure levels, dosing regimens, various scenarios of trial designs or subgroups of population that might not be well studied. Generally, these models can be further divided into empirical models and semimechanistic/mechanistic models. Empirical models are usually built using simple regression structures (e.g., assuming a linear or log-linear relationship) as an approximation of the association between responses and dose/exposure levels in the studied range. The model building is primarily driven by the clinical trial data. Although the relationship may be extrapolated to unstudied dose/exposure range for hypothesis generation, the reliability of prediction needs to be confirmed with further studies. Semimechanistic/mechanistic models are usually built using model structures (e.g., E_{max}, sigmoid E_{max} models, or combined multiple components) as an approximation of the integrated underlying key pharmacological processes, such as receptor binding or enzyme dynamics that may involve multiple intermediate bioprocesses/biomarkers and interactions. Model parameters are estimated using clinical trial data and should be physiologically plausible. The results of these analyses are usually reliable in the observed data range and their predictability generally is better than analyses that are based on purely empirical models. However, depending on the totality of evidence, the remaining uncertainty of the integrated pharmacological processes, and the risk of decisions, the predictions of these analyses may or may not need to be confirmed with additional studies [20, 21].

Given that dose/exposure-response analyses are generally conducted at the population level, it is important to adjust the analyses for individual difference [22]. Statistical mixed-effect modeling is commonly used for this situation. Subject's covariates (age, race, gender, body weight, disease severity, etc.) and trial or drug factors (country, food, formulation, etc.) that contribute to individual difference in drug exposure or response can be included as factors with fixed effects. The remained unexplained variability can be treated as random effects including between-subject variability (BSV) for model parameters and between-occasion variability (BOV) for model parameters or residual variability for observations. Various model structures for including fixed effects and random effects could be assessed: linear, power, or exponential functions for continuous covariates and dichotomous or polychotomous for discrete factors are commonly used covariate models; log-normal distributions are commonly assumed for BSV and BOV modeling; additive, proportional, exponential, or combined distributions are most common error models for residual variability.

Special considerations for minimizing bias in exposure-response analysis

Unlike dose-response analyses that are usually based on randomized data for different dose levels from a well-controlled trial, exposure-response analyses generally rely on both exposure and response data that are collected after the treatment. Therefore the exposure in a subject is generally not randomized and sample collection generally cannot cover the entire population and treatment duration of a trial. Moreover, assumptions based on our current best understanding for pharmacodynamics may still cause model misspecification. So, it is important to implement an appropriate exposure-response approach to minimize bias resulting from systematic differences between the structure, parameters, and estimates of the model and the underlying quantity of the pharmacodynamics and clinical outcomes.

The biases introduced by sample selection and data acquisition in a trial are common selection biases. Exposure-response analyses in a subgroup of subjects with pharmacokinetic data available may not reflect the underlying relationship in the general population because subjects in the pharmacokinetic subgroup may not adequately represent the entire population enrolled in the trial. If available, the demographics, treatment factors, response profiles, and dose-response relationships in the pharmacokinetic subgroup should always be compared with those in the entire population [23]. On the other hand, the biases introduced during exposure-response analyses are common assessment biases. These biases could include: (1) model misspecification due to inappropriate assumption of model structure (e.g., assuming a direct response relationship for a delayed effect or inadequately accounting for the effect of multiple moieties in a combination treatment) [24]; (2) missing a contribution to response from active metabolites; and (3) improper selection of exposure variables for analyses. The common issues with improper exposure variables for exposure-response analyses include: (a) using exposure estimated from nominal dosing without accounting for drug compliance or dosing interruption/modification; (b) a potential negatively biased relationship for time-to-event endpoints when using cumulative exposure, average cumulative exposure (i.e., cumulative exposure normalized by treatment duration), or exposure at an event time where a higher cumulative exposure could be the outcome of longer survival and high drug accumulation with longer treatment duration; (c) a potential positively biased relationship for time-to-event endpoints where the average cumulative exposure or exposure at an event time could be the outcome of more chance for dose reduction over time due to drug toxicity not related to the response outcome [25].

The ignorance of potential confounding factors that can affect both exposure and response variables is another major reason of assessment bias. The impact of these factors may vary across different disease areas and may be prominent for drugs whose pharmacokinetics are affected by disease status or responses to the treatment. For example, hepatic or renal function could simultaneously affect drug exposure and susceptibility to adverse effects or response to drugs targeting liver or kidney diseases. For a prevention therapy, a subject's behavior may also simultaneously alter treatment outcome by affecting adherence or risk of disease contact. In treating patients with late-stage cancer, disease burden at baseline and disease status change during treatment may affect drug clearance of some therapeutic proteins (e.g., due to association of cancer cachexia and catabolic clearance) [26, 27]. In this case, the disease burden may affect both exposure and treatment response independently and a high drug concentration at steady state might be the result, rather than the cause, of a good treatment response. Therefore the concentration-response relationships should always be compared with the dose-response if it is available.

Case studies

Dose-response and exposure-response analyses are ultimately tools aimed at answering drug development questions pertaining to the optimization of an individual patient's dosing regimen. The case studies described herein are intended to illustrate exposure-response analyses that have supported different dose optimization questions. It should become clear through these examples that dose-response and exposure-response analyses are critical throughout the entire drug development process to ultimately inform trial design and drug approval. Examples are shown across different therapeutic areas to emphasize that different benefit-risk profiles necessitate different approaches to select the approved dosing regimen.

Dapagliflozin

Dapagliflozin is indicated as an adjunct to diet and exercise to improve glycemic control in adults with type 2 diabetes mellitus. The starting dose is 5 mg/day and the dose can be increased to 10 mg/day in patients tolerating dapagliflozin who require additional glycemic control [28]. The clinical pharmacology development program was extensive with 8 Phase 1 PK/PD/safety studies, 13 pharmacokinetic drug-drug interaction studies, 4 studies in specific populations, a population pharmacokinetic and exposure-response analysis, and 4 biopharmaceutical studies being conducted. Of the Phase 1 studies, at least 6 were dose ranging (with doses anywhere between 0.001 and 500 mg). Of the specific population studies (i.e., renal impairment, hepatic impairment, Japanese single ascending dose, Japanese multiple ascending dose), 3 used doses ranging between 2.5 and 50 mg. Dose optimization was based on an exposure-response analysis of the relationship between dapagliflozin exposure and glycemic response [29].

As a result of the extensive clinical development program and the drug's mechanism of action, a clear dose-response relationship was confirmed for glycemic response in both patients and healthy subjects (Fig. 19.14). The wide range of doses that were evaluated is evident in this figure and the E_{max} model, derived from pharmacologic drug-receptor binding principles, fits the data well. The vertical line in Fig. 19.14 is for the 10-mg dose that the company intended to develop.

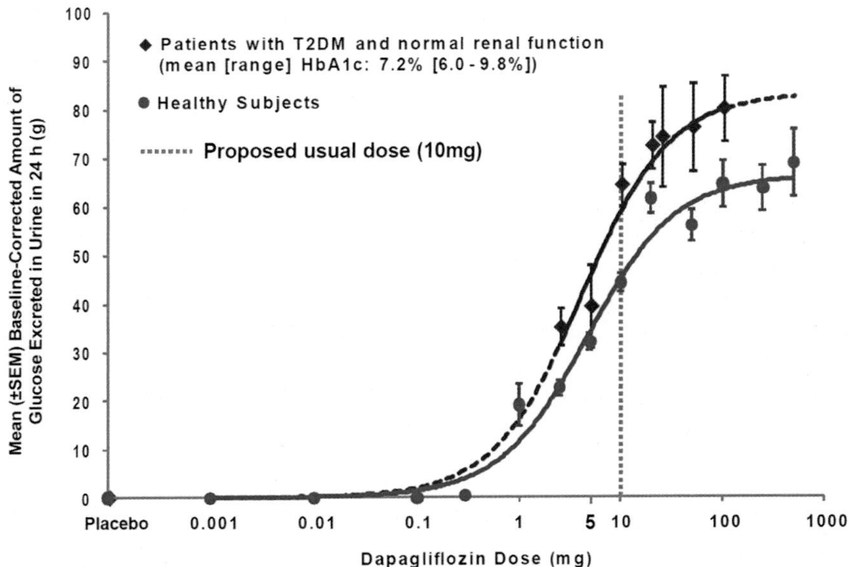

FIG. 19.14 Glycemic response to dapagliflozin was evaluated over a wide dose range. *(https://wayback.archive-it.org/7993/20170405215810/https://www.fda.gov/downloads/AdvisoryCommittees/CommitteesMeetingMaterials/Drugs/EndocrinologicandMetabolicDrugsAdvisoryCommittee/UCM379659.pdf.)*

A Phase 2 study in treatment naïve subjects with type 2 diabetes mellitus evaluated doses of 2.5, 5, 10, 20, and 50 mg/day as well as placebo to select doses for Phase 3 trials. After 12 weeks of treatment, all doses showed an improvement compared to placebo. Doses of 2.5, 5, and 10 mg/day were carried forward into Phase 3 because doses above 10 mg/day did not result in any additional incremental benefit. In the Phase 3 trials, the decrease from baseline in HbA1c was significantly greater for both the 5 and 10-mg dose arms than with placebo and was greater with the 10 mg than with the 5 mg/day dose. Thus daily doses of both 5 and 10 mg were approved with 5 mg as the starting dose and 10 mg reserved for patients who needed additional glycemic control and could tolerate this dose. This uptitration was not directly studied in the clinical trials but was approved since this option best fit the benefit-risk profile of dapagliflozin.

Edoxaban

Edoxaban is a novel anticoagulant (NOAC) indicated to reduce the risk of stroke and systemic embolism in patients with nonvalvular atrial fibrillation (NVAF) and for the treatment of deep vein thrombosis and pulmonary embolism. The following discussion focuses only on the NVAF indication. Both dose-response and exposure-response information were utilized during early drug development to select the Phase 3 doses for the ENGAGE-AF TIMI-48 trial in patients with NVAF [30].

Dose-response analysis of a Phase 2 dose-ranging study suggested that doses higher than 60 mg/day would yield more bleeding when compared to warfarin. This was particularly the case for the twice-daily edoxaban regimens where higher bleeding was noted with 30-mg BID dosing when compared to the 60 mg/day regimen. Combined with knowledge from Phase 1 PK/PD and drug-drug interaction studies of different intrinsic and extrinsic patient factors that impact edoxaban exposure, dose reductions were implemented in both the low-dose (30 mg/day) and high-dose edoxaban (60 mg/day) arms in the Phase 3 ENGAGE AF TIMI-48 trial in order to prevent unnecessary bleeding. The edoxaban dose was reduced by 50% for patients with moderate renal impairment, patients with low body weight ($\leq$60 kg), and patients receiving concomitant P-gp inhibitors. The Phase 3 ENGAGE AF TIMI-48 trial randomized 21,105 subjects to warfarin, low-dose edoxaban, or high-dose edoxaban. Edoxaban concentrations were assayed and reported from 95% of the 14,014 subjects randomized to either the low- or high-dose edoxaban arms.

Exposure-response analyses explained critical subgroup findings that suggested patients with normal renal function had higher stroke risk (HR) relative to warfarin (HR: 1.58 for high-dose edoxaban). However, in patients with mild renal function, edoxaban performed better than warfarin at reducing stroke (HR: 0.6 in favor of high-dose edoxaban relative to warfarin) and patients with moderate renal impairment edoxaban performed as well as warfarin (HR: 1.04), owing to a planned dose reduction to 30 mg for patients in the high-dose edoxaban arm. In each of the earlier mentioned subgroups, the HR relative to warfarin was correlated with the median edoxaban trough concentration, emphasizing that dose-response alone could not inform critical dose individualization to ensure stroke prevention. Thus multivariate time-to-event hazard analyses were performed to further consider dose individualization.

Multivariate time-to-event proportional hazards analyses were performed for both the occurrence of all stroke and bleeding to account for the effects of other patient factors that may influence interpretation of the exposure-efficacy or exposure-safety relationships. Model covariates tested included treatment (warfarin vs edoxaban), age, creatinine clearance, prior stroke/transient ischemic attack history, diabetes status, edoxaban trough concentrations, log-transformed edoxaban trough concentrations, body weight, concomitant aspirin use, the $CHADS_2$ (Congestive heart failure-Hypertension-Age-Stroke) score for atrial fibrillation stroke risk as a continuous variable, as well as the $CHADS_2$ score based on binary cut points between 2 and >2 or $\leq$3 and >3, and congestive heart failure. Covariates were included into a full model if their univariate assessment indicated significance of the parameter at $\alpha = 0.05$. Covariates were eliminated from the model during a backward elimination evaluation if based on a significance of the parameter at $\alpha = 0.05$. Final models for all stroke events and major bleeds are shown in Fig. 19.15 which highlights the need to optimize edoxaban concentrations to the point that gives the best benefit-risk profile.

The final model for all stroke/SEE events included prior stroke history, edoxaban trough concentration, body weight, age, and CHAD score. Of importance, among all the significant covariates that were evaluated, trough concentrations of edoxaban had the greatest impact on stroke risk. This analysis in combination with similar relationships for bleeding events was utilized to simulate stroke and bleeding risk for different patients based on their dose and renal function. The results suggested NVAF patients with normal kidney function would need to receive a dose of 90 mg/day to match exposures to patients with mild impairment who had better stroke outcomes. As the tolerability/bleeding risk of the 90-mg dose had not been established in patients with normal renal function, the labeled dosing of edoxaban does not include patients with

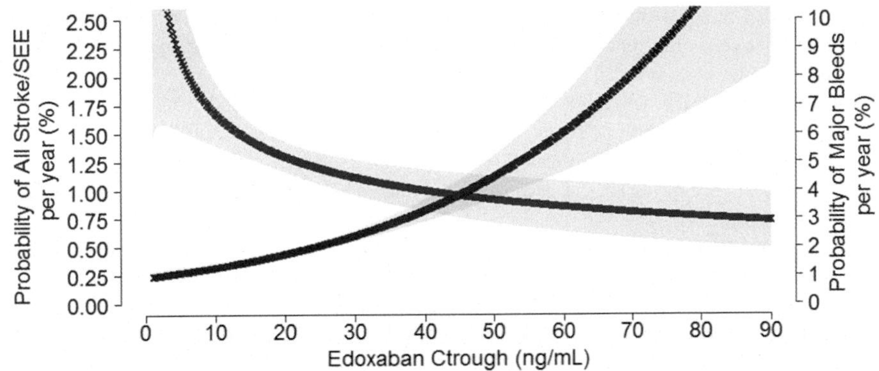

FIG. 19.15 Edoxaban exhibits concentration-dependent relationships for all stroke/SEE *(blue)* and major bleeds *(red)*. Analysis shown for "typical" patient population: Age: 72 years old, Renal Function: (70.4 mL/min), 28.3% with prior stroke, 29.2% with baseline aspirin use. *(https://wayback.archive-it.org/7993/20170405211258/https://www.fda.gov/downloads/AdvisoryCommittees/CommitteesMeetingMaterials/Drugs/CardiovascularandRenalDrugsAdvisoryCommittee/UCM421612.pdf.)*

normal renal function as defined by creatinine clearance of ≥95 mL/min and recommends dose reductions for reduced renal function for patients with NVAF, as well as with deep vein thrombosis or pulmonary embolism, as well as for all patients with low body weight or concomitant therapy with P-gp inhibitors.

Summary

As discussed in this chapter and as illustrated by the case studies on dapagliflozin and edoxaban, careful delineation of the dose-effect relationship over the expected dosing range for therapeutic and toxic effects is a high priority in the preclinical and clinical phases of drug development. Integration of our knowledge of pharmacokinetics and pharmacodynamics has contributed significantly to more rational and individualized dosing regimens in clinical practice.

References

[1] Eschbach JW, Egrie JC, Downing MR, Browne JK, Adamson JW. Correction of the anemia of end-stage renal disease with recombinant human erythropoietin: results of a combined phase I and II clinical trial. N Engl J Med 1987;316:73–78.

[2] Ferrante FM, Paggioli J, Cherukuri S, Arthur GR. The analgesic response to intravenous lidocaine in the treatment of neuropathic pain. Anesth Analg 1996;82:91–97.

[3] Garber AJ, Duncan TG, Goodman AM, Mills DJ, Rohlf JL. Efficacy of metformin in type II diabetes: results of a double-blind, placebo-controlled, dose–response trial. Am J Med 1997;102:491–497.

[4] Adamson PC, Poplack DG, Balis FM. The cytotoxicity of thioguanine vs mercaptopurine in acute lymphoblastic leukemia. Leuk Res 1994;18:805–810.

[5] Brackett LE, Shamim MT, Daley JW. Activities of caffeine, theophylline, and enprofylline analogs as tracheal relaxants. Biochem Pharmacol 1990;39:1897–1904.

[6] Piergies AA, Worwag EM, Atkinson AJ Jr. A concurrent audit of high digoxin plasma levels. Clin Pharmacol Ther 1994;55:353–358.

[7] Von Hoff DD, Layard MW, Basa P, Davis HL, Von Hoff AL, Rozencweig M, et al. Risk factors for doxorubicin-induced congestive heart failure. Ann Intern Med 1979;91:710–717.

[8] Johnston GD. Dose–response relationships with antihypertensive drugs. Pharmacol Ther 1992;55:53–93.

[9] Rolan P. The contribution of clinical pharmacology surrogates and models to drug development—a critical appraisal. Br J Clin Pharmacol 1997;44:219–225.

[10] Smith MA, Ungerleider RS, Horowitz ME, Simon R. Influence of doxorubicin dose intensity on response and outcome for patients with osteogenic sarcoma and Ewing's sarcoma. J Natl Cancer Inst 1991;83:1460–1470.

[11] CDER, CBER. Exposure–response relationships—study design, data analysis, and regulatory applications, In: Guidance for industry. Rockville, MD: FDA; 2003. Internet at www.fda.gov/downloads/Drugs/GuidanceComplianceRegulatoryInformation/Guidances/UCM072109.pdf.

[12] Holford NHG, Scheiner LB. Understanding the dose–effect relationship: clinical applications of pharmacokinetic– pharmacodynamic models. Clin Pharmacokinet 1981;6:429–453.

[13] Wang Y, Huang SM. Commentary on fit-for-purpose models for regulatory applications. J Pharm Sci 2019;108(1):18–20.

[14] ICH E4 guideline. https://www.ema.europa.eu/en/documents/scientific-guideline/ich-e-4-dose-response-information-support-drug-registration-step-5_en.pdf.

[15] Dykstra K, Mehrotra N, Tornøe CW, Kastrissios H, Patel B, Al-Huniti N, Jadhav P, Wang Y, Byon W. Reporting guidelines for population pharmacokinetic analyses, J Pharmacokinet Pharmacodyn 2015;42(3):301–314. https://doi.org/10.1007/s10928-015-9417-1. Epub 2015 Apr 30 25925797. PMC4432104.

[16] Liu X, Liu C, Huang R, Zhu H, Liu Q, Mitra S, Wang Y. Long short-term memory recurrent neural network for pharmacokinetic-pharmacodynamic modeling, Int J Clin Pharmacol Ther 2021;59(2):138–146. https://doi.org/10.5414/CP203800. 33210994.

[17] Huang R, Liu Q, Feng G, Wang Y, Liu C, Gopalakrishnan M, Liu X, Gong Y, Zhu H. A novel approach for personalized response model: deep learning with individual dropout feature ranking, J Pharmacokinet Pharmacodyn 2021;48(1):165–179. https://doi.org/10.1007/s10928-020-09724-x. Epub 2020 Oct 26 3310492.

[18] Liu Q, Zhu H, Liu C, Jean D, Huang SM, ElZarrad MK, Blumenthal G, Wang Y. Application of machine learning in drug development and regulation: current status and future potential, Clin Pharmacol Ther 2020;107(4):726–729. https://doi.org/10.1002/cpt.1771. Epub 2020 Feb 8 31925955.

[19] Zhang X, Yang Y, Grimstein M, Fan J, Grillo JA, Huang SM, Zhu H, Wang Y. Application of PBPK modeling and simulation for regulatory decision making and its impact on US prescribing information: an update on the 2018-2019 submissions to the US FDA's Office of Clinical Pharmacology. J Clin Pharmacol 2020;60(Suppl. 1):S160–S178.

[20] Thomas N, Sweeney K, Somayaji V. Meta-analysis of clinical dose–response in a large drug development portfolio. Stat Biopharm Res 2014;6 (4):302–317. https://doi.org/10.1080/19466315.2014.924876.

[21] Thomas N, Roy D. Analysis of clinical dose–response in small-molecule drug development: 2009–2014. Stat Biopharm Res 2017;9(2):137–146. https://doi.org/10.1080/19466315.2016.1256229.

[22] Garnett C, Bonate PL, Dang Q, Ferber G, Huang D, Liu J, Mehrotra D, Riley S, Sager P, Tornoe C, Wang Y. Scientific white paper on concentration-QTc modeling, J Pharmacokinet Pharmacodyn 2018;45(3):383–397. https://doi.org/10.1007/s10928-017-9558-5. Epub 2017 Dec 5. Erratum in: J Pharmacokinet Pharmacodyn. 2018 Jan 12 29209907.

[23] Yang J, Zhao H, Garnett C, Rahman A, Gobburu JV, Pierce W, Schechter G, Summers J, Keegan P, Booth B, Wang Y. The combination of exposure-response and case-control analyses in regulatory decision making, J Clin Pharmacol 2013;53(2):160–166. https://doi.org/10.1177/0091270012445206. Epub 2013 Jan 24 23436261.

[24] Zhu H, Wang Y. Evaluation of false positive rate based on exposure-response analyses for two compounds in fixed-dose combination products, J Pharmacokinet Pharmacodyn 2011;38(6):671–696. https://doi.org/10.1007/s10928-011-9214-4. Epub 2011 Sep 6 21898140.

[25] Wang Y, Harigaya Y, Cavaillé-Coll M, Colangelo P, Reynolds KS. Justification of noninferiority margin: methodology considerations in an exposure-response analysis, Clin Pharmacol Ther 2015;97(4):404–410. https://doi.org/10.1002/cpt.44. Epub 2015 Feb 13 25670256.

[26] Liu C, Yu J, Li H, Liu J, Xu Y, Song P, Liu Q, Zhao H, Xu J, Maher VE, Booth BP, Kim G, Rahman A, Wang Y. Association of time-varying clearance of nivolumab with disease dynamics and its implications on exposure response analysis, Clin Pharmacol Ther 2017;101(5):657–666. https://doi.org/10.1002/cpt.656. Epub 2017 Mar 22 28182273.

[27] Li H, Yu J, Liu C, Liu J, Subramaniam S, Zhao H, Blumenthal GM, Turner DC, Li C, Ahamadi M, de Greef R, Chatterjee M, Kondic AG, Stone JA, Booth BP, Keegan P, Rahman A, Wang Y. Time dependent pharmacokinetics of pembrolizumab in patients with solid tumor and its correlation with best overall response, J Pharmacokinet Pharmacodyn 2017;44(5):403–414. https://doi.org/10.1007/s10928-017-9528-y. Epub 2017 Jun 1 28573468.

[28] Anon, https://www.accessdata.fda.gov/drugsatfda_docs/label/2017/202293s011lbl.pdf.

[29] Anon, https://wayback.archive-it.org/7993/20170405215810/https://www.fda.gov/downloads/AdvisoryCommittees/CommitteesMeetingMaterials/Drugs/EndocrinologicandMetabolicDrugsAdvisoryCommittee/UCM379659.pdf.

[30] Anon, https://wayback.archive-it.org/7993/20170405211301/https://www.fda.gov/downloads/AdvisoryCommittees/CommitteesMeetingMaterials/Drugs/CardiovascularandRenalDrugsAdvisoryCommittee/UCM421613.pdf.

Chapter 20

Time course of drug response

Nicholas H.G. Holford
Department of Pharmacology and Clinical Pharmacology, University of Auckland, Auckland, New Zealand

Therapeutic drug responses are a consequence of drug exposure. Exposure describes the intensity and time course of drug concentration associated with treatment. Many clinicians and patients behave as if they believe drug exposure is defined by the drug dose. However, a central dogma of clinical pharmacology is that drug actions are determined by drug concentration. Events leading up to such concentrations include the therapeutic consultation between patient and prescriber, the patient's decision to obtain and take the medication, and the time course of delivery and loss of drug from the site of action. The act of taking a drug dose is only one step in this chain of events and provides only part of the information needed to predict the time course of response.

Pharmacokinetics provides a rational framework for understanding how the time course of observable drug concentration (usually in plasma) is related to the dose. The principles of pharmacodynamics described in Chapter 19 provide a companion framework for understanding the relationship between concentration and response. However, pharmacokinetics and pharmacodynamics are not enough by themselves to describe the time course of drug response for two main reasons:

1. Plasma is the reference site for describing drug concentrations, but it is not the site of action of most drugs, so responses will be delayed in relation to pharmacokinetic predictions of plasma concentrations. The only exceptions are a limited number of drugs whose action directly affects physical components of plasma (e.g., enoxaparin, apixaban).
2. The action of a drug is not the same as the drug response. In many cases, a network of events links receptor activation to physiological changes. These in turn are linked via complex pathophysiological mechanisms, often including homeostatic feedback, before the appearance of either therapeutic or adverse pharmacologic responses.

Recognizing these processes, it is useful to distinguish between the pharmacologic *action* (e.g., stimulation of a receptor, inhibition of an enzyme), the physiologic *effect* (e.g., bronchodilatation, lowering of cholesterol), and the clinical *outcome* (e.g., relief of an asthma attack, reduction of risk of a cardiovascular event).

These two reasons give rise to two basic conceptual approaches for describing the delay between plasma concentrations and changes in physiological effect [1]. In the first approach, the effect is considered to be an immediate consequence of drug action, and the delay is thought to reflect the time required for the drug to reach its site of pharmacologic action, or *biophase*. In the second approach, the drug is thought to alter the turnover (synthesis or degradation) of some factor, usually an endogenous compound, that mediates the physiological effect. With each approach, the basic relationships between drug concentration and intensity of effect that were described in Chapter 19 can be applied to the analysis of drug response. The relationship between drug-induced effects on pathophysiology and clinical outcome is often too complex to describe in detailed mechanistic terms and usually involves the pragmatic application of pharmacodynamic models linking observable biomarkers of drug effect to outcome as if the biomarkers, rather than drug concentrations, were themselves the driving force of drug response.

Pharmacokinetics and delayed pharmacologic effects

In some cases, it is biologically plausible to identify the site of drug action as one of the compartments used to characterize the kinetics of drug distribution. As described in Chapter 3, Sherwin et al. [2] noted that the time course of insulin-stimulated glucose utilization parallels expected insulin concentrations in the slowly equilibrating compartment of a three-compartment model of insulin distribution (fig. 3.4 in Chapter 3). Since the kinetics of drug in this compartment may correspond to insulin concentrations in skeletal muscle interstitial fluid [3], it is reasonable to use this pharmacokinetic compartment to predict the time course of this particular insulin effect. In a study of digoxin pharmacokinetics and inotropic

Atkinson's Principles of Clinical Pharmacology. https://doi.org/10.1016/B978-0-12-819869-8.00008-2

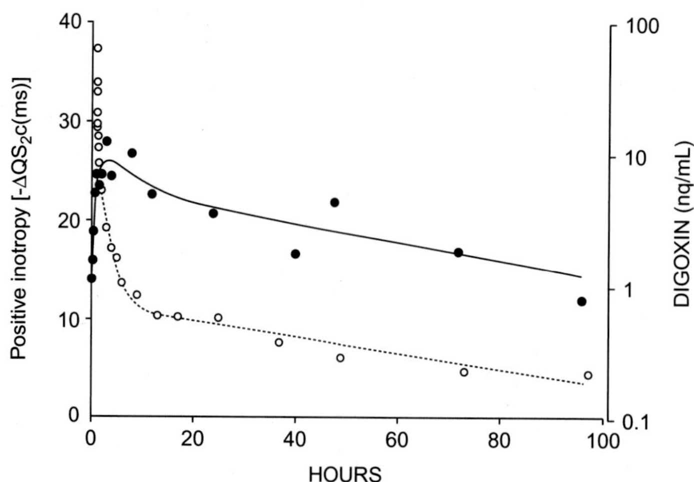

FIG. 20.1 An experiment in which a bolus injection of digoxin was administered and a model describing the slow binding of this drug to its receptor was used to fit the *solid and dotted lines* to average measurements of plasma digoxin concentration (○) and inotropic effect assessed from the heart-rate-corrected change in the QS_2 interval (●). *(Reproduced with permission from Weiss M, Kang W. Inotropic effect of digoxin in humans: mechanistic pharmacokinetic/pharmacodynamic model based on slow receptor binding. Pharm Res 2004;21:231–236, who based this analysis on plasma concentration and effect data taken from Kramer WG, Kolibash AJ, Lewis RP, Bathala MS, Visconti JA, Reuning RH. Pharmacokinetics of digoxin: relationship between response intensity and predicted compartmental drug levels in man. J Pharmacokinet Biopharm 1979;7:47–61.)*

effects, Kramer et al. [4] observed that there is a close relationship between the time course of these effects and estimated digoxin concentrations in the slowly equilibrating peripheral compartment of a three-compartment pharmacokinetic model (Fig. 20.1). Although the heart comprises only a small fraction of total body muscle mass, there is some physiological justification for identifying myocardium as a component of this compartment. The authors noted that the time course of inotropic response could also reflect a delay due to the time required for the chain of digoxin-initiated intracellular events to result in increased myocardial contractile force. However, it has been shown that neither the distribution of digoxin from plasma to the myocardium, nor the intracellular consequences of Na^+, K^+-ATPase inhibition are the key determinants of the slow onset of digoxin action. It is the slow dissociation of digoxin from Na^+, K^+-ATPase that best explains the slow equilibration between plasma digoxin and intensity of enzyme inhibition [5]. In this regard, models in which the effects of lysergic acid diethylamide on arithmetic performance are related to concentrations in a peripheral compartment of a pharmacokinetic model also appear to represent just a coincidence and do not have an obvious physiological rationale [6].

The biophase compartment

Because only a small fraction of an administered drug dose actually binds to receptors or in other ways produces an observed effect, it is reasonable to suppose that the biophase may have kinetic properties that are distinct from the bulk of other tissues that, as discussed in Chapter 3, are involved in the distribution of most of an administered drug dose. This was first appreciated by Segre [7], who introduced the concept of a separate biophase compartment to explain the fact that the pressor effects of norepinephrine lagged appreciably behind its concentration profile in blood. Hull et al. [8] and Sheiner et al. [9] independently incorporated a biophase compartment in their pharmacokinetic–pharmacodynamic models linking plasma concentrations of neuromuscular blocking drugs to their skeletal muscle paralyzing effects.

Fig. 20.2 is a schematic diagram of a pharmacokinetic–pharmacodynamic model in which a biophase compartment links drug concentrations in plasma to observed effects. The mathematical characteristics of this biophase compartment have been described in detail by Sheiner et al. [9] and by Holford and Sheiner [10].

If we make the assumptions that drug distribution to and from the site of action is first order (i.e., no active transport is involved) and that drug actions are directly determined by the unbound, unionized drug concentration in water at the site of action, then at steady state the drug concentration in plasma water will be directly proportional to its concentration at the site of action. From a practical viewpoint, the parameters estimated from biophase concentrations (such as the EC_{50}) to predict the drug effects will correspond to the concentrations (e.g., plasma) used for the pharmacokinetic forcing function.

The time course of drug concentration in the biophase to reach steady state is determined by the biophase elimination process. This can be understood in the simple case where the pharmacokinetic forcing function is a square wave achievable by a rapid loading dose and appropriate maintenance dose rate into the pharmacokinetic central compartment. With the

Dose = X_0

Baseline = E_0

V_f

k_{Bf}

Biophase V_B

ΔE

Effect

k_{01}

$t_{1/2eq}$

Pharmacokinetics

Effect Kinetics

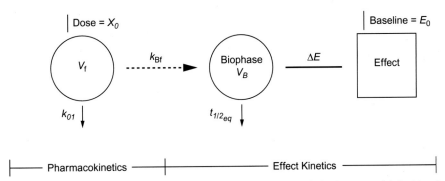

FIG. 20.2 A delayed pharmacodynamic model in which the kinetics of drug distribution and elimination are modeled with a single compartment (V_1), which receives a bolus input dose (X_0) and has an elimination clearance CL. Plasma concentrations are linked to a biophase compartment (V_B), and ΔE transduces drug concentrations in the biophase compartment into changes in the observed effect (E). The time course of the observed effects is governed by the rate constant k_{eq}. The arrow linking V_1 and V_B is dotted to indicate that no mass transfer occurs between these compartments and that k_{eq} is not an independent parameter of the system (see text).

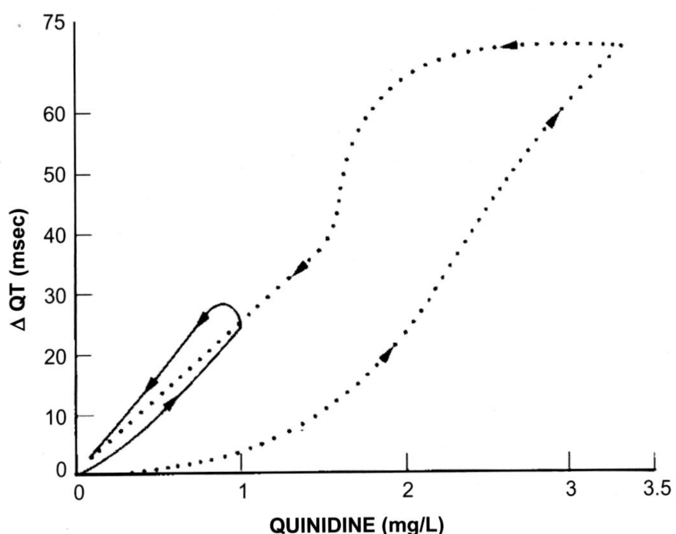

FIG. 20.3 Predicted changes in QT interval after administration of intravenous (*dotted line*) and oral (*solid line*) single doses of quinidine to healthy subjects [11]. The delay in effect with respect to plasma concentration causes *hysteresis* loops. The slope of the biophase concentration–effect relationship is greater after oral doses due to active metabolites formed during quinidine absorption. *(Reproduced with permission from Holford NH, Coates PE, Guentert TW, Riegelman S, Sheiner LB. The effect of quinidine and its metabolites on the electrocardiogram and systolic time intervals: concentration–effect relationships. Br J Clin Pharmacol 1981;11:187–195.)*

assumption of first-order input to the biophase this means the input rate to the biophase will be constant. Assuming first-order elimination, it is the half-life of the elimination process from the biophase that will determine the time to steady state.

A characteristic feature of delayed response is the existence of a hysteresis loop when plasma concentrations are plotted against effects occurring at the same time. This is shown in Fig. 20.3 in which plasma concentrations of quinidine have been related to changes in electrocardiographic QT intervals. When the effect of the drug increases with concentration, then the loop has a counterclockwise direction, but if the effect decreases with concentration, then the loop goes clockwise (e.g., if potassium channel conductance had been used to describe the effect of quinidine). In both cases the loop is described as showing hysteresis.

Incorporation of pharmacodynamic models

The models described in Chapter 19 that are used to relate steady-state plasma concentrations of drug to observed effects can also be applied to the time course of drug effects.

Linear response models

If the relationship between effect (E) and biophase concentration is linear, the change in E can be related to biophase concentrations (C_B) by a slope parameter (β) such that:

$$E = \beta \cdot C_B \tag{20.1}$$

Biophase concentrations then are related to observations as follows:

$$S = S_0 + E = S_0 + \beta \bullet C_B \tag{20.2}$$

where S is the observed state including the drug effect, S_0 is the baseline observed effect, termed baseline state in Chapter 21. The arithmetic sign of the value of β determines if the change in effect is either added to or subtracted from the baseline value.

A linear model was used to show that the blood pressure-lowering effects and blockade of transmission across sympathetic ganglia caused by *N*-acetylprocainamide (NAPA) followed a similar time course in dogs [12]. This pharmacokinetic–pharmacodynamic analysis was used to provide supporting evidence for the conclusion that the observed hypotensive effect of the drug was mediated by its ganglionic blocking action. This detailed analysis in dogs then was extended to demonstrate that the hypotensive effects of NAPA in a human subject were similar in intensity and time course.

A linear model was used also to relate biophase quinidine concentrations to the time course of electrocardiographic QT interval changes after intravenous and oral dosing [11]. As shown in Fig. 20.3, the slope was greater after oral than after intravenous doses. This phenomenon was attributed to the formation of active metabolites of quinidine during first-pass metabolism of the oral dose [13].

E_{max} models

The apparent linear relationship between biophase concentration and pharmacologic effect usually indicates that effects have been analyzed over only a limited concentration range [14]. In many cases, an E_{max} model is required to analyze more pronounced effects, such as the blood pressure response of cats to norepinephrine. This was the concentration–effect relationship initially analyzed by Segre [7] when he proposed a model for the time course of biophase concentrations. For the E_{max} model, E is described by:

$$E = \frac{E_{max} \bullet C_B}{EC_{50} + C_B} \tag{20.3}$$

where E_{max} is a presumed maximal effect that is predicted from the observed nonlinearity of response and EC_{50} is the biophase concentration (C_B) at which effects are half maximal. The linear effect model defines this relationship adequately as long as biophase drug concentrations, C_B, are substantially less than the EC_{50}. However, the decision to use an E_{max} rather than a linear model is usually determined by the available data rather than by theoretical considerations. For example, in one study of QT interval prolongation by an antiarrhythmic drug, a linear effect model was satisfactory for analyzing the response of four patients, but an E_{max} model was required to analyze the more pronounced effect seen in a fifth patient [15].

Although the mathematical form of the E_{max} model is pharmacologically realistic [7], no physiological significance has been assigned to E_{max} and EC_{50} estimates in most applications of this model. Nonetheless, E_{max} values in some cases may provide an indication of the maximal degree to which a particular intervention can affect enzyme or receptor activity. It also may be possible to find similarities between EC_{50} values and drug binding affinity. For example, ε-aminocaproic acid is a lysine analog that has clot-stabilizing antifibrinolytic effects because it binds to lysine binding sites on plasminogen, preventing its attachment to fibrin. A study of ε-aminocaproic acid kinetics and antifibrinolytic effects in human subjects provided an estimate of half-maximal inhibitory biophase concentration of 63 μg/mL which was similar to the in vitro estimate of 0.55 mM or 72 μg/mL for the ε-aminocaproic acid-plasminogen dissociation constant [16]. In fact, these in vivo and in vitro results both represent an oversimplification of physiological reality, since plasminogen has one high-affinity and four low-affinity sites that bind ε-aminocaproic acid, rather than a single binding site [17].

Sigmoid E_{max} models

In some cases, the pharmacodynamic model will need to be modified to account for the fact that the biophase concentration–effect relationship is sigmoid rather than hyperbolic. This modification was necessary in analyzing the pharmacokinetics and effects of *d*-tubocurarine [9]. In this case, the following equation was used to relate estimated biophase concentrations of *d*-tubocurarine to the degree of skeletal muscle paralysis (E), ranging from normal function to complete paralysis ($E_{max}=1$) caused by this drug:

$$E=\frac{E_{max}\bullet C_B^n}{EC_{50}^n+C_B^n} \tag{20.4}$$

The sigmoid E_{max} model was first developed by Hill [18] to analyze the oxygen-binding affinity of hemoglobin. For normal human hemoglobins and those of most other mammalian species, n has values ranging from 2.8 to 3.0 [19]. This reflects cooperative subunit interactions between the four heme elements of the hemoglobin tetramer. Proteins such as myoglobin that have a single heme subunit, and tetrameric hemoglobins such as hemoglobin H that lack subunit cooperativity, have n values of 1.0. On the other hand, if oxygenation of one hemoglobin subunit caused an infinite increase in the oxygen-binding affinity of the other subunits, n would equal 4. Therefore the n values for normal hemoglobins indicate that there is strong, but not infinite, cooperativity in oxygen binding by the four heme subunits.

Wagner [20] first proposed using the Hill equation to analyze the relationship between drug concentration and pharmacologic response. However, the physiologic significance of n values estimated in pharmacokinetic–pharmacodynamic studies is far less well understood than it is in the case of oxygen binding to hemoglobin. Accordingly, n is currently regarded in these studies as simply an empirical parameter that confers sigmoidicity and steepness to the relationship between biophase concentrations and pharmacologic effect. This is illustrated by Fig. 20.4 showing the relationship between tocainide plasma concentration and antiarrhythmic response [21]. It can be seen from this figure that the shape of the concentration–response curves approximates that of a step function as n values increase.

Sigmoid E_{max} models have been particularly useful in the pharmacokinetic–pharmacodynamic analysis of anesthetic drugs [22]. Waveform analyses of electroencephalographic (EEG) morphology have served as biomarkers for anesthetic effects and show characteristic changes that are different for barbiturates, benzodiazepines, and opiates. Since it often is impossible to conduct clinical studies of these agents at steady state, pharmacokinetic–pharmacodynamic investigations have been performed under conditions in which drug concentrations in plasma and effects are constantly changing. The time delay between changes in drug concentration and effect has been analyzed using a biophase compartment.

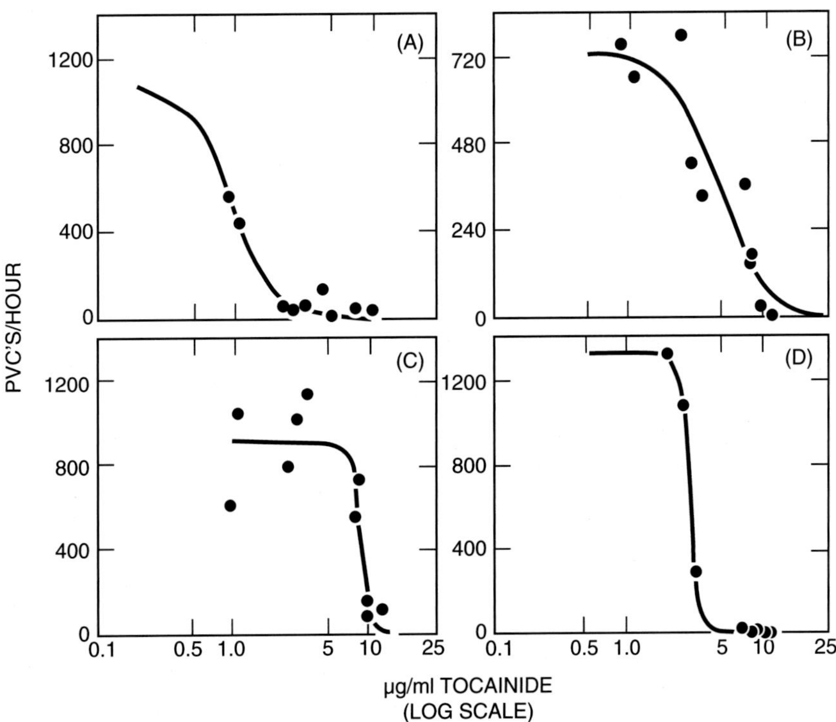

FIG. 20.4 Relationship between plasma concentrations of tocainide and suppression of ventricular premature beats (VPBs) for four representative patients. The relationship between VPB frequency and tocainide concentrations shown by the solid curves was obtained from a nonlinear least-squares regression analysis of the data using a sigmoid E_{max} model. The estimate of n for each patient can be compared with the shape of the tocainide concentration–antiarrhythmic response curve. *(Reproduced with permission from Meffin PJ, Winkle RA, Blaschke TF, Fitzgerald J, Harrison DC, Harapat SR, et al. Response optimization of drug dosage: antiarrhythmic studies with tocainide. Clin Pharmacol Ther 1977;22:42–57.)*

TABLE 20.1 Comparison of parameters describing midazolam and diazepam effect kinetics.

	t(1/2eq) (min)	E_{max} (μV)	EC_{50} (ng/mL)	N
Midazolam	5.6	141	171	1.8
Diazepam	1.9	137	946	1.7

Buhrer M, Maitre PO, Crevoisier C, Stanski DR. Electroencephalographic effects of benzodiazepines. II. Pharmacodynamic modeling of the electroencephalographic effects of midazolam and diazepam. Clin Pharmacol Ther 1990;48:555–567.

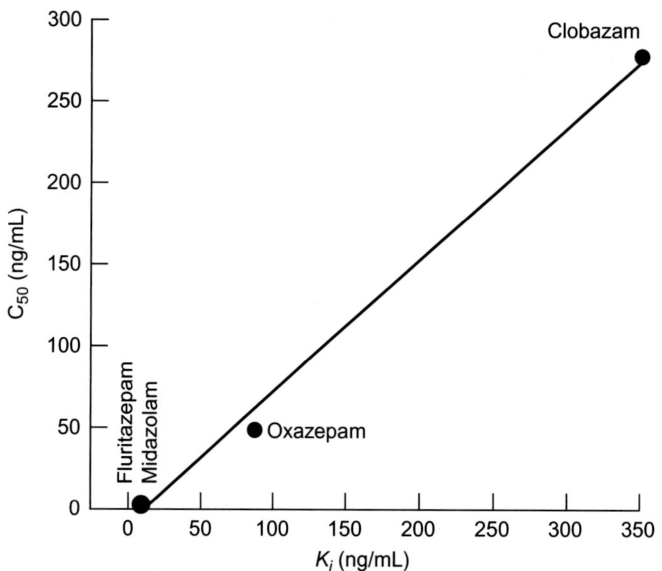

FIG. 20.5 Relationship in rats between the EC_{50} of EEG effects (averaged amplitude in the 11.5–30 Hz frequency band) and estimates of K_i obtained from in vitro studies of the ability of four benzodiazepines to displace [^{3}H]flumazenil from benzodiazepine receptors on brain tissue homogenates. Estimates of EC_{50} were based on free benzodiazepine concentrations not bound to plasma proteins. *(Data from Mandema JW, Sansom LN, Dios-Vieitez MC, Hollander-Jansen M, Danhof M. Pharmacokinetic-pharmacodynamic modeling of the electroencephalographic effects of benzodiazepines. Correlation with receptor binding and anticonvulsant activity. J Pharmacol Exp Ther 1991;257:472–478.)*

Of practical clinical importance is the role that pharmacokinetic–pharmacodynamic analysis played in optimizing dosing guidelines for using midazolam as an intravenous anesthetic agent [22]. Drug approval was based on results of traditional studies from which it was estimated that midazolam was no more than twice as potent as diazepam, the benzodiazepine with which clinicians had the greatest familiarity [23]. However, after considerable patient morbidity and mortality was encountered in routine clinical practice, pharmacokinetic–pharmacodynamic studies provided a significantly greater estimate of midazolam relative potency [24]. The EEG effect chosen in comparing midazolam with diazepam was total voltage from 0 to 30 Hz, as obtained from aperiodic waveform analysis. The results summarized in Table 20.1 show that the two agents have similar E_{max} values, indicating similar efficacy, but that the EC_{50} of midazolam is 5.5 times that of diazepam, demonstrating that midazolam is much more potent than diazepam. In addition, the equilibration half-life ($t_{1/2eq}$) between plasma and the biophase compartment is three times longer for midazolam (5.6 min) than for diazepam (1.9 min). This means that a longer time is needed after rapid injection for the effects of midazolam to become apparent [22]. No physiological significance has been attached to the values of the Hill coefficient, *n*, that were obtained in these studies. However, investigations in rats have demonstrated a correlation between the EC_{50} of EEG effects and estimates of K_i obtained from in vitro studies of the ability of a series of benzodiazepines to displace [^{3}H]flumazenil from benzodiazepine receptors (Fig. 20.5) [25].

Physiokinetics—The time course of effects due to physiological turnover processes

In almost all cases, effects are mediated by an endogenous substance, and drugs modulate these effects indirectly by affecting either the production or elimination of this effect mediator (Fig. 20.6). In addition to delays in drug effect

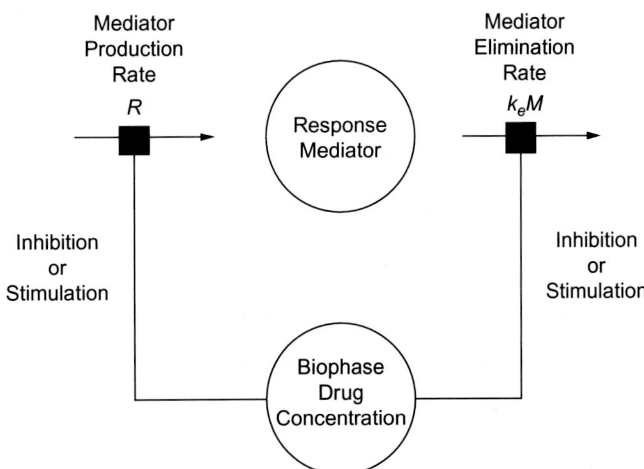

FIG. 20.6 Basic concept of physiological turnover or *physiokinetic* models. Observed effects are mediated by an endogenous substance (*effect mediator*). Drugs modulate these effects by either inhibiting or stimulating the production or elimination of this mediator. This accounts for the fact that the development of these drug effects is delayed beyond the time required for the drug to reach its pharmacologic site of action (*biophase*).

due to pharmacokinetic distribution to the site of action, there are delays determined by the turnover of these effect mediators. The time course of the physiological mediator can be described as *physiokinetics*. Delays of a few minutes, or perhaps an hour or so, might plausibly be explained by distribution of a drug to its site of action, but the rate limiting step for longer delays is likely to be physiokinetic rather than pharmacokinetic.

If the production rate (R) of the mediator (M) is regarded as a zero-order process and the elimination rate of the mediator is regarded as first order, the following equation describes the mass balance of the mediator:

$$\frac{dM}{dt} = R - k_e \cdot M \tag{20.5}$$

where k_e is a first-order elimination rate constant for the mediator. Drugs can be modeled as exerting their effects by altering either R or k_e from their initial values. Implicit in this turnover model is the fact that the time course of effect is governed by the elimination rate of the mediator following a step change in R.

Warfarin is a classic example of a drug with a delayed response that exerts its anticoagulant effects by blocking synthesis of vitamin K-dependent clotting factors (factors II, VII, IX, and X). This effect can be analyzed by including a forcing function, f_c, to relate the degree of inhibition of clotting factor production (R) to the plasma concentration of warfarin:

$$\frac{dM}{dt} = R \cdot f_c - k_e \cdot M \tag{20.6}$$

Nagashima et al. [26] developed an empirical model in which the pharmacodynamic function was modeled as proportional to the logarithm of the warfarin concentration in plasma. Subsequent studies of the effects of the S- and R-enantiomers of warfarin have indicated that an E_{max+} model is consistent with pharmacological theory of enzyme inhibition and can describe effects on clotting factor production [27].

Any of the pharmacodynamic models that we have described for other pharmacologic effects can serve to describe response, and model choice is guided best by an understanding of the mechanism of drug action and by the information content of the available data. In addition to warfarin, Sharma and Jusko [1] have listed a large number of other drugs with delays attributable to changes in mediator turnover. These range from H_2-receptor antagonists, diuretics, and bronchodilators to corticosteroids, nonsteroidal antiinflammatory drugs, and interferon.

Time varying changes in the relationship between concentration and drug effect

So far, we have considered examples in which the relationship between drug concentration at the site of action and the effect is time invariant. This is not the case for drugs that exhibit *pharmacologic tolerance*, in which the intensity of an effect after initial drug exposure subsequently declines despite maintenance of similar biophase drug concentrations. Pharmacologic tolerance is characteristically revealed by plotting plasma concentration against effect and observing a *proteresis* loop. The characteristic feature of proteresis is to see smaller drug effects at the same plasma concentration at later times.

There is now general agreement that tolerance develops rapidly to the cardiovascular and euphoric effects of cocaine [28, 29]. This phenomenon has been characterized by studies in which a bolus injection of cocaine was followed by an exponentially tapering infusion, so that relatively constant plasma concentrations were maintained while pharmacologic effects were observed [30]. Both the cardiovascular and euphoric effects of cocaine were analyzed with a biophase effect compartment and a linear pharmacodynamic model. Functions were used to characterize the acute development of tolerance by reducing the effect slope, β, over time. The increase in heart rate that followed cocaine administration decreased with a 31-min average half-life from its peak to a plateau that averaged 33% of peak values. Changes in blood pressure paralleled the increase and subsequent decline in heart rate [28]. However, subjective evaluation of cocaine-induced euphoria declined to baseline with an average half-life of 66 min. The slower development of tolerance to the euphoric response might reflect other phenomena such as a placebo response based on subjective expectations or a different physiological feedback system. Alternative models for tolerance have been evaluated by Gårdmark et al. [31]. Among the mechanisms proposed are the formation of a drug metabolite that acts as an antagonist and the depletion of a precursor substance when conversion to an active mediator is stimulated by the drug.

Sensitization refers to an increase in pharmacologic response despite maintenance of constant biophase concentrations of drug. Adverse clinical consequences of sensitization are commonly observed following abrupt withdrawal of β-adrenergic blocking drug therapy in patients with coronary heart disease and include ventricular arrhythmias, worsening of angina, and myocardial infarction [32]. Although several mechanisms have been proposed, these adverse events primarily reflect the fact that chronic therapy with β-adrenergic receptor-blocking drugs causes an increase in the number of available β-adrenergic receptors, a phenomenon termed *up-regulation* [32, 33]. When therapy with β-adrenergic receptor-blocking drugs is stopped abruptly, the decline in up-regulated receptors lags behind the elimination of the receptor-blocking drug, resulting in a period of exaggerated responses to normal circulating catecholamine levels.

Using data describing the time course of receptor upregulation in lymphocytes, Lima et al. [34] have developed a kinetic model of the fractional increase in β-adrenergic receptors that occurs with the institution of β-adrenergic receptor-blocking drug therapy, and of its subsequent decline when this therapy is stopped. A modification of Eq. (20.3) was used to characterize the initial intensity of β-adrenergic receptor agonist-induced chronotropic response in the presence of a β-adrenergic receptor antagonist. Supersensitivity was then modeled by simply multiplying this estimate of initial intensity by the expected increase in β-adrenergic receptor density.

Therapeutic response, cumulative drug effects, and schedule dependence

So far, we have focused our attention on the time course of drug effect. While the study of these effects can clarify the mechanism of drug action and factors affecting drug effectiveness and potency, it usually does not provide information on how drug exposure influences clinical outcome.

Clinical outcome can be defined as the effect of drug treatment on the clinical endpoint of how the patient feels, functions, or survives. Some clinical outcomes can be described by composite scales that are commonly used in drug development for regulatory approval [e.g., the Unified Parkinson's Disease Scale (UPDRS) and the Alzheimer's disease Assessment Scale (ADAS)]. These scales can be treated as if they were continuous measures of drug response and, as discussed in Chapter 21, are amenable to pharmacokinetic–pharmacodynamic modeling involving delayed effects even if no concentrations are available [35]. This seemingly broad definition of clinical outcome may exclude some of the drug effects we have discussed so far. For example, outcomes may be related to the cumulative effects of previous drug doses.

The acute treatment of congestive heart failure commonly involves the use of a diuretic to get rid of excess fluid that has accumulated as edema of the lungs and lower extremities. As shown in Fig. 20.7, a high-efficacy diuretic like furosemide has a steep concentration effect relationship, with a clearly defined maximum effect on sodium excretion. After an oral furosemide dose of 120 mg that causes almost maximal sodium excretion, the time course of drug concentrations reaches a peak of about 6 mg/L which is well above the EC_{50} of 1.5 mg/L (Fig. 20.8). A lower dose of 40 mg produces concentrations which are one-third of the 120-mg dose, but the natriuretic effects are not decreased in proportion to the dose. When three 40-mg doses are given over 12 h, the cumulative effect measured by total sodium excretion is 50% greater than that seen after a single 120-mg dose. Despite the same total dose and the same cumulative area under the concentration vs. time curve from the two patterns of dosing, the clinical outcome would be less with the single 120-mg dose. This is an example of the phenomenon of *schedule dependence*.

Schedule dependence occurs when the drug effect is reversible, the concentrations exceed the EC_{50} so that effects approach E_{max} with proportionately less drug effect at high concentrations, and the clinical outcome is related to the cumulative drug effect. The phenomenon is expected to be quite common but is not often recognized clinically, because of wide variability in response and other confounding factors such as disease progression.

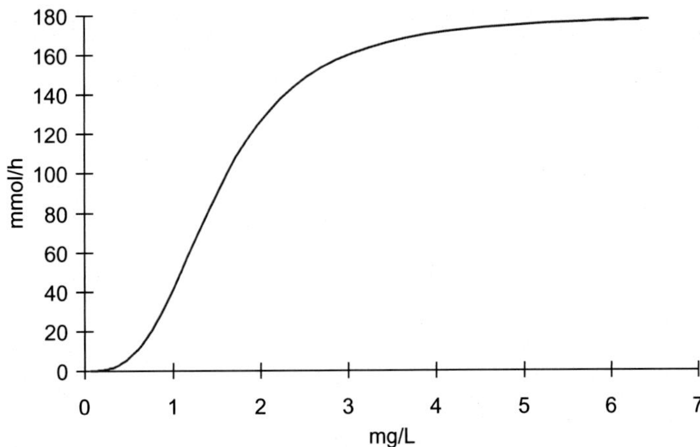

FIG. 20.7 The diuretic effect of furosemide is to increase the excretion rate of sodium. The pharmacodynamics of furosemide show a steep concentration–effect relationship with a clear maximum effect (180 mmol/h of Na^+). The EC_{50} is 1.5 mg/L and the Hill coefficient (n) is 3.

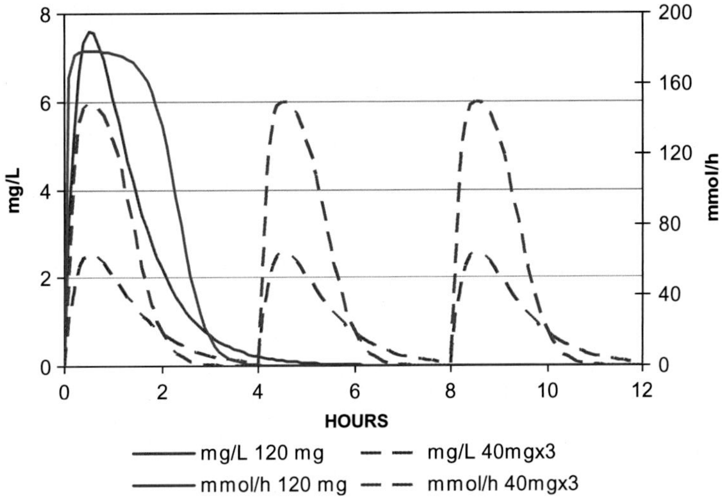

FIG. 20.8 The time course of furosemide concentration and natriuretic effect after 3 doses of 40 mg compared with those after a single 120-mg dose. Note that the concentrations after 120 mg are exactly three times higher than after 40 mg, but the peak effect after 40 mg is quite close to the peak after 120 mg because response to the 120-mg dose is limited by effects approaching E_{max}. The cumulative sodium loss after 120 mg is 400 mmol, while the three 40-mg doses produce a 600-mmol loss.

The reduction of pain and other symptoms due to peptic ulceration may be quite closely linked to the current effect of a drug on acid secretion, but the rate of healing and eventual disappearance of an ulcer is a slow process, determined in part by the extent and duration of gastric acid secretion suppression over several weeks. The clinical outcome of ulcer healing is therefore a consequence of the cumulative degree of acid inhibition. Proton pump inhibitors such as omeprazole bind irreversibly to the proton pump to suppress gastric acid secretion. The extent of inhibition is close to 100% and outcomes are related to cumulative effects, but the irreversible nature of the drug action means that schedule dependence is not observed.

Many clinical outcomes are described in terms of *events*. An event might be death, a stroke, a myocardial infarction, an epileptic seizure, admission to hospital, need for supplementary treatment, and so on. The occurrence of an event or the time to an event can be modeled using a survivor function. The word *survival* relates most obviously to a death event, but the term is commonly used in a much broader context to describe the probability that the event under study will not occur.

The hazard function approach allows complex pharmacokinetic–pharmacodynamic influences to affect the occurrence of an event. The hazard ($h(t)$, sometimes called instantaneous risk) of an event a time t is shown as:

$$h(t) = f(\Gamma, X) \tag{20.7}$$

where Γ is a set of parameters describing the hazard as a function of X (time, dose, etc.). The hazard is exactly equivalent to the elimination rate constant in a pharmacokinetic model [36]. Indeed, the time course of drug concentration can be described by thinking of each molecule as having a risk of "dying" when it is eliminated. It is the survival of the molecules that have yet to be eliminated that determines the drug concentration. Potential time-varying covariates for different event hazards are cholesterol concentrations (heart attack event), blood pressure (stroke event), or concentration of an anticonvulsant drug (seizure event). The chances of an event are related both to the size of the hazard and the time that the patient is exposed to the hazard. The cumulative hazard, $H(t)$, from 0 to t can be related to the probability of an event, as illustrated in the case of a constant hazard.

$$\begin{aligned} H(t) &= \int_0^t h(t) \\ &= \int_0^t \lambda_0 \\ &= \lambda_0 \cdot t \end{aligned} \tag{20.8}$$

In this equation, λ_0 is the instantaneous risk of an event when the hazard is constant. A constant hazard is not typically realistic for biological events and time-varying hazards are more commonly needed to describe clinical outcome events.

The probability of surviving from time 0 to time t is known as the survivor function, $S(t)$.

$$S(t) = \exp(-H(t)) \tag{20.9}$$

Note the exact similarity between survivor function and the equation describing the time course of drug concentration being eliminated from a one-compartment system. Cox et al. [37] describe the use of the hazard and the survivor function for modeling the likelihood of an event (L) whose time is known, $L(t)$:

$$L(t) = S(t) \cdot h(t) \tag{20.10}$$

More often an event is known to have occurred in an interval of time but the exact time is not known. The likelihood of an event in the interval $t[j-1]$ to $t[j]$ is given by:

$$L(t[j] - t[j-1]) = S(t[j-1]) - S(t[j]) \tag{20.11}$$

Hu and Sale [38] give interesting examples of applying this idea to simulating clinical trials with dropout events that may be determined by the underlying disease progress.

The use of a hazard function to describe the time-varying risk of an event is a flexible method for bringing together pharmacokinetics, changes in drug effects on biomarkers, and other risk factors such as concomitant changes in disease severity. It has been applied to understand the need for additional pain medication in clinical trials of analgesics [39] and the suppression of vomiting events caused by chemotherapy [37]. The hazard function idea can be extended to describe clinical outcomes that are described in terms of frequency (e.g., epileptic seizures per month) and categorical scales of severity (e.g., heartburn pain) [40]. Study of long-term drug effects requires incorporation of a disease progression model into the analysis, and this is the subject of Chapter 21.

References

[1] Sharma A, Jusko WJ. Characteristics of indirect pharmacodynamic models and applications to clinical drug responses. Br J Clin Pharmacol 1998;45:229–239.

[2] Sherwin RS, Kramer KJ, Tobin JD, Insel PA, Liljenquist JE, Berman M, et al. A model of the kinetics of insulin in man. J Clin Invest 1974;53:1481–1492.

[3] Steil GM, Meador MA, Bergman RN. Thoracic duct lymph. Relative contribution from splanchnic and muscle tissue. Diabetes 1993;42:720–731.

[4] Kramer WG, Kolibash AJ, Lewis RP, Bathala MS, Visconti JA, Reuning RH. Pharmacokinetics of digoxin: relationship between response intensity and predicted compartmental drug levels in man. J Pharmacokinet Biopharm 1979;7:47–61.

[5] Weiss M, Kang W. Inotropic effect of digoxin in humans: mechanistic pharmacokinetic/pharmacodynamic model based on slow receptor binding. Pharm Res 2004;21:231–236.

[6] Wagner JG, Aghajanian GK, Bing OH. Correlation of performance test scores with "tissue concentration" of lysergic acid diethylamide in human subjects. Clin Pharmacol Ther 1968;9:635–638.

[7] Segre G. Kinetics of interaction between drugs and biological systems. Farmaco Ed Sci 1968;23:907–918.

[8] Hull CJ, Van Beem HB, McLeod K, Sibbald A, Watson MJ. A pharmacodynamic model for pancuronium. Br J Anaesth 1978;50:1113–1123.

[9] Sheiner LB, Stanski DR, Vozeh S, Miller RD, Ham J. Simultaneous modeling of pharmacokinetics and pharmacodynamics: application to D-tubocurarine. Clin Pharmacol Ther 1979;25:358–371.

[10] Holford NH, Sheiner LB. Understanding the dose-effect relationship: clinical application of pharmacokinetic-pharmacodynamic models. Clin Pharmacokinet 1981;6:429–453.

[11] Holford NH, Coates PE, Guentert TW, Riegelman S, Sheiner LB. The effect of quinidine and its metabolites on the electrocardiogram and systolic time intervals: concentration–effect relationships. Br J Clin Pharmacol 1981;11:187–195.

[12] Eudeikis JR, Henthorn TK, Lertora JJ, Atkinson AJ Jr, Chao GC, Kushner W. Kinetic analysis of the vasodilator and ganglionic blocking actions of N-acetylprocainamide. J Cardiovasc Pharmacol 1982;4:303–309.

[13] Vozeh S, Bindschedler M, Ha HR, Kaufmann G, Guentert TW, Follath F. Pharmacodynamics of 3-hydroxyquinidine alone and in combination with quinidine in healthy persons. Am J Cardiol 1987;59:681–684.

[14] Holford NH, Sheiner LB. Pharmacokinetic and pharmacodynamic modeling in vivo. Crit Rev Bioeng 1981;5:273–322.

[15] Piergies AA, Ruo TI, Jansyn EM, Belknap SM, Atkinson AJ Jr. Effect kinetics of N-acetylprocainamide-induced QT interval prolongation. Clin Pharmacol Ther 1987;42:107–112.

[16] Frederiksen MC, Bowsher DJ, Ruo TI, Henthorn TK, Ts'ao CH, Green D, et al. Kinetics of epsilon-aminocaproic acid distribution, elimination, and antifibrinolytic effects in normal subjects. Clin Pharmacol Ther 1984;35:387–393.

[17] Markus G, DePasquale JL, Wissler FC. Quantitative determination of the binding of epsilon-aminocaproic acid to native plasminogen. J Biol Chem 1978;253:727–732.

[18] Hill AV. The possible effects of the aggregation of the molecules of hemoglobin on its dissociation curves. J Physiol (Lond) 1910;40:iv–vii.

[19] Bunn HF, Forget BG, Ranney HM. Human hemoglobins. Philadelphia: WB Saunders; 1977. p. 35–41.

[20] Wagner JG. Kinetics of pharmacologic response. I. Proposed relationships between response and drug concentration in the intact animal and man. J Theor Biol 1968;20:173–201.

[21] Meffin PJ, Winkle RA, Blaschke TF, Fitzgerald J, Harrison DC, Harapat SR, et al. Response optimization of drug dosage: antiarrhythmic studies with tocainide. Clin Pharmacol Ther 1977;22:42–57.

[22] Stanski DR. Pharmacodynamic modeling of anesthetic EEG drug effects. Annu Rev Pharmacol Toxicol 1992;32:423–447.

[23] Magni VC, Frost RA, Leung JW, Cotton PB. A randomized comparison of midazolam and diazepam for sedation in upper gastrointestinal endoscopy. Br J Anaesth 1983;55:1095–1101.

[24] Buhrer M, Maitre PO, Crevoisier C, Stanski DR. Electroencephalographic effects of benzodiazepines. II. Pharmacodynamic modeling of the electroencephalographic effects of midazolam and diazepam. Clin Pharmacol Ther 1990;48:555–567.

[25] Mandema JW, Sansom LN, Dios-Vieitez MC, Hollander-Jansen M, Danhof M. Pharmacokinetic-pharmacodynamic modeling of the electroencephalographic effects of benzodiazepines. Correlation with receptor binding and anticonvulsant activity. J Pharmacol Exp Ther 1991;257:472–478.

[26] Nagashima R, O'Reilly RA, Levy G. Kinetics of pharmacologic effects in man: the anticoagulant action of warfarin. Clin Pharmacol Ther 1969;10:22–35.

[27] Xue L, Holford N, Ding XL, Shen ZY, Huang CR, Zhang H, et al. Theory-based pharmacokinetics and pharmacodynamics of S- and R-warfarin and effects on international normalized ratio: influence of body size, composition and genotype in cardiac surgery patients. Br J Clin Pharmacol 2017;83:823–835.

[28] Ambre JJ. Acute tolerance to pressor effects of cocaine in humans. Ther Drug Monit 1993;15:537–540.

[29] Foltin RW, Fischman MW, Levin FR. Cardiovascular effects of cocaine in humans: laboratory studies. Drug Alcohol Depend 1995;37:193–210.

[30] Ambre JJ, Belknap SM, Nelson J, Ruo TI, Shin SG, Atkinson AJ Jr. Acute tolerance to cocaine in humans. Clin Pharmacol Ther 1988;44:1–8.

[31] Gardmark M, Brynne L, Hammarlund-Udenaes M, Karlsson MO. Interchangeability and predictive performance of empirical tolerance models. Clin Pharmacokinet 1999;36:145–167.

[32] Nattel S, Rangno RE, Van Loon G. Mechanism of propranolol withdrawal phenomena. Circulation 1979;59:1158–1164.

[33] Houston MC, Hodge R. Beta-adrenergic blocker withdrawal syndromes in hypertension and other cardiovascular diseases. Am Heart J 1988;116:515–523.

[34] Lima JJ, Krukemyer JJ, Boudoulas H. Drug- or hormone-induced adaptation: model of adrenergic hypersensitivity. J Pharmacokinet Biopharm 1989;17:347–364.

[35] Holford NH, Peace KE. Results and validation of a population pharmacodynamic model for cognitive effects in Alzheimer patients treated with tacrine. Proc Natl Acad Sci U S A 1992;89:11471–11475.

[36] Holford N. A time to event tutorial for pharmacometricians. CPT: Pharmacomet Syst Pharmacol 2013;2:1–8.

[37] Cox E, Veyrat-Follet C, Beal S, Fuseau E, Kenkare S, Sheiner L. A population pharmacokinetic-pharmacodynamic analysis of repeated measures time-to-event pharmacodynamic responses: the antiemetic effect of ondansetron. J Pharmacokinet Biopharm 1999;27:625–644.

[38] Hu C, Sale ME. A joint model for nonlinear longitudinal data with informative dropout. J Pharmacokinet Pharmacodyn 2003;30:83–103.

[39] Sheiner LB. A new approach to the analysis of analgesic drug trials, illustrated with bromfenac data. Clin Pharmacol Ther 1994;56:309–322.

[40] Plan EL, Karlsson KE, Karlsson MO. Approaches to simultaneous analysis of frequency and severity of symptoms. Clin Pharmacol Ther 2010;88 (2):255–259.

Chapter 21

Disease progress models

Diane R. Mould[a], Nicholas H.G. Holford[b], and Carl C. Peck[c]

[a]*Projections Research Inc, Phoenixville, PA, United States,* [b]*Department of Pharmacology and Clinical Pharmacology, University of Auckland, Auckland, New Zealand,* [c]*Department of Bioengineering and Therapeutic Sciences, University of California at San Francisco, San Francisco, CA, United States*

Clinical pharmacology and disease progress

Clinical pharmacology, like many disciplines, can be viewed from several perspectives. In the context of a clinical trial of a therapeutic agent, clinical pharmacology provides a conceptual framework for relating drug treatment to responses and differentiating possible mechanisms of drug action. Disease progression refers to the evolution of a disease over time. It typically implies worsening of the disease, but also may include spontaneous recovery. Disease progress on the other hand is a description of the disease and its response to treatment. In the context of simulation and modeling, it is useful to think of clinical pharmacology as itself a model that combines disease progression with drug action.

$$\text{Clinical pharmacology} = \text{Disease progression} + \text{Drug action} \tag{21.1}$$

Thus the study of clinical pharmacology is the study of disease progress during treatment. Disease progress models may be used to describe the time course of a disease biomarker or clinical outcome reflecting the status of a disease and the effects of drug treatment. The disease status in a clinical trial may also be modified by a placebo response which can occasionally be distinguished from the natural history of disease progression. Disease status is a reflection of the state of the disease at a point in time. The disease status may improve or worsen over time, or may be a cyclical phenomenon, e.g., malarial quartan fever or seasonal affective disorder. Therefore a model of disease progress is a quantitative expression that describes the expected changes in disease status over time.

Drug action refers to all the pharmacokinetic and pharmacodynamic processes involved in producing a drug effect on the disease. The effect of the drug is assumed to influence the disease status. Pharmacokinetic and pharmacodynamic drug properties are the major attributes determining drug action and its effect on the time course of progression of the disease. Disease progress models can be extended to include terms that account for the changes in disease progression that are affected by drug treatment. We call such a combined model the clinical pharmacology model for the drug (Eq. 21.1).

Disease progress models

In this chapter, we describe the basic elements of clinical pharmacology models for use in describing the time course of disease progression and the changes in disease progress in response to treatment. These models have two basic components: the first describes the disease progression without therapeutic intervention and the second defines the change in progress as a result of treatment.

"No Progress" model

The simplest model of disease progress assumes there is no change in disease status during the period of observation. Previously, this has been reflected in simple pharmacodynamic models, such as those described in Chapter 20, by the constant "baseline effect" parameter, often symbolized by E_0 [1]. The symbol E_0 is misleading because the "E" implies a drug effect but by definition the drug effect is zero at baseline before the drug has been administered. A constant baseline is a common assumption made in the design and analysis of clinical trials. Such an analysis ignores the progress of disease during the course of the trial by comparing the effect of drug treatment groups at similar points in time. This is a reflection of a "minimalist" approach to clinical trial design and analysis that seeks only to falsify the null hypothesis and thereby excludes learning by an informative description of the observed phenomena [2, 3]. The assumption that there is no change in disease status over time does not permit learning about the effect of the drug on the rate of disease progress.

Atkinson's Principles of Clinical Pharmacology. https://doi.org/10.1016/B978-0-12-819869-8.00017-3

Linear progression model

The linear disease progression model (Eq. 21.2) assumes a constant rate of change of a biomarker or clinical outcome that reflects the disease status (S) at any time, t, from the initial observation of the patient, for example, at the time of entry into a clinical trial. It can be defined in terms of a baseline disease status (S_0) and a slope (α), which reflects the change from baseline status over time.

$$S(t) = S_0 + \alpha \cdot t \tag{21.2}$$

S_0 is preferable to E_0 because it refers to the disease status before drug is given. Using this model as a basis to describe the effect of drug on the time course of disease progression, there are three drug effect patterns possible. Treatment can influence the patient's disease status without affecting the rate of progress (offset pattern), it can alter the rate of progression of the disease (slope pattern), or it can do both (combined slope and offset pattern).

Offset pattern

We define a drug-induced shift upward or downward without a change in slope of the disease status line as the offset pattern. The effect of the drug is a function of concentration ($C_{e,A}$) at the effect site, E_{OFF}, and can be thought of as modifying the baseline parameter S_0 as shown in Eq. (21.3):

$$S(t) = S_0 + E_{OFF}\left(C_{e,A}\right) + \alpha \cdot t \tag{21.3}$$

This model can be used to describe a nonpersistent drug effect (sometimes termed "symptomatic"), for example, lowering of blood pressure by an antihypertensive agent that persists during periods of exposure to the drug but with a return to pretreatment status on cessation of therapy. The onset of drug effect may be delayed by adding an effect compartment to the drug action part of the model, which incorporates more realism by delaying active drug concentrations at the effect site in relation to plasma drug concentrations [4].

Slope pattern

We define a drug-induced increase or decrease in the rate of progression of disease status as the slope pattern. The effect of the drug, E_{SLOPE}, can be thought of as modifying the slope parameter α as shown in Eq. (21.4):

$$S(t) = S_0 + \left[E_{SLOPE}\left(C_{e,A}\right) + \alpha\right] \cdot t \tag{21.4}$$

Compared to the offset pattern, this model can be used to describe a more permanent drug effect, such as slowing the progression of a disease such as rheumatoid arthritis. This kind of change in the rate of change of disease progression is called a "disease modifying" effect. In this case, the cessation of therapy would not be expected to result in a return to pretreatment status. In general, we might expect some delay in the onset of effect (predicted by $C_{e,A}$), but an instantaneous effect model to describe the drug effect on the slope parameter may be sufficient because changes in status tend to develop slowly when the slope changes.

Combined offset and slope pattern

Both an offset effect and a slope effect may be combined to describe the changes in disease status (Eq. 21.5):

$$S(t) = S_0 + E_{OFF}\left(C_{e,A}\right) + \left[E_{SLOPE}\left(C_{e,A}\right) + \alpha\right] \cdot t \tag{21.5}$$

Fig. 21.1 illustrates the offset and slope models and the combination of both types of effect. The offset pattern of drug effect provides an explicit definition of a temporary or symptomatic effect of a drug. In contrast, the slope pattern of drug effect defines a drug with a disease-modifying effect. The pattern of disease progress in the absence of drug is usually referred to as the natural history of the disease (Fig. 21.1).

A study by Griggs et al. [5] reporting temporary increases in muscle strength of muscular dystrophy patients treated with prednisone illustrates an application of the offset drug effect pattern (Fig. 21.2). Fig. 21.3 shows a similar offset pattern of the effect of zidovudine in CD4 cell measurements in HIV patients [6]. However, in this case, the model of disease progress is comprised of functions that are not simply straight lines (polynomial, Eq. 21.6) and zidovudine treatment (combined polynomial and exponential, Eq. 21.7):

$$NoTreatment(t) = CD4_0 - k_1 \cdot t - k_2 \cdot t^2 \tag{21.6}$$

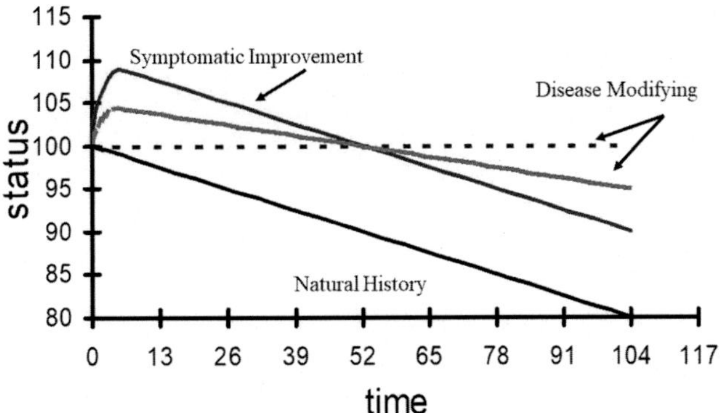

FIG. 21.1 The *thick black line* depicts the natural course of disease progress without therapeutic intervention (Eq. 21.2). The *thin red line* describes an offset pattern (symptomatic) as a consequence of treatment (Eq. 21.3). The *dotted blue line* reflects a slope pattern with a change in the rate of progress of the disease (disease modifying) (Eq. 21.4). The *dashed green line* shows the combination of both offset and slope patterns (Eq. 21.5).

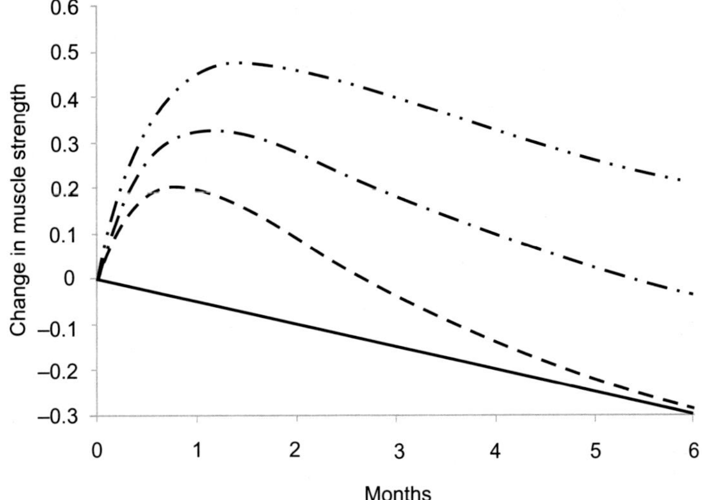

FIG. 21.2 Example of linear disease progress and offset drug effect pattern when prednisone is used to treat muscular dystrophy. The *solid line* is the expected natural history of progressive loss of muscle strength. The *dashed line* shows the transient improvement due to the placebo response. The *dotted lines* demonstrate the delayed offset pattern of drug effect at two doses of prednisone. *(Based on Griggs RC, Moxley RT, Mendell JR, Fenichel GM, Broooke MH, Pestronik A, et al. Prednisone in Duchenne dystrophy: a randomized, controlled trial defining the time course and dose response. Arch Neurol 1991;48:383–388.)*

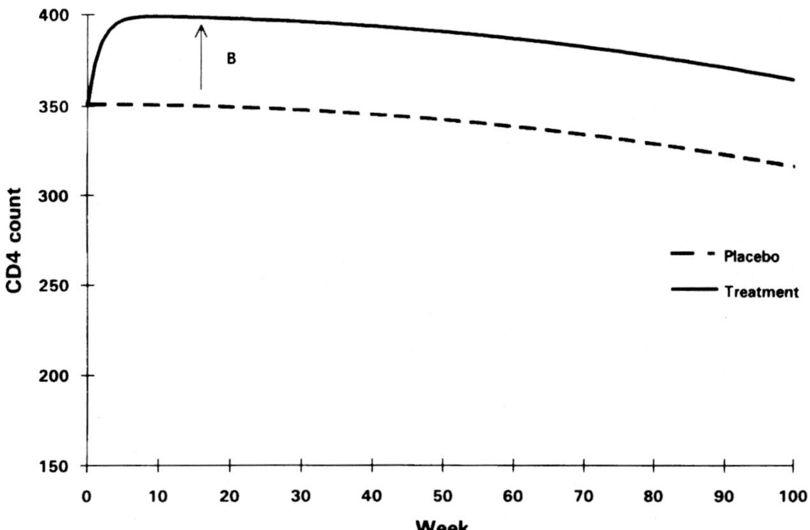

FIG. 21.3 Time course of CD4 count in placebo (*dashed line*) and zidovudine (*solid line*) treated patients. *(Reproduced with permission from Sale M, Sheiner LB, Volberding P, Blaschke TF. Zidovudine response relationships in early human immunodeficiency virus infection. Clin Pharmacol Ther 1993;54:556–566.)*

$$Treatment(t) = \left[B + (k_5 \cdot CD4_0) + \left(k_6 \cdot CD4_0{}^2\right)\right] \cdot \left(e^{-k_3 \cdot t} - e^{-k_4 \cdot t}\right) \tag{21.7}$$

The parameters B and k_1 through k_6 are used to describe how $CD4$ can be predicted from baseline $CD4_0$ and time. The model for the placebo group that did not receive treatment (*NoTreatment*) most likely reflects the natural history of HIV progression but it is not possible to distinguish a placebo response component in this case.

Models for multiple periods of treatment with placebo and active drug (with different doses) in a clinical trial have been used with a disease progress model to describe the response to tacrine in Alzheimer's disease. By assuming the disease progression model was linear, it was possible to identify a placebo response time course that was independent of the natural history of progression. Fig. 21.4 shows the placebo and active treatment components as well as the disease progression [7]. The predicted time course of response in patients with Alzheimer's disease in a complex clinical trial design combining disease progress, placebo, and tacrine effects is shown in Fig. 21.5 [8]. In this figure, the upper curve reflects the expected patient disease status, which would reflect a combination of disease progress and the effect of placebo on the time course of disease progress. In the lower curve, the sequential effects of varying treatments including doses of placebo (P), 40 and 80 mg/day of tacrine were simulated. The difference between the control and active groups increases notably over the duration of the trial. This underscores the need to incorporate appropriate models of disease progress as well as to account for placebo effect, if possible, in descriptions of clinical trials.

Finally, a disease progress model can reflect more complex drug action phenomena such as a drug concentration–effect delay, tolerance, and rebound to both placebo and active treatments [1]. For instance, a delay to onset can be accounted for

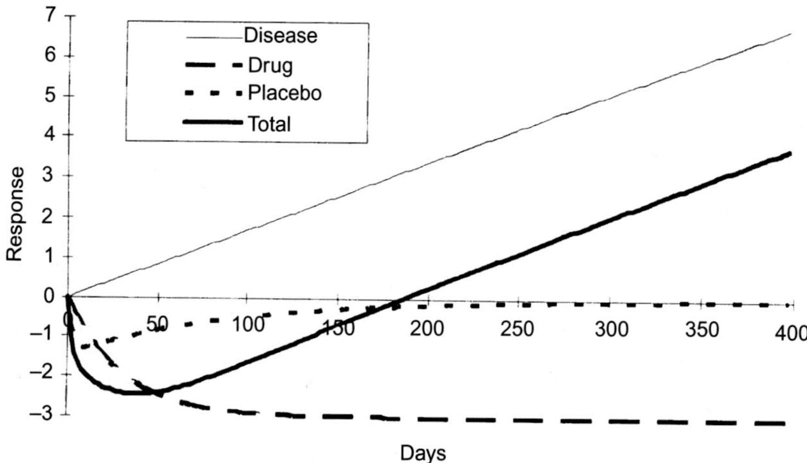

FIG. 21.4 Models of Alzheimer's disease progress (*thick line*), placebo effect (*dotted line*), and drug effect (*dashed line*) in absence of disease progress, and combined (drug plus placebo) response to active drug in the presence of disease progress (*thin line*). Drug effect is assessed by subtracting placebo response and disease progress from the combined response that is observed with drug therapy. *{Reproduced with permission from Holford NHG. Population models for Alzheimer's and Parkinson's disease. In: Aarons L, Balant LP, editors. The population approach: measuring and managing variability in response, concentration and dose. Brussels: COST B1 European Commission; 1997. 97–104.)*

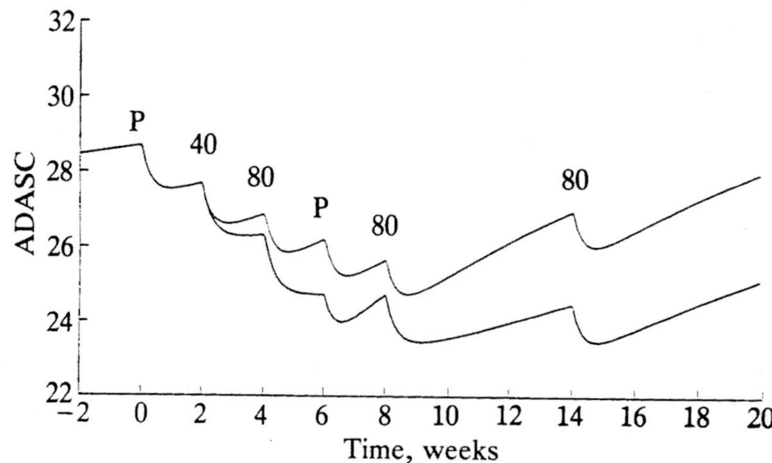

FIG. 21.5 The *upper curve* shows the time course of predicted responses in a patient receiving placebo treatments as part of the three-part trial design used to evaluate tacrine in Alzheimer's disease. The *lower curve* shows the simulated response in a patient receiving a particular sequence of placebo (P) followed by tacrine (40 or 80 mg/day). *{Reproduced with permission from Holford NHG, Peace KE. Methodologic aspects of a population pharmacodynamic model for cognitive effects in Alzheimer patients treated with tacrine. Proc Natl Acad Sci U S A 1992;89:11466–11470.)*

by the addition of an effect site compartment, and tolerance and rebound effects can be described by the addition of a precursor pool compartment, which would limit the effect of drug activity.

The offset and slope models account for open-ended monotonic disease progression in time, suitable for describing disease progression during a clinical trial comprising a brief time of observation relative to the duration of disease. The following asymptotic models provide for disease stabilization or return to a nondisease state, applicable to a clinical trial that encompasses disease progression to an eventual unchanging state.

Asymptotic progress model

Zero asymptote

A common pattern of disease progress provides for the patient's return to health or recovery. For example, the time course of postoperative pain can be expected to start at a baseline state, which involves intense levels of pain. However, over a few days the level of pain experienced by the patient usually decreases until eventually pain is no longer perceived. This recovery can be approximated by an exponential model with an asymptote of zero, indicating the absence of pain. As shown in Eq. (21.8), the parameters of this model are the baseline pain status S_0 and the half-life of progression, T_{prog}:

$$S(t) = S_0 \cdot e^{-\ln 2/T_{prog} \cdot t} \tag{21.8}$$

The asymptote model is particularly useful for illustrating one of the primary potential drawbacks of not accounting for disease progress. Because patients are expected to improve over time, a simple minimalist approach to the comparison of different drug effects would be expected to be dependent on the time of comparative assessment. If the comparison were made at a point in time where recovery has largely occurred, the difference between treatments would probably be undetectable.

As with the linear model of disease progress, the consequences of therapeutic intervention on the asymptotic model of disease progress can be described by including terms to account for the expected action of a drug. Drugs may exert an immediate and transient symptomatic effect, they may act to alter the progress of the disease, such as shortening the time to recovery, or they may do both.

Zero-asymptote offset model pattern

As shown in Eq. (21.9), drug action models based on the zero-asymptote model can be extended to include an offset term $[E_{OFF}\,(C_{e,A})]$ in the model of progress describing symptomatic benefit such as the relief of pain from a simple analgesic.

$$S(t) = E_{OFF}\left(C_{e,A}\right) + S_0 \cdot e^{-\ln 2/T_{prog} \cdot t} \tag{21.9}$$

As with the offset model for the linear disease progress model, the effect of drug would be expected to disappear on cessation of therapy in this offset model. Again, a delay to the onset of drug effect can be incorporated with the use of an effect site compartment component.

Zero-asymptote slope pattern

In addition, an exponentially progressing pattern of disease progress (parameterized by a half-life of progression) can reflect a disease-modifying benefit of drug treatment, if the therapeutic intervention accelerates the return to the normal state or shortens the half-life of the recovery process. Eq. (21.10) describes the disease-modifying benefit where $E_{TP}(C_{e,A})$ describes the time course of effect of concentration of A at the effect site $(C_{e,A})$ on the half-life of progression (T_{prog}):

$$S(t) = S_0 \cdot e^{-\ln 2/\left[E_{TP}\left(C_{e,A}\right) + T_{prog}\right] \cdot t} \tag{21.10}$$

Combined offset and slope pattern

The effects of a therapeutic agent on the progress of a disease may include both a symptomatic effect, E_{OFF}, and a disease modifying effect, E_{TP}. Eq. (21.11) describes the combination of these actions on the zero-asymptote disease progress model:

$$S(t) = E_{OFF}\left(C_{e,A}\right) + S_0 \cdot e^{-\ln 2/\left[E_{TP}\left(C_{e,A}\right) + T_{prog}\right] \cdot t} \tag{21.11}$$

Fig. 21.6 illustrates the expected changes in the progress of a disease, which can be described using the zero-asymptote model.

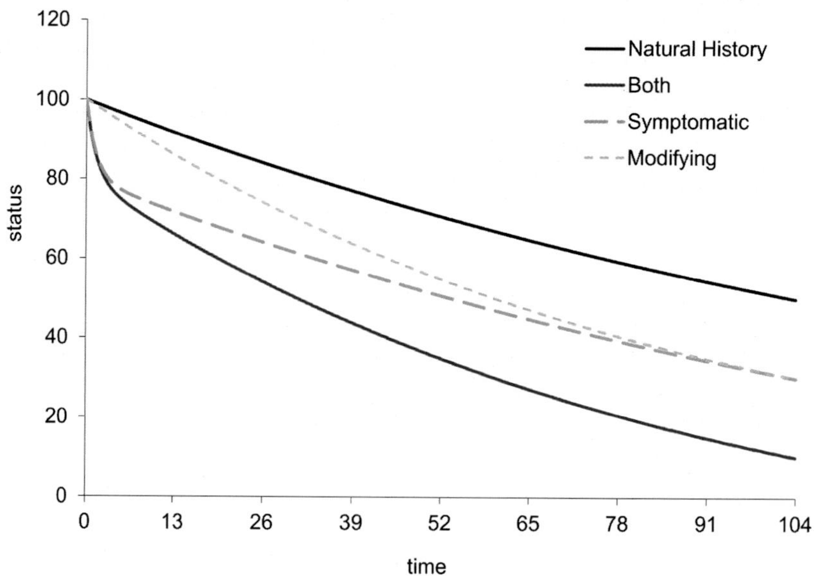

FIG. 21.6 Patterns of drug effect with the zero-asymptote progress model. The *black line* describes the natural history of disease without therapeutic intervention. The *red line* shows the change when a drug that affects symptoms with some delay in onset of effects. The *dotted yellow line* illustrates the expected time course of disease when an agent is given with immediate disease modifying effects and the *dashed green line* describes the expected results from administering an agent that exhibits both symptomatic and disease-modifying effects on the time course of disease progress.

Nonzero asymptote

Another pattern of disease progress encompasses reaching a "burned out" state (S_{SS}). This state is thought to happen when diseases, such as rheumatoid arthritis, reach a point when disease processes damage tissue beyond repair by any therapeutic means. This irreversibly damaged state can be described by another exponential model. The model can be expressed as follows (Eq. 21.12) where t is time after the start of observing the disease from a baseline state (S_0) and the half-life of progression is T_{prog}.

$$S(t) = S_0 \cdot e^{-\ln 2/T_{prog} \cdot t} + S_{SS} \cdot \left(1 - e^{-\ln 2/T_{prog} \cdot t}\right) \quad (21.12)$$

Offset pattern

Therapeutic treatment can affect disease status without altering the time to reach a burned-out steady-state status, S_{SS}. This improvement in status would be expected to be transient and dependent on continual drug exposure. (Eq. 21.13) describes the effect of adding a drug that has a symptomatic effect [$E_{OFF}(C_{e,A})$] on patient disease status:

$$S(t) = E_{OFF}\left(C_{e,A}\right) + S_0 \cdot e^{-\ln 2/T_{prog} \cdot t} + S_{SS} \cdot \left(1 - e^{-\ln 2/T_{prog} \cdot t}\right) \quad (21.13)$$

Slope pattern

Additional models for drug effects on the non-zero-asymptote model include two patterns of disease-modifying drug effects. These assume a drug effect changing either the burned-out state, S_{SS};

$$S(t) = S_0 \cdot e^{-\ln 2/T_{prog} \cdot t} + \left[E_{OFF}\left(C_{e,A}\right) + S_{SS}\right] \cdot \left(1 - e^{-\ln 2/T_{prog} \cdot t}\right) \quad (21.14)$$

or affecting the half-life of progression, T_{prog}.

$$S(t) = S_0 \cdot e^{-\ln 2/\left[E\left(C_{e,a}\right) + T_{prog}\right] \cdot t} + S_{SS} \cdot \left(1 - e^{-\ln 2/\left[E\left(C_{e,a}\right) + T_{prog}\right] \cdot t}\right) \quad (21.15)$$

Offset and slope patterns

Fig. 21.7 illustrates the non-zero-asymptote model with all three patterns of disease progress influenced by drug effect. Drug exposure starts at 1.0 time units and is stopped at 8.0 time units. In Eq. (21.16) the effects of symptomatic

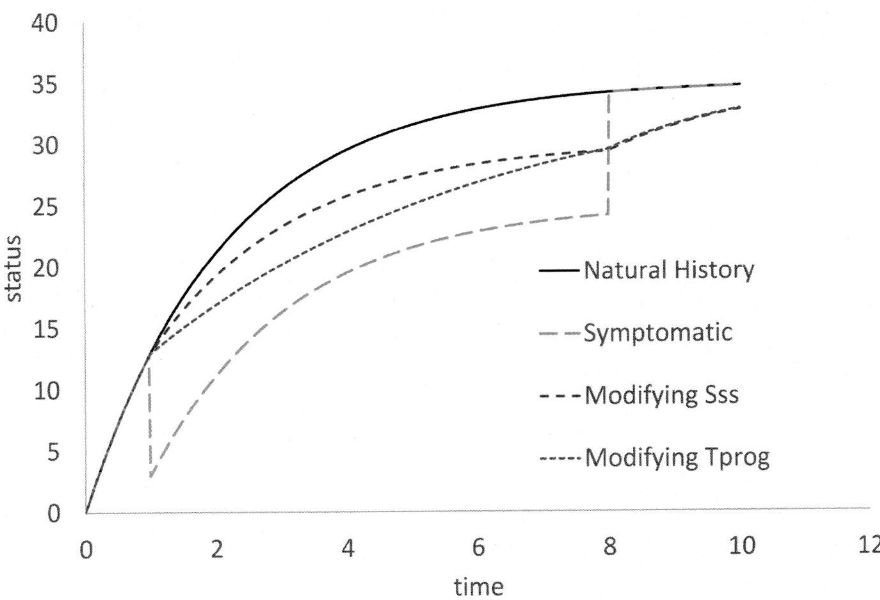

FIG. 21.7 Non-zero-asymptote model with natural history (*black line*), symptomatic drug effect (*dashed green line*) and two types of disease-modifying drug effects: S_{SS}—effect on steady-state burned-out state (*dashed red line*) and T_{prog}—effect on half-life of disease progress (*dotted purple line*). Drug treatment starts at time = 1 and stops at time = 8.

improvement and the two functions describing the action of drug on both the burned-out state and on the time to reach this state have been included.

$$S(t)=E_{OFF}\left(C_{e,A}\right)+S_0\cdot e^{-\ln 2/\left[E_{TP}\left(C_{e,a}\right)+T_{prog}\right]\cdot t}+\left[E_{SS}\left(C_{e,A}\right)+S_{SS}\right]\cdot\left(1-e^{-\ln 2/\left[E_{TP}\left(C_{e,a}\right)+T_{prog}\right]\cdot t}\right) \tag{21.16}$$

Eqs. (21.14)–(21.16) assume immediate onset of disease modifying effects with constant $C_{e,A}$. A system of differential equations is needed to predict $S(t)$ if $C_{e,A}$ varies with time.

The earlier mentioned models are descriptive and are not based on underlying biological mechanisms or pathophysiology. The following models employ physiological concepts and may be considered to be semiempirical models.

Physiological turnover models

The time course of drug effect can often be understood in terms of drug-induced changes in physiological turnover processes controlling synthesis rate (R_{syn}) or elimination of a physiological mediator [9, 10]. These models can be readily extended to describe disease progress by incorporating a time-varying inhibitory effect of the drug (Pharmaco Dynamic Inhibition, *PDI*) on either synthesis or elimination of the physiological mediator. For example, if the rate constant (k_{loss}) describing loss of a physiological mediator starts from a baseline state, $k_{loss\ 0}$, and decreases with a half-life of $T50_{loss}$, then the time course of the disease state can be described by solving the differential equation given in Eq. (21.17):

$$\frac{dS}{dt}=R_{syn}-k_{loss}\cdot PDI\cdot S \tag{21.17}$$

where

$$k_{loss}=k_{loss\ 0}\cdot\left[1+(\text{Max Prog}-1)\cdot\left(1-e^{\ln 2/T50_{loss}\cdot t}\right)\right] \tag{21.18}$$

MaxProg is a parameter that determines the fractional change in $k_{loss\ 0}$ at infinite time. The effect of a drug might be to inhibit loss, in which case *PDI* would be modeled by (Eq. 21.19), where $C_{e,A}$ is the effect site concentration and *C50* is the value of $C_{e,A}$ causing a 50% inhibition of loss.

$$PDI=1-\frac{C_{e,A}}{C50+C_{e,A}} \tag{21.19}$$

Fig. 21.8 illustrates the four basic drug effect patterns when the input or output parameter changes with an exponential time course. This type of mechanism for disease progression has subsequently been described as a model in which time-varying changes in the disease state model parameters comprise a disease progress model [11].

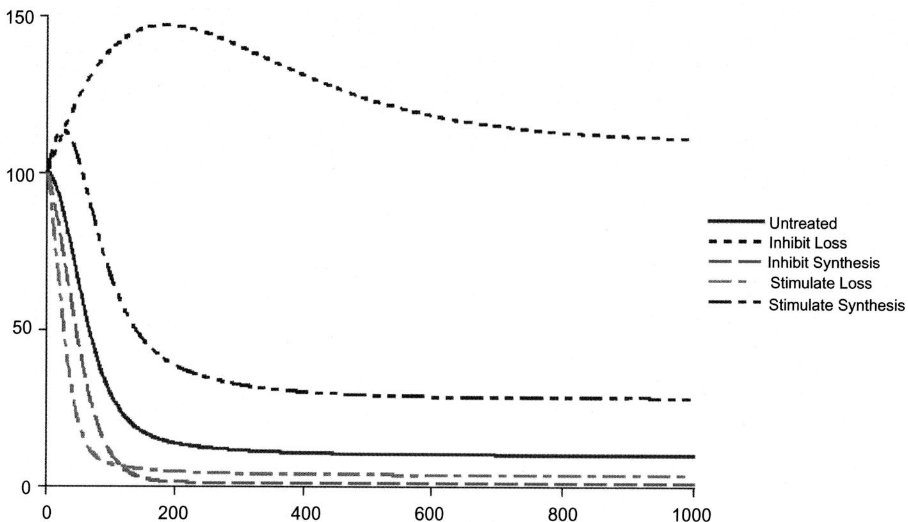

FIG. 21.8 Disease progression due to a time-varying increase in the rate of loss of a physiological mediator of the response. The *thick red line* shows the time course of response in the untreated state with an increase in the loss of physiological mediator. If the response was change in bone mass from a baseline of 100 at time 0 then the rate of bone loss would be increased by a factor of 10 reaching a new steady state after 200 time units. The time to steady state is determined both by the time course of change in rate of bone loss and the turnover time of bone. The other four lines show the patterns expected from four different kinds of drug effect. Potentially therapeutic effects are inhibition of bone loss (*thin brown dotted line*) and stimulation of bone synthesis (*upper blue broken line*). Deleterious drug effects are inhibition of synthesis (*lower green dashed line*) and stimulation of bone loss (*khaki broken line*).

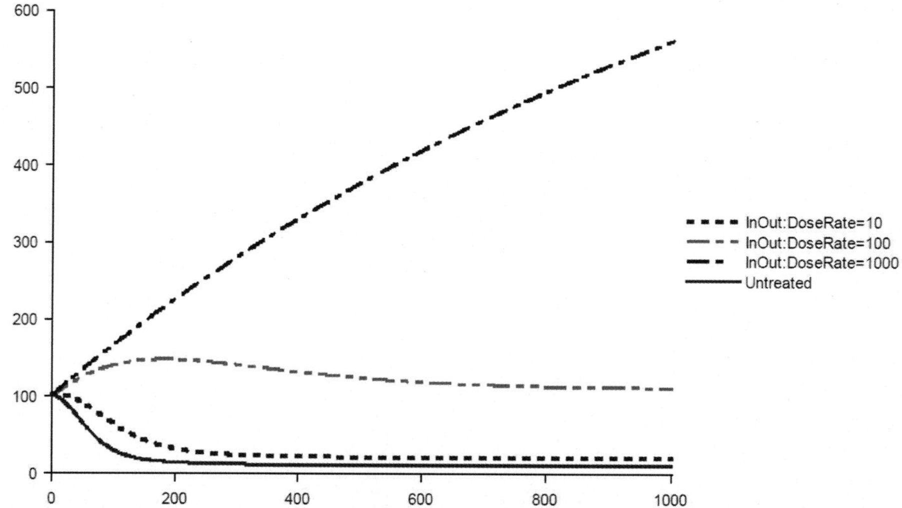

FIG. 21.9 The pattern and time course of response to treatment is crucially dependent on the dose. This shows the same model as that illustrated in Fig. 21.8 without treatment (*thick red line*) and with three different dose rates of a drug which reduces the rate of loss of physiological substance (*dotted purple line* = dose rate of 10, *broken green line* = dose rate of 100, *broken blue line* = dose rate of 1000).

As an example of this type of disease progression model, consider postmenopausal osteoporosis reflected by the net loss of bone mass that may be due to decreased formation or increased resorption of bone. Fig. 21.9 illustrates the time course of bone mass change due to increased bone loss and the effect of administering a drug to reduce that loss. For example, raloxifene has been shown to be beneficial in women with postmenopausal osteoporosis [12]. The pattern of increase in bone mineral density observed after treatment with raloxifene or placebo resembles the curves shown in Fig. 21.10. However, the treatment duration in this dataset was too short to identify the actual mechanism of raloxifene effect on disease progress.

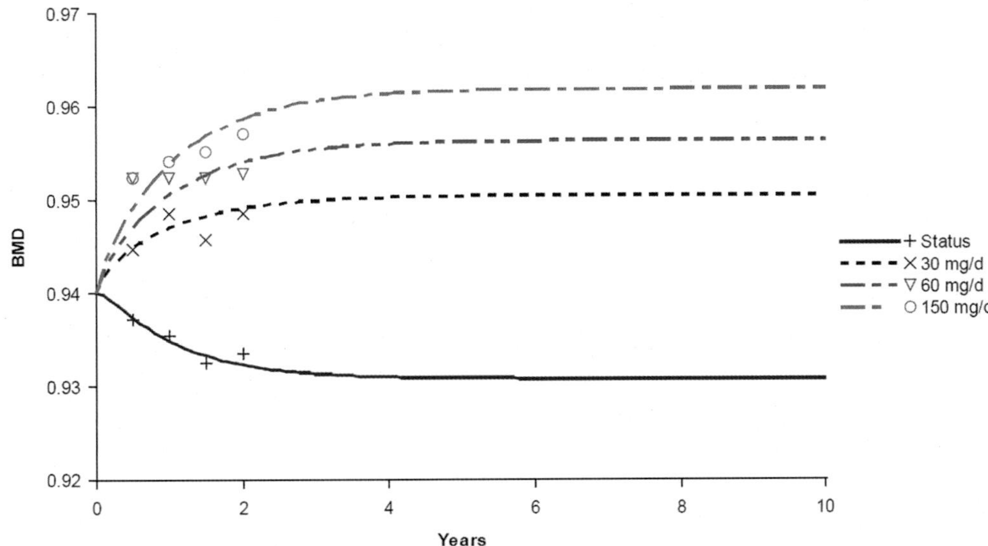

FIG. 21.10 Bone mineral density change with placebo and three doses of raloxifene. Symbols indicate observed responses to placebo (▲) and daily doses of 30mg (▪), 60mg (▼) and 150mg (●). *Curves* show predictions assuming disease progress is due to increased loss and raloxifene reduces loss. The model is the same as that shown in Fig. 21.8 and 21.9. *(Curves fit to lumbar spine data from Delmas PD, Bjarnason NH, Mitlak, BH, Ravoux A-C, Shah AS, Huster WJ, et al. Effects of raloxifene on bone mineral density, serum cholesterol concentrations, and uterine endometrium in postmenopausal women. N Engl J Med 1997;337:1641–1647.)*

Growth and decay models

Another semiempirical approach to modeling the course of disease progression is to use models originally developed to describe growth. The growth function might be used to describe something such as tumor growth or bacterial cell increase, where growth is dependent on the number of actively dividing cells. A simple function that can be used to describe the growth of a response R is given in Eq. (21.20) [13, 14].

$$\frac{dR}{dt} = k_{growth} \cdot R - k_{death} \cdot R \tag{21.20}$$

The solution to this equation describes an exponential increase in cell count with time.

As with the other physiological models, the effect of drug treatment may be realized by slowing the growth rate (k_{growth}) or increasing the cell death rate (k_{death}). In the latter case, this effect can be incorporated by including a term for the effect of drug concentration ($C_{e,A}$) on the rate constant for cell decrease, as shown in Eq. (21.21):

$$\frac{dR}{dt} = k_{growth} \cdot R - k_{death} \cdot R \cdot C_{e,A} \tag{21.21}$$

A more realistic refinement of the simple cell growth model would describe cells that, through mutation or other processes, may become resistant to drug treatment. The change of cell characteristic from a responsive to an unresponsive state can be either reversible or irreversible. Eqs. (21.22) and (21.23) describe the reversible case, which may be reflective of cells moving between sensitive phases (R_S) and phases that are not sensitive to therapeutic intervention (R_R) [15]:

$$\frac{dR_S}{dt} = k_{growth} \cdot R_S - k_{SR} \cdot R_S + k_{RS} \cdot R_R - k_{death} \cdot R_S \tag{21.22}$$

and

$$\frac{dR_R}{dt} = k_{SR} \cdot R_S - k_{RS} \cdot R_R \tag{21.23}$$

where the rates of transformation to and from the resistant state are indicated by k_{SR} and k_{RS}, respectively.

Another class of functions frequently used to describe growth kinetics are the Gompertz functions [16]. These functions are useful because they describe a rapid initial rapid rate of growth (β), followed by a slower phase of growth until a finite limit (β_{max}) is reached. This behavior makes the Gompertz functions particularly appropriate for describing disease progress where there is a maximum level of impairment associated with the disease (e.g., a burned-out state). Consequently, Gompertz functions have been used to describe the pharmacodynamics of antibacterial agents [17], as well as an empirical description of disease progression in Parkinson's disease [18]. Eqs. (21.24) and (21.25) describe a Gompertz function of cell growth in which the cells oscillate between a therapeutically sensitive state (R_S) and a resistant state (R_R). The effect of drug concentration ($C_{e,A}$) is described using an E_{max} equation that acts to reduce the number of responsive cells in the system by increasing loss (k_{SO}) independently of transformation to or from the resistant state:

$$\frac{dR_S}{dt} = k_{RS} \cdot R_R + \beta \cdot R_S \cdot (\beta_{\max} - R_S) - \left[k_{SR} + \left(1 + \frac{E_{\max} \cdot C_{e,A}}{EC50 + C_{e,A}}\right) \cdot k_{SO}\right] \cdot R_S \tag{21.24}$$

$$\frac{dR_{SR}}{dt} = k_{SR} \cdot R_S - k_{RS} \cdot R_R \tag{21.25}$$

Fig. 21.11 shows the expected pattern of cell growth in three different treatment groups. In the low-dose treatment group, cell regrowth is expected to be rapid, and there is some evidence of regrowth near the 20-day time point even in the high-dose group.

Weibull functions are used in another class of semiempirical models to describe disease progression (Fig. 21.12). Pennypacker et al. [19] first proposed using the Weibull function to describe the progression of plant diseases such as fungal infections and black rot.

Although commonly employed in epidemiology and in models of plant disease, Weibull functions have not been used widely to describe the time course of human disease. Freeman et al. [20] used this function to identify factors associated with rapid fibrosis progression in patients with hepatitis C. More rapid progression to cirrhosis was found to be correlated with alcohol consumption, elevated serum alanine aminotransferase, and histology demonstrating high-grade necroinflammatory activity. Similarly, Foucher et al. [21] implemented the Weibull function with a Markov chain to describe the progression of HIV through various states as life without disease, appearance of symptoms, disease progression, and eventual death.

The function was evaluated for numerical stability by Thal et al. [22]. The authors reported that the Weibull function was generally robust and allowed for a variety of inflection points that made this function suitable for describing a variety of disease progression scenarios. The authors, however, also pointed out that if the parameters exhibited high correlation, simplification of the Weibull function would provide more reasonable confidence intervals for the parameters. In order to maintain numerical plausibility, a modified Weibull function (Eq. 21.26) may be implemented. This function can take on several characteristics depending on the value of the shape function WE3. When all parameters are constrained to be positive and the parameter WE3 is at or below 1, the function mimics an exponential model, which describes a rapid fall off from a baseline value to a new lower plateau in the time course of response. However, as WE3 increases to values greater

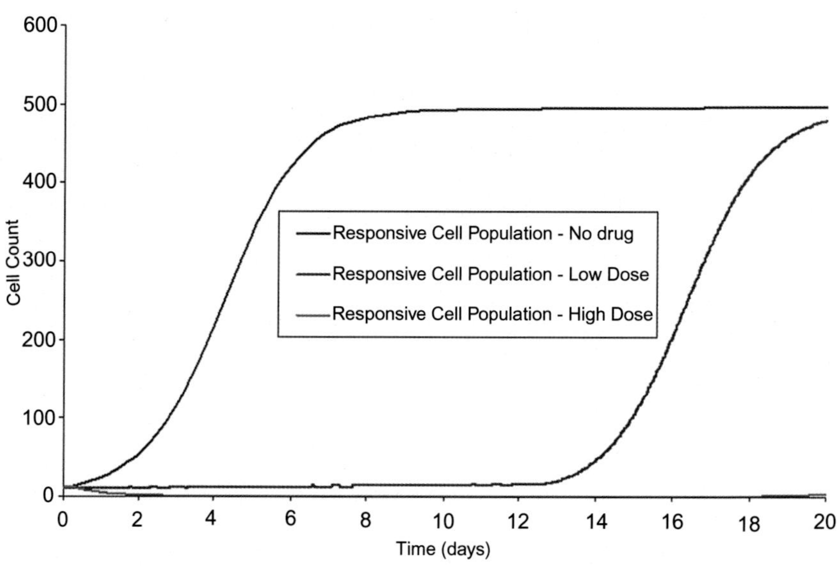

FIG. 21.11 Growth curves for responsive cells exposed to three different treatment regimens: untreated (*solid blue line*), inadequately treated with a low drug dose (*broken red line*), and adequately treated with a higher drug dose (*dotted green line*). The *curves* show that cell regrowth following inadequate treatment is rapid.

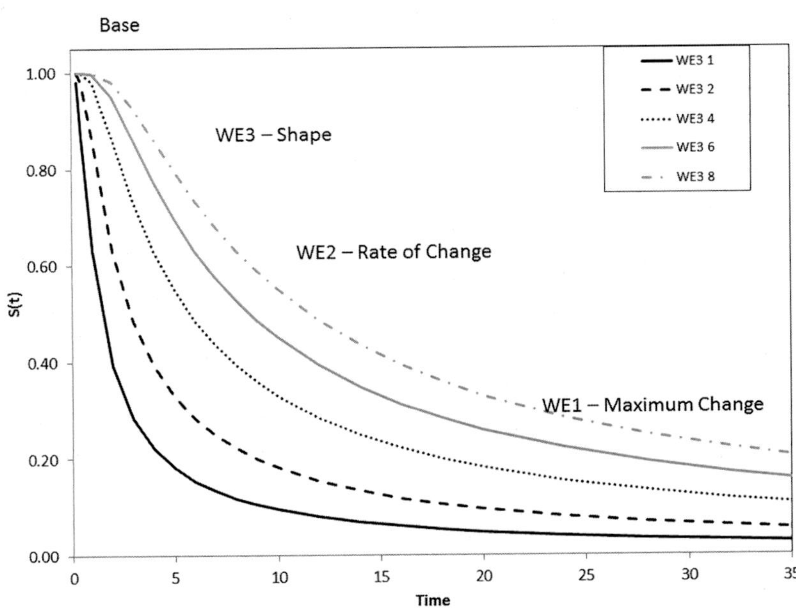

FIG. 21.12 Weibull decay curves for a variety of values of WE3 or shape parameter values. When the value of WE3 is low (≤1) the function mimics an exponential decay with a rapid fall off from its BASE level to a new lower plateau level. When the value of WE3 increases, there is a delay prior to the fall off and the rate of decline is slower. Although not shown here, ultimately all values for WE3 would eventually stabilize at the same new lower plateau value.

than 1, the function approximates a Weibull model, which allows for a delay in the onset of change before the function falls to a plateau. The rate of change of the score between baseline and plateau is controlled by the parameter WE2, and WE1 describes the maximum decrease from the baseline value. $S_i(t)$ is the Weibull function value at a given time "t."

$$S_i(t) = WE1 \cdot \left(1 - e^{-(WE2/t)^{WE3}}\right) \tag{21.26}$$

Depending on the Weibull parameter values, the function can either describe either a decay over time as shown in Fig. 21.11 or it can describe an increase in disease score over time to a new higher plateau. The application of a logit transform can be used to constrain the modified Weibull function to fall within the upper and lower bounds of a disease assessment score, thus ensuring that the disease progression model will not simulate inappropriate values.

$$\begin{aligned} &LGT = S_i(t) \\ &UB = 100 \\ &LB = 0 \\ &Score_i(t) = (UB - LB) \cdot \frac{e^{LGT}}{(1 + e^{LGT})} + LB \end{aligned} \tag{21.27}$$

In this equation, LGT is the Weibull function shown in Eq. (21.27), UB is the upper bound of the clinical disease assessment score, and LB is the lower bound of the disease score. Then, $Score_i(t)$ is the disease score at time t.

Physiologically based models of disease progression

Physiologically based (PB) and quantitative systems pharmacology (QSP) models are relatively new tools for modelers. A PBPK (physiologically based pharmacokinetic) model, as described in Chapters 3 and 31, refers to a model that incorporates parameters describing physiology, anatomy, and drug properties to simulate the changes of drug concentrations in organs and tissues over time. Typically, PBPK models incorporate both drug-dependent components reflecting the absorption, distribution, and elimination, and drug-independent system components (Fig. 21.13 Panel A from [23], Panel B from [24]). The latter components are based on knowledge of body fluid dynamics (e.g., blood and urine flow), tissue size and composition, abundance and distribution of drug receptors, drug-metabolizing enzymes, and membrane transporters in various organ and tissue compartments. Thus PBPK models can be used to predict the concentration time profile in target tissues after administration of drug. PBPK modeling and simulation can also be used to predict the pharmacokinetics of drugs in humans, including the effects of intrinsic (e.g., organ dysfunction, age, genetics) and extrinsic (e.g., drug–drug interactions) patient factors on drug exposure. PBPK models were initially primarily used to explore drug interaction potentials and the expected changes in concentration time profiles

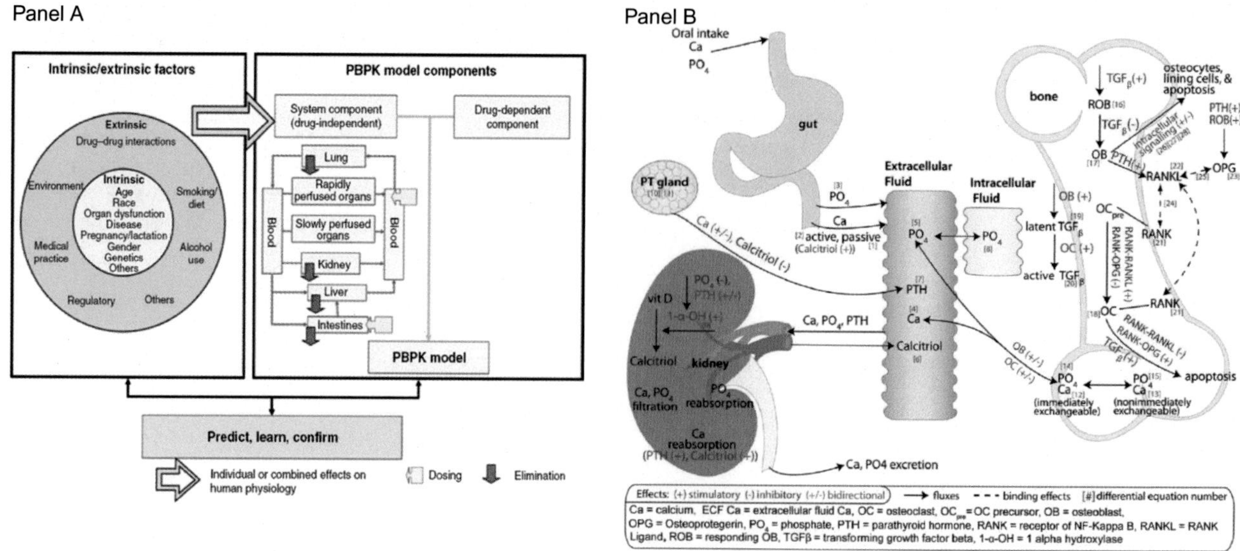

FIG. 21.13 (A) A PBPK model reflecting the effects of both intrinsic factors (e.g., age and genetics) and extrinsic factors (e.g., the presence of additional medications that cause drug–drug interactions and system factors including urine and blood flow). These models can be refined by incorporating values that represent specific populations and/or scenarios. (B) A QSP disease progress model reflecting the interrelations between bone process, renal function, and other components. *(Panel B: Figure reproduced from Peterson MC, Riggs MM. A physiologically based mathematical model of integrated calcium homeostasis and bone remodeling. Bone. 2010;46(1):49–63.)*

with drug formulation changes but their use is expanding. A recent publication from Zhou et al. reported that the use of PBPK simulation played a key role in several types of regulatory decisions: the need to conduct specific clinical pharmacology studies, specific study designs, and appropriate labeling language [23].

The expansion into physiologically based disease progression models, or QSP models, was prompted by the reality that the actual drug concentration at the site of action is not always known, and the fact that there is often a lag between drug reaching the site of action and a measurable effect. These facts have been most often described by semimechanistic models, such as effect compartment or turnover models. QSP models are based on physiological and anatomical principles to try to provide a mechanistic interpretation of drug effects based on first principles. Furthermore, a disease can differ between patients and can worsen, or regress, within a patient, making it more challenging to describe relationships between dose, serum, tissue drug concentrations and its resulting effects. Thus QSP modeling includes multifactorial functions describing the interrelationship between various processes within the body, and the expected response when these processes are altered by the administration of drug or the onset of disease (Fig. 21.13 Panel B [24]).

One of the earlier publications of a mechanistic disease progression model involved the development of a complex mechanistic model for blood pressure regulation developed by Guyton et al. [25] that took the impact of sodium and fluid intake on blood pressure into account, and was used to investigate the renin–angiotensin system in hypertension, as well as the role of aldosterone on blood pressure regulation. Their work was exhaustive, investigating a wide range of factors influencing blood pressure. The model was subsequently extended by Karaaslan et al. [26] to include a mechanistic model describing the effects of the renal sympathetic nerve activity (RSNA) on tubular sodium reabsorption and renin secretion. The resulting model was the first comprehensive model of the cardiovascular system accounting for the effects of RSNA on kidney function, which provided insights into RSNA-related mechanisms, which lead to mean arterial pressure increase in hypertension and total sodium amount increase (sodium retention) in congestive heart failure, nephrotic syndrome, and cirrhosis. The model was further refined by Hallow et al. to include a molecular-level model of the renin–angiotensin–aldosterone signaling pathway (RAAS) which allowed for the investigation of the effect of novel antihypertensive drugs targeting RAAS [27]. The model was then further extended to allow investigation of chronic kidney disease [28].

Another well-known QSP disease progression model was reported by Peterson and Riggs in 2010 to describe changes in bone mineral density over time [24]. This model was constructed from published data to integrate calcium homeostasis and bone biology. It included relevant cellular aspects with controlling mechanisms for bone remodeling and calcium homeostasis. The model was tested and found to describe a wide range of clinical and therapeutic conditions, including changes in parathyroid hormone, calcitriol, calcium and phosphate, and bone-remodeling markers as manifested in hypoparathyroidism and hyperparathyroidism, renal insufficiency, daily PTH 1–34 administration, and receptor activator of NF-kappaB ligand (RANKL) inhibition.

In a subsequent extension, this model was applied to investigate two classes of clinically relevant biomarkers, bone turnover markers, which provide information on bone formation produced by osteoblasts and bone resorption produced by osteoclasts. The activity of osteoblasts and osteoclasts impacts bone mineral density, which reflects bone mass that correlates with bone strength [29]. The model was used to evaluate changes in lumbar spine bone mineral density over a range of doses and regimens of denosumab and to provide guidance for the clinical development of this drug. A third extension of this model was used to address a bone safety question for gonadotropin-releasing hormone modulation therapies posed by FDA [30]. In 2014 the FDA Endocrine and Metabolic Drugs Advisory Committee reviewed a biologics license application for NATPARA (Recombinant Human Parathyroid Hormone (rDNA)), submitted as a replacement for endogenous parathyroid hormone and long-term treatment of hypoparathyroidism. The FDA reviewers' recommendations were based on their independent model qualification of the second-generation model using phase I data and subsequent simulations representative of the registration trial for NATPARA. This was not the first use of physiologically based models by FDA, however. The first involvement of FDA with this type of modeling occurred during the review of the teratogenic topical "wrinkle cream" active ingredient, tretinoin (Renova®) [31, 32]. In order to understand fetal exposure during early pregnancy, the FDA required a teratogenic risk assessment based on PBPK modeling and simulation, from which FDA concluded that the risk was acceptable, allowing its approval [33]. The involvement and acceptance of PBPK and QSP models has been expanding steadily.

Not all QSP models are developed from clinical data. Mathematical models built using data from xenograft animal models have been developed over the past 40 years. Such models were developed to predict the exposures at different doses and regimens in animals and to link that exposure to observed response. Mathematical modeling not only provides a robust way to summarize pharmacokinetic and pharmacodynamic properties of new agents, but can be even more important as a translational tool able to provide rational predictions of clinical findings. Thus a third example of a well-known QSP model is the semimechanistic model developed by Simeoni et al. to assess antitumor effects in xenograft mice assuming a delay in tumor response due to the duration of drug-induced cell death [34]. Threshold concentration was derived as secondary parameter, which defined the predicted concentration at which tumor stasis is achieved (e.g., drug-induced tumor kill rate is equal to tumor growth rate). Subsequently, Rocchetti et al. reported that the predicted threshold concentration derived from xenograft experiments using the Simeoni model correlated with the active dose in humans for several marketed drugs [35]. Modeling anticancer drugs often presents unique difficulties, such as limited (or no) pharmacokinetic sampling. In addition, biomarkers of clinical benefit such as tumor size are often ignored, oversimplified, or show high between-subject variability, resulting in poor insight of the clinical pharmacology necessary to better understand trial results and select appropriate treatment regimens. A discussion of various approaches used to model tumor growth and response to novel therapies is presented in Mould et al. [36].

Design of trials to study disease progress

The study of disease progress requires trial designs that can identify the time course of disease status. It is not sufficient just to measure a response at baseline and at the end of a period of treatment in order to describe the effect of a drug on disease progression. For example, the ELLODOPA study was intended to determine if levodopa affected the rate of progression of Parkinson's disease [37]. This study used a washout design which involved withdrawal of treatment and seeing if the disease status was the same in the placebo- and levodopa-treated groups after 2 weeks without levodopa. However, the results of the study were inconclusive, because the 2-week study period was not long enough to ensure that all the effects of prior therapy had been washed out and the primary analysis was based only on change from baseline. A prediction of the ELLDOPA results based on earlier studies [18, 38] accurately described the observed differences and also confirmed a disease-modifying effect of levodopa.

Another trial design, the delayed start design, has been proposed for identifying disease-modifying effects. The basic idea is that, if two groups of patients are observed in a trial in which treatment is delayed for one group, then if there is a disease-modifying effect, the disease status will show greater improvement (less progress) in the early start group. This trial design, like the washout design, requires an assumption about the time required for the effects of prior therapy to decline to asymptotic values. If this assumption is made a priori and is not borne out by the data, the prespecified analysis is invalidated. This is what happened with the ADAGIO trial which aimed to identify disease-modifying effects of rasagiline on Parkinson's disease [39]. A model-based analysis that uses the observed data to describe the time course of the symptomatic effect does not suffer from this limitation [40].

The importance of trial design for identifying disease-modifying effects may be studied by clinical trial simulation. For example, a simulation study has shown that a washout design is more powerful than a delayed start design for identifying symptomatic vs. disease-modifying drug effects in patients with Parkinson's disease [41]. The use of clinical trial simulation also is an important tool for understanding complex diseases and trial designs which try to distinguish the effects of treatments from natural disease progression [42]. In addition, the inclusion of quantitative models for disease progress in the regulatory and drug development process has been advocated as a means of sharing knowledge and improving trial design [43].

Conclusion

The use of models to describe disease progress is an important tool that allows the clinical pharmacologist and clinical trialist to evaluate the effects of drug treatment on the time course of disease. In the "learning and confirming" paradigm of drug development strategy [3], inclusion of models for disease progress can focus attention more clearly on the objectives of a clinical trial. In early, "learning phase" studies, the model of disease progress can be developed, and the mechanism of drug action elucidated. Subsequently, clinical trials can be designed to account for variability in the natural history of disease, which increases the statistical power to distinguish effects of different treatments and thus "confirm" the effectiveness of the drug. Once the disease progress model has been defined and an effect of the drug on progress has been accepted, study designs can be defined that optimize dosage regimens to achieve clinical benefit.

In this chapter, we have described some examples of models that can be used to describe the natural history of disease. We have also suggested modifications to these models that can be used to account for the effect of drug treatment. The development of an appropriate model for disease progress is ideally a team-based approach. It requires the input of clinical experts as to the validity of the status measure used to describe the progress of the disease, statisticians to advise on the inferences that can be drawn from clinical trial observations, and pharmacometricians to determine the appropriateness and utility of the clinical pharmacology model for predicting the response to treatment and to provide guidance to the patient and prescriber on how to use the drug safely and effectively.

References

[1] Holford NHG, Sheiner LB. Understanding the dose-effect relationship: clinical application of pharmacokinetic-pharmacodynamic models. Clin Pharmacokinet 1981;6:429–453.

[2] Sheiner LB. Clinical pharmacology and the choice between theory and empiricism. Clin Pharmacol Ther 1989;46:605–615.

[3] Sheiner LB. Learning versus confirming in clinical drug development. Clin Pharmacol Ther 1997;61:275–291.

[4] Holford NHG, Sheiner LB. Kinetics of pharmacologic response. Pharmacol Ther 1982;16:143–166.

[5] Griggs RC, Moxley RT, Mendell JR, Fenichel GM, Brooke MH, Pestronik A, et al. Prednisone in Duchenne dystrophy: a randomized, controlled trial defining the time course and dose response. Arch Neurol 1991;48:383–388.

[6] Sale M, Sheiner LB, Volberding P, Blaschke TF. Zidovudine response relationships in early human immunodeficiency virus infection. Clin Pharmacol Ther 1993;54:556–566.

[7] Holford NHG. Population models for Alzheimer's and Parkinson's disease. In: Aarons L, Balant LP, editors. The population approach: measuring and managing variability in response, concentration and dose. Brussels: COST B1 European Commission; 1997. p. 97–104.

[8] Holford NHG, Peace KE. Methodologic aspects of a population pharmacodynamic model for cognitive effects in Alzheimer patients treated with tacrine. Proc Natl Acad Sci U S A 1992;89:11466–11470.

[9] Holford NHG. Physiological alternatives to the effect compartment model. In: D'Argenio DZ, editor. Advanced methods of pharmacokinetic and pharmacodynamic systems analysis. New York: Plenum Press; 1991. p. 55–68.

[10] Dayneka NL, Garg V, Jusko WJ. Comparison of four basic models of indirect pharmacodynamic responses. J Pharmacokinet Biopharm 1993;21:457–478.

[11] Post TM, Freijer JI, DeJongh J, Danhof M. Disease system analysis: basic disease progression models in degenerative disease. Pharm Res 2005;22:1038–1049.

[12] Delmas PD, Bjarnason NH, Mitlak BH, Ravoux A-C, Shah AS, Huster WJ, et al. Effects of raloxifene on bone mineral density, serum cholesterol concentrations, and uterine endometrium in postmenopausal women. N Engl J Med 1997;337:1641–1647.

[13] Jusko W. Pharmacodynamics of chemotherapeutic effects: dose-time-response relationships for phase-nonspecific agents. J Pharm Sci 1971;60:892–895.

[14] Zhi J, Nightingale C, Quintiliani R. A pharmacodynamic model for the activity of antibiotics against microorganisms under non saturable conditions. J Pharm Sci 1986;25:1063–1067.

[15] Jusko W. A pharmacodynamic model for cell cycle-specific chemotherapeutic agents. J Pharmacokinet Biopharm 1973;1:175–200.

[16] Prior JC, Vigna YM, Schulzer M, Hall E, Bonen A. Determination of luteal phase length by quantitative basal temperature methods: validation against the midcycle LH peak. Clin Invest Med 1990;13:123–131.

[17] Yano Y, Oguma T, Nagata H, Sasaki S. Application of a logistic growth model to pharmacodynamic analysis of in vitro bacteriocidal kinetics. J Pharmacokinet Biopharm 1998;87:1177–1183.

[18] Holford NH, Chan PL, Nutt JG, Kieburtz K, Shoulson I. Disease progression and pharmacodynamics in Parkinson disease—evidence for functional protection with levodopa and other treatments. J Pharmacokinet Pharmacodyn 2006;33:281–311.
[19] Pennypacker SP, Knoble HD, Antle CE, Madden V. A flexible model for studying plant disease progression. Phytopathology 1980;70:232–235.
[20] Freeman AJ, Law MG, Kaldor JM, Dore GJ. Predicting progression to cirrhosis in chronic hepatitis C virus infection. J Viral Hepatol 2003;10:285–293.
[21] Foucher Y, Mathieu E, Saint-Pierre P, Durand JF, Daures JP. A semi-Markov model based on generalized Weibull distribution with an illustration for HIV disease. Biom J 2005;47:825–833.
[22] Thal WM, Campbell CL, Madden LV. Sensitivity of Weibull model parameter estimates to variation in simulated disease progression data. Phytopathology 1984;74:1425–1430.
[23] Zhao P, Zhang L, Grillo JA, Liu Q, Bullock JM, et al. Applications of physiologically based pharmacokinetic (PBPK) modeling and simulation during regulatory review. Clin Pharmacol Ther 2011;89(2):259–267.
[24] Peterson MC, Riggs MM. A physiologically based mathematical model of integrated calcium homeostasis and bone remodeling. Bone 2010;46 (1):49–63.
[25] Guyton AC, Coleman TG, Granger HJ. Circulation: overall regulation. Annu Rev Physiol 1972;34:13–46.
[26] Karaaslan F, Denizhan Y, Kayserilioglu A, Gulcur HO. Long-term mathematical model involving renal sympathetic nerve activity, arterial pressure, and sodium excretion. Ann Biomed Eng 2005;33(11):1607–1630.
[27] Hallow KM, Lo A, Beh J, Rodrigo M, et al. A model based approach to investigating the pathophysiological mechanisms of hypertension and response to antihypertensive therapies: extending the Guyton model. Am J Physiol Regul Integr Comp Physiol 2014;306(9):R647–R662.
[28] Helmlinger G, Al-Huniti N, Aksenov S, Peskov K, et al. Drug-disease modeling in the pharmaceutical industry—where mechanistic systems pharmacology and statistical pharmacometrics meet. Eur J Pharm Sci 2017;109S:S39–S46.
[29] Peterson MC, Riggs MM. Predicting nonlinear changes in bone mineral density over time using a multiscale systems pharmacology model. CPT Pharmacometrics Syst Pharmacol 2012 Nov 14;1. https://doi.org/10.1038/psp.2012.15, e14.
[30] Peterson MC, Riggs MM. FDA advisory meeting clinical pharmacology review utilizes a quantitative systems pharmacology (QSP) model: a watershed moment? CPT Pharmacometrics Syst Pharmacol 2015;4(3). https://doi.org/10.1002/psp4.20, e00020.
[31] Clewell 3rd HJ, Andersen ME, Wills RJ, Latriano L. A physiologically based pharmacokinetic model for retinoic acid and its metabolites. J Am Acad Dermatol 1997;36(3 Pt 2):S77–S85.
[32] Rowland M, Balant L, Peck C. Physiologically based pharmacokinetics in drug development and regulatory science: a workshop report (Georgetown University, Washington, DC, May 29–30, 2002). AAPS PharmSci 2004;6(1)E6.
[33] Ghosh TK (2000). Clinical pharmacology and biopharmaceutics review: NDA 21-108 0.02% Tretinoin emollient cream (RENOVA®). https://www.accessdata.fda.gov/drugsatfda_docs/nda/2000/21-108_Renova_BioPharmr.pdf. p. 19
[34] Simeoni M, Magni P, Cammia C, De Nicolao G, Croci V, Pesenti E, Germani M, Poggesi I, Rocchetti M. Predictive pharmacokinetic-pharmacodynamic modeling of tumor growth kinetics in xenograft models after administration of anticancer agents. Cancer Res 2004;64 (3):1094–1101.
[35] Bueno L, de Alwis DP, Pitou C, Yingling J, Lahn M, Glatt S, Trocóniz IF. Semi-mechanistic modelling of the tumour growth inhibitory effects of LY2157299, a new type I receptor TGF-beta kinase antagonist, in mice. Eur J Cancer 2008;44(1):142–150.
[36] Mould DR, Walz AC, Lave T, Gibbs JP, Frame B. Developing exposure/response models for anticancer drug treatment: special considerations. CPT Pharmacometrics Syst Pharmacol 2015;4(1). https://doi.org/10.1002/psp4.16, e00016.
[37] The Parkinson Study Group. Levodopa and the progression of Parkinson's disease. N Engl J Med 2004;351:2498–2508.
[38] Hauser RA, Holford NH. Quantitative description of loss of clinical benefit following withdrawal of levodopa-carbidopa and bromocriptine in early Parkinson's disease. Mov Disord 2002;17:961–968.
[39] Olanow CW, Rascol O, Hauser R, Feigin PD, Jankovic J, Lang A, et al. A double-blind, delayed-start trial of rasagiline in Parkinson's disease. N Engl J Med 2009;361:1268–1278.
[40] Holford NHG, Nutt J. Interpreting the results of Parkinson's disease clinical trials: time for a change. Mov Disord 2011;26(4):569–577.
[41] Ploeger BA, Holford NH. Washout and delayed start designs for identifying disease modifying effects in slowly progressive diseases using disease progression analysis. Pharm Stat 2009;8:225–238.
[42] Holford N, Ma SC, Ploeger BA. Clinical trial simulation: a review. Clin Pharmacol Ther 2010;88:166–182.
[43] Gobburu JVS, Lesko LJ. Quantitative disease, drug and trial models. Annu Rev Pharmacol Toxicol 2009;49:291–301.

Chapter 22

Sex-specific pharmacological differences

Karen D. Vo and Mary F. Paine

Department of Pharmaceutical Sciences, College of Pharmacy and Pharmaceutical Sciences, Washington State University, Spokane, WA, United States

Introduction

During the drug approval process, sponsors must submit data to the U.S. Food and Drug Administration (FDA) that demonstrates the safety and efficacy of the potential product in patient populations similar to those for whom the drug is intended [1]. Since the 1980s, the FDA has emphasized the need to include more females in clinical trials. Accordingly, the assessment of response differences between the sexes, as well as among population subgroups pertaining to age and race/ethnicity, has become an integral element of the approval process. In currently accepted usage, *sex* is defined by the biological and chromosomal variation between males and females, whereas *gender* is defined by cultural, social, and societal factors that influence an individual's identity as a man (boy), woman (girl), or nonbinary individual [2, 3]. Nonbinary individuals are those whose gender identity is not restricted solely to man or woman. This chapter focuses primarily on differences between males and females related to sex-based pharmacological response to drug therapy, then concludes with a brief summary of developments in the inclusion of transgender patients in pharmacokinetic (PK) and pharmacodynamic (PD) studies.

Reports during the 1960s of severe birth defects in infants born from females taking thalidomide, a drug that was used to treat nausea during pregnancy [4], led the FDA to recommend in 1977 that females of childbearing potential be excluded from Phase I and early Phase II clinical trials [5]. Females could still be included in further clinical studies, but only after adequate safety information from animal fertility and teratology studies and earlier clinical trials were assessed. Although established to protect females, this guidance led to a substantive underrepresentation of the sex in early clinical trials.

During the AIDS epidemic in the 1980s, this underrepresentation of females changed as concerns grew about the access of females to critical antiviral treatments, as well as potentially life-saving treatments for other diseases and conditions [6, 7]. Consequently, considerable efforts ensued during the 1990s to reverse the effects that the 1977 FDA guidance had on female representation in clinical trials. In 1992 the Government Accountability Office released a report highlighting the inadequate participation and representation of females in clinical trials [8]. The FDA released a new guidance in 1993, *Study and Evaluation of Gender Differences in the Clinical Evaluation of Drugs*, which outlined the use of PK and PD studies in females as tools to assess differences between sexes, including those pertaining to drug safety and efficacy [9]. The same year, the National Institutes of Health (NIH) established the Revitalization Act, which provided guidelines for including women and minorities in NIH-sponsored clinical research studies [10]. In 1994 the FDA established the Office of Women's Health with the goal of providing leadership and guiding policies relevant to women's health, as well as promoting the inclusion of women in clinical trials [11]. Despite these efforts, the underrepresentation of females in clinical trials remains evident today. Females and males are still prescribed the same doses for most drugs regardless of reports indicating that females are often overmedicated and are at a twofold higher risk of experiencing adverse drug reactions than males [12]. Additionally, females are more likely to be hospitalized for complications related to adverse drug reactions.

As discussed in other chapters, assessment of interindividual differences in drug PK and PD provides many benefits to patients and minimizes risks associated with pharmacotherapeutics. These considerations facilitate individualization of therapy based on drug, dose, and regimen, an approach termed *personalized medicine*. Sex differences can greatly influence drug safety and efficacy, leading to markedly different outcomes that can further complicate therapy. Sex differences can be specific to the time course of blood, plasma, and/or tissue concentrations of active drug and/or metabolites (PK) or biological responses (PD) due to underlying differences in physiology. Some of these differences are more readily detected and measurable in representative populations than others.

Atkinson's Principles of Clinical Pharmacology. https://doi.org/10.1016/B978-0-12-819869-8.00020-3

While evaluating these interindividual differences, other intrinsic and/or extrinsic factors must be considered. Such factors include hormone concentrations, exposure to concomitant drugs and other xenobiotics (e.g., prescription medicines, over-the-counter medicines, dietary supplements, and botanicals), healthcare utilization, and reporting bias. These additional factors can further complicate the evaluation of sex differences between males and females.

Pharmacokinetics

In 1971, the analgesic/antipyretic drug antipyrine was the first medication assessed for sex-based PK differences [13, 14]. Antipyrine is eliminated entirely by hepatic metabolism and was reported to have a 23% shorter half-life in females than in males [14]. Additional studies determining sex-based differences with respect to other drug products were completed throughout the 1970s and 1980s and provided increasing supportive evidence warranting further investigation into these differences. Notably, acetaminophen was shown to be cleared more rapidly in males than in females [15]. Several PK studies involving benzodiazepines concluded that the clearances for these drugs were higher in females than in males [16]. In the ensuing years, interest heightened in understanding sex differences and, as a result, reports of studies investigating PK (and PD) differences for new drugs in both sexes have grown.

A survey of new chemical entity small molecules and biologics approved by the FDA from September 2007 to August 2010 reported that more than 95% of systemically absorbed drugs were evaluated for sex differences in PK during that time period, with key results reported in regulatory reviews and product labels [17]. These PK studies typically involve 12–24 healthy volunteers and are conducted in the early phases of drug development, along with clinical pharmacology and early dose-ranging studies. Female participation in late-phase clinical trials also has increased over the years and has been analyzed for sex-based differences in both safety and efficacy [18].

As discussed in Chapter 2, the magnitude of response differences based on dose alone may exhibit higher variability than when response assessments are based on drug and metabolite concentrations in the systemic circulation. This discordance reflects interindividual and intraindividual differences in the processes of drug absorption, distribution, metabolism, and excretion determining the time course of systemic drug and/or metabolite concentrations after administration of a drug dose. These PK differences between subjects are due to both intrinsic (e.g., sex, genetic predisposition, disease state, hepatic function, renal function, body weight) and extrinsic (e.g., smoking, diet, concomitant drugs, and other xenobiotics) factors. The following sections describe sex-based differences in the various PK processes that govern drug disposition.

Transporters

Sex-specific differences in drug transporter expression and activity have been reported (Table 22.1). Because these ubiquitous proteins are involved in the absorption, distribution, metabolism, and excretion of drugs, such differences are discussed in the context of each of these biochemical processes in the corresponding sections.

TABLE 22.1 Sex-specific differences observed in human transporter activity.

Transporter	Sex difference (Y/N)	Substrate	Observations	References
P-gp	Y/N	N/A	Threefold higher hepatic protein expression in males compared to females ($P<.05$)	[19]
		N/A	No difference in intestinal protein expression detected	[20]
		N/A	No difference in hepatic protein expression detected	[21]
BCRP	N	N/A	No difference in hepatic protein expression detected	[22]
OATP1B1	N	N/A	No difference in hepatic protein expression detected	[21]
OATP1B3	N	N/A	No difference in hepatic protein expression detected	[21]
OATP2B1	N	N/A	No difference in hepatic protein expression detected	[21]

Absorption

Factors that influence sex differences in oral absorption include gastric pH, gastrointestinal (GI) motility, intestinal enzymatic activity, and intestinal transport activity. Research has shown that the gastric emptying rate of solids and liquids is slower in females than in males, which could delay drug absorption from distal GI sites [23]. One explanation for this difference in gastric emptying rate may be related to female sex hormones, such as progesterone and estradiol. Differences in hormone concentrations may also modify gastric acid secretion and gastric pH [24], but the exact mechanisms remain unknown.

Sex differences in absorption have been noted for several drugs, including rifampicin and benzylamine, prompting analysis of data for sex differences in the absorption of other drugs. One study assessing aspirin systemic exposure showed that, although not significant, the rate of absorption (i.e., mean absorption time) was more rapid in females than in males [25]. A sex difference in the extent of absorption (area under the plasma concentration vs. time curve) was not detected. Another study reported that aspirin systemic exposure in females was higher than that in males upon administration of the same aspirin doses [26]. The higher aspirin plasma concentrations in females were attributed to intrinsically lower blood concentrations of aspirin esterase activity rather than to sex differences in aspirin absorption.

Several GI enzymes may account for intestinal drug absorption differences between males and females. One of the most clinically relevant examples is alcohol. Exposure to alcohol can vary greatly between males and females, even when the same volume is consumed. This variability results in an uneven distribution of alcohol-related health complications between sexes. This sex disparity could be explained by differences in the expression of alcohol-metabolizing enzymes. For example, females have been reported to express less alcohol dehydrogenase, an enzyme responsible for alcohol oxidation, in the gut than males [27].

Gastric alcohol dehydrogenase is one of many drug-metabolizing enzymes involved in intestinal first-pass drug loss. Prominent among these enzymes are the cytochromes P450 (CYPs), of which sex-specific differences in expression and catalytic activity have been observed (Table 22.2). The CYPs have a major role in the first-pass metabolism of many drugs and thus influence the extent of absorption. Sex differences in both intestinal and hepatic CYP3A activity have been documented [48]. For example, the oral bioavailability of midazolam, a benzodiazepine and probe drug substrate for intestinal (and hepatic) CYP3A, has been reported to be higher in females compared to males [30]. However, CYP3A expression in the gut does not always correlate with that in the liver. Thus, sex differences noted after intravenous administration of CYP3A substrates may not parallel those after oral administration.

As with intestinal enzymes, sex-related differences in intestinal transporters can result in differences in systemic drug exposure between males and females. As discussed in Chapter 4, P-glycoprotein (P-gp), an efflux transporter expressed on the luminal membrane of enterocytes, facilitates back-transport of cellularly absorbed drugs, acting to hinder absorption into the systemic circulation. Although P-gp expression has been reported to be up to threefold higher in males than in females, several studies, including one involving duodenal pinch biopsies, reported large interindividual variability in overall P-gp expression and no sex differences between hepatic or intestinal expression (Table 22.1) [19, 20]. P-gp-facilitated efflux combined with CYP3A-mediated first-pass metabolism in the gut influence the systemic availability of many drugs. Due to the interplay between P-gp and CYP3A in the intestinal lumen and liver, differentiating the contribution of each pathway to the absorption of drugs that are cosubstrates is a challenging yet important consideration. Sex differences have also been noted for the efflux transporter breast cancer resistance protein (BCRP), which, like P-gp, is expressed on the luminal membrane of enterocytes and acts to hinder drug absorption [22, 49]. However, the data are conflicting, with some studies reporting significant sex differences in hepatic and intestinal expression and others lacking evidence to support this conclusion [22, 49–51].

Compared to P-gp, fewer sex-specific differences have been observed for uptake transporters, including the H^+/dipeptide transporter and organic anion transporting polypeptides (OATPs). These transporters mediate drug uptake into cells, including enterocytes and hepatocytes, acting to facilitate drug absorption [52]. Some studies have reported sex differences in Oatp protein and/or mRNA expression in animal models. However, such differences have not been observed in humans. Specifically, no differences were detected in hepatic protein expression of OATP1B1, OATP1B3, and OATP2B1 between males and females (Table 22.1) [53].

Although oral administration is the most common route for drugs, patients often require other means of drug administration based on their specific needs. Limited examples in the literature document sex differences in drug absorption from routes other than the GI tract, such as muscle, subcutaneous fat, and lung. One study evaluating the lysine salt of aspirin reported a slower rate of absorption but comparable bioavailability in females compared to males after intramuscular injection [25]. Although minor sex differences in regional blood flow have been reported and may have contributed to this observation, the more likely explanation was that the drug was injected into the subcutaneous fat of the females, rather than the gluteus muscle.

TABLE 22.2 Sex-specific differences observed in human drug-metabolizing enzyme activity.

Enzyme	Sex difference (Y/N)	Substrate	Observations	References
CYP3A4/5	Y	N/A	1.9-fold higher hepatic mRNA expression in females compared to males ($P<.05$)	[28]
		Verapamil	43% lower oral clearance in females compared to males ($P<.05$)	[29]
		Midazolam	1.7-fold higher oral clearance in females compared to males ($P<.05$) 38% shorter $t_{1/2}$ after oral administration in females compared to males ($P<.05$)	[30]
			2.3-fold higher increase in ratio of oral AUC in presence to absence of oral clarithromycin in females compared to males ($P<.05$)	
		Cortisol	1.4-fold higher ratio of 6β-hydroxycortisol to cortisol in females compared to males ($P<.05$)	[31]
		Triazolam	2.1-fold higher oral clearance in females compared to males ($P<.005$) 28% lower C_{max} in females compared to males ($P<.05$)	[32]
		Tirilazad	1.5-fold higher systemic clearance in females compared to males[a] ($P<.05$)	[33]
CYP2D6	Y	Dextromethorphan	60% lower dextromethorphan: dextrorphan metabolic ratio in females compared to males ($P<.0001$)	[34]
		Propranolol	39% lower oral clearance in females compared to males ($P<.02$)	[35]
CYP2C19	Y	Voriconazole	1.2-fold higher C_{max} in females compared to males 1.1-fold higher AUC_{τ} in females compared to males	[36, 37]
CYP2C9	N	Warfarin Phenytoin Tolbutamide	No difference in oral clearance detected	[38]
CYP1A2	Y/N	Caffeine	Lower in vivo catalytic activity in females than males[b]	[39]
		N/A	No difference in hepatic protein expression detected	[40, 41]
CYP2E1	N	Chlorzoxazone	No difference in oral clearance detected[c]	[42]
CYP2C8	N	N/A	No difference in hepatic protein or mRNA expression detected	[43]
CYP2B6	N	N/A	No difference in hepatic gene expression detected	[44, 45]
Aldehyde oxidase (AO)	N	N/A	No difference in in vitro catalytic activity detected[d]	[46]
Carboxylesterase (CES)	Y	Dabigatran	1.2-fold higher hepatic protein expression of CES1 in females compared to males ($P<.05$) 1.2-fold higher in vitro catalytic activity of CES1 in females compared to males ($P<.05$)	[47]

[a]*Observation in young subjects. Sex and age were considered in evaluation of pharmacokinetics.*
[b]*Activity defined by ratio of caffeine metabolites (5-acetyl-amino-6-formylamino-3-methyluracil, l-methylxanthine, 1-methyluric acid):caffeine.*
[c]*No difference in oral clearance was detected between sexes when normalized to body weight.*
[d]*Activity defined by intrinsic clearance.*

Distribution

The rate and extent of drug distribution are determined by multiple factors such as body mass index (BMI), body composition (i.e., muscle and fat content), blood/plasma volume, organ blood flow, and the extent of tissue and plasma protein binding. Compared to males, females have a higher body fat content and lower average BMI, blood/plasma volume, and organ blood flow [54]. These differences may contribute to sex differences in the rate and extent of drug distribution and should be considered when calculating loading or bolus doses to avoid unnecessary adverse events in females. Anesthetic agents are a notable example of drugs for which proper sex-specific dosing is critical to achieving the appropriate level of analgesia. Several studies highlight the importance of sex-based dosing modifications, particularly when rapid onset or short duration of action is required for rapid induction of anesthesia prior to a surgical procedure [55].

Regarding total body fat and total body water, significant differences in volume of distribution of lipophilic and hydrophilic drugs between sexes have been observed. Total body fat is estimated to be 13.5 kg in the adult male and 16.5 kg in the adult female [56]. As such, lipophilic drugs such as diazepam, nitrazepam, and chlordiazepoxide exhibit a relatively higher volume of distribution in females than in males when normalized to body mass [57–59]. Conversely, total body water constitutes a lower proportion of body mass in females than in males. Therefore the distribution volume of hydrophilic drugs such as ethanol is generally lower in females than in males when normalized to body mass [60]. These properties contribute to higher peak plasma concentrations and greater initial effects in females compared to males. Additional examples of hydrophilic drugs that exhibit a lower distribution volume in females include metronidazole, prednisolone, and the water-soluble fluoroquinolones [54].

Compared to males, females generally have a higher unbound ("free") drug concentration than males, which may correspond to sex-specific differences with respect to drug-binding proteins in plasma. Major drug-binding proteins in plasma include albumin, α_1-acid-glycoprotein (AAG), and globulins. Although drug binding to albumin is not greatly influenced by sex, sex-specific variation in AAG levels could influence unbound drug concentrations [61, 62]. Estrogens have been shown to decrease plasma concentrations of AAG by inducing hepatic glycosylation, presumably accounting for the fact that some drugs have a lower extent of plasma protein binding in females than in males [62]. Administration of exogenous estrogens could also increase concentrations of other proteins, such as sex hormone binding globulin, corticosteroid binding globulin, and thyroxine binding globulin, potentially contributing to observed sex differences in drug binding to plasma proteins [63].

Metabolism

The high interindividual variability associated with drug metabolism is influenced by both intrinsic and extrinsic factors. Important intrinsic factors include sex as well as age, race/ethnicity, body composition, disease states, genetic makeup, and hormonal status. The effects of hormonal status on PK are discussed later in this chapter. Extrinsic factors include smoking, alcohol use, diet, concomitant medications, and other environmental exposures. Although the metabolism of many drugs involves a single dominant pathway, multiple pathways operating in series or in parallel are equally prevalent. Therefore sex-specific observations in drug metabolism are often attributed to more than one enzyme, rendering difficulties in defining the magnitude of sex differences with respect to one enzyme. Sex-specific differences with respect to Phase I (Table 22.2) and Phase II metabolic pathways are described in the following sections.

Phase I metabolic pathways

Phase I metabolic reactions such as oxidation, reduction, and hydrolysis are primarily catalyzed by the CYP multigene superfamily of enzymes. Three major CYP families (CYP1, CYP2, CYP3) comprise multiple enzymes that are involved in drug metabolism, including CYP1A2, CYP2B6, CYP2C8, CYP2C9, CYP2C19, CYP2D6, CYP2E1, and CYP3A4/5 [54] (Fig. 22.1). Additional Phase I enzymes include aldehyde oxidase and carboxylesterases. Because these enzymes constitute major determinants of drug exposure, identifying and understanding potential sex differences and their clinical implications is imperative.

CYP1A2: CYP1A2 is responsible for metabolizing approximately 8% of the top 200 most prescribed drugs in the United States [64]. Many studies have reported higher CYP1A2 activity in males compared to females, as described by differences in metabolic ratios of CYP1A2 substrates (Table 22.2) [39]. However, some studies reported no difference in hepatic CYP1A2 protein expression, suggesting that a posttranslational mechanism underlies the sex difference in catalytic activity [40, 41].

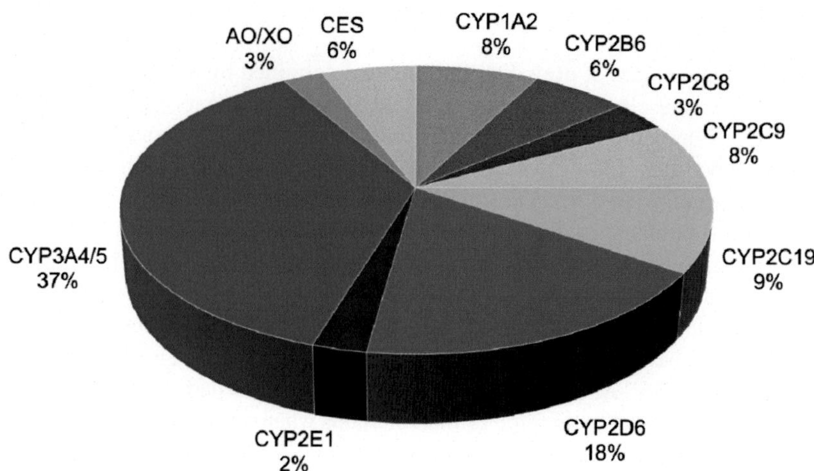

FIG. 22.1 Contribution of major Phase I drug-metabolizing enzymes to the metabolism of the top 200 most prescribed drugs in the United States. *(Based on Saravanakumar A, Sadighi A, Ryu R, Akhlaghi F. Physicochemical properties, biotransformation, and transport pathways of established and newly approved medications: a systematic review of the top 200 most prescribed drugs vs. the FDA-approved drugs between 2005 and 2016. Clin Pharmacokinet 2019;58:1281–1294.)*

CYP2B6: Although most studies report no differences in hepatic gene expression and protein content between sexes, results are controversial [44, 45]. An earlier study reported that females exhibit approximately fourfold higher CYP2B6 mRNA expression and twofold higher protein content compared to males [65]. Another study reported that females exhibit higher microsomal CYP2B6 protein content, but this effect was not significant in the absence of inducers [66].

CYP2C8: No differences in hepatic mRNA or protein expression or activity between sexes have been reported [43].

CYP2C9: Clinically relevant CYP2C9 substrates include *S*-warfarin, phenytoin, tolbutamide, and ketoprofen. No sex differences in the disposition of these drugs have been observed [38].

CYP2C19: CYP2C19 is responsible for the metabolism of several drugs, including citalopram, diazepam, proton pump inhibitors, and voriconazole. Regarding voriconazole, some studies have demonstrated higher C_{max} and AUC values in females compared to males, suggesting a lower clearance of voriconazole in females (Table 22.2) [36, 37]. However, these findings may have been confounded by other factors such as race/ethnicity and the use of oral contraceptives (OCs) by some of the females. For example, one study reported that females taking OCs exhibited 60% lower CYP2C19 activity compared to females not taking OCs. That is, when comparing CYP2C19 activity to that of males, females taking OCs exhibited a greater difference in enzyme activity than females not taking OCs. Evidence for the confounding effects of race/ethnicity on sex differences in CYP2C19 activity is more limited. Although sex differences in the metabolism of CYP2C19 substrates have been reported to be population specific, whether or not these observations were influenced by OC use is unclear as such use was not reported and most likely not considered [38].

CYP2D6: CYP2D6 is responsible for metabolizing roughly 18% of the top 200 most prescribed drugs in the United States and 15%–25% of all therapeutic agents, including dextromethorphan, paroxetine, aripiprazole, and propranolol [44, 64]. Current data support sex-specific differences with respect to CYP2D6 expression and activity, albeit the differences have been inconsistent. In a study using dextromethorphan to assess enzyme activity between sexes, the dextromethorphan to dextrorphan ratio was lower in females compared to males, indicating higher CYP2D6 activity in females compared to males (Table 22.2) [34]. A separate study assessing CYP2D6 activity using propranolol showed lower oral clearance in females than males [35]. These results suggest lower CYP2D6 activity in females compared to males, contrary to observations with dextromethorphan. The differences observed in CYP2D6 activity between the two substrates could be attributed to the contribution of other CYPs, particularly for propranolol. Specifically, in addition to CYP2D6, CYP1A2 has a major role in propranolol metabolism, and, as aforementioned, exhibits higher catalytic activity in males than females [39, 67].

CYP2E1: Limited information for CYP2E1 suggests an approximately 30% lower metabolic activity in females compared to males in studies using chlorzoxazone as a probe substrate [42]. However, when normalized to body weight, a sex difference was not detected.

CYP3A4/5: More than 50% of drugs are metabolized by CYP3A4/5, including midazolam, triazolam, cyclosporine, imatinib, and budesonide [68]. Females have been reported to exhibit approximately twofold higher hepatic mRNA expression than males, which correlates with a retrospective analysis concluding that females have approximately 20%–30% higher clearance of CYP3A4/5 substrates than males (Table 22.2) [28, 69]. Similar observations have been reported for other substrates such as verapamil, for which females show higher rates of verapamil metabolite formation compared to males [29]. Additionally, the ratio of 6β-hydroxycortisol to cortisol, an endogenous biomarker for CYP3A4/5 activity, was shown to be higher in females than in males [31]. Finally, CYP3A4/5 substrates including midazolam, triazolam, and tirilazad demonstrated higher oral or systemic clearance in females compared to males [30, 32, 33, 70].

These observations could also reflect sex-specific differences in transporter expression as discussed previously. Many drugs are substrates for both CYP3A4/5 and P-gp, rendering it difficult to distinguish the role of each in altering drug clearance, in as much as P-gp may lower intracellular drug concentrations available for CYP3A4/5 metabolism. Because males have higher hepatic P-gp content than females, this difference could result in lower intracellular drug concentrations available for metabolism in males, potentially explaining the lower clearance of CYP3A4/5 substrates in males compared to females [71, 72].

The unsuccessful attempt to develop the CYP3A4/5 substrate tirilazad to treat patients with aneurismal subarachnoid hemorrhage provides a cautionary example of the importance of designing clinical trials in which dosage adjustment is needed to account for sex differences in drug metabolism. In two large clinical trials intended to demonstrate the efficacy of tirilazad, male and female patients were treated with the same intravenous dose, yet only the male patients showed therapeutic response [73, 74]. PK studies indicated a 40%–60% higher systemic clearance in young premenopausal females compared to males. The clearance in middle-aged premenopausal females was approximately 10% lower than that in younger females, whereas the clearance in postmenopausal females was similar to that in males [33, 75]. Unfortunately, in these and subsequent failed clinical trials, plasma concentration monitoring of tirilazad was not used to adjust dosage to minimize the impact of either sex differences or CYP3A4 induction (e.g., by concurrent administration of phenobarbital or phenytoin) on tirilazad clearance [76].

Other CYPs: Although this chapter does not cover every CYP, others involved in drug disposition (e.g., CYP2A6 and CYP4F) merit discussion. CYP2A6 contributes to the metabolism of drugs such as nicotine, letrozole, efavirenz, and valproic acid [77]. Several studies have reported higher CYP2A6 activity in females compared to males, which was attributed to estrogen-mediated induction. In support of this observation, females express higher CYP2A6 mRNA and protein content than males. Similar observations have been made for the CYP4F subfamily, which metabolizes endogenous substrates such as arachidonic acid [78]. Studies in animal models have demonstrated higher Cyp4f mRNA and protein expression in females than in males [79].

Aldehyde oxidase: Aldehyde oxidase (AO), a cytosolic enzyme belonging to the molybdoflavoprotein family, is considered to have broad substrate specificity but is primarily responsible for oxidizing aliphatic and aromatic aldehydes and heteroaromatic rings and is capable of reducing a wide range of other functional groups [80]. Probe substrates for AO include vanillin, O^6-benzylguanine, and zoniporide. Examples of clinically relevant AO substrate drugs include lenvatinib, zaleplon, and methotrexate. Using cryopreserved human hepatocytes to predict total metabolic clearance, one study reported no sex-specific difference with respect to AO activity (Table 22.2) [46]. However, further investigation is needed to support this observation.

Carboxylesterases: Carboxylesterases (CESs) constitute a family of enzymes that catalyze the hydrolysis of molecules containing amides, esters, thioesters, and/or carbamates [81]. Several classes of drugs hydrolyzed by CESs include antiplatelet agents, HMG CoA-reductase inhibitors, central nervous system (CNS) stimulants, and immunosuppressants. In humans, CES1 and CES2 are involved in drug metabolism; both are expressed in the liver, whereas only CE2 is expressed in the intestine. A few studies have reported sex differences in CES expression and activity. Using the rate of dabigatran intermediate metabolite activation as a measure of CES activity, one in vitro study using human liver S9 fractions reported the metabolic activity of CES1 to be higher in females than males (Table 22.2) [47]. This observation supports a previous report in which oseltamivir was used as a substrate to demonstrate higher in vitro metabolic activity in normal liver tissue samples from females than from males [82]. Both studies further reported higher CES1 expression in females than in males [47, 82]. Neither study described the potential clinical implications of these sex-specific differences.

Phase II metabolic pathways

Phase II metabolic pathways include glucuronidation, sulfation, acetylation, and methylation. Metabolism of either a parent drug or its Phase I metabolite by these enzymes generally forms more polar conjugates that are readily excreted by the kidneys. Phase II enzymes include the UDP-glucuronosyltransferases (UGTs), sulfotransferases (SULTs), *N*-acetyltransferases (NATs), and methyltransferases, all of which have been assessed for sex differences.

Glucuronidation: Nearly 40%–70% of all therapeutic agents undergo conjugation by UGTs [83]. UGT substrates include bilirubin, raloxifene, morphine, and mycophenolic acid. Studies have shown that UGT conjugation of some substrates, including oxazepam and temazepam, is slower in females compared to males, contributing to slower oral clearance of these drugs in females [84, 85]. However, similar sex differences have not been observed for substrates such as clofibric acid and ibuprofen [86, 87]. OC use has been reported to increase glucuronidation rates in females, which could have confounded the lack of a sex difference in UGT activity observed in the latter studies [88, 89].

Sulfation: Limited and conflicting evidence exists for sex differences in sulfotransferase activity. Whereas some isoforms such as phenol sulfotransferase (SULT1A1) are reported to have approximately 70% lower activity in females than males, other isoforms such as catechol sulfotransferase (SULT1A3) exhibit no sex-specific differences [90]. Environmental and genetic factors have been thought to contribute to these inconsistent observations [90, 91].

Acetylation: In addition to hydralazine and procainamide, NAT substrates include caffeine, dapsone, isoniazid, mercaptopurine, and sulfamethazine [92]. No sex differences have been reported for NAT activity as assessed with isoniazid, caffeine, and sulfamethazine [92].

Methylation: Methyltransferases constitute a large class of enzymes that includes catechol-*O*-methyltransferases (COMTs) and thiopurine *S*-methyltransferase (TPMT). COMT content has been reported to be higher in males than in females [93]. Although COMT is responsible for the metabolism of norepinephrine, epinephrine, and dopamine, this sex difference does not appear to have clinically significant consequences [92]. Sex-specific differences in TPMT activity have also been reported. Using human liver biopsies or red blood cells, several studies have shown higher TPMT activity in males compared to females [94–96]. These studies suggested that sex may need to be considered in the dosing of some immunosuppressive agents, including azathioprine and 6-mercaptopurine [96]. Despite these findings, their clinical significance remains unclear, and no sex-based dosing recommendations have been established for drugs metabolized by TPMT.

Renal excretion

In general, females have a lower renal clearance for drugs that are predominantly excreted unchanged in urine, including vancomycin, ceftazidime, cefepime, and fleroxacin [38]. This sex difference partly reflects the fact that, after correcting for body surface area, glomerular filtration rate is about 10% lower in females than in males [21]. Sex differences with respect to transporters play a pivotal role in renal tubular secretion, as demonstrated for amantadine. The renal clearance of amantadine, which undergoes renal tubular secretion by organic cationic transporter 2 (OCT2), has been reported to be approximately 50% higher in males compared to females. Testosterone has been shown to upregulate Oct2 in rats and may explain this observation [38]. Digoxin, a P-gp substrate predominately excreted unchanged by the kidneys, has a 12%–14% lower oral clearance in females compared to males [38].

Pharmacodynamics

Major research interest has been generated in the analysis of sex differences in PD, as well as combined PK and PD, although published reports have focused on certain therapeutic areas more than others. Currently, a wealth of information is available about the cardiovascular effects of drugs, but there have also been studies involving analgesics, antidepressants, and immunosuppressants.

Cardiovascular effects

Clinical evidence has accumulated that demonstrates sex differences in both drug safety and efficacy with respect to the cardiovascular effects of drugs. Perhaps the most prominent and extensively discussed example related to safety is *torsades de pointes* (TdP), a rare life-threatening polymorphic ventricular tachycardia resulting from QT interval prolongation [97–99]. Females have twice the risk of developing drug-induced TdP compared to males [99–102]. As discussed in Chapter 1, TdP was observed with the nonsedating antihistamine terfenadine, attracting widespread attention to the severity of this adverse event, which eventually led to its market withdrawal in 1998. The 2001 GAO report, *Drug Safety: Most Drugs Withdrawn in Recent Years Had Greater Risks for Women*, drew further attention to the increased susceptibility of females to drug-induced TdP. This report lists the drugs withdrawn from the market during 1997–2000 [103]. Of the 10 drugs listed, 4 had high potential to induce TdP: astemizole, cisapride, grepafloxacin, and terfenadine.

Terfenadine and presumably other drugs that cause TdP block the delayed rectifier potassium current and lengthen the electrocardiographic QT interval [104]. However, TdP does not occur in every patient treated with these drugs and other factors may predispose patients to TdP, including bradycardia, hypocalcemia, hypokalemia, hypomagnesemia, and hypothyroidism [99, 105, 106]. Females appear to be at increased risk of TdP due to having a longer heart rate-corrected QT

(QTc) interval compared to males [101]. Other drugs known to increase the risk of TdP in females include dofetilide, probucol, quinidine, and sotalol [98,107–109]. No sex-specific differences in the PK of these drugs have been reported to contribute to the increased TdP risk in females.

Several underlying mechanisms have been proposed for the female-specific increased sensitivity to QTc interval prolongation and TdP. One proposal details the protective effects of testosterone in males. Baseline QTc assessments through puberty and the menstrual cycle revealed that prepubertal baseline QTc is similar between the sexes [110, 111]. However, at puberty, testosterone can contribute to the shortening of baseline QTc intervals in males. In contrast, baseline QTc intervals in females remain unchanged. Collectively, manifestation of this longer QTc interval in females is considered one cause of sex-related physiological divergence leading to higher arrhythmia and TdP risk in females [112].

The beta-blocker propranolol has shown sex differences in both PK and PD. For example, the Beta-Blocker Heart Attack Trial, in which male and female subjects received equal doses of propranolol, showed higher plasma propranolol concentrations in females than in males [35, 113]. However, when the subjects received an isoproterenol challenge infusion to assess the degree of β-adrenoreceptor blockade, females showed reduced sensitivity to propranolol, which offset the effect of their higher plasma concentrations [114, 115]. Although there are no sex-based recommendations for the use of propranolol, these offsetting PK and PD effects complicate potential sex-based drug decisions, as higher drug concentrations suggest a need for lower doses in females, whereas reduced sensitivity suggests a need for higher doses [114, 115].

Sex differences in patient response were observed in a trial designed to assess the efficacy of aspirin and dipyridamole in preventing recurrence of stroke [116]. The dosing regimen reduced the frequency of strokes and reduced mortality in males but was less effective in females. In vitro studies demonstrated that when the same amounts of aspirin were added to blood samples from males and females, platelet aggregation decreased by a greater extent in males than in females [117]. In addition, when aspirin was added to blood from orchiectomized males, the change in platelet aggregation was modest. However, when testosterone was added to these blood samples, platelet aggregation was similar to that observed with blood from nonorchiectomized males. These data indicate that testosterone contributes to the clinical sex differences in aspirin-mediated inhibition of platelet aggregation.

Analgesics

Studies of pain perception and response to analgesics have shown that females and males differ significantly with respect to pain threshold and tolerance to experimental pain [118, 119]. Specifically, higher degrees of pain intensity and pain prevalence have been reported for females [120–122]. However, various factors such as social behaviors, genetics, PK and PD differences, pain models used, and hormonal contributions complicate the reporting and interpretation of sex differences in pain response. In addition, phases of the female menstrual cycle have been reported to alter pain perception, with the periovulatory, luteal, and premenstrual phases yielding a lower pain threshold than the follicular phase [107]. These additional contributions, combined with inconsistencies in observed pain response, pose challenges for the future research that is needed to determine the clinical significance and underlying causes of sex differences in the response to and treatment of pain.

Several reports indicate substantial sex differences in the analgesic response to both opioid and nonsteroidal antiinflammatory drugs (NSAIDs). Using a clinical pain model in which morphine, a μ-opioid receptor agonist, was administered to males and females emerging from general anesthesia after surgical procedures, females experienced more intense pain than males [123]. Consequently, females required approximately 30% more morphine than males to achieve a similar degree of analgesia, despite the lack of a PK sex difference. This observation was made after adjusting for factors such as surgery type, age, and body weight. A study implementing an electric pain model reported that morphine provided higher μ-opioid analgesic potency but a slower onset and offset of analgesic effect in females than in males [124]. Consistent with these observations, the adverse events associated with opioid use, including respiratory depression, nausea, and vomiting, have been reported to be more pronounced in females than in males, further emphasizing the importance of dose adjustments in females [124–127]. The relative abundance of research on morphine has illuminated several important aspects of sex differences in analgesia; however, the data on nonmorphine μ-opioids and mixed μ-/κ-opioids are less conclusive and further research is needed [125].

Sex differences have been reported with κ-opioid receptor agonist-antagonists, such as pentazocine, butorphanol, and nalbuphine [128]. In the context of postoperative dental pain, a greater degree of analgesia was achieved in females compared to males. This sex difference may be a general characteristic of the κ-opioid drug class and could be partly responsible for the overall lower use of these drugs compared to the μ-opioid drug class. Compared to the opioids, there is only limited evidence that demonstrates a sex difference in analgesic response to NSAIDs. One study showed that standard doses of ibuprofen were more effective in males than in females when challenged with different degrees of ear lobe pain, despite no sex difference in PK profile [129].

Genotypic characteristics in pain response to analgesics have been reported. In a study in which κ-agonist-antagonist analgesic drugs were used to alleviate thermal and ischemic pain stimuli, females homozygous for a variant melanocortin-1 receptor (*MC1R*) allele exhibited a higher analgesic response to pentazocine compared to males or females harboring one or no variant *MC1R* alleles [130]. No sex differences were detected between males and females null for this variant allele.

Antidepressants

Depression is the most common mood disorder worldwide, afflicting more than 350 million people [131]. The underlying mechanism of depression is unclear; however, neurotransmitter imbalances are believed to play a critical role in its development. Many additional factors can significantly increase an individual's risk of developing depression, including genetics and traumatic life events. Compared to males, females are reported to be twice as likely to develop depression, especially during menopausal transition. Although largely attributed to major life event stress, the heritability of depression is also higher in females than in males. Finally, females present with different symptoms of depression and respond differently than males to antidepressants, which could be a manifestation of differences in antidepressant PK and PD.

Some studies have reported that young females tend to respond better to tricyclic antidepressants (TCAs) than to selective serotonin reuptake inhibitors (SSRIs), whereas no such response differences were observed in males [131]. These differences were believed to result from a lower drug clearance, thus higher plasma concentrations, of TCAs in females compared to males. For example, clearance of the TCA clomipramine is lower in females than males, potentially increasing the risk of adverse effects such as dizziness, drowsiness, headache, and insomnia [131, 132]. As a result, although evidence is conflicting, females appear to have a higher treatment withdrawal rate with respect to TCAs [133]. The clinical significance of these sex differences in exposure to TCAs remains equivocal, as another study described no differences in remission rate (i.e., posttreatment Hamilton depression scale score), treatment dropout rate, or adverse events [132].

As discussed later in this chapter, fluctuations in sex hormone concentrations are believed to be partly responsible for these sex differences in antidepressant PK and PD, and estrogen concentrations can shift markedly throughout the menstrual cycle. Because estrogen is a substrate and/or modulator of several CYPs, including CYP1A2 and CYP3A4 [131, 133], these fluctuations may alter the metabolic capacity of these enzymes [131, 133, 134]. One study described the inhibitory effects of sex hormones on the metabolism of antidepressants. Females were administered hormone replacement therapy (HRT; ethinyl estradiol and levonorgestrel) or an OC (ethinyl estradiol and desogestrel) and bupropion, a norepinephrine/dopamine reuptake inhibitor and CYP2B6 substrate [135]. Both HRT and OC administration led to a significant reduction in the systemic exposure to hydroxybupropion, a major active metabolite, in all subjects, suggesting inhibition of CYP2B6 by the sex hormones. These data suggest that females who receive HRT or take OCs may be at higher risk of therapeutic failure with bupropion and should consider either an alternative antidepressant or birth control method [135, 136].

Immunosuppressants

Although females are more susceptible to autoimmune diseases than males, there are few sex-analyzed studies of immunosuppressant therapy in patients with these diseases. However, several studies have identified differences between females and males in the risk of acute and chronic organ rejection following transplantation. For example, heart transplantation is followed by a higher incidence of organ rejection in females than in males [137]. Another study reported that females have a higher incidence of acute, but a lower incidence of chronic, renal graft rejection than males [138]. In this study, the immunosuppressant mycophenolate mofetil was reported to decrease the risk of chronic renal graft rejection in females to a greater extent than in males. Although the exact mechanisms contributing to these differences have not yet been determined, these results suggest that there may be clinically meaningful sex differences in the PK and PD of immunosuppressant drugs [96], although other factors such as organ sex mismatching may contribute.

Maintenance corticosteroids are often used to prevent organ rejection following solid organ transplantation. One study reported that the duration of survival following heart transplantation was inversely correlated with the time required to withdraw patients from maintenance corticosteroid therapy [139]. This relationship may reflect the increased difficulty of withdrawing females from corticosteroid therapy relative to males and the higher risk of posttransplantation mortality in females.

Cyclosporine, prednisolone, and methylprednisolone, all of which are CYP3A4/5 substrates, are frequently administered to organ transplant recipients for immunosuppression. As mentioned earlier, the clearance of CYP3A4/5 substrates tends to be higher in females compared to males. Further complexity emerged from a study of methylprednisolone PK and PD in healthy volunteers [140]. Although females were reported to clear the drug faster than males, they were more sensitive than males to suppression of endogenous cortisol production and had an IC_{50} for cortisol suppression that was 17 times lower than in males. However, these PK and PD sex differences were offsetting, so the observed clinical response to a given dose of methylprednisolone was similar in both sexes.

Other factors affecting sex differences in PK and PD

Defining sex-specific PK and PD differences is further complicated when they are impacted by other endogenous and exogenous factors. These factors can influence sex-specific drug PK and PD in a manner that leads to their amplification, reduction, or elimination. This section discusses the effects of age, race/ethnicity, menstrual cycle and menopause, dietary supplements, and lifestyle choices on sex differences in PK and PD.

Age

Although Chapter 25 deals specifically with the effects of aging on drug therapy, age should be considered in the context of sex differences in PK and PD. The body changes with increasing age, with individuals of advanced age experiencing an increase in body fat content, weight, and gastric pH, as well as a decrease in GI motility [141]. The elderly also tend to have lower drug clearance and decreased intravascular, muscle, and organ volumes than younger individuals. Less evidence in support of age-related effects on drug metabolism exists but there is consensus that sex differences generally persist with age and that there is a continuing need to evaluate sex effects on drug PK and PD in aging patients to better inform sex-based considerations in drug therapy for the elderly [141].

Race/ethnicity

Race/ethnicity is another factor to be considered in evaluating an individual's response to therapeutic agents. Differences in drug PK and PD have been reported for different racial/ethnic groups [142]. Despite these reports, potential synergistic effects of race/ethnicity and sex on drug PK and PD remain unclear. For example, black individuals are reported to have a higher incidence of angiotensin-converting enzyme (ACE) inhibitor-associated angioedema [143, 144]. Some studies also report female sex as a clinical risk factor for angioedema in patients taking ACE inhibitors [145]. In addition, ACE inhibitor-related angioedema is reported to be the most severe in elderly black females [146], suggesting the possibility of risk synergism [147]. However, there is limited research to fully support this conclusion.

The menstrual cycle and menopause

The menstrual cycle, consisting of the follicular, ovulatory, and luteal phases, is accompanied by substantial hormonal changes [148, 149] (Fig. 22.2). These changes are believed to result in PK differences for drugs administered during the various phases of the menstrual cycle. During the early follicular phase, estrogen, progesterone, follicle stimulating hormone (FSH), and luteinizing hormone (LH) concentrations are at a minimum and increase during the mid to late stages of the follicular phase [150]. The mid- to-late-follicular phase is characterized by a significant increase in hormone concentrations, with estrogen, followed by FSH, LH, and progesterone over a relatively short duration of approximately 2–3 days. Ovulation then occurs and is followed by the luteal phase, characterized by a decrease in estrogen concentrations and an increase in progesterone concentrations. At the end of the luteal phase, estrogen and progesterone concentrations decrease, and FSH concentrations begin to rise again.

Fluctuating hormone concentrations throughout the menstrual cycle can lead to functional changes in different organs, such as the kidneys and GI tract [150]. Data describing changes in renal function are conflicting, with some studies showing an increase in creatinine clearance during the luteal phase and others suggesting a lack of functional variation during the menstrual cycle. Data have also shown that changes in vasopressin, aldosterone, and renin concentrations throughout the menstrual cycle could influence the distribution and excretion of several therapeutic agents. However, changes have not been consistently observed. For example, tobramycin clearance and urine recovery were unaltered during different phases of the menstrual cycle.

Evidence is also conflicting regarding changes in the GI tract throughout the menstrual cycle [150]. GI motility is believed to be affected by sex hormones, with reports of a slower overall gastric emptying rate in females compared to males. Although this difference in gastric emptying rate could change with fluctuating concentrations of sex hormones,

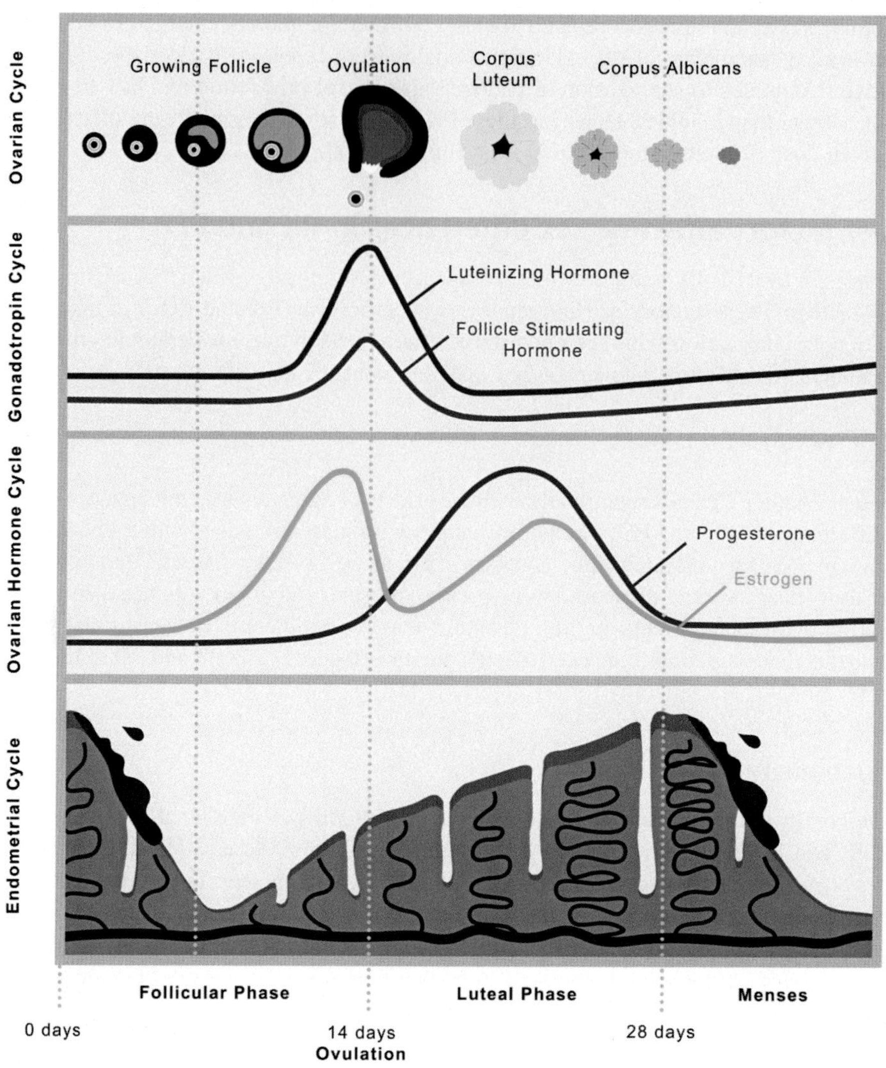

FIG. 22.2 Ovarian, hormonal, and endometrial changes throughout the menstrual cycle. *(Based on Carr B, Wilson J. Disorders of the ovary and female reproductive tract. In: Braunwald E, Isselbacher K, Petersdorf R, Wilson J, Martin J, Fauci A, editors. Harrison's principles of internal medicine. 11th ed. New York: McGraw-Hill; 1987. p. 1818–1837 and Huether S, McCance K, editors. Understanding pathophysiology. 5th ed. St. Louis, MO: Mosby; 2012. p. 785.)*

several studies failed to provide consistent evidence to support this notion. However, the rate of alcohol absorption has been reported to vary during the menstrual cycle, with the highest peak alcohol concentration occurring during the premenstrual phase.

In summary, few studies have encompassed the effects of all phases of the menstrual cycle on the PK of drugs. Although drugs including acetaminophen, caffeine, and theophylline have exhibited decreased clearance during the luteal phase, no effects of the menstrual cycle on the PK of drugs including propranolol, dextromethorphan, alprazolam, carbamazepine, midazolam, and methylprednisolone have been reported [150]. In addition, the changes in clearance with respect to acetaminophen, caffeine, and theophylline are not considered clinically important.

Females generally spend approximately one-third of their lives in menopause, when plasma concentrations of estrogen and progesterone are greatly reduced. These changes in female hormones are known to alter the PK of some drugs. Limited evidence suggests that drug absorption changes in response to menopausal hormonal changes. In one study, the GI absorption of calcium was decreased during menopause and could be reversed with estrogen HRT [151, 152]. The renal clearance of many drugs has been reported to decrease with age in parallel with a gradual decline in renal function.

In addition to renal clearance, the metabolic clearance of a number of drugs has been shown to decline in postmenopausal females, whereas similar changes have not been observed in males of corresponding age. One study reported a 20% decrease in intestinal CYP3A4 content in intestinal biopsy samples from postmenopausal females compared to premenopausal females [48]. In several other studies, the clearance of alfentanil, tirilazad, and intravenous midazolam was lower in older females compared to premenopausal females [153, 154]. Similar to the changes observed throughout the menstrual cycle, the effects of menopause on PK and PD require further investigation.

Dietary supplements, herbals, and other botanicals

According to data collected by the National Health and Nutrition Examination Survey, more than half of the US population uses dietary supplements, including vitamins, minerals, and nonvitamin and nonmineral natural products [155]. Although conventional drugs undergo rigorous testing prior to approval by regulatory authorities, dietary supplements and other natural products are not subject to the same processes [156]. These observations raise concern for adverse interactions between natural products and conventional drugs as more patients supplement their prescribed pharmacotherapeutic regimens with these alternative therapies [157, 158].

A textbook example of a dietary supplement that precipitates drug interactions is St. John's wort, which contains phytoconstituents with documented biological activity [159]. St. John's wort is a well-known inducer of hepatic and intestinal CYP3A4 and P-gp [160, 161]. These inductive effects can have clinical consequences, as evidenced by reports of graft rejection after organ transplantation when St. John's wort is coconsumed with the dual CYP3A/P-gp substrate cyclosporine [161]. Similar effects have been reported for sex steroids, several of which are metabolized by CYP3A4/5. More specifically, plasma concentrations of OCs can decrease in patients taking St. John's wort, which can further lead to breakthrough bleeding or an unintended pregnancy. Based on these observations, information regarding concomitant use of OCs and St. John's wort is included in the FDA-approved labels for these drugs [162]. These labels caution patients about the potential for lower efficacy and advise them to consider using alternative birth control methods [163].

Lifestyle choices

Lifestyle choice can significantly impact an individual's ability to absorb, metabolize, excrete, and respond to specific drugs. Such choices include the use of tobacco, alcohol, and illicit drugs, as well as poor diet and extent of physical activity. General changes to drug PK and PD have been identified, and studies have shown that these changes may differ between sexes.

In 2018, 12% of females in the United States smoked cigarettes [164, 165]. Smoking induces CYP1A2 activity, increasing the clearance of CYP1A2 substrates such as caffeine and theophylline. However, sex differences in the extent of this increase have been inconsistently observed. In general, smoking induces CYP1A2 activity to a greater extent in males than in females [38, 166, 167]. Some studies have reported that smoking induces caffeine clearance in males to a greater extent than in females, whereas the opposite was reported for theophylline [162, 168].

The antipsychotic drug olanzapine is a CYP1A2 substrate that exemplifies the overlapping effects of sex, age, and smoking status on drug clearance [169]. Olanzapine clearance in nonsmokers is reported to be higher in males than in females, consistent with CYP1A2 activity being higher in males. Age-specific differences have also been observed, with olanzapine clearance being lower in individuals $\geq$65 years compared to those <65 years old. Finally, olanzapine clearance is approximately 40% higher in smokers than in nonsmokers. Although each of these factors may not independently justify a dosing adjustment for olanzapine, the combined effects of sex, age, and smoking status could lead to substantial PK differences among different patients and increase the likelihood of suboptimal therapeutic response. Specific recommendations have not been made for females or smokers, but the labeling for olanzapine recommends a lower starting dose for patients who exhibit a combination of certain factors (e.g., nonsmoking female patients $\geq$65 years of age).

There is minimal evidence for sex-specific effects of alcohol on drug PK and PD. As discussed earlier, females express less alcohol dehydrogenase in the gut than males, potentially contributing to higher rates of alcohol-related health complications in females than males [27]. Such differences have not been observed with respect to drug metabolism. For example, a sex difference was not detected for CYP2E1 activity in human subjects under conditions of alcohol-induced CYP2E1 induction [42, 170].

Transgender considerations

As defined earlier, *sex* is biologically or chromosomally based, and the terms "male" and "female" have been used to designate the sexes. *Gender* was defined as one's identity as a man (boy), woman (girl), or nonbinary individual which is influenced by cultural, social, and societal factors. The term "transgender" is used to describe someone whose gender identity or expression differs from their assigned sex at birth [171]. In contrast to the abundance of studies that compare PK and PD differences between males and females, fewer studies have considered transgender men and women. In addition to the lack of research focused on this patient population, many transgender patients face discrimination and report being denied medical care [172]. Combined, these factors place this population at a higher risk of adverse drug reactions, therapeutic failure, and disease.

A study and meta-analysis from 2006 to 2017 estimated that approximately one million people in the United States identify as transgender [173]. The transgender population is considered to have a much higher risk of disease, particularly HIV, compared to the general population. Reports indicate that transgender women have a 49-fold increased HIV risk than the general population, with 25%–28% of the transgender population being HIV-positive [174]. Antiretrovirals are commonly prescribed to treat HIV. Preexposure prophylaxis (PrEP) is indicated to prevent HIV infection, especially for high-risk individuals. Despite the promise of PrEP in reducing patient risk of contracting HIV, the use of feminizing or masculinizing hormone therapy (FHT and MHT, respectively) in transgender patients complicates PrEP use.

FHT typically involves the use of an estrogen and antiandrogen to induce development of female secondary sexual characteristics in transgender women [174]. As discussed previously, sex hormones can significantly influence the PK and PD of some drugs. Therefore fluctuations in sex hormones due to FHT (or MHT) could lead to changes in drug absorption, distribution, metabolism, excretion, and response. In one study, transgender women who were administered FHT (estradiol valerate and cyproterone acetate) and PrEP (tenofovir disoproxil fumarate/emtricitabine) exhibited a 12% reduction in tenofovir blood plasma exposure between weeks 5 and 8 of the study. Changes in blood plasma estradiol concentrations were not detected, suggesting PrEP does not interfere with FHT. However, administering PrEP with FHT could decrease the efficacy of PrEP, placing transgender women at higher risk of contracting HIV. Clearly, more studies are needed to confirm this potential drug-drug interaction and identify others, as some reports failed to produce conclusive evidence supporting drug-drug interactions between FHT and PrEP [175].

Summary

Historically, sex differences in response to drug treatment were attributed to differences in body weight or alternatively, a higher propensity for females to report adverse events. However, evidence of sex-specific differences in drug PK and PD has accumulated considerably since the 1980s. Most PK and PD differences discussed in this chapter discount these variables as the only source of reported differences. Heightened interest in the underlying causes of variable inter- and intraindividual patient outcomes, combined with increasingly supportive NIH and FDA policies and practices, compelled researchers to investigate and understand sex differences through clinical research studies. Although some studies are conflicting, the available data highlight the importance of including females in all stages of drug development.

Continued attention to the influence of intrinsic and extrinsic factors on the physiological changes throughout a female's life cycle will further the mechanistic understanding of PK and/or PD changes associated with these factors. Additional studies are also needed to address the potential effects of endogenous hormones, exogenous hormone use (i.e., HRT, OCs, MHT, and FHT), and hormone fluctuations on drug PK and PD and to confirm prior observations. It is encouraging that a growing number of clinical studies now include a sex-based approach with respect to study design, enrollment, analysis, and data reporting [68]. These approaches need to be extended to the transgender population, which is at higher risk of treatment failure and disease complications due to limited data and study exclusions. Finally, potential interactions between race/ethnicity and sex should be evaluated to determine patient risk of adverse events and responsiveness to therapeutics. An increased understanding of the relationship between the physiological changes that occur throughout a female's life or with exogenous hormone use and therapeutic response, along with considerations of race/ethnicity, will further define sex-specific, as well as gender-specific, treatment needs to fulfill the realization of personalized medicine.

References

[1] CDER Small Business and Industry Assistance (SBIA). New drug development and approval process, Silver Spring, MD: FDA; June 1, 2020. Available from: https://www.fda.gov/drugs/development-approval-process-drugs.

[2] Kim J, Nafziger A. Is it sex or is it gender? Clin Pharmacol Ther 2000;68:1–3.

[3] Miller VM, Rice M, Schiebinger L, Jenkins MR, Werbinski J, Núñez A, et al. Embedding concepts of sex and gender health differences into medical curricula. J Women Heal 2013;22:194–202.

[4] Kim JH, Scialli AR. Thalidomide: the tragedy of birth defects and the effective treatment of disease. Toxicol Sci 2011;122:1–6.

[5] CDER. General considerations for the clinical evaluation of drugs. Guidance for industry, Rockville, MD: FDA; February 1997. Available from: https://www.fda.gov/media/71495/download.

[6] Merkatz R. Women in clinical trials: an introduction. Food Drug Law J 1993;48:161–166.

[7] McCarthy CR. Historical background of clinical trials involving women and minorities. Acad Med 1994;69:695–698.

[8] US Government Accountability Office. Women's health: FDA needs to ensure more study of gender differences in prescription drugs testing. Washington, DC. Publication No GAO/HRD-93-17; October 20, 1992. Available from: https://www.gao.gov/products/GAO/HRD-93-17.

[9] CDER. Guideline for the study and evaluation of gender differences in the clinical evaluation of drugs. Guidance for industry, Rockville, MD: FDA; February 1997. initially published as a Guideline in the Federal Register on July 22, 1993. Available from: https://www.fda.gov/media/71107/download.

[10] NIH. NIH policy and guidelines on the inclusion of women and minorities as subjects in clinical research, Bethesda, MD: NIH; October 2001. Available from: https://grants.nih.gov/policy/inclusion/women-and-minorities/guidelines.htm.

[11] FDA. Office of women's health, Silver Spring, MD: FDA; December 2019. Available from: https://www.fda.gov/about-fda/office-commissioner/office-womens-health.

[12] Zucker I, Prendergast BJ. Sex differences in pharmacokinetics predict adverse drug reactions in women. Biol Sex Differ 2020;11:32. https://doi.org/10.1186/s13293-020-00308-5.

[13] Berg M. Drugs, vitamins and gender. J Gend Specif Med 1999;2:18–20.

[14] O'Malley K, Crooks J, Duke E, Stevenson IH. Effect of age and sex on human drug metabolism. Br Med J 1971;3:607–609.

[15] Miners J, Attwood J, Birkett D. Influence of sex and oral contraceptive steroids on paracetamol metabolism. Br J Clin Pharmacol 1983;16:503–509.

[16] Cotreau MM, von Moltke LL, Greenblatt DJ. The influence of age and sex on the clearance of cytochrome P450 3A substrates. Clin Pharmacokinet 2005;44:33–60.

[17] Copeland V, Parekh A. FDA approved drug labels 2007–10: dose adjustments for women based on exposure, In: Drug Information Association 47th Annual Meeting; 2011.

[18] Poon R, Khanijow K, Umarjee S, Zhang L, Fadiran E, Yu M. Tracking women's participation and sex analyses in late-phase clinical trials of new molecular entity (NME) drugs and biologics approved by FDA between 2007–2009. In: Drug Information Association 47th Annual Meeting; 2011.

[19] Shuetz E, Furuya K, Shuetz J. Interindividual variation in expression of P-gp in normal human liver and secondary hepatic neoplasm. J Pharmacol Exp Ther 1995;275:1011–1018.

[20] Paine MF, Ludington SS, Chen M-L, Stewart PW, Huang S-M, Watkins PB. Do men and women differ in proximal small intestinal CYP3A or P-glycoprotein expression? Drug Metab Dispos 2005;33:426–433.

[21] Gross J, Friedman R, Azevedo M, Silveiro S, Pecis M. Effect of age and sex on glomerular filtration rate measured by 51Cr-EDTA. Braz J Med Biol Res 1992;25:129–134.

[22] Prasad B, Lai Y, Lin Y, Unadkat JD. Interindividual variability in the hepatic expression of the human breast cancer resistance protein (BCRP/ABCG2): effect of age, sex, and genotype. J Pharm Sci 2013;102:787–793.

[23] Datz F, Christian P, Moore J. Gender-related differences in gastric emptying. Nucl Med 1987;28:1204–1207.

[24] del Carmen Carrasco-Portugal M, Flores-Murrieta FJ. Gender differences in the pharmacokinetics of oral drugs. Pharmacol Pharm 2011;02:31–41.

[25] Aarons L, Hopkins K, Rowland M, Brossel S, Thiercelin J-F. Route of administration and sex differences in the pharmacokinetics of aspirin, administered as its lysine salt. Pharm Res 1989;6:660–666.

[26] Ho P, Triggs E, Bourne D, Heazlewood V. The effects of age and sex on the disposition of acetylsalicylic acid and its metabolites. Br J Clin Pharmacol 1985;19:675–684.

[27] Seitz HK, Egerer G, Simanowski UA, Waldherr R, Eckey R, Agarwal DP, et al. Human gastric alcohol dehydrogenase activity: effect of age, sex, and alcoholism. Gut 1993;34:1433–1437.

[28] Wolbold R, Klein K, Burk O, Nüssler AAK, Neuhaus P, Eichelbaum M, et al. Sex is a major determinant of CYP3A4 expression in human liver. Hepatology 2003;38:978–988.

[29] Krecic-Shepard M, Barnas CR, Slimko J, Schwartz J. Faster clearance of sustained release verapamil in men versus women: continuing observations on sex-specific differences after oral administration of verapamil. Clin Pharmacol Ther 2000;68:286–292.

[30] Gorski JC, Jones DR, Haehner-Daniels BD, Hamman MA, O'Mara EM, Hall SD. The contribution of intestinal and hepatic CYP3A to the interaction between midazolam and clarithromycin. Clin Pharmacol Ther 1998;64:133–143.

[31] Lutz U, Bittner N, Ufer M, Lutz WK. Quantification of cortisol and 6 beta-hydroxycortisol in human urine by LC-MS/MS, and gender-specific evaluation of the metabolic ratio as biomarker of CYP3A activity. J Chromatogr B Analyt Technol Biomed Life Sci 2010;878:97–101.

[32] Greenblatt DJ, Harmatz JS, Gouthro TA, Locke J, Shader RI. Distinguishing a benzodiazepine agonist (triazolam) from a nonagonist anxiolytic (buspirone) by electroencephalography: kinetic-dynamic studies. Clin Pharmacol Ther 1994;56:100–111.

[33] Hulst LK, Fleishaker JC, Peters GR, Harry JD, Wright DM, Ward P. Effect of age and gender on tirilazad pharmacokinetics in humans. Clin Pharmacol Ther 1994;55:378–384.

[34] Labbé L, Sirois C, Pilote S, Arseneault M, Robitaille NM, Turgeon J, et al. Effect of gender, sex hormones, time variables and physiological urinary pH on apparent CYP2D6 activity as assessed by metabolic ratios of marker substrates. Pharmacogenetics 2000;10:425–438.

[35] Walle T, Walle UK, Cowart TD, Conradi EC. Pathway-selective sex differences in the metabolic clearance of propranolol in human subjects. Clin Pharmacol Ther 1989;46:257–263.

[36] Theuretzbacher U, Ihle F, Derendorf H. Pharmacokinetic/pharmacodynamic profile of voriconazole. Clin Pharmacokinet 2006;45:649–663.

[37] Voriconazole label. n.d. Available from: https://www.accessdata.fda.gov/drugsatfda_docs/label/2015/021266s038,021267s047,021630s028lbl.pdf.

[38] Anderson GD. Sex and racial differences in pharmacological response: where is the evidence? Pharmacogenetics, pharmacokinetics, and pharmacodynamics. J Womens Health 2005;14:19–29.

[39] Relling MV, Lin J, Ayers GD, Evans WE. Racial and gender differences in n-acetyltransferase, xanthine oxidase, and CYP1A2* activities. Clin Pharmacol Ther 1992;52:643–658.

[40] George J, Byth K, Farrell GC. Age but not gender selectively affects expression of individual cytochrome P450 proteins in human liver. Biochem Pharmacol 1995;50:727–730.

[41] Shimada T, Yamazaki H, Mimura M, Inui Y, Guengerich FP. Interindividual variations in human liver cytochrome P-450 enzymes involved in the oxidation of drugs, carcinogens and toxic chemicals: studies with liver microsomes of 30 japanese and 30 caucasians. J Pharmacol Exp Ther 1994;270:414–423.

[42] Kim RB, O'Shea D, Wilkinson GR. Interindividual variability of chlorzoxazone 6-hydroxylation in men and women and its relationship to CYP2E1 genetic polymorphisms. Clin Pharmacol Ther 1995;57:645–655.

[43] Naraharisetti SB, Lin YS, Rieder MJ, Marciante KD, Psaty BM, Thummel KE, et al. Human liver expression of CYP2C8: gender, age, and genotype effects. Drug Metab Dispos 2010;38:889–893.

[44] Zanger UM, Schwab M. Cytochrome P450 enzymes in drug metabolism: regulation of gene expression, enzyme activities, and impact of genetic variation. Pharmacol Ther 2013;138:103–141.

[45] Hofmann MH, Blievernicht JK, Klein K, Saussele T, Schaeffeler E, Schwab M, et al. Aberrant splicing caused by single nucleotide polymorphism c.516g>t [q172h], a marker of CYP2B6*6, is responsible for decreased expression and activity of CYP2B6 in liver. J Pharmacol Exp Ther 2008;325:284–292.

[46] Hutzler JM, Yang Y-S, Brown C, Heyward S, Moeller T. Aldehyde oxidase activity in donor-matched fresh and cryopreserved human hepatocytes and assessment of variability in 75 donors. Drug Metab Dispos 2014;42:1090–1097.

[47] Shi J, Wang X, Nguyen J-H, Bleske BE, Liang Y, Liu L, et al. Dabigatran etexilate activation is affected by the CES1 genetic polymorphism G143E (rs71647871) and gender. Biochem Pharmacol 2016;119:76–84.

[48] Nicolas J-M, Espie P, Molimard M. Gender and interindividual variability in pharmacokinetics. Drug Metab Rev 2009;41:408–421.

[49] Merino G, van Herwaarden AE, Wagenaar E, Jonker JW, Schinkel AH. Sex-dependent expression and activity of the atp-binding cassette transporter breast cancer resistance protein (BCRP/ABCG2) in liver. Mol Pharmacol 2005;67:1765–1771.

[50] Gutmann H, Hruz P, Zimmermann C, Beglinger C, Drewe J. Distribution of breast cancer resistance protein (BCRP/ABCG2) mRNA expression along the human gi tract. Biochem Pharmacol 2005;70:695–699.

[51] Riches Z, Abanda N, Collier AC. BCRP protein levels do not differ regionally in adult human livers, but decline in the elderly. Chem Biol Interact 2015;242:203–210.

[52] Tamai I, Saheki A, Saitoh R, Sai Y, Yamada I, Tsuji A. Nonlinear intestinal absorption of 5-hydroxytryptamine receptor antagonist caused by absorptive and secretory transporters. J Pharmacol Exp Ther 1997;283:108–115.

[53] Prasad B, Evers R, Gupta A, Hop CECA, Salphati L, Shukla S, et al. Interindividual variability in hepatic organic anion-transporting polypeptides and p-glycoprotein (ABCB1) protein expression: quantification by liquid chromatography tandem mass spectroscopy and influence of genotype, age, and sex. Drug Metab Dispos 2014;42:78–88.

[54] Gandhi M, Aweeka F, Greenblatt RM, Blaschke TF. Sex differences in pharmacokinetics and pharmacodynamics. Annu Rev Pharmacol Toxicol 2001;44:499–523.

[55] Ueno K. Gender differences in pharmacokinetics of anesthetics. Jpn J Anesthesiol 2009;58:51–58.

[56] Soldin OP, Chung SH, Mattison DR. Sex differences in drug disposition. J Biomed Biotechnol 2011;2011:1–14.

[57] Ochs HR, Greenblatt DJ, Divoll M, Abernethy DR, Feyerabend H, Dengler HJ. Diazepam kinetics in relation to age and sex. Pharmacology 1981;23:24–30.

[58] Greenblatt DJ, Abernethy DR, Locniskar A, Ochs HR, Harmatz JS, Shader RI. Age, sex, and nitrazepam kinetics: relation to antipyrine disposition. Clin Pharmacol Ther 1985;38:697–703.

[59] Roberts RK, Desmond PV, Wilkinson GR, Schenker S. Disposition of chlordiazepoxide: sex differences and effects of oral contraceptives. Clin Pharmacol Ther 1979;25:826–831.

[60] Wedel M, Pieters JE, Pikaar NA, Ockhuizen T. Application of a three-compartment model to a study of the effects of sex, alcohol dose and concentration, exercise and food consumption on the pharmacokinetics of ethanol in healthy volunteers. Alcohol Alcohol 1991;26:329–336.

[61] Verbeeck R, Cardinal J, Wallace S. Effect of age and sex on the plasma binding of acidic and basic drugs. Eur J Clin Pharmacol 1984;27:91–97.

[62] Succari M, Foglietti M-J, Percheron F. Microheterogeneity of α1-acid glycoprotein: variation during the menstrual cycle in healthy women, and profile in women receiving estrogen-progestogen treatment. Clin Chim Acta 1990;187:235–241.

[63] Wiegratz I, Kutschera E, Lee JH, Moore C, Mellinger U, Winkler UH, et al. Effect of four different oral contraceptives on various sex hormones and serum-binding globulins. Contraception 2003;67:25–32.

[64] Saravanakumar A, Sadighi A, Ryu R, Akhlaghi F. Physicochemical properties, biotransformation, and transport pathways of established and newly approved medications: a systematic review of the top 200 most prescribed drugs vs. the FDA-approved drugs between 2005 and 2016. Clin Pharmacokinet 2019;58:1281–1294.

[65] Lamba V, Lamba J, Yasuda K, Strom S, Davila J, Hancock ML, et al. Hepatic CYP2B6 expression: gender and ethnic differences and relationship to CYP2B6 genotype and car (constitutive androstane receptor) expression. J Pharmacol Exp Ther 2003;307:906–922.

[66] Al Koudsi N, Tyndale RF. Hepatic CYP2B6 is altered by genetic, physiologic, and environmental factors but plays little role in nicotine metabolism. Xenobiotica 2010;40:381–392.

[67] Masubuchi Y, Hosokawa S, Horie T, Suzuki T, Ohmori S, Kitada M, et al. Cytochrome P450 isozymes involved in propranolol metabolism in human liver microsomes. The role of CYP2D6 as ring-hydroxylase and CYP1A2 as n-desisopropylase. Drug Metab Dispos 2014;171:580–594.

[68] Franconi F, Campesi I. Pharmacogenomics, pharmacokinetics and pharmacodynamics: interaction with biological differences between men and women. Br J Pharmacol 2014;171:580–594.

[69] Greenblatt DJ, von Moltke LL. Gender has a small but statistically significant effect on clearance of CYP3A substrate drugs. J Clin Pharmacol 2008;48:1350–1355.
[70] Sakuma T, Kawasaki Y, Jarukamjorn K, Nemoto N. Sex differences of drug-metabolizing enzyme: female predominant expression of human and mouse cytochrome P450 3A isoforms. J Health Sci 2009;55:325–337.
[71] Benet L, Cummins C, Wu C. Unmasking the dynamic interplay between efflux transporters and metabolic enzymes. Int J Pharm 2004;277:3–9.
[72] Benet LZ. The drug transporter – metabolism alliance: uncovering and defining the interplay. Mol Pharm 2009;6:1631–1643.
[73] Kassell NF, Haley EC, Apperson-Hansen C, Alves WM. Randomized, double-blind, vehicle-controlled trial of tirilazad mesylate in patients with aneurysmal subarachnoid hemorrhage: a cooperative study in Europe, Australia, and New Zealand. J Neurosurg 1996;84:221–228.
[74] Haley EC, Kassell NF, Apperson-Hansen C, Maile MH, Alves WM. A randomized, double-blind, vehicle-controlled trial of tirilazad mesylate in patients with aneurysmal subarachnoid hemorrhage: a cooperative study in North America. J Neurosurg 1997;86:467–474.
[75] Fleishaker JC, Hulst-Pearson LK, Peters GR. Effect of gender and menopausal status on the pharmacokinetics of tirilizad mesylate in healthy subjects. Am J Ther 1995;2:553–560.
[76] Lanzino G, Kassell NF, Dorsch NWC, Pasqualin A, Brandt L, Schmiedek P, et al. Double-blind, randomized, vehicle-controlled study of high-dose tirilazad mesylate in women with aneurysmal subarachnoid hemorrhage. Part I. A cooperative study in Europe, Australia, New Zealand, and South Africa. J Neurosurg 1999;90:1011–1017.
[77] Tanner J-A, Tyndale R. Variation in CYP2A6 activity and personalized medicine. J Pers Med 2017;7:18.
[78] Michaels S, Wang MZ. The revised human liver cytochrome P450 "pie": absolute protein quantification of CYP4F and CYP3A enzymes using targeted quantitative proteomics. Drug Metab Dispos 2014;42:1241–1251.
[79] Kalsotra A, Anakk S, Boehme CL, Strobel HW. Sexual dimorphism and tissue specificity in the expression of CYP4F forms in Sprague Dawley rats. Drug Metab Dispos 2002;30:1022–1028.
[80] Dalvie D, Di L. Aldehyde oxidase and its role as a drug metabolizing enzyme. Pharmacol Ther 2019;201:137–180.
[81] Casey Laizure S, Herring V, Hu Z, Witbrodt K, Parker RB. The role of human carboxylesterases in drug metabolism: have we overlooked their importance? Pharmacotherapy 2013;33:210–222.
[82] Shi J, Wang X, Eyler RF, Liang Y, Liu L, Mueller BA, et al. Association of oseltamivir activation with gender and carboxylesterase 1 genetic polymorphisms. Basic Clin Pharmacol Toxicol 2016;119:555–561.
[83] Jancova P, Anzenbacher P, Anzenbacherova E. Phase II drug metabolizing enzymes. Biomed Pap Med Fac Univ Palacky Olomouc Czech Repub 2010;154:103–116.
[84] Divoll M, Greenblatt DJ, Harmatz JS, Shader RI. Effect of age and gender on disposition of temazepam. J Pharm Sci 1981;70:1104–1107.
[85] Greenblatt D, Divoll M, Harmatz J, Shader R. Oxazepam kinetics: effects of age and sex. J Pharmacol Exp Ther 1980;215:86–91.
[86] Miners J, Robson R, Birkett D. Gender and oral contraceptive steroids as determinants of drug glucuronidation: effects on clofibric acid elimination. Br J Clin Pharmacol 1984;18:240–243.
[87] Greenblatt DJ, Abernethy DR, Matlis R, Harmatz JS, Shader RI. Absorption and disposition of ibuprofen in the elderly. Arthritis Rheum 1984;27:1066–1069.
[88] Macdonald JI, Herman RJ, Verbeeck RK. Sex-difference and the effects of smoking and oral contraceptive steroids on the kinetics of diflunisal. Eur J Clin Pharmacol 1990;38:175–179.
[89] Bock KW, Schrenk D, Forster A, Griese E-U, Mörike K, Brockmeier D, et al. The influence of environmental and genetic factors on CYP2D6, CYP1A2 and UDP-glucuronosyltransferases in man using sparteine, caffeine, and paracetamol as probes. Pharmacogenetics 1994;4:209–218.
[90] Meibohm B, Beierle I, Derendorf H. How important are gender differences in pharmacokinetics? Clin Pharmacokinet 2002;41:329–342.
[91] Song W, Qian Y, Li A. Estrogen sulfotransferase expression in the human liver: marked interindividual variation and lack of gender specificity. J Pharmacol Exp Ther 1998;284:1197–1202.
[92] Schwartz JB. The influence of sex on pharmacokinetics. Clin Pharmacokinet 2003;42:107–121.
[93] Campesi I, Romani A, Franconi F. The sex–gender effects in the road to tailored botanicals. Nutrients 2019;11:1637. https://doi.org/10.3390/nu11071637.
[94] Szumlanski CL, Honchel R, Scott MC, Weinshilboum RM. Human liver thiopurine methyltransferase pharmacogenetics: biochemical properties, liver-erythrocyte correlation and presence of isozymes. Pharmacogenetics 1992;148–159.
[95] Karas-Kuzelicki N, Milek M, Mlinaric-Rascan I. MTHFR and TYMS genotypes influence tpmt activity and its differential modulation in males and females. Clin Biochem 2010;43:37–42.
[96] Momper JD, Misel ML, McKay DB. Sex differences in transplantation. Transplant Rev 2017;31:145–150.
[97] Nicolson TJ, Mellor HR, Roberts RRA. Gender differences in drug toxicity. Trends Pharmacol Sci 2010;31:108–114.
[98] Parekh A, Fadiran EO, Uhl K, Throckmorton DC. Adverse effects in women: implications for drug development and regulatory policies. Expert Rev Clin Pharmacol 2011;4:453–466.
[99] Ebert SN, Liu X-K, Woosley RL. Female gender as a risk factor for drug-induced cardiac arrhythmias: evaluation of clinical and experimental evidence. J Womens Health 1998;7:547–557.
[100] Credible Meds. Drugs that prolong the QT interval and/or induce torsades de points, Available from: https://crediblemeds.org/; November 2020.
[101] Makkar RR, Fromm B, Steinman R, Meissner M, Lehmann M. Female gender as a risk factor for torsades de pointes associated with cardiovascular drugs. JAMA 1993;270:2590–2597.
[102] Drici M-D, Knollmann BC, Wang W-X, Woosley RL. Cardiac actions of erythromycin: influence of female sex. JAMA 1998;280:1774–1776.

[103] US Government Accountability Office. Drug safety: most drugs withdrawn in recent years had greater health risks for women. Washington, DC. Publication No GAO-01-286R; January 19, 2001. Available from: www.gao.gov/new.items/d01286r.pdf.

[104] Woosley RL, Chen Y, Freiman J, Gillis R. Mechanism of the cardiotoxic actions of terfenadine. JAMA 1993;269:1532–1536.

[105] Kumar A, Bhandari A, Rahimtoola S. Torsade de pointes and marked QT prolongation in association with hypothyroidism. Ann Intern Med 1987;106:712–713.

[106] Bagchi N, Brown T, Parish R. Thyroid dysfunction in adults over age 55 years. Arch Intern Med 1990;150:785–787.

[107] Roden DM, Woosley RL, Primm RK. Incidence and clinical features of the quinidine-associated long qt syndrome: implications for patient care. Am Heart J 1986;111:1088–1093.

[108] Lehmann MH, Hardy S, Archibald D, Quart B, MacNeil DJ. Sex difference in risk of torsade de pointes with d,l-sotalol. Circulation 1996;94:2535–2541.

[109] Pfizer, Inc. NDA 20-931 Tikosyn (dofetilide) risk evaluation and mitigation statements (REMS) document. Available from: https://www.fda.gov/media/81635/download; July 11, 2011.

[110] Drici M-D, Clément N. Is gender a risk factor for adverse drug reactions? Drug Saf 2001;24:575–585.

[111] Rodriguez I, Kilborn J, Liu X, Pezzullo J, Woosley R. Drug-induced QT prolongation in women during the menstrual cycle. JAMA 2001;285:1322–1326.

[112] Rautaharju P, Zhou S, Wong S, Calhoun H, Berenson G, Prineas R, et al. Sex differences in the evolution of electrocardiographic qt interval with age. Can J Cardiol 1992;8:690–695.

[113] Walle T, Byington RP, Furberg CD, McIntyre KM, Vokonas PS. Biologic determinants of propranolol disposition: results from 1308 patients in the beta-blocker heart attack trial. Clin Pharmacol Ther 1985;38:509–518.

[114] Flockhart DA, Dricit MD, Samuel C, Abernethy DR, Woosley RL. Effects of gender on propranolol pharmacokinetics and pharmacodynamics. FASEB J 1996;10:A429.

[115] Berg M. Pharmacokinetics and pharmacodynamics of cardiovascular agents. J Gend Specif Med 1999;2:22–24.

[116] Sivenius J, Laakso M, Penttila IM, Smets P, Lowenthal A, Riekkinen PJ. The European Stroke Prevention Study: results according to sex. Neurology 1991;41:1189–1192.

[117] Spranger M, Aspey BS, Harrison MJ. Sex difference in antithrombotic effect of aspirin. Stroke 1989;20:34–37.

[118] Riley JL, Robinson ME, Wise EA, Price D. A meta-analytic review of pain perception across the menstrual cycle. Pain 1999;81:225–235.

[119] Kest B, Sarton E, Dahan A. Gender differences in opioid-mediated analgesia. Anesthesiology 2000;93:539–547.

[120] Cepeda SM, Africano JM, Manrique AM, Fragoso W, Carr DB. The combination of low dose of naloxone and morphine in PCA does not decrease opioid requirements in the postoperative period. Pain 2002;96:73–79.

[121] Unruh AM. Gender variations in clinical pain experience. Pain 1996;65:123–167.

[122] Barsky A, Peekna H, Borus J. Somatic symptom reporting in women and men. J Gen Intern Med 2001;16:266–275.

[123] Cepeda MS, Carr DB. Women experience more pain and require more morphine than men to achieve a similar degree of analgesia. Anesth Analg 2003;1464–1468.

[124] Sarton E, Olofsen E, Romberg R, den Hartigh J, Kest B, Nieuwenhuijs D, et al. Sex differences in morphine analgesia. Anesthesiology 2000;93:1245–1254.

[125] Niesters M, Dahan A, Kest B, Zacny J, Stijnen T, Aarts L, et al. Do sex differences exist in opioid analgesia? A systematic review and meta-analysis of human experimental and clinical studies. Pain 2010;151:61–68.

[126] Dahan AM, Sarton E, Teppema L, Olievier C. Sex-related differences in the influence of morphine on ventilatory control in humans. Anesthesiology 1998;88:903–913.

[127] Sarton E, Teppema L, Dahan A. Sex differences in morphine-induced ventilatory depression reside within the peripheral chemoreflex loop. Anesthesiology 1999;90:1329–1338.

[128] Gear RW, Miaskowski C, Gordon NC, Paul SM, Heller PH, Levine JD. Kappa–opioids produce significantly greater analgesia in women than in men. Nat Med 1996;2:1248–1250.

[129] Walker JS, Carmody JJ. Experimental pain in healthy human subjects. Anesth Analg 1998;86:1257–1262.

[130] Mogil JS, Wilson SG, Chesler EJ, Rankin AL, Nemmani KVS, Lariviere WR, et al. The melanocortin-1 receptor gene mediates female-specific mechanisms of analgesia in mice and humans. Proc Natl Acad Sci U S A 2003;100:4867–4872.

[131] Damoiseaux VA, Proost JH, Jiawan VCR, Melgert BN. Sex differences in the pharmacokinetics of antidepressants: influence of female sex hormones and oral contraceptives. Clin Pharmacokinet 2014;53:509–519.

[132] Hildebrandt MG, Steyerberg EW, Stage KB, Passchier J, Kragh-Soerensen P. Are gender differences important for the clinical effects of antidepressants? Am J Psychiatry 2003;160:1643–1650.

[133] Kornstein SG, Schatzberg AF, Thase ME, Yonkers KA, McCullough JP, Keitner GI, et al. Gender differences in treatment response to sertraline versus imipramine in chronic depression. Am J Psychiatry 2000;157:1445–1452.

[134] Bigos KL, Pollock BG, Stankevich BA, Bies RR. Sex differences in the pharmacokinetics and pharmacodynamics of antidepressants: an updated review. Gend Med 2009;6:522–543.

[135] Palovaara S, Pelkonen O, Uusitalo J, Lundgren S, Laine K. Inhibition of cytochrome P450 2B6 activity by hormone replacement therapy and oral contraceptive as measured by bupropion hydroxylation. Clin Pharmacol Ther 2003;74:326–333.

[136] Golden RN, De Vane CL, Laizure SC, Rudorfer MV, Sherer MA, Potter WZ. Bupropion in depression. II. The role of metabolites in clinical outcome. Arch Gen Psychiatry 1988;45:145–149.

[137] Esmore D, Keogh A, Spratt P, Jones B, Chang V. Heart transplantation in females. J Heart Lung Transplant 1991;10:335–341.
[138] Meier-Kriesche H-U, Ojo AO, Leavey SF, Hanson JA, Leichtman AB, Magee JC, et al. Gender differences in the risk for chronic renal allograft failure. Transplantation 2001;71:429–432.
[139] Taylor D, Bristow M, O'Connell J, Price G, Hammond E, Doty D. Improved long-term survival after heart transplantation predicted by successful early withdrawal from maintenance corticosteroid therapy. J Heart Lung Transplant 1996;15:1039–1046.
[140] Lew KH, Ludwig EA, Milad MA, Donovan K, Middleton E Jr, Ferry JJ, et al. Gender-based effects on methylprednisolone pharmacokinetics and pharmacodynamics. Clin Pharmacol Ther 1993;54:402–414.
[141] Schwartz JB. The current state of knowledge on age, sex, and their interactions on clinical pharmacology. Clin Pharmacol Ther 2007;82:87–96.
[142] Johnson JA. Influence of race or ethnicity on pharmacokinetics of drugs. J Pharm Sci 1997;86:1328–1333.
[143] Gibbs CR, Lip GY, Beevers DG. Angioedema due to ACE inhibitors: increased risk in patients of African origin. Br J Clin Pharmacol 2001;48:861–865.
[144] Brown NJ, Ray WA, Snowden M, Griffin MR. Black Americans have an increased rate of angiotensin converting enzyme inhibitor-associated angioedema. Clin Pharmacol Ther 1996;60:8–13.
[145] Kostis JB, Kim HJ, Rusnak J, Casale T, Kaplan A, Corren J, et al. Incidence and characteristics of angioedema associated with enalapril. Arch Intern Med 2005;165:1637–1642.
[146] Kupfer Y, Ramachandran K, Tessler S. ACE inhibitor–induced angioedema in elderly African American females requiring tracheostomy. J Natl Med Assoc 2010;102:529–530.
[147] Kamil RJ, Jerschow E, Loftus PA, Tan M, Fried MP, Smith RV, et al. Case-control study evaluating competing risk factors for angioedema in a high-risk population. Laryngoscope 2016;126:1823–1830.
[148] Huether S, McCance K. Understanding pathophysiology. 5th ed. St. Louis, MO: Mosby; 2012. p. 785.
[149] Carr B, Wilson J. Disorders of the ovary and female reproductive tract. In: Braunwald E, Isselbacher K, Petersdorf R, Wilson J, Martin J, Fauci A, editors. Harrison's principles of internal medicine. 11th ed. New York: McGraw-Hill; 1987. p. 1818–1837.
[150] Kashuba ADM, Nafziger AN. Physiological changes during the menstrual cycle and their effects on the pharmacokinetics and pharmacodynamics of drugs. Clin Pharmacokinet 1998;34:203–218.
[151] Arjmandi BH, Salih MA, Herbert DC, Sims SH, Kalu DN. Evidence for estrogen receptor-linked calcium transport in the intestine. Bone Miner 1993;21:63–74.
[152] Gennari C, Agnusdei D, Nardi P, Civitelli R. Estrogen preserves a normal intestinal responsiveness to 1,25-dihydroxyvitamin D3 in oophorectomized women. J Clin Endocrinol Metab 1990;71:1288–1293.
[153] Lemmens HJM, Burm AGL, Hennis PJ, Gladines MPPR, Bovill JG. Influence of age on the pharmacokinetics of alfentanil. Clin Pharmacokinet 1990;19:416–422.
[154] Fleishaker J, Pearson L, Pearson P, Wienkers L, Hopkins N, Peters G. Hormonal effects on tirilazad clearance in women: assessment of the role of CYP3A. J Clin Pharmacol 1999;39:260–267.
[155] NCCIH. Using dietary supplements wisely. Bethesda, MD: NIH; Updated January 2019. Available from: https://www.nccih.nih.gov/health/using-dietary-supplements-wisely.
[156] Roe AL, Paine MF, Gurley BJ, Brouwer KR, Jordan S, Griffiths JC. Assessing natural product–drug interactions: an end-to-end safety framework. Regul Toxicol Pharmacol 2016;76:1–6.
[157] Paine MF, Shen DD, McCune JS. Recommended approaches for pharmacokinetic natural product-drug interaction research: a NaPDI Center commentary. Drug Metab Dispos 2018;46:1041–1045.
[158] Gurley BJ, Yates CR, Markowitz JS. "...Not intended to diagnose, treat, cure or prevent any disease." 25 years of botanical dietary supplement research and the lessons learned. Clin Pharmacol Ther 2018;104:470–483.
[159] Butterweck V. In: Cooper R, Kronenberg F, editors. St. John's wort: quality issues and active compounds. New York: Mary Ann Liebert; 2009. p. 785.
[160] Zhou S, Chan E, Pan S-Q, Huang M, Lee EJD. Pharmacokinetic interactions of drugs with St. John's wort. J Psychopharmacol 2004;18:262–276.
[161] Henderson L, Yue QY, Bergquist C, Gerden B, Arlett P. St john's wort (*Hypericum perforatum*): drug interactions and clinical outcomes. Br J Clin Pharmacol 2002;54:349–356.
[162] Carrillo JA, Benitez J. CYP1A2 activity, gender and smoking, as variables influencing the toxicity of caffeine. Br J Clin Pharmacol 2003;41:605–608.
[163] CDER. Labeling for combined oral contraceptives. Draft guidance for industry, Silver Spring, MD: FDA; December 2017. Available from: https://www.fda.gov/media/110050/download.
[164] Anon. The facts about women and tobacco, Washington, DC: Truth Initiative; February 2019. Available from: https://truthinitiative.org/research-resources/targeted-communities/facts-about-women-and-tobacco.
[165] CDC. Tobacco product use and cessation indicators among adults—United States. Available from: https://www.cdc.gov/mmwr/volumes/68/wr/mm6845a2.htm?s_cid=mm6845a2_w; 2018.
[166] Ereshefsky L, Saklad S, Watanabe M, Davis C, Jann M. Thiothixene pharmacokinetic interactions: a study of hepatic enzyme inducers, clearance inhibitors, and demographic variables. J Clin Psychopharmacol 1991;11:296–301.
[167] Bruno R, Vivier N, Montay G, Le Liboux A, Powe LK, Delumeau J-C, et al. Population pharmacokinetics of riluzole in patients with amyotrophic lateral sclerosis. Clin Pharmacol Ther 1997;62:518–526.
[168] Jennings T, Nafziger A, Davidson L, Bertino J Jr. Gender differences in hepatic induction and inhibition of theophylline pharmacokinetics and metabolism. J Lab Clin Med 1993;122:208–216.

[169] Olanzepine label. n.d. Available from: http://pi.lilly.com/us/zyprexa-pi.pdf.

[170] Lucas D, Ménez C, Girre C, Berthou F, Bodenez P, Joannet I, et al. Cytochrome P450 2E1 genotype and chlorzoxazone metabolism in healthy and alcoholic caucasian subjects. Pharmacogenetics 1995;5:298–304.

[171] Lake JE, Clark JL. Optimizing HIV prevention and care for transgender adults. AIDS 2019;33:363–375.

[172] Saleem F, Rizvi SW. Transgender associations and possible etiology: a literature review. Cureus 2017;9:e1984. https://doi.org/10.7759/cureus.1984.

[173] Becasen JS, Denard CL, Mullins MM, Higa DH, Sipe TA. Estimating the prevalence of HIV and sexual behaviors among the US transgender population: a systematic review and meta-analysis, 2006–2017. Am J Public Health 2019;109:e1–e8.

[174] Hiransuthikul A, Janamnuaysook R, Himmad K, Kerr SJ, Thammajaruk N, Pankam T, et al. Drug-drug interactions between feminizing hormone therapy and pre-exposure prophylaxis among transgender women: the iFACT study. J Int AIDS Soc 2019;22. https://doi.org/10.1002/jia2.25338, e25338.

[175] Anderson PL, Reirden D, Castillo-Mancilla J. Pharmacologic considerations for preexposure prophylaxis in transgender women. J Acquir Immune Defic Syndr 2016;72(Suppl. 3):S230–S234.

Chapter 23

Drug therapy in pregnant and nursing women

Catherine S. Stika and Marilynn C. Frederiksen

Department of Obstetrics and Gynecology, Northwestern University Feinberg School of Medicine, Chicago, IL, United States

The pregnant woman is perhaps the last true therapeutic orphan. Because of the ethical, medicolegal, and fetal safety concerns regarding pregnant women, few pharmacokinetic, pharmacodynamic, or clinical trials are conducted during pregnancy. Despite the new pregnancy labeling enacted by the FDA in July 2015, the majority of drugs that are marketed in the United States continue to carry statements such as the following in their labeling:

> *There are, however, no adequate and well-controlled studies in pregnant women. Because animal reproductive studies are not always predictive of human response, this drug should be used during pregnancy only if clearly needed.*
> *Zinacef (cefuoxine for injection) labeling, revised 2/2020 [1].*

This places the burden squarely on the practitioner to assess the risks and benefits of a particular agent in a given clinical situation. The risk most often considered is the fetal risk of teratogenesis, or drug-induced malformation, irrespective of the gestational age during the pregnancy when therapy is initiated. Pregnant women are more often than not left untreated in an attempt to avoid any perceived fetal risk related to use of a pharmacologic agent, and the effect of untreated maternal disease on either the pregnancy outcome or the offspring is not a usual consideration. On those occasions when pharmacotherapy is initiated, issues of appropriate dosage and frequency of administration are often not evaluated, so that the usual adult dose is prescribed without thought to any changes dictated by physiologic differences between nonpregnant and pregnant women.

There are two compelling reasons for studying drugs and drug therapy during pregnancy. The first relates to the changing age of reproduction. The age of a woman's first pregnancy has been steadily rising in the United States, with an increasing number of first pregnancies occurring after age 30 [2]. The occurrence of pregnancy later in life increases the number of women who may require drug therapy for diseases present prior to pregnancy and who may need to continue therapy during pregnancy. Knowledge of drug therapy during pregnancy is needed if these women with underlying diseases are to be optimally treated.

The second reason supporting the need to study drugs during pregnancy relates to the physiologic changes that occur with gestation. This altered physiology can affect the pharmacokinetics of drugs. For example, physiologic changes during pregnancy may affect drug absorption, decrease drug binding to plasma proteins, increase drug distribution volume, and cause variations in either renal and/or hepatic drug clearance. Mere extrapolation of pharmacokinetic data from drug studies largely conducted in nonpregnant subjects to pregnant women fails to account for the impact of the multiple physiologic changes that occur during pregnancy. This disregard for the changes in maternal physiology may affect drug efficacy or place the woman at increased risk for adverse drug effects and ultimately impact the overall pregnancy outcome.

These issues were addressed by the US Food and Drug Administration (FDA) in a lengthy process that began in 1997 and has led to a revamping of the sections of the drug label that address pregnancy, labor and delivery, and nursing mothers. To provide more human data on the use of drugs during pregnancy, the FDA has required the establishment of a pregnancy registry after initial marketing of a drug. In August 2002, an FDA guidance for industry was published regarding pregnancy registries and the incorporation of the data from registries into drug labels [3]. Subsequently, three additional guidances for industry have been published: the design and conduct of pharmacokinetic studies in pregnant women in November 2004 [4]; a guidance regarding clinical lactation studies in February 2005 (revised in May 2019) [5]; and scientific and ethical considerations for including pregnant women in clinical trials in April 2018. These new labeling requirements were

Atkinson's Principles of Clinical Pharmacology. https://doi.org/10.1016/B978-0-12-819869-8.00009-4

TABLE 23.1 Pregnancy information included in the new drug labels.

General information	
	Contact information if pregnancy registry available General statement about background risk
Fetal risk summary	
	Based on all available data, this section characterizes the likelihood that the drug increases the risk of developmental abnormalities in humans and other relevant risks
	More than one risk conclusion may be needed
	For drugs that are not systemically absorbed, there is a standard statement that maternal use is not expected to result in fetal exposure
	For drugs that are systemically absorbed, include: When there are human data, a statement about the likelihood of increased risk based on this data and a description of findings A standard statement about likelihood of increased risk based on animal data
Clinical considerations	
	Inadvertent exposure: known predicted risk to the fetus from inadvertent exposure to drug early in pregnancy
	Description of any known risk to the pregnant woman and fetus from the disease or condition the drug is intended to treat
	Information about dosing adjustments during pregnancy, labor and delivery, and postpartum; maternal adverse reactions unique to pregnancy or increased in pregnancy; effects of dose, timing, and duration of exposure to drug during pregnancy; potential neonatal complications and needed interventions
Data	
	Human and animal data presented separately, with human data presented first, including study type, exposure information (dose, duration, timing), and identified fetal developmental abnormality or other adverse effects
	For human data, include: positive and negative experiences, number of subjects and duration of study
	For animal data, include: species studied and description of doses in terms of human dose equivalents (provide basis for calculation)

published for comment in the Federal Register in May 2008 [6], approved as a final document on December 4, 2014 [7], and went into effect on June 30, 2015. The deadline for adapting these changes is June 2020. As detailed in Table 23.1, the new label removes the simplistic letter category and instead includes the following sections: general information, which will include pregnancy registry information; a fetal risk summary; clinical considerations, which will include inadvertent exposure and dosage adjustments during pregnancy; and a summary of the data available. Subsections on lactation and nursing mothers and exposure in women and men of reproductive potential are also included.

The importance of both expanding research and educating physicians and the public about medication use in pregnancy and lactation has been recognized by the federal government. In 2017 the 21st Century Cures Act included the establishment of a Task Force on Research Specific to Pregnant Women and Lactating Women (PRGLAC) whose purpose was to provide guidance to the Secretary of Health and Human Services on activities related to identifying and addressing gaps in knowledge and research about safe and effective therapies for pregnant women and lactating women. The PRGLAC report was published in September 2018 [8]. Chief among their recommendations were: (1) include and integrate pregnant women and lactating women in the clinical research agenda; (2) increase the quantity, quality, and timeliness of research on safety and efficacy of therapeutic products used by pregnant women and lactating women; (3) expand the workforce of clinicians and research investigators with expertise in obstetric and lactation pharmacology and therapeutics; (4) remove regulatory barriers to research in pregnant women; (5) create a public awareness campaign to engage the public and health care providers in research on pregnant women and lactating women. The PRGLAC Task Force clearly identified a critical need to change the cultural assumptions that have historically restricted inclusion of pregnant women in pharmacology research. Despite these recommendations and little more than one year later, as federal agencies and national organizations rapidly developed trials to identify therapeutic agents effective against the novel coronavirus SARS-CoV-2, pregnant women were, once again, excluded from funded studies with remdesivir [9] and hydroxychloroquine with azithromycin [10]. The only option to obtain remdesivir for a pregnant patient with COVID-19 was for each obstetrician to apply for individual compassionate use through the drug's manufacturer [11]. It is obvious that without evidence and data, our ability to appropriately care for this special population is severely limited.

Pregnancy physiology and its effects on pharmacokinetics

Rather than present a list of the many changes in maternal physiology that occur during pregnancy, the focus here is to select those changes which have the greatest potential to alter the absorption, distribution, and elimination of drugs in pregnant women.

Gastrointestinal changes

Because it decreases smooth muscle activity, progesterone has long been thought to delay gastric emptying and prolong gastrointestinal transit time during pregnancy. Pregnancy-induced changes in plasma levels of both relaxin and motilin may also contribute to decreased intestinal motility [12, 13]. In addition, gastric acid secretion is also decreased in pregnant women and their gastric pH is correspondingly higher [14], which theoretically could reduce the gastric absorption of weak acids. Although most of the early studies of gastrointestinal function were done in women during labor [15, 16], more recent studies of acetaminophen absorption in nonlaboring women using real-time ultrasonography have shown no differences in gastric emptying during the first and third trimesters of pregnancy, as compared with the postpartum period [17, 18]. Only in the third trimester are orocecal transit times prolonged. This effect is correlated with the decrease in plasma pancreatic polypeptide concentrations that occurs in the third trimester of pregnancy and results in reduced gastrointestinal motility [18].

Only a few studies have been conducted in pregnant women to evaluate the effects of these pregnancy-related gastrointestinal changes on the actual rate and extent of drug absorption. In all these studies, women received both intravenous and oral drug doses while they were pregnant as well as after pregnancy, thus serving as their own controls. Sotalol, a beta-adrenergic receptor antagonist, showed no significant difference in bioavailability between the two time periods [19]. The antibiotics cefazolin, ampicillin, and cephradine also were studied during pregnancy and in the postpartum period [20, 21]. Peak drug levels were found to be lower during pregnancy, but pregnancy did not appear to change the extent of drug absorption or the time to peak drug concentration (t_{max}). Similar results have been demonstrated for other medications, e.g., oral midazolam, for which time to peak drug concentration is not altered by gastric changes in pregnancy [22].

Cardiovascular effects

The cardiovascular effects which occur during pregnancy include plasma volume expansion, an increase in cardiac output, and changes in regional blood flow. By the sixth to eighth week of pregnancy, plasma volume has expanded, and continues to increase until approximately 32–34 weeks of pregnancy [23]. For a singleton gestation, this increase in plasma volume is 1200–1300 mL, or approximately 40% higher than the plasma volume of nonpregnant women. Plasma volume expansion is even greater for multiple gestations [24]. There are also significant increases in extracellular fluid space and total body water that vary somewhat with patient weight [25, 26]. These changes in body fluid spaces are summarized in Table 23.2.

The increase in plasma volume is accompanied by a gradual increase in cardiac output that begins in the first trimester of pregnancy. By 8 weeks' gestation, cardiac output can be as much as 50% greater, and by the third trimester it is at least 30%–50% greater, than in the nonpregnant state [27]. Early in pregnancy, an increase in stroke volume accounts for the increased cardiac output. In later pregnancy, the increase in cardiac output is the result of both elevated maternal heart rate and a continued increase in stroke volume [28]. These changes in cardiovascular parameters have shown to persist above preconception baselines until at least 12 weeks postpartum [29].

TABLE 23.2 Body fluid spaces in pregnant and nonpregnant women.

	Weight (kg)	Plasma volume (mL/kg)	ECF space (L/kg)	TBW (L/kg)
Nonpregnant	<0	49	0.189	0.516
	70–80		0.156	0.415
	>80		0.151	0.389
Pregnant	<70	67	0.257	0.572
	70–80		0.255	0.514
	>80		0.240	0.454

Modified from Frederiksen MC, Ruo TI, Chow MJ, Atkinson AJ Jr. Theophylline pharmacokinetics in pregnancy. Clin Pharmacol Ther 1986;40:321–328.

Regional blood flow changes also occur in pregnant women and can affect drug distribution and elimination. Blood flow increases to the uterus, kidneys, skin, and mammary glands, with a compensatory decrease in skeletal muscle blood flow. At full term, blood flow to the uterus represents about 20%–25% of cardiac output and renal blood flow is 20% of cardiac output [30]. There is increased blood flow to the skin to dissipate the additional heat produced by the fetus [31]. Blood flow to the mammary glands is increased during pregnancy in preparation for lactation postpartum [32]. As shown in Fig. 23.1, arterial hepatic blood flow is maintained relatively unchanged during pregnancy but constitutes a lower percentage of cardiac output than in the nonpregnant condition because of the increased proportion of blood flow to the uterus and kidneys [33]. Portal venous blood flow has been shown by Doppler ultrasonography to increase beginning at 28 weeks of pregnancy and has been measured to be 150%–160% over the nonpregnant portal blood flow [34]. As a result of these hemodynamic changes, there is a decreased proportion of cardiac output available to skeletal muscle and other vascular beds.

These multiple physiological changes in pregnant women may affect drug distribution. In some cases, it is possible to correlate pregnancy-associated changes in distribution volume (V_d) with changes in extracellular fluid space (ECF), total body water (TBW), and drug binding to plasma proteins using the following equation, which was developed in Chapter 3:

$$V_d = \text{ECF} + f_U\,(\text{TBW} - \text{ECF}) \tag{23.1}$$

where f_U is the fraction of unbound drug.

Blood composition changes

Plasma albumin concentration decreases during pregnancy [35–37]. The fall in albumin concentration from 4.2 g/dL in the nonpregnant woman to 3.6 g/dL in the midtrimester of pregnancy (Fig. 23.2) has long been erroneously attributed to a "dilutional effect" caused by plasma volume expansion. However, it follows from pharmacokinetic principles that this decrease in plasma albumin concentration represents either a reduction in the rate of albumin synthesis or an increase in the rate of albumin clearance (see Chapter 1, Eq. 1.2). Additional support for this explanation is provided by the fact that the plasma concentrations of total protein are relatively unchanged during pregnancy [36]. However, the plasma concentration of α_1-acid glycoprotein, which binds many basic drugs, is reduced by almost 50% during the third trimester of pregnancy and rapidly normalizes by the 4th day postpartum [38].

The reduction in both albumin and α_1-acid glycoprotein concentrations potentially can alter the binding of drugs commonly bound to these plasma proteins [37, 38]. In a study of theophylline pharmacokinetics during the second and third trimesters of pregnancy, theophylline protein binding to plasma proteins was reduced to only 11% and 13% of total plasma concentrations, respectively, compared with 28% 6 months postpartum [35]. Although the decrease in the serum concentration of albumin may be thought to account for these differences, a subsequent study showed that the albumin binding

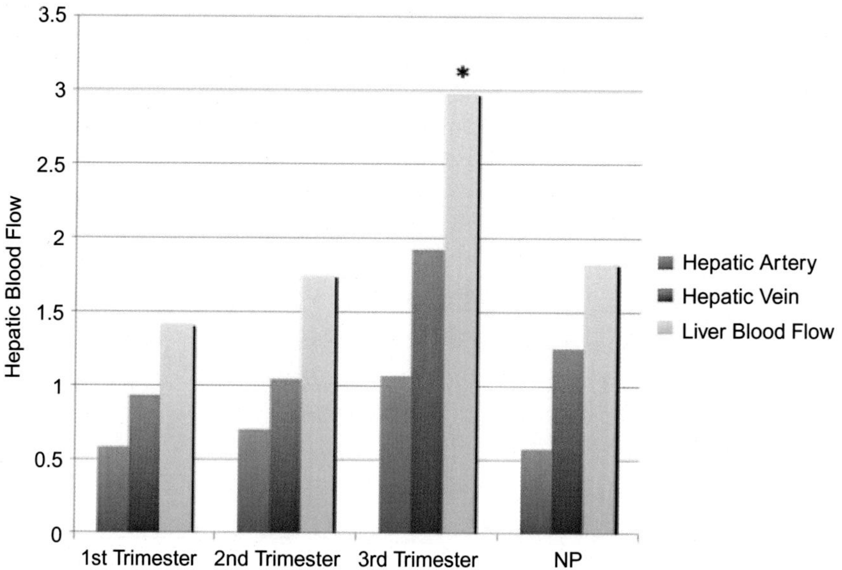

FIG. 23.1 Hepatic blood flow as measured by Doppler ultrasound. Portal venous blood flow is shown to be markedly increased in the third trimester of pregnancy as compared with hepatic blood flow in nonpregnant (NP) women (*$P < .5$). *Data from Nakai A, Sekiya I, Oya A, Koshino T, Araki T. Assessment of the hepatic arterial and portal venous blood flows during pregnancy with Doppler ultrasonography. Arch Gynecol Obste 2002;266:25–29.*

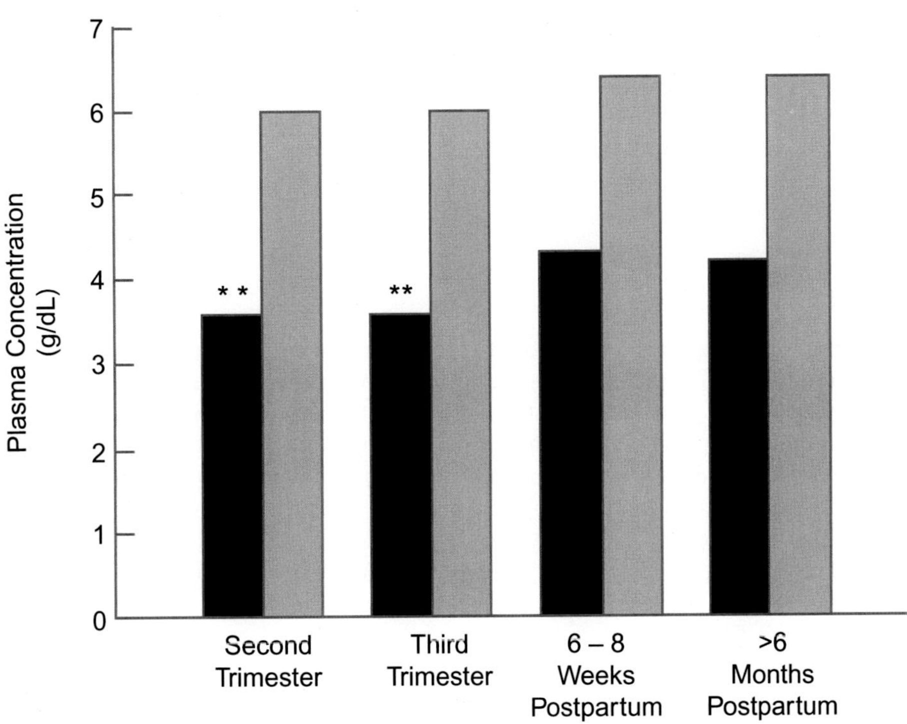

FIG. 23.2 Albumin (*black bars*) and total protein (*gray bars*) concentrations during the second and third trimesters of pregnancy and in the postpartum period. Albumin concentrations are reduced significantly during pregnancy when compared to >6months postpartum values (**$P < .01$). *Data from Frederiksen MC, Ruo TI, Chow MJ, Atkinson AJ Jr. Theophylline pharmacokinetics in pregnancy. Clin Pharmacol Ther 1986;40:321–328.*

sites for theophylline were actually increased during pregnancy, but the binding affinity constant was significantly lower during pregnancy than in the nonpregnant state [39].

Pregnancy is also associated with a partially compensated respiratory alkalosis that may affect the protein binding of some drugs. Respiratory changes in pregnancy include a decrease in arterial partial pressure of carbon dioxide to 30.9mmHg, most likely due to the effect of progesterone on increasing tidal volume by 30 to 50% beginning in the first trimester [40, 41]. In compensation, serum bicarbonate decreases and maternal serum pH increases slightly to 7.44 [40].

Renal changes

Accompanying the increased blood flow to the kidneys is an increase in glomerular filtration rate (GFR). This increase begins by the sixth week of gestation, gradually rises in the early portion of the third trimester [42], and plateaus or falls slightly until delivery. This increase in GFR is reflected in an increase in inulin and creatinine clearance during pregnancy. For drugs predominantly cleared by the kidney, the increase in drug clearance mirrors changes in GFR during pregnancy. Cefuroxime, a cephalosporin predominantly eliminated by the kidneys, has a significantly greater clearance in the midtrimester of pregnancy than during either delivery or the postpartum period [43]. Tobramycin clearance changes similarly, with the highest clearance and shortest half-life found in the midtrimester, followed by a fall in clearance and corresponding longer half-life in the third trimester [44].

Renal clearance of drugs in pregnancy can also be affected by pregnancy-induced changes in transporter-mediated renal tubular function which may affect net renal excretion by altering tubular reabsorption and/or tubular secretion. The increase in amoxicillin clearance observed in the second and third trimesters of pregnancy results from increases in both renal filtration and renal tubular secretion, of which the latter has been shown to increase by 60% over its postpartum baseline [45]. The beta lactam antibiotics are known substrates of human oligopeptide transporters 1 and 2 (hPepT1 and hPepT2), which are located on the apical surface of renal proximal tubular cells, and reabsorb these small molecules [46]. A suggested mechanism for the enhanced secretion of these antibiotics during pregnancy is that progesterone may decrease transcription of hPepT1 in renal tubular cells, as has been shown for intestinal cell lines [47]. By reducing renal hPepT1 reabsorption, renal secretion of amoxicillin also would be enhanced. In a study examining another renally cleared drug, digoxin renal clearance and secretion clearance were on average 61% and 120% higher, respectively, during the early third trimester of pregnancy compared to postpartum [22]. Digoxin renal secretion is mediated through activities of both the organic anion transporter polypeptides (OATPs), which are located on the basolateral surface of the renal tubular cell and move digoxin from blood into the cell [48], and the efflux transporter P-glycoprotein (P-gp), which is located on the apical, luminal facing cell surface and moves digoxin into the tubule [49]. The authors proposed that the enhanced renal secretion of digoxin observed in pregnancy resulted from upregulation in the activity of either one or both of these transporters.

Even for a drug primarily eliminated by hepatic metabolism in nonpregnant women, the increase in GFR can significantly affect total drug clearance during pregnancy. For example, the renal clearance of theophylline, a drug largely eliminated by CYP1A2 metabolism which is reduced during pregnancy, was found to increase during pregnancy so that its total elimination clearance was not significantly reduced but was maintained at 86% of its value 6 months postpartum [35].

Hepatic drug-metabolizing changes

The activity of hepatic drug-metabolizing enzymes also changes during pregnancy and can affect drug elimination clearance. Pregnancy is an estrogenic state with 100-fold increases in estradiol levels over a woman's nonpregnant baseline [50, 51]. Progesterone, the hormone responsible for sustaining gestation, also rises dramatically during pregnancy from luteal concentrations of 30–40 ng/mL to concentrations of 100–200 ng/mL in the third trimester [52–54]. Both estradiol and estrone, as well as the natural progestins, including progesterone, pregnenolone, 17-hydroxyprogesterone, and 5β-3-20-pregnanedione, have been shown to induce drug metabolism by activating the human orphan nuclear pregnane X receptor (PXR) and constitutive androgen receptor (CAR), the xenobiotic sensing receptors. As described in Chapter 11 (see Fig. 11.3), PXR forms a heterodimer complex with the 9-*cis*-retinoic acid receptor (RXR). This hPXR/RXR complex then binds to the promoter region of many of the hepatic enzymes and transporters, and serves as a key transcriptional regulator of that target gene [55, 56].

Earlier hypotheses that the dramatic hormonal changes that occur in pregnancy are responsible for the alterations in hepatic metabolism have been in part supported by recent studies with primary hepatic cell cultures. Hepatic cell cultures, in which environmental media can be manipulated, have been widely used to examine potential drug-drug interactions [57]. Similarly, adding estradiol and progesterone in concentrations comparable with pregnancy to hepatocytes from female donors has been shown to increase mRNA transcript levels and subsequent activity of several CYP enzymes, most prominently CYP2A6, CYP2B6, and CYP3A4 [58]. In another hepatocyte study, the induction of CYP2B6 activity by estradiol was commensurate with that produced by carbamazepine and rifampin [59]. Cortisol also increases in pregnancy, although less dramatically than the female hormones [60], and has been shown to significantly increase CYP3A4 activity in hepatic cell culture [61, 62]. Phase II glucuronidation has also been shown to be induced by female reproductive hormones. Estradiol, with the assistance of the transcription factor, protein-1 (Sp1), upregulates UGT1A4 activity in cultured hepatocytes [63]. On the other hand, progesterone is responsible for inducing UGT1A1 activity while UGT2B7 activity is not affected by any steroid hormone [64].

CYP3A4 substrates

Increased CYP3A4 activity in pregnancy has been shown to consistently accelerate the metabolism of many commonly used medications. Most studies have limited their evaluation to late second to third trimester pregnancy and have made comparisons with either postpartum or historical controls. Using dextromethorphan *N*-demethylation as a marker of CYP3A activity, Tracy et al. [65] demonstrated that CYP3A activity had already increased by early second trimester and remained consistently elevated by 35%–38% above baseline throughout the duration of pregnancy. However, because most authors have avoided drug studies in the first trimester, the exact onset of this increase has not been identified.

Because midazolam is exclusively eliminated by CYP3A4 metabolism [66, 67], midazolam clearance and the 1′-hydroxymidazolam to midazolam serum concentration ratio are recognized markers of CYP3A4 activity [68, 69]. Hebert et al. [22] compared midazolam pharmacokinetic parameters in pregnancy to 6–10 weeks postpartum in the same women. Apparent oral clearance of midazolam in the third trimester of pregnancy was increased by $108 \pm 62\%$ ($P = .002$) compared to postpartum.

Clearances of other CYP3A4 substrates have been shown to be similarly increased in pregnancy. The metabolic ratio of cortisol, a nonspecific probe of CYP3A4 activity, was increased in pregnant women near term when compared to the same women 1 week and 3 months postpartum [70]. The two corticosteroids, betamethasone and its stereoisomer, dexamethasone, which are administered antenatally to decrease the incidence of respiratory distress syndrome in neonates born prematurely, are metabolized predominantly by CYP3A4 [71–73]. Betamethasone clearance was found to be 1.2- to 1.6-fold higher in the third trimester of pregnancy as compared with nonpregnant women [73–75]. The area under the plasma concentration-time curve of the protease inhibitor, indinavir, another drug predominantly metabolized by CYP3A4, was 68% lower at 30–32 weeks of gestation in the same women compared to 6–8 weeks postpartum [76]. In a study of the extended release formulation of metronidazole, which is primarily metabolized by CYP3A4, the total oral clearance in pregnant women during the second and early third trimesters was 27% greater than in nonpregnant women and the mean maximum concentration of metronidazole was approximately 25% lower in pregnancy [77].

In 1992 the clearance of another CYP3A substrate, nifedipine, a frequently used tocolytic for preterm labor, was shown to be increased fourfold in women during the third trimester of pregnancy in comparison to historical controls [78]. More recently, Haas et al. [79] confirmed the increased clearance of nifedipine in pregnancy (128 L/h compared to 35–38 L/h in nonpregnant females), and also reported that nifedipine metabolism was further enhanced in women who carried the active CDYP3A5*1 variant as well as the CYP3A4*1B allele—both of which augment CYP3A activity. Of note, there are marked ethnic differences in CYP3A5*1 distribution, with approximately 75% of African Americans carrying the active allele compared to only 10%–20% of Caucasians [80]. The additional contribution of CYP3A5*1 to metabolism of CYP3A substrates also impacts the efficacy of the antimalarial drug, lumefantrine [81]. Pregnant women with the active CYP3A5 allele treated with lumefantrine for malaria have significantly lower day 7 drug concentrations and are at increased risk of treatment failure.

CYP1A2 substrates

The elimination clearance of caffeine, a marker of CYP1A2 enzymatic activity, has been shown to decrease by a factor of two by midgestation and by a factor of three by the third trimester compared to the postpartum period [82]. These findings were confirmed by Tracy et al. [65] who administered caffeine as part of his "probe cocktail" and demonstrated that CYP1A2 activity progressively decreases during pregnancy, with a 22% reduction in early second trimester and a 65% reduction in late third trimester, compared to postpartum activity in the same women. Although the intrinsic hepatic clearance of theophylline, another CYP1A2 substrate, was reduced during pregnancy, there was substantially less change in its hepatic clearance because of the pregnancy-associated decrease in theophylline binding to plasma proteins [35]. As a result of the offsetting changes in renal and hepatic clearance referred to previously, the total elimination clearance of theophylline was unchanged in the third trimester of pregnancy (Fig. 23.3).

CYP2B6 substrates

Assessing changes in the activity of CYP2B6 separate from that of CYP3A is often difficult because CYP2B6 activity contributes to the metabolism of approximately 25%–30% of the drugs metabolized by CYP3A4 and there are few drugs uniquely metabolized by CYP2B6 [83]. Although CYP2B6 activity was shown to be significantly induced by estradiol in

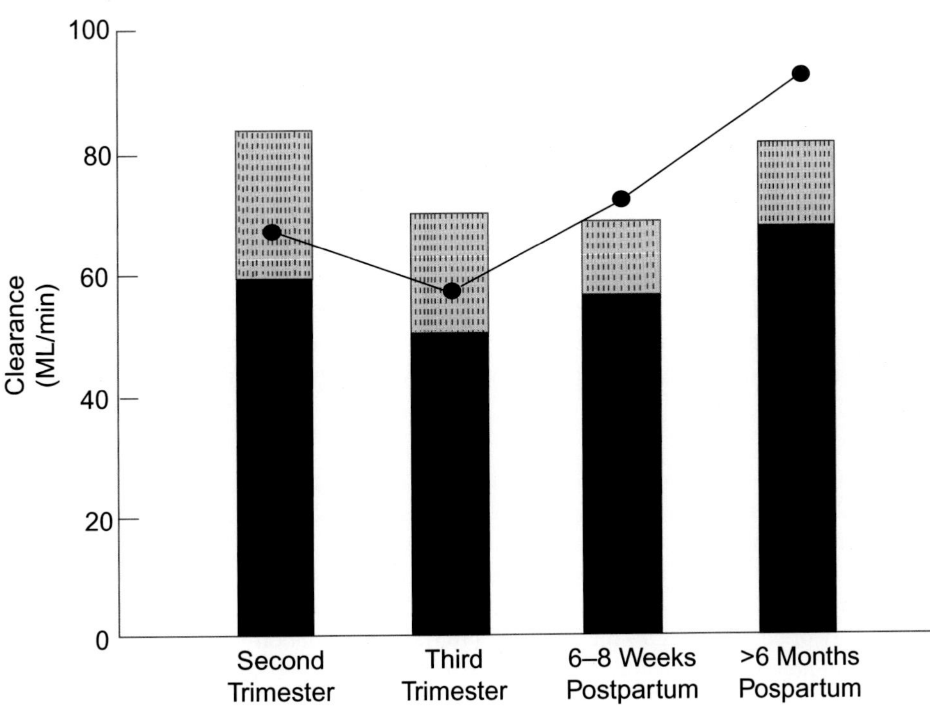

FIG. 23.3 Theophylline clearance measured during the second and third trimesters of pregnancy and in the postpartum period. During pregnancy, the substantial drop in the intrinsic hepatic clearance (●) of this CYP1A2 substrate is attenuated by decreased theophylline binding to plasma proteins and increased glomerular filtration rate so that overall elimination clearance, consisting of the sum of hepatic clearance (*solid bars*) and renal clearance (*stippled bars*), is relatively unaffected. *Data from Frederiksen MC, Ruo TI, Chow MJ, Atkinson AJ Jr. Theophylline pharmacokinetics in pregnancy. Clin Pharmacol Ther 1986;40:321–328.*

hepatocyte cultures [59], pharmacokinetic studies in pregnant women are less definitive. Methadone is metabolized by both CYP3A4 and CYP2B6 and its clearance significantly increases in pregnancy [84–89], but it is unclear how much each enzyme contributes to those changes. Efavirenz is predominantly metabolized by CYP2B6 to its hydroxy-metabolite with possible minor contributions by CYP3A4, CYP3A5, CYP1A2, and CYP2A6 [90]. In a study comparing the PK parameters in 25 women on efavirenz 600 mg once daily, there were no significant differences in AUC_{0-24} and C_{max} between the third trimester of pregnancy and postpartum, suggesting that CYP2B6 activity was not increased in pregnancy [91].

CYP2D6 substrates

Although, as detailed in Chapter 13, CYP2D6 activity is known to show considerable pharmacogenetic variation, this enzyme is not inducible by typical xenobiotics. However, in pregnancy, activity of CYP2D6 in extensive metabolizers is enhanced. Hogstedt et al. [92, 93] reported that the CYP2D6 substrate metoprolol had a four- to five-fold increase in clearance during pregnancy. Tracy et al. [65] used dextromethorphan *O*-demethylation as a marker of CYP2D6 activity and, limiting his analysis to only women known to be extensive and intermediate metabolizers, showed that CYP2D6 activity increases progressively during pregnancy, with a 25% increase in early second trimester, progressing to a 48% increase in the late third trimester. Wadelius et al. [94] also used dextromethorphan *O*-demethylation to characterize CYP2D6 activity in the late third trimester of pregnancy. He found that CYP2D6 activity increased during pregnancy in individuals who were homozygous and heterozygous extensive metabolizers but decreased in homozygous poor metabolizers. In the largest study to date examining the effects of pregnancy on CYP2D6 activity, Ververs et al. [95] assayed paroxetine concentrations across pregnancy in 74 women with depression. He demonstrated that in the 44 women who were extensive (EM) or ultra-rapid (UM) CYP2D6 metabolizers, paroxetine concentrations steadily decreased during pregnancy while in the poor (PM) and intermediate (IM) metabolizers, drug concentrations increased. He also found that depressive symptoms increased significantly in the EM/UM women, while in the IM/PM group they did not change.

CYP2C9 substrates

Although not as well studied as other hepatic Phase I enzymes, activity of CYP2C9 has been shown to increase during pregnancy for several medications primarily metabolized by this enzyme. The hepatic clearance of phenytoin, a restrictively eliminated drug that is predominantly a CYP2C9 substrate, increases during pregnancy, resulting in correspondingly lower total plasma concentration [96]. This is in large part a reflection of the decrease in protein binding that is well documented for phenytoin, as free plasma concentrations of this drug have been shown to remain relatively constant until late in pregnancy, when the intrinsic clearance of this drug does increase [97, 98].

Although glyburide can be metabolized by multiple pathways by different hepatic enzymes (CYP3A4, CYP2C9, CYP2C8, and CYP2C19) [99], in vivo studies in nonpregnant subjects support CYP2C9 as one of the primary enzymes [100]. Glyburide clearance was found to be twofold higher in pregnant women [101] and simulations predicted that compared to the standard twice-daily dosing range of 1.25–10.0 mg in nonpregnant women, doses would have to be increased to as much as 23.75 mg twice daily for optimal glucose control during pregnancy. However, the safety of glyburide for the fetus is open to question, since steady-state glyburide concentrations in serum from cord blood are approximately 70% of maternal serum concentrations [101].

Indomethacin, one of the nonsteroidal antiinflammatory drugs metabolized by CYP2C9, is prescribed in pregnancy for both its analgesic and tocolytic properties. In a pharmacokinetic study performed in 25 women who received oral indomethacin for either preterm labor or degenerating uterine fibroids during their second trimester of pregnancy, the apparent clearance of indomethacin was 14.5 ± 5.5 L/h, which was greater than the steady-state clearance of 6.5–9.8 L/h historically reported for nonpregnant subjects. The mean plasma concentration observed in these subjects for a 25-mg oral dose was also 37% lower than that reported following a similar dose in nonpregnant women who were approximately matched for age and weight [102].

CYP2C19 substrates

Even fewer studies have been performed that examine the influence of pregnancy on CYP2C19 activity; however, limited data indicate a decrease in its activity. The metabolism of proguanil, an antimalarial drug, to its active metabolite cycloguanil is dependent on CYP2C19 activity. The conversion of proguanil to cycloguanil has been shown to decrease by approximately 60% during the third trimester of pregnancy in women who were CYP2C19 extensive metabolizers. Pregnancy did not affect the metabolic activity of poor CYP2C19 metabolizers [103]. In a population-based study, CYP2C19-dependent clearance decreased by 50% in pregnancy, prompting the authors to recommend a dosing increase in pregnant women [104].

Phase II hepatic enzymes

Glucuronidation

Of the changes in drug metabolism that occur in pregnancy, none have been shown to change as dramatically as glucuronidation. This was first observed in studies with the anticonvulsant and mood-stabilizing drug, lamotrigine, which is primarily metabolized by uridine 5′-diphosphate glucuronosyltransferase 1A4 (UGT1A4). Multiple investigations have shown that enhanced lamotrigine clearance begins as early as 5 weeks' gestation and progressively increases until it peaks in the third trimester at 248–330% over baseline [105–110]. There is also prominent between-subject variability in lamotrigine clearance during pregnancy. When charting lamotrigine clearance by gestational age, Polepally et al. [111] identified two subpopulations: in 77% of 64 pregnancies, the third trimester lamotrigine clearance increased by 219% over baseline, whereas, in 23% of women, clearance rose by only 21%. However, these authors were not able to identify factors that differentiated these populations. Among the factors that have been proposed to contribute to the variability are polymorphisms in UGT1A4 and UGT2B7, which play a minor role in lamotrigine glucuronidation, variable changes in renal excretion, and even the sex of the fetus, as women carrying a female fetus may have more prominent increases in lamotrigine clearance later in pregnancy [112, 113]. As a result, serial dose increases are often necessary to maintain stable therapeutic lamotrigine concentrations and control of either maternal seizure activity or mood [110]. After delivery, clearance of lamotrigine falls rapidly and returns to nonpregnant levels by 3 weeks postpartum. So, tapering the dose should begin within the first week after delivery in order to prevent possible lamotrigine toxicity [106, 108, 110].

Potential drug-drug interactions that may occur when lamotrigine is administered with other anticonvulsant drugs during pregnancy have also been studied [114–116]. Coadministration with oxcarbazepine, whose active metabolite, 10-monohydroxy derivative (MHD), is also glucuronidated by at least UGT2B7 and UGT1A9 [117], does not affect the pregnancy-induced increase in lamotrigine clearance [116]. On the other hand, valproic acid, a known inhibitor of UGT1A4, partially blocks the pregnancy-associated increase in lamotrigine clearance, with the result that women receiving both lamotrigine and valproic acid during the third trimester have a lamotrigine clearance that is only 60% greater than baseline [114].

Glucuronidation of labetalol, an antihypertensive medication commonly used in pregnancy, also progressively increases during pregnancy [118, 119]. In 57 women taking labetalol for chronic hypertension, plasma samples were obtained from 12 weeks' gestation until 12 weeks after delivery. Using sparse sampling, population pharmacokinetic analysis, Fischer et al. [118] reported that the apparent oral clearance of labetalol at the end of the first trimester was 1.4-fold greater than postpartum and by term had increased to 1.6-fold greater. These results were consistent with those in an earlier study in which the elimination half-life of labetalol in the third trimester of pregnancy was significantly shorter than in nonpregnant controls, 1.7 h compared to 6–8 h, respectively [119]. Authors in both studies advised that the dosing interval of labetalol in pregnancy may need to be shortened to maintain hypertensive control.

Other phase II enzymes

Very little is known about the activity of other Phase II enzymes in pregnancy. Using caffeine metabolism, Bologna et al. [120] studied both pregnant and nonpregnant epileptic women and reported that the activity of *N*-acetyltransferase was decreased during pregnancy. In contrast, Tsutsumi et al. [121], also using caffeine, showed that the activity of *N*-acetyltransferase-2 (NAT-2) in pregnant women, all identified as fast acetylators, decreased by only 13% and only during early pregnancy; NAT-2 activity returned to nonpregnant levels during mid and late pregnancy. In the same study [121], the conversion of methylxanthine to 1-methyluric acid by xanthine oxidase was not affected by pregnancy.

Peripartum changes

The physiologic changes which begin early in gestation are most pronounced in the third trimester of pregnancy. Further physiologic changes occur during labor and delivery, when there is an even further increase in cardiac output, blood flow to muscle mass decreases, and there is a cessation of gastrointestinal activity [122]. The onset of labor decreases placental blood flow and drug distribution to the fetus during each contraction. There also may be a change in the pharmacodynamics of drugs during the intrapartum period, but this is largely unstudied.

Drugs are commonly studied during the intrapartum period, probably for no other reason than it is a time when pharmacologic intervention is indicated and the amount of drug distributed to the fetus can be estimated from cord blood obtained at delivery. However, the pharmacokinetics of drugs given during this period have been shown to be different from their pharmacokinetics during the antepartum period. An intrapartum study of cefuroxime showed that clearance was lower than during pregnancy but higher than in the remote postpartum period [43]. Morphine clearance has been shown to be markedly increased during labor, resulting in a shortening of its elimination half-life that reduces the dosing interval required for adequate pain relief during labor [123].

Postpartum changes

In the early postpartum period, maternal pregnancy physiologic changes are sustained with an elevated cardiac output, decreased plasma albumin concentration, and increased GFR [124, 125]. The cardiovascular changes of pregnancy are sustained as long as 12 weeks after delivery [29]. However, maternal hepatic enzymatic activity may either rapidly reverse within a few days of delivery or gradually return to normal during the first months after delivery [38, 106, 126].

The physiology of the postpartum period seems to have great interindividual variability, since pharmacokinetic studies during this period show greater between-subject variability than studies conducted in women who have not recently been pregnant. As shown in Fig. 23.4, a study of clindamycin pharmacokinetics in five postpartum women demonstrated that there was a 15-fold variation in peak drug concentrations and that t_{max} varied from 1 to 6 h after oral administration of this drug [127]. Similarly, a study of gentamicin in the postpartum period showed distribution volume estimates that varied from 0.1 to 0.5 L/kg, as compared with distribution volume estimates from studies in nonpregnant volunteers that only ranged from 0.2 to 0.3 L/kg [128].

Pharmacokinetic studies during pregnancy

Results of selected pharmacokinetic studies in pregnant women

Although an exhaustive survey of pharmacokinetic studies is not possible, the purpose here is to present illustrative studies that best demonstrate the effects of maternal physiologic changes on pharmacokinetics and potentially on drug dosing requirements and efficacy.

Ampicillin/amoxicillin

The pharmacokinetics of both intravenously and orally administered ampicillin were studied serially in 26 women who served as their own controls [20]. Perhaps because both intravenous and oral doses need to be administered, ampicillin is one of the few medications for which absolute bioavailability has been examined during pregnancy. No difference in the extent of ampicillin absorption or in time to peak drug concentrations was seen between pregnant and nonpregnant women, but peak levels were lower than in nonpregnant women. Although this study demonstrated an absolute increase in the distribution volume of ampicillin, it did not include an analysis of the effect of the change in maternal weight on the volume of distribution. Both renal and total elimination clearance of ampicillin increased by approximately 50% during pregnancy and resulted in correspondingly lower plasma concentrations. Unfortunately, the study combined data from

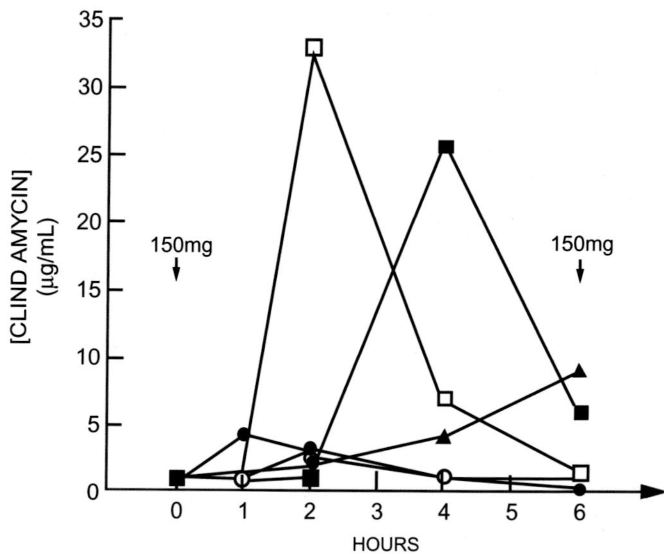

FIG. 23.4 Variability in plasma concentrations of clindamycin measured in five postpartum women over a 6-h period after oral administration of a 150-mg dose. *Reproduced with permission from Steen B, Rane A. Clindamycin passage into human milk. Br J Clin Pharmacol 1982;13:661–664.*

women whose pregnancies ranged from 13 to 33 weeks' gestation, which blurred assessment of the effects of the progression of changes in maternal physiology that is known to occur during the second and third trimesters of pregnancy. Another study of ampicillin pharmacokinetics in the third trimester of pregnancy showed an increase in the steady-state volume of distribution on a L/kg basis, but used results in male controls as an historic reference population [129].

A pharmacokinetic study of a similar antibiotic, amoxicillin, was conducted in 17 pregnant women during the second and third trimesters of pregnancy and again postpartum [45]. This was a single oral-dose study to evaluate whether the drug would be an appropriate therapy for anthrax infections during pregnancy. Both the *AUC*s and peak concentrations were lower and the elimination half-life was shorter during the second and third trimesters of pregnancy as compared with the postpartum period because of increased amoxicillin renal clearance. This increase in renal clearance consisted of an increase in renal filtration of amoxicillin and either a 50% increase in amoxicillin renal secretory transport or a similar decrease in its renal reabsorption. The authors concluded that amoxicillin would need to be dosed every 4 h to achieve adequate serum concentrations that would be effective against most strains of anthrax.

Cefuroxime

The pharmacokinetics of intravenously administered cefuroxime were studied serially in seven women during pregnancy, at delivery, and in the remote postpartum period [43]. Distribution volume ($V_{d(extrap)}$) during pregnancy and at delivery approximated the expected ECF volumes presented in Table 23.2. However, the difference in these volumes and the postpartum value was not statistically significant and there was no change in the weight-normalized distribution volumes. On the other hand, cefuroxime is largely eliminated by renal excretion, and renal clearance was significantly greater during pregnancy than that measured either at delivery or in nonpregnant women. As a result, plasma cefuroxime concentrations resulting from a 750-mg dose were significantly lower during pregnancy.

Caffeine

The pharmacokinetics of caffeine were studied serially during and after pregnancy [82]. Although only oral doses were administered, V_d/F showed no change when calculated on a L/kg basis to take into account the change in weight during and after pregnancy. On the other hand, CL/F was decreased by a factor of two by midgestation and by a factor of three in the third trimester compared to the postpartum period [82].

Theophylline

The pharmacokinetics of intravenously administered theophylline have been studied serially in women during and after pregnancy [35]. As described previously, theophylline binding to plasma proteins was reduced during the second and third trimesters of pregnancy to 11% and 13% of total plasma concentrations, respectively, compared with 28% 6 months postpartum. This appears to reflect the fact that the albumin binding affinity constant for theophylline is significantly lower during pregnancy than in the nonpregnant state, even though there is an increased number of albumin binding sites [29]. The steady-state distribution volume of theophylline was increased during the second and third trimesters of pregnancy. As presented in Table 23.3, the increases were similar to what was predicted from Eq. (23.1) (see also Chapter 3,

TABLE 23.3 Comparison of expected with measured values of theophylline distribution volume.

	$V_{d(SS)}$ [a]	
	Expected (L)	Measured (L)
Pregnant		
24–26 weeks	32.0 ± 2.0	30.3 ± 6.6
36–38 weeks	37.9 ± 1.9	36.8 ± 4.2
Postpartum		
6–8 weeks	28.0 ± 1.1	28.4 ± 3.0
> 6 months	26.9 ± 2.3	30.7 ± 4.4

[a] *Mean values for five women ± SD.*
Data from Frederiksen MC, Ruo TI, Chow MJ, Atkinson AJ Jr. Theophylline pharmacokinetics in pregnancy. Clin Pharmacol Ther 1986;40:321–328.

Fig. 3.1) using measured values for protein binding and the estimates of extracellular fluid volume and total body water presented in Table 23.2.

Renal clearance of theophylline paralleled the pregnancy-associated increase in creatinine clearance and accounted for 30% and 28% of total theophylline elimination in the second and third trimesters, respectively, compared to only 16% at 6 months postpartum. As shown in Fig. 23.3, the intrinsic clearance of theophylline was reduced substantially during pregnancy. Hepatic clearance showed substantially less change because of the pregnancy-associated decrease in theophylline binding to plasma proteins. As a result of the offsetting changes in renal and hepatic clearance, total elimination clearance of theophylline in the third trimester of pregnancy averaged 86% of its value 6 months postpartum. Although this reduction in elimination clearance was not statistically significant, it combined with the increase in theophylline distribution volume to significantly increase theophylline elimination half-life from an average of 4.4 h in the nonpregnant state (assessed 6 months postpartum) to 6.5 h in the third trimester of pregnancy.

Methadone

The pharmacokinetics of orally administered methadone were studied serially by Pond et al. [84] in nine women at 20–24 weeks and 35–40 weeks of pregnancy, and at 1–4 weeks and 8–9 weeks postpartum. There was no significant change in methadone binding to plasma proteins during pregnancy. Renal methadone clearance during pregnancy was approximately twice its value in the postpartum periods. However, renal clearance contributed only minimally to total methadone clearance, and this change did not reach statistical significance. On the other hand, estimates of *CL/F* during pregnancy also were doubled and this change was both statistically and clinically significant, resulting in a corresponding lowering of methadone plasma levels and symptoms of methadone withdrawal in some women near the end of gestation. Because the clearance of other CYP3A4 substrates is increased during pregnancy, the authors concluded that increased metabolic clearance rather than decreased bioavailability was responsible for the decrease in *CL/F*.

Since Pond's initial study of methadone in pregnancy in 1985, our understanding of the complexity of methadone metabolism has evolved with CYP2B6 playing an important role in supplementing CYP3A4 activity with additional contributions from CYP2D6, and possibly lesser contributions from CYP2C9, CYP2C19, and CYP1A2 [85, 86]. Individual pharmacogenetic differences in the activity of each of these enzymes also influence methadone metabolism [85]. Although large interindividual variability is observed, additional studies have confirmed the increase in methadone clearance during pregnancy and the need for dose escalation in many women [87–89].

An alternate method for assessing methadone metabolism and opioid status is to simultaneously measure trough concentrations of methadone and its pharmacologically inactive metabolite, EDDP (2-ethylidene-1,5-dimethyl-3,3-diphenylpyrrolidine) and then calculate the methadone/metabolite concentration ratio (MMR) [89]. At any given dose, larger ratios reflect decreased metabolism with greater opioid effect and smaller ratios, more rapid metabolism and less opioid activity. MMRs in nonpregnant adults are typically in the 11–12 range. In 23 pregnant women on methadone, dosed either twice daily or up to 6 times daily, trough serum concentrations and ratio data were collected every 4 to 6 weeks during pregnancy and within a week after delivery. Although considerable variability was seen in individual MMR trajectories, mean MMRs decreased as pregnancy progressed: (mean ± SD) first trimester 7.2, second trimester 5.9, third trimester 5.1, and postpartum 7.2). The percent of MMRs ≤4, indicating ultrarapid metabolism, increased from 8% in the first trimester, to 30% in the second, 38% in the third, and then decreased to 5% postpartum [89].

Anticonvulsants

The total plasma concentrations of some anticonvulsant drugs have been shown to decrease during pregnancy. This is in large part a reflection of the decrease in protein binding that is well documented for phenytoin [96, 97], carbamazepine [97], and phenobarbital [98]. However, these drugs are restrictively eliminated and unbound concentrations of carbamazepine [97, 130] and phenobarbital [98] remain unchanged during pregnancy, reflecting the fact that their intrinsic clearance is unchanged. As is the case for patients with impaired renal function (see Chapter 5), dosage of phenytoin and these other anticonvulsants should not be increased in pregnant women based solely on decreases in total plasma concentration. On the other hand, Tomson et al. [96] monitored phenytoin plasma levels serially in 36 women during pregnancy and in the nonpregnant state. Intrinsic clearance was increased only during the third trimester of pregnancy, resulting in unbound plasma concentrations that averaged 16% lower than in the nonpregnant woman (Fig. 23.5), and this may warrant increasing phenytoin doses for some women late in pregnancy.

Levetiracetam is a newer antiepileptic medication that is not appreciably protein bound and is eliminated primarily by renal excretion with approximately 30% of the dose metabolized by enzymatic hydrolysis [131]. Several small studies have been performed that have shown significant reductions in levetiracetam plasma concentrations in pregnant women. Tomson et al. [131] obtained trough plasma concentrations from seven women who were maintained on a fixed levetiracetam dose

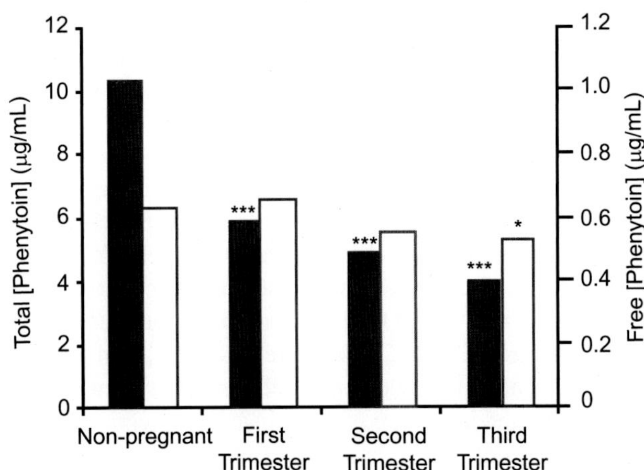

FIG. 23.5 Total (*solid bars*) and free (*open bars*) plasma concentrations of phenytoin in nonpregnant and pregnant women ($^{*}P<.05$, $^{***}P=.001$). *Data from Tomson T, Lindbom U, Ekqvist B, Sundqvist A. Epilepsy and pregnancy: a prospective study of seizure control in relation to free and total plasma concentrations of carbamazepine and phenytoin. Epilepsia 1994;35:122–130.*

during each trimester, at delivery, and postpartum. An additional 5 women were sampled only in the third trimester and postpartum. Compared to mean (±SD) postpartum values of 69.1 ± 37.9 μmol/L, mean first and second trimester levetiracetam concentrations were somewhat lower (each approximately 35 μmol/L), but dropped even more in the third trimester to 27.5 ± 15.7 μmol/L, which was a statistically significantly decrease ($P<.01$). Two of the seven women developed seizures during the third trimester. Using trough dose/plasma concentrations to represent apparent levetiracetam clearance for all 12 women, mean apparent clearance was significantly higher during the third trimester, 427.3 ± 211.3 L/day compared to postpartum baseline, 124.7 ± 57.9 L/day ($P<.0001$). The authors recommended that levetiracetam levels should be monitored during pregnancy with appropriate dosing adjustments. In another study by Westin et al. [132] 19 pregnant women receiving levetiracetam were followed with fasting trough blood samples obtained prior to pregnancy, during each trimester, and at several points postpartum. Plasma concentration to dose ratios were calculated to adjust for dose changes during pregnancy. Concentration to dose ratios (*C/D* ratios), representing the inverse of clearance, progressively decreased as pregnancy progressed, although they did not become significantly different from prepregnancy baseline ratios until the third trimester. By 3–5 days after delivery, the *C/D* ratios had returned to baseline. During the third trimester seizures either occurred for the first time or increased in frequency in 7 of the 19 women. In 2019, in the largest cohort of patients studied, Berlin et al. [133] followed 59 women on levetiracetam during 66 pregnancies and collected plasma concentrations prior to pregnancy, during each of the trimesters, and again postpartum. They reported that the mean apparent oral clearance increased during the first trimester by approximately 43% and remained elevated at approximately this same level throughout pregnancy until postpartum. They recommended that therapeutic drug monitoring with appropriate dose escalation begins in the first trimester.

Antiretrovirals

Of all drug classes, more pharmacokinetic studies in pregnancy have been performed with antiretroviral medications than any other category. Obstetrical care of this maternal-fetal dyad has benefitted from the efforts of two large research networks: the International Maternal Pediatric Adolescent AIDS Clinical Trial Network (IMPAACT) and Pharmacokinetics of Newly Developed Antiretroviral Agents in HIV Infected Pregnant Women (PANNA). Two of the numerous drugs studied will be reviewed.

Tenofovir disoproxil fumarate is a nucleoside reverse transcriptase inhibitor (NRTI) commonly used in pregnancy as one of the medications in an antiretroviral cocktail. It is only 7.2% protein bound and undergoes phosphorylation to its active metabolite, tenofovir diphosphate. Neither tenofovir nor its metabolites are substrates of CYP enzymatic metabolism; both molecules are eliminated by a combination of glomerular filtration and active renal tubular secretion. In nonpregnant adults after a single, orally administered dose, the terminal elimination half-life is approximately 17 h [134]. In 2013 the PANNA network [135] published the results of a pharmacokinetic study of oral tenofovir 300 mg and emtricitabine 200 mg daily in 34 pregnant women. Pharmacokinetic studies were performed in 24 women in the third trimester and again 4 to 6 weeks postpartum. Compared to the postpartum period, in the third trimester there was a 30% increase in tenofovir clearance ($P<.001$), a 23% decrease in $AUC_{0\text{–}24}$ ($P<.001$), a 19% decrease in C_{max} ($P=.001$), and a 21% decrease in C_{min} ($P=.003$). Although 9 of the women (26%) did not meet the tenofovir *AUC* dosing target of 2 mg h/L, all but one had an undetectable viral load close to delivery. Tenofovir was well transferred to the fetus; at delivery in 14 paired samples the median ratio of cord blood-to-maternal blood concentrations was 0.82 (0.64–1.10). The authors concluded that although tenofovir exposure during pregnancy was reduced, this was not associated with vertical transmission and no change in dosing was recommended.

In addition to two NRTI drugs, most multidrug antiretroviral regimens contain either a protease inhibitor or an integrase inhibitor. Darunavir, together with low dose ritonavir, is one of the two protease inhibitors that are currently recommended for treating pregnant women who are infected with HIV. Darunavir is approximately 95% protein bound, mostly to alpha-1-acid glycoprotein, and is metabolized to inactive metabolites primarily through CYP3A4 oxidation [136]. It also is a known P-gp substrate [137]. Because of its first-pass metabolism via intestinal and hepatic CYP3A4, augmented by intestinal P-gp efflux transport, bioavailability of darunavir is poor [136]. Coadministration with ritonavir, a strong CYP3A4 inhibitor, increases the bioavailability of darunavir from 37% to 82%, increases its C_{max} and AUC by approximately 40%, and prolongs its elimination half-life to 15h. In nonpregnant women, combining the two medications allows for once-daily dosing.

Studies in pregnancy have shown that the induction of CYP3A4 with pregnancy increases the clearance of both darunavir and ritonavir, making once-daily dosing less reliably effective. Once-daily dosing with a higher dose of darunavir/ritonavir 800/100mg was compared to darunavir/ritonavir 600/100mg twice daily in a prospective nonblinded study in 64 HIV-infected pregnant women with intensive 12- or 24-h pharmacokinetic analyses performed during the second and third trimesters and postpartum [138]. Mean darunavir AUC and C_{max} were significantly reduced during pregnancy compared with postpartum for both dosing regimens. With once-daily dosing of 800/100mg, darunavir AUC was reduced by 38% during the second trimester and by 39% during the third trimester. In contrast, with twice-daily dosing of 600/100mg, darunavir AUC was reduced by 26% in both trimesters. The authors concluded that twice-daily dosing was preferred but that larger doses needed to be studied.

In a similarly designed nonrandomized, open-label, multicenter, PANNA network study of pregnant women with HIV, 17 women received darunavir/ritonavir 800/100mg once daily and 6 women received 600/100mg twice daily [139]. Pharmacokinetic parameters were analyzed in the third trimester and postpartum the geometric mean ratios (GMR) of third trimester versus postpartum to total darunavir $AUC_{0\text{-}\tau}$ were 0.78 (90% CI, 0.60–1.00) after 600/100mg twice-daily dosing and 0.67 (0.56–0.82) after 800/100mg once-daily dosing. All children were HIV-negative. The authors concluded that a single daily dose of darunavir/ritonavir in pregnancy was appropriate for antiretroviral-naïve women. However, for other HIV-infected pregnant women, the twice-daily dose of 600/100mg was recommended. In a third pharmacokinetic study in 17 pregnant women taking darunavir/ritonavir 800/100mg once daily, 24-h pharmacokinetic analyses were performed in the second and third trimesters and postpartum [140]. The mean free fraction of darunavir, the ratio of unbound plasma concentration to total plasma concentration, was 0.2257 ± 0.0330 ($\pm$S.D.) in the second trimester and 0.2277 ± 0.343 in the third trimester, compared to 0.1843 ± 0.0245 postpartum, reflecting in part the impact of a 42% reduction in α1-acid glycoprotein during pregnancy. Compared to postpartum, the unbound darunavir $AUC_{0\text{–}24}$ was only 24% and 20% reduced during the second and third trimesters, whereas darunavir total plasma concentrations were 34% and 35% lower. Despite these reductions, all the women had undetectable HIV RNA at the time of delivery.

More recently, investigators increased the darunavir/ritonavir dose further to 800/100mg twice daily in 24 pregnant women infected with HIV [141]. They performed intensive pharmacokinetic evaluations at steady state during the second and third trimesters and in the postpartum period when the dose had been reduced to 600/100mg twice daily. Despite the increased dosing, darunavir $AUC_{0\text{–}12}$ values were still lower during pregnancy; the GMR during the second trimester was 0.62 (IQR: 0.44–0.88, $P = .055$) and during the third trimester it was 0.64 (IQR: 0.55–0.73, $P = 0 < .001$), compared with postpartum. The $AUC_{0\text{–}12}$ of ritonavir during the third trimester was also significantly reduced compared to postpartum, with a GMR of 0.65 (IQR: 0.52–0.82. $P = .007$). The authors suggested that the ritonavir dose should be increased during pregnancy in subsequent studies to further inhibit the increase in CYP3A4 metabolism of darunavir.

Other drugs

The clearance of a number of other drugs that are eliminated primarily by renal excretion has also been shown to increase during pregnancy. For example, the pharmacokinetics of subcutaneously administered enoxaparin, a low molecular weight heparin, were studied serially in 13 women at 12–15 weeks' and 30–33 weeks' gestation, and at 6–8 weeks postpartum [142]. Compared to postpartum values, elimination clearance was increased by approximately 50% in the first gestational study period but was not significantly increased in the later period. In another study, the clearance of tobramycin was shown to peak in the midtrimester and fall during the third trimester [44].

Metformin is an orally effective hypoglycemic agent used to treat women with polycystic ovarian disease and women with gestational, as well as preexisting, diabetes during pregnancy. Metformin is a small molecule not bound to plasma proteins [143] and is a substrate for organic cation transporters (OCT) [144–146]. It is primarily eliminated by renal clearance at a rate that is correlated with creatinine clearance but exceeds GFR, thus indicating net renal tubular secretion [147, 148]. Pharmacokinetic studies in pregnant women have shown that metformin clearance is increased by 49% during the second trimester and by 29% during the third trimester of pregnancy. The increase in clearance was found to be the result of a combination of the increased GFR known to occur during pregnancy, and also to an increase in the tubular secretion of the drug which increased by 45% in the second trimester and by 38% during the third trimester. In fact, the renal clearance of metformin was better correlated with tubular secretion ($r = 0.97$) than with creatinine clearance ($r = 0.80$). This increased clearance was thought to be due to an increase in renal plasma flow during pregnancy, but a change in the expression and/or function of the OCT during pregnancy could also be possible [149].

Plasma concentrations of orally administered nifedipine, another CYP3A4 substrate, have been reported to be decreased in 15 women with pregnancy-induced hypertension who were studied during the third trimester of pregnancy but not subsequently postpartum [78]. Estimates of *CL/F* averaged 2.0 L/h per kg, compared to a value of 0.49 L/h per kg that was reported in a study of nonpregnant subjects. Another study of nifedipine pharmacokinetics in eight patients with pre-eclampsia indicated that *CL/F* remains elevated in the immediate postpartum period, averaging 3.3 L/h per kg in this clinical setting [150].

First-pass conversion of a prodrug to an active drug has been studied in pregnancy with the drug valacyclovir [151]. Orally administered valacyclovir produced three times higher plasma levels of acyclovir than when acyclovir was administered orally. However, the levels achieved with valacyclovir are somewhat lower than that reported in normal volunteers. On the other hand, acyclovir pharmacokinetics were, overall, similar to what have been reported in nonpregnant women.

Guidelines for the conduct of drug studies in pregnant women

Although abstinence from the use of pharmacologic agents is held forth as the ideal during pregnancy, studies have shown that most pregnant women use either prescribed or over-the-counter drugs during pregnancy and this creates the need for careful pharmacokinetic studies to be conducted in this subset of patients [152, 153]. Studying drugs in pregnancy requires special considerations, and guiding principles for these studies were formally published in October 2004 by the Pharmacokinetics in Pregnancy Working Group of the Pregnancy Labeling Task Force in the Guidance for Industry—Pharmacokinetics in Pregnancy—Study Design, Data Analysis, and Impact on Dosing and Labeling [4]. Ethically, because it is difficult to justify performing drug studies in pregnancy in normal pregnant "volunteers," most trials are performed in women who require a drug for a clinical reason. For this reason, study design for these trials must include the ethical justification that the woman would be using the particular agent during pregnancy to treat a medical condition. FDA approval of drugs specific to pregnancy, such as tocolytic agents, oxytocic agents, and a drug to treat preeclampsia, requires that studies be done during pregnancy. However, drugs commonly used by women of childbearing potential, such as antidepressants, asthma medications, antihypertensive agents, and antihistamines, also can be justifiably studied during pregnancy. Drugs can be studied not only when given for maternal indications (e.g., hypertension or asthma) but also when given for fetal indications (e.g., fetal supraventricular tachycardia).

Some subpopulations of pregnant women, however, often have disease-related alterations in physiology that may affect pharmacokinetics. Therefore pharmacokinetic studies in these women should be designed so that maximal information is obtained that separates the effects of their pathophysiology from those resulting from more general pregnancy-related changes. As a first step, population pharmacokinetic techniques can serve as a screening tool to establish the need for further intensive pharmacokinetic studies. For drugs that are chronically administered, these intensive studies should be conducted serially during the second and third trimesters of pregnancy and in the postpartum period, so that each woman serves as her own control. Ideally, both an early and a remote postpartum evaluation should be included. However, drugs used only during the peripartum period need only be studied at that time. Studies should incorporate in vitro measurements of drug binding to plasma proteins, and use established tracer substances or concurrent noninvasive measures of physiology as reference markers. For bioavailability evaluations, the stable isotope method described in Chapter 4 would decrease the number of studies necessary and decrease the biologic variation between studies. As shown in Fig. 23.6, caffeine has been used as a probe to assess the effects of pregnancy on a number of drug metabolic pathways [120]. This has the advantage over the "cocktail" approaches described in Chapter 7 in that only a single drug is needed to simultaneously assess a number of metabolic pathways. A multiprobe study has also been conducted to assess the effects of pregnancy on drug metabolism [65]. However, in evaluating the effect of pregnancy on the metabolism of a drug, it is important to note that a change in one enzymatic pathway may alter the proportion of drug metabolized through another pathway without reflecting a true change in the enzyme activity of that pathway.

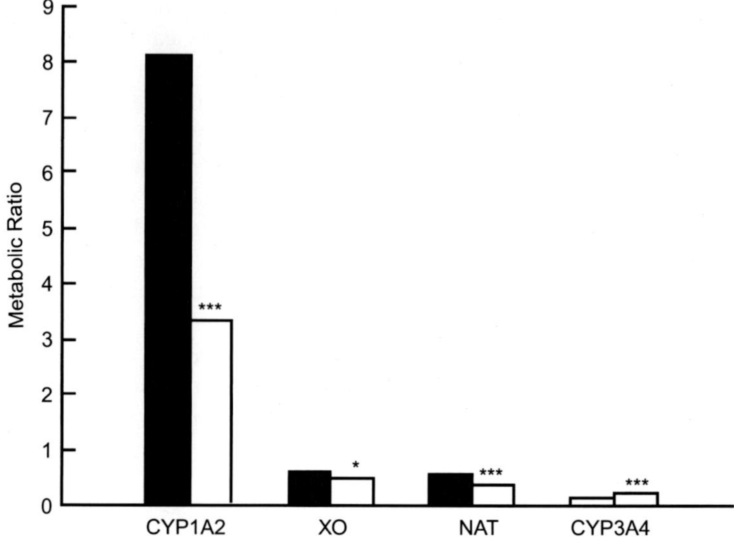

FIG. 23.6 Paired comparisons of measured ratios of caffeine metabolites to parent drug in nonpregnant (*solid bars*) and pregnant (*open bars*) women. Comparisons were made of the metabolic activities of CYP 1A2, xanthine oxidase (XO), *N*-acetyltransferase (NAT), and CYP3A4 (*P <.05, ***P <.005). *Data from Bologa M, Tang B, Klein J, Tesoro A, Koren G. Pregnancy-induced changes in drug metabolism in epileptic women. J Pharmacol Exp Ther 1991;257: 735–740.*

Placental transfer of drugs

The placenta was long thought to be a barrier that protected the fetus from drugs and chemicals administered to the mother. However, the thalidomide tragedy, reported independently by McBride [154] and Lenz [155], showed that the placenta was capable of transferring drugs ingested by the mother to the fetus, with the potential for great harm. On the other hand, placental transfer of drugs administered to the mother has been used beneficially to treat fetal arrhythmias, congestive heart failure, and other conditions [156].

The placenta develops from a portion of the zygote, and thus has the same genetic endowment as the developing fetus [157]. The embryonic/fetal component consists of trophoblastic-derived chorionic villi, which invade the maternal endometrium and are exposed directly to maternal blood in lake-like structures called lacunae. These villi create the large surface area necessary for maternal-fetal transfer in what becomes the intervillous space of the placenta. Here, the maternal blood pressure supplies pulsatile blood flow in jet-like streams from the spiral arteries of the endometrium to bathe the chorionic villi and allow for transfer of gases, nutrients, and metabolic products. Biologically, the human placenta is classified as a hemochorial placenta because maternal blood is in direct contact with the fetal chorionic membrane. It is this membrane that determines what is transferred to the fetus.

For the most part, drugs and other substances given to the mother will be transferred to the fetus. Drugs cross the placenta largely by simple diffusion. Factors affecting drug transfer are similar to those affecting transfer across other biological membranes, and include the molecular weight, lipid solubility, protein binding, and degree of ionization of the compound. Generally, drugs and chemicals with a molecular weight of less than 600 Da traverse the placenta readily, while drugs with a molecular weight larger than 1000 Da transfer less readily, if at all. Compounds that are uncharged and more lipid soluble are also more readily transferred.

There are factors which affect the transfer of drugs and chemicals that are unique to the placenta. The placenta has a pore system which allows for bulk water flow across the placenta and can be responsible for small drugs and chemicals crossing the membrane by solvent drag. Within the placenta there is also a process of endocytosis that is capable of transferring large immunoglobulins to the fetus. Placental tissue has a full complement of cytochrome enzymes capable of metabolizing drugs and chemicals, and some of these metabolites may then transfer more readily to the fetus than the parent drugs. The permeability and diffusion properties of the placenta may increase as the placenta matures due to a decrease in thickness of the trophoblastic epithelium forming the chorionic membrane from more than 50 μm in the first trimester to less than 5 μm at term [158, 159].

One of the factors affecting drug transfer to the fetus is the amount of drug delivered to the intervillous space by utero-placental blood flow. Blood flow to the uterus and placenta increases during pregnancy from 50 mL/min at 10 weeks' gestation to 500–600 mL/min at term [157]. Maternal blood flow to the uterus is also influenced by posture, diseases affecting maternal vasculature (such as hypertension and diabetes), placental size, and uterine contractions. For example, maternal cardiac output and utero-placental blood flow are reduced in the supine position and placental perfusion virtually ceases during a contraction. Placentas that are small for gestational age, or those with diffuse calcifications, are less efficient at transferring any maternal compounds to the fetus. Diseases, such as diabetes, which can thicken the chorionic membrane may also potentially affect diffusion of drugs into the fetal circulation.

In addition to passive and facilitated diffusion, the placenta contains a rich complement of numerous drug transporters that actively move compounds against their concentration gradient into and out of the fetus. Transporters are found on both surfaces of the syncytiotrophoblast. Those on the apical brush border facing maternal blood include ATP-binding cassette transporters: multidrug resistance protein (MDR-1/P-gp), breast cancer resistance protein (BCRP/ABCG2), and the multidrug resistance-associated proteins MRP-2 and MRP-3; plus serotonin transporter SERT, organic anion-transporter polypeptide OATP-E, and organic cation transporter OATN2. Among those on the basolateral membrane adjacent to fetal capillaries are multidrug resistance protein MDR-3, multidrug resistance-associated proteins MRP-1 and MRP-5, organic anion transporter polypeptide OATP-2B1, OATP-B, organic cation transporter OCT-3, and noradrenalin transporter NET. Additional transporters that have been identified on fetal capillary endothelium are multidrug resistance-associated proteins MRP-1, MRP-3, MRP-5, and brain cancer resistance protein (BRCP) [160]. Because these membranes express different transporters, polarized movement of compounds can occur, sometimes with efflux and uptake transporters in different locations working synergistically [160–165].

The P-gp placental transporter

Of the placental transporters, the most extensively studied is P-gp, which has been shown to play a critical role in transporting a large number of maternally administered drugs back into maternal circulation and away from the fetus. As described in Chapter 13, P-gp is a large 140–70-kDa transmembrane phospho-glycoprotein whose role as an energy-dependent efflux transporter was first elucidated in the investigation of cellular multidrug resistance. Coded for by the *MDR1* gene, P-gp belongs to a superfamily of ATP-binding cassette transporters which are present in all organisms from bacteria to humans [166–168]. Actively excreting absorbed molecules from the cytoplasm, the evolutionary job of P-gp has been to reduce exposure to xenobiotics, or foreign, natural toxins [169, 170]. Numerous seemingly structurally unrelated drugs are substrates for this transporter.

In humans, although P-gp is expressed on trophoblastic cells throughout pregnancy, it undergoes a twofold decline in expression between late first trimester and term [171–174]. P-gp has been located in the vesicles of the maternal-facing, apical brush-border membrane of the syncytiotrophoblast that directly abuts human maternal blood, but not within maternal vascular endothelium [160, 172, 175]. Actively transporting molecules in a basolateral-to-apical direction, the role of P-gp within the placenta is similar to its function at other sites: it extrudes drugs from the placenta back into maternal circulation, thereby protecting the developing fetus from potential toxic factors within the maternal circulation [175].

In genetically altered *mdr1a/b(−/−)* knockout mice without P-gp, both transplacental transport of P-gp substrates and the incidence of fetal malformations increase [176]. Transplacental transport of the P-gp substrates digoxin, saquinavir, and paclitaxel was increased 2.4-, 7-, and 16-fold, respectively, in the knockout mice compared to transport in the wild-type animals. In another murine study, *mdr1a/b(−/−)* fetuses were susceptible to cleft palate malformation induced by prenatal exposure to a photoisomer of the naturally occurring avermectin B1a, whereas their wild-type littermates were protected from this teratogen [163].

An active transport mechanism has long been suspected to account for the placental barrier that causes maternal and fetal concentrations for many drugs to differ [159, 177]. Studies of maternal-fetal transport of medications used during pregnancy in HIV-positive women have shown variable penetration into the fetus [178, 179]. Whereas the maternal–fetal drug ratios for zidovudine, lamivudine, and nevirapine (approximately 0.85, 1.0, and 0.9, respectively) demonstrate good fetal penetration, darunavir penetrates to a lesser extent with a median ratio of 0.13 (range: 0.08–0.35) [139], and most other protease inhibitors, including nelfinavir, ritonavir, saquinavir, lopinavir, and indinavir, also are known P-gp substrates and do not cross the placenta in detectable levels [179–181].

Several studies have examined the interaction between selective serotonin reuptake inhibitors (SSRIs) and P-gp and have shown that not all members of this class of drugs are P-gp substrates. Concentrations of paroxetine and venlafaxine, but not fluoxetine, were significantly increased in the brains of *mdr1a/b −/−* knockout mice compared to concentrations in the wild-type mice [182]. In cell culture studies, sertraline, its metabolite, desmethylsertraline, and paroxetine were shown to be potent inhibitors of P-gp; however, citalopram and venlafaxine were only weak inhibitors [183, 184]. P-glycoprotein polymorphisms may also alter drug transport across the placenta and influence fetal exposure. Whereas the P-gp SNP C3435T allele has no effect on saquinavir placental transport [185], its presence is associated with significantly increased maternal to fetal transfer of quetiapine [186]. Both the C3435T and G2677T alleles have also been associated with lower levels of placental P-gp expression [187, 188].

The BCRP placental transporter

BCRP is another ATP-binding cassette transporter that is located on the apical brush border of the syncytiotrophoblast and the chorionic villi fetal vessels. It also has been shown to play a critical role in limiting fetal drug exposure [189–192]. CRP mRNA expression is higher in the human placenta than any other organ [193], its expression may increase with advancing gestation [190], and the expression of BCRP transcripts in the human term placenta is 10-fold higher than its expression of P-gp [192]. Using pregnant mice and a specific inhibitor of Bcrp1 (the murine homolog of human BCRP), Jonker et al. [194] demonstrated that Bcrp1 limited fetal exposure to topotecan and both reduced maternal to fetal passage of cimetidine and actively removed existing drug from the fetal circulation [195]. Other studies with Bcrp1 knockout mice have shown that this transporter reduces fetal exposure to phytoestrogens [196] and nitrofurantoin [197, 198]. Fetal exposure to the oral hypoglycemic glyburide has been shown to be limited by BCRP efflux transport in human [199, 200] and rat [201] placental perfusion models, in human placental tissue [202], in pregnant mice [203], and in fetal umbilical cord samples [101]. Maternal to fetal transport of bupropion is also restricted by BCRP, but its primary active metabolite, OH-bupropion, freely passes across the placenta [204].

The precise function and significance of additional transporters is currently under active study [160, 164]. Similarly not yet well understood is how environmental factors, including steroid hormones, growth factors, and inflammation and infection may influence the expression and activity of these transporters which can then alter placental drug disposition and fetal exposure [205–208].

Teratogenesis

During the 38 weeks that comprise human gestation the human conceptus develops from a one-cell zygote to a fully developed newborn infant. This complicated process has a high degree of wastage, with approximately 65% of conceptions lost prior to implantation, 20% lost from spontaneous abortion, and 15% born prematurely. Major congenital abnormalities that are recognized at birth occur in approximately 2–3 infants per 100. Minor anomalies occur in another 7–14 infants per 100. Major birth defects cause 20% of infant mortality and are responsible for the majority of childhood hospitalizations.

From the patient's perspective, a birth defect may be any abnormality of the infant found at birth. This may include birth injuries, such as a cephalohematoma or a brachial plexus injury. However, birth defects are usually considered to be structural defects of the newborn. Structural defects have been broken down into four major categories: a *malformation*, which is a structural defect caused by an intrinsic problem in embryologic differentiation and/or development; a *disruption*, which is an alteration in shape or structure of a normally differentiated part, such as a limb amputation from an amniotic band or a vascular event; a *deformation*, which is an alteration in the shape or structure of a normally differentiated part, such as a Potter's facies or metatarsus adductus, which is often due to a mechanical constraint; and a *dysplasia*, which is a primary defect in cellular organization into tissues [209]. A *teratogen* is a chemical substance which can induce a malformation during development. An expansion of the definition includes an adverse effect on the developing fetus either in causing a structural abnormality or in altering organ function. This should be distinguished from a *mutagen*, which causes a genetic mutation whose effects cannot be seen for at least a generation.

Underlying causes of birth defects are presented in Table 23.4. It should be appreciated that approximately 90% of birth defects have a genetic component. Birth defects caused by drugs represent the one group of anomalies that can potentially be prevented. However, there is only a small list of drugs that have been proven to cause human anomalies (Table 23.5).

TABLE 23.4 Human reproductive risk.

Causes of anomalies	Percent of total anomalies
Chromosomal	5
Single gene	20
Polygenic/multifactorial	65
Environmental	10
Irradiation	<1
Maternal disease	1–2
Infection	2–3
Drugs and chemicals	4–5

TABLE 23.5 Known human teratogens.

Agent	Teratogenic effect
Carbamazepine	Facial dysmorphogenesis, neural tube defect
Phenytoin	Facial dysmorphogenesis, mental retardation, growth retardation, distal digital hypoplasia
Valproate	Lumbosacral spina bifida, facial dysmorphogenesis
Trimethadione	Facial dysmorphogenesis, intrauterine growth retardation, intrauterine fetal demise, neonatal demise
Coumadin	Nasal hypoplasia, epiphyseal stippling, optic atrophy
Alcohol	Facial dysmorphogenesis, growth retardation, mental retardation
Diethylstilbestrol	Vaginal adenosis, uterine anomalies, vaginal carcinogenesis
Androgens	Masculinization of the female genitalia
Methyl mercury	Growth retardation, severe mental retardation
ACE inhibitors	Oligohydramnios, potential lung hypoplasia, postnatal renal failure
Folic acid antagonists (aminopterin, methotrexate)	Abortion, intrauterine growth retardation, microcephaly, hypoplasia of frontal bones
Thalidomide	Phocomelia
Isotretinoin	CNS anomalies, including optic nerve abnormalities; craniofacial anomalies; cardiovascular malformations, thymic abnormalities
Inorganic iodides	Fetal goiter
Tetracycline	Bone deposits, teeth discoloration
Lithium	Ebstein's anomaly

Potential effects of drugs on the developing fetus include altered structural development during the first trimester, producing a dysmorphic infant; altered fetal growth during the second and third trimesters of pregnancy; and altered function of organ systems.

Principles of teratology

The general principles of teratology have been articulated by Wilson [210]. The first principle is that teratogens act with specificity. A teratogen produces a specific abnormality or constellation of abnormalities. For example, thalidomide produces phocomelia, and valproic acid produces neural tube defects. This specificity also applies to species, because drug effects may be seen in one species and not another. The best example is cortisol, which produces cleft palate in mice but not in humans.

The next principle is that teratogens demonstrate a dose-effect relationship. Given to the mother at a specific time during gestation, low doses can produce no effect, intermediate doses can produce the characteristic pattern of malformation, and higher doses will be lethal to the embryo. Dose-effect curves for most teratogens are steep, changing from minimal to maximal effect by dose doubling. Increasing the dose beyond that found to be lethal to the embryo will eventually lead to maternal death. This is used as an endpoint in animal teratogenicity studies.

The third principle is that teratogens must reach the developing conceptus in sufficient amounts to cause their effects. The extent of fetal exposure to drugs and other xenobiotics is determined not only by maternal dose, route of elimination, and placental transfer, but also by fetal elimination mechanisms. Because the fetal liver is interposed between the umbilical vein and systemic circulation, drugs transferred across the placenta are subject to fetal first-pass metabolism [156]. This protective mechanism is compromised by ductus venosus shunting, which enables 30%–70% of umbilical venous blood flow to bypass the liver. After drugs reach the fetal systemic circulation, hepatic metabolism constitutes the primary elimination mechanism and renal excretion is relatively ineffective, because the fetal kidney is immature and fetal urine passing into the amniotic fluid is swallowed by the fetus. CYP3A7 is a fetal-specific enzyme that accounts for about one-third of fetal hepatic cytochrome P450. CYP1A1, CYP2C8, CYP2D6, and CYP3A3/4 have also been identified in fetal liver. These enzymes are not only protective, but, as described in Chapter 15, their presence in fetal tissues other than liver is also capable of converting drugs into electrophilic reactive teratogenic intermediates, such as phenytoin epoxide, or to reactive free radical intermediates or free radicals.

The fourth principle is that the effect that a teratogenic agent has on a developing fetus depends upon the stage during development when the fetus is exposed. From conception to implantation there is an all-or-nothing effect, in that the embryo, if exposed to a teratogen, either survives unharmed or dies. This concept developed from Brent's studies of the effects of radiation on the developing embryo, and may or may not apply to fetal exposure to chemicals [211]. After implantation, during the process of differentiation and embryogenesis, the embryo is very susceptible to teratogens. However, since teratogens are capable of affecting many organ systems, the pattern of anomalies produced depends on which organ systems are differentiating at the time of teratogenic exposure. A difference of 1 or 2 days can result in a slightly different pattern of anomalies. After organogenesis, a teratogen can affect the embryo by producing growth retardation, or by changing the size or function of a specific organ. Giving a teratogen after the fetus has developed normally has no effect on the development of organs already formed. For example, beginning lithium after cardiac development, or valproic acid after the closure of the neural tube, will not produce either drug's characteristic anomalies. However, of particular interest is the effect of psychoactive agents, such as cocaine, crack, or antidepressants, on the developing central nervous system during the second and third trimesters of pregnancy, as these drugs can potentially affect the function and behavior of the infant after delivery.

The fifth principle is that susceptibility to teratogens is influenced by the genotype of the mother and fetus. Animal studies have shown that certain animal strains are more susceptible to the production of malformations when exposed to a teratogen compared to other animal strains. In humans, the fetus homozygous for the recessive allele associated with decreased epoxide hydrolase activity has an increased risk of developing the full fetal hydantoin syndrome [212]. Maternal smoking increases the risk for the development of cleft lip and palate in a fetus carrying the atypical allele for transforming growth factor α [213]. Single mutant genes or polygenic inheritance may explain why certain fetuses are unusually susceptible to teratogens.

Mechanisms of teratogenesis include genetic interference, gene mutation, chromosomal breakage, interference with cellular function, enzyme inhibition, and altered membrane characteristics. The response of the developing embryo to these insults is failure of cell-cell interaction crucial for development, interference with cell migration, or mechanical cellular disruption. The common endpoint is cell death-teratogenesis causing fewer cells. Most mechanisms of teratogenesis are theoretical, not well understood, and imply a genetic component. An example is the mechanism of thalidomide teratogenesis for which three theories are currently favored [214]. In the most recent theory, which was explained in Chapter 15, the binding of thalidomide to the ubiquitin ligase cereblon (CRBN) induces the degradation of SALL4, a developmental transcription factor that regulates limb development (see Fig. 15.12). This effect of thalidomide only occurs in thalidomide sensitive species, e.g. rabbits but not mice, but how this molecular interaction results in malformations has not been demonstrated. A second theory relates to the antiangiogenic properties of thalidomide. As demonstrated with CPS49, a tetrafluorinated analog of thalidomide that induces limb defects in a chick limb model, the antiangiogenic effects on newly formed or newly forming blood vessels occur before changes in the expression patterns of important limb development genes. In the third theory, thalidomide is metabolized by prostaglandin H synthase in susceptible species to free radical intermediates that form reactive oxygen species that cause oxidative DNA damage and result in phocomelia among other teratogenic malformations. Pretreatment with acetylsalicylic acid or a free radical spin trapping agent prevents both the DNA damage and teratogenicity [215]. These theories are not mutually exclusive and they all may be involved in some aspect of the pathogenesis of thalidomide's teratogenic effects.

Measures to minimize teratogenic risk

All new drug applications filed with the FDA include data from developmental and reproductive toxicology (DART) studies. These studies examine the effects of the particular agent on all aspects of reproduction, including oogenesis, spermatogenesis, fertility, and fecundity, as well as effects on litter size, spontaneous resorption, fetal malformation, fetal size, and newborn pup function. Most studies are conducted in mice, rats, and rabbits. All studies are designed with dose escalations, with maternal death as the stopping point. Information from these teratologic experiments is included in the drug labeling. Some, but not all, human teratogenic reactions of new drugs have been predicted from animal studies, in large part because most animals have a shorter gestational clock than humans. In addition, species vary in their susceptibility to teratogens, with some animal models being either more or less susceptible to teratogenesis than humans. Thus if an agent does not produce an anomaly in animal studies, it does not necessarily prove that it is safe for humans.

Safety of a drug for use in human pregnancy is demonstrated by observational studies conducted after the drug is marketed. Better studies are conducted prospectively with an exposed and unexposed control population selected before pregnancy outcome is known. Although population-based large cohort studies begun prior to pregnancy are considered the best type, they are expensive to conduct and limited to those agents used at the time of the study. Epidemiologic clues to teratogenesis are often found in case reports of abnormal infants, but these are biased in that an abnormal infant is more likely reported than a normal infant, and the background rate of malformations is high. Proof of teratogenicity in humans is supported by the following criteria: a recognizable pattern of anomalies; a higher prevalence of the particular anomaly or anomalies in patients exposed to an agent than in a control population; presence of the agent during the stage of organogenesis of the organ system affected; increased incidence of the anomaly after introduction of the agent; and production of the anomaly in experimental animals by administration of the agent during the appropriate stage of organogenesis.

A general approach to reduce the risk of human teratogenesis includes planning for pregnancy. Prior to conception, women with medical problems should be counseled about the medications they chronically use, which ones can safely be continued throughout pregnancy, and which ones should be discontinued. Medications should be evaluated and changed if necessary, to decrease teratogenic risk. Plasma level monitoring of unbound concentrations of anticonvulsant drugs may be helpful in optimizing seizure control, decreasing the need for multiple drug therapy, and minimizing dosage and fetal risk. Since more than 50% of pregnancies in the United States are unplanned, all women of childbearing potential should be treated as antenatal patients and counseled regarding use of any new drug in a potential pregnancy. Therefore when a woman of childbearing potential develops a new medical problem, counseling for pregnancy should be included in management. In general, the use of agents that are already widely used during pregnancy is preferred to use of newer agents. Just stopping pharmacologic therapy or leaving the issue up to the woman does not help her and may place both the mother and fetus at risk for adverse pregnancy outcome or an uncontrolled medical condition during pregnancy.

When using a known human teratogen, particular attention should be given to preventing pregnancy. This includes counseling the patient on the fetal effects of the drug being used and on the use of one or more effective forms of contraception. Therapy should be begun with a normal menstrual period, or no more than 2 weeks from a negative pregnancy test. Pregnancy tests bear repeating every 2–4 weeks, depending upon the form of contraception being used and the woman's menstrual history. When renewing prescriptions for these drugs, it is necessary to repeat a pregnancy test to verify that the patient is not pregnant.

To allow thalidomide, a known teratogen on the market, the FDA required the development of a program called System for Thalidomide Education and Prescribing Safety (STEPS) which ensures that pregnant women will not be exposed to the drug [216]. All patients, physicians, and pharmacists involved in thalidomide usage must be registered with the program. Women who can become pregnant must have a negative pregnancy test within 24 h before therapy is begun. Pregnancy tests are then required once per week for the first 4 weeks of therapy and every 2–4 weeks while on therapy. Two forms of acceptable contraception must be used for 4 weeks prior to use, during use, and for 4 weeks after use.

Drug therapy in nursing mothers

Transfer of drugs into breast milk is bidirectional, reflecting passive diffusion of unbound drug between plasma and blood rather than active secretion. Factors which affect the milk concentration include binding to maternal plasma proteins, protein binding in milk, lipid content of milk, and physiochemical properties of the drug [217]. Infant blood levels can be monitored and are usually less than those required for pharmacologic effects. For most drugs, an important clinical point that is a consequence of the bidirectional transfer of drug between plasma and breast milk, is that infant dosage can be minimized by breast-feeding just prior to drug administration, when drug concentrations in milk are lowest [218].

As shown for theophylline in Fig. 23.7, drug concentrations in breast milk are usually lower than plasma concentrations and there usually is a fixed ratio between milk and plasma concentrations [218]. In the usual case, drug concentrations measured in plasma and breast milk can be used to calculate a milk:plasma ratio (*M/P*), from which the daily drug dose to the infant is estimated as follows:

$$\text{Infant dose}/\text{Day} = C_{maternal} \times M/P \times V_{milk} \tag{23.2}$$

where $C_{maternal}$ is the average maternal plasma concentration of drug during nursing and V_{milk} is the volume of maternal milk ingested each day, usually estimated as 150 mL/kg [217]. This estimate of infant dose is often reported as a percentage of administered maternal dose. However, concentration-dependent saturation of the plasma protein binding precludes calculation of a fixed *M/P* ratio for a few drugs as shown for prednisolone in Fig. 23.8 [219]. In addition, there are drugs that because of physiochemical properties or their active transport into milk can give a higher dose to the infant than would otherwise be expected. For example, cimetidine has been shown to be actively transported into human breast milk, giving

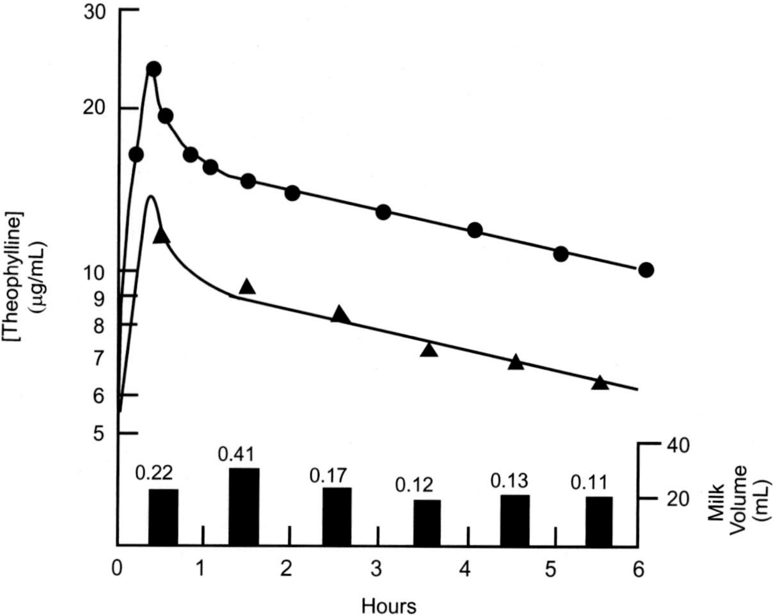

FIG. 23.7 Kinetic analysis of theophylline plasma (●) and milk (▲) concentrations after intravenous administration of a 3.2- to 5.3-mg/kg aminophylline dose. The solid lines represent the least-squares fit of the measured concentrations. The interval and volume of each milk collection are shown by the solid bars. The milligram recovery of theophylline in each breast-milk collection is shown by the numbers above the bars. *Reproduced with permission from Stec GP, Greenberger P, Ruo TI, Henthorn T, Morita Y, Atkinson AJ Jr, et al. Kinetics of theophylline transfer to breast milk. Clin Pharmacol Ther 1980;28:404–408.*

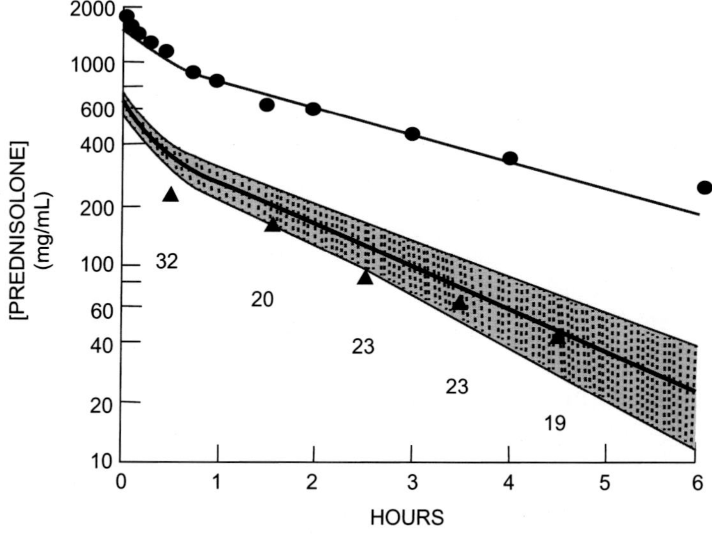

FIG. 23.8 Kinetic analysis of prednisolone plasma (●) concentrations after intravenous administration of a 50-mg prednisolone dose. The solid lines represent the least-squares fit of the measured plasma concentrations. Measured milk concentrations (▲) are plotted along with the range (*shaded area*) of unbound prednisolone plasma concentrations expected if serum transcortin binding capacity is allowed to vary ±1 SD from its reported mean. The volume (in milliliters) of each breast-milk sample is shown by the numbers below the milk concentrations. *Reproduced with permission from Greenberger PA, Odeh YK, Frederiksen MC, Atkinson AJ Jr. Pharmacokinetics of prednisolone transfer to breast milk. Clin Pharmacol Ther 1993;53:324–328.*

a *M/P* ratio of 5.5—far higher than expected on the basis of passive diffusion, binding to milk proteins, ion trapping, or lipid solubility [220]. Despite this high *M/P* ratio, the estimated infant dose is still low and no infant toxicity has been reported. Dapsone, used in the therapy of dermatitis herpetiformis, is a weak base with a pKb of 13, is highly protein bound at physiologic pH, and has a half-life of 20 h that ensures significant serum concentrations during the entire 24-h dosing period. These physiochemical properties result in infants receiving dapsone doses that are higher than expected, and use of the drug with breast-feeding has been reported to cause hemolytic anemia in infants [221].

The prodrug codeine and its active metabolite morphine have been shown to pass into breast milk in generally insignificant amounts, and short-term use of codeine for postpartum pain relief has been considered safe for mothers breast-feeding their infants [222, 223]. However, a report of an infant death secondary to maternal codeine use prompted a reappraisal of the use of codeine in breast-feeding mothers [224]. In this case, the mother was found to be heterozygous for a CYP2D6*2A allele with CYP2D6*2X2 gene duplication, and was therefore an ultra-rapid metabolizer who converted codeine to morphine at an increased rate. The incidence of ultra-rapid CYP2D6 metabolizers ranges from 1% in the Scandinavian population to as high as 29% in the Ethiopian population. In addition, although morphine is metabolized through

TABLE 23.6 Drug information sources for breastfeeding women.

Information source	Description	URL or source
LactMed	A database of information on drugs and chemicals to which a breastfeeding mother may be exposed. The database is administered by the NIH, peer-reviewed, and is free of charge	https://toxnet.nlm.nih.gov/newtoxnet/lactmed.htm
Mother-to-Baby	A division of the nonprofit Organization of Teratology Information Specialists (OTIS) that provides information about drugs and teratogens to both consumers and health care providers through phone and online contact	http://mothertobaby.org
Briggs GG, Freeman RK, Towers CV, Forinash AB. Drugs in Pregnancy and Lactation: A Reference Guide to Fetal and Neonatal Risk. 11th ed. 2017; Philadelphia: Wolters Klewer	Hardcover reference book or ebook available	www.lww.com

glucuronidation mainly to the inactive metabolite morphine-3-glucuronide, it also is metabolized to a lesser extent by UGT2B7 to morphine-6-glucuronide (M6G), which is equipotent to morphine [225]. A UGT2B7*2 variant has been reported that increases the proportion of morphine that is metabolized to M6G [226]. So an infant whose mother is an ultra-rapid CYP2D6 metabolizer and also carries the UGT2B7*2 variant would be at a particularly high risk of life-threatening CNS depression from maternal codeine usage [227]. To put the case report into perspective, a population-based retrospective cohort study of 15,608 postnatal women who either received or did not receive codeine failed to demonstrate an association between maternal codeine use and adverse neonatal outcomes [228].

Drugs considered safe for pregnancy are usually safe during the lactation period. Often women who need medications chronically are discouraged from nursing or told to avoid taking medications while nursing because of concerns about possible adverse effects in the nursing infant [229]. Such advice may be based upon inability to find good information. Some sources of information are listed in Table 23.6, a particularly good source of current, comprehensive, and peer-reviewed information being that now available online at LactMed. Adverse events in nursing infants are not as common as many think, occurring more often in neonates younger than 2 months and rarely in infants older than 6 months [230]. Actually, there are few drugs that are contraindicated during lactation. These include antineoplastics, ergot alkaloids, some anticonvulsants, gold, iodine, radiopharmaceuticals, and social drugs of abuse. Because of differences in codeine metabolism, codeine should be administered at the lowest effective dose for the shortest period of time during lactation and the infant monitored for drowsiness and difficulty feeding. Clinical monitoring of infants exposed to amiodarone, lithium carbonate, and cyclosporine through breast milk is recommended.

In 2014 the FDA published a final rule that specified requirements for pregnancy and lactation labeling [231]. The part of the rule dealing with lactation was expanded and now includes three sections: Risk Summary, Clinical Considerations, and Data. In the Risk Summary section is a discussion regarding data or lack of data on the effect of a drug on breast milk production, the drug concentration in breast milk, the relative infant dose, any known short-term or long-term effect on the breastfeeding child, and a risk–benefit statement. If a drug does not adversely affect milk production or the nursing child, the drug is compatible with breast-feeding. Under the Clinical Considerations section, dosing modifications, strategies to minimize exposure of the child, and interventions for monitoring adverse effects of the drug on the child are included. The Data section includes data from a variety of sources, both animal and human studies, with results from each listed separately. To augment the new labeling rules and correct the current paucity of human data, the FDA has issued guidance on the design and conduct of clinical lactation studies. It is hoped that these efforts will improve the quality and quantity of scientific data that is available to guide drug therapy in nursing women [5].

References

[1] Zinacef® (cefuroxime for injection) labeling. Buena, NJ: Teligent, Inc. Revised 02/2020. Available from: https://www.accessdata.fda.gov/drugsatfda_docs/label/2020/050558s075lbl.pdf.

[2] Anon. CDC Births: Preliminary data for 1999. National Vital Statistics Reports 48(14). Atlanta, GA: Centers for disease control; 2000.

[3] CDER, CBER. Establishing pregnancy exposure registries. Guidance for industry, Rockville, MD: FDA; August 2002. Available from:https://www.fda.gov/media/75607/download.

[4] CDER. Pharmacokinetics in pregnancy—study design, data analysis, and impact on dosing and labeling. Draft guidance for industry, Rockville, MD: FDA; October 2004. Available from: www.fda.gov/media/71353/download.

[5] CDER, CBER. Clinical lactation studies – Considerations for study design. Draft guidance for industry, Silver Spring, MD: FDA; May 2019. Available from: https://www.fda.g-ov/media/124749/download.

[6] Content and format of labeling for human prescription drug and biological products; requirements for pregnancy and lactation labeling. Proposed Rule in the US Code of Federal Regulations: 21 CFR Part 201. Available from: https://www.regulations.gov/document?D=FDA-2006-N-0515-0001 [29 May 2008].

[7] Content and format of labeling for human prescription drug and biological products; requirements for pregnancy and lactation labeling. Final rule in the US Code of Federal Regulations: 21 CFR Part 201 Rules and Regulations. Available from: https://www.regulations.gov/document?D=FDA-2006-N-0515-0068 [04 December 2014].

[8] NICHD. Task force on research specific to pregnant women and lactating women. Report to secretary, Washington, DC: Health and Human Services, Congress; 2018. Available from: https://www.nichd.nih.gov/sites/default/files/2018-09/PRGLAC_Report.pdf.

[9] CDC. Information for clinicians on investigational therapeutics for patients with COVID-19. Available from: https://www.cdc.gov/coronavirus/2019-ncov/hcp/therapeutic-options.html [25 April 2020].

[10] Clinical trials.gov. Information for clinicians on investigational therapeutics for patients with COVID-19. Available from: https://clinicaltrials.gov/ct2/show/NCT04339816 [Accessed 30 April 2020].

[11] Gilead Sciences, Inc. Emergency access to remdesivir outside of clinical trials. Available from: https://www.gilead.com/purpose/advancing-global-health/covid-19/emergency-access-to-remdesivir-outside-of-clinical-trials; 2020. [Accessed 30 April 2020].

[12] Verrengia M, Sachdeva P, Gaughan J, Fisher RS, Parkman HP. Variation of symptoms during the menstrual cycle in female patients with gastroparesis. Neurogastroenterol Motil 2011;23:625–e254.

[13] Cullen G, O'Donoghue D. Constipation and pregnancy. Best Pract Res Clin Gastroenterol 2007;21:807–818.

[14] Gryboski WA, Spiro HM. The effect of pregnancy on gastric secretion. N Engl J Med 1956;255:1131–1134.

[15] Hunt JN, Murray FA. Gastric function in pregnancy. J Obstet Gynaecol Br Emp 1958;65:78–83.

[16] Parry E, Shields R, Turnbull AC. Transit time in the small intestine in pregnancy. J Obstet Gynaecol Br Commonw 1970;77:900–901.

[17] Wong CA, Loffredi M, Ganchiff JN, Zhao J, Wang Z, Avram MJ. Gastric emptying of water in term pregnancy. Anesthesiology 2002;96:1395–1400.

[18] Chiloiro M, Darconza G, Piccioli E, De Carne M, Clemente C, Riezzo G. Gastric emptying and orocecal transit time in pregnancy. J Gastroenterol 2001;36:538–543.

[19] O'Hare MF, Leahey W, Murnaghan GA, McDevitt DG. Pharmacokinetics of sotalol during pregnancy. Eur J Clin Pharmacol 1983;24:521–524.

[20] Philipson A. Pharmacokinetics of ampicillin during pregnancy. J Infect Dis 1977;136:370–376.

[21] Philipson A, Stiernstedt G, Ehrnebo M. Comparison of the pharmacokinetics of cephradine and cefazolin in pregnant and non-pregnant women. Clin Pharmacokinet 1987;12:136–144.

[22] Hebert MF, Easterling TR, Kirby B, Carr DB, Buchanan ML, Rutherford T, et al. Effects of pregnancy on CYP3A and P-glycoprotein activities as measured by disposition of midazolam and digoxin: a University of Washington specialized center of research study. Clin Pharmacol Ther 2008;84:248–253.

[23] Lund CJ, Donovan JC. Blood volume during pregnancy. Significance of plasma and red cell volumes. Am J Obstet Gynecol 1967;98:394–403.

[24] Hytten F. Blood volume changes in normal pregnancy. Clin Haematol 1985;14:601–612.

[25] Petersen VP. Body composition and fluid compartments in normal, obese and underweight human subjects. Acta Med Scand 1957;158:103–111.

[26] Plentl AA, Gray MJ. Total body water, sodium space, and total exchangeable sodium in normal and toxemic pregnant women. Am J Obstet Gynecol 1959;78:472–478.

[27] Lees MM, Taylor SH, Scott DB, Kerr MG. A study of cardiac output at rest throughout pregnancy. J Obstet Gynaecol Br Commonw 1967;74:319–328.

[28] Robson SC, Hunter S, Boys RJ, Dunlop W. Serial study of factors influencing changes in cardiac output during human pregnancy. Am J Physiol 1989;256:H1060–H1065.

[29] Capeless EL, Clapp JF. When do cardiovascular parameters return to their preconception values? Am J Obstet Gynecol 1991;165:883–886.

[30] Metcalfe J, Romney SL, Ramsey LH, Reid DE, Burwell CS. Estimation of uterine blood flow in normal human pregnancy at term. J Clin Invest 1955;34:1632–1638.

[31] Ginsburg J, Duncan SL. Peripheral blood flow in normal pregnancy. Cardiovasc Res 1967;1:132–137.

[32] Thoresen M, Wesche J. Doppler measurements of changes in human mammary and uterine blood flow during pregnancy and lactation. Acta Obstet Gynecol Scand 1988;67:741–745.

[33] Robson SC, Mutch E, Boys RJ, Woodhouse KW. Apparent liver blood flow during pregnancy: a serial study using indocyanine green clearance. Br J Obstet Gynaecol 1990;97:720–724.

[34] Nakai A, Sekiya I, Oya A, Koshino T, Araki T. Assessment of the hepatic arterial and portal venous blood flows during pregnancy with Doppler ultrasonography. Arch Gynecol Obste 2002;266:25–29.

[35] Frederiksen MC, Ruo TI, Chow MJ, Atkinson AJ Jr. Theophylline pharmacokinetics in pregnancy. Clin Pharmacol Ther 1986;40:321–328.

[36] Mendenhall HW. Serum protein concentrations in pregnancy. I. Concentrations in maternal serum. Am J Obstet Gynecol 1970;106:388–399.

[37] Dean M, Stock B, Patterson RJ, Levy G. Serum protein binding of drugs during and after pregnancy in humans. Clin Pharmacol Ther 1980;28:253–261.

[38] Bardy AH, Hiilesmaa VK, Teramo K, Neuvonen PJ. Protein binding of antiepileptic drugs during pregnancy, labor, and puerperium. Ther Drug Monit 1990;12:40–46.

[39] Connelly TJ, Ruo TI, Frederiksen MC, Atkinson AJ Jr. Characterization of theophylline binding to serum proteins in pregnant and nonpregnant women. Clin Pharmacol Ther 1990;47:68–72.

[40] Lucius H, Gahlenbeck H, Kleine HO, Fabel H, Bartels H. Respiratory functions, buffer system, and electrolyte concentrations of blood during human pregnancy. Respir Physiother 1970;9:311–317.

[41] Elkus R, Popovich J Jr. Respiratory physiology in pregnancy. Clin Chest Med 1992;13:555–565.

[42] Davison JM, Hytten FE. Glomerular filtration during and after pregnancy. J Obstet Gynaecol Br Commonw 1974;81:588–595.

[43] Philipson A, Stiernstedt G. Pharmacokinetics of cefuroxime in pregnancy. Am J Obstet Gynecol 1982;142:823–828.

[44] Bourget P, Fernandez H, Delouis C, Taburet AM. Pharmacokinetics of tobramycin in pregnant women. Safety and efficacy of a once-daily dose regimen. J Clin Pharm Ther 1991;16:167–176.

[45] Andrew MA, Easterling TR, Carr DB, Shen D, Buchanan ML, Rutherford T, et al. Amoxicillin pharmacokinetics in pregnant women: modeling and simulations of dosage strategies. Clin Pharmacol Ther 2007;81:547–556.

[46] Li M, Anderson GD, Phillips BR, Kong W, Shen DD, Wang J. Interactions of amoxicillin and cefaclor with human renal organic anion and peptide transporters. Drug Metab Dispos 2006;34:547–555.

[47] Watanabe K, Jinriki T, Sato J. Effects of progesterone and norethisterone on cephalexin transport and peptide transporter PEPT1 expression in human intestinal cell line Caco-2. Biol Pharm Bull 2006;29:90–95.

[48] Ivanyuk A, Livio F, Biollaz J, Buclin T. Renal drug transporters and drug interactions. Clin Pharmacokinet 2017;56:825–892.

[49] Hori R, Okamura N, Aiba T, Tanigawara Y. Role of P-glycoprotein in renal tubular secretion of digoxin in the isolated perfused rat kidney. J Pharmacol Exp Ther 1993;266:1620–1625.

[50] Buster JE, Abraham GE. The applications of steroid hormone radioimmunoassays to clinical obstetrics. Obstet Gynecol 1975;46:489–499.

[51] Devroey P, Camus M, Palermo G, Smitz J, Van Waesberghe L, Wisanto A, et al. Placental production of estradiol and progesterone after oocyte donation in patients with primary ovarian failure. Am J Obstet Gynecol 1990;162:66–70.

[52] Schneider MA, Davies MC, Honour JW. The timing of placental competence in pregnancy after oocyte donation. Fertil Steril 1993;59:1059–1064.

[53] Mishell DR Jr, Thorneycroft IH, Nagata Y, Murata T, Nakamura RM. Serum gonadotropin and steroid patterns in early human gestation. Am J Obstet Gynecol 1973;117:631–642.

[54] Tulchinsky D, Hobel CJ. Plasma human chorionic gonadotropin, estrone, estradiol, estriol, progesterone, and 17 alpha-hydroxyprogesterone in human pregnancy. 3. Early normal pregnancy. Am J Obstet Gynecol 1973;117:884–893.

[55] Lehmann JM, McKee DD, Watson MA, Willson TM, Moore JT, Kliewer SA. The human orphan nuclear receptor PXR is activated by compounds that regulate CYP3A4 gene expression and cause drug interactions. J Clin Invest 1998;102:1016–1023.

[56] Goodwin B, Hodgson E, Liddle C. The orphan human pregnane X receptor mediates the transcriptional activation of CYP3A4 by rifampicin through a distal enhancer module. Mol Pharmacol 1999;56:1329–1339.

[57] Jeong H, Stika CS. Methods to study mechanisms underlying altered hepatic drug elimination during pregnancy. Semin Perinatol 2020;151228. https://doi.org/10.1016/j.semperi.2020.151228.

[58] Choi SY, Koh KH, Jeong H. Isoform-specific regulation of cytochromes P450 expression by estradiol and progesterone. Drug Metab Dispos 2013;41:263–269.

[59] Dickmann LJ, Isoherranen N. Quantitative prediction of CYP2B6 induction by estradiol during pregnancy: potential explanation for increased methadone clearance during pregnancy. Drug Metab Dispos 2013;41:270–274.

[60] Soldin OP, Guo T, Weiderpass E, Tractenberg RE, Hilakivi-Clarke L, Soldin SJ. Steroid hormone levels in pregnancy and 1 year postpartum using isotope dilution tandem mass spectrometry. Fertil Steril 2005;84:701–710.

[61] Papageorgiou I, Grepper S, Unadkat JD. Induction of hepatic CYP3A enzymes by pregnancy-related hormones: studies in human hepatocytes and hepatic cell lines. Drug Metab Dispos 2013;41:281–290.

[62] Zhang Z, Farooq M, Prasad B, Grepper S, Unadkat JD. Prediction of gestational age-dependent induction of in vivo hepatic CYP3A activity based on HepaRG cells and human hepatocytes. Drug Metab Dispos 2015;43:836–842.

[63] Chen H, Yang K, Choi S, Fischer JH, Jeong H. Up-regulation of UDP-glucuronosyltransferase (UGT) 1A4 by 17beta-estradiol: a potential mechanism of increased lamotrigine elimination in pregnancy. Drug Metab Dispos 2009;37:1841–1847.

[64] Jeong H, Choi S, Song JW, Chen H, Fischer JH. Regulation of UDP-glucuronosyltransferase (UGT) 1A1 by progesterone and its impact on labetalol elimination. Xenobiotica 2008;38:62–75.

[65] Tracy TS, Venkataramanan R, Glover DD, Caritis SN, National Institute for Child Health and Human Development Network of Maternal-Fetal-Medicine Units. Temporal changes in drug metabolism (CYP1A2, CYP2D6 and CYP3A activity) during pregnancy. Am J Obstet Gynecol 2005;192:633–639.

[66] Gorski JC, Hall SD, Jones DR, VandenBranden M, Wrighton SA. Regioselective biotransformation of midazolam by members of the human cytochrome P450 3A (CYP3A) subfamily. Biochem Pharmacol 1994;47:1643–1653.

[67] Kronbach T, Mathys D, Umeno M, Gonzalez FJ, Meyer UA. Oxidation of midazolam and triazolam by human liver cytochrome P450IIIA4. Mol Pharmacol 1989;36:89–96.

[68] Thummel KE, O'Shea D, Paine MF, Shen DD, Kunze KL, Perkins JD, et al. Oral first-pass elimination of midazolam involves both gastrointestinal and hepatic CYP3A-mediated metabolism. Clin Pharmacol Ther 1996;59:491–502.

[69] Thummel KE, Shen DD, Podoll TD, Kunze KL, Trager WF, Hartwell PS, et al. Use of midazolam as a human cytochrome P450 3A probe: I. *In vitro-in vivo* correlations in liver transplant patients. J Pharmacol Exp Ther 1994;271:549–556.

[70] Ohkita C, Goto M. Increased 6-hydroxycortisol excretion in pregnant women: implication of drug-metabolizing enzyme induction. DICP 1990;24:814–816.

[71] Varis T, Kivisto KT, Backman JT, Neuvonen PJ. The cytochrome P450 3A4 inhibitor itraconazole markedly increases the plasma concentrations of dexamethasone and enhances its adrenal-suppressant effect. Clin Pharmacol Ther 2000;68:487–494.

[72] Gentile DM, Tomlinson ES, Maggs JL, Park BK, Back DJ. Dexamethasone metabolism by human liver in vitro. Metabolite identification and inhibition of 6-hydroxylation. J Pharmacol Exp Ther 1996;277:105–112.

[73] Petersen MC, Nation RL, McBride WG, Ashley JJ, Moore RG. Pharmacokinetics of betamethasone in healthy adults after intravenous administration. Eur J Clin Pharmacol 1983;25:643–650.

[74] Della Torre M, Hibbard JU, Jeong H, Fischer JH. Betamethasone in pregnancy: influence of maternal body weight and multiple gestation on pharmacokinetics. Am J Obstet Gynecol 2010;203:254 e1–254 e12.

[75] Petersen MC, Collier CB, Ashley JJ, McBride WG, Nation RL. Disposition of betamethasone in parturient women after intravenous administration. Eur J Clin Pharmacol 1983;25:803–810.

[76] Unadkat JD, Wara DW, Hughes MD, Mathias AA, Holland DT, Paul ME, et al. Pharmacokinetics and safety of indinavir in human immunodeficiency virus-infected pregnant women. Antimicrob Agents Chemother 2007;51:783–786.

[77] Stika CS, Andrews W, Frederiksen MC, Mercer B, Sabai B, Antal E. Steady state pharmacokinetic study of Flagyl® ER in pregnant patients during the second to third trimester of pregnancy [Abstract]. Clin Pharmacol Ther 2004;75:24.

[78] Prevost RR, Akl SA, Whybrew WD, Sibai BM. Oral nifedipine pharmacokinetics in pregnancy-induced hypertension. Pharmacotherapy 1992;12:174–177.

[79] Haas DM, Quinney SK, Clay JM, Renbarger JL, Hebert MF, Clark S, et al. Nifedipine pharmacokinetics are influenced by CYP3A5 genotype when used as a preterm labor tocolytic. Am J Perinatol 2013;30:275–281.

[80] Xie HG, Wood AJ, Kim RB, Stein CM, Wilkinson GR. Genetic variability in CYP3A5 and its possible consequences. Pharmacogenomics 2004;5:243–272.

[81] Mutagonda RF, Minzi OMS, Massawe SN, Asghar M, Färnert A, Kamuhabwa AAR, et al. Pregnancy and CYP3A5 genotype affect day 7 plasma lumefantrine concentrations. Drug Metab Dispos 2019;47:1415–1424.

[82] Aldridge A, Bailey J, Neims AH. The disposition of caffeine during and after pregnancy. Semin Perinatol 1981;5:310–314.

[83] Walsky RL, Astuccio AV, Obach RS. Evaluation of 227 drugs for in vitro inhibition of cytochrome P450 2B6. J Clin Pharmacol 2006;46:1426–1438.

[84] Pond SM, Kreek MJ, Tong TG, Raghunath J, Benowitz NL. Altered methadone pharmacokinetics in methadone-maintained pregnant women. J Pharmacol Exp Ther 1985;233:1–6.

[85] Eap CB, Buclin T, Baumann P. Interindividual variability of the clinical pharmacokinetics of methadone: implications for the treatment of opioid dependence. Clin Pharmacokinet 2002;41:1153–1193.

[86] Ferrari A, Coccia CP, Bertolini A, Sternieri E. Methadone—metabolism, pharmacokinetics and interactions. Pharmacol Res 2004;50:551–559.

[87] Wolff K, Boys A, Rostami-Hodjegan A, Hay A, Raistrick D. Changes to methadone clearance during pregnancy. Eur J Clin Pharmacol 2005;61:763768.

[88] Bogen DL, Perel JM, Helsel JC, Hanusa BH, Romkes M, Nukui T, et al. Pharmacologic evidence to support clinical decision making for peripartum methadone treatment. Psychopharmacology (Berl) 2013;225:441–451.

[89] McCarthy JJ, Vasti EJ, Leamon MH, Graas J, Ward C, Fassbender C. The use of serum methadone/metabolite ratios to monitor changing perinatal pharmacokinetics. J Addict Med 2018;12:241–246.

[90] Ward BA, Gorski JC, Jones DR, Hall SD, Flockhart DA, Desta Z. The cytochrome P450 2B6 (CYP2B6) is the main catalyst of efavirenz primary and secondary metabolism: implication for HIV/AIDS therapy and utility of efavirenz as a substrate marker of CYP2B6 catalytic activity. J Pharmacol Exp Ther 2003;306:287–300.

[91] Cressey TR, Stek A, Capparelli E, Bowonwatanuwong C, Prommas S, Sirivatanapa P, et al. Efavirenz pharmacokinetics during the third trimester of pregnancy and postpartum. J Acquir Immune Defic Syndr 2012;59:245–252.

[92] Högstedt S, Lindberg B, Peng DR, Regardh CG, Rane A. Pregnancy-induced increase in metoprolol metabolism. Clin Pharmacol Ther 1985;37:688–692.

[93] Högstedt S, Lindberg B, Rane A. Increased oral clearance of metoprolol in pregnancy. Eur J Clin Pharmacol 1983;24:217–220.

[94] Wadelius M, Darj E, Frenne G, Rane A. Induction of CYP2D6 in pregnancy. Clin Pharmacol Ther 1997;62:400–407.

[95] Ververs FF, Voorbij HA, Zwarts P, Bowonwatanuwong C, Prommas S, Sirivatanapa P, et al. Effect of cytochrome P450 2D6 genotype on maternal paroxetine plasma concentrations during pregnancy. Clin Pharmacokinet 2009;48:677–683.

[96] Tomson T, Lindbom U, Ekqvist B, Sundqvist A. Epilepsy and pregnancy: a prospective study of seizure control in relation to free and total plasma concentrations of carbamazepine and phenytoin. Epilepsia 1994;35:122–130.

[97] Tomson T, Lindbom U, Ekqvist B, Sundqvist A. Disposition of carbamazepine and phenytoin in pregnancy. Epilepsia 1994;35:131–135.

[98] Chen SS, Perucca E, Lee JN, Richens A. Serum protein binding and free concentration of phenytoin and phenobarbitone in pregnancy. Br J Clin Pharmacol 1982;13:547–552.

[99] Zharikova OL, Fokina VM, Nanovskaya TN, Hill RA, Mattison DR, Hankins GD, et al. Identification of the major human hepatic and placental enzymes responsible for the biotransformation of glyburide. Biochem Pharmacol 2009;78:1483–1490.

[100] Niemi M, Cascorbi I, Timm R, Kroemer HK, Neuvonen PJ, Kivisto KT. Glyburide and glimepiride pharmacokinetics in subjects with different CYP2C9 genotypes. Clin Pharmacol Ther 2002;72:326–332.

[101] Hebert MF, Ma X, Naraharisetti SB, Hill RA, Mattison DR, Hankins GD, et al. Are we optimizing gestational diabetes treatment with glyburide? The pharmacologic basis for better clinical practice. Clin Pharmacol Ther 2009;85:607–614.

[102] Rytting E, Nanovskaya TN, Wang X, Vernikovskaya DI, Clark SM, Cochran M, et al. Pharmacokinetics of indomethacin in pregnancy. Clin Pharmacokinet 2014;53:545–551.

[103] McGready R, Stepniewska K, Seaton E, Cho T, Cho D, Ginsberg A, et al. Pregnancy and use of oral contraceptives reduces the biotransformation of proguanil to cycloguanil. Eur J Clin Pharmacol 2003;59:553–557.

[104] McGready R, Stepniewska K, Edstein MD, Cho T, Gilveray G, Looareesuwan S, et al. The pharmacokinetics of atovaquone and proguanil in pregnant women with acute falciparum malaria. Eur J Clin Pharmacol 2003;59:545–552.

[105] Öhman I, Beck O, Vitols S, Tomson T. Plasma concentrations of lamotrigine and its 2-N-glucuronide metabolite during pregnancy in women with epilepsy. Epilepsia 2008;49:1075–1080.

[106] Öhman I, Vitols S, Tomson T. Lamotrigine in pregnancy: pharmacokinetics during delivery, in the neonate, and during lactation. Epilepsia 2000;41:709–713.

[107] Tomson T, Öhman I, Vitols S. Lamotrigine in pregnancy and lactation: a case report. Epilepsia 1997;38:1039–1041.

[108] Pennell PB, Newport DJ, Stowe ZN, Helmers SL, Montgomery JQ, Henry TR. The impact of pregnancy and childbirth on the metabolism of lamotrigine. Neurology 2004;62:292–295.

[109] Karanam A, Pennell PB, French JA, Cho T, Gilveray G, Looareesuwan S, et al. Lamotrigine clearance increases by 5 weeks gestational age: relationship to estradiol concentrations and gestational age. Ann Neurol 2018;84:556–563.

[110] Fotopoulou C, Kretz R, Bauer S, Schefold JC, Schmitz B, Dudenhausen JW, et al. Prospectively assessed changes in lamotrigine-concentration in women with epilepsy during pregnancy, lactation and the neonatal period. Epilepsy Res 2009;85:60–64.

[111] Polepally AR, Pennell PB, Brundage RC, Stowe ZN, Newport DJ, Viguera AC, et al. Model-based lamotrigine clearance changes during pregnancy: clinical implication. Ann Clin Transl Neurol 2014;1:99–106.

[112] Petrenaite V, Öhman I, Ekström L, Sæbye D, Hansen TF, Tomson T, et al. UGT polymorphisms and lamotrigine clearance during pregnancy. Epilepsy Res 2018;140:199–208.

[113] Reimers A, Helde G, Brathen G, Brodtkorb E. Lamotrigine and its N2-glucuronide during pregnancy: the significance of renal clearance and estradiol. Epilepsy Res 2011;94:198–205.

[114] Tomson T, Luef G, Sabers A, Pittschieler S, Öhman I. Valproate effects on kinetics of lamotrigine in pregnancy and treatment with oral contraceptives. Neurology 2006;67:1297–1299.

[115] Reimers A, Skogvoll E, Sund JK, Spigset O. Drug interactions between lamotrigine and psychoactive drugs: evidence from a therapeutic drug monitoring service. J Clin Psychopharmacol 2005;25:342–348.

[116] Wegner I, Edelbroek P, de Haan GJ, Lindhout D, Sander JW. Drug monitoring of lamotrigine and oxcarbazepine combination during pregnancy. Epilepsia 2010;512:500–502.

[117] Lin WW, Li XW, Jiao Z, Zhang J, Rao X, Zeng DY, et al. Population pharmacokinetics of oxcarbazepine active metabolite in Chinese paediatric epilepsy patients and its application in individualised dosage regimens. Eur J Clin Pharmacol 2019;75:381–392.

[118] Fischer JH, Sarto GE, Hardman J, Endres L, Jenkins TM, Kilpatrick SJ, et al. Influence of gestational age and body weight on the pharmacokinetics of labetalol in pregnancy. Clin Pharmacokinet 2014;53:373–383.

[119] Rogers RC, Sibai BM, Whybrew WD. Labetalol pharmacokinetics in pregnancy-induced hypertension. Am J Obstet Gynecol 1990;162:362–366.

[120] Bologa M, Tang B, Klein J, Tesoro A, Koren G. Pregnancy-induced changes in drug metabolism in epileptic women. J Pharmacol Exp Ther 1991;257:735–740.

[121] Tsutsumi K, Kotegawa T, Matsuki S, Tanaka Y, Ishii Y, Kodama Y, et al. The effect of pregnancy on cytochrome P4501A2, xanthine oxidase, and N-acetyltransferase activities in humans. Clin Pharmacol Ther 2001;70:121–125.

[122] Lees MM, Scott DB, Kerr MG. Haemodynamic changes associated with labour. J Obstet Gynaecol Br Commonw 1970;77:29–36.

[123] Gerdin E, Salmonson T, Lindberg B, Rane A. Maternal kinetics of morphine during labour. J Perinat Med 1990;18:479–487.

[124] Ueland K, Metcalfe J. Circulatory changes in pregnancy. Clin Obstet Gynecol 1975;18:41–50.

[125] Sims EA, Krantz KE. Serial studies of renal function during pregnancy and the puerperium in normal women. J Clin Invest 1958;37:1764–1774.

[126] Dam M, Christiansen J, Munck O, Mygind KI. Antiepileptic drugs: metabolism in pregnancy. Clin Pharmacokinet 1979;4:53–62.

[127] Steen B, Rane A. Clindamycin passage into human milk. Br J Clin Pharmacol 1982;13:661–664.

[128] Del Priore G, Jackson-Stone M, Shim EK, Garfinkel J, Eichmann MA, Frederiksen MC. A comparison of once-daily and 8-hour gentamicin dosing in the treatment of postpartum endometritis. Obstet Gynecol 1996;87:994–1000.

[129] Kubacka RT, Johnstone HE, Tan HS, Reeme PD, Myre SA. Intravenous ampicillin pharmacokinetics in the third trimester of pregnancy. Ther Drug Monit 1983;5:55–60.

[130] Yerby MS, Friel PN, Miller DQ. Carbamazepine protein binding and disposition in pregnancy. Ther Drug Monit 1985;7:269–273.

[131] Tomson T, Palm R, Källén K, Ben-Menachem E, Söderfeldt B, Danielsson B, et al. Pharmacokinetics of levetiracetam during pregnancy, delivery, in the neonatal period, and lactation. Epilepsia 2007;48:1111–1116.

[132] Westin AA, Reimers A, Helde G, Nakken KO, Brodtkorb E. Serum concentration/dose ratio of levetiracetam before, during and after pregnancy. Seizure 2008;17:192–198.

[133] Berlin M, Barchel D, Gandelman-Marton R, Brandriss N, Blatt I, Ziv-Baran T, et al. Therapeutic levetiracetam monitoring during pregnancy: "mind the gap". Ther Adv Chronic Dis 2019;10. https://doi.org/10.1177/2040622319851652. 2040622319851652.

[134] Anon. Viread® (tenofovir disoproxil fumarate) labeling, Foster City, CA: Gilead Sciences, Inc.; 2001. revised August 2012. Available from: https://www.accessdata.fda.gov/drugsatfda_docs/label/2012/021356s042,022577s002lbl.pdf. [Accessed April 2020].

[135] Colbers AP, Hawkins DA, Gingelmaier A, Kabeya K, Rockstroh JK, Wyen C, et al. The pharmacokinetics, safety and efficacy of tenofovir and emtricitabine in HIV-1-infected pregnant women. AIDS 2013;27:739–748.

[136] Anon. Prezista® (darunavir) labeling, N.V. Beerse, Belgium: Janssen Pharmaceutica; 2006. revised 2016. Available from: https://www.accessdata.fda.gov/drugsatfda_docs/label/2017/021976s045_202895s020lbl.pdf. [Accessed April 2020].

[137] Fujimoto H, Higuchi M, Watanabe H, Koh Y, Ghosh AK, Mitsuya H, et al. P-glycoprotein mediates efflux transport of darunavir in human intestinal Caco-2 and ABCB1 gene-transfected renal LLC-PK1 cell lines. Biol Pharm Bull 2009;32:1588–1593.

[138] Stek A, Best BM, Wang J, Capparelli EV, Burchett SK, Kreitchmann R, et al. Pharmacokinetics of once versus twice daily darunavir in pregnant HIV-infected women. J Acquir Immune Defic Syndr 2015;70:33–41.

[139] Colbers A, Molto J, Ivanovic J, Kabeya K, Hawkins D, Gingelmaier A, et al. Pharmacokinetics of total and unbound darunavir in HIV-1-infected pregnant women. J Antimicrob Chemother 2015;70:534–542.

[140] Crauwels H, Baugh B, Ryan B, Zorrilla C, Osiyemi OO, Yasin, et al. Total and unbound pharmacokinetics of once-daily darunavir/ritonavir in HIV-1 infected pregnant women. HIV Med 2016;17:643–652.

[141] Eke AC, Stek AM, Wang J, Kreitchmann R, Shapiro DE, Smith E, et al. Darunavir pharmacokinetics with an increased dose during pregnancy. J Acquir Immune Defic Syndr 2020;83:373–380.

[142] Casele HL, Laifer SA, Woelkers DA, Venkataramanan R. Changes in the pharmacokinetics of the low-molecular-weight heparin enoxaparin sodium during pregnancy. Am J Obstet Gynecol 1999;1811113–1811117.

[143] Scheen AJ. Clinical pharmacokinetics of metformin. Clin Pharmacokinet 1996;30:359–371.

[144] Wang DS, Jonker JW, Kato Y, Kusuhara H, Schinkel AH, Sugiyama Y. Involvement of organic cation transporter 1 in hepatic and intestinal distribution of metformin. J Pharmacol Exp Ther 2002;302:510–515.

[145] Kimura N, Okuda M, Inui K. Metformin transport by renal basolateral organic cation transporter hOCT2. Pharm Res 2005;22255–22259.

[146] Zhou M, Xia L, Wang J. Metformin transport by a newly cloned proton-stimulated organic cation transporter (plasma membrane monoamine transporter) expressed in human intestine. Drug Metab Dispos 2007;35:1956–1962.

[147] Pentikainen PJ, Neuvonen PJ, Penttila A. Pharmacokinetics of metformin after intravenous and oral administration to man. Eur J Clin Pharmacol 1979;16:195–202.

[148] Tucker GT, Casey C, Phillips PJ, Connor H, Ward JD, Woods HF. Metformin kinetics in healthy subjects and in patients with diabetes mellitus. Br J Clin Pharmacol 1981;12:235–246.

[149] Eyal S, Easterling TR, Carr D, Umans JG, Miodovnik M, Hankins GD, et al. Pharmacokinetics of metformin during pregnancy. Drug Metab Dispos 2010;38(5):833–840.

[150] Barton JR, Prevost RR, Wilson DA, Whybrew WD, Sibai BM. Nifedipine pharmacokinetics and pharmacodynamics during the immediate postpartum period in patients with preeclampsia. Am J Obstet Gynecol 1991;165:951–954.

[151] Kimberlin DF, Weller S, Whitley RJ, Andrews WW, Hauth JC, Lakeman F, et al. Pharmacokinetics of oral valacyclovir and acyclovir in late pregnancy. Am J Obstet Gynecol 1998;179:846–851.

[152] Nelson MM, Forfar JO. Associations between drugs administered during pregnancy and congenital abnormalities of the fetus. Br Med J 1971;1:523–527.

[153] Bonati M, Bortolus R, Marchetti F, Romero M, Tognoni G. Drug use in pregnancy: an overview of epidemiological (drug utilization) studies. Eur J Clin Pharmacol 1990;38:325–328.

[154] McBride WG. Thalidomide and congenital abnormalities [Letter]. Lancet 1961;ii:1358.

[155] Lenz W. Kindliche missbildungen nach medicament während der gravidität. Deutsch Med Wschr 1961;86:2555–2556.

[156] Morgan DJ. Drug disposition in mother and foetus. Clin Exp Pharmacol Physiol 1997;24:869–873.

[157] Martin CB. The anatomy and circulation of the placenta. In: Barnes AC, editor. Intra-uterine development. Philadelphia, PA: Lea & Febiger; 1968. p. 35–67.

[158] Castellucci M, Kaufmann P. Basic structure of the villous trees. In: Benirschke K, Kaufmann P, Baergen R, editors. Pathology of the human placenta. New York, NY: Springer; 2006. p. 50–120.

[159] van der Aa EM, Peereboom-Stegeman JH, Noordhoek J, Gribnau FW, Russel FG. Mechanisms of drug transfer across the human placenta. Pharm World Sci 1998;20:139–148.

[160] Vahakangas K, Myllynen P. Drug transporters in the human blood-placental barrier. Br J Pharmacol 2009;158:665–678.

[161] Evseenko D, Paxton JW, Keelan JA. Active transport across the human placenta: impact on drug efficacy and toxicity. Expert Opin Drug Metab Toxicol 2006;2:51–69.

[162] Grube M, Reuther S, Meyer Zu Schwabedissen H, Köck K, Draber K, Ritter CA, et al. Organic anion transporting polypeptide 2B1 and breast cancer resistance protein interact in the transepithelial transport of steroid sulfates in human placenta. Drug Metab Dispos 2007;35:30–35.

[163] Lankas GR, Wise LD, Cartwright ME, Pippert T, Umbenhauer DR. Placental P-glycoprotein deficiency enhances susceptibility to chemically induced birth defects in mice. Reprod Toxicol 1998;12:457–463.

[164] Prouillac C, Lecoeur S. The role of the placenta in fetal exposure to xenobiotics: importance of membrane transporters and human models for transfer studies. Drug Metab Dispos 2010;38:1623–1635.

[165] Syme MR, Paxton JW, Keelan JA. Drug transfer and metabolism by the human placenta. Clin Pharmacokinet 2004;43:487–514.

[166] Gottesman MM, Pastan I, Ambudkar SV. P-glycoprotein and multidrug resistance. Curr Opin Genet Dev 1996;6:610–617.

[167] Higgins CF. ABC transporters: from microorganisms to man. Annu Rev Cell Biol 1992;8:67–113.

[168] Schinkel AH, Wagenaar E, Mol CA, van Deemter L. P-glycoprotein in the blood-brain barrier of mice influences the brain penetration and pharmacological activity of many drugs. J Clin Invest 1996;97:2517–2524.

[169] Mylona P, Glazier JD, Greenwood SL, Sides MK, Sibley CP. Expression of the cystic fibrosis (CF) and multidrug resistance (MDR1) genes during development and differentiation in the human placenta. Mol Hum Reprod 1996;2:693–698.

[170] Nakamura Y, Ikeda S, Furukawa T, Sumizawa T, Tani A, Akiyama S, et al. Function of P-glycoprotein expressed in placenta and mole. Biochem Biophys Res Commun 1997;235:849–853.

[171] Gil S, Saura R, Forestier F, Farinotti R. P-glycoprotein expression of the human placenta during pregnancy. Placenta 2005;26:268–270.

[172] MacFarland A, Abramovich DR, Ewen SW, Pearson CK. Stage-specific distribution of P-glycoprotein in first-trimester and full-term human placenta. Histochem J 1994;26:417–423.

[173] Mathias AA, Hitti J, Unadkat JD. P-glycoprotein and breast cancer resistance protein expression in human placentae of various gestational ages. Am J Physiol Regul Integr Comp Physiol 2005;289:R963–R969.

[174] Sun M, Kingdom J, Baczyk D, Lye SJ, Matthews SG, Gibb W. Expression of the multidrug resistance P-glycoprotein, (ABCB1 glycoprotein) in the human placenta decreases with advancing gestation. Placenta 2006;27:602–609.

[175] Ushigome F, Takanaga H, Matsuo H, Tsukimori K, Nakano H, Ohtani H, et al. Human placental transport of vinblastine, vincristine, digoxin and progesterone: contribution of P-glycoprotein. Eur J Pharmacol 2000;408:1–10.

[176] Smit JW, Huisman MT, van Tellingen O, Wiltshire HR, Schinkel AH. Absence or pharmacological blocking of placental P-glycoprotein profoundly increases fetal drug exposure. J Clin Invest 1999;104:1441–1447.

[177] Pacifici GM, Nottoli R. Placental transfer of drugs administered to the mother. Clin Pharmacokinet 1995;28:235–269.

[178] Casey BM, Bawdon RE. Placental transfer of ritonavir with zidovudine in the ex vivo placental perfusion model. Am J Obstet Gynecol 1998;179:758–761.

[179] Marzolini C, Rudin C, Decosterd LA, Telenti A, Schreyer A, Biollaz J, et al. Transplacental passage of protease inhibitors at delivery. AIDS 2002;16:889–893.

[180] Sudhakaran S, Ghabrial H, Nation RL, Kong DC, Gude NM, Angus PW, et al. Differential bidirectional transfer of indinavir in the isolated perfused human placenta. Antimicrob Agents Chemother 2005;49:1023–1028.

[181] Marzolini C, Kim RB. Placental transfer of antiretroviral drugs. Clin Pharmacol Ther 2005;78:118–122.

[182] Uhr M, Steckler T, Yassouridis A, Holsboer F. Penetration of amitriptyline, but not of fluoxetine, into brain is enhanced in mice with blood-brain barrier deficiency due to mdr1a P-glycoprotein gene disruption. Neuropsychopharmacology 2000;22:380–387.

[183] Weiss J, Dormann SM, Martin-Facklam M, Kerpen CJ, Ketabi-Kiyanvash N, Haefeli WE. Inhibition of P-glycoprotein by newer antidepressants. J Pharmacol Exp Ther 2003;305:197–204.

[184] Weiss J, Kerpen CJ, Lindenmaier H, Dormann SM, Haefeli WE. Interaction of antiepileptic drugs with human P-glycoprotein in vitro. J Pharmacol Exp Ther 2003;307:262–267.

[185] Rahi M, Heikkinen T, Hakkola J, Hakala K, Wallerman O, Wadelius M, et al. Influence of adenosine triphosphate and ABCB1 (MDR1) genotype on the P-glycoprotein-dependent transfer of saquinavir in the dually perfused human placenta. Hum Exp Toxicol 2008;27:65–71.

[186] Rahi M, Heikkinen T, Härtter S, Hakkola J, Hakala K, Wallerman O, et al. Placental transfer of quetiapine in relation to P-glycoprotein activity. J Psychopharmacol 2007;21:751–756.

[187] Hitzl M, Schaeffeler E, Hocher B, Slowinski T, Halle H, Eichelbaum M, et al. Variable expression of P-glycoprotein in the human placenta and its association with mutations of the multidrug resistance 1 gene (MDR1, ABCB1). Pharmacogenetics 2004;14:309–318.

[188] Tanabe M, Ieiri I, Nagata N, Inoue K, Ito S, Kanamori Y, et al. Expression of P-glycoprotein in human placenta: relation to genetic polymorphism of the multidrug resistance (MDR)-1 gene. J Pharmacol Exp Ther 2001;297:1137–1143.

[189] Evseenko DA, Paxton JW, Keelan JA. ABC drug transporter expression and functional activity in trophoblast-like cell lines and differentiating primary trophoblast. Am J Physiol Regul Integr Comp Physiol 2006;290:R1357–R1365.

[190] Yeboah D, Sun M, Kingdom J, Baczyk D, Lye SJ, Matthews SG, et al. Expression of breast cancer resistance protein (BCRP/ABCG2) in human placenta throughout gestation and at term before and after labor. Can J Physiol Pharmacol 2006;84:1251–1258.

[191] Maliepaard M, Scheffer GL, Faneyte IF, van Gastelen MA, Pijnenborg AC, Schinkel AH, et al. Subcellular localization and distribution of the breast cancer resistance protein transporter in normal human tissues. Cancer Res 2001;61:3458–3464.

[192] Ceckova M, Libra A, Pavek P, Nachtigal P, Brabec M, Fuchs R, et al. Expression and functional activity of breast cancer resistance protein (BCRP, ABCG2) transporter in the human choriocarcinoma cell line BeWo. Clin Exp Pharmacol Physiol 2006;33:58–65.

[193] Allikmets R, Schriml LM, Hutchinson A, Romano-Spica V, Dean M. A human placenta-specific ATP-binding cassette gene (ABCP) on chromosome 4q22 that is involved in multidrug resistance. Cancer Res 1998;58:5337–5339.

[194] Jonker JW, Smit JW, Brinkhuis RF, Maliepaard M, Beijnen JH, Schellens JH, et al. Role of breast cancer resistance protein in the bioavailability and fetal penetration of topotecan. J Natl Cancer Inst 2000;92:1651–1656.

[195] Staud F, Vackova Z, Pospechova K, Pavek P, Ceckova M, Libra A, et al. Expression and transport activity of breast cancer resistance protein (Bcrp/Abcg2) in dually perfused rat placenta and HRP-1 cell line. J Pharmacol Exp Ther 2006;319:53–62.

[196] Enokizono J, Kusuhara H, Sugiyama Y. Effect of breast cancer resistance protein (Bcrp/Abcg2) on the disposition of phytoestrogens. Mol Pharmacol 2007;72:967–975.

[197] Zhang Y, Wang H, Unadkat JD, Mao Q. Breast cancer resistance protein 1 limits fetal distribution of nitrofurantoin in the pregnant mouse. Drug Metab Dispos 2007;35:2154–2158.

[198] Merino G, Jonker JW, Wagenaar E, van Herwaarden AE, Schinkel AH. The breast cancer resistance protein (BCRP/ABCG2) affects pharmacokinetics, hepatobiliary excretion, and milk secretion of the antibiotic nitrofurantoin. Mol Pharmacol 2005;67:1758–1764.

[199] Pollex E, Lubetsky A, Koren G. The role of placental breast cancer resistance protein in the efflux of glyburide across the human placenta. Placenta 2008;29:743–747.

[200] Elliott BD, Langer O, Schenker S, Johnson RF. Insignificant transfer of glyburide occurs across the human placenta. Am J Obstet Gynecol 1991;165:807812.

[201] Cygalova LH, Hofman J, Ceckova M, Staud F. Transplacental pharmacokinetics of glyburide, rhodamine 123, and BODIPY FL prazosin: effect of drug efflux transporters and lipid solubility. J Pharmacol Exp Ther 2009;331:1118–1125.

[202] Gedeon C, Anger G, Piquette-Miller M, Koren G. Breast cancer resistance protein: mediating the trans-placental transfer of glyburide across the human placenta. Placenta 2008;29:39–43.

[203] Zhou L, Naraharisetti SB, Wang H, Unadkat JD, Hebert MF, Mao Q. The breast cancer resistance protein (Bcrp1/Abcg2) limits fetal distribution of glyburide in the pregnant mouse: an Obstetric-fetal Pharmacology Research Unit Network and University of Washington Specialized Center of Research Study. Mol Pharmacol 2008;73:949–959.

[204] Hemauer SJ, Patrikeeva SL, Wang X, Abdelrahman DR, Hankins GD, Ahmed MS, et al. Role of transporter-mediated efflux in the placental biodisposition of bupropion and its metabolite, OH-bupropion. Biochem Pharmacol 2010;80:1080–1086.

[205] Evseenko DA, Paxton JW, Keelan JA. Independent regulation of apical and basolateral drug transporter expression and function in placental trophoblasts by cytokines, steroids, and growth factors. Drug Metab Dispos 2007;35:595–601.

[206] Morgan ET, Goralski KB, Piquette-Miller M, Renton KW, Robertson GR, Chaluvadi MR, et al. Regulation of drug-metabolizing enzymes and transporters in infection, inflammation, and cancer. Drug Metab Dispos 2008;36:205–216.

[207] Wang H, Lee EW, Zhou L, Leung PC, Ross DD, Unadkat JD, et al. Progesterone receptor (PR) isoforms PRA and PRB differentially regulate expression of the breast cancer resistance protein in human placental choriocarcinoma BeWo cells. Mol Pharmacol 2008;73:845–854.

[208] Wang H, Unadkat JD, Mao Q. Hormonal regulation of BCRP expression in human placental BeWo cells. Pharm Res 2008;25:444452.

[209] Jones KL, Jones MC, del Campo M. Smith's recognizable patterns of human malformation. Philadelphia, PA: Elsevier Saunders; 2013.

[210] Wilson JG. Current status of teratology – General principles and mechanisms derived from animal studies. In: Wilson JG, Fraser FC, editors. Handbook of teratology. Vol. 1 general principles and etiology. New York, NY: Plenum Press; 1977. p. 47–74.

[211] Brent RL. Radiation teratogenesis. Teratology 1980;21:281–298.

[212] Buehler BA, Delimont D, van Waes M, Finnell RH. Prenatal prediction of risk of the fetal hydantoin syndrome. N Engl J Med 1990;322:1567–1572.

[213] Shaw GM, Wasserman CR, Lammer EJ, O'Malley CD, Murray JC, Basart AM, et al. Orofacial clefts, parental cigarette smoking, and transforming growth factor-alpha gene variants. Am J Hum Genet 1996;58:551–561.

[214] Vargesson N. The teratogenic effects of thalidomide on limbs. J Hand Surg Eur Vol 2019;44:88–95.

[215] Parman T, Wiley MJ, Wells PG. Free radical-mediated oxidative DNA damage in the mechanism of thalidomide teratogenicity. Nat Med 1999;5:582–585.

[216] Thalidomide product information. Summit NJ: Celgene Corporation. Available from: https://media2.celgene.com/content/uploads/sites/23/Thalomid-Product_Monograph_-_English_Version.pdf.

[217] Begg EJ, Atkinson HC, Duffull SB. Prospective evaluation of a model for the prediction of milk:plasma drug concentrations from physicochemical characteristics. Br J Clin Pharmacol 1992;33:501–505.

[218] Stec GP, Greenberger P, Ruo TI, Henthorn T, Morita Y, Atkinson AJ Jr, et al. Kinetics of theophylline transfer to breast milk. Clin Pharmacol Ther 1980;28:404–408.

[219] Greenberger PA, Odeh YK, Frederiksen MC, Atkinson AJ Jr. Pharmacokinetics of prednisolone transfer to breast milk. Clin Pharmacol Ther 1993;53:324–328.

[220] Oo CY, Kuhn RJ, Desai N, McNamara PJ. Active transport of cimetidine into human milk. Clin Pharmacol Ther 1995;58:548–555.

[221] Sanders SW, Zone JJ, Foltz RL, Tolman KG, Rollins DE. Hemolytic anemia induced by dapsone transmitted through breast milk. Ann Intern Med 1982;96:465–466.

[222] Kwit NT, Hatcher RA. Excretion of drugs in milk. Am J Dis Child 1935;49:900–904.

[223] Meny RG, Naumburg EG, Alger LS, Brill-Miller JL, Brown S. Codeine and the breastfed neonate. J Hum Lact 1993;9:237–240.

[224] Koren G, Cairns J, Chitayat D, Gaedigk A, Leeder SJ. Pharmacogenetics of morphine poisoning in a breastfed neonate of a codeine-prescribed mother. Lancet 2006;368:704.

[225] Coffman BL, Rios GR, King CD, Tephly TR. Human UGT2B7 catalyzes morphine glucuronidation. Drug Metab Dispos 1997;25:1–4.

[226] Sawyer MB, Innocenti F, Das S, Cheng C, Ramírez J, Pantle-Fisher FH, et al. A pharmacogenetic study of uridine diphosphate-glucuronosyltransferase 2B7 in patients receiving morphine. Clin Pharmacol Ther 2003;73:566–574.

[227] Madadi P, Ross CJ, Hayden MR, Carleton BC, Gaedigk A, Leeder JS, et al. Pharmacogenetics of neonatal opioid toxicity following maternal use of codeine during breastfeeding: a case-control study. Clin Pharmacol Ther 2009;85:31–35.

[228] Juurlink DN, Gomes T, Guttmann A, Hellings C, Sivilotti ML, Harvey MA, et al. Postpartum maternal codeine therapy and the risk of adverse neonatal outcomes: a retrospective cohort study. Clin Toxicol (Phila) 2012;50:390–395.

[229] Berlin CM, Briggs GG. Drugs and chemicals in human milk. Semin Fetal Neonatal Med 2005;10:149–159.

[230] Anderson PO, Pochop SL, Manoguerra AS. Adverse drug reactions in breastfed infants: less than imagined. Clin Pediatr (Phila) 2003;42:325–340.

[231] Anon. FDA pregnancy and lactation Labeling final rule. Fed Registry 2014;79(233):72064–72103.

Chapter 24

Pediatric clinical pharmacology and therapeutics

Bridgette L. Jones[a], John N. Van Den Anker[b], Gilbert J. Burckart[c], and Gregory L. Kearns[d]
[a]*Department of Pediatrics, University of Missouri-Kansas City School of Medicine, Children's Mercy, Kansas City, MO, United States,* [b]*Division of Pediatric Clinical Pharmacology and Medical Toxicology, Children's National Hospital, Washington, DC, United States,* [c]*Office of Clinical Pharmacology, U.S. Food and Drug Administration, Silver Spring, MD, United States,* [d]*Department of Medical Education and Pediatrics, Texas Christian University and UNTHSC School of Medicine, Fort Worth, TX, United States*

Children younger than 15 years old account for 28% of the population worldwide and about one quarter of the U.S. population. As one must undergo the developmental trajectory of childhood to reach adulthood, any discussion of clinical pharmacology would be incomplete without inclusion of how development, the most dynamic period of human life, influences drug disposition, action, and creates unique therapeutic scenarios that are not seen in adults.

Development, despite being a continuum of physiologic events that culminate in maturity, is often arbitrarily divided into the stages of infancy, childhood, adolescence, and even early adulthood. During development, organ size and function change as does body composition, protein expression, and cellular function. Some cellular components are active during early development and subsequently lose function with age, and vice versa. Some tissues may be more sensitive to pharmacologic effects early in life, whereas later in life function may decline. As these developmental changes in function and form occur, their implications with respect to the clinical pharmacology of drugs and to their appropriate place in pediatric therapy must be considered.

History of pediatric clinical pharmacology

The practice of pediatrics developed out of the realization that illness affects children differently than adults. The same realization regarding the need to "individualize" drug therapy for infants and children fostered the birth of pediatric clinical pharmacology. In 1968 Dr. Harry Shirkey wrote in an editorial the following: "By an odd and unfortunate twist of fate, infants and children are becoming therapeutic or pharmaceutical orphans" [1]. Many of the laws regulating drug manufacturing, testing, and distribution, which were often the result of therapeutic tragedies in children, had the unfortunate result that relatively few drugs being labeled for use in children. One specific pediatric tragedy was the death from renal failure of nearly 100 children who had ingested an elixir of sulfanilamide preparation made with diethylene glycol. As discussed in Chapter 35, this precipitated the U.S. Food, Drug and Cosmetic Act of 1938. This Act required that drugs and cosmetics sold in the U.S. be tested for toxicity before marketing. In 1962 the Kefauver-Harris Amendment was brought about by another tragic event that affected children. In the late 1950s and early 1960s, more than 10,000 children in 46 countries were born with limb deformities as a consequence of thalidomide exposure in utero, the drug being taken by pregnant women for nausea. The German pediatrician Widukind Lenz suspected a link between birth defects and the drug, which he subsequently proved in 1961. Prior to this knowledge, Dr. Frances Oldham Kelsey, a clinical pharmacologist serving as a medical officer at the FDA, became an unknown hero at the time by denying approval and subsequent marketing of thalidomide in the United States due to a lack of safety data. Dr. Kelsey's apprehension regarding the drug was partly spurred by her previous research in which she found that pregnant rabbits and embryonic rabbits metabolized quinine differently than nonpregnant mature rabbits. She also had suspicions that thalidomide might be toxic in developing fetuses after hearing of reports that the drug was a possible cause of nerve damage in adults [2]. Thus it was her understanding of developmental and clinical pharmacology that led Dr. Kelsey to a decision which prevented this pediatric drug tragedy from reaching the US. Dr. Kelsey was later awarded the medal for Distinguished Federal Civilian Service by President John F. Kennedy.

Atkinson's Principles of Clinical Pharmacology. https://doi.org/10.1016/B978-0-12-819869-8.00014-8

The bitter irony of the early regulatory laws and decisions is that they put forward the practice of therapeutic restriction as the primary means to maximize drug safety in pediatric patients. Thus these laws did not actually benefit children as much as they could have because pediatric patients were excluded from the study of therapeutic drugs, many of which even were intended for pediatric use. In fact, the laws actually led to drug labeling that included warnings for most new drugs, stating that, due to inadequate (or nonexistent) data in children, they were not recommended for pediatric use. This led Dr. Shirkey to describe children as "therapeutic orphans" and to issue a call to academia, industry, and government to actively take responsibility for prudently including children in the development programs of drugs intended for pediatric use [1]. Despite this profound unmet need, little progress in making safe and effective drugs for children was made for almost three decades after this call to action was issued.

In fact, all of the regulatory preparation for pediatric drug development was accomplished in the 1970s by the FDA, the American Academy of Pediatrics, and the NIH. In 1974 Congress passed the National Research Act and established the National Commission for the Protection of Human Subjects of Medical and Behavioral Research. The same year the American Academy of Pediatrics issued a report commissioned by the FDA on "*General Guidelines for the Evaluation of Drugs to be Approved for Use during Pregnancy and for Treatment of Infants and Children.*" In 1977 the FDA issued a Pediatric Guidance, "*General Considerations for the Clinical Evaluation of Drugs in Infants and Children.*" Finally, in 1979 FDA issued a Regulation on the *Pediatric Use* Subsection of Product Package Insert *Precautions* Section (21 CFR 201.57 (f)(9)). In this way, the stage was set for pediatric drug development, but formal studies in infants and children would not take place for another 20 years.

However, the decades of the 1970s, 1980s, and 1990s were not devoid of pediatric clinical pharmacology activity, and some might consider that the pediatric studies performed during this period were critical to the initiation of formal pediatric drug development studies after 1997. One of the most notable pediatric clinical pharmacologists during this time was Dr. Sumner Yaffe, regarded as the "Father of Pediatric Clinical Pharmacology" by many in the United States. Dr. Yaffe was a Harvard-trained physician who became the Director of the Clinical Research Center for Premature Infants at Stanford University. Dr. Yaffe moved to Buffalo Children's Hospital in the early 1960s and found valuable collaborators in a group of pharmaceutical scientists that were engaged in a new field of study called pharmacokinetics. These early pharmacokinetic studies in infants and children provided the basis for an understanding of pediatric ontogeny and established pharmacokinetics as a primary tool used by subsequently pediatric clinical pharmacologists.

Evolution of pediatric drug development regulations

In the mid-1990s, government mandates were initiated that provided provisions to ensure future progress in pediatric drug development. In 1994 the FDA issued the Pediatric Rule stating that if the course of the disease and/or the response to a given drug is similar in children and adults, labeling of drugs for pediatric use would be allowed based on extrapolation of efficacy in adults and additional pharmacokinetic (PK), pharmacodynamic (PD), and safety studies in pediatric populations. Unfortunately, this rule prompted the conduct of only a small number of well-designed and well-conducted studies. For this reason, the FDA Modernization Act (FDAMA) was passed in 1997 which provided for a six months of extended market exclusivity for new drugs in exchange for pediatric studies that were completed in accordance with a written request issued by the FDA. This Act also mandated that a list be compiled of already approved drugs for which additional information was needed for pediatric labeling, and again provided additional market exclusivity if pediatric studies were performed for these drugs [3]. In 2002 The Best Pharmaceuticals for Children Act was signed which provided mechanisms for studying on- and off-patent drugs in children. This Act extended the 6 months' marketing exclusivity provided in 1997 under the FDAMA to include pediatric studies of drugs currently under patent in addition to nonpatent drugs in which studies were initiated under the provisions of an FDA Written Request. In 2003 The Pediatric Research Equity Act (PREA) was passed into US law, and mandated the conduct of pediatric clinical trials for drugs under development that had the potential for significant pediatric use. The BPCA and PREA provisions were renewed in the 2007 Food and Drug Administration Amendments Act (FDAAA) and sections were added pertaining to the study of pediatric devices, requiring the FDA to actively monitor safety for all drugs studied under the provisions of this legislation and to establish an FDA Pediatric Review Committee to standardize pediatric drug development programs. After another five years, BPCA and PREA were finally made permanent under the 2012 FDA Safety and Innovation Act (FDASIA). FDASIA also focused attention on neonates, which previously had been neglected as a pediatric group in drug development.

In 2017 the FDA Reauthorization Act (FDARA) focused on another neglected pediatric patient group in drug development, namely pediatric oncology patients. Since cancer indications in adults frequently do not pertain to pediatric patients, studies cannot be required under PREA which is indication based. Therefore the Research to Accelerate Cures and Equity (RACE) for Children Act was passed as part of FDARA. This act changed the basis for PREA inclusion in pediatric oncology to be based on molecular target instead of indication. The RACE Act for Children also removed the PREA exemption for orphan drug products, which is critically important for small pediatric oncology patient groups. This change to PREA-based pediatric drug development study requirements will take effect in August of 2020.

Pediatric regulatory science

Collectively, these regulatory initiatives have brought about a marked increase in the number of pediatric clinical trials that have characterized the clinical pharmacology of both the old and new drugs that are used in pediatric patients and have led to improvements in pediatric dosing and labeling. As of December 2019, 841 pediatric labeling changes have been made which included new dosing, dosing changes, or pharmacokinetic information, new safety data, lack of efficacy data, new formulations, and dosing instructions that extend the age limits for use in children [4].

These initiatives also had global impact in creating the framework for similar European regulations which require that children be included in clinical trials of drugs intended to be used in their treatment. Comparisons to FDA labeling for pediatric use may also encourage other international regulatory agencies to reconsider approaches to pediatric drug use [5]. Despite the improvements in pediatric therapeutics over the past 20 years that have been driven by these regulations, a significant number of drugs, particularly many that have been used for years in pediatric practice, have both insufficient pediatric labeling and incomplete knowledge regarding their pharmacologic properties. Thus significant gaps in pediatric drug development still exist in assessing pediatric drug–drug interactions, pediatric dosing in renal and hepatic impairment, bioequivalence with new pediatric dosage forms, and long-term drug safety concerns [6].

Developmental clinical pharmacology

Normal human development represents a dynamic continuum with aspects that are overtly evident (e.g., acquisition of speech, mobility, linear growth, accretion of body weight, pubertal onset) and others that are not (e.g., maturation of renal and hepatic function, neuronal development). Throughout development, the impact of ontogeny on pharmacokinetics and pharmacodynamics is, to a great degree, predictable and follows definable physiologic "patterns." Examples are illustrated in Fig. 24.1 [7] and are described in greater detail in the sections that follow.

Ontogeny of pharmacokinetics in children

Oral absorption

As in adults, most medications administered to infants and children are given via the peroral route and development can influence both the rate and extent of drug absorption. During the first few years of life there are significant changes in gastric pH related to the density and function of parietal cells which are present early in fetal life in the antrum and body of the stomach. However, at term only about 20% of neonates possess the proportion of parietal cells in the antrum observed in adults [8]. The highest gastric pH levels [6–8] occur in the neonate immediately after birth and are influenced by amniotic fluid in the stomach [9]. It is not clear what happens after birth as available data vary between describing a neutral gastric pH at 1–3 days after birth followed by a progressive decrease over several weeks to years to reach adult values (Fig. 24.1, panel C), or an acidic gastric pH soon after birth that persists even in the most preterm infants [10, 11]. Thus there currently is no clear consensus about the ontogeny of gastric acid production and secretion in newborn infants and during early infancy [12]. In the case of drugs that are weak organic acids and with a narrow therapeutic index (e.g., phenytoin), these developmental changes in pH may result in the need for more frequent dose adjustments to achieve desired therapeutic plasma concentrations in younger children. During the neonatal period and infancy, the oral bioavailability of acid labile drugs (e.g., beta-lactam antibiotics) may be increased because higher gastric pH results in their reduced degradation. Moreover, it is important to consider the impact of feeding on gastric pH and its effects on drug absorption. Feedings with infant formula have been found to increase gastric pH, buffering it to levels > 4 for up to 90 minutes after a feeding. Finally, human breast milk contains large amounts of epidermal growth factor, a peptide that inhibits gastric acid secretion.

Until very recently it was assumed that gastric emptying was much slower below the age of 6-8 months because neuroregulation of gastric motility had not matured [13]. This assumption was substantiated in several clinical investigations involving drugs such as acetaminophen and cisapride [14, 15]. However, in a recent meta-analysis of 49 published studies including 1500 participants between the age of 29 weeks of gestation and adults, variation in gastric emptying was not explained by differences in age but seemed to reflect the type of food (water, milk, solid) consumed [16]. There is currently very limited understanding of the effect of age on the rate and extent of gastric emptying in neonates and during early

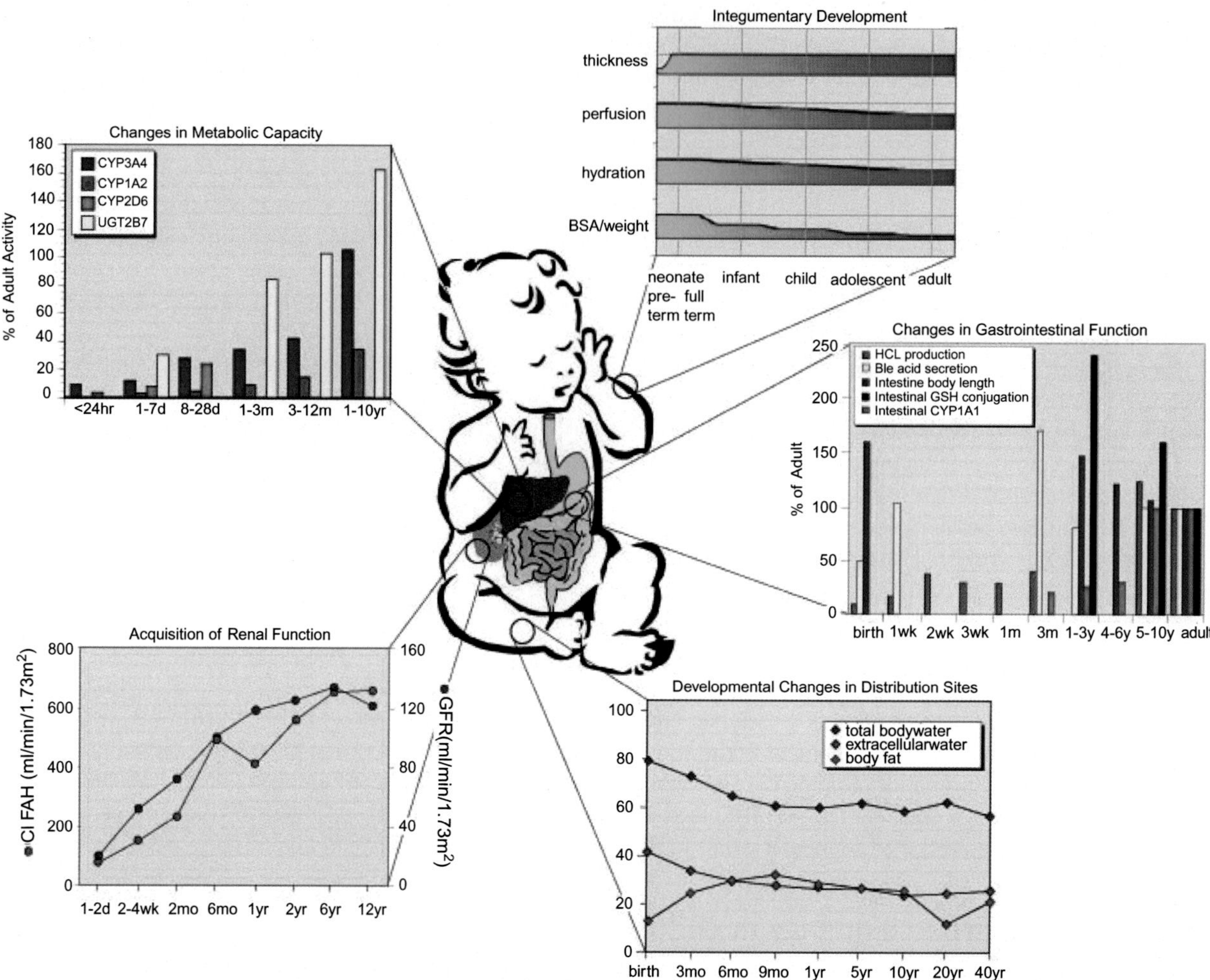

FIG. 24.1 Physiologic changes in multiple organs and organ systems during development are responsible for age-related differences in drug disposition. *Panel A* shows that the activity of many cytochrome P-450 (CYP) isoforms and a single glucuronosyltransferase (UGT) isoform is markedly diminished during the first 2 months of life. The acquisition of adult activity over time also is enzyme- and isoform-specific. *Panel B* shows age-dependent changes in body composition, which influence the apparent distribution volume for drugs. Infants in the first 6 months of life have markedly expanded TBW and ECF relative to total body weight than older infants and adults. *Panel C* shows the age-dependent changes in gastrointestinal tract structure and function. As with hepatic drug-metabolizing enzyme, the activity of CYP1A in the intestine is low during early life. *Panel D* summarizes the effect of postnatal development on the GFR and active renal tubular secretion, both of which approximate adult activity by 6-12 months of age. *Panel E* shows age dependence in the thickness, extent of perfusion, and extent of hydration of the skin and the relative size of the skin-surface area which are reflected in the ratio of body-surface area to body weight. *Modified from Kearns GL, Abdel-Rahman SM, Alander SW, Blowey DL, Leeder JS, Kauffman RE. Developmental pharmacology—drug disposition, action, and therapy in infants and children. N Engl J Med 2003;349:1157–1167.*

infancy. However, it appears that gastrointestinal functions achieve adult values by the age of 2 years. In contrast, it seems that age has minimal influence on transit time through the small intestine and colon [17].

Finally, intestinal drug-metabolizing enzymes (e.g., CYP3A4/5, CYP1A, *N*-acetyltransferase, xanthine oxidase, glutathione-*S*-transferase) and transporters (e.g., P-glycoprotein, organic anion, and cation transporters) whose activity likely varies with developmental stage may also alter the bioavailability of drugs [18]. In humans, the expression of these proteins appears to reach adult levels between 6 and 12 months of age; however, data are limited [19]. Very few clinical investigations have provided additional insight into the possible impact of CYP3A4 maturation on the clearance of any of its substrates. Very recently a physiological population PK model was developed that also incorporated PK data on midazolam and 1-OH-midazolam concentrations from 37 preterm infants who were given both intravenous and oral doses of this drug [20]. This model made it possible to distinguish between intestinal and hepatic intrinsic clearance of midazolam and showed that a very low first-pass effect by intestinal and hepatic metabolism resulted in an intestinal and hepatic bioavailability of this CYP3A substrate that was much higher than in adults. Glutathione-*S*-transferase activity and bile acid secretion also exhibit developmental differences that may affect drug exposure (Fig. 25.1, panel C). Other factors, such as differences in intestinal microbial flora, have also been proposed to affect intestinal drug absorption in infants.

Extravascular drug absorption

Development can also alter the systemic exposure to drugs given by extravascular routes of administration (e.g., dermal, subcutaneous, buccal, intramuscular, rectal, intraosseous, intrapulmonary). For example, differences in perfusion and hydration status of the stratum corneum in young infants (Fig. 24.1, panel E) can facilitate transdermal absorption of specific drugs, thereby, predisposing neonates and young infants to potential systemic toxicity as has been reported for corticosteroid and diphenhydramine containing drug products [21]. Such toxicity can be exacerbated by conditions (e.g., eczema) that disrupt the integumentary barrier.

The rate of absorption of intramuscularly administered drugs can be reduced in neonates, compared to older children and adults, consequent to reduced skeletal muscle blood flow and inefficient muscular contractions, which work together to disperse drug within large muscles. However, the density of skeletal muscle capillaries is higher in infants in comparison to older children and adults, and appears to lead to a more efficient intramuscular absorption of specific agents (e.g., amikacin and cephalothin) in this age group.

Absorption of rectally administered agents may be reduced in infants because they have a greater number of high-amplitude pulsatile contractions in the rectum than adults and are prone to premature expulsion of solid rectal drug formulations (e.g., suppositories). In contrast, rectal solutions of drugs such as diazepam (which is commonly prescribed for outpatient emergency treatment of seizures) are readily and rapidly absorbed in children, achieving therapeutic plasma concentrations within 4 minutes of administration [22]. On the other hand, the bioavailability of some rectally administered drugs is greater in neonates and young infants than in older infants (i.e., >6–12 months) and children because the activity of their hepatic drug-metabolizing enzymes is reduced (Fig. 24.1, panel A).

Drug distribution

Changes in drug distribution during development are largely associated with changes in body composition and the quantity and nature of plasma proteins capable of drug binding. As reflected by Fig. 24.1, panel B, significant age-dependent changes in body composition occur. When expressed as a percentage of total body mass, neonates and young infants have significantly higher extracellular fluid (ECF) and total body water (TBW) spaces (80% in infants vs. 60% in adults). In contrast, the percentage of intracellular water (ICW) as a function of body mass remains stable from the first months of life through adulthood (Fig. 24.1, panel B). Age-dependent changes in body composition can alter the apparent volume of distribution (V_d) for both hydrophilic and lipophilic drugs. For example, as described in Chapter 3, aminoglycoside antibiotics distribute in a central compartment that corresponds to ECF, so the corresponding V_d of these drugs is increased in neonates (e.g., 0.4–0.7 L/kg) relative to adults (usually ~0.2 L/kg). While higher relative body fat is observed in infants and children (Fig. 24.1, panel B), this does not appear to markedly alter the V_d for most therapeutic drugs, although it must be considered under certain circumstances (e.g., obesity) and for extremely lipophilic agents (see Chapter 3). Although neonates tend to have a lower percentage of total body fat than older infants, lipid content in the developing central nervous system (CNS) is high and this situation has implications for the distribution of lipophilic drugs and their CNS effects (e.g. propranolol) in neonates. Special considerations must also be made for overweight and obese children, particularly as the prevalence of obesity in children continues to increase [23]. Studies have found that obese children had significantly higher body volume, lean mass, fat mass, and TBW than nonobese children [24]. Drug dose adjustments for obesity, especially for agents with a narrow therapeutic index (e.g., aminoglycosides, cancer chemotherapeutic agents), must therefore be made in obese children so as to prevent either under- or overdosing and thus provide the optimal systemic exposure for the desired drug effects [25, 26].

Circulating plasma protein concentrations, albumin and α_1-acid glycoprotein, are influenced by disease state, nutrition, and age. The proteins are present in relatively low concentrations (~80% of adult) in young infants and neonates but usually reach adult levels by 1 year of age. Similar patterns are also observed for α_1-acid glycoprotein, where neonatal plasma concentrations are approximately three times lower than in maternal plasma and attain adult values by approximately 1 year of age. These proteins are not only quantitatively diminished but are also functionally immature and, compared to adults, neonates have a larger concentration of fetal albumin which has a lower binding capacity for weak acids. For example, 88 is more extensively (~94%–98%) bound to albumin in healthy adults than in neonates (80%–85%), and, as described in Chapter 5 for adults with impaired renal function, the resultant 6- to 8-fold difference in the free fraction can result in CNS adverse effects in the neonate when total plasma phenytoin concentrations are within the generally accepted "therapeutic range" of 10–20 mg/L. Endogenous substances in the neonate, such as bilirubin and free fatty acids, may also displace drugs from their albumin binding sites and vice versa. For example, sulfonamides have an albumin binding affinity that exceeds that of bilirubin, and their administration to neonates can lead to excess free bilirubin concentrations that have the potential to produce CNS injury (e.g., kernicterus).

Drug transport

Drug transporters, such as P-glycoprotein (P-gp), multidrug resistance protein 1 (MRP1), and breast cancer resistance protein (BCRP) may also influence drug distribution and elimination. Limited data in humans suggest that both P-gp and MRP1 expression follow a developmental pattern [27]. Pgp is expressed in the human central nervous system as early as 27 weeks of gestation with expression intensity during the neonatal period becoming most prevalent at 33 weeks of gestation. Within the CNS there is also differential expression within various regions of the brain in relation to age [27]. P-gp in the liver also follows a developmental pattern of expression in which activity increases during the first few months of life and adult levels are reached by 2 years of age [28].

Drug metabolism

Drug metabolism also exhibits marked developmental dependence, especially during fetal and early postnatal life. The liver undergoes significant changes during fetal life and early childhood after its origin in the fourth week of gestation as a duodenal diverticulum. By the sixth week of fetal life hepatic lobules are present, and the organ represents 10% of fetal weight by the ninth week of gestation [29]. As the architecture of the liver develops, so do the families of enzymes responsible for the biosynthesis and metabolism of both endogenous and exogenous substrates.

Cytochrome P450 enzymes

The cytochrome P450 family of enzymes (CYPs) is responsible for the biotransformation of numerous endogenous substrates (e.g., adrenal steroids) and therapeutic agents, and there are considerable changes in the expression and activity of these enzymes during development. At birth the total hepatic CYP concentration is approximately 30% that of adults, and there are variable rates of both quantitative and functional maturation [30, 31]. In early studies CYP1A1 was not detected in fetal liver during the second and third trimester, but very low levels have been detected more recently [32, 33]. This discrepancy may reflect a dynamic expression pattern whereby low levels of this enzyme are expressed during organogenesis early in fetal development but decline to undetectable levels later in gestation. As illustrated by Fig. 24.1 (panel A), CYP1A2 activity is minimal during the fetal period and begins to rise at 8-28 days of postnatal life before reaching adult activity by one year of age [34]. Diet has also been shown to affect the ontogeny of CYP1A2 activity, and formula-fed infants acquire function of this enzyme more rapidly than do breast-fed infants [35].

The CYP3A subfamily is the most abundant of the hepatic CYP450s and is responsible for the biotransformation of approximately 50% of the therapeutic drugs that are administered to pediatric patients (e.g., salmeterol, cyclosporine, tacrolimus, midazolam, fentanyl, macrolide antibiotics). The subfamily consists of four genes, *CYP3A4*, *CYP3A5*, *CYP3A7*, and *CYP3A43*, which are located on chromosome 7q21.1. CYP3A4, CYP3A5, and CYP3A7 are the most clinically relevant enzymes for pharmacotherapy as CYP3A43 has little xenobiotic metabolizing activity. CYP3A7 was found to be the most abundant CYP3A isoform in fetal liver samples obtained from 76 days to 32 weeks gestation and continues to be the predominant isoform during the first one to two months of life [36]. A "switch" from CYP3A7 to CYP3A4 predominance begins at birth, with the activity of the former progressively declining toward adult levels during the first year of life to activity that is approximately 7% of fetal levels [37]. The high activity of this enzyme early in fetal life is associated with its function in forming a precursor for estriol biosynthesis, a hormone that is important in fetal growth and timing of parturition. In contrast, the activity of CYP3A4 is minimal in the fetus and only 10% of adult levels at birth, but rises steadily during the neonatal period and early childhood, probably reaching adult levels by early adolescence (Fig. 24.1 panel A) [37, 38]. CYP3A4 and CYP3A5 have overlapping substrate specificities and in the case of the latter, polymorphic expression with racial differences in the genotype-phenotype relationship that can have significant effects on the biotransformation of drugs that are substrates for this isoform [39, 40]. While CYP3A5 has been demonstrated across the developmental continuum, a clear developmental pattern for its expression has not yet been fully elucidated.

As discussed in Chapter 12, CYP2D6, a polymorphically expressed enzyme in humans, is responsible for the biotransformation of approximately 12% of clinically relevant drugs used in pediatric practice (e.g., ß-antagonists, antiarrhythmics, antidepressants, morphine derivatives, antipsychotics, dextromethorphan, diphenhydramine, atomoxetine, metoclopramide).

CYP2D6 has not been consistently detected in the fetal period, and its activity remains low (approximately 5%–10% of adult activity) during the first few weeks of life. Interestingly, expression of this enzyme appears to be independent of gestational age in newborns, which suggests that there is a birth-dependent process that activates its expression. After birth there is a steady increase in CYP2D6 activity with levels approximating 30% and 70% of adult activity at 1 month and 1-5 years of life, respectively [41]. However, in vivo longitudinal phenotyping studies have revealed that genotype-phenotype relationships are present as early as 2 weeks postnatal age and that genotype is a more important contributor than ontogeny to the interindividual variability of CYP2D6 enzyme activity [42].

CYP2C9 is a polymorphically expressed enzyme which catalyzes the biotransformation of several important drugs used in pediatrics (e.g., phenytoin, ibuprofen, indomethacin). CYP2C9 has been detected at very low levels (1% of adult levels) in early gestation (earliest at 8 weeks). At term, activity increases to approximately 10% of that observed in adults and is approximately 25% of adult levels by 5-6 months of age. A similar pattern of developmental expression is demonstrated for CYP2C19, an enzyme that is also polymorphically expressed and is largely responsible for the biotransformation of proton pump inhibitors (e.g., lansoprazole, omeprazole, pantoprazole, esomeprazole, rabeprazole)—a drug class used extensively in neonates and infants with gastroesophageal reflux. As illustrated in Fig. 24.2, CYP2C19 activity increases quickly after birth and reaches adult levels at approximately 6 months postnatally [43]. As is the case for CYP2C9, genotype-phenotype concordance is expected at this point and predictive relationships appear between the *CYP2C19* genotype and the activity of the enzyme [43]. In examining the ontogeny of both CYP2C9 and CYP2C19, as is the case with most all of the cytochrome P450 isoforms, significant intersubject variability occurs across the developmental continuum (Fig. 24.2). Also, when constitutive activity of the enzyme is normally low shortly after birth, genotype-phenotype discordance can lead to erroneous classification of metabolizer.

Of the cytochrome P450 isoforms quantitatively important for drug metabolism in human, all studied to date appear to have a developmental pattern with respect to the attainment of activity. It is beyond the scope of this chapter to provide a detailed description for each enzyme, this has been accomplished in recent reviews on the topic [44], and an overview is summarized in Table 24.1 [45].

Phase II biotransformations

A historical catastrophe in pediatric clinical pharmacology, the chloramphenicol-associated "Grey Baby Syndrome," was a sentinel event that demonstrated the impact of development on the activity of a Phase II drug-metabolizing enzyme (UDP glucuronosyltransferase or UGT). More importantly this event illustrated how failure to recognize these differences and account for them in the determination of age-appropriate drug doses can lead to unnecessary morbidity and mortality. As with chloramphenicol, morphine, acetaminophen, and zidovudine, are all UGT substrates that also have a requirement for dosing regimen alterations to compensate for reduced enzyme activity in the first weeks and months of life. In premature infants (gestational age 24–37 weeks) the plasma clearance of morphine was found to be fivefold lower than in older children and generally reaches adult levels between 2 and 6 months of life, although considerable variability exists

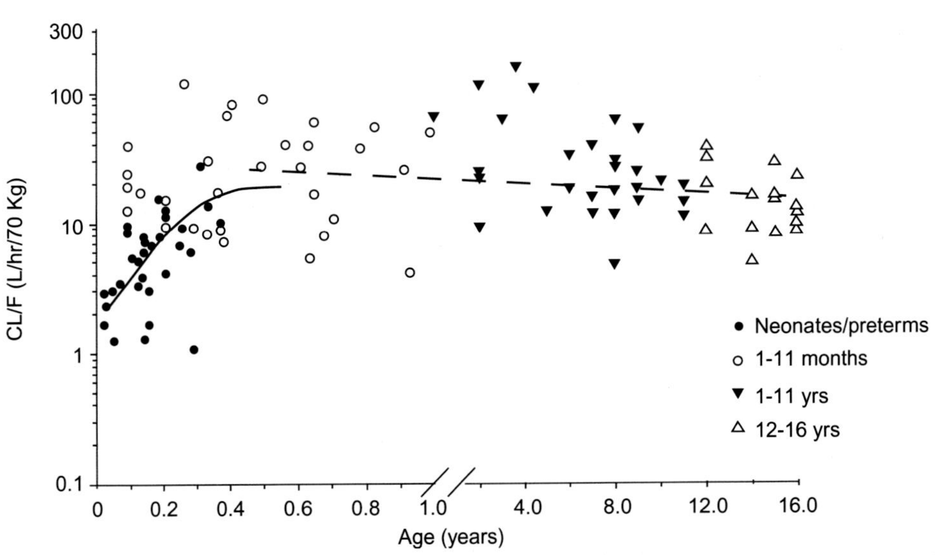

FIG. 24.2 In vivo assessment of CYP2C19 activity as a function of age, using oral clearance of pantoprazole as a marker for CYP2C19 activity. The activity of this enzyme is considerably reduced in neonates and preterm infants relative to older age groups. *Reproduced from Kearns GL, Leeder JS, Gaedigk A. Impact of the CYP2C19*17 allele on the pharmacokinetics of omeprazole and pantoprazole in children: evidence for a differential effect. Drug Metab Dispos 2010;38:894–897.*

TABLE 24.1 Developmental patterns for the ontogeny of phase I drug-metabolizing enzymes in humans.

Enzymes	Known developmental pattern
Phase I Enzymes	
CYP2D6	Low to absent in fetal liver but present at 1 week of age. Poor activity (i.e., 20% of adult) by 1 month. Adult competence by 3–5 years of age
Substrates	SSRIs (fluoxetine, paroxetine, sertraline), risperidone, atomoxetine, promethazine, dextromethorphan, diphenhydramine, chlorpheniramine
CYP2C19	Apparently absent in fetal liver. Low activity in first 2–4 weeks of life with adult activity reached by approximately 6 months. Activity may exceed adult levels during childhood and declines to adult levels after conclusion of puberty
Substrates	Proton pump inhibitors (omeprazole, pantoprazole, lansoprazole), propranolol
CYP2C9	Detected at very low levels (1% of adult levels) in early gestation (earliest at 8 weeks). At term, activity increases to approximately 10% of that observed in adults and by 5 to 6 months of age, is approximately 25% of adult levels
Substrates	Warfarin, phenytoin, ibuprofen, indomethacin
CYP1A2	Not present in appreciable levels in human fetal liver. Adult levels reached by approximately 4 months and exceeded in children at 1–2 years of age. Adult activity reached after puberty
Substrates	Clozapine, clomipramine, caffeine, haloperidol, ondansetron, theophylline
CYP3A7	Fetal form of CYP3A which is functionally active (and inducible) during gestation. Virtually disappears by 1 to 4 weeks of postnatal when CYP3A4 activity predominates, but remains present in approximately 5% of individuals
CYP3A4	Extremely low activity at birth reaching approximately 30 to 40% of adult activity by 1 month and full adult activity by 6 months. May exceed adult activity between 1 and 4 years of age, decreasing to adult levels after puberty
Substrates (3A7 and 3A4)	Cyclosporine, erythromycin, lidocaine, midazolam, nifedipine, tacrolimus, verapamil, zolpidem
CYP2E1	Undetectable expression in the fetal liver. In newborn livers levels are 10% of adults. Steady increase of expression with age. Adult levels are reached in children between 1 and 10 years of age. There is a strong association between protein levels and activity along the developmental spectrum
Substrates	Anesthetics (halothane, isoflurane, enflurane), acetaminophen
CYP2B6	Variable detection in fetal liver and at low levels relative to adults (median levels approximately 15% of adult). There is an approximate 2-fold increase in median expression after the neonatal period (birth to 30 days postnatal) with considerable variability. Expression is less variable in infants and children with median levels reported at approximately 40% of adults

Abbreviations: *CYP*, cytochrome P450; *SSRIs*, serotonin selective reuptake inhibitors.
Adapted from Leeder JS, Kearns GL. Pharmacogenetics in pediatrics. Implications for practice. Pediatr Clin North Am 1997;44:55–77.

[46]. Acetaminophen glucuronidation, mediated by UGT1A6 and UGT1A9, is present in the fetus and newborn at very low levels (1%–10% of adults). Following birth, activity steadily increases, with levels approaching ~50% of adult levels by 6 months of age and with full maturation by puberty. A similar maturation pattern is seen for zidovudine, a substrate for UGT2B7. Zidovudine clearance is significantly reduced in children <2 years of age relative to older children, with the result that they have a higher risk for hematologic toxicity (anemia) from this drug [47]. Similar to what is seen for the UGT isoforms, ontogenic profiles also exist for glutathione *S*-transferase (GST), *N*-acetyltransferase (NAT), epoxide hydroxylase (EPHX), and the sulfotransferases (SULT). These are summarized in Table 24.2 [48] and are discussed in a previously published authoritative review [44].

Drug elimination

Drug elimination in pediatric patients can occur via multiple routes, including exhalation via the respiratory tract, biliary secretion, and renal clearance. However, the kidney is the primary organ responsible for the excretion of drugs and their metabolites. The development of renal function begins during early fetal development and is complete by early childhood (Fig. 24.1, panel D). From a developmental perspective, renal function is highly dependent on gestational age and postnatal

TABLE 24.2 Ontogeny of phase II drug-metabolizing enzymes in the neonate.

	Prenatal trimester			Neonate	1 month to 1 year
Enzyme	**1**	**2**	**3**		
GSTA1/A2	+	+	+	+	+
GSTM	+	+	+	+	+
GSTP1	+	+	+	+	0
NAT2	+	+	+	+	+
UGT1A1	0	0	0	+	+
UGT1A3	?	+	+	+	+
UGT1A6	0	0	0	+	+
UGTB7	?	+	+	+	+
UGTB17	?	+	+	+	+
EPHX1	+	+	+	+	+
EPHX2	?	+	+	+	+
SULT1A1	?	+	+	+	+
SULT1A3	?	+	+	+	+
SULT2A1	0	0	+	+	+

+, activity or protein detectable; 0, activity or protein not detectable; ?, undetermined.
Abbreviations: *EPHX*, epoxide hydrolase; *GST*, glutathione S-transferase; *NAT*, *N*-acetyltransferase; SULT, sulfotransferase; *UGT*, uridine 5′-diphospho-glucuronosyltransferase.
Adapted from Blake MJ, Castro L, Leeder JS, Kearns GL. Ontogeny of drug metabolizing enzymes in the neonate. Semin Fetal Neonatal Med 2005;10:123–138.

adaptations. Renal function begins to mature early during fetal organogenesis and is complete by early childhood. Increases in glomerular filtration rate (GFR) result from both nephrogenesis, a process that is completed by 34 weeks of gestation, and changes in renal and intrarenal blood flow [49]. GFR varies widely among different postconceptional ages and ranges from approximately 2–4 mL/min/1.73 m^2 in term neonates to a low of 0.6–0.8 mL/min/1.73 m^2 in preterm neonates. GFR increases rapidly during the first 2 weeks of life, then more slowly until adult values are reached by 8–12 months of postnatal age [50, 51] (Table 24.3). Development impacts not only GFR but also tubular secretion, which is immature at birth and reaches adult capacity during the first year of life (Fig. 25.1, panel D).

TABLE 24.3 Glomerular filtration rate (GFR) according to age.

Age (sex)	Mean GFR ± SD (mL/min/1.73 m^2)
1 week (males and females)	40.6 ± 14.8
2-8 weeks (males and females)	65.8 ± 24.8
>8 weeks	95.7 ± 21.7
2–12 years (males and females)	133.0 ± 27.0
13–21 years (males)	140.0 ± 30.0
13–21 years (females)	126.0 ± 22.0

Reproduced with permission from National Kidney Foundation. Clinical practice guidelines. Available from: http://www.kidney.org/professionals/kdoqi/guidelines_ckd/Gif_File/kck_t24.gif.

Developmental changes that occur in renal function are better characterized than for any other organ system. For drugs that have substantial renal clearance, kidney function serves as a major determinant of age-specific drug dosing regimens. Failure to account for the ontogeny of renal function and adjust dosing regimens accordingly can result in a degree of systemic exposure that increases the risk of drug-associated adverse events. For example, digoxin is predominantly eliminated by the kidneys and its plasma clearance is markedly reduced in neonates and young infants, approaching adult values only when both GFR and active tubular secretory capacity mature (Fig. 24.1, panel D) [52]. Failure to adjust the digoxin dose and dosing interval to compensate for developmentally associated differences in its plasma clearance can result in significant toxicity, especially given the low therapeutic index for this drug [53]. Another example is provided by gentamicin for which a starting dosage interval of 12 hours in infants of any gestational age, or a starting dosage interval of 24 h for infants of less than 30 weeks gestational age, has been shown to lead to serum gentamicin trough levels in the toxic range [54]. It is also important to note that use of some medications concomitantly (i.e., betamethasone and indomethacin) may alter the normal progress of renal maturation in the neonate [55]. Therefore both maturation and the effects of concomitant drug treatment can affect renal function and are important to consider when selecting appropriate drug treatments for neonates and infants.

As denoted before, development produces profound differences in processes that collectively can influence all facets of drug disposition (i.e., absorption, distribution, metabolism, and excretion). Knowledge of the impact of ontogeny on the physiologic determinants of these processes enables prediction of how development per se can impact PK, and also enables prescribers to use this information as a tool to design age-appropriate pediatric drug regimens. A review by Rakhmanina and van den Anker describes the implications of developmental PK on pediatric therapeutics, and the information presented is summarized in Table 24.4 [56].

Developmental pharmacodynamics

As with drug disposition, drug action appears in many instances to have a profound dependence upon development. Developmental PD has been described as the study of age-related maturation of the structure and function of biologic systems and how this affects drug response. Relative to PK data, there is paucity of information regarding developmental PD. However, studies in animals and the few studies that have been conducted in children provide important insight into some of the potential differences that must be considered in the pediatric age group.

Drug receptors

There is evidence that differences in receptor number, density, distribution, function, and ligand affinity differ among children of differing ages and adults. Much of the data demonstrating these differences has been acquired from studies of the central and peripheral nervous systems. Specifically, receptors for γ-aminobutyric acid (GABA), the most prevalent inhibitory neurotransmitter, have been found in animals to be reduced early in infancy [57]. A study in humans found that the $GABA_A$ receptor, which binds benzodiazepines and barbiturates, has significantly higher CNS expression levels at the age of 2 years as compared to older children and adults [58]. These data suggest that the GABA receptors have a rapid increase in expression early in infancy that subsequently declines with age. In addition, there is evidence in animal models that GABA actually has excitatory functions early in development because neurons have relatively high chloride concentrations when GABA opens chloride channels, and this leads to neuronal depolarization and excitation. With maturation, intracellular chloride concentrations decrease when GABA opens these channels, causing neuronal hyperpolarization and inhibition of excitation. These changes may explain why infants require relatively larger doses of antiepileptic medications (e.g., midazolam) to control seizures and furthermore explain why some infants experience seizures when treated with benzodiazepines. In animal studies, neonatal exposure to GABAergic agents (anticonvulsants, IV and inhaled anesthetics) during synaptogenesis accelerates apoptotic cell death in the CNS [59]. On the other hand, GABA has a trophic role early in brain development, so interference with the neurotransmitter early in life may affect neurodevelopment and cognitive deficits such as reported in children who were exposed to phenobarbital in utero [58].

Another example of CNS receptor development is provided by the μ-opioid receptor, the numbers of which are markedly reduced by >50% in newborn as compared to adult rats [60, 61]. Regional opioid receptor distribution in the brain also exhibits developmental differences. In neonates, receptor density is lower in the areas of the brain responsible for analgesic effect (e.g., cortex, thalamus, hippocampus) as compared to those areas of the brain responsible for autonomic side effects (e.g., pons, medulla, hypothalamus) where receptor density approximates that observed in adults [60, 62]. These findings suggest that the analgesic efficacy of opiates in neonates is limited by their side-effect profile because the relatively higher doses required for desired effect may not be tolerated. Finally, CNS developmental changes have been suggested for the glutamate receptors, and

TABLE 24.4 Summary of developmentally dependent changes in drug disposition.

Physiologic system	Age-related trends	Pharmacokinetic implications	Clinical implications
Gastrointestinal tract	Neonates and young infants: reduced and irregular peristalsis with prolonged gastric emptying time. Neonates: greater intragastric pH (>4) relative to infants. Infants: enhanced lower GI motility	Slower rate of drug absorption (e.g., increased T_{max}) without compensatory compromise in the extent of bioavailability. Reduced retention of suppository formulations	Potential delay in the onset of drug action following oral administration. Potential for reduced extent of bioavailability from rectally administered drugs
Integument	Neonates and young infants: thinner stratum corneum (neonates only), greater cutaneous perfusion, enhanced hydration and greater ratio of total BSA to body mass	Enhanced rate and extent of percutaneous drug absorption. Greater relative exposure of topically applied drugs as compared to adults	Enhanced percutaneous bioavailability and potential for toxicity. Need to reduce amount of drugs applied to skin
Body compartments	Neonates and infants: decreased fat, decreased muscle mass, increased extracellular and total body water spaces	Increased apparent volume of distribution for drugs distributed to body water spaces and reduced apparent volume of distribution for drugs that bind to muscle and/or fat	Requirement of higher weight normalized (i.e., mg/kg) drug doses to achieve therapeutic plasma drug concentrations
Plasma protein binding	Neonates: decreased concentrations of albumin and α1-acid glycoprotein with reduced binding affinity for albumin bound weak acids	Increased unbound concentrations for highly protein-bound drugs with increased apparent volume of distribution and potential for toxicity if the amount of free drug increases in the body	For highly bound (i.e., >70%) drugs, need to adjust dose to maintain plasma levels near the low end of the recommended "therapeutic range"
Drug metabolizing enzyme (DME) activity	Neonates and young infants: immature isoforms of cytochrome P450 and phase II enzymes with discordant patterns of developmental expression. Children 1-6 years: apparent increased activity for selected DMEs over adult normal values. Adolescents: attainment of adult activity after puberty	Neonates and young infants: decreased plasma drug clearance early in life with an increase in apparent elimination half-life. Children 1-6 years: increased plasma drug clearance (i.e., reduced elimination half-life) for specific pharmacologic substrates of DMEs	Neonates and young infants: increased drug dosing intervals and/or reduced maintenance doses. Children 1-6 years: for selected drugs, need to increase dose and/or shorten dose interval in comparison to usual adult dose
Renal drug excretion	Neonates and young infants: decreased glomerular filtration rates (first 6 months) and active tubular secretion (first 12 months) with adult values attained by 24 months	Neonates and young infants: accumulation of renally excreted drugs and/or active metabolites with reduced plasma clearance and increased elimination half-life, greatest during first 3 months of life	Neonates and young infants: increased drug dosing intervals and/or reduced maintenance doses during the first 3 months of life

Reproduced with permission from Rakhmanina NY, van den Anker JN. Pharmacological research in pediatrics: from neonates to adolescents. Adv Drug Deliv Rev 2006;58:4–14.

acetylcholine receptors, and for the serotonin and norepinephrine neurotransmitter systems (Fig. 24.3), which have potential implications for the pharmacodynamics of drugs whose action involves their modulation [58].

Immune function

The ontogenic pathway by which the human immune system acquires full immunocompetence has been well described. As might be expected, age-dependent differences in the action of immunomodulatory drugs have also been reported. For example, cyclosporine, a calcineurin inhibitor has an EC_{50} (measured using an in vitro monocyte proliferation assay and IL-2 expression) in infants less than 1 year of age which is approximately 50% of that in older children and adults (Fig. 24.4) [63]. Furthermore, T-lymphocyte sensitivity to dexamethasone has been found to be greater in preterm infants and term infants than in adults. Specifically, concentrations of dexamethasone resulting in suppression of T-lymphocyte

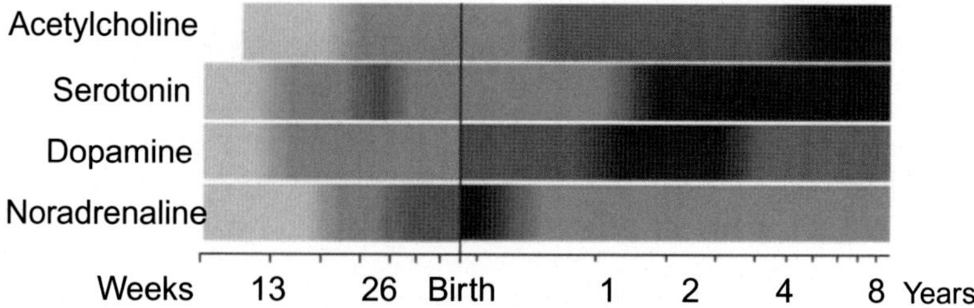

FIG. 24.3 Differences in expression of CNS neurotransmitters in humans along the developmental spectrum. Lighter shading indicates decreased expression and darker shading indicates increased expression. *Reproduced from Herlenius E, Lagercrantz H. Development of neurotransmitter systems during critical periods. Exp Neurol 2004;190 (Suppl. 1): S8–S21.*

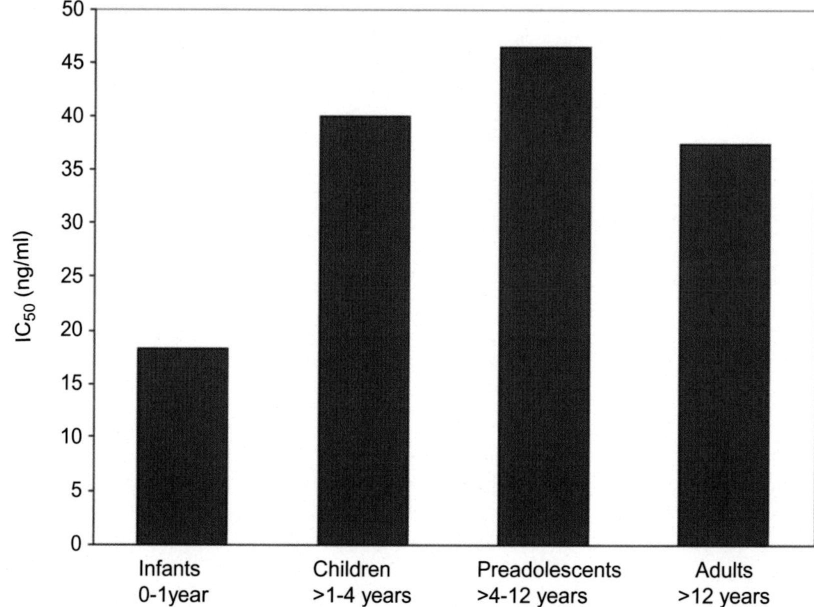

FIG. 24.4 Differences in IC_{50} of cyclosporine across the developmental spectrum. *Based on data from Marshall JD, Kearns GL. Developmental pharmacodynamics of cyclosporine. Clin Pharmacol Ther 1999;66:66–75.*

proliferation in newborns are significantly lower in preterm newborns (0.29 nM) compared to adults (1.90 nM) [63]. Consequently, young children exposed to immunomodulatory medications may be at a greater risk of side effects than older children and adults.

Pharmacodynamic biomarkers

A recent review summarized the PK and PD factors that must be considered in evaluating drug action across the developmental spectrum (Fig. 24.5) [64]. A hindrance in accomplishing this goal is the greater difficulty in defining and validating PD endpoints in pediatric patients than in adults [65]. Simply stated, there are some procedures and evaluations used to assess drug action in adults that, for a variety of reasons (e.g., technical, ethical, lack of conformity with usual clinical care procedures), cannot be performed in children. For example, early in the pediatric development of proton pump inhibitors, it was realized that the efficacy endpoint chosen for studies in adults (e.g., histologic improvement assessed by repeated esophageal biopsy) could not be for ethical reasons (e.g., inability of an infant or child to consent to repeated assessments, risks associated with sedation/anesthesia for procedures) be used in children, so the effect endpoints needed to be different in these two populations [66].

Table 24.5 lists examples of failed pediatric drug registration trials in the U.S. in which pediatric and adult endpoints were not the same. This does not mean that a given drug did not work in pediatric patients but rather that the extrapolation of efficacy assessment between pediatric and adult populations could not be reliably made for regulatory purposes because the marked disparity in effect/efficacy endpoint rendered them incomparable. To address this disparity, there is a need to develop PD biomarkers that are sufficiently noninvasive and robust that they can be used to assess the relationship of drug exposure and response across the developmental continuum [65, 67]. Table 24.6 lists several biomarkers that have been used in pediatrics to assess disease progression or response to treatment, explore systemic drug exposure or effect, or to

Neonate
Adolescent
Pharmacokinetics:
• Absorption, distribution, excretion, metabolism
• Genetics
Pharmacodynamics:
• Receptor numbers and affinity- mode of action
• Disease progression/natural history
• Disease severity
• Co-morbidities
• Impact of growth and normal developmental processes
• Age-specific aspects of disease
• Differences in microbiome
• Genetics

FIG. 24.5 Impact of developmental and age-related changes on pharmacodynamics. *Adapted from Conklin LS, Hoffman EP, van den Anker J. Developmental pharmacodynamics and modeling in pediatric drug development. J Clin Pharmacol 2019;59 (Suppl. 1):S87–S94.*

TABLE 24.5 Examples of failed drug registration trials in the U.S. where pediatric and adult endpoints were not the same.

Indication	Pediatric age group	Pediatric endpoint	Adult endpoint
Pulmonary arterial hypertension	1–17 years	Percent change in V02 peak	6-min walk
Chronic HBV	2–17 years	HBV DNA <1000 copies/mL and ALT normalization	Histological improvement (biopsy)
Bronchospasm	0–5 years	Daily asthma severity score. Pediatric asthma caregiver assessment	FEV1
Prevention or treatment of thrombosis	0–16 years	aPTT and ACT	Death and amputation and new thrombosis
Postoperative nausea and vomiting	2–16 years	Complete control (no nausea, vomiting, or use of rescue medications) within 2 hours following extubation	Complete control (no nausea, vomiting, or use of rescue medications) within 24 h after surgery
Ulcerative colitis	5–17 years	Treatment success defined by Pediatric Ulcerative Colitis Activity Index	Physician global assessment

Data provided by Dr. Gilbert Burkhart, U.S. Food and Drug Administration, 2018 (used with permission).

TABLE 24.6 Examples of pediatric biomarkers with therapeutic implications.

Disease progression or response	Systemic drug exposure or effect	Pharmacodynamic biomarkers
Hemoglobin A1C (diabetes)	CYP2D6 (codeine response)	Plasma drug concentrations
C-reactive protein (inflammation)	TPMT (azathioprine or 6-mercaptopurine effect)	PET imaging and functional MRI
Alanine aminotransferase (hepatitis C)	VKORC1 (warfarin response)	Blood pressure
Exhaled nitric oxide (asthma)	CYP2C9 (warfarin metabolism)	Epicutaneous histamine response
MYCN (neuroblastoma)	Methotrexate polyglutamates (JIA response)	Esophageal pH monitoring (gastroesophageal reflux)
C reactive protein (inflammation)	CYP2C19 (proton pump inhibitors)	AUC/MIC ratio (antimicrobial effect)

Adapted from Kearns GL, Artman M. Curr Pharm Dev 2015;21:5636–5642.

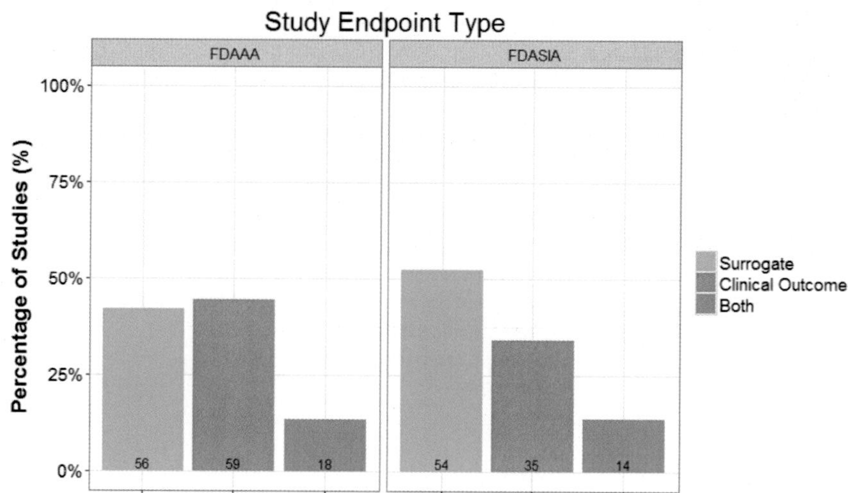

FIG. 24.6 Impact on surrogate endpoint use resulting from enactment of the Food and Drug Administration Amendments Act of 2007 (FDAAA) and Food and Drug Administration Safety and Innovation Act of 2018 (FDASIA). The number of studies submitted to the FDA is indicated by the numbers at the bottom of each bar in the graph. *Data provided by Dr. Gilbert Burkhart, U.S. Food and Drug Administration; 2019. Used with permission.*

directly explore drug action or drug effect. While the majority of these have been used clinically in pediatrics and have occasionally been applied to clinical trials of drugs in infants and children, they have largely not been validated for use in pediatrics. Consequently, this currently limits their application in regulated drug development programs.

In response to the need for more PD information in pediatric patients, an increased number of exposure-response (E-R) analyses are being conducted during drug development [68]. Pediatric drug development programs have applied E-R evaluations primarily to 3 areas: (1) to support the extrapolation of efficacy from adults to pediatric patients when the E-R relationships are similar between the populations; (2) to aid dose selection in balancing the risk benefit profile; and (3) to support approval of a new formulation, new dosing regimen, or new route of administration. These studies illustrate the utility of obtaining E-R information in pediatric patients, especially when interpretation can be supported by similar adult information.

Creative and selective use of noninvasive biomarkers that are appropriately qualified for their intended use, as described in Chapter 17, can add to the current body of knowledge pertaining to the ontogeny of PD response. This is essential to facilitate and expedite expansion of pediatric drug development when E-R relationships are used to determine age-appropriate drug doses and therapeutic regimens. The increased acceptance of surrogate endpoints for pediatric investigations being undertaken as part of the drug approval process is illustrated in Fig. 24.6 [69]. When data from studies undertaken under the provisions of the 2007 Food and Drug Administration Amendments Act (FDAAA) are compared to those conducted under the provisions of the 2018 Food and Drug Administration Safety and Innovation Act (FDASIA), it is evident that the use of surrogate endpoints in pediatric studies appears greater than the use of clinical outcome alone for assessing drug response in clinical regulatory trials.

Finally, it is important to note that pediatric PD biomarkers must have several properties. These include: (1) a predictive association with normal growth and development; (2) sufficient sensitivity to discriminate between time-dependent changes in disease pathogenesis and/or response to treatment; (3) reasonable proximity to a drug's mechanism of action; (4) demonstrated accuracy and precision with repeated measurement, and sensitivity and specificity of quantitation and discrimination; (5) not be subject to epigenetic changes that could influence phenotypic expression of disease and/or drug response; (6) ability to be accurately and repeatedly assessed in a pediatric patient so as to enable time- and concentration-dependent study of PD; and (7) be noninvasive and nonnoxious so as to be well tolerated by the patient and parents [65].

Therapeutic considerations

Formulation

In addition to the inadequate labeling of medications for children, there is also a significant lack of drug formulations that are suitable for use in all pediatric patients. As in adults, oral drug administration represents the most common route of administration. However in 2008, the US Pharmacopeia collected data that identified over 70 drug products that lacked an appropriate formulation for use in children. The Food and Drug Administration, under mandate of the Best

TABLE 24.7 Drugs that lack a suitable formulation for use in children.

Isoniazid	Methotrexate
Benznidazole	Prednisone
Nifurtimox	Isotretinoin
Albendazole	Baclofen
Mefloquine	l-Thyroxine
Sulfadoxine	Zinc sulfate
Pyrimethamine	Sildenafil
Dapsone	Famciclovir
Hydroxyurea	Saquinavir
6-Mercaptopurine	Lisinopril

Adapted from the Best Pharmaceuticals for Children Act (BPCA) Priority List of Needs in Pediatric Therapeutics. Available from: http://bpca.nichd.nih.gov/about/process/upload/2009-Summary-091509-1-rev.pdf.

Pharmaceuticals for Children Act, has also compiled a priority list of medications that lack an appropriate pediatric formulation (Table 24.7) [70, 71]. Many times it is not practical and not feasible to use conventional solid oral dosage forms in children because of the need to administer weight-based doses, or a child's inability or refusal to swallow tablets or capsules. When compared to other routes of administration used in infants and children (e.g., transdermal, rectal, inhalation), age-appropriate oral formulations (e.g., solutions, suspensions, chewable tablets, rapidly disintegrating oral tablets) offer the greatest flexibility and accuracy in dosing.

Even a formulation that is elegant from the standpoint of physicochemical characteristics (e.g., stability, disintegration/dissolution properties) may not provide successful treatment unless it is palatable and has a flavor that is not objectionable. Flavor results from an interaction between the five basic tastes (i.e., bitter, sweet, salty, sour, umami) and odor or smell [72]. Flavor is linked to an oral medication via a basic taste (e.g., sweet) combined with an odor (e.g., cherry) which is transmitted retro-nasally from the back of the oral cavity to the nasal pharynx and subsequently to the olfactory receptors. A large number of receptors on the tongue, oral cavity, pharynx, and esophagus transmit a bitter taste that is commonly associated with potentially toxic or harmful substances found in nature. This taste can be effectively masked by preparing bitter tasting drugs in an oral solid formulation (e.g., tablet, granule, microcapsules).

Because these formulations are of limited utility in infants and younger children, amelioration of bitter tastes has mainly focused on two methods: blocking through pharmacologic antagonism of bitter pathways, and psychological masking to interfere with bitter perception. Sodium salts are one method of reducing bitter taste, and studies have shown that children prefer salty tastes more than adults [73]. Salty tastes also enhance the flavor of sweet in liquid formulations, presumably by blocking bitter perception.

Taste and olfactory preferences are also influenced by developmental stage of the child. Rejection of bitter tastes and preference for sweet and umami tastes are present hours after birth. Preference for salty tastes is not acquired until around 4 months of age. Children in general have a much stronger preference than adults for tastes that are sweet, salty, and even sour [73, 74]. Sweet-tasting solutions have even been found to produce an analgesic effect in both infants and children. Preference for sweets declines during childhood and appears near adult preference levels during adolescence [75]. The olfactory system is well developed at birth, and there is evidence that an infant's preferences for certain odors/flavors are influenced by flavors experienced *in utero* and with breast feeding as well as by culture and dietary experience [76]. For example, children in the United States prefer medications that are cherry- or bubblegum-flavored, while those in other parts of the world prefer different flavors (e.g., lemon in England and Australia, licorice in The Netherlands).

Given the complexity and cost of preparing pediatric drug formulations and the relatively small market offered by the pediatric population, age-specific drug formulations are often prepared extemporaneously by pharmacists. In a few instances (e.g., captopril, benazepril hydrochloride, clonazepam, lisinopril, losartan potassium, rifampin) the approved product labeling contains specific instructions on how to prepare an oral liquid formulation of the drug from the marketed tablets [71]. There also are established compendia (e.g., the European Paediatric Formulations Initiative, the American

Society of Health-Systems Pharmacists guidance on extemporaneous formulations) and primary medical literature which describe methods to prepare extemporaneous formulations of many drugs. When these are used, the practitioner should determine that appropriate data on stability, purity/sterility, and storage conditions are present for the extemporaneous formulation. Unfortunately, the most common practice is to prepare an extemporaneous formulation at the time of dosing by mixing the powdered content of a tablet or capsule (either through emptying a capsule or pulverizing a solid dosage form) with a liquid or foodstuff that is known to be generally palatable to patients of similar age (e.g., formula or breastmilk for infants; cherry syrup, apple sauce, or puddings for children). In these situations, stability of the drug with the vehicle is an important consideration as is accuracy of preparation/dosing and the potential adverse effects associated with excipients in tableted drug formulations. Other limitations associated with this "point of administration" approach to extemporaneous drug formulation include the inaccuracy in dose delivery associated with dividing a solid formulation (i.e., tablet, capsule, or suppository), insuring equal dispersion of the solid phase into the liquid phase of the vehicle, and the accuracy of the device chosen for drug administration (e.g., oral dosing syringe vs. kitchen teaspoon). Finally, it is important to note that, in most instances, extemporaneous formulations have not been evaluated in controlled trials for efficacy or safety. Consequently, it is important to monitor children who are given these medications for efficacy and adverse effects.

Variability in drug absorption by inhaled routes exists along the developmental continuum and is related to anatomical changes through the continuum of life and overall development. The availability and appropriate use of effective inhaled drug delivery devices is essential to the safety and efficacy of inhaled medications in children [77]. However, considerable variability exists in clinical practice with respect to both the suitability of the delivery device and its adequate operation for drug delivery [78]. Effective drug delivery by inhalation also relies on a child's cooperation and coordination. These factors are often dependent on age and cognitive/psychomotor development, which may not be congruent.

Adherence/compliance

Adherence is the medically preferred term to describe a patient's willingness to take medications as prescribed. However, the term compliance, defined as to conform, submit, or adapt, may actually be more appropriate in pediatrics as most children are dependent upon the actions and directions of caregivers who are responsible for oversight of their medical treatment. Until a child reaches an age at which they can self-administer a drug in an accurate, proficient fashion, and can mentally assume responsibility for doing this (generally from 7 to 14 years of age), adherence with a drug regimen is the responsibility of an adult who is able to insure that age-appropriate doses and dosing regimens are followed. Developmental challenges to adherence are observed in school-aged-children (e.g., ensuring adequate access to treatment that may be too complicated to execute in a normal school environment) and during puberty, especially in the face of chronic medical conditions where the adolescent must increasingly assume responsibility for his or her treatment in order for it to be effective (e.g., asthma, type I diabetes, cystic fibrosis).

Difficulties with adherence in the adolescent patient can be the result of normal psychological development whereby children seek to gain independence, question values of parents/institutions, may participate in risk taking and/or acting out, and have strong concerns about views of peers [79]. Average adherence rates in children with chronic diseases are approximately 50% and are similar to rates observed in adults. However, rates have been shown to decrease with increasing age as children enter into adolescence, presumably due to less parent supervision [80]. Several strategies for improving adherence have been evaluated in the pediatric population, and strategies that provide families with individualized and group education have met some success. Involvement of schools and other social supports is also valuable in facilitating adherence in children. New technologies, such as text messaging and automated audiovisual alerts via cell phone and electronic device applications, may also be used in older children and adolescents to foster good adherence practices, and have great promise to "personalize" therapeutics given that they enable real-time monitoring and intervention by physicians, health professionals, and caregivers.

Adverse drug reactions in children

Due to the paucity of controlled clinical trials in children, data regarding adverse drug reactions (ADRs) are generally lacking in this population. Spontaneous ADR reporting is also much less than for adult patients for various reasons, which include: (1) greater off-label use of drugs in pediatric patients; (2) an underappreciation for ADRs that appear to have a predilection for infants and children (e.g., hepatotoxicity associated with valproic acid, weight gain from the use of psychoactive medications, paradoxical CNS responses to commonly used drugs) and cannot always be reliably predicted from adult ADR profiles; (3) the relative inability of young children (especially those that are nonverbal) to report symptoms that may be associated with an ADR; and (4) the fact that available reporting systems are largely designed to capture ADRs in adults. The incidence of ADRs in children has been reported to be between 14% and 17% and to be responsible for 2%–4% of all pediatric hospitalizations. Moreover, 12.3% of pediatric ADRs have been reported to be classified as severe [81, 82]. So despite a lack of systematic data, it is well known that ADRs in children represent a significant public health concern.

The incidence of ADRs is particularly likely to be significantly increased in specific populations, such as the sick newborn, children with chronic disease, and/or in children with multiorgan dysfunction, as these children often have simultaneous exposure to multiple medications. Infants and children are also at increased risk of ADRs during the maturation of organs and biological processes that collectively are responsible for drug disposition, consequent to either inappropriate systemic exposure (i.e., associated with improper individualization of dose) or, potentially, developmentally based PD differences. For example, a recent study has demonstrated an increased incidence of sedation and weight gain in children who are exposed to antipsychotic and antidepressant medications, compared to the incidence of these ADRs in adults [83]. The potential impact of sedation and weight gain is particularly concerning in children as they have potential long-term consequences such as learning disability and obesity-related chronic disease. Other well-known ADRs in children that have life-long consequences include aminoglycoside-associated hearing loss in neonates, developmental delay in infants treated for seizures with phenobarbital, and linear growth retardation associated with corticosteroid use for lung disease. Other ADRs appear to be relatively unique to children, such as aspirin-associated Reye's syndrome, serum sickness-like reactions produced by cefaclor, and behavioral adverse events (increased activity, impulsivity, disinhibition, and insomnia) with serotonin selective reuptake inhibitor (SSRI) exposure. In most instances, the specific mechanisms which underlie these "pediatric-specific" ADRs are not known (e.g., the "neonatal SSRI syndrome" produced by exposure). Enhanced reporting is needed to establish the true incidence of pediatric ADRs, as is the use of current technology (e.g., pharmacogenomics, metabolomics) to understand the biological basis of their genesis and, eventually, to enable their prediction and avoidance.

Special therapeutic considerations in the neonate

In addition to growth and development, there are several other major variables that will influence the PK and PD of drugs used in the neonatal nursery. These include inborn or acquired diseases, patent ductus arteriosus (PDA), extracorporeal membrane oxidation (ECMO), and environmental influences such as therapeutic hypothermia. While a complete description of these variables is outside the scope of this chapter, several of the more predominant therapeutic considerations in these special populations can be highlighted.

Patent ductus arteriosus (PDA)

The ductus arteriosus is a normal fetal vascular connection between the left pulmonary artery and the descending aorta. In utero, the ductus serves to allow the majority of blood flow leaving the right ventricle to circumvent the high resistance pulmonary circulation and flow directly into the descending aorta. This directs oxygen-deprived blood to the placenta, the fetal source for reoxygenation. After birth, the elimination of the low-resistance placenta results in an increase in systemic vascular resistance, and the exchange of air for fluid in the lungs creates decreased pulmonary resistance. Constriction of the ductus arteriosus and functional closure generally are spontaneous after birth, so that blood flow is redirected toward the lungs. Factors crucial to the closure of the ductus arteriosus are oxygen tension, concentrations of circulating prostanoids, and available muscle mass in the ductus. In preterm infants, higher circulating concentrations of prostaglandins, an immature ductus, or an immature respiratory system contribute to continued patency of the ductus [84].

The primary physiological consequences of a PDA result from hypoxia, hypoperfusion, fluid overload, and acidosis. As a consequence, the apparent V_d of drugs may be altered in neonates with a PDA [84, 85]. Thus drugs that distribute into body water may demonstrate an increased V_d as the result of fluid overload. The presence of acidosis may decrease protein binding of some drugs and thereby increase their apparent V_d [86]. Acidosis may also reduce the ionization of agents with a pK_a close to 7.4, permitting an increased concentration of unionized molecules available to cross biological membranes more freely and potentially distribute more extensively into tissue [87]. PK studies in neonates with a PDA have shown that the V_d of several drugs is increased [88–90]. In addition to changes in V_d, a PDA decreases renal and hepatic blood flow, and this may reduce drug elimination capacity [85]. However, the interpretation of drug clearance in neonates with a PDA is often confounded by the effects of pharmacological (e.g., indomethacin, ibuprofen) or surgical treatment of the PDA, which both significantly alter blood flow to the liver and kidneys [88–92]. Therefore the increase in digoxin, gentamicin, amikacin, and vancomycin plasma concentrations with concurrent use of indomethacin appears to be the consequence of the dual effects of decreasing renal elimination secondary to indomethacin and decreased V_d once the PDA closes. As either or both interactions may play a role, drug concentrations should be monitored closely, both when indomethacin or ibuprofen therapy is initiated and after it has been completed.

Extracorporeal membrane oxygenation (ECMO)

ECMO is used in a variety of conditions and is another example in neonatal therapeutics where physiologic intervention can alter drug disposition. ECMO support is used in a variety of conditions and neonatal indications include congenital diaphragmatic hernia, meconium aspiration syndrome, persistent pulmonary hypertension of the newborn, congenital heart defects, and sepsis. ECMO provides extracorporeal gas exchange and circulatory support by pumping blood from the patient through an extracorporeal circuit that includes a pump, a heater, and an oxygenator to oxygenate the blood and extract carbon dioxide. Blood is drawn from a venous access site, preferably the right atrium, and returned either into the right atrium via a double lumen catheter (venovenous ECMO) for respiratory support, or via the carotid artery (venoarterial ECMO) for cardiopulmonary support. Alternatively, access can be achieved via the femoral vein or artery.

On average, neonates on ECMO generally receive more than 10 different drugs per day. All patients on ECMO must be heparinized to prevent the ECMO circuit from clotting, and often receive sedatives and analgesics to alleviate pain and discomfort, diuretics to manage fluid overload, and antibiotics or antiviral medication to treat infections [93]. As only sparse PK and PD data are available for neonates treated with ECMO, drug therapy must be individualized using a combination of existing knowledge of the drug (e.g., expected "normal" PK data in neonates and knowledge of how renal and/or hepatic compromise would impact normal drug disposition), the physical properties of the ECMO circuit (e.g., composition of tubing and oxygenator membrane and their capacity to adsorb drugs to their surface, the volume and type of fluids used to prime the ECMO circuit), and therapeutic drug monitoring data. For example, circuit material, size, and priming fluid composition could affect the increase in V_d that occurs with cannulation [94–98]. Silicone membranes have a higher capacity for drug adsorption compared to the newer microporous membranes, presenting a potential problem for highly lipophilic drugs. While the extent of drug adsorption to ECMO circuit components can be predicted based upon in vitro data, its significance with regard to the in vivo PK profile can only be discerned by measuring drug concentrations simultaneously directly from both the patient and the ECMO circuit. The volume of the ECMO circuit also increases the total circulating volume of a patient by between 5% and 100%, which in turn, influences not only V_d but blood composition, coagulation, and circulation as well as organ perfusion and function. These ECMO effects can compound the innate alterations in function that are expected in critically ill patients treated with this modality. When all these factors are considered in the context of how ontogeny influences drug disposition, it is easy to understand many of the reasons that neonates and young infants have altered PK when they are treated with ECMO [7, 99–102]. The few studies that have been published report that ECMO alters PK for a variety of drugs, including antibiotics (gentamicin, vancomycin), sedative agents, and opiate analgesics [103–110]. Most of these studies have demonstrated changes in V_d as well as total plasma clearance [93]. A recent overview of the currently available evidence on drug disposition during neonatal ECMO has identified the main determinants of altered PK and PD and elaborated on evidence-based recommendations for optimal pharmacotherapy [111].

Therapeutic hypothermia

Therapeutic hypothermia is being used in some centers to treat acute perinatal asphyxia. The exact mechanism of neuroprotection produced by hypothermia is unknown, but is believed to occur via a reducing apoptosis and thus interrupting early necrosis. In asphyxiated neonates, hypothermia reduces metabolic rate and decreases release of nitric oxide and endogenous "excitotoxins," thereby reducing the likelihood that neonatal encephalopathy will develop. The effects of hypothermia on neonatal PK and PD are incompletely understood because there are only limited pediatric clinical data and most research has been done in animals and in adults [112]. Some of these studies were done under conditions of severe hypothermia (28°C), rather than the moderate hypothermia (33–34°C) that is used to treat neonatal asphyxia.

Therapeutic hypothermia causes a redistribution of regional blood flow that may significantly alter drug distribution and clearance [113]. Previous reports illustrate that hypothermia increases the V_d of phenobarbital and midazolam and reduces the V_d of gentamicin, fentanyl, morphine, and pancuronium. Since most enzymatic processes exhibit temperature dependency, alterations in the activity of drug-metabolizing enzymes also are expected [114]. This likely explains why the clearance of morphine in asphyxiated neonates treated with hypothermia is prolonged when compared to a normothermic control group [115]. Decreased renal blood flow may also decrease the clearance of some drugs. However, a recent study in neonates showed that the effects of asphyxia on renal function overwhelm any changes in gentamicin clearance related to hypothermia [116]. In recent years the PK of many drugs (phenobarbital, midazolam, topiramate, morphine) have been investigated in neonates treated with therapeutic hypothermia [117–119].

Pediatric dose and regimen selection

Historically, pediatric dose selection was driven by allometric scaling, in that the dose for a child was determined from their weight relative to that of an adult. Thus if the dose of a drug for a 100-kg adult was 500 mg, the pediatric dose for a child weighing 20 kg would be 100 mg. However, this approach does not consider known developmental differences in drug disposition, and has, in almost all cases, been demonstrated to not be effective in producing a degree of systemic drug exposure for a pediatric patient which would approximate that in an adult. Unfortunately, incomplete developmental profiles for hepatic and extrahepatic drug-metabolizing enzymes and drug transporters that may influence drug clearance and/or bioavailability also prevent simple formulas and/or allometric scaling from being used effectively for pediatric dose prediction. While these approaches may have some potential clinical utility in older children (i.e., >8 years of age) and adolescents whose organ function and body composition approximates that of young adults, their utility is severely limited in neonates, infants, and young children where ontogeny produces dramatic differences in drug disposition. This is especially problematic for drugs whose doses cannot be easily individualized using patient-specific PK data obtained from therapeutic drug monitoring. In the absence of such data and/or established pediatric dosing guidelines, alternate methods must often be employed.

To date, more than 20 different approaches have been described for initial selection of a drug dose for pediatric patients. The majority of these utilize either total body weight (BW) or body surface area (BSA) as surrogates that reflect the developmental changes in either body composition or the function of those organs that collectively determine drug disposition. Selection based on BW or BSA will generally produce similar relationships between drug dose and resultant plasma concentration, except for those drugs whose apparent V_d approximates ECF (i.e., $V_d \sim 0.3$ L/kg), in which case a BSA-based approach is preferable. In contrast, a BW-based approach is preferable for drugs whose apparent V_d exceeds the ECF (i.e., $V_d > 0.3$ L/kg), and this method is most frequently used in pediatrics. When the pediatric dose for a given drug is not known, these principles can be used to best approximate a proper dose for the initiation of treatment as is illustrated by the following equations:

$$\text{Child dose (if } V_d < 0.3\text{L/kg}) = \left(\text{child BSA in m}^2/1.73\text{m}^2\right) \times \text{adult dose} \tag{24.1}$$

$$\text{Infant dose (if } V_d \geq 0.3\text{L/kg}) = (\text{infant BW in kg}/70\,\text{kg}) \times \text{adult dose} \tag{24.2}$$

It should be noted that this approach assumes that the child's weight, height, and body composition are age appropriate and normal, and that the "reference" normal adult has a BW and BSA of 70 kg and 1.73 m^2, respectively.

This V_d-based approach is useful only for selecting dose size and additional factors need to be considered in order to estimate an appropriate dosing interval. For example, when administering multiple doses of drugs with significant (i.e., >50%) renal elimination to neonates and young infants with developmental immaturity in either glomerular filtration and/or active tubular secretion, it is often necessary to increase the dosing interval normally used for older infants and children who have attained more developed renal function so as to prevent excessive drug accumulation and possible associated toxicity. To accomplish this therapeutic goal, it is necessary to estimate the apparent elimination half-life of the drug and to use this estimate, along with age-appropriate estimates of the apparent V_d, to calculate an appropriate drug dose and dosing interval for a given patient.

The primary approaches for pediatric dose selection in drug development continue to be based on allometric scaling and the use of sparse population pharmacokinetic data, but the use of in silico approaches is increasing (see Chapter 31) [120]. Model-informed drug development in pediatric patients is now being used frequently for dose selection and optimization, clinical trial design, and to bridge our gap in knowledge between age groups [121].

Application of pediatric pharmacology to clinical study design

The accumulated knowledge of how ontogeny influences both PK and PD should be used together with available pharmacogenetic information to guide the design of ethical and rational clinical drug trials in neonates, infants, children, and adolescents. The application of these clinical pharmacology principles to the study of drugs in pediatrics is, in most respects, similar to what must be done in adults. What is different are the approaches and, in some instances, the restrictions that are superimposed by facets of normal human development.

Increasingly, in silico approaches are used to design pediatric clinical trials and, specifically, predict dose-exposure relationships. This is particularly useful for drugs for which effective plasma concentration ranges and/or systemic exposure (i.e., area under the curve) are known from adult data and can be plausibly extrapolated to produce similar PD effects in pediatric patients. Approaches to accomplish these objectives range from using simple allometric models to the use of known and/or approximated PK parameter estimates, obtained by applying known profiles for maturation of specific drug-metabolizing enzymes, transporters, renal function ontogeny, and body composition. These estimates are particularly helpful in that they can support modeling and simulation that incorporates the impact of ontogeny on the PK-PD interface.

One such approach is that afforded by the application of physiologically based PK (PBPK) modeling. As described in Chapter 31, these models draw together the physiological and biochemical information that determines drug disposition, and then link it in a physiologically based systems model which incorporates additional information on developmental physiology and relevant biochemistry. The value of PBPK models in pediatric drug development resides with their ability to refine initial dose projection, and thereby improve safety by a more adaptive approach to control systemic exposure. PBPK models also can be used to elucidate mechanistic reasons underlying altered PK during development, to explore the potential impact of development on important drug-drug interactions, and to improve the efficiency of pediatric clinical trials by reducing the number of subjects needed to characterize the role of development and disease on drug disposition and action. About 15% of all PBPK submissions to the FDA are now pediatrics related. These PBPK models can not only help to optimize the design of pediatric clinical trials, but recently have been shown to help estimate fetal exposure from maternal drug administration [122, 123].

References

[1] Shirkey H. Therapeutic orphans. J Pediatr 1968;72:119–120.

[2] Frances BL, Kelsey O. FDA medical reviewer leaves her mark on history. FDA Consum 2001;35:24–29.

[3] Food and Drug Administration Modernization Act of 1997. Public Law 105-115. In the US Code of Federal Regi;atopms 21 CFR 355a.111 Stat 2296, Nov 21, 1997. Available from: www.fda.gov/cber/fdama.htm.

[4] US Food and Drug Admiinistration. New Pediatric Labeling Information Database. Silver Spring, MD. Available from: https://www.accessdata.fda.gov/scripts/sda/sdNavigation.cfm?sd=labelingdatabase.

[5] Song YK, Han N, Burckart GJ, Oh JM. International coherence of pediatric drug labeling for drug safety: comparison of approved labels in Korea and the United States. Clin Pharmacol Ther 2020;107:530–540.

[6] Salerno SN, Burckart GJ, Huang SM, Gonzalez D. Pediatric drug-drug interaction studies: barriers and opportunities. Clin Pharmacol Ther 2019;105:1067–1070.

[7] Kearns GL, Abdel-Rahman SM, Alander SW, Blowey DL, Leeder JS, Kauffman RE. Developmental pharmacology—drug disposition, action, and therapy in infants and children. N Engl J Med 2003;349:1157–1167.

[8] Kelly EJ, Newell SJ. Gastric ontogeny: clinical implications. Arch Dis Child 1994;71:F136–F141.

[9] Avery GB, Randolph JG, Weaver T. Gastric acidity in the first day of life. Pediatrics 1966;37:1005–1007.

[10] Batchelor HK, Marriott JF. Paediatric pharmacokinetics: key considerations. Br J Clin Pharmacol 2015;79:395–404.

[11] Yu G, Zheng QS, Li GF. Similarities and differences in gastrointestinal physiology between neonates and adults: a physiologically based pharmacokinetic modeling perspective. AAPS J 2014;16:1162–1166.

[12] Van den Anker J, Reed MD, Allegaert K, Kearns GL. Developmental changes in pharmacokinetics and pharmacodynamics. J Clin Pharmacol 2018;58(Suppl. 10):S10–S25.

[13] Allegaert K, van den Anker J. Neonatal drug therapy: the first frontier of therapeutics for children. Clin Pharmacol Ther 2015;98:288–297.

[14] Anderson BJ, Woollard GA, Holford NH. A model for size and age changes in the pharmacokinetics of paracetamol in neonates, infants and children. Br J Clin Pharmacol 2000;50:125–134.

[15] Kearns GL, Robinson PK, Wilson JT, Wilson-Costello D, Knight GR, Ward RM, et al. Cisapride disposition in neonates and infants: in vivo reflection of cytochrome P450 3A4 ontogeny. Clin Pharmacol Ther 2003;74:312–325.

[16] Johnson TN, Bonner JJ, Tucker GT, Turner DB, Jamei M. Development and applications of a physiologically-based model of paediatric oral drug absorption. Eur J Pharm Sci 2018;115:57–67.

[17] Maharaj AR, Edginton AN. Examining small intestinal transit time as a function of age: is there evidence to support age-dependent differences among children? Drug Metab Dispos 2016;44:1080–1089.

[18] Fakhoury M, Litalien C, Medard Y, Cave H, Ezzahir N, Peuchmaur M, et al. Localization and mRNA expression of CYP3A and P-glycoprotein in human duodenum as a function of age. Drug Metab Dispos 2005;33:1603–1607.

[19] Mooij MG, Schwarz UI, de Koning BA, Leeder JS, Gaedigk R, Samsom JN, et al. Ontogeny of human hepatic and intestinal transporter gene expression during childhood: age matters. Drug Metab Dispos 2014;42:1268–1274.

[20] Brussee JM, Yu H, Krekels EHJ, de Roos B, Brill MJE, van den Anker JN, et al. First-pass CYP3A-mediated metabolism of midazolam in the gut wall and liver in preterm neonates. CPT Pharmacometrics Syst Pharmacol 2018;7:374–383.

[21] Turner JW. Death of a child from topical diphenhydramine. Am J Forensic Med Pathol 2009;30:380–381.

[22] Choonara IA. Giving drugs per rectum for systemic effect. Arch Dis Child 1987;62:771–772.

[23] Skinner AC, Ravanbakht SN, Skelton JA, Perrin EM, Armstrong SC. Prevalence of obesity and severe obesity in US children, 1999–2016. Pediatrics 2018;141. https://doi.org/10.1542/peds.2017-3459, e20173459.

[24] Wells JC, Fewtrell MS, Williams JE, Haroun D, Lawson MS, Cole TJ. Body composition in normal weight, overweight and obese children: matched case-control analyses of total and regional tissue masses, and body composition trends in relation to relative weight. Int J Obes 2006;30:1506–1513.

[25] Van Rongen A, Vaughns JD, Moorthy GS, Barrett JS, Knibbe CA, Van den Anker JN. Population pharmacokinetics of midazolam and its metabolites in overweight and obese adolescents. Br J Clin Pharmacol 2015;80:1185–1196.
[26] Vaughns JD, Conklin LS, Long Y, Zheng P, Faruque F, Green DJ, et al. Obesity and pediatric drug development. J Clin Pharmacol 2018;58:650–661.
[27] Daood M, Tsai C, Ahdab-Barmada M, Watchko JF. ABC transporter (P-gp/ABCB1, MRP1/ABCC1, BCRP/ABCG2) expression in the developing human CNS. Neuropediatrics 2008;39:211–218.
[28] Johnson TN, Thomson M. Intestinal metabolism and transport of drugs in children: the effects of age and disease. J Pediatr Gastroenterol Nutr 2008;47:3–10.
[29] Miethke AG, Balistreri WF. Morphogenesis of the liver and biliary system. In: Kliegman RM, Stanton BF, Schor NF, St Geme III JW, Behram RE, editors. Nelson textbook of pediatrics. 19th ed. Philadelphia, PA: Elsevier; 2011.
[30] Treluyer JM, Cheron G, Sonnier M, Cresteil T. Cytochrome P-450 expression in sudden infant death syndrome. Biochem Pharmacol 1996;52:497–504.
[31] Treluyer JM, Gueret G, Cheron G, Sonnier M, Cresteil T. Developmental expression of CYP2C and CYP2C-dependent activities in the human liver: in-vivo/in-vitro correlation and inducibility. Pharmacogenetics 1997;7:441–452.
[32] Cresteil T, Beaune P, Kremers P, Celier C, Guengerich FP, Leroux JP. Immunoquantification of epoxide hydrolase and cytochrome P-450 isozymes in fetal and adult human liver microsomes. Eur J Biochem 1985;151:345–350.
[33] Cresteil T, Beaune P, Kremers P, Flinois JP, Leroux JP. Drug-metabolizing enzymes in human foetal liver: partial resolution of multiple cytochromes P 450. Pediatr Pharmacol (New York) 1982;2:199–207.
[34] Sonnier M, Cresteil T. Delayed ontogenesis of CYP1A2 in the human liver. Eur J Biochem 1998;251:893–898.
[35] Blake MJ, Abdel-Rahman SM, Pearce RE, Leeder JS, Kearns GL. Effect of diet on the development of drug metabolism by cytochrome P-450 enzymes in healthy infants. Pediatr Res 2006;60:717–723.
[36] Leeder JS, Gaedigk R, Marcucci KA, Gaedigk A, Vyhlidal CA, Schindel BP, et al. Variability of CYP3A7 expression in human fetal liver. J Pharmacol Exp Ther 2005;314:626–635.
[37] Lacroix D, Sonnier M, Moncion A, Cheron G, Cresteil T. Expression of CYP3A in the human liver—evidence that the shift between CYP3A7 and CYP3A4 occurs immediately after birth. Eur J Biochem 1997;247:625–634.
[38] Stevens JC, Hines RN, Gu C, Koukouritaki SB, Manro JR, Tandler PJ, et al. Developmental expression of the major human hepatic CYP3A enzymes. J Pharmacol Exp Ther 2003;307:573–582.
[39] Min DI, Ellingrod VL, Marsh S, McLeod H. CYP3A5 polymorphism and the ethnic differences in cyclosporine pharmacokinetics in healthy subjects. Ther Drug Monit 2004;26:524–528.
[40] Kuehl P, Zhang J, Lin Y, Lamba J, Assem M, Schuetz J, et al. Sequence diversity in CYP3A promoters and characterization of the genetic basis of polymorphic CYP3A5 expression. Nat Genet 2001;27:383–391.
[41] Treluyer JM, Jacqz-Aigrain E, Alvarez F, Cresteil T. Expression of CYP2D6 in developing human liver. Eur J Biochem 1991;202:583–588.
[42] Blake MJ, Gaedigk A, Pearce RE, Bomgaars LR, Christensen ML, Stowe C, et al. Ontogeny of dextromethorphan O- and N-demethylation in the first year of life. Clin Pharmacol Ther 2007;81:510–516.
[43] Kearns GL, Leeder JS, Gaedigk A. Impact of the CYP2C19*17 allele on the pharmacokinetics of omeprazole and pantoprazole in children: evidence for a differential effect. Drug Metab Dispos 2010;38:894–897.
[44] Hines RN. The ontogeny of drug metabolism enzymes and implications for adverse drug events. Pharmacol Ther 2008;118:250–267.
[45] Leeder JS, Kearns GL. Pharmacogenetics in pediatrics. Implications for practice. Pediatr Clin North Am 1997;44:55–77.
[46] Choonara IA, McKay P, Hain R, Rane A. Morphine metabolism in children. Br J Clin Pharmacol 1989;28:599–604.
[47] Capparelli EV, Englund JA, Connor JD, Spector SA, McKinney RE, Palumbo P, et al. Population pharmacokinetics and pharmacodynamics of zidovudine in HIV-infected infants and children. J Clin Pharmacol 2003;43:133–140.
[48] Blake MJ, Castro L, Leeder JS, Kearns GL. Ontogeny of drug metabolizing enzymes in the neonate. Semin Fetal Neonatal Med 2005;10:123–138.
[49] Robillard J, Petershack J. Renal function during fetal life. In: Barratt T, Avner E, Harmon W, editors. Pediatric nephrology. 4th ed. Baltimore: Lippincott Williams & Wilkins; 1999. p. 21–37.
[50] Arant BS Jr. Developmental patterns of renal functional maturation compared in the human neonate. J Pediatr 1978;92:705–712.
[51] van den Anker JN, Schoemaker RC, Hop WC, van der Heijden BJ, Weber A, Sauer PJ, et al. Ceftazidime pharmacokinetics in preterm infants: effects of renal function and gestational age. Clin Pharmacol Ther 1995;58:650–659.
[52] Steinberg C, Notterman DA. Pharmacokinetics of cardiovascular drugs in children. Inotropes and vasopressors. Clin Pharmacokinet 1994;27:345–367.
[53] Wells TG, Young RA, Kearns GL. Age-related differences in digoxin toxicity and its treatment. Drug Saf 1992;7:135–151.
[54] Davies MW, Cartwright DW. Gentamicin dosage intervals in neonates: longer dosage interval- -less toxicity. J Paediatr Child Health 1998;34:577–580.
[55] van den Anker JN, Hop WC, de Groot R, van der Heijden BJ, Broerse HM, Lindemans J, et al. Effects of prenatal exposure to betamethasone and indomethacin on the glomerular filtration rate in the preterm infant. Pediatr Res 1994;36:578–581.
[56] Rakhmanina NY, van den Anker JN. Pharmacological research in pediatrics: from neonates to adolescents. Adv Drug Deliv Rev 2006;58:4–14.
[57] Brooksbank BW, Atkinson DJ, Balazs R. Biochemical development of the human brain. III. Benzodiazepine receptors, free gamma-aminobutyrate (GABA) and other amino acids. J Neurosci Res 1982;8:581–594.
[58] Herlenius E, Lagercrantz H. Development of neurotransmitter systems during critical periods. Exp Neurol 2004;190(Suppl 1):S8–21.
[59] Henschel O, Gipson KE, Bordey A. GABAA receptors, anesthetics and anticonvulsants in brain development. CNS Neurol Disord Drug Targets 2008;7:211–224.
[60] Kretz FJ, Reimann B. Ontogeny of receptors relevant to anesthesiology. Curr Opin Anaesthesiol 2003;16:281–284.
[61] Georges F, Normand E, Bloch B, Le Moine C. Opioid receptor gene expression in the rat brain during ontogeny, with special reference to the mesostriatal system: an in situ hybridization study. Brain Res Dev Brain Res 1998;109:187–199.

[62] Freye E. Development of sensory information processing—the ontogenesis of opioid binding sites in nociceptive afferents and their significance in the clinical setting. Acta Anaesthesiol Scand Suppl 1996;109:98–101.

[63] Marshall JD, Kearns GL. Developmental pharmacodynamics of cyclosporine. Clin Pharmacol Ther 1999;66:66–75.

[64] Conklin LS, Hoffman EP, van den Anker J. Developmental pharmacodynamics and modeling in pediatric drug development. J Clin Pharmacol 2019;59(Suppl. 1):S87–S94.

[65] Dinh JC, Hosey-Cojocari CM, Jones BL. Pediatric clinical endpoint and pharmacodynamic biomarkers: limitations and opportunities. Paediatr Drugs 2020;22:55–71.

[66] Ward RM, Kearns GL. Proton pump inhibitors in pediatrics: mechanism of action, pharmacokinetics, pharmacogenetics, and pharmacodynamics. Paediatr Drugs 2013;15:119–131.

[67] Kearns GL. Beyond biomarkers: an opportunity to address the 'pharmacodynamic gap' in pediatric drug development. Biomark Med 2010;4:783–786.

[68] Zhang Y, Wang Y, Khurana M, Sachs HC, Zhu H, Burckart GJ, et al. Exposure-response assessment in pediatric drug development studies submitted to the US FDA. Clin Pharmacol Ther 2020;108:90–98.

[69] Green DJ, Sun H, Burnham J, Liu XI, van den Anker J, Temeck J, et al. Surrogate endpoints in pediatric studies submitted to the US FDA. Clin Pharmacol Ther 2019;105:555–557.

[70] NIH Eunice Kennedy Shriver NICHD Priority list of needs in pediatric therapeutics. Available from: http://bpca.nichd.nih.gov/about/process/upload/2009-Summary-091509-1-rev.pdf.

[71] Nahata MC, Allen LV Jr. Extemporaneous drug formulations. Clin Ther 2008;30:2112–2119.

[72] Mennella JA, Beauchamp GK. Optimizing oral medications for children. Clin Ther 2008;30:2120–2132.

[73] Beauchamp GK, Cowart BJ. Preferences for high salt concentrations among children. Dev Psychol 1990;26:539–545.

[74] Segovia C, Hutchinson I, Laing DG, Jinks AL. A quantitative study of fungiform papillae and taste pore density in adults and children. Brain Res Dev Brain Res 2002;138:135–146.

[75] Desor JA, Beauchamp GK. Longitudinal changes in sweet preferences in humans. Physiol Behav 1987;39:639–641.

[76] Mennella JA, Jagnow CP, Beauchamp GK. Prenatal and postnatal flavor learning by human infants. Pediatrics 2001;107:E88.

[77] DiBlasi RM. Clinical controversies in aerosol therapy for infants and children. Respir Care 2015;60:894–914. discussion-6.

[78] Erzinger S, Schueepp KG, Brooks-Wildhaber J, Devadason SG, Wildhaber JH. Facemasks and aerosol delivery in vivo. J Aerosol Med 2007;20 (Suppl. 1):S78–S83. discussion S-4.

[79] Hazen E, Scholzman S, Beresin E. Adolescent psychological development: a review. Pediatr Rev 2008;29:161–168.

[80] Bender B, Wamboldt FS, O'Connor SL, Rand C, Stanley S, Milgrom H, et al. Measurement of children's asthma medication adherence by self report, mother report, canister weight, and Doser CT. Ann Allergy Asthma Immunol 2000;85:416–421.

[81] Martinez-Mir I, Garcia-Lopez M, Palop V, Ferrer JM, Rubio E, Morales-Olivas FJ. A prospective study of adverse drug reactions in hospitalized children. Br J Clin Pharmacol 1999;47:681–688.

[82] Gonzalez-Martin G, Caroca CM, Paris E. Adverse drug reactions (ADRs) in hospitalized pediatric patients. a prospective study. Int J Clin Pharmacol Ther 1998;36:530–533.

[83] Liu XI, Schuette P, Burckart GJ, Green DJ, La J, Burnham JM, et al. A comparison of pediatric and adult safety studies for antipsychotic and antidepressant drugs submitted to the United States Food and Drug Administration. J Pediatr 2019;208:236–242.

[84] Bhatt V, Nahata MC. Pharmacologic management of patent ductus arteriosus. Clin Pharm 1989;8:17–33.

[85] Huhta JC. Patent ductus arteriosus in the preterm neonate. In: Long WA, editor. Fetal and neonatal cardiology. Philadelphia, PA: WB Sanders; 1990. p. 389–400.

[86] Vallner JJ, Speir WA Jr, Kolbeck RC, Harrison GN, Bransome ED Jr. Effect of pH on the binding of theophylline to serum proteins. Am Rev Respir Dis 1979;120:83–86.

[87] Waddell WJ, Butler TC. The distribution and excretion of phenobarbital. J Clin Invest 1957;36:1217–1226.

[88] Collins C, Koren G, Crean P, Klein J, Roy WL, MacLeod SM. Fentanyl pharmacokinetics and hemodynamic effects in preterm infants during ligation of patent ductus arteriosus. Anesth Analg 1985;64:1078–1080.

[89] Watterberg KL, Kelly HW, Johnson JD, Aldrich M, Angelus P. Effect of patent ductus arteriosus on gentamicin pharmacokinetics in very low birth weight (less than 1,500 g) babies. Dev Pharmacol Ther 1987;10107–10117.

[90] Gal P, Ransom JL, Weaver RL, Schall S, Wyble LE, Carlos RQ, et al. Indomethacin pharmacokinetics in neonates: the value of volume of distribution as a marker of permanent patent ductus arteriosus closure. Ther Drug Monit 1991;13:42–45.

[91] van den Anker JN, Hop WC, Schoemaker RC, van der Heijden BJ, Neijens HJ, de Groot R. Ceftazidime pharmacokinetics in preterm infants: effect of postnatal age and postnatal exposure to indomethacin. Br J Clin Pharmacol 1995;40:439–443.

[92] Van Overmeire B, Touw D, Schepens PJ, Kearns GL, van den Anker JN. Ibuprofen pharmacokinetics in preterm infants with patent ductus arteriosus. Clin Pharmacol Ther 2001;70:336–343.

[93] Buck ML. Pharmacokinetic changes during extracorporeal membrane oxygenation: implications for drug therapy of neonates. Clin Pharmacokinet 2003;42:403–417.

[94] Buylaert WA, Herregods LL, Mortier EP, Bogaert MG. Cardiopulmonary bypass and the pharmacokinetics of drugs. An update. Clin Pharmacokinet 1989;17:10–26.

[95] D'Arcy PF. Drug interactions with medicinal plastics. Adverse Drug React Toxicol Rev 1996;15:207–219.

[96] Mulla H, Lawson G, von Anrep C, Burke MD, Upton DU, Firmin RK, et al. In vitro evaluation of sedative drug losses during extracorporeal membrane oxygenation. Perfusion 2000;15:21–26.

[97] Rosen DA, Rosen KR, Silvasi DL. In vitro variability in fentanyl absorption by different membrane oxygenators. J Cardiothorac Anesth 1990;4:332–335.

[98] Yahya AM, McElnay JC, D'Arcy PF. Drug sorption to glass and plastics. Drug Metabol Drug Interact 1988;6:1–45.

[99] de Wildt SN. Profound changes in drug metabolism enzymes and possible effects on drug therapy in neonates and children. Expert Opin Drug Metab Toxicol 2011;7:935–948.

[100] Lopez SA, Mulla H, Durward A, Tibby SM. Extended-interval gentamicin: population pharmacokinetics in pediatric critical illness. Pediatr Crit Care Med 2010;11:267–274.

[101] Peeters MY, Bras LJ, DeJongh J, Wesselink RM, Aarts LP, Danhof M, et al. Disease severity is a major determinant for the pharmacodynamics of propofol in critically ill patients. Clin Pharmacol Ther 2008;83:443–451.

[102] Vet NJ, de Hoog M, Tibboel D, de Wildt SN. The effect of critical illness and inflammation on midazolam therapy in children. Pediatr Crit Care Med 2012;13:48–50.

[103] Bhatt-Mehta V, Johnson CE, Schumacher RE. Gentamicin pharmacokinetics in term neonates receiving extracorporeal membrane oxygenation. Pharmacotherapy 1992;12:28–32.

[104] Buck ML. Vancomycin pharmacokinetics in neonates receiving extracorporeal membrane oxygenation. Pharmacotherapy 1998;18:1082–1086.

[105] Mulla H, Lawson G, Peek GJ, Firmin RK, Upton DR. Plasma concentrations of midazolam in neonates receiving extracorporeal membrane oxygenation. ASAIO J 2003;49:41–47.

[106] Mulla H, McCormack P, Lawson G, Firmin RK, Upton DR. Pharmacokinetics of midazolam in neonates undergoing extracorporeal membrane oxygenation. Anesthesiology 2003;99:275–282.

[107] Peters JW, Anderson BJ, Simons SH, Uges DR, Tibboel D. Morphine pharmacokinetics during venoarterial extracorporeal membrane oxygenation in neonates. Intensive Care Med 2005;31:257–263.

[108] Peters JW, Anderson BJ, Simons SH, Uges DR, Tibboel D. Morphine metabolite pharmacokinetics during venoarterial extra corporeal membrane oxygenation in neonates. Clin Pharmacokinet 2006;45:705–714.

[109] Wells TG, Fasules JW, Taylor BJ, Kearns GL. Pharmacokinetics and pharmacodynamics of bumetanide in neonates treated with extracorporeal membrane oxygenation. J Pediatr 1992;121:974–980.

[110] Wells TG, Heulitt MJ, Taylor BJ, Fasules JW, Kearns GL. Pharmacokinetics and pharmacodynamics of ranitidine in neonates treated with extracorporeal membrane oxygenation. J Clin Pharmacol 1998;38:402–407.

[111] Raffaeli G, Pokorna P, Allegaert K, Mosca F, Cavallaro G, Wildschut ED, et al. Drug disposition and pharmacotherapy in neonatal ECMO: from fragmented data to integrated knowledge. Front Pediatr 2019;7:360.

[112] Zanelli S, Buck M, Fairchild K. Physiologic and pharmacologic considerations for hypothermia therapy in neonates. J Perinatol 2011;31:377–386.

[113] van den Broek MP, Groenendaal F, Egberts AC, Rademaker CM. Effects of hypothermia on pharmacokinetics and pharmacodynamics: a systematic review of preclinical and clinical studies. Clin Pharmacokinet 2010;49:277–294.

[114] Tortorici MA, Kochanek PM, Poloyac SM. Effects of hypothermia on drug disposition, metabolism, and response: a focus of hypothermia-mediated alterations on the cytochrome P450 enzyme system. Crit Care Med 2007;35:2196–2204.

[115] Roka A, Melinda KT, Vasarhelyi B, Machay T, Azzopardi D, Szabo M. Elevated morphine concentrations in neonates treated with morphine and prolonged hypothermia for hypoxic ischemic encephalopathy. Pediatrics 2008;121:e844–e849.

[116] Liu X, Borooah M, Stone J, Chakkarapani E, Thoresen M. Serum gentamicin concentrations in encephalopathic infants are not affected by therapeutic hypothermia. Pediatrics 2009;124:310–315.

[117] Favie LMA, Groenendaal F, van den Broek MPH, Rademaker CMA, de Haan TR, van Straaten HLM, et al. Pharmacokinetics of morphine in encephalopathic neonates treated with therapeutic hypothermia. PLoS ONE 2019;14:e0211910.

[118] Nunez-Ramiro A, Benavente-Fernandez I, Valverde E, Cordeiro M, Blanco D, Boix H, et al. Topiramate plus cooling for hypoxic-ischemic encephalopathy: a randomized, controlled, multicenter, double-blinded trial. Neonatology 2019;116:76–84.

[119] Favie LMA, Groenendaal F, van den Broek MPH, Rademaker CMA, de Haan TR, van Straaten HLM, et al. Phenobarbital, midazolam pharmacokinetics, effectiveness, and drug-drug interaction in asphyxiated neonates undergoing therapeutic hypothermia. Neonatology 2019;116:154–162.

[120] Abernethy DR, Burckart GJ. Pediatric dose selection. Clin Pharmacol Ther 2010;87:270–271.

[121] Bi Y, Liu J, Li L, Yu J, Bhattaram A, Bewernitz M, et al. Role of model-informed drug development in pediatric drug development, regulatory evaluation, and labeling. J Clin Pharmacol 2019;59(Suppl. 1):S104–S111.

[122] Grimstein M, Yang Y, Zhang X, Grillo J, Huang SM, Zineh I, et al. Physiologically based pharmacokinetic modeling in regulatory science: an update from the U.S. Food and Drug Administration's Office of Clinical Pharmacology. J Pharm Sci 2019;108:21–25.

[123] Liu XI, Momper JD, Rakhmanina N, van den Anker JN, Green DJ, Burckart GJ, et al. Physiologically based pharmacokinetic models to predict maternal pharmacokinetics and fetal exposure to emtricitabine and acyclovir. J Clin Pharmacol 2020;60:240–255.

Chapter 25

Medication therapy in older adults

S.W. Johnny Lau[a], Danijela Gnjidic[b], and Darrell R. Abernethy[a,†]

[a]*Office of Clinical Pharmacology, Food and Drug Administration, Silver Spring, MD, United States,* [b]*School of Pharmacy, Faculty of Medicine and Health, and Charles Perkins Centre, The University of Sydney, Sydney, NSW, Australia*

Introduction

A hallmark of aging in humans is the development of multiple, coexisting physiological and pathophysiological changes which may benefit from drug therapy. Multimorbidity is the coexistence of two or more chronic conditions and is highly prevalent among older adults across the world [1]. The most common chronic conditions observed in older adults include hypertension, hyperlipidemia, ischemic heart disease, diabetes, arthritis, and heart failure [2]. Overall, the number of older adults with multimorbidity varies from country to country, with studies reporting prevalence rates of >50% [3, 4], with higher prevalence reported in certain populations, such as nursing home residents (82%) [5] and among people with intellectual disabilities (99%) [6]. By 2035, it is anticipated that the number of people living with two or more chronic conditions will increase by 86.4%, with the largest increases observed for cancer (a 179.4% increase) and diabetes (a 118.1% increase) [7]. As the number of individuals aged 85 years and over dramatically increases, the prevalence of chronic conditions such as dementia, including Alzheimer's disease and other subtypes of dementia, will increase as well (Fig. 25.1). This will result in increased concurrent use of multiple medications, commonly termed *polypharmacy* [8], and an even greater potential increase in drug interactions (see Chapter 14) [9]. In addition to multimorbidity, geriatric syndromes are also highly prevalent in older adults. Geriatric syndromes are defined as "multifactorial health conditions that occur when the accumulated effects of impairments in multiple systems render an older person vulnerable to situational challenges," and include pressure ulcers, falls, frailty, urinary incontinence, and delirium [10]. Thus, with the availability of medications to treat many of the medical conditions and syndromes associated with aging, it is imperative to understand the consequences of the high drug burden that polypharmacy imposes on older individuals.

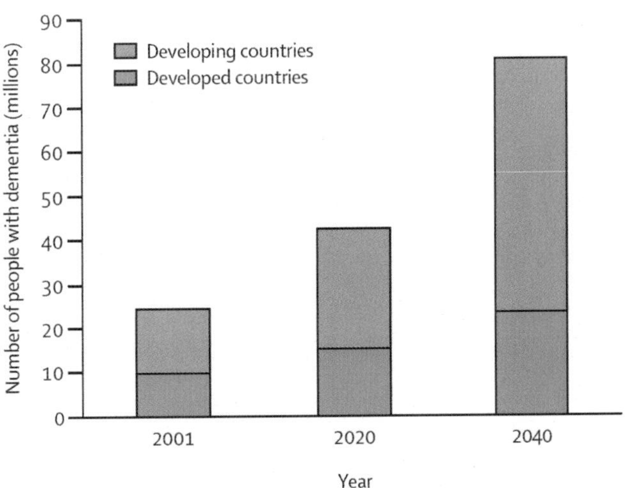

FIG. 25.1 Projections for numbers of people with dementia in developing and developed countries. *(Reproduced with permission from Ferri, et al. Lancet 2005;366:2112–2117.)*

†. Deceased.

Atkinson's Principles of Clinical Pharmacology. http://doi.org/10.1016/B978-0-12-819869-8.00006-9

A number of studies over the past three decades have demonstrated that the likelihood of an adverse drug reaction (ADR) increases with the number of drugs prescribed [11, 12]. The World Health Organization defines ADR as "a response to a drug which is noxious and unintended, and which occurs at doses normally used in man for the prophylaxis, diagnosis, or therapy of disease, or for the modifications of physiological function" [13]. The number of regularly prescribed medications is directly correlated with the risk of an adverse drug event (ADE), defined as an injury resulting from medical intervention related to a drug. Thus ADEs are a broad category of adverse drug effects that encompass medication errors and overdose, as well as ADRs. Compared to patients taking a single drug, those taking five to six medications had twice the likelihood of an ADE [odds ratio (OR) = 2; 95% CI: 1.2–3.2], those taking seven to eight medications had an OR of 2.8 (95% CI: 1.7–4.7), and those taking nine or more medications had OR of 3.3 (95% CI: 1.9–5.6) [14]. Older patients using certain drugs such as warfarin, theophylline, or digoxin are more likely to experience ADRs. However, the absolute number of drugs the patient concurrently receives is probably the best predictor of ADR risk (Fig. 25.2) [12, 15]. This risk is likely to increase as the proportion of older adults in the United States taking five or more medications has tripled from 13.8% to 42.4% from 1994 to 2014 [16], with recent data suggesting half of the US adults older than 65 years of age take five or more medications [17].

Further complicating this issue is the relative therapeutic benefit of treatments such as thrombolytic therapy, hypocholesterolemic therapy, postmyocardial infarction β-blocker treatment, and angiotensin-converting enzyme inhibitor treatment in patients with congestive heart failure over the age of 75, compared to that seen in younger patients. Disease-specific clinical practice guidelines reflect this by including age-specific recommendations for treatment. However these practice guidelines do not adequately account for the presence of multiple comorbid diseases in older patients, with the result that contradictory medication regimens and polypharmacy may occur if all pertinent guidelines are followed for a given patient [18, 19]. This has led the geriatric medicine community to call for patient-centered, not disease-centered treatment guidelines that make adequate provision for older patients with multiple comorbid conditions. Unfortunately, this creates a dilemma in that the dramatic therapeutic advances for many illnesses that afflict older patients have led to the coadministration of multiple medications thereby increasing the likelihood of ADEs.

Polypharmacy in older adults

Older adult patients usually have more diseases and thus take multiple medications, which result in polypharmacy. Polypharmacy is most commonly defined as the concurrent use of five or more medications [20]. However, regardless of how polypharmacy is defined, high rates of polypharmacy have been consistently reported for several decades despite clear recognition of unsafe medication practices [21]. From 1999–2000 to 2011–12, the coadministration of five or more medications increased from 24% to 39% among Americans aged 65 years and older [22]. Because of the dramatic increase in medication use, the term hyperpolypharmacy has been introduced to describe the concurrent use of 10 or more medications. Among older Australian adults living in the community, the prevalence of hyperpolypharmacy is 4.5% [23]. Similarly, about half of the population aged 65 and above in Sweden is exposed to five or more concurrent medications, 11.7% of this population is exposed to hyperpolypharmacy [24].

Polypharmacy should be separated from potentially inappropriate medication (PIM) use which describes situations in which the risks generally outweigh the benefits, whereas polypharmacy usually defines the number of concurrent

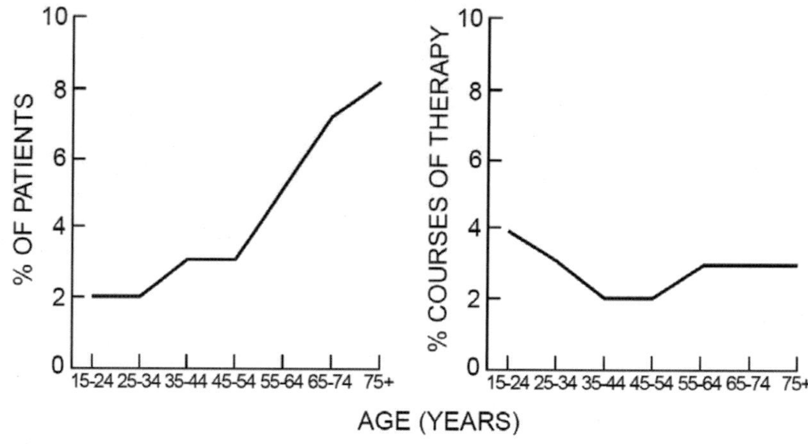

FIG. 25.2 The relationship of increasing age and likelihood of adverse drug reactions *(left panel)*, and the relationship of increasing age and adverse drug reactions when corrected for number of drugs per patient *(right panel)*. *(Reproduced with permission from Gurwitz JH, Avorn J. Ann Intern Med 1991;114:956–966.)*

medications regardless of appropriateness [20]. However, polypharmacy is correlated with the prevalence of PIM use [25]. Polypharmacy in older adults increases the risk of ADRs, inappropriate prescriptions, drug interactions, number of hospitalizations, costs, and even death [26]. Polypharmacy can also be a major contributor to the development of frailty in older adults [27]. Frailty in older adults is a condition characterized by the loss of biological reserves, failure of homeostatic mechanisms, and vulnerability to adverse outcomes [28]. Frailty eventually leads to disability and loss of an individual's independence [29].

Deprescribing, a systematic process of identifying and tapering or discontinuing medications in instances in which existing or potential harms outweigh existing or potential benefits, may help in reducing inappropriate polypharmacy and ADEs [30]. Deprescribing is an emerging and promising approach to manage the use of unnecessary or inappropriate medications in older adults. Deprescribing will be an important way forward in optimizing the management of polypharmacy [20]. Interindividual differences in drug response are substantial and difficult to predict in older adult patients. Thus patient-centered care that considers patient preferences can also be a way to minimize unnecessary polypharmacy and guide prioritization for deprescribing medications [20]. However, a multidisciplinary team approach is recommended to detect, manage, and prevent drug interactions as well as optimize medication therapy in older adult patients [31]. Readers may follow up on two programs that aim to address the challenges of polypharmacy, namely the Scottish polypharmacy guidance on realistic prescribing and the European Union SIMPATHY project [32].

Pathophysiology of aging

Although it is useful to think of the aging process in physiological, not chronological terms, a chronological definition is still often used to stratify the aging population into three groups: *young old*, age 65–75; *old*, age 75–85 years; and *old old*, age ≥85 years [33]. Nearly all of the research which describes pharmacokinetics and pharmacodynamics in older individuals has been obtained from studying young old individuals ≤75 years. Therefore the validity of extrapolating these findings to even older age groups may be questioned. In contrast, the data describing ADEs and ADRs in older as compared to younger patients are obtained from patient populations and databases that include the full age spectrum of older adults. The general physiological changes that occur with aging can be characterized as a decrease in maximum performance capacity and loss of homeostatic reserve [34]. Although these changes occur to different degrees for each organ system or function, they are present in individuals who are in good health and are accentuated during illness.

Placed in the context of response to drugs, it is most useful to discuss age-related physiological changes that occur in integrated functions. Systemic drug responses are the result of the complex interaction of specific and nonspecific drug effects, and the direct and indirect physiological or pathological responses to these drug effects. The sum of these effects is the observed pharmacodynamic response, whether therapeutic or toxic. Therefore the age-related changes that occur in physiological or psychological function prior to drug exposure are helpful in predicting and describing a particular drug response.

The observed pharmacodynamic response is the result of extent of drug exposure, determined by drug pharmacokinetics (Table 25.1) [35, 36], and sensitivity to a given drug exposure, determined by the state of function of the effectors of drug response such as receptor-cellular transduction processes (Fig. 25.3). In this chapter, we will discuss the age-related changes that have been described for renal drug elimination and hepatic and extrahepatic drug biotransformations, and then briefly review the age-related changes that have been described for central nervous system function, autonomic nervous system function, cardiovascular function, and renal function. These functions are selected as each has been evaluated in healthy older adults and because many diverse medications can have adverse as well as beneficial effects on these functions. We will describe and/or predict the effect of these changes on drug pharmacodynamics for drug groups commonly used in older patients. Due to the high incidence and prevalence of cancer in older patients, we will review the information available to guide cancer chemotherapy in this patient group. Similarly, osteoporosis is prevalent in older individuals and we will discuss therapeutic alternatives. Finally, we will discuss drug groups for which increased age confers greater risk for drug toxicity, along with the mechanism when known.

Age-related changes in pharmacokinetics

Age-related changes in drug distribution

With aging, body fat increases as a proportion of total body weight whereas lean body mass and total body water decrease [37]. Accordingly, the volume of distribution per unit total body weight decreases for polar drugs such as digoxin, theophylline, and aminoglycosides and increases for lipophilic drugs such as diazepam [38]. Assuming that the therapeutic goal is

TABLE 25.1 Pharmacokinetic and pharmacodynamics changes in the older adults.

Pharmacology	Change with age	Example drug
Pharmacokinetics		
Gastrointestinal absorption (passive)	—	Penicillins and metronidazole
(Carrier mediated)	— or ↓	Glucose, calcium, vitamin B12
Drug distribution		
Central compartment volume	— or ↓	
Peripheral compartment volume		
Lipophilic drugs	↑↑	Diazepam
Hydrophilic drugs	↓↓	Theophylline and aminoglycosides
Plasma protein binding		
Binding to albumin	↓	Acidic drugs
Binding to α_1-acid glycoprotein	— or ↑	Basic drugs
Drug Elimination		
Renal excretion	↓↓	Digoxin
Hepatic metabolism		
Phase I reactions		
CYP3A	↓	Midazolam
CYP1A2	— or ↓	Theophylline
CYP2D6	— or ↓	Nortriptyline
CYP2C9	— or ↓	Ibuprofen
CYP2C19	— or ↓	Diazepam
CYP2E1	— or ↓	Chlorzoxazone
Phase II reactions		
Glucuronidation	—	Oxazepam
Sulfation	—	Acetaminophen
Acetylation	—	Procainamide

— = no change, ↓ = reduced, and ↑ = increased.

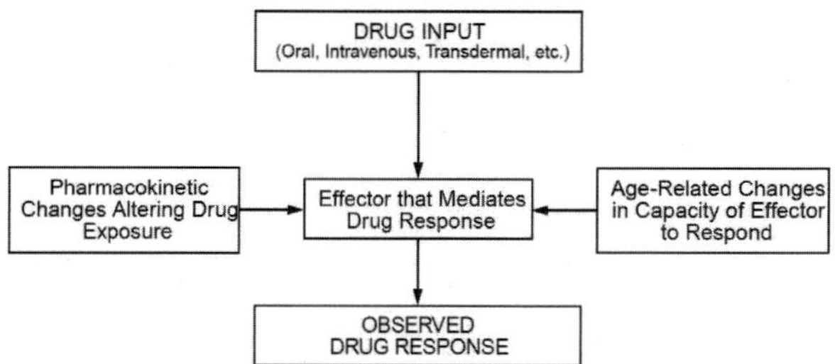

FIG. 25.3 Observed drug responses in older adult patients represent the combined effects of drug input and age-related pharmacokinetic and pharmacodynamic changes.

to achieve average plasma concentrations in older adults that are similar to those in younger patients, the changes in drug volume of distribution will generally be relevant only for drugs which are administered as a single dose or for the determination of a loading dose for drugs in which use of a loading dose is appropriate. However, as discussed in Chapter 2, distribution volume changes will also affect the observed elimination-phase half-life, as well as the peak and trough drug concentrations that are achieved during a dosing interval, and the changes described before may, for example, adversely affect the response of older adult patients to therapy with sedative-hypnotic drugs (see Fig. 2.7).

Serum albumin concentrations may slightly decrease or be unchanged, whereas α_1-acid glycoprotein tends to increase with age. These changes in plasma proteins are generally not attributed to age *per se*, but to pathophysiological changes or disease states that may occur more frequently in older patients. Again, these changes affect unbound drug exposure only for drugs administered as a single dose or with a loading dose [39]. However, the change of unbound drug exposure is particularly important when therapeutic drug monitoring is limited to measurement of just total drug concentrations, such as total phenytoin concentration in anephric patients (see Chapter 5 and Fig. 5.3).

Age-related changes in renal clearance

The most consistent and predictable age-related change in pharmacokinetics is that of renal drug clearance. Renal function, including renal blood flow, glomerular filtration rate (GFR), and active renal tubular secretory processes, all decline with increasing age [40]. Measured GFR is the best overall index of renal function, but it is cumbersome to collect urine over an extended period of time and this procedure is prone to measurement error. For this reason, as described in Chapter 1, the following three formulae are commonly used to estimate GFR based on serum creatinine:

- The Cockcroft-Gault (CG) equation [41]
- The Modification of Diet in Renal Disease (MDRD) equation [42]
- The Chronic Kidney Disease Epidemiology Collaboration (CKD-EPI) equation shown as follows [43]:

$$\text{eGFR} = 141 \times \min(S_{Cr}/\kappa, 1)^{\alpha} \times \max(S_{Cr}/\kappa, 1)^{-1.209} \times 0.993^{\text{Age}} \times 1.018\,(\text{if female}) \times 1.159\,(\text{if Black}) \qquad (25.1)$$

where eGFR = estimated glomerular filtration rate (mL/min/1.73 m^2), S_{Cr} = standardized serum creatinine (mg/dL), $\kappa = 0.7$ for females, 0.9 for males, $\alpha = -0.329$ for females, -0.411 for males, min = minimum of S_{Cr}/κ or 1, max = maximum of S_{Cr}/κ or 1.

The CG equation systematically underestimates creatinine clearance because the decline in kidney function with age is expressed linearly with the CG equation and exponentially with the MDRD equation. On the other hand, the MDRD equation underestimates measured GFR at the higher range, around 60 mL/min/1.73 m^2. Thus the National Kidney Foundation currently recommends replacing the MDRD Study equation with the CKD-EPI equation by clinical laboratories and in clinical practice for those over 70 years of age [43, 44]. The CKD-EPI equation also is the recommended for monitoring kidney function in CKD. However, it has not yet been determined which method is optimal for determining drug dosage in patients with kidney dysfunction and there is a legacy of drug dosing recommendations that is based on the CG equation. The performance of CG, MDRD, and CKD-EPI equations in older adults is often suboptimal. Therefore the recommendation has been made to base dosing decisions as described in Chapter 5 on the results from several creatinine clearance estimation methods and on an assessment of the risks and benefits of providing a subtherapeutic *vs* supratherapeutic dose for a specific patient and clinical scenario [45].

Drugs that are eliminated primarily by glomerular filtration, including aminoglycoside antibiotics, lithium, and digoxin, have an elimination clearance that decreases with age in parallel with the decline in measured or calculated creatinine clearance [46–48]. The renal clearance of drugs undergoing active renal tubular secretion also decreases with aging (Table 25.2). For example, the decrease in renal tubular secretion of cimetidine has been shown to parallel the decrease in creatinine clearance in older patients [49]. On the other hand, the renal clearance/creatinine clearance *ratio* of both procainamide and *N*-acetylprocainamide decreases in older adults, indicating that with aging, the renal tubular secretion of these drugs declines more rapidly than creatinine clearance does [50].

Age-related changes in hepatic and extrahepatic drug biotransformations

Drug biotransformation occurs in quantitatively important amounts in the liver, gastrointestinal tract, kidneys, lung, and skin. However, nearly all organs have some metabolic activity. As described in Chapter 10, in vivo drug biotransformations are commonly separated into Phase I and Phase II biotransformations. In general, the rate of Phase I biotransformation via

TABLE 25.2 Examples of drugs with decreased clearance in older adults.

Route of clearance	Representative drugs	
Renal	All aminoglycosides Vancomycin Digoxin Procainamide Lithium	Sotalol Atenolol Dofetilide Cimetidine
Single Phase I metabolic pathway		
CYP3A	Alprazolam Midazolam Triazolam Verapamil Diltiazem Dihydropyridine calcium channel blockers Lidocaine	
CYP2C	Diazepam Phenytoin Celecoxib	
CYP1A2	Theophylline	
Multiple Phase I metabolic pathways	Imipramine Desipramine Trazodone Hexobarbital Flurazepam	

cytochrome P450 (CYP) enzymes in humans is reduced with increasing age, especially for drugs with high extraction ratios [35]. This reduction in metabolizing enzyme activity may primarily reflect the 20%–30% reduction in liver mass and 20%–50% reduction in liver blood flow that have been described in older adults [51]. However, drugs with low extraction ratio and high protein binding also have shown reduced unbound clearance of 20%–60% in older adults that may be due to reduced liver size and age-related pseudocapillarization which reduces oxygen availability within hepatocytes and limits CYP-mediated Phase I oxidative reactions [35, 52].

Phase II biotransformations are little changed with aging, based on studies of glucuronidation, sulfation, and acetylation [35, 38]. Prototype substrates studied for glucuronidation have been lorazepam, oxazepam, and acetaminophen; for sulfation, acetaminophen; and for acetylation, isoniazid and procainamide. It has been proposed that the activity of these metabolic pathways is maintained with aging because Phase II enzymes are not directly dependent on oxygen for energy production [52]. However, some Phase II biotransformations, such as glucuronidation and sulfation, are reduced in frail older adults [51].

There is limited information on the pharmacodynamic consequences of changes in drug clearance. However, when altered drug effects have been reported in older individuals, they most likely result from a combination of age-related pharmacokinetic and physiologic changes [53]. Frailty in particular is associated with greater exposure to polypharmacy and medications with anticholinergic and sedative effects, which may increase the risk of adverse outcomes including falls. People who are frail experience a higher incidence and severity of ADEs because of their medication use and potential changes in pharmacokinetics and pharmacodynamics [54]. Changes in pharmacokinetics and pharmacodynamics in frailty are likely to affect the efficacy and safety of medications. Indeed, there is uncertainty about the benefits of many medications in frail older people due to a lack of direct clinical trial data.

Age-related changes in effector system function

Central nervous system

It is important to separate age-related and disease-related changes in central nervous system (CNS) function. A number of changes have been noted in the absence of dementia, Parkinson's disease, and primary psychiatric disease. Brain aging proceeds in a relatively selective fashion, with the prefrontal cortex and the subcortical monoaminergic nuclei most affected. In the case of the prefrontal cortex, progressive loss of volume with aging is consistently shown. Age-related slowing in mental-processing function is a consistent finding, but the mechanism is uncertain. Aging has been associated with changes in brain activation during encoding and retrieval processes of memory function. Older individuals have more widespread task-related brain activation to conduct the same tasks as compared to younger individuals. One postulate has been that older individuals need to recruit greater brain resources to conduct the same memory function [55]. Even in the absence of Parkinsonism, the dopaminergic systems are diminished as a function of age, as has been most clearly defined for processes related to dopamine D2 receptors [56].

An important pharmacodynamic principle is that older individuals have increased sensitivity to a given exposure to some CNS depressant drugs. After accounting for age-related pharmacokinetic changes that may cause greater drug exposure at a given dose, the aged individual is more sensitive to the opiate anesthetic induction agents propofol, fentanyl, and alfentanil [57–59]. In the case of propofol, the concentration needed to induce anesthesia in a 75-year-old healthy individual was approximately one-half that required for a 25-year-old individual [57, 58]. A similar increase in pharmacodynamic sensitivity to fentanyl and alfentanil has been described, with a 50% decrease in the dose necessary to induce the same degree of drug effect in older individuals (up to 89 years) as compared to younger individuals [59]. The mechanism for the increased pharmacodynamic sensitivity to these opiates is unknown.

These findings for opiates are in contrast to findings with the barbiturate thiopental and the benzodiazepines midazolam and triazolam [53, 60, 61]. Although a substantially lower dose of these drugs is needed to induce anesthesia or the same degree of sedation in older than younger individuals, this is the result of the pharmacokinetic changes of aging. When drug effect is related to arterial drug concentration, the concentration-effect relationship is similar in young and older adults. For ambulatory older adult patients, the clinical consequences of increased exposure to benzodiazepines due to decreased Phase I metabolic clearance can be devastating, with an increased incidence of hip fracture noted in older patients taking long half-life benzodiazepines [62]. These drugs (e.g., flurazepam and diazepam) undergo Phase I biotransformation, and the decreased clearance observed in older adults results in markedly greater drug accumulation, even when taken once daily as a sedative-hypnotic [63, 64].

There are fewer data on adverse drug effects caused by neuroleptic and antidepressant drugs in older patients. However, as shown in Fig. 25.4, older patients have three- to fivefold higher incidence of tardive dyskinesia than younger patients when "typical" neuroleptics (e.g., phenothiazines and haloperidol) are administered [65–67]. The incidence of neuroleptic-induced tardive dyskinesia is lower among younger individuals (3%–5% per year) and higher in middle-aged and older adult patients, particularly women in whom incidence rates are as high as 30% after 1 year of cumulative exposure to neuroleptics [68]. Across studies, 10%–20% of younger patients develop tardive dyskinesia after 3 years or more of neuroleptic treatment, while 40%–60% of older patients are affected within the same treatment period [67]. It is unknown if this is related to age-dependent pharmacokinetic or pharmacodynamic changes. The relatively newer neuroleptics, such as risperidone and olanzapine, have a much lower incidence of tardive dyskinesia in all patient groups studied and may be of greater clinical utility for this reason [69]. However, it should be noted that all neuroleptics are associated with increased mortality in older patients [70, 71], and, although they are often prescribed for behavioral and psychological symptoms in dementia, there is no evidence for their efficacy for this indication [72].

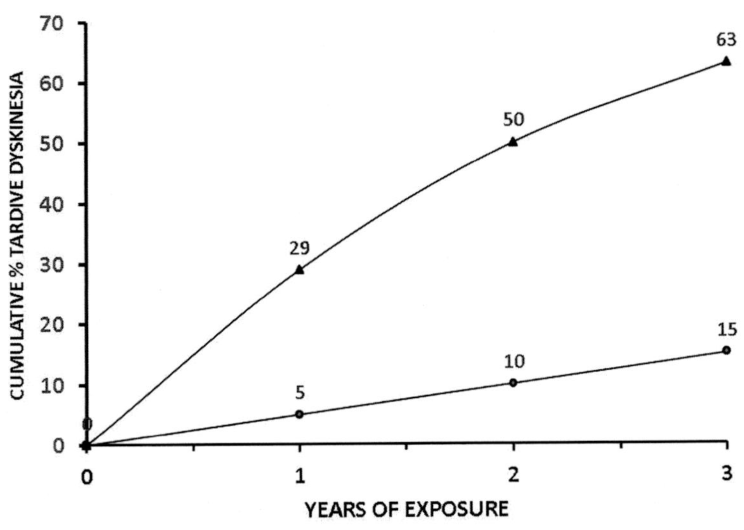

FIG. 25.4 Cumulative incidence of neuroleptic-induced tardive dyskinesia in old (▲) and young (•) adults. *(Data from Jeste DV, Rockwell E, Harris MJ, Lohr JB, Lacro J. Am J Geriatr Psychiatry 1999;7:70–6; Kane JM, Woerner M, Lieberman J. J Clin Psychopharmacol 1988;8:52S–6S.)*

There has been less comprehensive analysis of other classes of CNS active drugs, but the general clinical impression is that older patients are more sensitive to side effects and require a lower dose of drug to achieve similar therapeutic benefit. Pharmacokinetic studies of lithium, which undergoes renal elimination, and tricyclic antidepressants, which undergo Phase I biotransformation, show decreased clearance on the basis of age-related decrease in renal function and age-related decrease in Phase I drug-metabolizing capacity, respectively [47, 73]. In addition, drugs in a wide range of therapeutic classes, such as antihypertensives, antiarrhythmics, antihistamines, antidepressants, and neuroleptics, have "off-target" anticholinergic and sedative drug effects, and sensitivity to these drug effects is also greater in older patients. This is at least partly due to their increased central nervous system depressant effects in older patients. The need for tools and methods to evaluate anticholinergic and sedative drug effects on functional impairment in older individuals has prompted development of a *Drug Burden Index* that links extent of anticholinergic and sedative drug exposure to physical functional status [74, 75]. Although not conclusively established, this tool also may help predict future decreased functional status in the context of anticholinergic and/or sedative drug exposure [76, 77].

Autonomic nervous system

The age-related changes in autonomic nervous system (ANS) function are very diverse and are likely to be associated with many of the age-related changes observed in drug response and toxicity across many therapeutic classes of drugs. Thermoregulatory homeostasis is impaired in older adults who have a higher thermoreceptor threshold with decreased sweating when perspiration is initiated and are thus more susceptible to heatstroke [78]. Cardiovagal function is diminished, as indicated by age-related decreases in resting heart rate and beat-to-beat heart rate variability. Older individuals have lower vagal tone, as indicated by a reduced increase in heart rate increase when atropine is administered. Other findings consistent with this conclusion are that older individuals have decreased heart rate variation with deep breathing and reduced increases in heart rate in response to standing. Baroreflex function is also impaired in healthy older adults, and this is accentuated in the presence of illnesses such as hypertension and diabetes mellitus that are common in older patients [78]. Cardiac sympathetic function is also altered, as demonstrated by decreased tachycardic response to isoproterenol and increased circulating plasma norepinephrine concentrations [79, 80]. Orthostatic hypotension is substantially increased in older individuals and is an integrated response that reflects many of these age-related ANS changes [81]. Orthostatic hypotension may be particularly evident in older patients in the postprandial state [82] and may be exacerbated when older patients are treated with diuretics [83] or antihypertensive medications, which have recently been shown to be associated in older adults with an increased risk of serious injuries such as falls and hip fractures [84, 85].

Data that conclusively establish that altered drug effects result from impaired ANS function are sparse, perhaps due to the difficulty in ascribing a particular drug effect to a particular ANS function. However, the administration of drugs that cause sympathetic blockade, such as typical neuroleptics and tricyclic antidepressants, to patients with increased baseline orthostatic hypotension is likely to be a contributing factor to the increased incidence of hip fracture noted in patients receiving these drugs [86]. Similarly, the anticholinergic effects of many drugs, including antihistamines and neuroleptics, may not only accentuate orthostatic blood pressure changes, but may also be associated with greater cognitive impairment in older individuals. Impaired thermoregulation under baseline conditions may also be accentuated by administration of these drugs because their potent anticholinergic effects further disable thermoregulatory responses. It is unclear at this time how age-related ANS changes may relate to the cardiac proarrhythmic effects of drugs that prolong the electrocardiographic QT interval. However, there is a clear association of increasing age with the proarrhythmic effects of neuroleptic drugs [87]. It is clear that these ANS changes markedly alter systemic cardiovascular responses to a drug such as the α- and β-adrenergic blocking drug labetalol, which, as shown in Fig. 25.5, lowers blood pressure to a greater extent in older than in younger hypertensive patients while decreasing heart rate to a much lesser extent [88].

Cardiovascular function

The age-related changes in cardiovascular function that relate to drug responses are typically separated into changes in cardiac function and changes in peripheral vascular function. However, this separation must be made with the understanding that the pharmacodynamic responses seen are generally an integrated function of ANS, cardiac, and peripheral vascular function.

Cardiac output at rest is not substantially changed with age in the absence of superimposed cardiac disease. However, components of the cardiac cycle are indeed changed. Heart rate is decreased, reflecting the decrease in parasympathetic withdrawal noted previously, and perhaps impaired β-adrenergic and sinoatrial function. Left ventricular mass and left ventricular stroke volume are increased, which allows cardiac output to be maintained in the face of a decreased heart rate. However, diastolic relaxation is slowed, making the late left ventricular filling that is associated with atrial contraction a

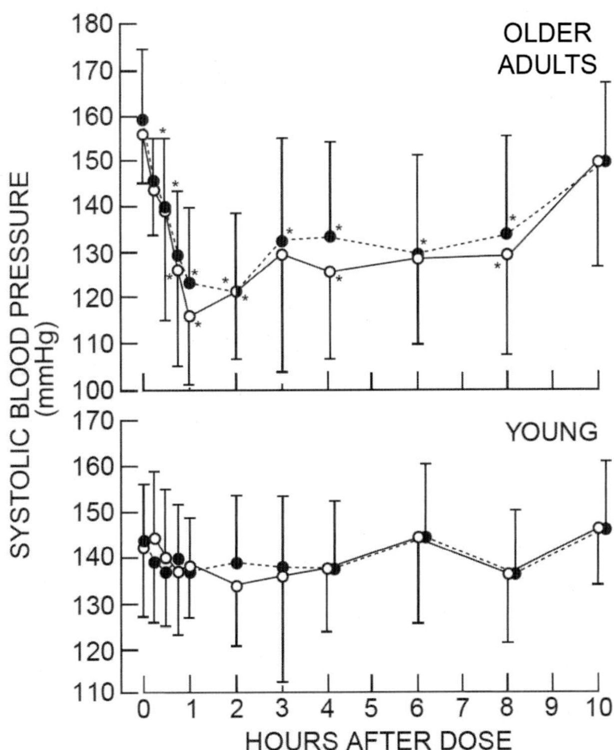

FIG. 25.5 Comparison of changes in erect (○——○) and sitting (●– –●) systolic blood pressures between older adults *(upper panel)* and young *(lower panel)* hypertensive patients treated with a daily oral labetalol 200mg dose. *Bars* represent the standard deviation from the mean and *asterisks* indicate values that are significantly different ($P < .05$) from the baseline in that posture for the respective group. No differences were noted between sitting and standing blood pressure for either group. *(Reproduced with permission from Abernethy, et al. Am J Cardiol 1987;60:697–702.)*

more important determinant of stroke volume in older adults. Chronotropic response to β-adrenergic stimulation is impaired, but it is uncertain if this is the cause or the result of increased circulating norepinephrine levels [89]. Cellular and molecular mechanisms for these changes have been studied in some detail in animal models and may offer some insight into drug responses. The prolonged left ventricular contraction period and slowed diastolic relaxation may be associated with decreased uptake of calcium by the sarcoplasmic reticulum [90]. Many potential mechanisms for the impairment in β-adrenoceptor function have been suggested, but this remains controversial.

The pharmacodynamic consequences of these age-related changes can be substantial. Impaired β_1-adrenergic responsiveness results in a decreased tachycardic response to both direct pharmacologic stimulation by drugs, such as isoproterenol [79], and indirect reflex sympathetic stimulation induced by vasodilating drugs, such as the calcium antagonist nisoldipine [91]. Conversely, the decrease in heart rate caused by β_1-adrenoceptor blockade is reduced in older adult patients [88]. Although diastolic relaxation is slowed as a usual consequence of aging, this slowing progresses in many older patients to the extent that symptoms of congestive heart failure occur. As many as 40% of older adult patients with clinical congestive heart failure have normal left ventricular function when it is defined as left ventricular ejection fraction ≥40% [92, 93]. When these patients with diastolic dysfunction are treated with loop diuretics, they are particularly susceptible to intravascular volume depletion that is manifest clinically as increased orthostatic hypotension [94]. If the volume depletion is sufficient to decrease vital organ perfusion, other symptoms may occur, such as central nervous system depression and decreased renal function [95].

Vascular stiffness increases with age, even in the absence of disease. This may be due to both structural and functional changes, with increased deposition of collagen and other ground substance evident on microscopic or molecular examination [96]. In addition, advanced age by itself decreases endothelial-mediated relaxation, even in the absence of concurrent diseases, such as hypertension and hypercholesterolemia, and environmental exposures, such as cigarette smoking, that are associated with impaired vascular endothelial relaxation [97]. Not only is β-adrenergic function impaired, but β_2-adrenergic-mediated peripheral vasodilatation is impaired as well, due to decreased β-adrenergic vascular relaxation [98]. The clinical result of these changes is an increase in pulse pressure, with systolic blood pressure disproportionately increased relative to diastolic blood pressure.

The pharmacodynamic consequences of these age-related cardiovascular changes are quite diverse. With initial administration of a nonselective β-adrenoceptor blocking drug, the decrease in heart rate is diminished. However, one would predict as well that the β_2-adrenoceptor blockade-mediated increase in peripheral vascular resistance would be diminished simultaneously. Clinical data indicate that β-blocker therapy for hypertension may indeed be somewhat less effective in older hypertensive patients. However, the available data indicate that β-blocker therapy is as efficacious in older as in younger patients when administered after myocardial infarction or for the treatment of congestive heart failure. Administration of an α-adrenergic blocking drug (e.g., terazosin for the treatment of urinary retention due to prostate hypertrophy) results in greater hypotensive response in the older individual due to lack of reflex β-adrenergic stimulation [99].

The clinical response of older individuals to calcium channel antagonists reflects a combination of changes in direct drug effects and age-related alterations in reflex responses to drug effect. Hypotensive responses are maintained because direct arterial vasodilatation remains intact, even though there is the previously noted age-related impairment in reflex sympathetic stimulation [100]. For verapamil and diltiazem, atrioventricular nodal conduction delay is less in older than in younger individuals, while sinoatrial suppression is greater in older adults [101, 102]. Mechanisms for these changes are unclear but are thought to entail a complex summation of changes in direct drug effects and age-related ANS and cardiac function changes.

Angiotensin-converting enzyme inhibitors may be less effective in treating hypertension in older than in younger patients [103]. The mechanism for this is probably related to the low-renin state and resulting decreased role of the circulating renin-angiotensin-aldosterone axis in maintaining blood pressure in older hypertensive patients [104, 105]. Conversely, available data indicate that angiotensin-converting enzyme inhibitors are an extremely effective treatment for congestive heart failure in older as well as younger patients [106].

Renal function

Kidney morphology and renal function change markedly with aging. These changes have been associated with pharmacokinetic changes (decreased renal drug clearance) and also changes in pharmacodynamics for three drug classes important for older adults—nonsteroidal antiinflammatory drugs, angiotensin-converting enzyme inhibitors, and diuretics—and each may have responses altered by renal aging.

The anatomic changes associated with aging include a decrease in kidney weight that, from the fourth to the ninth decade of life, may fall by as much as one-third. This loss of renal mass occurs primarily from the renal cortex, and results in decreased numbers and size of glomeruli. The remaining renal blood vessels may then produce shunts between afferent and efferent arterioles. The functional result is a decline in GFR that averages 0.75 mL/min/year, but is quite variable. Perhaps as many as one-third of individuals have no decrease in GFR while others have more rapid decreases. Renal plasma flow, measured by para-aminohippurate clearance, decreases more with age than GFR as measured by inulin clearance, and may be decreased as much as 50% in individuals in the ninth decade as compared to the fourth decade of life. The result is that filtration fraction (GFR/renal plasma flow) increases in older adults [34, 107]. These findings also may be related to intrarenal impairment in vascular endothelial vasodilating function as demonstrated by an attenuated vasodilatory response to acetylcholine. Consistent with findings in other vascular beds, intrarenal vasoconstrictive responses to angiotensin II are maintained in older adults. Circulating atrial natriuretic hormone is increased in older individuals, and this may be responsible for suppressing renal renin secretion. This suppression leads to decreased basal activation of the renin-angiotensin-aldosterone axis [108]. As mentioned previously, the age-associated decrease in renal tubular secretion parallels the decrease in GFR for some drugs [47], but occurs more rapidly for others [48]. The decrease in renal tubular reabsorption, at least as measured by glucose reabsorption, appears to parallel the decline in GFR. A final impairment in renal tubular function that occurs with aging is manifest as a decreased capacity to concentrate or dilute urine that results in an impaired ability to excrete a free-water load and to excrete sodium during states of volume depletion [109].

Altered or accentuated responses to nonsteroidal antiinflammatory drugs in older adult patients include decreased GFR with azotemia, sodium retention, and hyperkalemia [110, 111]. A common basis for these effects is likely to rest in part on the increased dependence of the aging kidney on vasodilating prostaglandins that results from the age-related decrease in renal plasma flow. Furthermore, selective inhibition of cyclooxygenase-2 in older patients may decrease GFR to the same extent as occurs with nonselective cyclooxygenase inhibitors [112, 113]. The increased likelihood of sodium retention in older patients may also be associated with the loss of action of vasodilating prostaglandins, decreased glomerular filtration, and decreased renal tubular capacity to concentrate sodium in the decreased urine volume. The increased likelihood of hyperkalemia may reflect a preexisting state of relative hyporeninemic hypoaldosteronism in older individuals, exacerbated either by loss of prostaglandin effect on renin secretion or by increased effective intravascular volume due to drug-induced sodium retention [108–113].

Treatment with angiotensin-converting enzyme inhibitors is also more likely to be associated with hyperkalemia in older individuals [114]. Impaired angiotensin II formation limits this potent stimulus for aldosterone secretion, and this is superimposed on the already age-related decrease in activity of the renin-angiotensin-aldosterone axis. The same drug-induced hyporeninemic hypoaldosteronism is predicted for the angiotensin receptor blockers. However, to date this has not been documented clinically.

Thiazide diuretic-induced hyponatremia is much more common in older than in younger patients, most likely due to thiazide-mediated impairment in renal diluting capacity superimposed on the already present age-related decrease in capacity to dilute urine. Older studies indicated this was an extremely common cause of moderate to severe hyponatremia. However, this may occur less frequently now that lower doses of thiazide diuretics are used to treat hypertension [115–117].

Hematopoietic system and the treatment of cancer

Available data suggest that the antitumor therapeutic response of older patients is optimal when exposure to appropriate chemotherapy is the same as for younger patients. For example, the treatment of non-Hodgkin's lymphoma with cyclophosphamide, doxorubicin, vincristine, and prednisone (CHOP) or etoposide, mitoxantrone, and prednimustine (VMP) is less effective in older patients when dose reductions are made [118, 119]. Similarly, treatment of metastatic breast cancer in younger and older patients with the same dose intensity of doxorubicin-based chemotherapy results in similar outcomes as measured by time to progression of disease and overall survival [120].

However, these findings must be coupled with the known increased risk of hematopoietic toxicity in older patients undergoing cancer chemotherapy. The risk of myelosuppression is increased in patients over the age of 70 [121], leading to the recommendation that these patients receive hematopoietic growth factor treatment during cancer chemotherapy [121, 122]. Such treatment also has been associated with a decrease in febrile neutropenia and sepsis-related mortality [121, 123, 124]. Anemia, defined as a hemoglobin concentration of less than 13 g/dL in men and 12 g/dL in women, is common in older adults [125], and its presence is an independent risk factor for myelotoxicity associated with anthracycline, epipodophyllotoxin, and camptothecin chemotherapy [126]. This is at least in part due to changes in the tissue distribution of these drugs that are highly bound to red blood cells. These findings have led to a recommendation that hemoglobin levels should be maintained at 12 g/dL in older patients undergoing chemotherapy [127]. Irrespective of the age of cancer patients, functional status and the presence of comorbid conditions, such as heart disease, renal dysfunction, and hepatobiliary disease, are the most important predictors of survival [128, 129]. Identification of comorbid conditions by clinical and laboratory assessment and of functional status using comprehensive geriatric assessment has been proposed as the most effective way to target therapeutic interventions in older cancer patients [130].

With respect to the pharmacokinetics and pharmacodynamics of specific cancer chemotherapy drugs in older patients, the goal is to achieve a desired tissue exposure to the drug(s) in the context of the age-related changes in drug disposition described in other sections of this chapter. Specific for anticancer agents is the role of erythrocyte and platelet binding of these drugs. Chemotherapy itself may cause anemia and/or thrombocytopenia in older patients. In the case of anemia, a diminished response to chemotherapy has been described that perhaps is due to decreased tissue delivery of drugs [131]. A summary of reported age-associated pharmacokinetic and pharmacodynamic changes for specific drugs is presented in Table 25.3 [132–139]. However, for many anticancer drugs and tumors, similar information is not available to guide therapy despite the demonstration that such information can be used to treat older patients more effectively.

Musculoskeletal system and the treatment of osteoporosis

Osteoporosis is a highly prevalent disease in older individuals, affecting as many as 75% of women and 50% of men over the age of 80 years in the United States [140]. In addition, it is present as a comorbid condition in a number of other diseases that occur commonly in older adults, including renal impairment, cardiovascular disease, and stroke [141]. Bone homeostasis is the result of a balance between osteoblastic bone formation and osteoclastic bone resorption. Mesenchymal stem cells differentiate either into osteoblasts or adipocytes in the bone, while osteoclasts are of hematopoietic origin. Age-related increases in PPAR-γ2 may decrease the differentiation of mesenchymal stem cells to osteoblasts and increase the formation of bone adipocytes [142]. Other local regulatory factors including IGF-1 are positively correlated with bone mass, and age-related decreases in IGF-1 have been associated with age-related bone loss [143]. Also important is local "cross-talk" between osteoblasts and osteoclasts that involves ephrinB2 on osteoclasts and EphB4, its receptor, on osteoblasts [144]; receptor activator of nuclear factor kappa B (NF-κB) ligand (RANKL), and macrophage colony stimulating factor (M-CSF) [145]. A number of these modulators of osteoblast and osteoclast function have been therapeutic targets for treating patients with osteoporosis in order to prevent bone fractures.

TABLE 25.3 Summary of age-related changes in disposition and effect of chemotherapeutic agents.

Drug	Pharmacokinetic change in older patients[a]	Pharmacodynamic change in older patients	Reference
Cyclophosphamide	–	↑ myelosuppression	[114]
Ifosfamide	↑ V_d, ↓ CL, ↑ $t_{1/2}$ (Dose reduction for decreased renal function)[b]	?	[115]
Melphalan	Dose reduction for decreased renal function[b]	?	[115]
Chlorambucil	–	–?	[114]
Dacarbazine	Dose reduction for decreased renal function[b]	–?	[115]
Temozolomide	–	↑ hematotoxicity	[114]
Busulfan	–	?	[114]
Carmustine	? ↑ Vd, Dose reduction for decreased renal function[b]	?	[115]
Cisplatin	Dose reduction for decreased renal function[b]	↑ hematotoxicity, ↑ nausea	[114, 115]
Carboplatin	Dose reduction for decreased renal function[b]	?	[114]
Oxaliplatin	?	?	[114, 115]
Vincristine	?	?	[114]
Vinblastine	?	?	[114]
Vinorelbine	–	–	[114]
Paclitaxel	–	–	[116]
Docetaxel	↓ CL (CYP3A4)	?	[114]
Etoposide	↓ CL, Dose reduction for decreased renal function[b]	?	[114]
Teniposide	?	?	[114]
Irinotecan	↑ AUC	?	[117]
Topotecan	↓ CL, Dose reduction for decreased renal function[b]	–?	[114, 118]
Methotrexate	↓ CL, ↑ $t_{1/2}$, Dose reduction for decreased renal function[b]	–	[114, 119]
5-Fluorouracil	–	? –	[114]
Capecitabine	? –	–	[114]
Cytarabine	↓ CL, Dose adjustment for decreased renal function[b]	–	[114]
Gemcitabine	↓ CL, ↑ $t_{1/2}$	–	[120]
Fludarabine	Dose adjustment for decreased renal function[b]	–	[114]
Hydroxyurea	Dose adjustment for decreased renal function[b]	–	[114]
Doxorubicin	–	↑ cardiotoxicity	[114]
Daunorubicin	–	?	[114]
Idarubicin	Dose adjustment for decreased renal function[b]	?	[114]
Epirubicin	–	?	[114]
Mitoxantrone	–	? ↑ hematotoxicity	[114]
Bleomycin	–	–	[114, 115]
Mitomycin C	? ↑ AUC	? ↑ myelosuppression	[121]

[a] *Indicates no change, often based on steady-state plasma concentration rather than full pharmacokinetic analysis.*
[b] *Dose adjustment for renal function is in some cases recommended based on clinical experience rather than documented pharmacokinetic changes.*

The primary treatment for osteoporosis is physical activity combined with calcium and vitamin D supplementation. There is evidence that older individuals require a higher daily intakc of vitamin D and calcium than do younger individuals, so the Institute of Medicine's Recommended Dietary Allowance (IOM-RDA) for vitamin D is 600 IU/day for individuals younger than 70 years of age and 800 IU/day for individuals older than 70 years of age [146]. For individuals older than 50 years who have a decreased amount of 7-dehydrocholesterol (precursor of vitamin D) in their skin, recommended measures to avoid vitamin D deficiency also include intake of 800–1000 IU of vitamin D_3 per day [147]. The IOM-RDA for calcium intake is 1000 mg/day for men between 51 and 70 years of age, but is increased to 1200 mg/day for women between 51 and 70 years of age and for anyone older than 70 years of age [146].

Pharmacological therapies for the treating patients with postmenopausal osteoporosis in the United States include bisphosphonates, raloxifene, estrogen, calcitonin, denosumab, teriparatide, abaloparatide, and romosozumab. An effort to review comparative effectiveness among the various agents concluded that although these agents individually have been demonstrated to decrease bone fracture incidence, there are insufficient data to rank the effectiveness of specific agents [148]. However, bisphosphonates (alendronate, risedronate, ibandronate, and zoledronic acid) have become the mainstay for the treatment of osteoporosis. Though as a group they clearly decrease incidence of bone fracture, there are limitations to their use in older patients. Because they are renally eliminated, they should not be used in patients with marked renal impairment (creatinine clearance <35 mL/min). In addition, nephrotoxicity occurs with excessive bisphosphonate exposure, so renal function needs to be monitored during bisphosphonate treatment [149].

The selective estrogen receptor modulator raloxifene slightly increases spine bone mineral density and decreases the risk of vertebral fracture by 40% in osteoporotic women, but it has no effect on the risk of nonvertebral fracture [150]. Raloxifene may be the most appropriate choice for patients at high risk for vertebral fractures who cannot tolerate bisphosphonate therapy, but a primary concern is that it is associated with an increased risk of deep vein thrombosis and pulmonary embolism. Older patients with additional comorbidities that result in low mobility may be at a particularly high risk of developing deep vein thrombosis during raloxifene therapy [149]. Estrogen (estradiol and conjugated estrogens), which act by blocking cytokine signaling to osteoclasts, have also been used to slow bone resorption in older adult patients [151, 152]. Although estrogens continue to be used to prevent postmenopausal osteoporosis and the Women's Health Initiative study confirmed that estrogen plus progestin increased both hip and vertebral bone mineral density. This study also documented that estrogen plus progestin increased the incidence of breast cancer and cardiovascular disease to the extent that these risks are generally considered to outweigh therapeutic benefit [153]. These risks appear to increase with increasing age as older women tend to have higher breast cancer and thromboembolic event rates while receiving postmenopausal hormone replacement therapy [154].

Alternate therapeutic options are available but are not as widely used as other treatments. Calcitonin (salmon calcitonin) has been shown in a single randomized trial to reduce the incidence of vertebral, but not nonvertebral, fracture [155]. Denosumab is a fully humanized monoclonal antibody against receptor activator of NF-κB ligand (RANKL) that inhibits osteoclastic bone resorption [156]. In individuals at high risk of fracture, its benefit versus risk profile is likely to be favorable for up to 10 years of treatment [157].

Teriparatide is the N-terminal chain 34-amino acid fragment of parathyroid hormone. It requires intermittent administration to obtain its anabolic effects [158, 159]. The usual adverse effect is mild hypercalcemia, which occurs in 1%–3% of patients and is usually corrected by reducing calcium or vitamin D supplementation. Abaloparatide is identical to the parathyroid hormone-related peptide through the first 22 residues but with significantly different amino acids between residues 22 and 34 [160]. Teriparatide and abaloparatide are ligands that bind to and activate the parathyroid hormone receptor type 1. However, abaloparatide favors the transient, more anabolic configuration of the receptor. Romosozumab, a monoclonal antibody that binds to and inhibits sclerostin, appears to have dual actions via stimulating bone formation and reducing bone resorption [157]. Both abaloparatide and romosozumab have been approved in the US to treat postmenopausal women with osteoporosis at high risk for fracture.

Drug classes for which age confers increased risk for toxicity

In contrast to the adverse pharmacodynamic consequences described, for which there is at least a potential mechanistic understanding, it is more difficult to formulate a mechanistic explanation for a number of drug toxicities that are more frequent in older than younger patients.

Evidence from clinical studies is uniform in identifying age as a major contributing risk factor for theophylline toxicity, although it is unclear whether decreased theophylline clearance and increased exposure in older patients fully explain this apparent sensitivity [161, 162]. This has resulted in much less use of theophylline in older patients.

Isoniazid-induced hepatotoxicity is more likely to occur in individuals who are more than 35 years of age [163]. Possible mechanisms by which isoniazid causes hepatotoxicity are discussed in Chapter 15, but attempts to establish a pharmacokinetic or pharmacogenetic explanation for the increased susceptibility of older individuals to this reaction have been unsatisfactory. Nevertheless, this clinical finding had led to the subsequent recommendation that isoniazid be withheld from chemoprophylactic therapy of individuals older than 35 years of age who have a positive tuberculin skin test ($\geq$15 mm) but no other risk factors [164]. Because approximately 5%–10% of patients with a positive tuberculin test will develop active tuberculosis and older adult individuals are at highest risk, there currently is concern that appropriate chemoprophylaxis is not being made available to individuals who are $\geq$50 years of age [165]. However, routine patient monitoring has reduced the risk of severe isoniazid hepatotoxicity in recent years, so current guidelines do not put an age limit on using isoniazid to treat latent tuberculosis but simply discourage tuberculin testing in low-risk individuals [166].

Neuroleptic-induced tardive dyskinesia has been discussed. However, the mechanism for tardive dyskinesia is not well established. It is clear that increased patient age contributes significantly to the risk of developing tardive dyskinesia with the "typical" neuroleptics [65–68].

Nonsteroidal antiinflammatory drugs are probably more likely to induce gastric ulceration in older than in younger patients [167]. This may be the result of decreases in gastric mucosal prostaglandins in older adults [168], with drug-induced inhibition of gastric prostaglandins compounding the age-related decrease.

Oral anticoagulation therapy with vitamin K antagonists is more likely to be associated with bleeding, and, particularly with intracranial hemorrhage, in older as compared to younger patients. This may be in part related to impaired drug clearance [169]. Although the potential therapeutic benefit of oral anticoagulation for the treatment of venous thromboembolism or atrial fibrillation (AF) is maintained in older patients, their risk from these adverse events is higher, even when the extent of their anticoagulation is controlled by maintaining the INR in the therapeutic range of 2–3 [170, 171]. Due to these risks and the difficulty in treating older patients with vitamin K antagonists, there has been considerable interest in the thrombin and factor Xa inhibitors that are direct acting oral anticoagulants (DOAC). Consequently, the use of warfarin to treat nonvalvular AF (NVAF) is decreasing, whereas the use of DOAC to treat NVAF is on the rise [172].

Conclusion

Older adults with multiple chronic diseases, polypharmacy, and complex health needs are a major consumer of health care. Although there is little doubt that the risk of a specific drug therapy, such as the ADR of cough for angiotensin-converting enzyme inhibitor treatment of patients with congestive heart failure, is in most instances far outweighed by the benefit of therapy. However, the concurrent presence of multiple diseases in older patients results in their being treated with multiple medications, which itself is a risk factor for ADEs. Therefore it is an appropriate generalization to assume that the risk/benefit ratio, or the therapeutic index, of any given therapy is narrowed for older patients. Understanding age-related pathophysiology can in some instances allow for prediction of age-related changes in drug disposition and effect. The following concepts may optimize medication therapy to care for our growing aging population [173]:

- Recognize the imperative for increased attention to the needs of older adults.
- Continue to explore the development of biomarkers for biological aging and frailty to expand our understanding beyond chronologic age.
- Develop the evidence for likelihood of benefit/harm and time to benefit/harm of drugs for older adults by including more older adults and a population more representative of anticipated actual clinical use (multimorbidity and polypharmacy) in clinical trials.
- Investigate deprescribing of medications as part of drug development to reduce withdrawal-associated side effects and include this information in product labels.
- Assess drug dosage forms for the ease of use and appropriateness in older populations and their caregivers.
- Apply quantitative approaches for model-informed drug development to convert theoretical concepts to quantitative predictions, thereby helping to optimize dosing for older persons and those with multimorbidity.
- Align resources and incentives in the regulatory drug development process, as has been successfully implemented with other patient populations, such as pediatrics, to accelerate innovation.

Disclaimer

The views expressed in this chapter are the personal views of the first author and may not be understood or quoted as being made on behalf of or reflecting the position of the Food and Drug Administration.

References

[1] Garin N, Koyanagi A, Chatterji S, Tyrovolas S, Olaya B, Leonardi M, Lara E, Koskinen S, Tobiasz-Adamczyk B, Ayuso-Mateos JL, Haro JM. Global multimorbidity patterns: a cross-sectional, population-based, multi-country study. J Gerontol A Biol Sci Med Sci 2016;71:205–14.

[2] Salive ME. Multimorbidity in older adults. Epidemiol Rev 2013;35:75–83.

[3] Barnett K, Mercer SW, Norbury M, Watt G, Wyke S, Guthrie B. Epidemiology of multimorbidity and implications for health care, research, and medical education: a cross-sectional study. Lancet 2012;380:37–43.

[4] Palladino R, Lee JT, Ashworth M, Triassi M, Millett C. Associations between multimorbidity, healthcare utilisation and health status: evidence from 16 European countries. Age Ageing 2016;45:431–5.

[5] Schram MT, Frijters D, van de Lisdonk EH, Ploemacher J, de Craen AJ, deWaal MW, van Rooij FJ, Heeringa J, Hofman A, Deeg DJH, Schellevis FG. Setting and registry characteristics affect the prevalence and nature of multimorbidity in the elderly. J Clin Epidemiol 2008;61:1104–12.

[6] Kinnear D, Morrison J, Allan L, Henderson A, Smiley E, Cooper SA. Prevalence of physical conditions and multimorbidity in a cohort of adults with intellectual disabilities with and without Down syndrome: cross-sectional study. BMJ Open 2018;8:e018292.

[7] Kingston A, Robinson L, Booth H, Knapp M, Jagger C. MODEM project. Projections of multi-morbidity in the older population in England to 2035: estimates from the Population Ageing and Care Simulation (PACSim) model. Age Ageing 2018;47:374–80.

[8] Gnjidic D, Hilmer SN, Blyth FM, Naganathan V, Waite L, Seibel MJ, McLachlan AJ, Cumming RG, Handelsman DJ, Le Couteur DG. Polypharmacy cutoff and outcomes: five or more medicines were used to identify community-dwelling older men at risk of different adverse outcomes. J Clin Epidemiol 2012;65:989–95.

[9] Kaufman DW, Kelly JP, Rosenberg L, Anderson TE, Mitchell AA. Recent patterns of medication use in the ambulatory adult population of the United States. The Slone Survey. JAMA 2002;287:337–44.

[10] Inouye SK, Studenski S, Tinetti ME, Kuchel GA. Geriatric syndromes: clinical, research, and policy implications of a core geriatric concept. J Am Geriatr Soc 2007;55:780–91.

[11] Smith JW, Seidl LG, Cluff LE. Studies on the epidemiology of adverse drug reactions. V. Clinical factors influencing susceptibility. Ann Intern Med 1966;65:629–40.

[12] Hutchinson TA, Flegel KM, Kramer MS, Leduc DG, Kong HH. Frequency, severity and risk factors for adverse drug reactions in adult outpatients. J Chronic Dis 1986;39:533–42.

[13] World Health Organization. International drug monitoring—The role of the national centres. Tech Rep Series no 498, Geneva: WHO; 1972.

[14] Field TS, Gurwitz JH, Avorn J, McCormick D, Jain S, Eckler M, Benser M, Bates DW. Risk factors for adverse drug events among nursing home residents. Arch Intern Med 2001;161:1629–34.

[15] Gurwitz JH, Avorn J. The ambiguous relation between aging and adverse drug reactions. Ann Intern Med 1991;114:956–66.

[16] Anon. Medication overload: America's other drug problem. How the drive to prescribe is harming older adults. LOWN Institute; April 2019. https://lowninstitute.org/reports/medication-overload-americas-other-drug-problem/.

[17] Reeve E, Wolff JL, Skehan M, Bayliss EA, Hilmer SN, Boyd CM. Assessment of attitudes toward deprescribing in older Medicare beneficiaries in the United States. JAMA Intern Med 2018;178:1673–80.

[18] Tinetti ME, Bogardus ST, Agostini JV. Potential pitfalls of disease-specific guidelines for patients with multiple conditions. N Engl J Med 2004;351:2870–4.

[19] Boyd CM, Darer J, Boult C, Fried LP, Boult L, Wu AW. Clinical practice guidelines and quality of care for older patients with multiple comorbid diseases. JAMA 2005;295:716–24.

[20] Johnell K. The controversies surrounding polypharmacy in old age—where are we? Expert Rev Clin Pharmacol 2018;11:825–7.

[21] Gnjidic D, Tinetti M, Allore HG. Assessing medication burden and polypharmacy: finding the perfect measure. Expert Rev Clin Pharmacol 2017;10:345–7.

[22] Kantor ED, Rehm CD, Haas JS, Chan AT, Giovannucci EL. Trends in prescription drug use among adults in the United States from 1999-2012. JAMA 2015;314:1818–31.

[23] Gnjidic D, Hilmer SN, Blyth FM, Naganathan V, Cumming RG, Handelsman DJ, McLachlan AJ, Abernethy DR, Banks E, Le Couteur DG. High-risk prescribing and incidence of frailty among older community-dwelling men. Clin Pharmacol Ther 2012;91:521–8.

[24] Morin L, Johnell K, Laroche ML, Fastbom J, Wastesson JW. The epidemiology of polypharmacy in older adults: register-based prospective cohort study. Clin Epidemiol 2018;10:289–98.

[25] Morin L, Laroche ML, Texier G, Johnell K. Prevalence of potentially inappropriate medication use in older adults living in nursing homes: a systematic review. J Am Med Dir Assoc 2016;17:862. e1–9.

[26] Maher RL, Hanlon J, Hajjar ER. Clinical consequences of polypharmacy in elderly. Expert Opin Drug Saf 2014;13:57–65.

[27] Gutiérrez-Valencia M, Izquierdo M, Cesari M, Casas-Herrero Á, Inzitari M, Martínez-Velilla N. The relationship between frailty and polypharmacy in older people: a systematic review. Br J Clin Pharmacol 2018;84:1432–44.

[28] Clegg A, Young J, Iliffe S, Rikkert MO, Rockwood K. Frailty in elderly people. Lancet 2013;381:752–62.

[29] Hoogendijk EO, Afilalo J, Ensrud KE, Kowal P, Onder G, Fried LP. Frailty: implications for clinical practice and public health. Lancet 2019;394:1365–75.

[30] Scott IA, Hilmer SN, Reeve E, Potter K, Le Couteur D, Rigby D, Gnjidic D, Del Mar CB, Roughead EE, Page A, Jansen J, Martin JH. Reducing inappropriate polypharmacy: the process of deprescribing. JAMA Intern Med 2015;175:827–34.

[31] Mallet L, Spinewine A, Huang A. The challenge of managing drug interactions in elderly people. Lancet 2007;370:185–91.

[32] Mair A, Wilson M, Dreischulte T. Addressing the challenge of polypharmacy. Annu Rev Pharmacol Toxicol 2020;60:661–81.

[33] Klotz U. The elderly—a challenge for appropriate drug treatment. Eur J Clin Pharmacol 2008;64:225–6.

[34] Hall DA. The biomedical basis of gerontology. Littleton, MA: John Wright PSG, Inc.; 1984.
[35] Reeve E, Wiese MD, Mangoni AA. Alterations in drug disposition in older adults. Expert Opin Drug Metab Toxicol 2015;11:491–508.
[36] Ginsberg G, Hattis D, Russ A, Sonawane B. Pharmacokinetic and pharmacodynamic factors that can affect sensitivity to neurotoxic sequelae in elderly individuals. Environ Health Perspect 2005;113:1243–9.
[37] Borkan GA, Hults DE, Gerzof SG, Robbins AH, Silbert CK. Age changes in body composition revealed by computed tomography. J Gerontol 1983;38:673–7.
[38] Shi S, Klotz U. Age-related changes in pharmacokinetics. Curr Drug Metab 2011;12:601–10.
[39] Benet LZ, Hoener B-A. Changes in plasma protein binding have little clinical significance. Clin Pharmacol Ther 2002;71:115–21.
[40] Davies DF, Shock NW. Age changes in glomerular filtration rate, effective renal plasma flow, and tubular excretory capacity in adult males. J Clin Invest 1950;29:496–507.
[41] Cockcroft DW, Gault MH. Prediction of creatinine clearance from serum creatinine. Nephron 1976;16:31–41.
[42] Levey AS, Bosch JP, Lewis JB, Greene T, Rogers N, Roth D. A more accurate method to estimate glomerular filtration rate from serum creatinine: a new prediction equation. Modification of Diet in Renal Disease Study Group. Ann Intern Med 1999;130:461–70.
[43] Stevens LA, Li S, Kurella Tamura M, Chen SC, Vassalotti JA, Norris KC, Whaley-Connell AT, Bakris GL, McCullough PA. Comparison of the CKD Epidemiology Collaboration (CKD-EPI) and Modification of Diet in Renal Disease (MDRD) study equations: risk factors for and complications of CKD and mortality in the Kidney Early Evaluation Program (KEEP). Am J Kidney Dis 2011;57(Suppl. 2):S9–16.
[44] College of American Pathologists. Current status of reporting eGFR, http://www.cap.org/apps/docs/committees/chemistry/current_ status_reporting_egfr_09.pdf; 2010.
[45] Hart LA, Anderson GD. Methods of estimating kidney function for drug dosing in special populations. Clin Pharmacokinet 2018;57:943–76.
[46] Bauer LA, Blouin RA. Age and phenytoin kinetics in adult epileptics. Clin Pharmacol Ther 1982;31:301–4.
[47] Sproule BA, Hardy BG, Shulman KI. Differential pharmacokinetics of lithium in elderly patients. Drugs Aging 2000;16:165–77.
[48] Cusack B, Kelly J, O'Malley K, Noel J, Lavan J, Horgan J. Digoxin in the elderly: pharmacokinetic consequences of old age. Clin Pharmacol Ther 1979;25:772–6.
[49] Drayer DE, Romankiewicz J, Lorenzo B, Reidenberg MM. Age and renal clearance of cimetidine. Clin Pharmacol Ther 1982;31:45–60.
[50] Reidenberg MM, Camacho M, Kluger J, Drayer DE. Aging and renal clearance of procainamide and acetylprocainamide. Clin Pharmacol Ther 1980;28:732–5.
[51] Reeve E, Trenaman SC, Rockwood K, Hilmer SN. Pharmacokinetic and pharmacodynamic alterations in older people with dementia. Expert Opin Drug Metab Toxicol 2017;13:651–68.
[52] McLean AJ, Le Couterur D. Aging biology and geriatric clinical pharmacology. Pharmacol Rev 2004;56:163–84.
[53] Greenblatt DJ, Harmatz JS, Shapiro L, Engelhardt N, Gouthro TA, Shader RI. Sensitivity to triazolam in the elderly. N Engl J Med 1991; 324:1691–8.
[54] Hilmer SN, Gnjidic D. Prescribing for frail older people. Aust Prescr 2017;40:174–8.
[55] Raz N. Aging of the brain and its impact on cognitive performance: integration of structural and functional findings. In: Craik FIM, Salthouse TA, editors. The handbook of aging and cognition. 2nd ed. Mahwah, NJ: Lawrence Erlbaum Associates; 2000. p. 1–90.
[56] Volkow ND, Gur RC, Wang G-J, Fowler JS, Moberg PJ, Ding Y-S, Hitzemann R, Smith G, Logan J. Association between decline in brain dopamine activity with age and cognitive and motor impairment in healthy individuals. Am J Psychiatry 1998;155:344–9.
[57] Schnider TW, Minto CF, Shafer SL, Gambus PL, Andresen C, Goodale DB, Youngs EJ. The influence of age on propofol pharmacodynamics. Anesthesiology 1999;90:1502–16.
[58] Olmos M, Ballester JA, Vidarte A, Elizalde JL, Escobar A. The combined effect of age and premedication on the propofol requirements for induction by target controlled infusion. Anesth Analg 2000;90:1157–61.
[59] Scott JC, Stanski DR. Decreased fentanyl and alfentanil dose requirements with age. A simultaneous pharmacokinetic and pharmacodynamic evaluation. J Pharmacol Exp Ther 1987;240:159–66.
[60] Stanski DR, Maitre PO. Population pharmacokinetics and pharmacodynamics of thiopental: the effect of age revisited. Anesthesiology 1990;72:412–22.
[61] Jacobs JR, Reves JG, Marty J, White WD, Bai SA, Smith LR. Aging increases pharmacodynamic sensitivity to the hypnotic effects of midazolam. Anesth Analg 1995;80:143–8.
[62] Ray WA, Griffin MR, Downey W. Benzodiazepines of long and short elimination half-life and the risk of hip fracture. JAMA 1989;262:3303–7.
[63] Greenblatt DJ, Shader RI, Abernethy DR. Drug therapy. Current status of benzodiazepines. N Engl J Med 1983;309:354–8. 410–6.
[64] Greenblatt DJ, Allen MD, Shader RI. Toxicity of high-dose flurazepam in the elderly. Clin Pharmacol Ther 1977;21:355–61.
[65] Saltz BL, Woerner MG, Kane JM, Lieberman JA, Alvir JMJ, Bergmann KJ, Blank K, Koblenzer J, Kahaner K. Prospective study of tardive dyskinesia incidence in the elderly. JAMA 1991;266:2402–6.
[66] Jeste DV, Caligiuri MP, Paulsen JS, Heaton RK, Lacro JP, Harris J, Bailey A, Fell RL, McAdams LA. Risk of tardive dyskinesia in older patients: a prospective longitudinal study of 266 outpatients. Arch Gen Psychiatry 1995;52:756–65.
[67] Woerner MG, Alvir JMJ, Saltz BL, Lieberman JA, Kane JM. Prospective study of tardive dyskinesia in the elderly: rates and risk factors. Am J Psychiatry 1998;155:1521–8.
[68] Waln O, Jankovic J. An update on tardive dyskinesia: from phenomenology to treatment. Tremor Other Hyperkinet Mov (NY) 2013;3:e1–e11.
[69] Jeste DV, Lacro JP, Bailey A, Rockwell E, Harris MJ, Caligiuri MP. Lower incidence of tardive dyskinesia with risperidone compared with haloperidol in older patients. J Am Geriatr Soc 1999;47:716–9.

[70] Ballard C, Creese B, Corbett A, Aarsland D. Atypical antipsychotics for the treatment of behavioral and psychological symptoms in dementia, with a particular focus on longer term outcomes and mortality. Expert Opin Drug Saf 2011;10:35–43.

[71] Rochon PA, Normand S-L, Gomes T, Gill SS, Anderson GM, Melo M, Sykora K, Lipscombe L, Bell CM, Gurwitz JH. Antipsychotic therapy and short-term serious events in older adults with dementia. Arch Intern Med 2008;168:1090–6.

[72] Schneider LS, Tariot PN, Dagerman KS, Davis SM, Hsaio JK, Ismail S, Leibowitz BD, Lyketsos CG, Ryan JM, Stroup TS, Sultzer DL, Weintraub D, Lieberman JA, for the CATIE-AD Study Group. Effectiveness of atypical antipsychotic drugs in patients with Alzheimer's disease. N Engl J Med 2006;355:1525–38.

[73] Abernethy DR, Greenblatt DJ, Shader RI. Imipramine and desipramine disposition in the elderly. J Pharmacol Exp Ther 1985;232:183–8.

[74] Hilmer SN, Mager DE, Simonsick EM, Cao Y, Ling SM, Windham BG, Harris TB, Hanlon JT, Rubin SM, Shorr RI, Bauer DC, Abernethy DR. A drug burden index to define the functional burden of medications in older people. Arch Intern Med 2007;167:781–7.

[75] Cao Y-J, Mager DE, Simonsick EM, Hilmer SN, Ling SM, Windham BG, Crentsil V, Yaser S, Fried LP, Abernethy DR. Physical and cognitive performance and burden of anticholinergics, sedatives, and ACE inhibitors. Clin Pharmacol Ther 2008;83:422–9.

[76] Hilmer SN, Mager DE, Simonsick EM, Ling SM, Windham BG, Harris TB, Shorr RI, Bauer DC, Abernethy DR, for the Health ABC Study. Drug burden index and functional decline in older people. Am J Med 2009;122:1142–9.

[77] Gnjidic D, Le Couteur DG, Abernethy DR, Hilmer SN. A pilot randomized clinical trial utilizing the drug burden index to reduce exposure to anticholinergic and sedative medications in older people. Ann Pharmacother 2010;44:1725–32.

[78] Low PA. The effect of aging on the autonomic nervous system. In: Low PA, editor. Clinical autonomic disorders. 2nd ed. Philadelphia: Lippincott-Raven; 1977. p. 161–75.

[79] Vestal RE, Wood AJJ, Shand DG. Reduced beta-adrenoceptor sensitivity in the elderly. Clin Pharmacol Ther 1979;26:181–6.

[80] Ziegler MG, Lake CR, Kopin IJ. Plasma noradrenaline increases with age. Nature 1976;261:333–5.

[81] Rodstein M, Zeman FD. Postural blood pressure changes in the elderly. J Chronic Dis 1957;6:581–8.

[82] Lipsitz LA, Nyquist RP, Wei JY, Rowe JW. Postprandial reduction in blood pressure in the elderly. N Engl J Med 1983;309:81–3.

[83] van Kraaij DJW, Jansen RWMM, Gribnau FWJ, Hoefnagels WHL. Diuretic therapy in elderly heart failure patients with and without left ventricular systolic dysfunction. Drugs Aging 2000;16:289–300.

[84] Tinetti ME, Han L, Lee DSH, McAvay GJ, Peduzzi P, Gross CP, Zhou B, Lin H. Antihypertensive medications and serious fall injuries in a nationally representative sample of older adults. JAMA Intern Med 2014;174:588–95.

[85] Butt DA, Mamdani M, Austin PC, Tu K, Gomes T, Glazier RH. The risk of hip fracture after initiating antihypertensive drugs in the elderly. Arch Intern Med 2012;172:1739–44.

[86] Ray WA, Griffin MR, Schaffner W, Baugh DK, Melton LJ. Psychotropic drug use and the risk of hip fracture. N Engl J Med 1987;316:363–9.

[87] Reilly JG, Ayis SA, Ferrier IN, Jones SJ, Thomas SHL. QT_c-interval abnormalities and psychotropic drug therapy in psychiatric patients. Lancet 2000;355:1048–52.

[88] Abernethy DR, Schwartz JB, Plachetka JR, Todd EL, Egan JM. Comparison in young and elderly patients of pharmacodynamics and disposition of labetalol in systemic hypertension. Am J Cardiol 1987;60:697–702.

[89] Lakatta EG. Cardiovascular aging research: the next horizons. J Am Geriatr Soc 1999;47:613–25.

[90] Maciel LMZ, Polikar R, Rohrer D, Popovich BK, Dillmann WH. Age-induced decreases in the messenger RNA coding for the sarcoplasmic reticulum Ca^{2+}-ATPase of the rat heart. Circ Res 1990;67:230–4.

[91] van Harten J, Burggraaf J, Ligthart GJ, van Brummelen P, Breimer DD. Single- and multiple-dose nisoldipine kinetics and effects in the young, the middle-aged, and the elderly. Clin Pharmacol Ther 1989;45:600–7.

[92] Hunt SA, Baker DW, Chin MH, Cinquegrani MP, Feldman AM, Francis GS, et al. ACC/AHA Task Force Report: Guidelines for the evaluation and management of chronic heart failure in the adult. Circulation 2001;104:2996–3007.

[93] Tresch DD. The clinical diagnosis of heart failure in older patients. J Am Geriatr Soc 1997;45:1128–33.

[94] Bonow RO, Udelson JE. Left ventricular diastolic dysfunction as a cause of congestive heart failure: mechanisms and management. Ann Intern Med 1992;117:502–10.

[95] van Kraaij DJW, Jansen RWMM, Bouwels LHR, Hoefnagels WHL. Furosemide withdrawal improves postprandial hypotension in elderly patients with heart failure and preserved left ventricular systolic function. Arch Intern Med 1999;159:1599–605.

[96] Cangiano JL, Martinez-Maldonado M. Isolated systolic hypertension in the elderly. In: Martinez-Maldonado M, editor. Hypertension and renal disease in the elderly. Oxford: Blackwell Scientific Publications; 1992. p. 79–94.

[97] Andrawis NS, Jones DS, Abernethy DR. Aging is associated with endothelial dysfunction in the human forearm vasculature. J Am Geriatr Soc 2000;48:193–8.

[98] Pan HYM, Hoffman BB, Porshe RA, Blaschke TF. Decline in beta-adrenergic receptor mediated vascular relaxation with aging in man. J Pharmacol Exp Ther 1986;239:802–7.

[99] Hosmane BS, Maurath CJ, Jordan DC, Laddu A. Effect of age and dose on the incidence of adverse events in the treatment of hypertension in patients receiving terazosin. J Clin Pharmacol 1992;32:434–43.

[100] Abernethy DR, Gutkowska J, Winterbottom LM. Effects of amlodipine, a long-acting dihydropyridine calcium antagonist in aging hypertension: pharmacodynamics in relation to disposition. Clin Pharmacol Ther 1990;48:76–86.

[101] Abernethy DR, Schwartz JB, Todd EL, Luchi R, Snow E. Verapamil pharmacodynamics and disposition in young versus elderly hypertensive patients. Ann Intern Med 1986;105:329–36.

[102] Schwartz JB, Abernethy DR. Responses to intravenous and oral diltiazem in elderly versus younger patients with systemic hypertension. Am J Cardiol 1987;59:1111–7.
[103] Verza M, Cacciapuoti F, Spiezia R, D'Avino M, Arpino G, D'Errico S, Sepe J, Varricchio M. Effects of the angiotensin converting enzyme inhibitor enalapril compared with diuretic therapy in elderly hypertensive patients. J Hypertens 1988;6(Suppl. 1):S97–9.
[104] Crane MG, Harris JJ. Effect of aging on renin activity and aldosterone excretion. J Lab Clin Med 1976;87:947–59.
[105] Hall JE, Coleman TG, Guyton AC. The renin-angiotensin system: normal physiology and changes in older hypertensives. J Am Geriatr Soc 1989;37:801–13.
[106] Agency for Health Care Policy and Research (AHCPR). Heart failure: evaluation and treatment of patients with left ventricular systolic dysfunction. J Am Geriatr Soc 1998;46:525–9.
[107] Lindeman RD. Overview: renal physiology and pathophysiology of aging. Am J Kidney Dis 1990;26:275–82.
[108] Miller M. Hyponatremia: age-related risk factors and therapy decisions. Geriatrics 1998;53:32–48.
[109] Rowe JW, Minaker KL, Levi M. Pathophysiology and management of electrolyte disturbances in the elderly. In: Martinez-Maldonado M, editor. Hypertension and renal disease in the elderly. Boston: Blackwell Scientific Publications; 1992. p. 170–84.
[110] Gurwitz JH, Avorn J, Ross-Degnan D, Lipsitz LA. Nonsteroidal anti-inflammatory drug associated azotemia in the very old. JAMA 1990; 264:471–5.
[111] Field TS, Gurwitz JH, Glynn RJ, Salive ME, Gaziano JM, Taylor JO, Hennekens CH. The renal effects of nonsteroidal anti-inflammatory drugs in older people: findings from the Established Populations for Epidemiologic Studies of the Elderly. J Am Geriatr Soc 1999;47:507–11.
[112] Whelton A, Schulman G, Wallemark C, Drower EJ, Isakson PC, Verburg KM, Geis S. Effects of celecoxib and naproxen on renal function in the elderly. Arch Intern Med 2000;160:1465–70.
[113] Swan SK, Rudy DW, Lasseter KC, Ryan CF, Buechel KL, Lambrecht LJ, Pinto MB, Dilzer SC, Obrda O, Sundblad KJ, Gumbs CP, Ebel DL, Quan H, Larson PJ, Schwartz JI, Musliner TA, Gertz BJ, Brater DC, Yao S-L. Effect of cyclooxygenase-2 inhibition on renal function in elderly persons receiving a low salt diet. Ann Intern Med 2000;133:1–9.
[114] Reardon LC, Macpherson DS. Hyperkalemia in outpatients using angiotensin-converting enzyme inhibitors. Arch Intern Med 1998;158:26–32.
[115] Sunderam SG, Mankikar GD. Hyponatremia in the elderly. Age Ageing 1983;12:77–80.
[116] Fichman M, Vorherr H, Kleeman G. Diuretic-induced hyponatremia. Ann Intern Med 1971;75:853–63.
[117] Ashraf N, Locksley R, Arieff A. Thiazide-induced hyponatremia associated with death or neurologic damage in outpatients. Am J Med 1981;70:1163–8.
[118] Dixon DO, Neilan B, Jones SE, Lipschitz DA, Miller TP, Grozea PN, Wilson HE. Effect of age on the therapeutic outcome in advanced diffuse histiocytic lymphoma: the Southwest Oncology Group experience. J Clin Oncol 1986;4:295–305.
[119] Tirelli U, Errante D, Van Glabbeke M, Teodorovic I, Kluin-Nelemans JC, Thomas J, Bron D, Rosti G, Zagonel V, Noordijk EM. CHOP is the standard regimen in patients > or = 70 years of age with intermediate-grade and high-grade non-Hodgkin's lymphoma: results of a randomized study of the European Organization for Research and Treatment of Cancer Lymphoma Cooperative Study Group. J Clin Oncol 1998;16:27–34.
[120] Ibrahim NK, Frye DK, Buzdar AU, Walters RS, Hortobagyi GN. Doxorubicin-based chemotherapy in elderly patients with metastatic breast cancer. Tolerance and outcome. Arch Intern Med 1996;156:882–8.
[121] Balducci L, Lyman GH. Patients aged ≥ 70 are at high risk for neutropenic infection and should receive hemopoietic growth factors when treated with moderately toxic chemotherapy. J Clin Oncol 2001;19:1583–5.
[122] Balducci L, Yates J. General guidelines for the management of older patients with cancer. Oncology (Huntingt) 2000;14:221–7.
[123] Lyman GH, Kuderer NM, Djulbegovic B. Prophylatic granulocyte colony-stimulating factor in patients receiving dose-intensive cancer chemotherapy: a meta-analysis. Am J Med 2002;112:406–11.
[124] Lyman GH, Kuderer N, Agboola O, Balducci L. Evidence-based use of colony-stimulating factors in elderly cancer patients. Cancer Control 2003;10:487–99.
[125] Ania BJ, Suman VJ, Fairbanks VF, Rademacher DM, Melton 3rd LJ. Incidence of anemia in older people: an epidemiologic study in a well defined population. J Am Geriatr Soc 1997;45:825–31.
[126] Schrijvers D, Highley M, De Bruyn E, Van Oosterom AT, Vermorken JB. Role of red blood cells in pharmacokinetics of chemotherapeutic agents. Anticancer Drugs 1999;10:147–53.
[127] Winn RJ, McClure J. The NCCN clinical practice guidelines in oncology: a primer for users. J Natl Compr Cancer Netw 2003;1:5–13.
[128] Satariano WA, Ragland DR. The effect of comorbidity on 3-year survival of woman with primary breast cancer. Ann Intern Med 1994;120:104–10.
[129] Extermann M, Overcash J, Lyman GH, Parr J, Balducci L. Comorbidity and functional status are independent in older cancer patients. J Clin Oncl 1998;16:1582–7.
[130] Ferrucci L, Guralnik JM, Cavazzini C, Bandinelli S, Lauretani F, Bartali B, Reppetto L, Longo DL. The frailty syndrome: a critical issue in geriatric oncology. Crit Rev Oncol Hematol 2003;46:127–37.
[131] Eisenhauer EA, Vermorken JB, van Glabbeke M. Predictors of response to subsequent chemotherapy in platinum pretreated ovarian cancer: a multivariate analysis of 704 patients. Ann Oncol 1997;8:963–8.
[132] Wildiers H, Highley MS, de Bruijn EA, van Oosterom AT. Pharmacology of anticancer drugs in elderly population. Clin Pharmacokinet 2003;42:1213–42.
[133] Kintzel PE, Dorr RT. Anticancer drug renal toxicity and elimination: dosing guidelines for altered renal function. Cancer Treat Rev 1995;21:33–64.
[134] Nakamura Y, Sekine I, Furuse K, Saijo N. Retrospective comparison of toxicity and efficacy in phase II trials of 3-h infusions of paclitaxel for patients 70 years of age or older and patients under 70 years of age. Cancer Chemother Pharmacol 2000;46:114–8.

[135] Miya T, Goya T, Fujii H, Ohtsu T, Itoh K, Igarashi T, Minami H, Sasaki Y. Factors affecting the pharmacokinetics of CPT-11: the body mass index, age and sex are independent predictors of pharmacokinetic parameters of CPT-11. Invest New Drugs 2001;19:61–7.
[136] O' Reilly S, Rowinsky EK, Slichenmyer W, Donehower RC, Forastiere AA, Ettinger DS, Chen TL, Sartorius S, Grochow LB. Phase I and pharmacologic study of topotecan in patients with impaired renal function. J Clin Oncol 1996;14:3062–73.
[137] Gelman RS, Taylor SG. Cyclophosphamide, methotrexate, and 5-fluorouracil chemotherapy in women more than 65 years old with advanced breast cancer: the elimination of age trends in toxicity by using doses based on creatinine clearance. J Clin Oncol 1984;2:1404–13.
[138] Lichtman SM, Skirvin JA. Pharmacology of antineoplastic agents in older cancer patients. Oncology (Huntingt) 2000;14:1743–55.
[139] Miya T, Sasaki Y, Karato A, Saijo N. Pharmacokinetic study of mitomycin C with emphasis on the influence of aging. Jpn J Cancer Res 1992;83:1382–5.
[140] Looker AC, Johnston CC, Wahner HW, Dunn WL, Calvo MS, Harris TB, Heyse SP, Lindsay RL. Prevalence of low femoral bone density in older US women from NHANES III. J Bone Miner Res 1995;10:796–802.
[141] Colon-Emeric C, O'Connell MB, Haney E. Osteoporosis piece of the multi-morbidity puzzle in geriatric care. Mt Sinai J Med 2011;78:515–26.
[142] Moerman EJ, Teng K, Lipschitz DA, Lecka-Czernik B. Aging activates adipogenic and suppresses osteogenic programs in mesenchymal marrow stroma/stem cells: the role of PPAR-γ2 transcription factor and TGF-β/BMP signaling pathways. Aging Cell 2004;3:379–89.
[143] Lecka-Czernik B, Rosen CJ, Kawai M. Skeletal aging and the adipocyte program. Cell Cycle 2010;9:3648–54.
[144] Mundy GR, Elefteriou F. Boning up on ephrin signaling. Cell 2006;126:441–3.
[145] Teitelbaum SL, Ross FP. Genetic regulation of osteoclast development and function. Nat Rev Genet 2003;4:638–49.
[146] Institute of Medicine. Dietary reference intakes for calcium and vitamin D. Report Brief, Washington DC: IOM; 2011. Revised March 2011 https://pubmed.ncbi.nlm.nih.gov/21796828/.
[147] Holick MF. Vitamin D deficiency. N Engl J Med 2007;357:266–81.
[148] MacLean C, Newberry S, Maglione M, McMahon M, Ranganath V, Suttorp M, Mojica W, Timmer M, Alexander A, McNamara M, Desai SB, Zhou A, Chen S, Carter J, Tringale C, Valentine D, Johnsen B, Grossman J. Systematic review: comparative effectiveness of treatments to prevent fractures in men and women with low bone density or osteoporosis. Ann Intern Med 2008;148:197–213.
[149] Gates BJ, Sonnett TE, DuVall CA, Dobbins EK. Review of osteoporosis pharmacotherapy for geriatric patients. Am J Geriatr Pharmacother 2009;7:293–323.
[150] Ettinger B, Black DM, Mitlak BH, Knickerbocker RK, Nickelsen T, Genant HK, Christiansen C, Delmas PD, Zanchetta JR, Stakkestad J, Gluer CC, Krueger K, Cohen FJ, Eckert S, Ensrud KE, Avioli LV, Lips P, Cummings SR. Reduction of vertebral fracture risk in postmenopausal women with osteoporosis treated with raloxifene: results from a 3-year randomized clinical trial. JAMA 1999;282:637–45.
[151] Miyaura C, Kusano K, Masuzawa T, Chaki O, Onoe Y, Aoyagi M, Sasaki T, Tamura T, Koishihara Y, Ohsugi Y, Suda T. Endogenous bone-resorbing factors in estrogen deficiency: cooperative effects of IL-1 and IL-6. J Bone Miner Res 1995;10:1365–73.
[152] Giuliani N, Sansoni P, Girasole G, Vescovini R, Passeri G, Passeri M, Pedrazzoni M. Serum interleukin-6, soluble interleukin-6 receptor and soluble gp130 exhibit different patterns of age- and menopause-related changes. Exp Gerontol 2001;36:547–57.
[153] Cauley JA, Robbins J, Chen Z, Cummings SR, Jackson RD, LaCroix AZ, LeBoff M, Lewis CE, McGowan J, Neuner J, Pettinger M, Stefanick ML, Wactawski-Wende J, Watts NB, Women's Health Initiative Investigators. Effects of estrogen plus progestin on risk of fracture and bone mineral density: the Women's Health Initiative Randomized Trial. JAMA 2003;290:1729–38.
[154] Nelson HD, Humphrey LL, Nygren P, Teutsch SM, Allan JD. Postmenopausal hormone replacement therapy: scientific review. JAMA 2001;288:872–81.
[155] Chesnut CH, Silverman S, Andriano K, Genant H, Gimona A, Harris S, Kiel D, LiBoff M, Maricic M, Miller P, Moniz C, Peacock M, Richardson P, Watts N, Baylink D, for the PROOF Study Group. A randomized trial of nasal spray salmon calcitonin in postmenopausal women with established osteoporosis: the Prevent Recurrence of Osteoporotic Fractures Study. Am J Med 2000;109:267–76.
[156] Cummings SR, San Martin J, McClung MR, Siris ES, Eastell R, Reid IR, Delmas P, Zoog HB, Austin M, Wang A, Kutilek S, Adami S, Zanchetta J, Libanate C, Siddhanti S, Christiansen C. The FREEDOM Trial: denosumab for prevention of fractures in postmenopausal women with osteoporosis. N Engl J Med 2009;361:756–65.
[157] Compston JE, McClung MR, Leslie WD. Osteoporosis. Lancet 2019;393:364–76.
[158] Jilka RL. Molecular and cellular mechanisms of the anabolic effect of intermittent PTH. Bone 2007;40:1434–6.
[159] Canalis E, Giustina A, Bilezikian JP. Mechanisms of anabolic therapies for osteoporosis. N Engl J Med 2007;357:905–16.
[160] Tabacco G, Bilezikian JP. Osteoanabolic and dual action drugs. Br J Clin Pharmacol 2019;85:1084–94.
[161] Shannon M, Lovejoy FH. The influence of age vs. peak serum concentration on life-threatening events after chronic theophylline intoxication. Arch Intern Med 1990;150:2045–8.
[162] Schiff GD, Hegde HK, LaCloche L, Hryhoczuk DO. Inpatient theophylline toxicity. Preventable factors. Ann Intern Med 1991;114:748–53.
[163] Kopanoff DE, Snider DE Jr, Caras GJ. Isoniazid-related hepatitis: a U.S. Public Health Service cooperative surveillance study. Am Rev Respir Dis 1979;117:992–1001.
[164] American Thoracic Society. Treatment of tuberculosis and tuberculosis infection in adults and children. Am J Respir Crit Care Med 1994; 149:1359–74.
[165] Sorresso DJ, Mehta JB, Harvil LM, Bently S. Underutilization of isoniazid chemoprophylaxis in tuberculosis contacts 50 year of age and older. A prospective analysis. Chest 1995;108:706–11.
[166] American Thoracic Society. Targeted tuberculin testing and treatment of latent tuberculosis infection. MMWR 2000;49(RR-6):1–51.

[167] Gabriel SE, Jaakkimainen L, Bombardier C. Risk for serious gastrointestinal complications related to use of nonsteroidal anti-inflammatory drugs. Ann Intern Med 1991;115:787–96.

[168] Cryer B, Lee E, Feldman M. Factors influencing gastroduodenal mucosal prostaglandin concentrations: roles of smoking and aging. Ann Intern Med 1992;116:636–40.

[169] Shepherd AMM, Hewick DS, Moreland TA, Stevenson IH. Age as a determinant of sensitivity to warfarin. Br J Clin Pharmacol 1977;4:315–20.

[170] Fang MC, Chang Y, Hylek EM, Rosand J, Greenberg SM, Go AS, Singer DE. Advanced age, anticoagulation intensity, and risk for intracranial hemorrhage among patients taking warfarin for atrial fibrillation. Ann Intern Med 2004;141:745–52.

[171] Palareti G, Hirsch J, Legnani C, Manotti C, D'Angelo A, Pengo V, Moia M, Guazzaloca G, Musolesi S, Coccheri S. Oral anticoagulation treatment in the elderly: a nested, prospective, case-control study. Arch Intern Med 2000;160:470–8.

[172] Rose AJ, Goldberg R, McManus DD, Kapoor A, Wang V, Liu W, Yu H. Anticoagulant prescribing for non-valvular atrial fibrillation in the Veterans Health Administration. J Am Heart Assoc 2019;8:e012646.

[173] Lau SWJ, Schlender JF, Slattum PW, Heald DL, O'Connor-Semmes R. Geriatrics 2030: developing drugs to care for older persons-a neglected and growing population. Clin Pharmacol Ther 2020;107:53–6.

Chapter 26

Clinical analysis of adverse drug reactions and pharmacovigilance

Christine Chamberlain, Cindy Kortepeter, and Monica Muñoz
Food and Drug Administration Office of Surveillance and Epidemiology, Division of Pharmacovigilance, Silver Spring, MD, United States

Introduction

Drugs are developed for a specific purpose based on their pharmacology or drug action, to cure or control a disease or to aid in diagnosis of a disease. Although a drug may have a targeted effect, it may cause some undesirable effects during its clinical use. All drugs have risks. Throughout the drug development and approval process, adverse drug reactions (ADRs) are monitored and assessed to determine a benefit-risk profile for the drug. Even so, the risk profile of a drug is often not fully delineated at the time of regulatory approval as very rare adverse events may be undetected and the risk in vulnerable populations is often unknown, as was shown with chloramphenicol and development of blood dyscrasias in the 1950s [1]. As a result, ADR assessment, monitoring, and surveillance are necessary throughout a drug's entire life cycle in order to enhance our knowledge about its risks and safety. The term drug as used in this chapter refers to both human drugs and therapeutic biological products.

ADRs are an important public health issue that can cause significant morbidity and mortality. It has been estimated that approximately 5% of hospital admissions are related to ADRs and about 10%–20% of hospitalized patients experience an ADR while in the hospital [2–4]. The true incidence of ADRs may be higher because ADRs are often underreported; in addition, health care providers and patients may not recognize the relatedness of symptoms to a drug. A systematic review of data from 12 countries estimated underreporting of ADRs to spontaneous reporting systems to exceed 90% [5]. There is also some confusion when comparing incidence estimates because medical literature often groups ADRs with adverse drug events (ADEs) that may include medication errors, inappropriate use, or overdoses and may not be directly related to the mechanism of drug action [6].

ADRs are costly and involve the use of significant resources. ADRs may present as minor symptoms or cause serious harm or death and therefore should be identified early in the course of therapy to prevent further harm. Depending on the severity of the ADR, patients may require hospitalization or extension of hospitalization, significantly increasing health care expenditures. When ADRs are not recognized, additional medications may be added to treat symptoms and present added risks. Clinical diagnosis may not be apparent and require additional testing, procedures, or readmission. Besides direct costs, indirect costs may be incurred such as missed days of work or loss of employment [7]. The economic impact of an ADR varies depending on outpatient or inpatient setting, severity of the reaction, and length of time and resources necessary for appropriate diagnosis and treatment. Therefore health care providers need to have an adequate understanding of ADRs and consider an ADR as a potential cause of a patient's symptoms instead of attributing it to their underlying illness.

For newly approved drugs, our knowledge and understanding of ADRs is primarily based on the premarketing development program (i.e., animal, pharmacology, and clinical studies). Because of the limitations of these data sources, ADR knowledge continues to mature in the postmarketing setting through spontaneous reporting, observational studies, registries, and other information sources that reflect experience from broader utilization. *Pharmacovigilance*, as defined by the World Health Organization (WHO), includes the science and activities relating to the detection, assessment, understanding, and prevention of adverse effects or any other possible drug-related problems [8]. Pharmacovigilance efforts are necessary to ensure a well-informed risk profile. Unfortunately, many health care providers are not aware that drug labels are continuously updated with safety information as it arises and that their clinical experience in reporting ADRs is an important element of postmarket safety surveillance [9].

Atkinson's Principles of Clinical Pharmacology. https://doi.org/10.1016/B978-0-12-819869-8.00036-7

Definitions and classification

Definitions

The terms "adverse event" or "adverse drug event" are often used interchangeably with "adverse drug reaction"; however, these terms have different meanings. An *adverse event* is a broader term defined by the WHO as a "medical occurrence temporally associated with the use of a medicinal product, but not necessarily causally related." Regulatory agencies such as the Food and Drug Administration (FDA) define an *adverse event* (also referred to as *an adverse experience*) as any untoward medical occurrence associated with the use of a drug in humans, whether or not considered drug related [10]. These definitions include an adverse event occurring under any circumstance in the course of a drug's use in professional practice: from drug overdose whether accidental or intentional, from drug abuse, from drug withdrawal, or with any failure of expected pharmacological action, and do not require a causal relationship [11]. According to the WHO, an *adverse drug reaction* is a response to a drug that is noxious and unintended and which occurs at doses normally used for prophylaxis, diagnosis, or therapy of a disease or for modification of physiologic function [12]. Edwards and Aronson [13] further distinguished an ADR as "an appreciably harmful or unpleasant reaction, resulting from an intervention related to the use of a medicinal product, which predicts hazard from future administration and warrants prevention or specific treatment, or alteration of the dosage regimen or withdrawal of the product." Essentially, an ADR is a subset of adverse drug events (ADE) that represents harm from appropriate drug use, often directly attributed to a drug's properties (suspected causal association) and *not* related to inappropriate dosing, misuse, or overdose [6].

Classification by type

ADRs can be classified by type, onset, or severity to aid in comparisons among drugs and to guide treatment strategies. As described in Chapter 15, the traditional classification system introduced by Rawlins and Thompson [14] classifies ADRs into Type A and Type B. Type A ADRs are dose related and often predictable as they are a known augmentation of a drug's pharmacologic effects. Type B ADRs are not dose related and are unpredictable (bizarre) and often rare. Our current understanding of the mechanistic basis of Type B reactions is extensively discussed in Chapter 15. The Type A and B classification system evolved over the years as new drug adverse events became apparent to include Type C through E that incorporate time-related ADRs, withdrawal, and failure of therapy reactions [13, 15]. Type C reactions relate to both dose and time with chronic use and correlate with a cumulative dose (e.g., hypothalamic-pituitary adrenal axis suppression with corticosteroid use) [13]. Type D reactions are time delayed, becoming apparent some time after drug use, such as carcinogenesis [13, 16]. Type E or end-of-use reactions are a consequence of withdrawing a drug such as the withdrawal syndrome that occurs when opiates are suddenly removed [13]. Table 26.1 lists the types of ADRs with additional examples. Although these expanded classification types may not be commonplace, they provide knowledge on possible mechanisms and management [17].

ADR classification systems continue to evolve and another classification system known as **Do**se, **T**ime, **S**usceptibility (DoTS) similarly classifies reactions based on dose and time and also includes genetic, pathological, and other biological differences to provide a more clinical pharmacological approach [18, 19]. Additionally, a mechanistic classification system known as EIDOS was established to complement the DoTS system and describes mechanisms for the adverse effect: **e**xtrinsic chemical species that initiates the effect, **i**ntrinsic chemical species that it affects, **d**istribution in the body, the physiologic **o**utcome, and **s**equela (the adverse effect) [20]. These systems have been used together to assess preventability of an ADR [21].

The traditional classification systems described by Rawlins and Thompson, and others, were formulated based on ADRs induced by small molecule drugs and are not well suited for larger molecules such as biological products (biologics). These biologic therapies include cytokines, antibodies, and fusion proteins. They differ from small molecule drugs because they are larger sized proteins, similar in structure to naturally occurring proteins, administered parenterally, and not metabolized, but rather they are processed [22]. With the increasing use of biologics to treat various diseases, a new classification scheme is warranted to accommodate the different characteristics of these products. Pichler et al. [17] proposed a unique classification of adverse reactions to biologics based on their immune target or mechanism of action. To distinguish it from the traditional classifications, Greek letters are used for the five types as presented in Table 26.2 [22]. This classification system can be used in surveillance of adverse reactions as new biological products are marketed.

TABLE 26.1 Types of adverse drug reactions.

Type	Description	Example
Type A[a]	Extend directly from a drug's pharmacologic action Dose related Predictable Avoidable	Hypoglycemia from insulin Bleeding with anticoagulants
Type B	No relationship to the usual pharmacologic effect of a drug Relatively uncommon Difficult to predict Not dose related, host dependent Includes idiosyncratic reactions, drug allergies	Drug-induced rashes Increased vulnerability of erythrocytes to oxidative injury by several drugs in G6PD-deficient individuals
Type C	Related to the duration of therapy and to some extent, the dose Long-term exposure required	Tardive dyskinesia seen with antipsychotic medications
Type D	Observed with prolonged exposure to a drug or exposure at a critical time	Increased risk of endometrial cancer with tamoxifen
Type E	Observed on abrupt discontinuation of long-term therapy	Delirium tremens on alcohol withdrawal Rebound hypertension with clonidine withdrawal

[a]*Most common type.*
Modified from reference: Rehan HS, Chopra D, Kakkar AK. Physician's guide to pharmacovigilance: terminology and causality assessment. Eur J Intern Med 2009;20(1):3–8 and Pichler W.J. Adverse side-effects to biological agents. Allergy. 2006;61:912–920 (anticoagulation example).

TABLE 26.2 Proposed classification of adverse reactions to biologic agents.

Type	Terminology	Example of reaction and (medication)
α	High cytokine and cytokine release syndrome	Cytokine release syndrome (Muromonab-CD3)
β	Hypersensitivity	Common acute infusion reactions (Rituximab) Delayed reactions (Etanercept) Anaphylaxis (Omalizumab)
γ	Immune or cytokine imbalance: Immunodeficiency	Increased risk of tuberculosis (TNF inhibitors) Hypogammaglobulinemia (Rituximab)
	Autoimmunity	Systemic lupus erythematosus (Interferon-γ)
	Atopic disorders	Atopic dermatitis (TNF inhibitors)
δ	Cross-reactivity	Acne from anti-EGFR (Cetuximab)
ε	Nonimmunological side effects	Neuropsychiatric side effects including confusion or depression (Interferon-α)

Abbreviations: *EGFR*, epidermal growth factor receptor; *TNF*, tumor necrosis factor.
Modified from reference: Pichler W.J. Adverse side-effects to biological agents. Allergy. 2006;61:912–920.

Classification by severity

Classification of ADRs by severity is helpful in guiding acute treatment and future medication therapy decisions. *Severity* is used to describe the intensity of an ADR that may or may not be serious [13]. For example, a headache may be severe in intensity but may not be life threatening. A severity grading system initially established by the National Cancer Institute for clinical trials with oncology drugs, known as NCI Common Terminology Criteria for Adverse Events (CTCAE) is a descriptive grading system that is used for Adverse Event (AE) reporting [23]. A scale for grading severity is provided for each AE that is listed under the Medical Dictionary for Regulatory Activities (MedDRA) hierarchy System Organ Class (SOC), with each grade referring to the severity of the AE [24]. The grading scale has a range from 1 through 5 with unique clinical descriptions of severity for each AE. Not all AEs are assigned every grade, for example Stevens-Johnson Syndrome can only be assigned grades 3 through 5. Although initially established for comparing AEs for oncology drugs, this severity system can be applied to other drug categories as well. This severity scale can be used to describe any AE regardless of whether or not the AE is causally related to the drug.

Regulatory authorities classify ADEs based on seriousness. FDA defines a *serious adverse drug experience* as one "occurring at any dose that results in any of the following outcomes: Death, a life-threatening adverse drug experience, inpatient hospitalization or prolongation of existing hospitalization, a persistent or significant disability/incapacity, or a congenital anomaly/birth defect" [11]. Important medical events that do not result in death, are not life threatening, or do not require hospitalization may also be considered a serious adverse drug experience when, based upon appropriate medical judgment, they may jeopardize the patient and may require medical or surgical intervention to prevent one of the outcomes listed in the earlier definition. An example of an important medical event is allergic bronchospasm requiring intensive treatment in an emergency department that may not result in inpatient hospitalization. Other regulatory authorities use similar definitions: for example, the European Medicines Agency defines a serious adverse reaction as "an adverse reaction that results in death, is life-threatening, requires hospitalisation or prolongation of existing hospitalisation, results in persistent or significant disability or incapacity, or is a birth defect" [25]. International regulatory authorities often use standardized terminology, such as defined by MedDRA, to improve reporting consistency and research regarding ADEs and ADRs [24]. Seriousness of an ADE or ADR is used to prioritize safety issues and determine regulatory action.

The aim of classifying ADRs is to better characterize them for detection, monitoring, and management in clinical trials and subsequent patient care. Some ADRs are predictable and potentially avoidable, such as Type A reactions which comprise about 80% of ADRs [3,26]. Our understanding of a majority of Type B reactions is evolving as described in Chapter 15. Additionally, biological products differ from small molecule drugs and have their own mechanistic ADR classification system (Table 26.2) [17]. General knowledge of ADR mechanisms is helpful in facilitating their detection, treatment, and prevention.

Assessing ADRS

ADR detection

Recognizing ADRs in the clinical setting is challenging because drug-induced illness may closely resemble natural disease. A patient's new symptom, an abnormal laboratory value, or a directly observed event can potentially be an ADR, but it may also be attributable to alternative etiologies such as comorbidity or other treatments. Electronic health records (EHR) and other health technologies provide opportunities to actively detect ADRs [27]. The first step is to conduct a thorough medication history and include ADRs in the differential diagnosis when evaluating a patient with new onset symptoms [20]. In a recent analysis, the prevalence of ADEs was approximately 6% in patients hospitalized for a cardiovascular event, pneumonia, or conditions requiring surgery [28]. Elucidating additional details related to the symptoms before instituting treatment with an additional medication may uncover an ADR that is responsible for the symptoms and prevent adding unnecessary medications or prolonging the ADR.

Some methods of retrospectively detecting ADRs in the inpatient and outpatient setting include medication order screening for specific medication changes or alert drugs. Abrupt discontinuation of a drug and an order for a corticosteroid or diphenhydramine may indicate a drug allergy. A dose reduction or an order to "hold" a drug may prompt a pharmacist to check for an abnormal drug level and screen for a potential ADR or drug interaction. Trigger tools have been developed to detect ADRs, to help characterize the most frequent AEs and to develop priorities for quality improvement and prevention [29,30]. These methods involve a two-stage process: a screening process for the detection of criteria or triggers, and subsequent in-depth manual review of the medical record for an ADE [30]. Additionally, newly approved medications can be targeted for medication order screening for safety concerns identified during premarketing trials and noted in drug labeling that may not have been fully characterized. Other strategies for ADR detection and reporting include targeting medication classes most commonly associated with ADEs such as antibiotics, corticosteroids, antineoplastics, anticoagulants, NSAIDS, and narcotics [31,32]. Tools have also been developed to identify patients at higher risk for certain ADRs based on EHR information. These tools incorporate patient demographics, medications, medical history, and laboratory results into predictive models that may facilitate ADE prevention and mitigation in real time [33–35].

An abnormal laboratory value or diagnostic test can alert a health care provider to review the patient's EHR for an ADR. EHRs can be programmed to compile reports of laboratory values that are outside a predetermined range. For example, alanine aminotransferase (ALT) elevation of three times the reference range can alert a health care provider to review for any drug-related causes such as a statin. Baseline laboratory testing and subsequent laboratory monitoring is used to monitor for ADRs with certain drugs. Changes in laboratory values do not necessarily mean that an ADR has occurred but can alert a health care provider to review a patient's medication record and ask the patient pertinent questions to assess for an ADR.

Another way of identifying ADRs is through review of daily inpatient multidisciplinary notes or screening of outpatient clinic notes. Reviewing notes for lethargy, oversedation, and cognitive decline may be a sign of an ADR caused by a sedative, analgesic, or hypoglycemic agent. Multidisciplinary notes may provide additional information on how an event was managed and if an ADR was considered or if an alternative medication was added to treat the event, which could present opportunity for additional ADRs. This process is time consuming and may be an opportunity for new technologies to enhance detection using natural language processing [36].

Special populations such as infants, children, pregnant women, and the elderly are susceptible to ADRs. These populations are often not well studied during premarket clinical trials and changes in development, reduced drug clearance secondary to impaired renal or hepatic function, and new onset comorbidities can increase the risk of an ADR [19]. Mitigation strategies can be implemented to circumvent ADRs such as routine screening of prescription orders for appropriate dose when administering medications requiring renal dose adjustments (e.g., gabapentin, ganciclovir, ranitidine, and rivaroxaban) to a patient with changing renal function. Computerized physician order entry (CPOE) systems with decision support that incorporates laboratory data can alert health care providers to adjust the dose of renally and hepatically eliminated drugs during the ordering process thus preventing an ADR. Knowing a drug's dose-related ADRs and monitoring for them can avoid harm.

Assessing risk and causality

Determining if a patient's AE is an ADR is complex and requires a causality assessment. Patients often take more than one drug and have several comorbidities making causality assessment challenging. Causal association assessment in the clinical setting is focused on a particular individual who experienced the AE and often it is not possible to know with a high level of certainty whether the AE was caused by the drug. Clinical data from the patient, pertinent laboratory results, and extensive drug information review aid in determining whether there is a causal association between a drug and an AE. Ultimately the determination is based on the strength of evidence from all available data. The Bradford Hill criteria for causation, originally presented to demonstrate epidemiologic evidence of a causal relationship between an exposure and outcome, is useful in deciding if some level of causal association is present [37]. Table 26.3 is a causality checklist with some of the principles from the Bradford Hill criteria, which include temporality (the event occurs after drug initiation), positive dechallenge (the event resolves with drug discontinuation), positive rechallenge (event reappears with drug reinitiation), and ruling out other plausible causes. Edwards and Aronson [13] outlined steps to assess causality that include (1) thorough medication history (including over-the-counter medications), (2) timing of medications to the event (latency), (3) pattern of the AE to the known pharmacology or allergy pattern of suspected drugs, (4) background frequency of the event, (5) investigations (drug levels, organ function tests, biopsies) to aid in diagnosis or rule out alternative causes, and (6) consideration of rechallenge if appropriate and if patient will directly benefit from knowledge gained. When assessing a potentially drug-related AE or symptom, review for latency of development of the AE after drug initiation in the clinical context of the event, and the known pharmacokinetics (PK) and pharmacodynamics (PD) of the drug, for plausibility. For example, the onset of the reaction should be clinically reasonable such as an anaphylactic reaction, which usually occurs within a few minutes to several hours after the drug is administered versus agranulocytosis, which may take days to weeks to develop. If a drug is suspected of causing cancer, which may take a much longer time to develop, a latency of less than a month would exclude causality. Additionally, it is necessary to review recognized adverse reactions of the drug, or related drugs in the same class, and if the AE under assessment is similar or involves similar mechanisms, because a causal association would be more likely.

TABLE 26.3 Causality considerations.
Patient-level data (intrinsic evidence considerations)
Temporality
Dechallenge/rechallenge
Response to antidote/reversal agents
Alternative causes
Drug levels in body fluids or tissues
Dose-response relationship
Prior adverse event experience with the same or a similar drug
Existing knowledge about the potential ADR (extrinsic evidence considerations)
Known association with drug or drug class
Strength of association
Disease/event epidemiology
Biologic and pharmacologic plausibility

A thorough review of available drug information is needed to assess the possible role of a drug in causing an AE. It is logical to start with a review of the safety information in the Boxed Warning, Warnings and Precautions, and Adverse Reaction sections of the drug's labeling (also known as the package insert or the prescribing information), which can be found at Drugs@FDA or DailyMed [38, 39]. Drugs@FDA, which contains the most recent FDA-approved drug labeling, also contains redacted premarketing review documents from FDA medical, chemistry, and pharmacology reviewers as well as other disciplines that may contain information to establish biologic plausibility for a drug-AE association. DailyMed, sponsored by the National Library of Medicine, contains drug labeling but may also contain any labeling changes that have been recently submitted to the FDA by the drug manufacturer[a] that are under review. MedWatch safety alerts contain information from reports submitted to the FDA Adverse Event Reporting System (FAERS) from health professionals, patients, consumers, and drug manufacturers [40]. Additionally, FDA posts potential signals of serious risks/new safety information identified from FAERS in quarterly reports [41]. A review of published medical literature for similar case reports can provide additional evidence to support an association.

Causality assessment is needed to classify the relationship between a drug and AE at two levels: the individual patient case and the overall drug-AE level. Assessment of a causal association at the drug-AE level considers the strength of evidence collectively from various sources of data and is discussed later in this chapter. Causality assessment at the individual patient level uses clinical judgment based on assessment of the AE in the context of what is known about the patient and the drug [42]. Methods have been developed to standardize assessment in the clinical setting, which use different causality categories and are assessed using different criteria. Some methods are specific to a particular ADR while other methods are more general, and some can be complex and time consuming [43]. Two approaches that are easy to use are WHO-Uppsala Monitoring Centre (WHO-UMC) Causality Categories (Table 26.4) and the Naranjo probability scale (Table 26.5). The WHO-UMC Causality Assessment relies on expert judgment in considering the clinical and pharmacological aspects of the case and the quality of the observation [43]. This system assigns one of six category terms to the drug–event combination based on several assessment criteria: certain, probable/likely, possible, unlikely, conditional/unclassified, and unassessable/unclassifiable [44]. AEs with a probable/likely or certain causal association are likely to recur, therefore knowing an event is probable/likely, may help prevent future episodes [45]. In practice, few ADRs are classified as "certain" because information relevant to assessing all alternative etiologies may not be available and it may not be practical to obtain confirmatory evidence (e.g., biopsy); therefore, most drug-event combinations with a causal association deemed greater than unlikely are considered possible or probable.

a. Throughout this chapter the term "drug manufacturer" is used for simplicity, but is intended to encompass sponsors, applicants, licensed manufacturers, packers, distributors, and other responsible persons subject to FDA's requirements for postmarketing safety reporting.

TABLE 26.4 WHO-UMC causality categories.

Causality term	Assessment criteria[a]
Certain	• Event or laboratory test abnormality, with plausible time relationship to drug intake • Cannot be explained by disease or other drugs • Response to withdrawal plausible (pharmacologically, pathologically) • Event definitive pharmacologically or phenomenologically (i.e., an objective and specific medical disorder or a recognized pharmacological phenomenon) • Rechallenge satisfactory, if necessary
Probable/likely	• Event or laboratory test abnormality, with reasonable time relationship to drug intake • Unlikely to be attributed to disease or other drugs • Response to withdrawal clinically reasonable • Rechallenge not required
Possible	• Event or laboratory test abnormality, with reasonable time relationship to drug intake • Could also be explained by disease or other drugs • Information on drug withdrawal may be lacking or unclear
Unlikely	• Event or laboratory test abnormality, with a time to drug intake that makes a relationship improbable (but not impossible) • Disease or other drugs provide plausible explanations
Conditional/ unclassified	• Event or laboratory test abnormality • More data for proper assessment needed, or • Additional data under examination
Unassessable/ unclassifiable	• Report suggesting an adverse reaction • Cannot be judged because information is insufficient or contradictory • Data cannot be supplemented or verified

[a]*All points should be reasonable complied with.*
Reproduced from World Health Organization. The use of the WHO-UMC system for standardised case causality assessment. https://www.who.int/publications/m/item/WHO-causality-assessment. WHO 5 June 2013 [Accessed 30 June 2020].

The Naranjo probability scale is a quantitative instrument for causality assessment that is commonly used in the hospital setting and utilizes similar principles as the WHO-UMC system. By answering 10 questions regarding onset of the reaction, investigations, dechallenge and rechallenge information, alternative causes, and prior exposure, an ADR numeric probability score is assigned and classified based on the total score (Table 26.5) [46]. Unfortunately, no scale can provide a definitive causality ascertainment and some tools may not work well for certain ADRs such as Stevens-Johnson Syndrome (SJS) and toxic epidermal necrolysis (TEN) [47]. However, they can guide health care providers through the thought process for assessing ADRs. Determining if the patient is experiencing an ADR by using causality assessment tools can prevent patient exposure to additional often unnecessary medications, determine appropriate treatment, ensure proper documentation of the ADR diagnosis, and lead to measures to prevent future occurrences (e.g., use a lower dose or pretreat with an antihistamine) [6, 48].

Managing and reporting ADRS

Managing ADRs

Despite efforts to avoid or minimize ADRs, they still occur and may require swift action to avoid harm. For serious, life-threatening ADRs such as toxic epidermal necrolysis, the offending drug should be stopped and supportive care provided [49]. ADR management can be guided by the type of ADR, for example, Type A reactions are dose dependent and may respond to a dose reduction whereas Type C reactions that occur with long-term use can be managed by using the lowest effective dose or the shortest duration of therapy for the clinical condition, such as with corticosteroids and adrenal axis suppression. Some ADRs may require specific reversal agents such as idarucizumab for the treatment of uncontrolled bleeding with dabigatran [19]. Information on how to treat or otherwise manage an ADR that has occurred may be found in a drug's prescribing information [50, 51]. While information may be acquired from multiple sources, answers are often

TABLE 26.5 The Naranjo Adverse Drug Reaction Probability Scale.

To assess the adverse drug reaction, please answer the following questionnaire and give the pertinent score	Yes	No	Do not know	Score
1. Are there previous *conclusive* reports on this reaction?	+1	0	0	
2. Did the adverse event occur after the suspected drug was administered?	+2	−1	0	
3. Did the adverse reaction improve when the drug was discontinued or a *specific* antagonist was administered?	+1	0	0	
4. Did the adverse reaction reappear when the drug was readministered?	+2	−1	0	
5. Are there alternative causes (other than the drug) that could have on their own caused the reaction?	−1	+2	0	
6. Did the reaction reappear when a placebo was given?	−1	+1	0	
7. Was the medication detected in the blood (or other fluids) in concentrations known to be toxic?	+1	0	0	
8. Was the reaction more severe when the dose was increased or less severe when the dose was decreased?	+1	0	0	
9. Did the patient have a similar reaction to the same or similar drugs in *any* previous exposure?	+1	0	0	
10. Was the adverse event confirmed by any objective evidence?	+1	0	0	
The ADR is assigned to a probability category from the total score as follows: *definite* if the overall score is 9 or greater, *probable* for a score of 5–8, *possible* for 1–4 and *doubtful* if the score is 0.			Total	

Reproduced with permission from Naranjo CA, Busto U, Sellers EM, Sandor P, Ruiz I, Roberts EA, Janecek E, Domecq C, and Greenblatt DJ. A method for estimating the probability of adverse drug reactions. Clin Pharmacol Ther 1981;30:239–245.

lacking to many practical questions regarding management, such as if continued use will lead to progression or regression of an ADR, or how long after drug discontinuation will it take for an ADR to resolve. Insight to answer some of these questions may be provided by a drug's clinical pharmacology and a search of the medical literature for case reports of similar drug-events for possible management options. Whenever it is reasonably clear that a specific drug is causal, there should be a reevaluation for its need and consideration of therapeutic alternatives with an unlikely risk of the ADR [13]. Although one might assume an ADR to a drug might translate to avoidance of all drugs in the same class, this is dependent on the type of reaction, underlying mechanism of the reaction, and availability of alternative therapies. For example, drug allergy with a penicillin does not automatically mean the patient is allergic to all beta-lactam antibiotics as new generations of beta-lactam containing molecules with dissimilar side chains, such as cephalosporins exhibit less (or no) cross-reactivity [52]. If certain drug hypersensitivity reactions occur with a drug that is needed and for which there is no alternative, desensitization can be attempted under supervision of an allergist/immunologist [53]. When a patient is taking multiple drugs that could cause the ADR, eliminating those drugs (dechallenge) that are least essential to care is a reasonable approach.

Reporting ADRs

It is necessary to document and report ADRs in order to evaluate the benefit-risk profile of a drug and develop mitigation strategies. Various accrediting organizations, societies, and regulatory authorities, both in the United States and internationally, have developed guidelines for reporting ADRs [54–56]. As it may be impractical to report every ADR that is encountered in clinical practice, some authors have encouraged reporting just those ADRs that are serious, associated with a drug that was recently marketed (1–3 years), and considered high risk by regulatory and medical institution accreditation organizations, such as anticoagulants, insulins, and narcotics [57]. Nonetheless, spontaneous reporting of ADRs by health care providers, patients, and caretakers continues to be an important source of drug safety signals. Publishing case reports of ADRs also disseminates information to other health care providers, regulatory authorities, and stakeholders and provides for detailed information about the AE and drug association.

The FDA supports direct reporting of observed or suspected adverse events to the Agency via the MedWatch program. FDA launched the MedWatch program in 1993 as part of a medical product safety reporting program [58]. The program is still active today with over 21 million reports of adverse events, medication errors, and drug quality complaints captured in the FAERS database as of 2020. The MedWatch program enables submission of voluntary reports via phone (toll-free: 1-800-FDA (332)-1088), fax (1-800-FDA(332)-0178), or online via the MedWatch website https://www.fda.gov/safety/medwatch-fda-safety-information-and-adverse-event-reporting-program [59]. The original goals of the MedWatch program were to make it easier for health care providers to report serious events for any FDA-regulated medical product, clarify which types of reports the FDA wants to receive, disseminate information on the FDA's actions that have resulted from AE reporting, and increase understanding and awareness of drug and device-induced disease [58]. In the years since its inception, MedWatch has broadened its reach with expanded tools and processes for disseminating safety information to both health care providers and consumers [60].

Because spontaneous reporting systems depend upon voluntary participation, FAERS is limited by underreporting, selection bias, and variability in report quality. Factors influencing AE reporting tend to relate to motivations and attitudes. Inman [61] proposed the "seven deadly sins" theoretical basis for the underreporting of AEs among health care providers (financial incentives, legal aspects, complacency, diffidence, indifference, ignorance, and lethargy). A systematic review of the determinants of underreporting of adverse reactions by Lopez-Gonzalez et al. [62] confirmed that Inman's model can account for factors influencing ADR underreporting. Barriers to reporting include lack of awareness of the reporting system, inadequate skills needed to report, erroneous beliefs about consequences, motivation and goals, social influences, and environmental constraints [63]. Moreover, spontaneous reports may have significant variability in the quality of information in the report as some reports have detailed information while others may be missing the critical information needed to assess a causal relationship. Nonetheless, spontaneous reporting of ADRs has enabled the detection of drug-related risks.

Pharmacovigilance: Postmarketing surveillance of adverse drug reactions

Pharmacovigilance, as defined by the WHO, is the science and activities relating to the detection, assessment, understanding, and prevention of adverse effects or any other possible drug-related problem [8]. Pharmacovigilance systems are designed to detect ADRs that were not noted during a drug's preapproval clinical development program and to identify medication errors and problems with drug quality [64]. In the United States, the FDA is responsible for protecting the public health by ensuring the safety, efficacy, and security of human and veterinary drugs, biological products, and medical devices. As part of this charge, FDA conducts surveillance of data for new safety information or potential signals of a serious risk [65]. Other countries have developed ADR reporting systems to assist and identify ADRs which include: Canada Vigilance Program; United Kingdom Yellow Card Scheme operated by the Medicines and Healthcare Products Regulatory Agency (MHRA); Australia's Blue Card system; the French Pharmacovigilance Spontaneous Reporting System database; the Adverse Drug Reaction Information Management System of the Pharmaceutical and Medication Devices Agency; Ministry of Health, Labor, and Welfare (Japan); the Lareb database (Netherlands); and the BiSi database (Sweden). These ADR reporting systems as well as other pharmacovigilance activities have expanded over the years in response to tragic events resulting from drug toxicity [66]. The FAERS will be used as an example throughout the remainder of this chapter.

A safety signal is information that arises from one or multiple sources (including observations or experiments), which suggests a new, potentially causal association between a drug and an AE. Signals can also be a new aspect of a known association between an intervention and an event or set of related events, either adverse or beneficial [67]. Signals can arise from various postmarket data sources (e.g., case reports, observational studies), preclinical data, and events associated with other drugs in the same pharmacologic class [64]. Identifying safety signals in these data sources is known as signal detection. Even a single well-documented case report can provide a safety signal, particularly if the report describes a positive rechallenge (i.e., following drug discontinuation and recovery from an event, the drug is restarted and the event reoccurs) or if the event is extremely rare in the absence of drug use [68]. Once a safety signal is identified, further evaluation of a theoretical association is warranted.

Experience drawn from the postmarketing setting can lead to regulatory actions such as revising the drug's labeling to include new information on drug risks and benefits to health care providers and patients. This information may affect a health care provider's decision to prescribe a drug or a patient's willingness to take the drug. A review of drugs approved by the FDA between 2002 and 2014 determined labeling updates occur frequently following a drug's approval with the period between the second and eighth postapproval years being the most active [9]. Importantly, labeling updates for drugs also occur outside of this time period, signifying that surveillance must continue throughout the drug's life cycle [69].

Postmarketing surveillance principles from an FDA perspective

FDA monitors the benefits and risks of drugs throughout their life cycle and takes regulatory action(s) when there is a new or increased risk. FDA's safety surveillance starts early in the drug's life cycle as part of the drug application review process that may lead up to FDA approval. A multidisciplinary team evaluates the drug applications filed with the FDA, and considers appropriate measures to assess the safety of the drug in the postmarketing period. Multidisciplinary team members bring their expertise in medicine, pharmacology, epidemiology, safety surveillance, medication error prevention, risk management, product quality, and statistical analysis together to develop a postmarketing surveillance strategy that is drug specific using a risk-based approach [70,71].

The principles of risk-based safety surveillance consider the drug's characteristics and use and incorporate this information in making decisions on the appropriate frequency and extent of monitoring. Drugs that generally are subject to more extensive monitoring are included in Table 26.6. When conducting surveillance, safety specialists prioritize their review of information that suggests a safety signal or broadly describes safety concerns (i.e., important identified risk(s), important potential risk(s), and important missing information) for the drug being evaluated [72]. Safety information of interest to safety specialists during surveillance is listed in Table 26.7 [71].

After identifying a suspected new risk with a drug, the FDA evaluates the potential risk using available evidence from various data sources. Evaluations may include analyses of drug utilization data, the FDA's Sentinel system (see

TABLE 26.6 **Drug characteristics that may require extensive postmarketing surveillance [71].**

New molecular entities and original biological license applications
Biosimilar biological products
First in class approvals
Newly approved formulation(s)
Newly approved indication(s)
Extension into new patient populations
Drugs with complex pharmacokinetic (PK) or pharmacodynamic (PD) characteristics
Drugs with complex compositions or manufacturing processes

TABLE 26.7 **Safety information aspects used in postmarket surveillance of drugs [71].**

Important potential risks of the drug recognized at the time of or after approval
Apparent increase in the severity or frequency of reporting of a labeled AE
Deaths, particularly in populations or in patients using the drug for indications for which there would not be the expectation of death
AEs for which causal attribution to the drug is biologically plausible, based on the product's known pharmacological action
Reports of unlabeled, serious AEs
Serious AEs thought to be rare in the general population and associated with a high drug-attributable risk
Interactions among different drugs (e.g., drug-drug, drug-device, drug-food, or drug-dietary supplement)
Reports of reduced effectiveness or efficacy
Medication errors resulting from confusion about a drug's name, labeling, packaging, use
Off-label use, misuse, abuse, and other intentional uses of a drug in a manner that is inconsistent with the FDA-approved labeling
AEs reported or observed in a specific patient population
AEs for which a Risk Evaluation and Mitigation Strategy (REMS) is intended to mitigate the risk

AE, adverse event.

"Epidemiologic assessments" later in this chapter), clinical pharmacology data, mechanistic studies, or other population-based approaches to support or refute the risk [71]. The FDA can also ask drug manufacturers to perform additional studies if the information is unknown and a study is feasible [73]. The next section discusses additional data sources.

Data sources for signal identification

FAERS

For several decades, spontaneous reporting systems such as FAERS and its predecessor systems have been the main sources of ADR information. An analysis of all US drug labeling changes occurring in 2010 found that 52% of labeling changes were informed by spontaneous reports [74]. Similarly, an evaluation of all FDA-issued Drug Safety Communications between 2007 and 2009 found that 57% were informed by FAERS data [75]. FAERS relies on health care providers, consumers, patients, and others to report (AEs) voluntarily either to the drug's manufacturer, which will subsequently report them to the FDA according to regulations, or to the FDA directly via the MedWatch program. FAERS is a computerized database containing over 21 million AE individual case safety reports (ICSRs) received from 1969 through 2020 [76]. ICSRs in FAERS contain narrative text describing an AE, a list of suspected drugs involved in that event, and information identifying the reporter. Reporters may elect to supply additional information such as past medical history, laboratory data, details about the suspect drug, concomitant medications, event dates, exposure dates, and the event outcome (e.g., hospitalization, death). The structure of FAERS complies with international safety reporting guidance by the International Council for Harmonization of Technical Requirements for Pharmaceuticals for Human Use (ICH) [77].

Data mining

Multiple similar case reports or even a single well-documented case report can indicate a signal, especially if the report describes a positive rechallenge or if the event is extremely rare in the absence of drug use. Because of the increasingly large volume of ICSRs received annually (e.g., >2 million in 2020), FDA screens ICSRs and uses disproportionality analyses as a data mining tool to identify potential signals. Data mining refers to the use of statistical or mathematical tools to discover patterns of associations or unexpected occurrences in large databases [78]. It involves the systematic examination of reported AEs to estimate if the AE is reported at a higher frequency for a particular drug relative to other drugs in the database (disproportionality). Unexpectedly high reporting associations may generate a hypothesis that there may be an association between the particular AE and the drug, but it is not a confirmation of a causal association. Similarly, the absence of disproportionality does not confirm the absence of a safety signal or disprove a signal detected by other methods.

Limitations of spontaneous reporting systems

While FAERS is an important source of postmarketing safety information, it does have limitations. Because of the voluntary nature of reporting, the magnitude or incidence of risks cannot be determined from FAERS data. Various factors such as the duration of drug marketing, severity of the AE, reporting regulations, and publicity influence whether an AE will be reported [79]. Comparisons between drugs can be challenging particularly if their marketing periods differ and if certain factors influencing reporting are present. For example, drug manufacturer-sponsored programs, such as patient support programs, have increasingly contributed to the number of ICSRs in the FAERS database [80]. FDA issued a final rule in 2014 requiring drug manufacturers to submit postmarketing safety reports in an electronic format that the Agency can process, review, and archive [81]. Implementation of the electronic reporting rule resulted in the electronic submission of ICSRs that may have previously been submitted on paper [82]. The quality of ICSRs in terms of the completeness of the report and relevance of information provided varies among reports. An analysis of all ICSRs reporting an outcome of death received in FAERS as of 2017 demonstrated that key information needed to assess the role of a drug in a patient's death was frequently missing (e.g., patient's past medical history and concomitant medications) [80]. Bohn et al. [83] demonstrated that it was difficult to accurately identify a drug's manufacturer when multiple generic drugs with the same active ingredient are marketed, therefore making it difficult to evaluate potential drug quality issues with FAERS data. So, techniques are being developed to identify ICSRs with more robust information and differentiate them from less informative cases to improve timeliness in assessing safety signals [84]. Lastly, ICSRs describing the same occurrence of an AE in a patient reported by more than one reporter can result in duplicate reports in FAERS. The reporter could be drug manufacturers of the different drugs when there are multiple suspect drugs, different drug manufacturers of a single suspect drug (e.g., brand and generic drug manufacturers), or reports directly from the public to the FDA that were also reported by a drug manufacturer. During case series evaluation, it is not unusual for 10%–25% of ICSRs for a case series to be duplicate reports [84]. These limitations need to be considered in the evaluation of potential safety signals.

Other data sources for signal identification

There are many other information sources for safety signal identification which can include medical literature monitoring, review of a drug manufacturer's Periodic Safety Reports (PSR), postmarketing studies, and communications with international regulators. Routine screening of the medical literature is helpful to identify emerging safety signals that are not submitted as ICSRs to FDA or other regulatory authorities. Screening is accomplished by searching the medical literature by the drug name, drug class, or by an AE of interest. The principles underlying how safety specialists select drugs and AEs for medical literature screening are listed in Tables 26.6 and 26.7 [71]. Safety specialists supplement their screening of published AE case reports with additional data sources, such as studies completed by academic institutions or other researchers outside of FDA, studies performed by other Government agencies, and results from randomized controlled clinical trials that were required of the drug manufacturer or the drug manufacturer voluntarily performed in the postmarket setting. Information on the use of the drug in special populations (e.g., pediatrics, geriatrics, patients with chronic kidney disease) may be available in postmarketing studies. These may be presented in peer-reviewed or online journals or as abstracts at conferences. Safety specialists also communicate with international regulators on any trends in AE reporting especially if the drug was approved earlier in another country. Additionally, drug manufacturers submit PSRs, which may include safety assessments of previously unknown risks that they are monitoring. The drug manufacturer is required to submit PSRs to FDA on a recurring basis for review [85]. These PSRs provide summary information directly from the drug manufacturer, which may include clinical and nonclinical study reports and the drug manufacturer's assessment of the marketed drug's benefit-risk profile. In reviewing PSRs, reviewers pay particular attention to drugs with recently approved new indications or worldwide safety data with findings that might suggest an emerging safety signal.

Signal evaluation

Safety signal identification merely establishes a hypothesis that an ADR exists and requires subsequent evaluation and understanding of the safety risk. Identified safety signals are prioritized based on the AE, the seriousness of the outcome, how long the drug has been marketed, and the public health impact. Evaluations are conducted to see if the benefit–risk profile of a drug has changed based on the new information. A multidisciplinary team evaluates the prioritized safety signal using various data sources to determine whether regulatory action(s) are indicated. The data sources that are collected and analyzed can include, but are not limited to, ICSRs submitted to FAERS, medical literature case reports, observational studies, drug utilization data, and epidemiologic assessments.

Case reports often play a critical role in evaluating a safety signal [74]. Case reports with the AE of interest are retrieved from FAERS and the medical literature to formulate a case series. The search for case reports requires pharmacovigilance expertise and includes consideration of the safety signal to be evaluated, whether or not to include all drugs in the class, and a specified time period in order to retrieve the most pertinent data. Because the case reports that form a case series may derive from different sources (FAERS or medical literature) and from various reporters with varying medical expertise, it is usually necessary to develop a *case definition*. The case definition includes clinical characteristics of the event of interest, without taking into account the causal role of the drug with the AE being investigated [64]. A case definition is developed using information from medical literature and clinical practice guidelines and consists of criteria for determining whether a person should be identified as having a particular disease, injury, or other health condition [70]. Case definitions provide a consistent and reproducible approach to identifying cases of interest. Each report is then reviewed for inclusion in the case series if the case definition criteria are met. As medical literature reports may also be submitted to FAERS and multiple reporters can submit reports for the same patient, these duplicate reports need to be identified and removed. Assessment of causal association is the final step in developing a case series. Specific features that are evaluated include (1) chronologic data (e.g., plausible temporal sequence, dechallenge, rechallenge), (2) precedents (e.g., similar AEs with the same drug or related drug), (3) biological or pharmacological plausibility (e.g., toxic drug concentration in body fluid, occurrence of a recognized pharmacodynamic phenomenon), (4) information quality, and (5) alternative etiologies (e.g., concurrent diseases or conditions, concomitant medications) [71]. Assessing for potential causal association can be challenging; however, it is useful in excluding cases with no temporal relationship such as if the adverse event occurred prior to initiation of a drug. The causal assessment tools presented in Tables 26.4 and 26.5 can be used to strongly suggest an association; however, rarely can information from spontaneous reporting systems provide definitive answers [86]. In addition, summaries for select ICSRs that contain a majority of the elements of a good case report (e.g., time to onset, comorbid conditions, concomitant medications, documentation of diagnosis, response to dechallenge and rechallenge) and best represent the cases in the series are often discussed in detail. The evaluation of the developed case series may reveal important trends, risk factors, vulnerable subpopulations, or other attributes that may provide supportive evidence for the safety signal.

Drug utilization

New ADRs may emerge with increased use of a drug, when used in patients with more comorbidities, or when a drug is used off-label for other conditions or in other patient populations (e.g., in a pediatric patient). Consequently, it is important to know utilization patterns and how the patient and prescriber characteristics may differ from those included in the pre-approval clinical trials. Information from drug utilization analyses aid in identification and evaluation of safety signals and are useful in designing ways to mitigate identified risks. For example, a utilization analysis may identify specific prescribers that may benefit from enhanced communication (e.g., Dear Health Care Provider Letter) about a particular risk.

National utilization data is available in countries with a single-payer system; however, this is not available in the United States and use of data from other countries may not be generalizable to the US population. Sources of drug utilization data include drug manufacturer sales, outpatient prescription transactions, unique patient exposures, office-based physician surveys, hospital discharge billing, and longitudinal health care claims. Depending on the data sources used, the multidisciplinary team can obtain information about patient demographics, prescriber specialty, diagnoses and procedures associated with the patient visit, directions for use, prescribed dosing, dosage form or route of administration, duration of drug use, drugs taken concurrently, and use during pregnancy. Drug utilization data can be used to provide an estimate of the number of prescriptions dispensed and help put FAERS reports into context (e.g., low number of prescriptions dispensed but there are many reports of Stevens-Johnson syndrome or other very rare event) [64]. Each utilization data source has limitations that can impact appropriate interpretation and application of the data. Overall, drug utilization analyses can provide context for other pharmacovigilance activities and provide insight into real-world use.

During evaluation of a safety signal from a postmarketing spontaneous reporting system (e.g., FAERS), a *reporting ratio* (sometimes called a reporting rate) can be estimated by using drug utilization data as a surrogate measure of drug exposure. Reporting ratios are not incidence rates, but can be used to provide context and generate hypotheses using real-world data. Although reporting ratios are useful in supporting safety signal evaluation, they have limitations. The numerator (representing the number of cases of an AE) and the denominator (obtained from the approximate use of a drug in a population) are from different data sources; in addition, there may be underreporting of the AE, and the size of the exposed population is in itself an estimate [70, 71]. For these reasons, reporting ratios are not considered in isolation; safety specialists must take into account all available data and the strength of such evidence. Nonetheless, reporting ratios can be useful crude estimates for providing context and are exploratory theories to the extent that inherent limitations from each data source are considered appropriately (e.g., both numerator and denominator are aligned by date, time period, indication for use, setting of care, and reporting requirement considerations) [71].

Epidemiologic assessments

Other data sources, including well-designed pharmacoepidemiology or clinical studies, may be necessary to assess safety signals if information from a case series is insufficient or additional information is needed to strengthen the evidence. Epidemiologic assessments are often an integral part of the signal evaluation process. In the past, epidemiology studies were conducted in single health care systems to evaluate a given safety issue with a drug; however, with the passing of the FDA Amendments Act (FDAAA) in 2007, FDA was required to develop methods to gain access to a variety of data sources and validate methods for the establishment of a system to link and analyze safety data from multiple sources [87]. This is known as the Sentinel Initiative and the sources include data from public, academic, and private entities. Through the Sentinel Initiative, FDA accesses information from large electronic health care databases, such as electronic health records, insurance claims data, and registries [88, 89]. These health care databases are made available through a distributed data system that enables FDA to actively monitor the safety of marketed drugs. The Sentinel Initiative began as a pilot (Mini-Sentinel) and has since evolved into a fully integrated system that allows for both active surveillance and methodological innovation and serves as a platform to advance the science of real-world evidence. Hundreds of safety analyses have been conducted by FDA since the official launch of Sentinel's Active Risk Identification and Analysis (ARIA) system in 2016 [90]. While FDA considers the totality of available information when taking a regulatory decision such as drug withdrawal, analyses from ARIA have provided significant contributions.

Regulatory actions

Based on the totality of evidence evaluated from the various data sources mentioned before, the FDA may take regulatory action to reduce the potential for harm or communicate new risk information to health care providers and the public. The multidisciplinary team may determine certain actions are necessary such as (1) requiring a change to the drug labeling, (2) issuing a drug safety communication, (3) gathering additional data through requiring a postmarketing study or trial with the aim of better characterizing the risk, and (4) requiring a new or modifying an existing Risk Evaluation and Mitigation Strategy (REMS) to better mitigate the risk.

If insufficient evidence exists to support a causal association between the drug and an AE, the AE can be considered an AE of interest for continued close monitoring. Regardless of regulatory action taken, FDA continues to monitor for new safety information. Other regulatory authorities have their own risk communication and mitigation strategies [91]. Some of the strategies FDA uses are briefly described as follows.

Drug labeling changes

FDA-approved drug labeling for health care providers summarizes in an easy-to-read format the essential scientific information that is needed for the safe and effective use of a drug. All new human prescription drugs approved since June 2001 and certain new human prescription drugs approved before June 2001 (e.g., those approved for new uses after June 2001) must have prescribing information in the Physician Labeling Rule format. This effort standardizes the content and format of labeling to make information in the labeling (including safety related information) easier for health care providers to access, read, and use when making prescribing decisions [92]. When new safety information about a drug is identified, FDA can require drug manufacturers to make safety-related labeling changes [93]. FDA guidance documents describe how new safety information is implemented including the location of the information in labeling (e.g., Adverse Reactions, Warnings and Precautions, Boxed Warning sections) [94–96].

Safety communications

Important drug safety issues, including emerging drug safety information, is communicated to health care providers, patients, consumers, and other interested persons in a timely fashion so that they have the most current information about potential risks and benefits of a marketed drug [97]. This information is disseminated as a Drug Safety Communication (DSC), a specific tool used by FDA to communicate important new and emerging safety information. The FDA website contains the most recent Drug Safety Communications as well as links for Early Communications, Follow-Up Early Communications, and Information for Healthcare Professional sheets (https://www.fda.gov/drugs/drug-safety-and-availability/drug-safety-communications).

FDA considers issuing a DSC when the information can help with prescribing decisions, affect a patient's decision to use the drug, or indicate whether actions can be taken to avoid, prevent, or minimize harm. For example, eszopiclone, zaleplon, and zolpidem, prescription drugs used for insomnia, received a Boxed Warning for serious injuries caused by sleepwalking, which was communicated as a DSC [98]. DSCs may relate to previously unknown safety concerns including drug interactions, a potential medication error, or updated information about a known AE and highlight potentially serious or life-threatening risks. DSCs include information regarding:

- The safety issue and the nature of the risk being communicated.
- The approved indication or use of the drug.
- The established benefit(s) and risks of the drug being discussed.
- Recommended actions for health care professionals and patients, when appropriate.
- A summary of the data reviewed or being reviewed by FDA.

In addition to DSCs issued by the FDA, the drug manufacturers may be requested or required by FDA to issue a Dear Health Care Provider letter to disseminate information regarding a significant health risk, to highlight important changes in prescribing information, or to communicate corrections to prescription drug advertising or prescribing information.

Postmarketing studies and trials

When new safety information becomes available, the FDA Amendments Act (FDAAA) authorizes FDA to require that drug manufacturers of approved drugs conduct additional studies or clinical trials and establish timelines for their completion [99]. Before requiring a postmarketing study, FDA must find that AE reporting under section 505(k)(1) of the FD&C Act and the postmarket ARIA system, a component of FDA's Sentinel System, will not by themselves be sufficient to meet the purposes of assessing a safety signal [100]. In this situation, FDA can require that an observational pharmacoepidemiologic study or a randomized clinical trial be conducted. For example, upon approval of remdesivir the drug manufacturer was required to conduct a clinical trial to evaluate the pharmacokinetics and safety of remdesivir in subjects with mild, moderate, and severe renal impairment to establish appropriate dosage recommendations in patients with COVID-19 with impaired renal function [101].

Additional pharmacovigilance activities

In an effort to enhance FDA's ability to perform safety surveillance of any AEs of interest, FDA may request that the drug manufacturer:

- Use a targeted data collection tool to gather detailed case information specific to the drug and AE of interest (e.g., liver injury specific questionnaire).
- Submit reports of labeled AEs of interest more frequently and beyond minimum reporting requirements.
- Summarize and assess AEs of interest at a frequency defined by FDA (e.g., in PSRs or on a yearly basis).

Web posting of potential safety signals

In accordance with statutory requirements and established policies and procedures, FDA has a website posting of *potential* signals of serious risks or new safety information that were identified from FAERS, or for which FAERS data were contributory [102]. A new report is made available each quarter. Listing of a drug and potential safety issue on this quarterly posting enables this information to be shared with the public at an early stage of FDA's evaluation, while simply indicating that the FDA has identified a potential safety signal for further evaluation. Therefore the FDA may not have determined or communicated what type of regulatory action, if any, is appropriate for the issue at the time of posting. Information from previous quarters is updated and the drug safety issue remains active until an FDA regulatory action has been taken or a determination is made that no regulatory action may be required. Types of regulatory action can include: modifying the drug labeling, gathering additional data to characterize the risk, development or a modification of a REMS, or suspending or withdrawing a drug from the market. In addition to the quarterly posting, a separate website posting includes signals evaluated under the Sentinel program [90]. The information posted on the Sentinel website is provided as part of FDA's commitment to make knowledge acquired from the Sentinel system readily available to the public.

Risk evaluation and mitigation strategies (REMS)

Some drugs may require additional measures to mitigate risks and ensure benefits are achieved. FDAAA amended the FD&C Act to authorize FDA to require a REMS when FDA determines that a REMS is necessary to ensure that the benefits of a drug outweigh its risks [103]. A REMS utilizes risk minimization strategies beyond the drug labeling and can provide safe access to drugs with known serious risks that would otherwise be unavailable to patients. Even after a drug is approved, new safety information may become available that requires the use of a REMS to ensure the benefits of the drug continue to outweigh the risks. An FDA guidance for drug manufacturers is available for determining when a REMS may be necessary [103]. Some of the considerations used to determine if a REMS is needed for a new safety issue include estimated size of the population using the drug, seriousness of the disease or condition being treated, expected benefit of the drug, duration of treatment, and seriousness of the AE [103].

After determining that a REMS is necessary, the goals of the REMS and specific strategies to meet the goals are considered. A REMS can include (1) a medication guide [104]; (2) a communication plan; (3) additional safety precautions, termed ETASU (**e**lements **t**o **a**ssure **s**afe **u**se); (4) an implementation system, and requires a timetable for assessment of the REMS. Medication guides are patient-friendly labeling and can be required if it could help prevent serious adverse events. A communication plan to health care providers may be required to support implementation of the REMS, to disseminate information to health care providers regarding REMS requirements and about serious risks, or to explain certain safety protocols, such as medical monitoring through periodic laboratory tests. ETASU can be required as part of a REMS to mitigate a specific serious risk listed in the drug labeling if, in the absence of an ETASU, the drug would otherwise not be approved or would be withdrawn. The following are specific elements that may be part of an ETASU: certification and specialized training of health care providers who prescribe the drug, ongoing periodic patient monitoring in order to continue drug therapy, enrollment of treated patients in a registry, or that the drug be dispensed or administered to patients with evidence or other documentation of safe use conditions [103]. Table 26.8 lists some examples of REMS components for selected drugs [105].

Manufacturers of drugs with a REMS are required to periodically assess the REMS to determine if the goals of the REMS are being met and to modify them if they are not. These assessments are submitted to FDA and reviewed by specialists. The drug manufacturer and FDA collaborate to modify the REMS throughout the life cycle of the drug as new information becomes available with expanded use.

TABLE 26.8 Examples of risk evaluation and mitigation strategies components.

Component	Drug example	Purpose
Medication guide	Qsymia (weight loss)	– Informs of congenital malformation risk and the importance of pregnancy prevention
Communication plan	Bydureon (diabetes)	– Dear Health care provider Letter informs health care providers of acute pancreatitis risk
Elements to ensure safe use	Revlimid (multiple myeloma)	– Certifies and enrolls health care providers and pharmacies in the REMS program – Pregnancy testing must occur within a certain time of prescribing – Drug dispensed to enrolled patients with evidence of safe-use conditions
Implementation system	Revlimid (multiple myeloma)	– Requires that drug manufacturer maintain a secure database of certified physicians, pharmacies, and enrolled patients and monitor compliance with elements to ensure safe use

Disclaimer

The views expressed are those of the authors and do not necessarily represent the position of, nor imply endorsement from, the US Food and Drug Administration or the US Government.

References

[1] Best WR. Choramphenicol-associated blood dyscrasias. JAMA 1967;201:181–188.

[2] Kongkaew C, Noyce PR, Ashcroft DM. Hospital admissions associated with adverse drug reactions: a systematic review of prospective observational studies. Ann Pharmacother 2008;42:1017–1025.

[3] Pirmohamed M, Breckenridge AM, Kitteringham NR, Park BK. Adverse drug reactions. BMJ 1998;316:1295–1298.

[4] Lazarou J, Pomeranz BH, Corey PN. Incidence of adverse drug reactions in hospitalized patients: a meta-analysis of prospective studies. JAMA 1998;279:1200–1205.

[5] Hazell L, Shakir SA. Under-reporting of adverse drug reactions : a systematic review. Drug Saf 2006;29:385–396.

[6] Nebeker JR, Barach P, Samore MH. Clarifying adverse drug events: a clinician's guide to terminology, documentation, and reporting. Ann Intern Med 2004;140:795–801.

[7] Lundkvist J, Jönsson B. Pharmacoeconomics of adverse drug reactions. Fundam Clin Pharmacol 2004;18:275–280.

[8] Uppsala Monitoring Centre/World Health Organization Centre for International Drug Monitoring. Glossary of pharmacovigilance terms. https://www.who-umc.org/global-pharmacovigilance/publications/glossary/. (Accessed 24 June 2020).

[9] Pinnow E, Amr S, Bentzen SM, Brajovic S, Hungerford L, St George DM, et al. Postmarket safety outcomes for new molecular entity (NME) drugs approved by the Food and Drug Administration between 2002 and 2014. Clin Pharmacol Ther 2018;104:390–400.

[10] FDA. Guidance for Industry and Investigators. Safety reporting requirements for INDs and BA/BE studies. Available from: https://www.fda.gov/regulatory-information/search-fda-guidance-documents/safety-reporting-requirements-inds-investigational-new-drug-applications-and-babe; 2012. (Accessed 26 July 2020).

[11] Anon. 21CFR314.80 Postmarketing reporting of adverse drug experiences. Available from: https://www.accessdata.fda.gov/scripts/cdrh/cfdocs/cfcfr/CFRSearch.cfm?fr=314.80; April 2019. (Accessed 15 June 2020).

[12] WHO Definition. Council for International Organizations of Medical Sciences (CIOMS), pharmacovigilance definition, history, results. Available from: https://cioms.ch/pharmacovigilance/; 1972. (Accessed 26 July 2020).

[13] Edwards IR, Aronson JK. Adverse drug reactions: definitions, diagnosis, and management. Lancet 2000;356:1255–1259.

[14] Rawlins MD, Thomas SHL. Mechanisms of adverse drug reactions. In: Davies DM, Ferner RE, de Glanville H, editors. Davies's textbook of adverse drug reactions. 5th ed. London: Chapman & Hall Medical; 1998. p. 40–64.

[15] Rohilla A, Singhraj Y. Adverse drug reactions: an overview. Int J Pharmacol Res 2013;3:53–56.

[16] Rehan HS, Chopra D, Kakkar AK. Physician's guide to pharmacovigilance: terminology and causality assessment. Eur J Intern Med 2009;20:3–8.

[17] Pichler WJ. Adverse side-effects to biological agents. Allergy 2006;61:912–920.

[18] Aronson JK, Ferner RE. Joining the DoTS: new approach to classifying adverse drug reactions. BMJ 2003;327:1222–1225.

[19] Coleman JJ, Pontefract SK. Adverse drug reactions. Clin Med (Lond) 2016;16:481–485.

[20] Ferner RE, Aronson JK. EIDOS: a mechanistic classification of adverse drug effects. Drug Saf 2010;33:15–23.

[21] Aronson JK, Ferner RE. Preventability of drug-related harms - part II: proposed criteria, based on frameworks that classify adverse drug reactions. Drug Saf 2010;33(11):995–1002.

[22] Patel SV, Khan DA. Adverse reactions to biologic therapy. Immunol Allergy Clin North Am 2017;37:397–412.

[23] National Cancer Institute. Common terminology criteria for adverse events. Available from: https://ctep.cancer.gov/protocolDevelopment/electronic_applications/ctc.htm. (Accessed 15 June 2020).
[24] Medical Dictionary for Regulatory Activities (MedDRA). https://www.meddra.org/. (Accessed 16 March 2021).
[25] European Medicines Agency. About us, glossary of regulatory terms. https://www.ema.europa.eu/en/about-us/about-website/glossary/name_az/S. (Accessed 10 November 2020).
[26] Warrington R, Silviu-Dan F, Wong T. Drug allergy. Allergy Asthma Clin Immunol 2018;14(Suppl. 2):60.
[27] Morimoto T, Gandhi TK, Seger AC, Hsieh TC, Bates DW. Adverse drug events and medication errors: detection and classification methods. Qual Saf Health Care 2004;13:306–314.
[28] Furukawa MF, Eldridge N, Wang Y, Metersky M. Electronic health record adoption and rates of in-hospital adverse events. J Pat Saf 2020;16:137–142.
[29] Classen DC, Resar R, Griffin F, Federico F, Frankel T, Kimmel N, et al. 'Global trigger tool' shows that adverse events in hospitals may be ten times greater than previously measured. Health Aff (Millwood) 2011;30:581–589.
[30] Hibbert PD, Molloy CJ, Hooper TD, Wiles LK, Runciman WB, Lachman P, et al. The application of the Global Trigger Tool: a systematic review. Int J Qual Health Care 2016;28:640–649.
[31] Poudel DR, Acharya P, Ghimire S, Dhital R, Bharati R. Burden of hospitalizations related to adverse drug events in the USA: a retrospective analysis from large inpatient database. Pharmacoepidemiol Drug Saf 2017;26:635–641.
[32] Sakuma M, Kanemoto Y, Furuse A, Bates DW, Morimoto T. Frequency and severity of adverse drug events by medication classes: the JADE study. J Patient Saf 2020;16:30–35.
[33] Winterstein AG, Jeon N, Staley B, Xu D, Henriksen C, Lipori GP. Development and validation of an automated algorithm for identifying patients at high risk for drug-induced hypoglycemia. Am J Health Syst Pharm 2018;75(21):1714–1728. https://doi.org/10.2146/ajhp180071.
[34] Winterstein AG, Staley B, Henriksen C, Xu D, Lipori G, Jeon N, et al. Development and validation of a complexity score to rank hospitalized patients at risk for preventable adverse drug events. Am J Health Syst Pharm 2017;74:1970–1984.
[35] Muñoz MA, Jeon N, Staley B, Henriksen C, Xu D, Weberpals J, et al. Predicting medication-associated altered mental status in hospitalized patients: development and validation of a risk model. Am J Health Syst Pharm 2019;76:953–963.
[36] Luo Y, Thompson WK, Herr TM, Zeng Z, Berendsen MA, Jonnalagadda SR, et al. Natural language processing for EHR-based pharmacovigilance: a structured review. Drug Saf 2017;40:1075–1089.
[37] Hill AB. The environment and disease: association or causation? Proc R Soc Med 1965;58:295–300.
[38] Drugs@FDA: FDA-approved drugs. Available from: https://www.accessdata.fda.gov/scripts/cder/daf/. (Accessed 31 January 2021).
[39] DailyMed. Available from: https://dailymed.nlm.nih.gov/dailymed/. (Accessed 31 January 2021).
[40] MedWatch: the FDA safety information and adverse event reporting program. Available from: https://www.fda.gov/safety/medwatch-fda-safety-information-and-adverse-event-reporting-program. (Accessed 10 November 2020).
[41] Potential signals of serious risks/new safety information identified from the FDA Adverse Event Reporting System (FAERS). https://www.fda.gov/drugs/questions-and-answers-fdas-adverse-event-reporting-system-faers/potential-signals-serious-risksnew-safety-information-identified-fda-adverse-event-reporting-system. (Accessed 10 November 2020).
[42] Johnson J. Reasonable possibility: causality and postmarketing surveillance. Drug Inf J 1992;26:553–558.
[43] Agbabiaka TB, Savović J, Ernst E. Methods for causality assessment of adverse drug reactions: a systematic review. Drug Saf 2008;31:21–37.
[44] Uppsala Monitoring Centre. The use of the WHO-UMC system for standardised case causality assessment. https://www.who.int/medicines/areas/quality_safety/safety_efficacy/WHOcausality_assessment.pdf. (Accessed 30 June 2020).
[45] Kakkar A. Physician's guide to pharmacovigilance: terminology and causality assessment. Eur J Intern Med 2008;20:3–8.
[46] Naranjo CA, Busto U, Sellers EM, Sandor P, Ruiz I, Roberts EA, et al. A method for estimating the probability of adverse drug reactions. Clin Pharmacol Ther 1981;30:239–245.
[47] Goldman JL, Chung WH, Lee BR, Chen CB, Lu CW, Hoetzenecker W, et al. Adverse drug reaction causality assessment tools for drug-induced Stevens-Johnson syndrome and toxic epidermal necrolysis: room for improvement. Eur J Clin Pharmacol 2019;75:1135–1141.
[48] Schiff GD, Galanter WL, Duhig J, Lodolce AE, Koronkowski MJ, Lambert BL. Principles of conservative prescribing. Arch Intern Med 2011;171:1433–1440.
[49] Ferner RE. Adverse drug reactions. BMJ 2018;363:1–9.
[50] Boehringer Ingelheim. Pradaxa (dagigatran etexilate mesylate) prescribing information, Ridgefield, CT: Boehringer Ingelheim Pharmaceuticals, Inc.; 2020. Drugs@fda label update 07/01/2020. https://www.accessdata.fda.gov/scripts/cder/daf/index.cfm?event=overview.process&ApplNo=022512 (Accessed 10 November 2020).
[51] FDA. Guidance for industry: warnings and precautions, contraindications, and boxed warning sections of labeling for human prescription and drug and biological products—content and format; October 2011. https://www.fda.gov/media/71866/download (web archive link, 01 July 2020). (Accessed 31 January 2021).
[52] Bonfiglio MF, Weinstein DM. Allergic reactions to small-molecule drugs: will we move from reaction to prediction? Am J Health Syst Pharm 2019;76(9):574–580.
[53] de Las Vecillas Sánchez L, Alenazy LA, Garcia-Neuer M, Castells MC. Drug hypersensitivity and desensitizations: mechanisms and new approaches. Int J Mol Sci 2017;18:1316.
[54] American Society of Health-Systems Pharmacists. ASHP guidelines on adverse drug reaction monitoring and reporting. Am J Health Syst Pharm 1995;52:417–419.
[55] The Joint Commission. Available from: https://www.jointcommission.org/standards/. (Accessed 20 June 2020).

[56] How to report product problems and complaints to the FDA. https://www.fda.gov/consumers/consumer-updates/how-report-product-problems-and-complaints-fda. (Accessed 6 November 2020).

[57] Pushkin R, Frassetto L, Tsourounis C, Segal ES, Kim S. Improving the reporting of adverse drug reactions in hospital setting. Postgrad Med 2010;122:154–164.

[58] Kessler DA. Introducing MEDWatch. A new approach to reporting medication and device adverse effects and product problems. JAMA 1993;269:2765–2768.

[59] Reporting serious problems to FDA. https://www.fda.gov/safety/medwatch-fda-safety-information-and-adverse-event-reporting-program. (Accessed 6 November 2020).

[60] Rose BJ, Fritsch BF. FDA's MedWatch program turns 20: what's new? American Pharmacist Association: Pharmacy Today; 2013. p. 68–69. Available from: https://www.pharmacytoday.org/article/S1042-0991(15)31139-7/abstract.

[61] Inman WH. Attitudes to adverse drug reaction reporting. Br J Clin Pharmacol 1996;4:434–435.

[62] Lopez-Gonzalez E, Herdeiro MT, Figueiras A. Determinants of under-reporting of adverse drug reactions: a systematic review. Drug Saf 2009;32:19–31.

[63] Mirbaha F, Shalviri G, Yazdizadeh B, Gholami K, Majdzadeh R. Perceived barriers to reporting adverse drug events in hospitals: a qualitative study using theoretical domains framework approach. Implement Sci 2015;10:110.

[64] Dal Pan GJ, Lindquist M, Gelperin K. Postmarketing spontaneous pharmacovigilance reporting systems. In: Strom BL, Kimmel SE, Hennessy S, editors. Pharmacoepidemiology. Wiley; 2019. p. 169–201.

[65] FDA website for the 21st Century Cures Act. Available from: https://www.fda.gov/regulatory-information/selected-amendments-fdc-act/21st-century-cures-act. (Accessed 2 February 2021).

[66] Fornasier G, Francescon S, Leone R, Baldo P. An historical overview over pharmacovigilance. Int J Clin Pharmacol 2018;40:744–747.

[67] CIOMS Working Group VIII. Practical aspects of signal detection in pharmacovigilance. Report of CIOMS Working Group VIII. Geneva; 2010.

[68] Edwards IR, Lindquist M. First, catch your signal! Drug Saf 2010;33:257–260.

[69] Bulatao I, Pinnow E, Day B, Cherkaoui S, Kalaria M, Brajovic S, et al. Postmarketing safety-related regulatory actions for new therapeutic biologics approved in the U.S. 2002–2014: similarities and differences with new molecular entities. Clin Pharmacol Ther 2020;108:1243–1253.

[70] FDA. Guidance for industry good pharmacovigilance practices and pharmacoepidemiologic assessment, https://www.fda.gov/regulatory-information/search-fda-guidance-documents/good-pharmacovigilance-practices-and-pharmacoepidemiologic-assessment; March 2005. (Accessed 10 November 2020).

[71] FDA. Best practices in drug and biological product postmarket safety surveillance for FDA Staff, draft. Available from: https://www.fda.gov/media/130216/download; November 2019. (Accessed 31 January 2021).

[72] FDA. Guidance for industry E2E pharmacovigilance planning. Available from: https://www.fda.gov/downloads/Drugs/GuidanceComplianceRegulatoryInformation/Guidances/UCM073107.pdf. (Accessed 31 January 2021).

[73] FDA. Postmarketing studies and clinical trials—implementation of Section 505(o)(3) of the Federal Food, Drug, and Cosmetic Act, guidance for industry draft guidance. Available from: https://www.fda.gov/media/131980/download; October 2019. (Accessed 4 February 2021).

[74] Lester J, Neyarapally GA, Lipowski E, Graham CF, Hall M, Dal Pan G. Evaluation of FDA safety-related drug label changes in 2010. Pharmacoepidemiol Drug Saf 2013;22:302–305.

[75] Ishiguro C, Hall M, Neyarapally GA, Dal Pan G. Post-market drug safety evidence sources: an analysis of FDA drug safety communications. Pharmacoepidemiol Drug Saf 2012;21:1134–1136.

[76] FDA. Adverse Event Reporting System (FAERS) public dashboard. Available from: https://www.fda.gov/drugs/questions-and-answers-fdas-adverse-event-reporting-system-faers/fda-adverse-event-reporting-system-faers-public-dashboard. (Accessed 20 June 2020).

[77] International Council for Harmonisation of Technical Requirements for Pharmaceuticals for Human Use (ICH). https://www.ich.org/. (Accessed 10 November 2020).

[78] Duggirala HJ, Tonning JM, Smith E, Bright RA, Baker JD, Ball R, et al. Use of data mining at the Food and Drug Administration. J Am Med Inform Assoc 2016;23:428–434.

[79] U.S. Food & Drug Administration Questions and Answers on FDA's Adverse Event Reporting System (FAERS). Available from: https://www.fda.gov/drugs/surveillance/questions-and-answers-fdas-adverse-event-reporting-system-faers. (Accessed 18 March 2021).

[80] Marwitz K, Jones SC, Kortepeter CM, Dal Pan GJ, Muñoz MA. An evaluation of postmarketing reports with an outcome of death in the US FDA adverse event reporting system. Drug Saf 2020;43:457–465.

[81] U.S. Department of Health and Human Services. Guidance for industry providing submissions in electronic format—postmarketing safety reports draft guidance. Available from: https://www.fda.gov/regulatory-information/search-fda-guidance-documents/providing-submissions-electronic-format-postmarketing-safety-reports; June 2014. (Accessed 23 March 2021).

[82] FDA issues final rule on postmarketing safety report in electronic format. Available from: http://wayback.archive-it.org/7993/20170111002213/http://www.fda.gov/Drugs/DrugSafety/ucm400526.htm (Accessed 15 August 2020).

[83] Bohn J, Kortepeter C, Muñoz MA, Simms K, Dal Pan G. Patterns in spontaneous adverse event reporting among branded and generic antiepileptic drugs. Clin Pharmacol Ther 2015;97:508–517.

[84] Muñoz MA, Dal Pan GJ, Wei YJ, Delcher C, Xiao H, Kortepeter CM, et al. Towards automating adverse event review: a prediction model for case report utility. Drug Saf 2020;43:329–338.

[85] FDA. Guidance for industry postmarketing safety reporting for human drug and biological products including vaccines. https://www.fda.gov/media/73593/download. (Accessed 10 November 2020). FDA's postmarketing safety reporting regulations require applicants to submit PSRs in the form of a periodic adverse drug experience report (PADER) (for drugs) or a periodic adverse experience report (PAER) (for biologics) (21 CFR 314.80(c)(2) and 600.80(c)(2)).

[86] Edwards RI. Causality assessment in pharmacovigilance: still a challenge. Drug Saf 2017;40:365–372.

[87] FDA's Sentinel Initiative—background. https://www.fda.gov/safety/fdas-sentinel-initiative/fdas-sentinel-initiative-background. (Accessed 13 November 2020).

[88] Platt R, Brown JS, Robb M, McClellan M, Ball R, Nguyen MD, et al. The FDA Sentinel Initiative—an evolving national resource. N Engl J Med 2018;379:2091–2093.

[89] Dal Pan GJ. Real-world data, advanced analytics, and the evolution of postmarket drug safety surveillance. Clin Pharmacol Ther 2019;106:28–30.

[90] Sentinel Initiative. https://www.sentinelinitiative.org/. (Accessed 31 January 2021).

[91] Insani WN, Pacurariu AC, Mantel-Teeuwisse AK, Gross-Martirosyan L. Characteristics of drugs safety signals that predict safety related product information update. Pharmacoepidemiol Drug Saf 2018;27:789–796.

[92] Department of Health and Human Services. FDA 21 CFR parts 201, 314, and 601 requirements on content and format of labeling for human prescription drug and biological products and draft guidances and two guidances for industry on the content and format of labeling for human prescription drug and biological products; final rule and notices. Available from: https://www.govinfo.gov/content/pkg/FR-2006-01-24/pdf/06-545.pdf. (Accessed 3 February 2021).

[93] Under Section 505(o)(4) of the FD&C Act. https://www.fda.gov/regulatory-information/laws-enforced-fda/federal-food-drug-and-cosmetic-act-fdc-act.

[94] FDA. Guidance for industry safety labeling changes—implementation of Section 505(o)(4) of the FD&C Act. Available from: https://www.fda.gov/RegulatoryInformation/Guidances/default.htm; July 2013. (Accessed 10 November 2020).

[95] Guidance for industry adverse reactions section of labeling for human prescription drug and biological products—content and format. Available from: https://www.fda.gov/RegulatoryInformation/Guidances/default.htm.

[96] FDA. Guidance for industry drug safety information—FDA's communication to the public. Available from: https://www.fda.gov/RegulatoryInformation/Guidances/default.htm; March 2012.

[97] Woodcock J, Behrman RE, Dal Pan GJ. Role of postmarketing surveillance in contemporary medicine. Annu Rev Med 2011;62:1–10.

[98] FDA adds Boxed Warning for risk of serious injuries caused by sleepwalking with certain prescription insomnia medicines. Available from: https://www.fda.gov/drugs/drug-safety-and-availability/fda-adds-boxed-warning-risk-serious-injuries-caused-sleepwalking-certain-prescription-insomnia. (Accessed 1 February 2021).

[99] FDA. Guidance for industry postmarketing studies and clinical trials—implementation of Section 505(o)(3) of the Federal Food, Drug, and Cosmetic Act. Available from: https://www.fda.gov/RegulatoryInformation/Guidances/default.htm.

[100] Active Risk Identification and Analysis (ARIA) overview. Available from: https://www.sentinelinitiative.org/assessments/aria-overview. (Accessed 31 January 2021).

[101] Veklury (remdesivir), NDA 214787 approval letter issued on October 22, 2020. https://www.accessdata.fda.gov/drugsatfda_docs/appletter/2020/214787Orig1s000ltr.pdf. (Accessed 1 February 2021).

[102] Potential signals of serious risks/new safety information identified from the FDA Adverse Event Reporting System (FAERS). Available from: http://www.fda.gov/Drugs/GuidanceComplianceRegulatoryInformation/Surveillance/AdverseDrugEffects/ucm082196.htm.

[103] FDA. Guidance for industry REMS: FDA's application of statutory factors in determining when a REMS is necessary. Available from: https://www.fda.gov/RegulatoryInformation/Guidances/default.htm; April 2019. (Accessed 31 January 2021).

[104] FDA. Guidance for industry medication guides—distribution requirements and inclusion in Risk Evaluation and Mitigation Strategies (REMS). Available from: https://www.fda.gov/RegulatoryInformation/Guidances/default.htm.

[105] Approved Risk Evaluation and Mitigation Strategies (REMS). Available from: https://www.accessdata.fda.gov/scripts/cder/rems/index.cfm. (Accessed 31 January 2021).

Chapter 27

Quality assessment of drug therapy

Charles E. Daniels
Skaggs School of Pharmacy and Pharmaceutical Sciences, University of California, San Diego, CA, United States

Introduction

Dozens of new drugs, new combinations, and new dosage forms are approved each year in the United States and Europe. The availability of valuable new agents creates opportunities for improved therapeutic outcomes, but also creates increased opportunities for inappropriate medication use. The clinical pharmacologist must have generalized expertise in the use of medications that can be applied across the organization in clinical practice and in independent and collaborative research activities. Quality assessment and improvement of medication use constitute an important skill set.

The objective of this chapter is to review medication use quality issues from an institutional perspective and highlight their impact on patient care and clinical research. The focus is on three themes: understanding the medication use system and organizational priorities in medication use, understanding the application of drug use monitoring as a tool to improve medication use, and understanding processes to identify and improve medication errors. Improvement in quality of medication use revolves around identifying and minimizing systematic risk of error, and improving outcomes through the use of relevant guidelines and benchmarking tools.

Adverse drug events

In 2001 Ernst [1] estimated that costs of $177 billion a year are attributable to medication misuse that projects to approximately $260 billion in 2020. Adverse drug events (ADEs) are instances in which patient harm results from the use of medication. This includes both adverse drug reactions, which are not preventable, and medication errors, which are inherently preventable. A 1999 Institute of Medicine (IOM) report estimated that 98,000 Americans die each year due to medical error [2]. This includes diagnostic mistakes, wrong-site surgery, and other categories of error, including medication errors. A supplemental IOM report in 2007 estimated that hospitals experienced up to 450,000 preventable ADEs each year and long-term care facilities experienced an estimated 800,000 per year. It further concluded that up to $3.5 billion is added to hospital costs due to preventable ADEs [3]. Approximately 20% of all medical errors are medication related [4, 5].

A medication error is any preventable event that may cause or lead to inappropriate medication use or patient harm while medication is in the control of a healthcare professional, patient, or consumer [6]. Not all medication errors reach the patient. These are sometimes referred to as "near misses." They are not usually considered to be ADEs only because no harm was done. Preventable ADEs are a subset of medication errors that cause harm to a patient [7]. Fig. 27.1 depicts the relationship between ADEs, medication errors, and adverse drug reactions [8]. Because adverse drug reactions are generally unexpected, they are not presently considered to be a reflection of medication use quality in a classic sense. However, as genetic variances become a more prominent consideration in drug selection and monitoring, it may be possible to predict and avoid some of the reactions that have been previously unexpected. This offers an opportunity to improve the quality of medication use.

Medication errors are costly and are a diversion from the intended therapeutic objective. Morbidity or mortality are possible outcomes of medication errors. A 1997 study by Bates et al. [9] found that 6.5 ADEs occurred for every 100 non-obstetric hospital admissions, and that 28% of them were preventable. It also was determined that 42% of life-threatening and serious ADEs were preventable. Preventable ADEs were responsible for an increased length of hospital stay of 4.6 days and $5857 per event. The cost for all ADEs was projected to be $5.6 million per year just for the institution in which the study was conducted. McDonnell [10] concluded from a separate data set that ADE-related admissions resulted in a 6.1 day length of stay. Anderson et al. [11] conducted a simulation of the impact of an integrated medication use system and

Atkinson's Principles of Clinical Pharmacology. https://doi.org/10.1016/B978-0-12-819869-8.00004-5

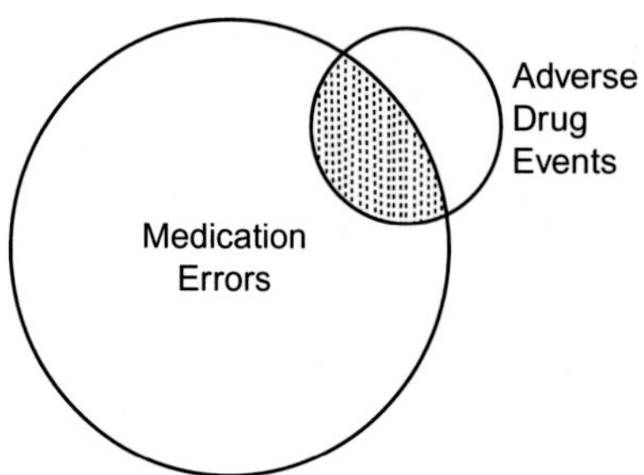

FIG. 27.1 Diagram showing the relationship between medication errors and adverse drug events. Because some adverse drug events are preventable, they are also considered to be medication errors *(shaded area). (Based on Bates DW, Boyle DL, Vander Vliet MB, Schneider J, Leape L. Relationship between medication errors and adverse drug events. J Gen Intern Med 1995;10:199–205.)*

projected $1.4 million in excess costs that might have been saved had the components of the system been effectively integrated. These findings imply that safer medication use, with fewer adverse medication events, is a cost-effective strategy.

Medication use process

Medications are prescribed, distributed, and consumed under the assumption that the therapeutic plan will work as intended to provide the expected outcome. It is clear from previous chapters that there are many biological system issues that will influence the success of the plan. Other organizational and societal system issues also influence the success of the therapeutic plan as profoundly as do those biological systems issues. A prescriber writes an order for a medication based on the best available information, the likely diagnosis, and the expected outcome. A pharmacist reviews the requested medication order (prescription), clarifies it based upon additional information about the patient or medication (allergies, drug interactions, etc.), prepares the medication for use, counsels the patient about the drug, and gives it to the patient. The patient is responsible for understanding the therapeutic objective, knowing about the drug, creating a daily compliance plan (deciding when to take the drug), watching for good or bad results, and providing feedback to the prescriber or pharmacist regarding planned or unplanned outcomes. This process occurs over a variable period of time, in a system where the key participants of the process seldom speak with each other. Each action creates an opportunity for success or failure. Is there any wonder that the quality and integrity of the system are compromised on a regular basis?

The medication use system in a hospital or long-term care setting offers even more complexity, with more chances for error. The five subsystems of the medication system in a hospital are selection and procurement of drugs, drug prescribing, preparation and dispensing, drug administration, and monitoring for medication or related effects [12]. Evaluation and improvement of medication use quality require consideration of all of these subsystems.

Fig. 27.2 is a flowchart of appropriate, safe, effective, and efficient use of medications in the hospital setting [13]. It incorporates the role of the prescriber, nurse, pharmacist, and patient in a typical inpatient environment. It also depicts the role of the organization's pharmacy and therapeutics committee and quality improvement functions, which will be discussed later in this chapter. The decision to treat a patient in a hospital or extended-care facility typically adds a nurse or other healthcare provider (respiratory therapist, etc.) to the trio described in the ambulatory care setting. Every time that individual has to read, interpret, decide, or act is yet another opportunity for a mistake to occur. Each of the steps in the medication use process provides an opportunity for correct or incorrect interpretation and implementation of the tactics that support the therapeutic plan. With this many opportunities for medication misadventures to occur, it is easy to understand why tracking and improving quality are important aspects of medication use.

Phillips and colleagues [14] found a 236% increase in medication error-related deaths for hospitalized patients between 1983 and 1993. The same study showed an increase of over 800% for outpatient medication error deaths. The reported growth in medication error deaths may be partially attributed to more accurate reporting, but clearly represents a growth in the problem of medication errors from potent drugs. Phillips [15] has further proposed that impediments to reductions in medical error include perceptual, legal, and medical barriers. Winterstein [16] conducted a metaanalysis of 15 studies and concluded that 4.3% of hospital admissions were drug related and that greater than 50% of them were preventable. A study by Bates et al. [17] determined that the 56% of medication errors in a hospital setting were associated with the ordering process, 6% with transcription of written orders, 4% with pharmacy dispensing, and 34% with administration of medications. Another study by Barker et al. [18] of medication administration in 36 healthcare settings identified a 19% total error rate during medication administration. Based on these findings it is easily concluded that there is room for improvement in how medications are used in both the inpatient and outpatient setting.

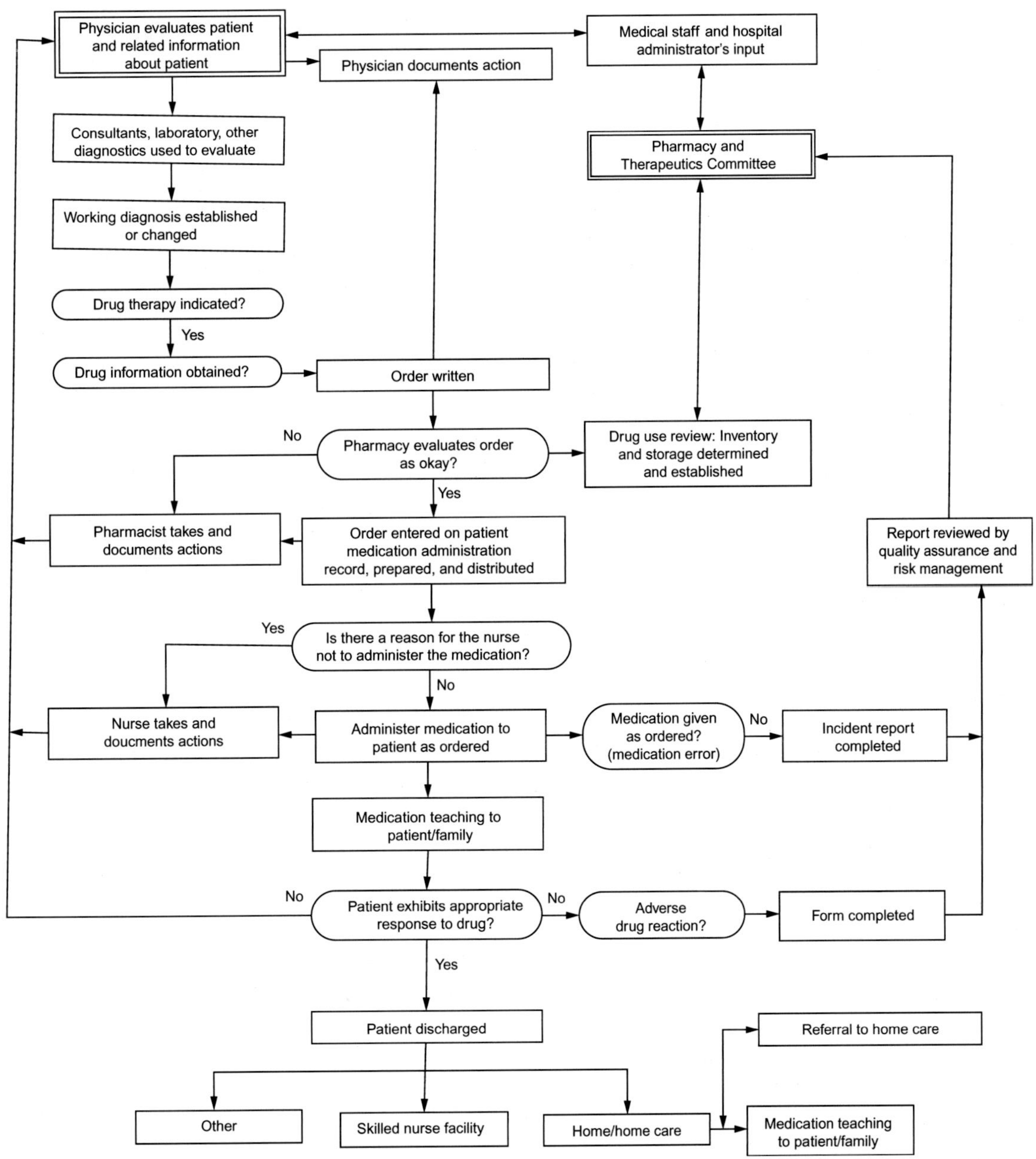

FIG. 27.2 Flowchart of the inpatient medication use process showing the start and end points *(double-boxed rectangles)*, intervening actions *(rectangles)*, and decision-making steps *(ovals)* required for appropriate, safe, effective, and efficient medication use. *(Reproduced with permission from Atkinson AJ Jr, Nadzam DM, Schaff RL., An indicator-based program for improving medication use in acute care hospitals. Clin Pharmacol Ther 1991;50:125–128.)*

Improving the quality of medication use

There are multiple facets to be considered in assessing the quality of medication use. Among them are the monitoring adverse medication event and medication use evaluation programs. To improve medication use, Berwick [19] has applied the industrial principles of continuous quality improvement to the healthcare setting. The critical elements of this approach are collection and use of data with a system focus. Deming [20] has championed the use of the Shewhart Cycle in continuous quality improvement. As shown in Fig. 27.3, the Shewhart Cycle is an approach for implementing systematic change, based on data collection and evaluation with each iteration of the cycle. Each time the work cycle is completed, the result is compared to the expected outcome or ideal target. Modifications that improve the result are permanently

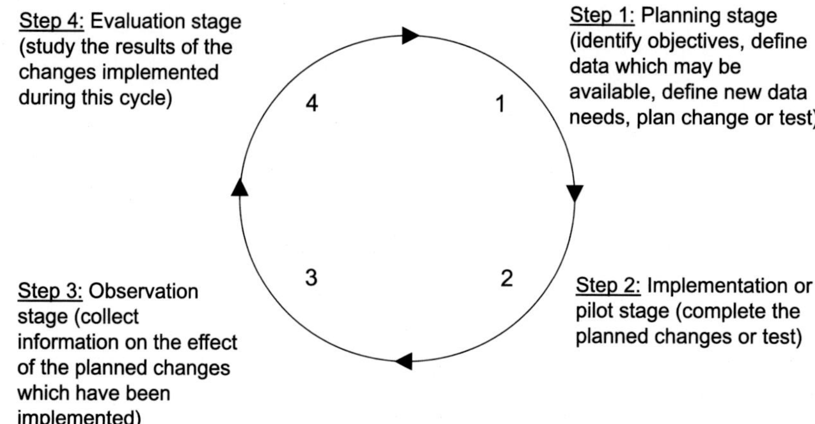
Step 4: Evaluation stage (study the results of the changes implemented during this cycle)
Step 1: Planning stage (identify objectives, define data which may be available, define new data needs, plan change or test)
4
1
3
2
Step 3: Observation stage (collect information on the effect of the planned changes which have been implemented)
Step 2: Implementation or pilot stage (complete the planned changes or test)
The Shewhart cycle is repeated multiple cycles with expected improvements implemented in each new cycle

FIG. 27.3 The Shewhart cycle. The cycle is repeated with desired improvements implemented with each iteration and the measured results used to guide the design of the next cycle. *(Reproduced with permission from Deming WE. Out of the crisis. Cambridge, MA: MIT Press; 2000. p. 87–89.)*

incorporated into the process. Changes with no impact or a negative result will be deleted in the next iteration. Deming's message is that ongoing process and system change, along with measurement of the result, provide the feedback loop that is needed to support continuous improvement of the product or service.

Organizational influences on medication use quality

Several external organizations and internal elements of the healthcare system have an interest in optimizing medication use. These include the hospital or health system, the medical staff, the group purchasing organization with which the hospital participates for the contractual purchase of drugs, and external regulatory or accreditation organizations (e.g., the Joint Commission on Accreditation of Healthcare Organizations (TJC), Center for Medicare and Medicaid Services, National Council on Quality Assurance, state and local public health agencies). There is interest in what drugs are used, when and how they are used, the economic impact of drug selection, and outcomes that result in safe and effective use of medications.

TJC is the organization that accredits many hospitals, health systems, and home care agencies. A significant element of the overall TJC review of patient care involves medication use quality and medication system safety. Accreditation standards for medication-related activities are applied across the organization. Organizations are expected to present evidence that ordering, dispensing, administering, and monitoring of medications are overseen by the medical staff. The organization must be able to demonstrate that policies for safe medication use practices are in place. Quality-directed medication use is a key performance element for accreditation. Ongoing medication use evaluation, adverse medication event investigation, medication use performance improvement, and compliance with National Patient Safety Goals are required to meet the standards. The National Council on Quality Assurance accredits many managed care organizations. State professional boards (medicine, nursing, or pharmacy) provide oversight of specialized domains such as prescribing, dispensing, and administering medications. Most healthcare facilities are also regulated by state or local health departments that often have additional regulations on medication-related issues.

It is the shared responsibility of the medical staff and executive administration in a healthcare organization to oversee medication use activities, ranging from product selection to long-term monitoring. This includes development of medication use policies, selection of drug products that are appropriate to the needs of the patient population being served, and oversight of the quality of medication use. The pharmacy and therapeutics committee is frequently the focal point for medication-related activities within the organization. The pharmacy and therapeutics committee develops policies for managing drug use and administration, manages the formulary system, and evaluates the clinical use of drugs [21].

The structure of the pharmacy and therapeutics committee may vary to meet the unique needs and structure of the organization. It routinely reports to the medical staff executive committee or other leadership group within the medical staff organization. The committee is made up of representatives from the principal medication using services (internal medicine, surgery, pediatrics, etc.) within the organization, plus representatives from the nursing services, pharmacy services, quality improvement program, and hospital administration. The chair of the committee is most frequently a clinician with experience in system-wide activities, and most important, an interest in quality use of medications. It is customary for the director of the pharmacy department to serve on the committee to assure a working link between pharmacy department and committee activities.

Pharmacy and therapeutics committees meet as frequently as needed to accomplish their mission, typically monthly. The schedule is dependent on the traditions of the organization and the amount of work included during the full committee meeting. The agenda should be prepared under the supervision of the committee chair and distributed well in advance of the meeting to allow all participants to read formulary drug monographs and drug use reports before the meeting. Ongoing elements of many committees are special standing subcommittees or focused task force workgroups. Typical standing subcommittees focus on drug formulary management, antimicrobial agents, and medication use evaluation. Standing subcommittees are appropriate for providing ongoing special expertise on matters that can be referred back to the full committee for action. A task force workgroup also may be used to address special limited-scope issues, such as ad hoc evaluations of agents within a given therapeutic drug class.

Medication policy issues

The pharmacy and therapeutics committee is expected to oversee important policies and procedures associated with the use of medications. Medication policy includes a wide range of issues, from stipulating who may prescribe or administer drugs, to specifying what prescribing direction and guidance are appropriate to assure safe and appropriate use of high-risk, high-volume, high-cost, or problem-prone drugs. Additional policies are often needed to assure consistent supply or quality of drug products, or to allocate drugs in times of shortage. Responsibility for developing policies to address special circumstances or issues is often delegated to the pharmacy and therapeutics committee by the organization. Examples of this type of policy are special drug class restriction (e.g., antimicrobial agents) and use of agents for sedation during medical procedures.

Formulary management

The objective of an active formulary program is to direct medication use to preferred agents, which offer a therapeutic or safety benefit or an economic advantage. When optimally implemented, this serves as an important quality/benefit-driven opportunity. A statement of principles of a Sound Drug Formulary System was developed in 2000, by a consortium composed of the U.S. Pharmacopeia, the Department of Veterans Affairs, the American Medical Association, the American Society of Health-System Pharmacists, the Academy of Managed Care Pharmacists, and the National Business Coalition on Health [22]. In this statement, a formulary is defined as "a continually updated list of medications and related information, representing the clinical judgment of physicians, pharmacists, and other experts in the diagnosis and or treatment of disease and promotion of health." A specific formulary is intended for use in a defined population. The defined population may consist of patients in a single hospital, patients seen within a group practice, a managed care patient population (local, regional, or national), or even an entire community.

Historically, formulary drug inclusion or exclusion has been used as an administrative barrier to discourage prescribers from using nonpreferred drugs. The historical approach to formulary decision making was based on a simple "on formulary" or "not-on formulary" classification of drugs. Formulary drugs were available immediately with no special requirements. Not-on-formulary drugs were not immediately available and might even need administrative review before requests to dispense them could be approved. So, a formulary drug often was selected by the prescriber to avoid a prolonged waiting period for the nonformulary item to be ordered and made available for the patient. This approach has been most effective when the array of effective drug choices was somewhat limited, and the principal cost and quality management need was to reduce the number of "me-too" products.

With the advent of many of the newest generation of products, including monoclonal antibodies and cytokine agents, it is not logical to simply deny the formulary availability of these novel agents. Accordingly, the standard for most institutions has been to include these novel drugs with committee approved restrictions and guidelines for use. Continued expansion of prescriber order entry within an electronic medical record system offers growing opportunity for enhanced clinical decision support and evidence-based, diagnosis-specific formulary management. Individual patient pharmacogenetic and pharmacogenomic characteristics have begun to influence our understanding of drug toxicity and effectiveness and can be expected to play an enhanced role in formulary drug management going forward. As discussed in previous chapters, the ability to use this information to better customize and optimize patient-specific drug therapy will require an increasingly sophisticated approach in selecting the most appropriate drug.

Drug selection process

Effective formulary development is based upon the scientific evaluation of drug safety, clinical effectiveness, and cost impact. That information is used by the pharmacy and therapeutics committee, to determine the specific value and risk of the drug for the patient population to whom the drug will be administered. The committee evaluates a given drug relative to the disease states typically treated in this population. For instance, the presence or absence of certain tropical diseases may impact on the need to include some antimicrobial agents on the formulary. The evaluation of a drug should include discussion of what doses and duration of therapy might be most appropriate in order to establish guidelines for measuring prescribing quality. In some cases, it may be necessary to determine which healthcare professionals are appropriately trained or qualified to prescribe a particular drug. The committee may elect to restrict the use of a drug to certain specialists (e.g., board-trained oncologists for some cancer drugs) or the drug may be restricted by the manufacturer or FDA to those prescribers who have received some drug-specific training and been approved by the supplier (e.g., thalidomide). Risk Evaluation and Mitigation Strategies (REMS) have become common as drugs have come to the market since this FDA program was begun in 2007. REMS are intended to help reduce the occurrence and severity of specific risks through information or actions in prescribing, dispensing, or administering the drug [23].

Economic evaluation of medications is a routine element of formulary review. The development of many effective but expensive drugs, which may cost thousands of dollars for a single short course of therapy or tens of thousands for long-term therapy, has placed financial impact at center stage in product selection. The availability of these high-cost agents has created a specialty discipline called pharmacoeconomics. A growing list of academic medical centers have established units that focus research and practice efforts on outcomes measurement of drug therapy. These programs often provide sophisticated evaluations of the economic or quality-of-life elements of drug use.

Drug costs, and their impact, are perceived differently from different perspectives in the healthcare system. Each component of the healthcare system (hospital, home care, ambulatory provider, and patient) may have a different perspective on the cost of therapy. Hospitals are usually responsible for all drug-related costs (drug purchase, medication administration, laboratory monitoring, etc.) for the finite period of time that a patient is hospitalized. A stand-alone outpatient drug benefit manager might only worry about the drug cost for the nonhospitalized portion of the therapy. The integrated delivery network may be at financial risk for all elements of covered outpatient and inpatient care. Patient copay responsibility for a fractional portion of a high-cost therapy is now recognized as an element in the decision of what drugs have what role in therapy.

Because each element of the system may be responsible for a different component of the total cost of care, the cost impact of a given drug product selection may be different for each of them. The "societal perspective" often represents yet another view of drug costs in that it incorporates nonhealthcare costs and the value of lost days of work and disability. Formulary inclusion is not routinely based on that level of evaluation, but public policy may be influenced by that information.

The cost-impact analysis of two hypothetical drug choices shown in Fig. 27.4 demonstrates the role of cost perspective in the formulary selection process. Both regimens offer the same long-term clinical result and adverse reaction profile. This analysis shows that the decision as to which drug is the lower-cost option will vary with the perspective of the organization that is responsible for the different inpatient and outpatient components of care. This dilemma is a regular element of the formulary selection process in many institutions. The puzzle becomes more complex when trying to decide what elements of cost (e.g., laboratory tests or other monitoring activities) should be included. Despite this lack of clarity, the cost impact of drug therapy on different stakeholders requires that this issue be considered in the decision process, and some hospitals have begun to use both expert guidelines and benchmarking data to guide formulary decision making.

Most healthcare provider organizations participate in a purchasing group to leverage volume-driven price advantages. The makeup and operations of these groups vary widely, but the price agreements and changing landscape of drug pricing add an additional dimension to the drug price factor. A specific drug may be the lowest price option for a given contract period, after which the choice may change. In another variation, a package of prices for bundled items may cause the price for a given item to change, depending on the use of yet another item. How these added dimensions influence formulary decisions is a function of the drug and many other factors.

Formulary tactics

In addition to drug selection, the pharmacy and therapeutics committee is responsible for considering formulary tactics to support the overall goal of optimal medication use. Several of these tactics have been successfully used to direct drug use toward preferred agents. The most obvious tactic to direct use away from a given agent is to exclude it from the formulary. The use of nonformulary agents usually triggers some required override, or post hoc review of use by the committee or

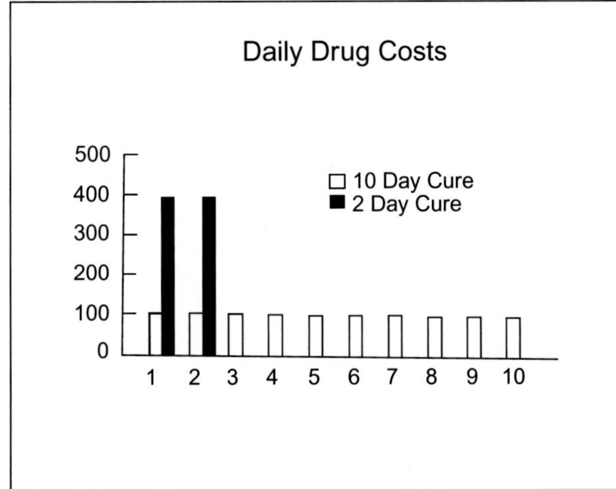

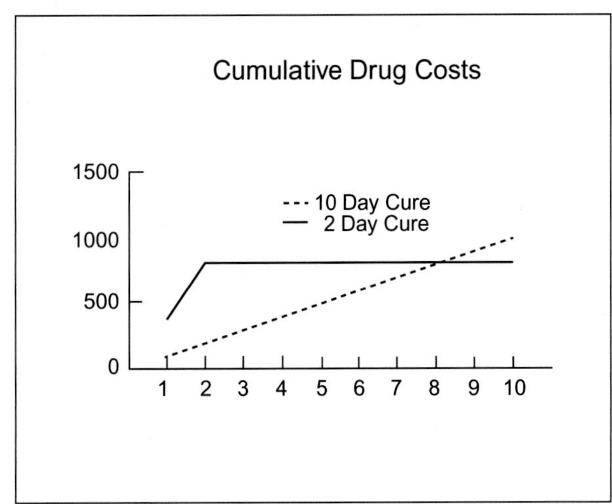

Financial Responsibility at Discharge

	Daily Cost	10 Day Total	Total at Hospital Discharge
2 Day Cure	$400	$800	$800
10 Day Cure	$100	$1000	$300

Perspective Based Financial Responsibility

	2 Day Cure	10 Day Cure
Hospital	$800	$300
Outpatient Payer	$0	$700
Total	$800	$1000

FIG. 27.4 Financial perspective in formulary decision making. Comparison of two treatment options: 2-day cure at $400 per day versus 10-day cure at $100 per day, with an anticipated hospital stay of 3 days.

designated individual. A second tactic involves a global management of medication use by therapeutic class. This tactic can be employed to minimize the use of drugs with a less clear profile of therapeutic efficacy or safety. A decision to limit the number of agents from a given drug class can also provide some advantages in price contracting, if formulary inclusion is effective in directing medication use to lower cost agents.

Limiting prescribing access for some specific drugs to a subset of prescribers who possess special expertise that qualifies them to use these drugs can improve the quality of their use. In many cases, drug restriction is managed by one or more gatekeepers whose approval is required prior to beginning therapy with the drug (e.g., infectious disease approval prior to starting a specified antibiotic). In some cases, direct financial incentives have been used to encourage use of a given drug or group of drugs. These formulary tactics have been used to influence decision making by prescribers, pharmacists, and patients.

Analysis and prevention of medication errors

Reason [24] has described a model for looking at human error that portrays a battle between the sources of error and the system-based defenses against them. This model is often referred to as the "Swiss cheese model" because the defenses against error are displayed as thin layers with holes that are described as latent error in the system. Fig. 27.5 demonstrates the model as applied to medication error. Each opportunity for error is defended by the prescriber, pharmacist, nurse, and patient. When a potential error is identified and corrected (e.g., dose error, route of administration error) the event becomes

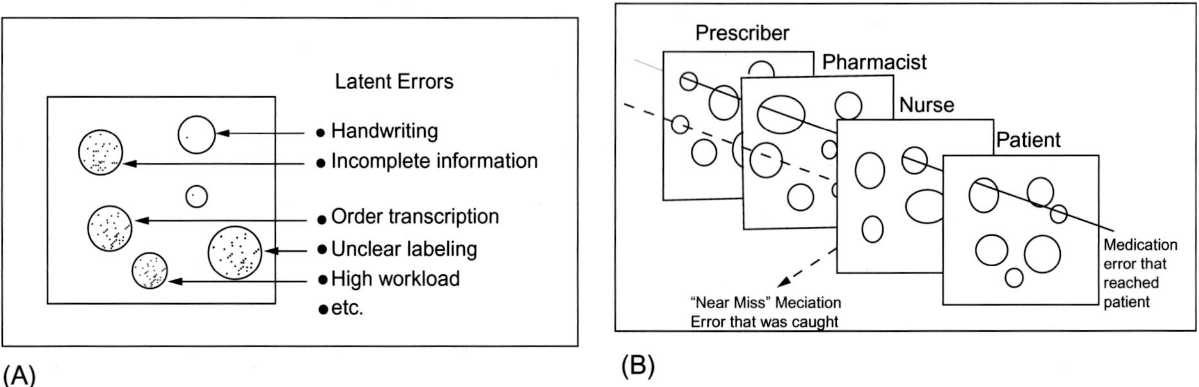

FIG. 27.5 Latent medication system errors (*Panel A*) and defensive layers against error (*Panel B*) in the medication system.

a "near miss" rather than an ADE. In those cases in which the holes in the Swiss cheese line up, a preventable medication error occurs. The Swiss cheese model provides an interesting framework for research in this field.

The latent errors in the medication use system have been described in several studies. Major contributors to errors in medication use were found to be knowledge gap related to drug therapy (30%); knowledge gap related to patient factors (30%); errors in dose calculations, placement of decimal points, and dosage units (18%); nomenclature failures such as wrong drug name or misinterpreted abbreviation (13%) [25]. Cohen [26] described six common causes of medication error based on his review of events reported to public reporting databases. These causes of errors include failed communication practices (including verbal orders), poor drug distribution, dose miscalculations, drug and device-related problems (such as name confusion, labeling, or poor design), and lack of patient education on the drugs that are prescribed for their use. Leape et al. [27] identified 13 proximal causes of medication errors in an academic medical center. They are detailed in Table 27.1.

Medication error data

The rate and nature of medication errors has been studied by several authors. Nightingale et al. [28] found a medication error rate of 0.7% in a British National Health Service general hospital. Phillips et al. [29] evaluated all medication events reported to the FDA from 1993 through 1998 that were associated with a patient death and found that 41% were associated with a wrong dose, 16% with the wrong drug, and 9.5% with the wrong route of administration. Rothschild et al. [30] found a rate of 36.2% preventable ADEs plus an additional 149.7 serious errors per 1000 patient days. Medication ordering or execution represented 61% of the serious errors. Slips and lapses rather than rule-based or knowledge errors were most common. Lesar et al. [25] describe the results of a review of 2103 clinically significant medication errors in an academic medical center. It was determined that 0.4% of medication orders were in error: 42% of the errors were overdosage, and 13% were the result of drug allergies that were not accounted for prior to prescribing. This work showed that medication errors result most frequently from failure to alter dose or drug after changes in renal or hepatic status, missed allergies,

TABLE 27.1 Proximal causes of medication errors.

Lack of knowledge of the drug	Faulty dose checking
Lack of information about the patient	Infusion pump and parenteral delivery problems
Violation of rules	Inadequate monitoring
Slips and memory lapses	Drug stocking and delivery problems
Transcription errors	Preparation errors
Faulty checking of identification	Lack of standardization
Faulty interaction with other services	

Based on Leape LL, Bates DW, Cullen DJ, Cooper J, Demonaco HJ, Gallivan T, et al. Systems analysis of adverse drug events. JAMA 1995;274:35–43.

wrong drug name, wrong dosage form (e.g., IV for IM), use of abbreviations, or incorrect calculation of a drug dose. They concluded that an improved organizational focus on technological risk management and training should reduce errors and patient risk of ADEs.

Given the latent errors associated with some elements of human performance, it seems likely that automation may reduce error. Several studies have demonstrated the value of computer assistance in the medication order entry process. Rules-based prescriber order entry systems have been shown to identify and reduce the chances of adverse medication events due to drug duplication, calculation errors, and drug-drug interactions [11, 31–36]. Despite these demonstrated advantages to computer-assisted medication ordering, the process is still far from error free. MedMARx data from 2003 showed that nearly 20% of the medication errors reported to that national database were associated with problems in computerization and automation [37]. A large number of these were order entry errors associated with interruptions during order entry. Another study showed that an early generation computerized prescriber order entry system facilitated some error types due to formatting and display limitations [38]. In still another study, Nebeker et al. [39] found that ADEs continued to occur following the implementation of a computerized prescriber order entry system. They concluded that effective decision support functions are required to prevent order entry-related medication errors associated with computerized prescribing systems. Dreischulte et al. [40] identified 11 high-priority topics for quality improvement initiatives in primary care: 7 topics related to medication use *quality* (e.g., omission of beta blocker therapy in patients with a history of chronic heart failure), and 4 topics related to medication use *safety* (e.g., using oral nonsteroidal antiinflammatory drugs in patients at increased risk of renal failure).

Some therapeutic categories of medications might be predicted to be prone to error due to narrow therapeutic index, complexity of therapy, or other factors. Phillips et al. [14] found that analgesics, central nervous system agents, and nontranquilizer psychotropic drugs were most frequently associated with deaths due to medication errors. Lesar et al. [25] found antimicrobials and cardiovascular drugs to be the most error-prone therapeutic categories in an academic medical center. Calabrese et al. [41] found vasoactive drugs and sedative/analgesics to be most problematic in the intensive care unit (ICU) setting. Hicks [42] found that opioid drugs were most frequently associated with reported errors causing patient harm. Based on these nonconverging findings, it might be concluded that the specific drugs of concern are unique to the institution or practice setting, a conclusion that is partially true. The Joint Commission [43] has identified a list of drugs and drug practices that are associated with high risk for significant error based upon high-report rates, and the Institute for Safe Medication Practices [44] also has identified drugs which should generate a high alert due to risk for medication errors. Lambert and colleagues [45, 46] have described a series of experiments that test the likelihood of drug name confusion based on fixed similarity patterns. This theoretical concept is providing the basis for selecting drug names that minimize the chance of sound-alike errors [47].

Research methods on medication error data are not standardized. Therefore they are subject to some limitations in generalizability. Because widespread interest in developing scientific approaches for reducing medication error is relatively recent, there are few well-established methods for conducting research in this field. However, funding for research in safe medication use and error reduction is available from several public and private sources, including the Agency for Healthcare Research and Quality.

Medication error data collection and analysis for clinical use and quality improvement are also complex activities. Observational data, post hoc review of medical records, and self-reporting have all been used with varying degrees of success for research and functional applications. Each offers strengths and weaknesses, and the appropriate method for data collection is in large part a function of its intended use and the resources available to collect it. Most hospitals collect internal medication error data through a voluntary reporting mechanism. This system is used as the backbone of error reporting because it requires minimal resources for data collection and is supported by organizational risk management programs. Voluntary reporting is presumed to underreport total errors. It is widely believed that most significant errors are reported when they are identified, but many mistakes are never recognized. Many other errors are determined to be insignificant and, therefore, not formally reported. For these reasons, it is difficult to determine in the hospital setting if changes in a given series of numbers represent a real change or simply a different level of reporting.

Fig. 27.6 illustrates a typical presentation of aggregated or high-level medication error data in an institutional setting. This presentation allows for general trends in total numbers to be plotted and tracked over time. Review of high-level data shows trends and provides a framework for the first level of error analysis. Major changes can be seen, which may trigger more intense analysis. However, this high-level data approach does not provide any detail to the analyst regarding the subcomponents of the composition of the reported errors. As a result, there are pitfalls in drawing conclusions from aggregated high-level data that can make these conclusions problematic. For instance, one might presume that administration of medication to the wrong patient is generally more serious than administration of a medication at the wrong time. However, an increase of five "wrong patient" errors and a decrease of five "wrong time" errors for a specific time period will register as a

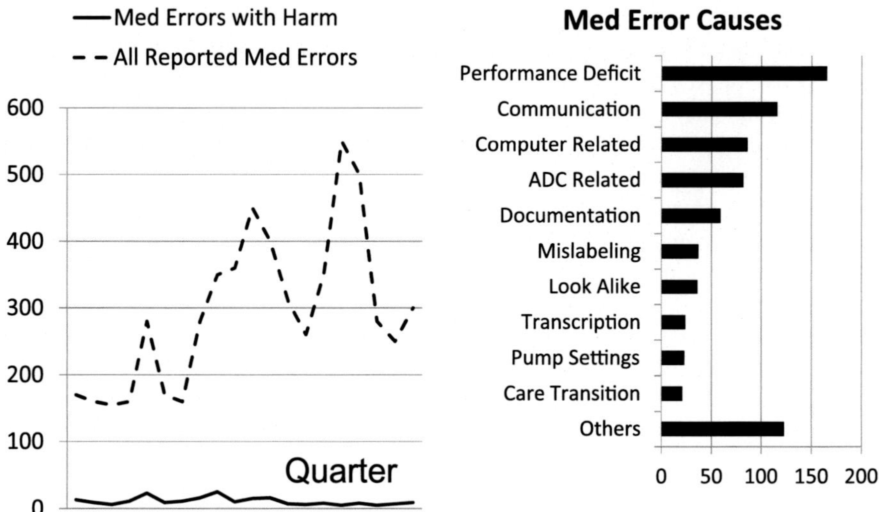

FIG. 27.6 Presentation of a typical approach to tracking medication error data. (A) Tracking data in aggregate form, separating errors that result in harm *(solid line)* from total reported errors *(broken line)*. (B) Summary of medication errors categorized by error type.

zero change for that period if only aggregated data is used. If fact, it may represent a serious degradation in some element of the medication system that will not be seen through this level of error analysis.

Classification and analysis of medication error data by error type is recommended as a method to spot potentially important changes in system performance. The National Coordinating Council for Medication Error Reporting and Prevention system for classifying medication errors may be used [6]. Commercial systems for cataloging and analyzing medication errors are available. A potentially valuable element of some programs is the ability to share anonymous data with other hospitals for comparison with similar institutions [48]. Regardless of the system used to classify and analyze medication error data, clear and consistent classification must be made to avoid confounding conclusions regarding underlying problems.

Reducing medication errors

Collection and use of medication error data at the hospital level are challenging but important functions. A key organizational principle in quality improvement is to make reporting errors a nonpunitive process. This usually increases the number of errors that will be reported, but not the number occurring. Making errors visible is an important step in the process of finding and fixing system-related problems [48]. The ongoing monitoring of ADE data (both medication errors and adverse drug reactions) is an important responsibility of the pharmacy and therapeutics committee. The committee is the organization's only convergence point for all medication-related issues. This convergence allows for a full review of the medication use process for system adjustments.

To identify opportunities for reducing medication errors, it is important that each error be carefully reviewed by a limited number of individuals to gain intimate knowledge of each reported incident. Collection and classification of error data must be followed by use of a careful epidemiological approach to problem solving at the system level. Narrative data, which may not be seen by looking at the categorical data alone, can be used to provide important details about proximal causes and latent error that may have contributed to the event. Success in this type of error reduction requires the reviewers to read between the lines, look for common threads between reports, and link multiple errors which are the result of system weaknesses.

There is still work to be done in understanding errors in the medication use process. However, available information provides suggestions on how to reduce medication errors. Bates's [49] ongoing studies of medication errors led to eight specific error prevention strategies: (1) unit-dose medication dispensing, (2) targeted physician education on optimal medication use, (3) inclusion of the clinical pharmacist in decision-making patient activities, (4) computerized medication checking, (5) computerized order entry by the prescriber, (6) standardized processes and equipment, (7) automated medication dispensing systems, (8) bar-coded medications for dispensing and administration. In addition, the IOM study on preventing medication errors [3] recommended a stronger role for consumers/patients in self-management, enhanced consumer information sources, complete patient information for providers, enhanced decision support, improved labeling, and standardization of technologies. They also encouraged further research in the field of medication error prevention.

The more complex a patient's drug therapy regimen, the greater the likelihood that adverse medication events will occur. Cullen et al. [50] determined that the rate of preventable and potential adverse drug events was twice as high in intensive care units, compared to non-ICUs. This was attributed to the higher number of drugs used in the ICU. Lesar et al. [51] reviewed medication prescribing errors over a 9-year period and concluded that the incidence of prescribing errors increased as intensity of care increased and new drugs became available. Koecheler et al. [52] reported that greater than 5 current medications, 12 or more doses per day, or medication regimen changes four or more times in a year were all predictors for drug therapy problems in ambulatory patients. Transition between levels of care or components of the healthcare system put patients at-risk for medication errors. Cornish [53] found that 53% of the patients they studied had at least one medication unintentionally not ordered during the transition from home status to inpatient admission, but that dose errors were also a significant problem. Gray et al. [54] determined that the occurrence of an ADE was positively related to the number of new medications received at hospital discharge. The knowledge that some patients are at higher risk for ADEs suggests possible high-return intervention targets. When selecting improvement opportunities, it is wise to look for those areas most likely to yield results.

Examples of system improvements to reduce medication errors have been reported by several authors. Leape et al. [55] reduced medication errors in an ICU by including a pharmacist on the clinical rounding team. Flynn et al. [56] identified interruptions (telephone calls, conversations, etc.) during critical phases of pharmacist drug preparation activities as significant contributors to errors in medication preparation. Comprehensive efforts to prevent medication errors include the four-pronged medication error analysis program from the Institute for Safe Medication Practices [57]. This four-pronged approach includes evaluation of specific medication errors, evaluation of aggregated error data and near-miss data for the hospital, as well as evaluation of error reports from other hospitals. In addition, effective medication error prevention includes ongoing monitoring of drug therapy trends, changes in medication use patterns, information from the hospital quality improvement or risk management program, and general hospital programmatic information.

Monitoring institutional trends in medication use can provide clues to possible high-risk or error-prone therapies. Increased use of drugs with a history of medication errors, such as patient-controlled analgesia, should alert organizations to develop safeguards to protect against errors before, rather than after, they become problems. Cohen and Kilo [44] describe a framework for improving the use of high-alert drugs, which is based on reducing or eliminating the possibility of error, making errors visible, and minimizing the consequences of errors. Table 27.2 presents change concepts for safeguarding against errors when using high-risk drugs.

Medication error prevention opportunities also may present themselves in unusual hospital programmatic information from sources not routinely applied to medication safety. For instance, reports of laboratory-related incidents or hospital information system problems may be indicators that medication-related problems can be expected. Thoughtful use of this information may prevent medication-related errors attributed to supplemental systems that are critical to safe and appropriate medication use. Reports of staff shortages within an institution (e.g., critical care nurses, nurse anesthetists) can be used to identify potential problem areas prior to medication error reports. Likewise, reports of planned construction or information system conversions may be an indicator that routines will be interrupted. Thus use of hospital program information in a prospective way can be used to provide safe alternatives that avoid medication errors before they occur.

System improvements may improve the quality of prescribing by standardizing to an expert level. Morris [58] described the development, testing, and use of computerized protocols for managing intravenous fluid and hemodynamic factors in patients with acute respiratory distress syndrome. Evans et al. [59] used a computerized antiinfectives management program to improve the quality of medication use and reduce costs. In consideration of what is currently known, Leape [60] provided a simple set of recommendations to reduce medical error: reduce reliance on memory, improve access to information, error-proof critical tasks, standardize processes, and instruct healthcare providers on possible errors in processes. These simple but thoughtful recommendations are important components of an overall concept that can help to reduce medication errors.

Medication use evaluation

Medication use evaluation (also referred to as MUE or drug use evaluation) is a required component of the medication use quality improvement process. It is a performance improvement method with the goal of optimizing patient outcomes [61]. The first element of drug use tracking is the global monitoring of organizational drug use. This can be completed by routine evaluation of totals and changes in drug use within a therapeutic drug category. The American Hospital Formulary Service Drug Information (AHSF-DI) has created a comprehensive therapeutic classification system that is often used for drug use monitoring [62], but other commercial medication databases are also available.

TABLE 27.2 Safeguarding against errors in high risk drugs.

Concept	Example
Build in system redundancies	Independent calculation of pediatric doses by more than one person (e.g., prescriber and pharmacist)
Use fail-safes	IV pumps with clamps that automatically shut off flow during power outage
Reduce options	Use of a single concentration of heparin for infusion (e.g., 25,000 units in 250 mL of saline)
Use forcing functions	Preprinted order forms for chemotherapy drugs which require patient height and weight information before preparation and dispensing
Externalize or centralize error-prone processes	Prepare IV admixtures in the pharmacy instead of on nursing units
Use differentialization	Supplemental labels for dosage forms which are not appropriate for intravenous use without dilution
Store medications appropriately	Store dopamine and dobutamine in separate locations
Screen new products	Review new formulary requests for labeling, packaging, and medication use issues which may be error prone
Standardize and simplify order communication	Avoid use of verbal orders
Limit access	Restrict access to the pharmacy during "non-staffed" hours and follow-up on all medications removed from the pharmacy during this time
Use constraints	Require approval before beginning therapy (e.g., attending signature on chemotherapy orders)
Use reminders	Place special labels on products when they are dispensed by the pharmacy to remind of special procedures for use (e.g., double check rate calculation of insulin infusions)
Standardize dosing procedures	Develop standardized dose and rate charts for products such as vasoactive drugs (e.g., infusion rate expressed as micrograms per kilogram per minute)

Based on Cohen MR, Kilo CM. High-alert medications: safeguarding against errors. In: Cohen MR, editor. Medication errors. Washington, DC: American Pharmaceutical Association; 1999. p. 5.3–5.11.

Fig. 27.7 is an example of a global drug use report that may be used to look for trends and variations in medication use. This report should be examined for changes that represent increases or decreases in comparison to previous reporting periods. A change in any specific category or group of drugs may be important and worthy of specific follow-up. Smaller changes that support a trend over time can demonstrate ongoing changes in drug use patterns. Changes seen in global level monitoring may trigger a focused evaluation to further assess the appropriateness with which certain medications are used.

Medication use evaluation has historically been categorized with regard to how and when data collection or intervention occurs (Table 27.3). Most medication use evaluations are retrospective, as exemplified by an analysis of 8 years of emergency department prescribing data by Caterino et al. [63]. These authors found that, despite the availability of published lists of medications that are not generally appropriate for geriatric patients, one or more of those inappropriate medications were prescribed for 12.6% of elderly patients during their emergency department visits. Table 27.3 also describes concurrent and prospective reviews, classified based on the use and timing of intervention as part of the process that is used for screening and incorporating data.

Focused medication use evaluation

Focused or targeted medication use evaluation follows a reasonably well-established cycle: identification of a potential problem in the use of a specific drug or therapy, collection and comparison of data, determination of compliance with a preestablished guideline/expectation, and action as needed to improve discrepancies between expected and measured results. This type of medication use evaluation provides an excellent opportunity to apply the Shewhart Cycle for continuous quality improvement (Fig. 27.3). Focused medication use projects are typically selected for a specific reason. Table 27.4 lists reasons to consider drugs for focused evaluation projects. A well-planned medication use evaluation program includes a balance of high-volume, high-risk, high-cost, and problem-prone drugs.

E	F	G	SPENT FY 15	SPENT FY 16	SPENT FY 17	SPENT FY 18	SPENT FY 19
4:00:00	ANTIHISTAMINE		$21,175	$28,185	$41,918	$54,237	$64,221
8:00:00	ANTI-INFECTIVE AGENTS						
	80400	AMEBICIDES	$1,522	$332	$884	$1,321	$746
	80800	ANTHELMINTICS	$996	$2,623	$1,231	$1,834	$2,702
	81202	AMINOGLYCOSIDES	$13,457	$10,351	$35,468	$47,014	$35,272
	81204	ANTIFUNGAL ANTIBIOTICS	$320,884	$357,206	$946,657	$1,082,165	$1,056,544
	81206	CEPHALOSPORINS	$197,231	$162,850	$180,186	$188,435	$146,069
	81207	B-LACTAMS	$77,722	$77,703	$90,073	$112,235	$81,442
	81208	CHLORAMPHENICOLS	$204	$172	$771	$1,331	$34
	81212	ERYTHROMYCINS	$69,377	$89,793	$112,984	$109,499	$92,816
	81216	PENICILLINS	$41,427	$65,243	$46,314	$61,153	$89,200
	81224	TETRACYCLINES	$4,427	$4,788	$4,569	$8,820	$5,962
	81228	MISCELLANEOUS ANTIBIOTICS	$35,347	$35,261	$37,811	$41,473	$80,727
	81600	ANTITUBERCULOSIS AGENTS	$27,937	$42,335	$53,318	$46,223	$39,438
	81800	ANTIVIRALS	$1,399,246	$2,472,982	$3,251,543	$3,417,004	$3,775,675
	82000	ANTIMALARIAL AGENTS	$60,942	$20,848	$19,051	$20,577	$17,524
	82200	QUINOLONES	$113,064	$94,705	$117,380	$116,301	$119,356
	82400	SULFONAMIDES	$6,730	$3,425	$3,660	$2,770	$4,579
	82600	SULFONES	$4,839	$4,651	$4,972	$5,366	$3,735
	83200	ANTITRICHOMONAL AGENTS	$3,923	$677	$924	$1,454	$1,627
	83600	URINARY ANTI-INFECTIVES	$2,009	$2,142	$1,632	$2,836	$763
	84000	MISCELLANEOUS ANTI-INFECTIVES	$34,661	$30,211	$27,401	$19,394	$23,766
		TOTAL ANTI-INFECTIVE AGENTS	$2,415,944	$3,478,297	$4,936,828	$5,287,206	$5,577,978
16:00:00	BLOOD DERIVATIVIES TOTAL		$188,350	$204,843	$236,087	$348,825	$11,095
20:00:00	BLOOD FORMATION AND COAGULATION						
	200404	IRON PREPARATIONS	$2,687	$2,402	$2,240	$2,012	$6,150
	201204	ANTICOAGULANTS	$66,851	$75,294	$114,764	$179,357	$146,496
	201208	ANTIHEPARIN AGENTS	$237	$83	$182	$156	$52,186
	201216	HEMOSTATICS	$21,246	$27,266	$48,408	$75,817	$65,886
	201600	HEMATOPOIETIC AGENTS	$1,526,711	$1,471,910	$1,515,326	$2,027,767	$1,406,002
	202400	HEMORRHEOLOGIC AGENTS	$2,717	$2,046	$3,014	$6,683	$1,109
	204000	THROMBOLYTIC AGENTS	$72,684	$58,657	$87,678	$72,382	$51,789
		TOTAL BLOOD FORMATION AND COAG.	$1,693,133	$1,637,657	$1,771,613	$2,142,912	$1,729,616
24:00:00	CARDIOVASCULAR DRUGS						
	240400	CARDIAC DRUGS	$185,225	$179,912	$197,914	$258,000	$264,424
	240600	ANTILIPEMIC AGENTS	$237,827	$298,091	$269,520	$298,957	$333,476
	240800	HYPOTENSIVE AGENTS	$89,871	$106,383	$112,858	$122,181	$117,703
	241200	VASODILATING AGENTS	$21,023	$28,385	$39,040	$26,947	$25,841
	241600	SCLEROSING AGENTS	$0	$0	$0	$0	$220
24:00:00		TOTAL CARDIOVASCULAR DRUGS	$533,946	$612,771	$619,332	$706,085	$741,664

FIG. 27.7 Sample therapeutic category drug monitoring report based upon therapeutic classifications used by the American Hospital Formulary Service.

TABLE 27.3 Drug use review categories.

Review category	Data collection model (s)	Typical application	Comments
Retrospective	Data is collected for a fixed period which may be archival or accumulation of new patients for a fixed period of time	Data archive review of emergency department prescribing for geriatric patients [63]	Supports large-scale epidemiologic approach No active intervention to change medication use patterns occurs due to the post hoc data collection process
Concurrent	Each new order generates an automatic review of previously approved criteria for use within a specified period of the initiation of therapy	Review of naloxone to investigate possible nosocomial adverse medication event	
	Laboratory or other monitoring criteria are reported for all patients on the drug Abnormal Laboratory or other monitoring criteria are reported for all patients on the drug on a regular basis	Digoxin monitoring based upon daily review of digoxin serum levels [64] Regular review of serum creatinine for patients on aminoglycosides	
Prospective	Each new order for the drug is evaluated for compliance with previously approved criteria for use. Variance to the criteria require intervention prior to initiation of therapy	Medication use guidelines for ketorolac Restricted antibiotics	

TABLE 27.4 Selection of targets for focused medication use review.

• Medication is known or suspected to cause adverse reactions or drug interactions	• Medication is used in patients at high risk for adverse reactions
• Medication use process affects large number of patients or medication is frequently prescribed	• Medication or process is a critical component of care for a specific disease, condition, or procedure
• Medication is potentially toxic or causes discomfort at normal doses	• Medication is most effective when used in a specific way
• Medication is under consideration for formulary retention, addition, or deletion	• Medication or process is one for which suboptimal use would have a negative effect on patient outcomes or system costs
• Medication use is expensive	

Data from American Society of Health-System Pharmacists. ASHP guidelines on medication-use evaluation. Am J Health Syst Pharm 1996;53:1953–1955. (Internet at https://www.ashp.org/-/media/assets/policy-guidelines/docs/guidelines/medication-use-evaluation 5/9/2020; http://www.ashp.org/DocLibrary/BestPractices/FormGdlMedUseEval.aspx).

Concurrent or prospective focused medication use review

Concurrent or prospective focused medication use review activities can be used to prevent medication-related adverse events and improve the quality of medication use. Focused concurrent review of potentially toxic digoxin concentration measurements has been used to monitor potential ADEs from this drug [64]. Information system support also has been used to warn of abnormalities in coagulation, or of predefined changes in renal function, blood glucose, and electrolytes which are all potential indicators of medication use problems in individual patients. When such laboratory test results are reported along with specific drugs, it is possible to respond to potential medication-related problems before serious negative outcomes occur. Kuperman et al. [65] concluded that incorporation of an automatic alerting system in the laboratory data system resulted in a 38% shorter response to appropriate treatment following alert to a critical value. Awdishu et al. [66] reported that a real-time clinical decision support improved appropriate dose adjustments for 20 medications that were prescribed for patients with renal impairment.

Approaches for improving medication use

Identification of best medication use practices and benchmarking against best performers has become feasible over the last decade. Development and implementation of medication use guidelines is one way for individual healthcare provider organizations to apply evidence-based medicine to improve medication use quality. This evidential approach to the use of medications is designed to rely on the best available clinical evidence to develop a treatment plan for a specific illness or use of a specific drug or drugs. Simple medication use guidelines can be developed based on literature and the best judgment of inhouse experts. Development of more formal clinical practice guidelines is a complex process that relies on well-defined methods to combine the results of multiple studies to draw statistically valid conclusions. These sophisticated products are often addressed by professional or governmental organizations such as the National Institutes of Health (NIH) as well as by many professional medical societies. These help to provide the guidance required to set best practices in healthcare provider organizations. A typical clinical practice guideline contains systematically developed statements that include recommendations, strategies, or information to assist physicians, other healthcare practitioners, and patients to make appropriate decisions about healthcare for specific clinical circumstances. These vetted guidelines are a valuable resource when considering plans for quality medication use.

The CMS Hospital Compare.gov website [67] provides access to detailed information about an organization's performance on standardized performance measures, such as compliance with specific national patient safety goals. For instance, it is feasible to see how a particular organization compares with other nearby organizations on patient satisfaction, emergency room time until treatment, or other measures. It is also possible to compare multiple organizations to look for best performers. Many organizations (e.g., Kaiser, VA Health System, Vizient) have focused internal benchmarking systems to support improvements in medication use. Benchmarking use and outcome results and sharing of best medication use practices provide among the strongest tools for quality improvement in medication use.

The use of "counter-detailing" by designated hospital staff [68] to offset the impact of pharmaceutical sales forces also has been an effective strategy for improving medication use. The objective of this category of quality improvement program is to educate prescribers regarding the organization's approved and preferred medication use guidelines. This has been implemented by providing literature and prescriber contact from a pharmacist or other staff member to support the desired medication use objective.

Several approaches have been described for improving medication use through the use of dosing service teams. Demonstrated enhancements in the quality of medication use have been reported for anticoagulants, antimicrobials, anticonvulsants, and other drugs. The common method of these programs is the use of expert oversight (physicians or pharmacists) to manage therapy with the targeted drug. Therapeutic management may rely on algorithms, pharmacokinetic models, or preapproved collaborative plans [69–79].

Adoption of standardized medication order forms has been demonstrated to increase the quality of medication use and the effectiveness of medications that are prone to error [80, 81]. Chemotherapy, patient-controlled analgesia, and antimicrobial drug therapy are likely candidates for order standardization. Yet another approach to improved medication use is implementation of alert systems for sudden, unexpected actions, such as medication stop orders, or use of antidote-type drugs, such as diphenhydramine, hydrocortisone, or naloxone. A computerized application of this method was described by Classen et al. [82]. Another computerized system described by Paltiel et al. [83] improved outcomes by using a flashing alert on a computer monitor to highlight low potassium levels, thereby increasing the rate of therapeutic interventions and decreasing hypokalemia in patients at discharge.

Summary

The medication use process is a complex system intended to optimize patient outcomes within organizational constraints. Quality medication use involves selection of the optimal drug, avoidance of adverse medication events, and completion of the therapeutic objective. Safe medication practices focus on the avoidance of medication errors. Medication use review and ongoing medication monitoring activities focus on optimizing medication selection and use. These two approaches are important means of assessing and optimizing the quality of medication use.

References

[1] Ernst FR, Grizzle AJ. Drug-related morbidity and mortality: updating the cost-of-illness model. J Am Pharm Assoc 2001;41:192–199.

[2] Committee on Quality of Health Care in America. In: Kohn LT, Corrigan JM, Donaldson MS, editors. To err is human: building a safer health system. Washington, DC: National Academy Press; 1999. p. 223.

[3] Preventing Medication Errors. Committee on identifying and preventing medication errors. Washington, DC: National Academies Press; 2007.

[4] Leape LL, Brennan TA, Laird N, Lawthers AG, Localio AR, Barnes BA, et al. The nature of adverse events in hospitalized patients. Results of the harvard medical practice study II. N Engl J Med 1991;324:377–384.

[5] Thomas EJ, Brennan TA. Incidence and types of preventable adverse events in elderly patients: population based review of medical records. BMJ 2000;320:741–744.

[6] Anon. National coordinating council for medication error reporting and prevention, Rockville, MD: U.S. Pharmacopoeia; 1999. Internet at https://www.nccmerp.org/sites/default/files/algorBW2001-06-12.pdf.

[7] American Society of Health-System Pharmacists. Suggested definitions and relationships among medication misadventures, medication errors, adverse drug events, and adverse drug reactions. Am J Health Syst Pharm 1998;55:165–166.

[8] Bates DW, Boyle DL, Vander Vliet MB, Schneider J, Leape L. Relationship between medication errors and adverse drug events. J Gen Intern Med 1995;10:199–205.

[9] Bates DW, Spell N, Cullen DJ, Burdick E, Laird N, Petersen LA, et al. The costs of adverse drug events in hospitalized patients. JAMA 1997;277:307–311.

[10] McDonnell PJ, Jacobs MR. Hospital admissions resulting from preventable adverse drug reactions. Ann Pharmacother 2002;36:1331–1336.

[11] Anderson JG, Jay SJ, Anderson M, Hunt TJ. Evaluating the capabilities of information technology to prevent adverse drug events: a computer simulation approach. J Am Med Inform Assoc 2002;9:479–490.

[12] Nadzam DM. A systems approach to medication use. In: Cousins DD, editor. Medication use: a systems approach to reducing errors. Oakbrook Terrace, IL: Joint Commission on Accreditation of Healthcare Organizations; 1998. p. 5–17.

[13] Atkinson AJ Jr, Nadzam DM, Schaff RL. An indicator-based program for improving medication use in acute care hospitals. Clin Pharmacol Ther 1991;50:125–128.

[14] Phillips DP, Christenfeld N, Glynn LM. Increase in US medication-error deaths between 1983 and 1993. Lancet 1998;351:643–644.

[15] Phillips P, Breder C. Morbidity and mortality from medical errors: an increasingly serious public health problem. Annu Rev Public Health 2002;23:135–150.

[16] Winterstein A, Sauer BC, Hepler CD, Poole C. Preventable drug-related hospital admissions. Ann Pharmacother 2002;36:1238–1248.

[17] Bates DW, Cullen DJ, Laird N, Petersen LA, Small SD, Servi D, et al. Incidence of adverse drug events and potential adverse drug events. Implications for prevention. JAMA 1995;274:29–34.

[18] Barker KN, Flynn EA, Pepper GA, Bates DW, Mikeal RL. Medication errors observed in 36 health care facilities. Arch Intern Med 2002;162:1897–1903.

[19] Berwick DM. Continuous improvement as an ideal in health care. N Engl J Med 1989;320:53–56.

[20] Deming WE. Out of the crisis. Cambridge, MA: MIT Press; 2000. p. 87–89.

[21] American Society of Health-System Pharmacists. ASHP statement on the pharmacy and therapeutics committee and the formulary system, Am J Health Syst Pharm 2008;65:2384–2386. Also available through Internet at http://www.ashp.org/DocLibrary/BestPractices/FormStPTCommFormSyst.pdf.

[22] Coalition Working Group. Principles of a sound formulary system, Rockville, MD: US Pharmacopoeia; 2000. Internet at https://www.ashp.org/-/media/assets/policy)guidelines/docs/endorsed-documents/endorsed-documents-principles-sound-drug-formulary-system.

[23] Anon. Risk evaluation and mitigation strategies, Silver Spring: FDA; August 8, 2019. Internet at https://www.fda.gov/drugs/drug-safety-and-availability/risk-evaluation-and-mitigation-strategies-rems.

[24] Reason J. Human error. Cambridge: Cambridge University Press; 1990.

[25] Lesar TS, Briceland L, Stein DS. Factors related to errors in medication prescribing. JAMA 1997;77:312–317.

[26] Cohen MR. Causes of medication errors. In: Cohen MR, editor. Medication errors. Washington, DC: American Pharmaceutical Association; 1999. p. 198–212.

[27] Leape LL, Bates DW, Cullen DJ, Cooper J, Demonaco HJ, Gallivan T, et al. Systems analysis of adverse drug events. JAMA 1995;274:35–43.

[28] Nightingale PG, Adu D, Richards NT, Peters M. Implementation of rules based computerised bedside prescribing and administration: intervention study. BMJ 2000;320:750–753.

[29] Phillips J, Beam S, Brinker A, Holquist C, Honig P, Lee LY, et al. Retrospective analysis of mortalities associated with medication errors. Am J Health Syst Pharm 2001;58:1835–1841.

[30] Rothschild JM, Landrigan CP, Cronin JW. The critical care safety study: the incidence and nature of adverse events and serious medical errors in intensive care. Crit Care Med 2005;33:1694–1700.

[31] Bates DW, Leape LL, Cullen DJ, Laird N, Petersen NA, Teich JM, et al. Effect of computerized physician order entry and a team intervention on prevention of serious medication errors. JAMA 1998;280:1311–1316.

[32] Bates DW, Teich JM, Lee J, Seger D, Kuperman GJ, Ma'Luf N, et al. The impact of computerized physician order entry on medication error prevention. J Am Med Inform Assoc 1999;6:313–321.

[33] Pestotnik SL, Classen DC, Evan RS, Burke JP. Implementing antibiotic practice guidelines through computer-assisted decision support: clinical and financial outcomes. Ann Intern Med 1996;124:884–890.

[34] Raschke RA, Gollihare B, Wunderlich TA, Guidry JR, Leibowitz AI, Peirce JC, et al. A computer alert system to prevent injury from adverse drug events: development and evaluation in a community teaching hospital. JAMA 1998;280:1317–1320.

[35] Feldstein AC, Smith DH, Perrin N, Yang X, Simon SR, Krall M, et al. Reducing warfarin medication interactions: an interrupted time series analysis. Arch Intern Med 2006;166:1009–1015.

[36] Taylor JA, Loan LA, Kamara J, Blackburn S, Whitney D. Medication administration variances before and after implementation of computerized physician order entry in a neonatal intensive care unit. Pediatrics 2008;121:123–128.

[37] Zhan C, Hicks RW, Blanchette CM, Keyes MA, Cousins DD. Potential benefits and problems with computerized prescriber order entry: analysis of a voluntary medication error-reporting database. Am J Health Syst Pharm 2006;63:353–358.

[38] Koppel R, Metlay JP, Cohen A, Abaluck B, Localio AR, Kimmel SE, Strom BL. Role of computerized physician order entry systems in facilitating medication errors. JAMA 2005;293:1197–1203.

[39] Nebeker JR, Hoffman JM, Weir R, Bennett CL, Hurdle JF. High rates of adverse drug events in a highly computerized hospital. Arch Intern Med 2005;165:1111–1116.

[40] Dreischulte T, Grant AM, McCowan C, McAnaw J, Guthrie B. Quality and safety of medication use in primary care: consensus validation of a new set of explicit medication assessment criteria and prioritization of topics for improvement. BMC Clin Pharmacol 2012;12. https://doi.org/10.1186/1472-6904-12-5.

[41] Calabrese AD, Erstad BL, Brandl K, Barletta JF, Kane SL, Sherman DS. Medication administration errors in adult patients in the ICU. Intensive Care Med 2001;27:1592–1598.

[42] Hicks RW, Becker SC, Cousins DD. Harmful medication errors in children: a 5-year analysis of data from the USP MedMARx program. J Pediatr Nurs 2007;21:290–298.

[43] Joint Commission. High-alert medications and patient safety. Sentinel event alert 11 (Nov 19). Internet at http://www.jointcommission.org/sentinel_event_alert_issue_11_high-alert_medications_and_patient_safety/; 1999.

[44] Cohen MR, Kilo CM. High-alert medications: safeguarding against errors. In: Cohen MR, editor. Medication errors. Washington, DC: American Pharmaceutical Association; 1999. p. 5.3–5.11.

[45] Lambert BL. Predicting look-alike and sound-alike medication errors. Am J Health Syst Pharm 1997;54:1161–1171.

[46] Lambert BL, Lin SJ, Chang KY, Gandhi SK. Similarity as a risk factor in drug-name confusion errors: the look-alike (orthographic) and sound-alike (phonetic) model. Med Care 1999;37:1214–1225.

[47] Lambert BL, Lin SJ, Tan H. Designing safe drug names. Drug Saf 2005;28:495–512.

[48] Nolan TW. System changes to improve patient safety. BMJ 2000;320:771–773.

[49] Bates DW. Medication errors. How common are they and what can be done to prevent them? Drug Saf 1996;15:303–310.

[50] Cullen DJ, Sweitzer BJ, Bates DW, Burdick E, Edmonson A, Leape LL. Preventable adverse drug events in hospitalized patients: a comparative study of intensive care and general care units. Crit Care Med 1997;25:1289–1297.

[51] Lesar TS, Lomaestro BM, Pohl H. Medication-prescribing errors in a teaching hospital. A 9-year experience. Arch Intern Med 1997;157:1569–1576.

[52] Koecheler JA, Abramowitz PW, Swim SE, Daniels CE. Indicators for the selection of ambulatory patients who warrant pharmacist monitoring. Am J Hosp Pharm 1989;46:729–732.

[53] Cornish PL, Knowles SR, Marchesano R, Tam V, Shadowitz S, Juurlink DN, Etchells EE. Unintended medication discrepancies at the time of hospital admission. Arch Intern Med 2005;165:424–429.

[54] Gray SL, Mahoney JE, Blough DK. Adverse drug events in elderly patients receiving home health services following hospital discharge. Ann Pharmacother 1999;33:1147–1153.

[55] Leape LL, Cullen DJ, Clapp MD, Burdick E, Demonaco HJ, Erickson JI, et al. Pharmacist participation on physician rounds and adverse drug events in the intensive care unit. JAMA 1999;282:267–270.

[56] Flynn EA, Barker KN, Gibson JT, Pearson RE, Berger BA, Smith LA. Impact of interruptions and distractions on dispensing errors in an ambulatory care pharmacy. Am J Health Syst Pharm 1999;56:1319–1325.

[57] Gaunt MJ. The "best practice" is a four-pronged error analysis. Pharm Times 2006-09-01. Internet at https://www.pharmacytimes.com/publications/issue/2006/2006-09/2006-09-5869.

[58] Morris AH. Developing and implementing computerized protocols for standardization of clinical decisions. Ann Intern Med 2000;132:373–383.

[59] Evans RS, Pestotnik SL, Classen DC, Clemmer TP, Weaver LK, Orme JF, et al. A computer-assisted management program for antibiotics and other antiinfective agents. N Engl J Med 1998;338:232–238.

[60] Leape LL. Error in medicine. JAMA 1994;272:1851–1857.

[61] American Society of Health-System Pharmacists. ASHP guidelines on medication-use evaluation, Am J Health Syst Pharm 1996;53:1953–1955. Internet at https://www.ashp.org/-/media/assets/policy-guidelines/docs/guidelines/medication-use-evaluation. 5/9/2020.

[62] American Society of Health-System Pharmacists n.d. AHFS drug information. Bethesda, MD.: American Society of Health-System Pharmacists (Internet at https://www.ahfsdruginformation.com/ahfs-pharmacologic-therapeutic-classification.).

[63] Caterino JM, Emond JA, Camargo CA Jr. Inappropriate medication administration to the acutely ill elderly: a nationwide emergency department study, 1992-2000. J Am Geriatr Soc 2004;52:1847–1855.

[64] Piergies AA, Worwag EM, Atkinson AJ Jr. A concurrent audit of high digoxin plasma levels. Clin Pharmacol Ther 1994;55:353–358.

[65] Kuperman GJ, Teich JM, Tanasijevic MJ, Ma'Luf N, Rittenberg E, Jha A, et al. Improving response to critical laboratory results with automation: results of a randomized controlled trial. J Am Med Inform Assoc 1999;6:512–522.

[66] Awdishu L, Coates CR, Lyddane A, Tran K, Daniels CE, Lee J, et al. The impact of real-time alerting on appropriate prescribing in kidney disease; a cluster randomized controlled trial. J Am Med Inform Assoc 2016;23:609–616.

[67] Medicare.gov. Hospital compare. Internet at https://www.medicare.gov/hospitalcompare/search.html. (Accessed 9 May 2020).

[68] Soumerai SB, Avorn J. Predictors of physician prescribing change in an educational experiment to improve medication use. Med Care 1987;25:210–221.

[69] Ellis RF, Stephens MA, Sharp GB. Evaluation of a pharmacy-managed warfarin-monitoring service to coordinate inpatient and outpatient therapy. Am J Hosp Pharm 1992;49:387–394.

[70] Dager WE, Branch JM, King JH, White RH, Quan RS, Musallam NA, et al. Optimization of inpatient warfarin therapy: impact of daily consultation by a pharmacist-managed anticoagulation service. Ann Pharmacother 2000;34:567–572.

[71] Destache CJ, Meyer SK, Bittner MJ, Hermann KG. Impact of a clinical pharmacokinetic service on patients treated with aminoglycosides: a cost-benefit analysis. Ther Drug Monit 1990;12:419–426.

[72] Cimino MA, Rotstein CM, Moser JE. Assessment of cost-effective antibiotic therapy in the management of infections in cancer patients. Ann Pharmacother 1994;28:105–111.

[73] Okpara AU, Van Duyn OM, Cate TR, Cheung LK, Galley MA. Concurrent ceftazidime DUE with clinical pharmacy intervention. Hosp Formul 1994;29:392–394. 399, 402–4.

[74] Kershaw B, White RH, Mungall D, Van Houten J, Brettfeld S. Computer-assisted dosing of heparin. Management with a pharmacy-based anticoagulation service. Arch Intern Med 1994;154:1005–1011.

[75] De Santis G, Harvey KJ, Howard D, Mashford ML, Moulds RF. Improving the quality of antibiotic prescription patterns in general practice. The role of educational intervention. Med J Aust 1994;160:502–505.

[76] Donahue T, Dotter J, Alexander G, Sadaj JM. Pharmacist-based i.v. theophylline therapy. Hosp Pharm 1989;24:440. 442–8, 460.

[77] Ambrose PJ, Smith WE, Palarea ER. A decade of experience with a clinical pharmacokinetics service. Am J Hosp Pharm 1988;45:1879–1886.

[78] Li SC, Ioannides-Demos LL, Spicer WJ, Spelman DW, Tong N, et al. Prospective audit of an aminoglycoside consultative service in a general hospital. Med J Aust 1992;157:308–311.

[79] McCall LJ, Dierks DR. Pharmacy-managed patient-controlled analgesia service. Am J Hosp Pharm 1990;47:2706–2710.

[80] Lipsy RJ, Smith GH, Maloney ME. Design, implementation, and use of a new antimicrobial order form: a descriptive report. Ann Pharmacother 1993;27:856–861.

[81] Frighetto L, Marra CA, Stiver HG, Bryce EA, Jewesson PJ. Economic impact of standardized orders for antimicrobial prophylaxis program. Ann Pharmacother 2000;34:154–160.

[82] Classen DC, Pestotnik SL, Evans RS, Burke JP. Description of a computerized adverse drug event monitor using a hospital information system. Hosp Pharm 1992;27:774. 776–9, 783.

[83] Paltiel O, Gordon L, Berg D, Israeli A. Effect of a computerized alert on the management of hypokalemia in hospitalized patients. Arch Intern Med 2003;163:200–204.

Chapter 28

Portfolio and project planning and management in the drug discovery, evaluation, development, and regulatory review process

Charles Grudzinskas[a], Michael Dyszel[b], Khushboo Sharma[c], and Charles T. Gombar[d]

[a]*NDA Partners LLC, Rochelle, VA, United States,* [b]*Global Portfolio & Program Management, Mallinckrodt Pharmaceuticals, Bedminster, NJ, United States,* [c]*Office of New Drugs, CDER, US FDA, Silver Spring, MD, United States,* [d]*HIV Drugs, Bill & Melinda Gates Foundation, Seattle, WA, United States*

Introduction

Drug discovery, evaluation, development, and regulatory reviews are complex, lengthy, and costly processes that involve in excess of 10,000 interdependent activities. In order to be successful in biopharmaceutical new product development, one needs a set of general principles that provide guidance in (1) the construction of a *Research and Development (R&D) Portfolio*, (2) the construction of individual *Product Development Plans*, and (3) the subsequent tracking and controls required to keep the portfolio and product development plans current as learning occurs. The following five *Principles of Optimal Product Development* [1] form the basis for defining a decision-based operational model, identifying and quantifying the critical information required at each major decision point, projecting the probabilities of various outcomes, and informing key stakeholders (management, board, investors, etc.) with clear and concise status information that is needed for effective product development governance. These five principles are as follows:

Principle I: Market advantage

The Product Development Program must produce data that clearly differentiate the new product from current therapies, products, or practices and demonstrate that the product will compete effectively in the market. The product must address a clear medical need, and the data generated in the development program must justify the cost of the product. The cost benefit of a product is sometimes referred to as the fourth hurdle. Traditionally products were valued based on hurdles 1, 2, and 3 (safety, efficacy, and quality). In today's healthcare environment, cost-effectiveness plays a significant role in adoption and coverage.

Principle II: Product readiness

Prior to commencing each phase of clinical studies, the appropriate in vitro, nonclinical, and clinical ADME, efficacy, pharmacokinetic, pharmacodynamic, toxicological, Chemistry, Manufacturing and Controls (CMC), and clinical knowledge will be available, reviewed, verified, and integrated into a single coherent picture of the product's properties, with due emphasis on the types and magnitudes of key remaining uncertainties.

Principle III: Value-driven program execution

All studies (in vitro, nonclinical, clinical, and CMC) must be designed to produce knowledge that directly impacts expected product value, as specified in the target product profile (TPP), along with the data that need to be generated to support the intended indications and claims that will become the approved product labeling.

Principle IV: Learning and confirming

Predictive knowledge of product properties is essential to a decision theory-driven development program. Knowledge will be derived primarily from scientific learning studies which will form the knowledge needed to design the appropriate confirming studies, such as Proof of Concept. Use of study designs that allow "Learning while Confirming" should be maximized.

Atkinson's Principles of Clinical Pharmacology. https://doi.org/10.1016/B978-0-12-819869-8.00033-1

Principle V: Regulatory collaboration

Satisfaction of requirements and constraints from both US and non-US regulatory authorities must be addressed, coordinated and integrated into the program design, and revisited at every milestone and major decision point.

These principles are applicable to all medical product development programs regardless of technology, therapeutic area, or indication, and can be applied to the development of devices and diagnostics as well. However, not all of these principles are fully applicable to all product development programs, nor are they applied in precisely the same manner and to the same extent from program to program. Consequently, their use must be guided by adequate experience and judgment so that these principles can be adapted to the specific needs of each program based on informed interpretation of study results and mid-course corrections can be made on the basis of accumulating knowledge. Each organization will need to develop corollaries for these principles that provide more specific guidance and help keep the product development effort focused on the critical success factors and key data and knowledge needed to support major decisions.

To operationalize these five principles and to manage and optimize the returns of this complex, lengthy, and costly product development process, the biopharmaceutical enterprise has embraced the concept of portfolio and project management. What do the terms portfolio, program, platform, and project management mean and how are they different? *Projects* are typically subsets of programs. A typical project might be installing a new tablet press and validating its use. *Programs* are broader in scope. The tablet press project mentioned earlier could be in support of the development, approval, and launch of a new therapy. All of the activities and subprojects needed to develop a product through to launch are captured under a program. Multiple programs may be combined into a Platform. *Platforms* can be clusters of drugs based on a novel drug delivery method. Platforms can also consist of multiple indications for the same molecule or therapy. Some companies use platform management, others do not. The *portfolio* is comprised of all programs and platforms that exist in an organization. Most organizations simply combine the management of these elements under the term project management. This is fine most of the time, but for those heavily involved in the teams, it is important to understand the different levels of project, program, platform, and portfolio management as the levels of authority, governance, team remit, and goals are quite different for each element. Different organizations may use different terminology, for the sake of this chapter, we will use the definition stated before and as shown in Fig. 28.1.

In the past, biopharmaceutical companies typically executed programs in a siloed environment. The concept of value-driven portfolio management was introduced in the 1990s and has become the standard method for managing a diverse pipeline containing multiple development assets. The obvious benefits of good portfolio and project planning and management are presented in Table 28.1. Achieving approval from global regulatory authorities to market a new biopharmaceutical product is no longer the only endgame for R&D organizations. Increasingly, the major hurdle to being able to deliver new medicines to patients is formulary access and/or reimbursement, be it by a government or private insurers. There are more and more pressures to contain healthcare spending. For a new product to be successful it must address a true medical need, thereby bringing true "value" to patients, healthcare providers, and payers.

The expected market advantage is often referred to as the "differentiation" of the new product, and the establishment of differentiation points is an important goal that drives the design and construction of the product development plan. Estimating the value dimensions of the differentiation points adds even more complexity to an already complex process. The level of complexity also demands a new level of collaboration between the R&D and the commercial groups such as marketing and manufacturing, as well as improved interaction between drug development organizations and payers. Understanding and operating within this reality of complexity and collaboration increases the importance of portfolio planning and management and the role of project planning and management in ensuring effective, efficient, and timeline-driven development of new products. Over the past decade, it has become very common for biopharmaceutical companies to have an internal group focused on the economics and outcomes related to a product with the purpose of building a body of evidence to convince payers and other stakeholders that the cost of the drug is justified by an offset in other costs or a significant improvement in health outcomes. In the past, Health Economics and Outcomes Research was done as a lifecycle management activity after a product was approved. However, Health Economics and Outcomes Research must now be an integral part of the full development program so that, at time of approval, data can be provided to establish or at least justify pricing and coverage in the market.

What is R&D portfolio design, planning, and management?

A *well-planned and managed* pharmaceutical R&D portfolio can be defined as: "The combination of *all* R&D programs, that based on past company, industry, and regulatory agency performance, *will predictably yield* valuable new products at the *rate needed* to support the planned growth of the organization." The portfolio needs to be continually compared with the

Portfolio Management

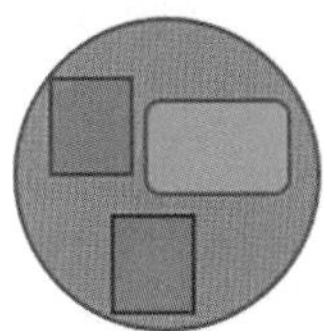

Managing resources across multiple programs. Ensuring governance and business practices are in place and adhered to. Strategic decision making, tracking, controls and reporting on entire portfolio. Very cross functional at senior levels of the organization.

Platform Management

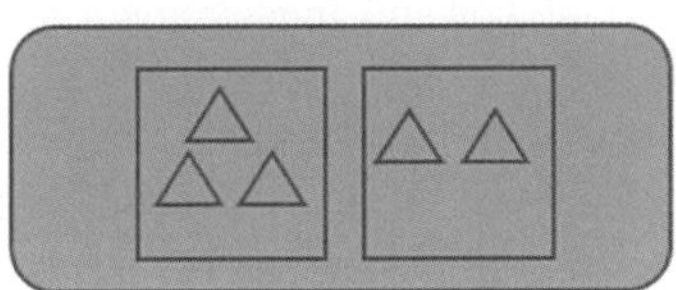

Managing resources across multiple programs that are connected by technology, therapeutic area or other factors. Ensuring multiple programs within the platform are prioritized and complimentary to each other.

Program Management

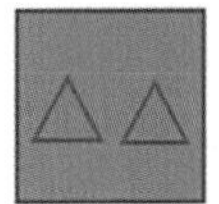
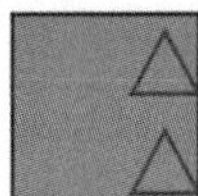
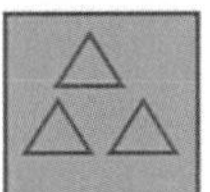
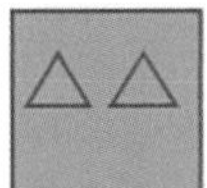

Product development team tasked with efficiently advancing a development program. Focus on program strategy, major decisions, risks and mitigations, following program governance.
Very cross functional in nature containing representatives from research & development, engineering, operations and commercial

Project Management

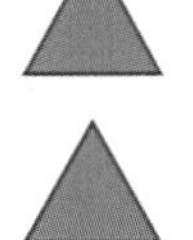
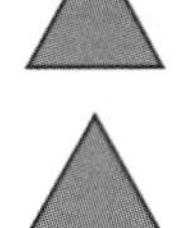
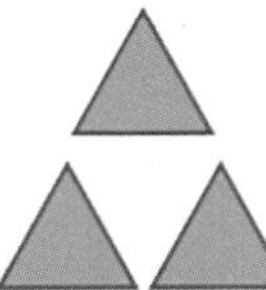

Individual projects led at sub-team level (facility expansions, document management systems, CMC initiatives, individual clinical trials...) that support program team objectives. Usually contained within a specific discipline with some cross functional involvement.

FIG. 28.1 Illustration of the hierarchy of project, program, platform, and portfolio management.

TABLE 28.1 Benefits of good portfolio and project planning and management.
The organization is able to do more with less
The organization is able to optimize the value of a portfolio of projects
Better planning
Better decision-making
Projects meet expected outcomes
Projects finish on time
Projects finish within budget

strategic plan of the enterprise to ensure new product development activities support the long-term vision of the enterprise. Portfolio design, planning, and management are the processes that are used to ensure a well-balanced and value-optimized R&D pipeline. Balancing a portfolio now is far more challenging than in the past and requires more diversification in the products being developed. This means not only diversification across therapeutic areas, but also a mix of traditional small molecule drugs, biological agents (large molecules such as proteins, peptides, monoclonal antibodies, and vaccines), diagnostics, including companion diagnostics, devices, and services. Diversification must expand even further as new technologies yield new types of products (e.g., gene and cellular therapies).

The lifespan of pharmaceutical products is limited by intellectual property duration, regulatory data exclusivity, and the competitive landscape. Loss of market exclusivity for products poses a major challenge to individual companies and to the industry as a whole. This limited product lifespan is being addressed by incorporating lifecycle management much earlier into product development programs. The variety of generic products now available across the therapeutic spectrum has led some to believe that pharmaceuticals are now a commodity market. We reject that view as there remain numerous unmet medical needs and the understanding of disease pathophysiology continues to expand at a staggering rate, creating new opportunities for developing improved therapeutic agents. The stakes for effective decision-making on *which products to develop* have never been higher—indeed, the survival of many companies will depend on how well they design and manage their respective portfolios. Therefore better, more sophisticated portfolio design and management, along with highly efficient and rapid product development, is a requirement for sustainability.

Multiple pressures combine to constantly threaten the overall value for a product development program and the subsequent lifecycle management program, constituting what can be thought of as "The AUC Value Problem." This is diagrammed in Fig. 28.2, which depicts a typical revenue vs time forecast for a product under development, although the lifecycle management enhancement of additional indications and formulations is not represented. The figure illustrates that once a product receives regulatory approval, revenues are realized, and the revenues then increase as the new product gains market share. At a certain point, sales will flatten and the revenues remain constant or might even decrease depending on the competitive landscape. The sharp decline in revenues at the right side of the value curve is due to loss of patent protection, through either expiration or a successful patent challenge. This results in loss of market exclusivity, subsequent generic competition, and a sharp decline in revenues, termed the "generic cliff." Indeed, it has been reported that in some cases 90% of a product's annual sales are lost to generic competition within 6 months after patent protection is lost. The figure also shows the potential loss of market exclusivity and revenue that might be associated with increased regulatory requirements or the inability of the company that is developing the product to achieve a "First-Cycle" marketing approval in major markets. In addition, there is the combined potential loss in revenue and product value due to pressures from government and other third-party payers to force down the overall cost of biopharmaceuticals. It is the role of a Product Development Team (PDT) to identify and quantify these threats (see discussion of a "Risk register" later in this chapter) and to develop proactive contingency plans that will ensure optimization of the product's value.

What is project planning and management?

Project planning is an integral part of project management, which is defined in the Project Management Institute's *Guide to the Project Management Body of Knowledge* [2] as "the application of knowledge, skills, tools, and techniques to project activities in order to meet or exceed stakeholder needs and expectations from a project." As we will see later in this chapter, a project is defined by the specifications (i.e., a product label which drives product value), the required resources needed to achieve the desired specification, and the timelines, which are dependent on the combination of the specifications and resources.

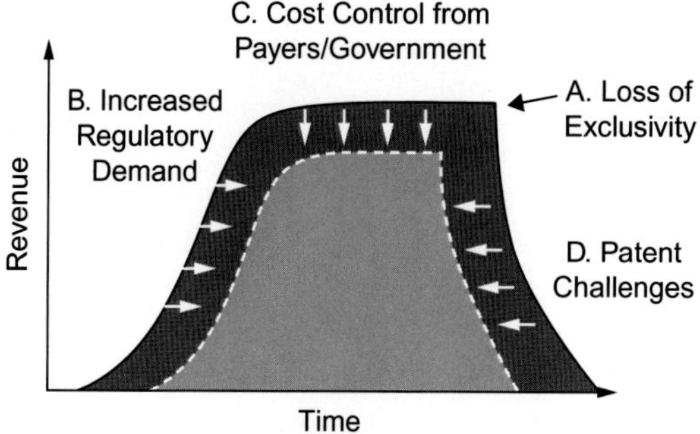

FIG. 28.2 "The AUC Value Problem" illustrates how the combined pressures of (A) Loss of Exclusivity, (B) Increased Regulatory Demand, (C) Cost Control from Payers/Government, and (D) Patent Challenges could affect the overall lifecycle value of a product.

Portfolio design, planning, and management (PDPM)

Portfolio management is the term used to describe the overall process of platform, program, and franchise management. This process includes the three dimensions of portfolio design, portfolio planning, and portfolio management. Each of these three dimensions is described in this section. The five components needed for the successful use of PDPM are identified in Table 28.2. If any one (or more) of the five components is missing or not fully operational, then the likelihood of successful PDPM will be low.

Most large organizations have now adopted the portfolio management team (PMT) concept. PMT membership consists of the senior management of the organization, and the mission of the PMT is to oversee the successful design, planning, and management of the organization's portfolio. The PMT usually has several working groups that focus on specific therapeutic areas. The ultimate responsibility of the PMT is to ensure that the portfolio has been optimized to maximize the potential expected value of the individual R&D programs and to meet the strategic growth goals of the organization. Most organizations have a business planning process that begins with the enterprise *strategic plan*. The strategic plan drives initiatives for platforms and therapeutic areas. PMTs are accountable for selecting and developing programs that will meet the expectations given by the strategic plan. The development programs will be tracked and controlled by cross-functional teams that operate with the guidance of a program manager who will use schedule, cost, scope, and risk tools to track and communicate essential metrics back to the PMT and senior management.

Maximizing portfolio value

Portfolio value is maximized by appropriately prioritizing the programs and the program value drivers within the portfolio based on the future potential financial value of each program and program value driver, multiplied by its probability of technical and regulatory success (i.e., regulatory approval). *For* established biopharmaceutical companies with a self-sustaining cash flow, the focus is typically on the programs with the highest potential value. The future value of each development program is typically based on a calculation of its net present value (NPV). In this calculation, the anticipated financial return from the program is compared with that of an alternative investment of an equivalent amount of capital [3]. The general equation for calculating NPV is as follows:

$$\text{NPV} = I_0 + \frac{I_1}{1+r} + \frac{I_1}{(1+r)^2} + \cdots + \frac{I_n}{(1+r)^n} \tag{28.1}$$

where the I values are given a negative sign for annual net cash outflow and a positive sign for projected net annual income. The subscripts and exponents correspond to the number of years of projected development and marketing time, and r, termed the *discount rate*, is the rate of return of an alternate investment, such as US Treasury Bills. The discount rate will be company specific as it is related to how the company gets its funds. Hence it is the rate of return that the investors expect or the cost of borrowing money. In some smaller organizations, time to market may be a stronger driver than potential financial value. Especially for investor-funded startups, minimizing time to market, even at the cost of a lower value indication for the drug, may be a necessity to keep the company financially viable.

A NPV analysis using a 5% discount rate is summarized for a hypothetical drug in Table 28.3. It is assumed that the drug will be developed within 4 years at a total cost of $500 million. Because this investment is spread over 4 years, development funds budgeted for this program that are unexpended after year zero are assumed to be earning 5% interest until spent, and are discounted accordingly. Marketing begins in Year 4 but income is similarly discounted as shown in Eq. (28.1) and is assumed to be negligible when patent protection expires after Year 7. The NPV for the program is the sum of the discounted

TABLE 28.2 The five components of successful portfolio design, planning, and management.
Portfolio design
Portfolio planning
Portfolio management
Portfolio management teams (PMTs)
Portfolio optimization using sensitivity analysis

TABLE 28.3 Discounted cash flows for a hypothetical drug development project.[a]

	Year	0	1	2	3
Development	Expense	($25)	($75)	($200)	($200)
	Discounted expense	($25)	($71.4)	($181.4)	($172.8)
	Year	**4**	**5**	**6**	**7**
Marketing	Income	$50	$100	$200	$300
	Discounted income	$41.1	$78.4	$149.2	$213.2

[a]*Dollar amounts are in millions.*

cash inflows and outflows over the life of the product, and in this case is $31.3 million. The NPV is far less than the $150 million difference between total income and expenditures for the program because this latter difference makes no allowance for potential alternative use of the money and the time cost of money. The *internal rate of return* is another metric that may be helpful in evaluating different programs in a portfolio [3]. The internal rate of return is defined simply as the discount rate needed to yield an NPV of zero and would be 6.78% for the hypothetical program presented in Table 28.3.

A note of caution is necessary in using NPV analyses because they are based on the *forecasted* value of products and the associated product value drivers (i.e., differentiation points). For whatever reason, the forecasted values of pharmaceutical products are notoriously inaccurate. The sales of new products frequently are over- or underestimated, sometimes by orders of magnitude. So it is important to factor this into value calculations used for portfolio prioritization and to rely on no *single* metric to prioritize programs.

The probability of success is the second factor used to estimate portfolio value and is calculated as the product of the probability of technical success, the probability of regulatory success, and the probability of commercial success. The criteria for these probabilities of success need to be clearly defined and characterized so that future PMTs can translate the impact of program progress and decisions, as well as the ever-changing regulatory and competitive landscapes, on the value of the programs in the portfolio (see section on "Portfolio optimization using sensitivity analysis"). Decision trees are a useful tool to estimate the probability of technical and regulatory success (see later).

It is easy to assess that programs for which application for marketing have been submitted to worldwide regulatory review bodies for review will most commonly have the highest probability of success. Therefore they are likely to have the highest overall financial value in the portfolio (overall value equals possible future value times the probability of success), whereas programs that are in the discovery stage will have the lowest overall value in the portfolio but are the lifeblood of the organization 4–6 years in the future.

It is the role of the PMT to develop a "balanced portfolio" that supports the near-term, mid-term, and long-term needs of the organization. One must be careful to not put all bets on the highest probability programs and handicap novel therapies that will determine the longer-term future of the enterprise. The R&D and commercial senior management teams need to ensure that organizational resources are properly allocated according to the agreed-upon program prioritization.

Portfolio design

It is not an overstatement to say that the near-term and long-term future of a biopharmaceutical company depends on the size and likelihood of success of its R&D pipeline. The pipeline is the totality of a company's portfolio, consisting of programs ranging from very early discovery to marketed products that are ending their current lifecycle and will need a line extension (new formulation or expanded indications) to remain competitive, or pharmacoeconomic data to continue to support the product's value proposition. A pharmaceutical R&D portfolio begins with a vision of the intended growth rate of the organization. Based on the envisioned growth rate, a portfolio can be developed that is based on what the future pipeline will need to look like at each of the four phases of the drug development process described in Chapter 34, and the factors associated with successful transition between these phases, termed *phase transition*. The size of the pipeline needed at each phase of drug development is estimated from both past industry and regulatory experiences and reported metrics.

The probability of a drug candidate maturing to an approved drug, as well as the average duration of development until approval, has been extensively studied by the Center for the Study of Drug Development (CSDD) at Tufts University. In 2011 CSDD reported that on average only one compound reaches the market for every six (16% success rate) that enter the clinical development process [4]. While the overall success rate for drugs varies somewhat from decade to decade, it does not vary much from the "rule of thumb" of 1 successful drug for every 10 that enter clinical development. As shown in Fig. 28.3, the likelihood of overall clinical success rate (regulatory approval) for NCEs (new chemical entities) varies by therapeutic area. In this example from an analysis published in 2010, the highest success rate observed for systemic anti-biotics (23.9%) and the lowest success rate observed for CNS (central nervous system) (8.2%) [5].

In recent analyses, the clinical success rate for cancer compounds was 13.4% [6], 3.7% for cardiovascular drugs [7], and 7.7% for diabetes drugs [8]. Development time until marketing approval for a new drug also depends on therapeutic area and can range from 6 to 10 years [5].

Therefore, as shown in the portfolio pyramid in Fig. 28.4, a company that wants to produce one new approved product (NDA/BLA and MAA) each year would have to initiate on average a minimum of six new First-in-Human (FIH) clinical studies, and would need to adjust the size of the portfolio depending upon the likelihood for success of individual development programs, based on the compound type, therapeutic area, and whether self-originated or licensed-in. Naturally, if a company wanted to develop two or three new NDAs/BLAs and MAAs each year, it would have to have a pipeline portfolio that is, respectively, two or three times as large as is illustrated in Fig. 28.4. However, this "shots-on-goal" approach has its limitations in that it must be supplemented by a robust assessment of the potential technical, regulatory, and commercial success of each product in the portfolio.

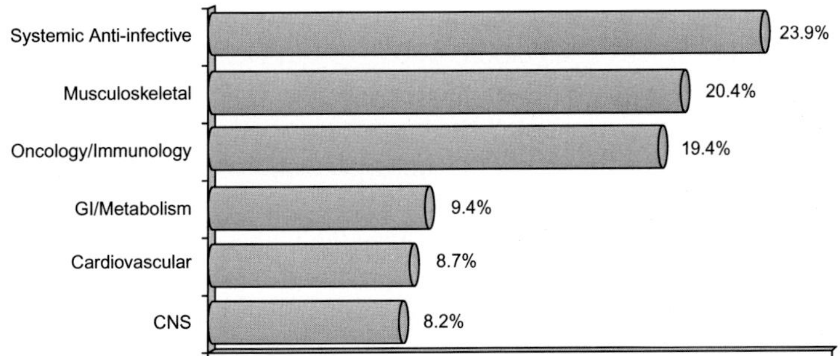

FIG. 28.3 Influence of the therapeutic class being studied upon the likely success rate from initiation of a first-in-human (FIH) study to regulatory approval for compounds with FIH studies between 1993 and 2004. *(Based on data from DiMasi JA, Feldman L, Seckler A, Wilson A. Trends in risks associated with new drug development: Success rates for investigational drugs. Clin Pharmacol Ther 2010;87:272–277.)*

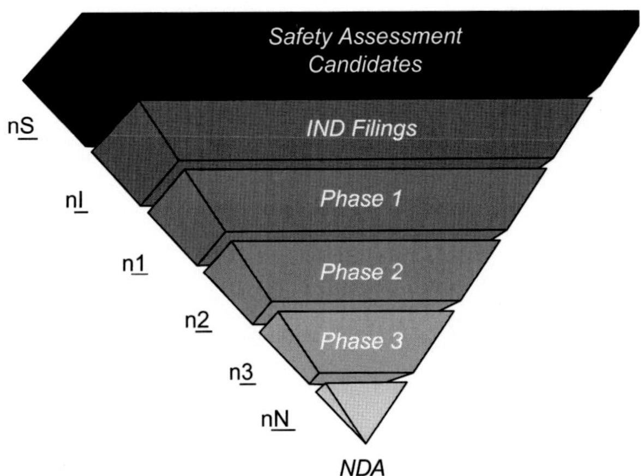

FIG. 28.4 Size of the drug development portfolio needed to support an NDA/BLA/MAA pipeline. (*nS*, number of compounds that will need to be screened each year; *nI*, number of INDs/CTCs that will need to be submitted each year for approval of a FIH clinical study; *n1*, number of Phase 1 projects that will need to be initiated each year; *n2*, number of Phase 2I projects that will need to be initiated each year; *n3*, number of Phase 3 projects that will need to be initiated each year; and *nN*, number of NDAs/BLAs/MAAs that will need to be submitted each year based on the portfolio of compounds screened, INDs/CTCs filed and Phase 1-Phase 3 projects initiated each year.)

Portfolio planning

Once the portfolio vision and design have been defined, the organization can focus on how to build that portfolio. As programs mature from one stage to the next, or are terminated for lack of success, additional programs will need to be added to the various stages of the portfolio to ensure that a portfolio of adequate size exists at each stage. To maintain an aggressive portfolio, companies have acknowledged that it is nearly impossible to fill the pipeline by being dependent solely on self-originated research. There are many sources for new products in addition to the organization's own discovery program. For example, companies can fill out their portfolios by entering into joint ventures and alliances with both established and startup organizations. Additional sources of new products include in-licensing early stage research from the National Institutes of Health (NIH), universities, and foundations (e.g., the Juvenile Diabetes Foundation). Thus the planning process includes both the identification and successful in-licensing of the candidates needed to populate the stages of the drug development process that we saw in Fig. 28.4.

Portfolio management

Portfolio management is primarily focused on the prioritization of programs within an ever-changing portfolio, and the associated resource allocation decisions. Several consulting groups and software programs are available to aid in the management of a dynamic portfolio. These same tools can be used to evaluate "what-if" scenarios to determine how the addition or deletion of programs to the portfolio either increases or decreases the portfolio's overall value based on the trade-offs of program values, resource requirements, and development timelines. As with most processes of this nature, the most important consideration is the quality of the information regarding the potential value and probability of success of each program. Precise evaluations of the commercial, regulatory, and technical probabilities need to come from those within the organization, as well as those outside of the organization, who have sufficient experience to be able to provide informed, realistic estimates of both expected values and probabilities of success.

As illustrated in Fig. 28.5, organizations can graph the value that is expected to be gained vs the cost of the R&D needed to achieve the overall value that is calculated for each program. Organizations can then make decisions as to how to allocate resources based on the "steepness" of the slope of each program, which represents the ratio of added value per resource unit, keeping in mind that programs closest to the market (which have the highest probability of success) will likely have the steepest slope. In the next section, we examine how to avoid the pitfall of assuming that programs (such as the one identified in the oval in Fig. 28.5) necessarily need to be terminated because they have less than acceptable expected value vs cost slopes.

Naturally, organizations will want to populate their portfolio with programs that balance potential value and probability of success, as illustrated in Fig. 28.6 and described in Table 28.4. Clearly the most desirable programs are in Quadrant I (high value with a high probability of success). Programs in Quadrant IV, with low value and low probability of success, should either be examined for ways to increase the expected program value or probability of success, or be recommended

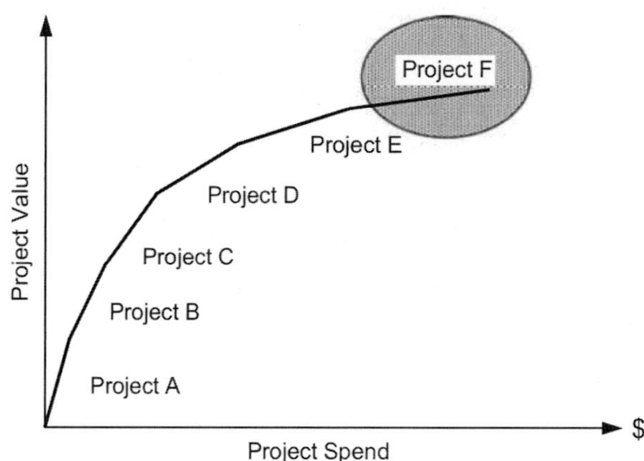

FIG. 28.5 Relationship between project value and R&D funds invested in their clinical development (project spend). The value of this hypothetical portfolio would be the cumulative value of its constituent projects. Project F clearly has the lowest expected value per "project spend." These low-value projects are usually considered as candidates for termination. In addition to termination as a possibility, effective companies evaluate the low-expected-value projects to identify the drivers that would lead to a significant increase in the project's expected value (see Fig. 28.7 and discussion of "Portfolio optimization using sensitivity analysis").

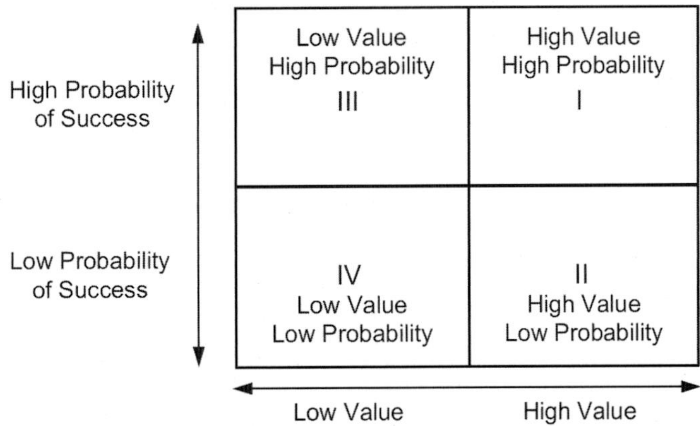

FIG. 28.6 Four-quadrant table used for portfolio analysis in which projects are evaluated on the basis of their potential financial return (value) and probability of development success.

TABLE 28.4 The four portfolio quadrants.

Quadrant I	A diamond mine
Quadrant II	Betting the ranch
Quadrant III	A sure bet
Quadrant IV	A turkey ranch

for termination. Unfortunately, few programs fall into Quadrant I, so a typical portfolio is composed of programs mostly from Quadrants II and III (most organizations try to avoid Quadrant IV-type programs).

Portfolio optimization using sensitivity analysis

Sensitivity analysis is used to identify and quantify program characteristics that are major factors in the expected commercial value of a program, and is one of the most powerful tools of modern portfolio management. Sensitivity analyses serve two goals. The first goal is to identify the program characteristics that were used to determine the program value—the so-called value drivers—and ensure that the program plan developed by the product development team solidly supports these value drivers. For example, a value driver for a potential sedative hypnotic might be that it has no potentiation or interaction with alcohol. Because much of the value of this program depends on this product characteristic, the product development team will design a development plan to assess this expected value driver as early as possible in the development cycle. Indeed, the absence of an interaction with alcohol could be adopted as a "Proof of Concept" milestone.

The second goal is to identify "differentiation" characteristics that, *if added* to the already existing program characteristics, would significantly increase the expected value of the program. This type of sensitivity analysis is important for all programs in the portfolio, but is critically important for those programs that are in danger of being terminated from the portfolio for lack of adequate value. The results of a sensitivity analysis are plotted with broad ranges of value for each criterion and are called tornado charts because their shape resembles that of the meteorological phenomenon. As an example, Table 28.5 lists a set of "as planned" goals for a hypothetical antibiotic. We see from the tornado chart in Fig. 28.7 that the portfolio analysis has determined that the "as planned" NPV for the program is $1 billion (represented by the dotted vertical axis on the chart). The stipulation of "as planned" underscores an important caveat, for the value determined was based on the program goals presented in Table 28.5.

What one can learn from this sensitivity analysis is that the scenario with the highest probability of occurring ("most likely") is the one that incorporates the following:

- The NDA will be submitted in 12 months.
- Evidence supporting twice-a-day dosing will be established.

TABLE 28.5 Example of "as planned" goals for a hypothetical oral antibiotic.

NDA submission	In 12 months
Dose regimen	Twice a day
Concomitant use	With some (but not all) drugs likely to be used by this population
Diagnostic kit	Available at launch
Cost of goods	~$25,000/kg
IV formulation	Not available at launch

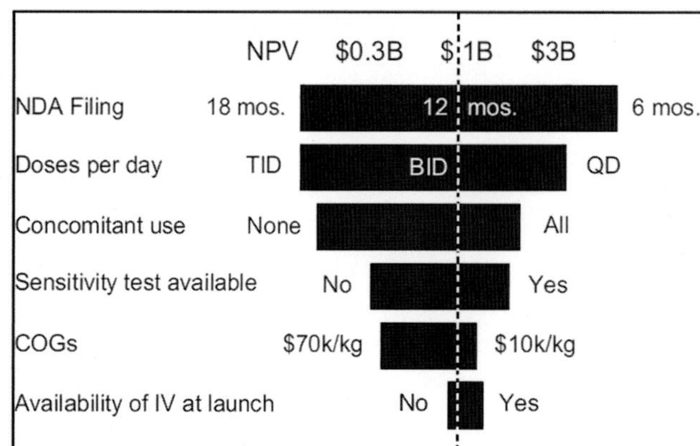

FIG. 28.7 "Tornado" chart illustrating a sensitivity analysis for the development of a hypothetical antibiotic. (*COGs*, cost of goods; *NPV*, net present value.)

- The product can be administered concomitantly with many, but not all, of the drugs that might be expected to be used by this patient population.
- A diagnostic kit for antibiotic sensitivity will not be widely available at the time that product marketing is launched.
- The cost of goods will be in the range of $25,000/kg.
- It is unlikely that an intravenous form of the drug will be available at launch.

This "most likely" scenario values the oral antibiotic at $1 billion. The bars for each of the critical goals indicate that product value would be increased by $2 billion if the NDA could be submitted in 6 months. Likewise, the value would be reduced to $0.3 billion if the time required for NDA submission slips to 18 months. The sensitivity analysis also indicates that the product could have an increased value of $2.5 billion if a once-a-day formulation could be developed and made available at product launch. Although other changes would also increase the NPV of the product, the first two (a NDA submission within 6 months and a once-a-day formulation) provide the greatest increase in value. Clearly, the PMT and the senior management board would focus resources on these two high-value areas. If there were limited resources, then the program team would be asked which of the two increased value goals (a NDA submission within 6 months or once-a-day formulation) would be the most likely to be achieved. Similar sensitivity assessments would be conducted for each of the development programs within the R&D portfolio, and a decision would be made as to which of the subprograms that would significantly increase the portfolio value should be funded.

Project planning and management

Once the portfolio has been designed, planned, and managed for optimization, it is the job of the PDT to manage each development program. Project planning and management for the biopharmaceutical industry began in the early 1980s and quickly became an integral part of the R&D organization by the mid-1980s. Project planning and management have progressed to the point that there are now six dimensions of project planning and management that are routinely used to plan and manage biopharmaceutical programs (Table 28.6). An overview of each of these dimensions will be provided.

TABLE 28.6 Project management dimensions in the biopharmaceutical industry.
Project planning
Project scheduling
Team management
Resource allocation
Decision-making
Process leadership and benchmarking

Defining a program

Biopharmaceutical projects within a program, like all R&D projects, consist of three components, which must be planned and managed in an integrated manner. These three components are *project specifications*, *project timelines*, and *project resources* and can be thought of as "the what?," "the when?," and "the how/where?" of a project, respectively. Recently, "project specification" has focused on the assessment of value, which, as described earlier, is a requirement for commercial success. Once these three components have been defined and agreed upon, they become known as the *baseline specifications*, the *baseline resource requirement*, and the *baseline timelines*.

Project specifications (the what?)

Target product profile

Project specifications include (1) the projected efficacy, safety, and especially the differentiation criteria (i.e., Market Advantage) of a program; (2) drug substance and formulation (e.g., oral, parenteral, transdermal, modified release); and (3) package styles (e.g., bottles, ampoules, blister packs). Drug development organizations typically use a *target product profile* (TPP) to define and communicate the expectations of a particular development program. In some cases, TPPs are used as early as drug discovery to define the selection criteria for identifying "development leads" (e.g., orally active, does not inhibit CYP3A4, can be used in combination with drug X, etc.). The TPP frequently will include both the "optimal" criteria to drive the design of a development plan and "threshold" criteria for minimal acceptability. The threshold metric is identified as the criteria that if not achieved will prompt serious review of the program for possible termination. Although many different functions provide input into the TPP, the commercial group is typically the ultimate owner of the TPP.

Target package insert and target summary of product characteristics

A companion planning and decision-making tool to the TPP is the *target package insert* (TPI) for US programs and the *target summary of product characteristics* (TSPC) for non-US programs. The TPI and TSPC reflect the target labeling that the organization hopes to achieve (see Fig. 28.8). The TPP is used as a tool for planning the clinical and nonclinical activities needed to generate evidence of safety, efficacy, and quality, and to inventory the new knowledge that has been generated. This inventory of knowledge, along with the organization's level of confidence in the likelihood for product success, is used to assess whether adequate scientific evidence will exist to convince regulatory authorities that the product is deserving of market approval with the desired label. Thus the TPI/TSPC serves as a baseline for the desired labeling. A *Draft Package Insert* (DPI) and the corresponding *Draft Summary of Product Characteristics* (DSPC) begins to evolve as new knowledge is generated, and these drafts are constantly compared to the baseline TPI/TSPC to assess whether the drug candidate is still likely to achieve the prespecified value level that was initially used to justify the selection of the drug candidate and the continued allocation of the organization's resources to the program.

In March 2007, the FDA issued a draft *Guidance for Industry and Review Staff Target Product Profile—A Strategic Development Process Tool* to encourage TPP-focused meetings with sponsors at the FDA [9]. The following is stated in the FDA TPP Guidance:

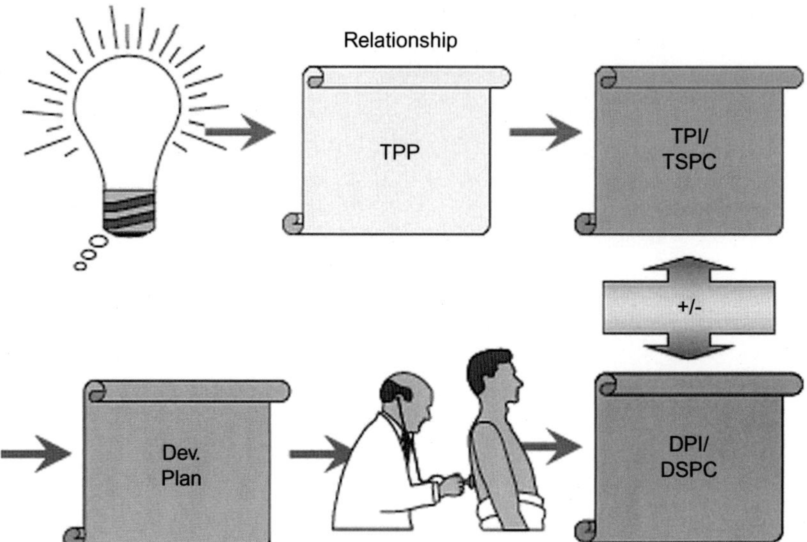

FIG. 28.8 The target product profile (TPP) is a driver for the program development plan and is a tool for assessing whether the program is achieving the intended expectations and value. (*DPI*, draft package insert; *DSPC*, draft summary of product characteristics; *TPI*, target package insert; *TSPC*, target summary of product characteristics.)

An efficient dialogue between a sponsor and the FDA during the drug development process can minimize the risk of late-stage drug development failures, increase the probability that optimal safety and efficacy data are available in a timely manner, improve labeling content, and possibly decrease the total time involved with drug development.

The major value of the FDA guidance on target product profiles was to give a format and structure for sponsor companies to outline key product attributes. As it provides a valuable framework for the organization to set expectations around key product attributes, the biopharmaceutical industry has subsequently embedded target product profiles into their portfolio management practices. The TPP also serves as a guide to help sponsors format and drive questions and briefing books to be used at Pre-IND, End of Phase 2, pre-NDA/BLA, or other meetings. Examples for product profile templates can be found at:

a. https://www.covance.com/content/dam/covance/pdf/Drug-Target-Profile-Template-Fillable-Web.pdf
b. See Appendix C of FDA Guidance at https://www.fda.gov/media/72566/download

Project timelines (the when?)

Project timelines consist of the timelines for both the overall program and for the subproject goals. In the context of drug development, time is a resource. However, time is the one resource that cannot be replaced. An organization can provide additional staff, funds, animals, clinical sites, and subjects, but the organization cannot recapture time once it has been consumed. Project timelines can be established by three processes. The first process of establishing timelines is by the forward planning process based on project specifications and available (usually limited) resources. The second process for establishing timelines is by an impending deadline, which the organization uses to define the balance between (1) project specifications that can be accomplished within the specified timeline and (2) the available resources. The third process for establishing project timelines is to set a deadline, define what must be accomplished, and then resource accordingly to ensure the defined project can be completed by the deadline.

It needs to be noted that project planning and project scheduling are two separate, but interdependent, dimensions. The ideal way to craft a drug development program is to first define the goals of the project. This is often described as "label driven-question based" development planning, since the desired approved product label is used to define and drive the program goals. Once the goals are defined, it is the role of a PDT to (1) develop both a strategic plan and a tactical plan that define and support the major program objectives; (2) define the program Go/No-Go decisions with prespecified decision-making criteria; (3) identify the individual activities, the supporting tasks, and the required resources (funding, people, and facilities) that will be needed to accomplish the program objectives; and (4) identify both the order (precedence) in which these tasks need to be carried out and any interdependencies between activities.

There are at least two approaches for defining the order of the activities. The first is the "plan for success" approach, in which as many activities as possible are conducted in parallel to provide the shortest timeline to the Go/No-Go decisions [e.g., proof of mechanism (PoM), proof of concept (PoC), risk evaluation and mitigation studies (REMS)] and program completion. The second approach is used when there are very scarce resources or when there is a *low probability of success*. This second approach defers resource-intensive activities until a PoC has been achieved, thereby reducing the risk of the program. At that point, a plan-for-success style approach for the program will be developed and implemented. One can also stage the development of lower prioritized programs in a portfolio, if resources are limited, or if the risk is still high and the programs need to be managed more conservatively by the organization.

Project resources (the how/where?)

An example of program definition:

An example of a program definition in the biopharmaceutical industry would be the development of a drug–device combination product for treating patients post cardiac arrest. The product will have two configurations, one designed for an in-hospital treatment and one designed for use in an emergency vehicle. There is an overarching Product Development team who operate at the program level, ensuring that appropriate strategic decision-making and governance is followed. There will also be functional project teams that support the overall program.

The time to develop the in-hospital device is 3 years to get to a Pre-Market Authorization (PMA) filing at a cost of $48 million. Based on successful prior PMA filing, the time to develop the portable device is 5 years to get to a 510k submission at a cost of $68 million. The drug product will take 4 years to get to an NDA filing at a cost of $570 million.

This example incorporates many subprojects that need to run in parallel. A *device development team* needs to not only plan the development work for both devices and go through all required testing and design controls, but they also need to work hand in hand with customer service, operations, and commercial to ensure that the devices are reasonable to manufacture, serviceable, and meet the needs of the end customer. To meet anticipated launch timelines, the organization will need to execute a $240-million capital project to build a manufacturing facility for the devices before the clinical outcomes of the Phase 3 trials are known. A *clinical development team* will need to design and execute two parallel Phase 3 clinical trials using the drug in the intended device to gather clinical information to support the intended target product claims. A *CMC group* will need to develop manufacturing methods, testing methods, and establish stability of the drug product in the intended final packaging. A *preclinical team* will need to continue studying long-term toxicity, carcinogenicity, and mechanism of action in support of a regulatory dossier submission.

All of these teams need to interface regularly to ensure that both the drug and the device are available for clinical trials and also for commercial readiness. It is imperative to finalize formulations and device characteristics prior to entering Phase 3 trials as posttrial changes create regulatory challenges and often the need to repeat studies, or at a minimum perform costly bridging studies to show comparability of previous formulations/devices to the formulations/devices that will be marketed.

The integration of all these teams is critical to the success of the program and is typically done at the PDT level. It also is important to strategically evaluate and plan to secure intellectual property rights, potential future indications, and geographic expansions to ensure maximization of value. To accomplish this effectively, key opinion leaders need to be engaged and primary market research carried out, using either internal or external resources.

In summary, the program will need internal resources, external resources, and extensive capital investment. The summation of all resources required along with the stated deliverables is typically captured in a *program charter*. The program charter is a commitment to stakeholders that states what will be delivered, when it will be delivered, and at what cost and risk. The charter is usually developed by a program manager working with all subteams and is approved by senior leaders from each of the respective areas. Different organizations may take a different approach. Top-down directive development of the charter ensures senior leaders are aligned, but may not have the same team buy-in as an organization that uses a bottom-up method to gain stronger commitment.

The project management triangle

Project components can be represented as the three sides of a triangle, as illustrated in Fig. 28.9. This representation is quite useful, since once the project components have been established, the length of each side (component) of the project management triangle is locked in and represents the baseline specifications. As usually happens with any project, changes constantly occur. If the project is changed by expanding the number of indications or formulations, then we realize from the geometric analogy that one or both of the other two components will need to change. Either the project resource component must be increased to adhere to the original timeline, or the project timeline component must be lengthened to maintain the project resource component as originally defined, or a balance needs to occur, involving a change in both the project

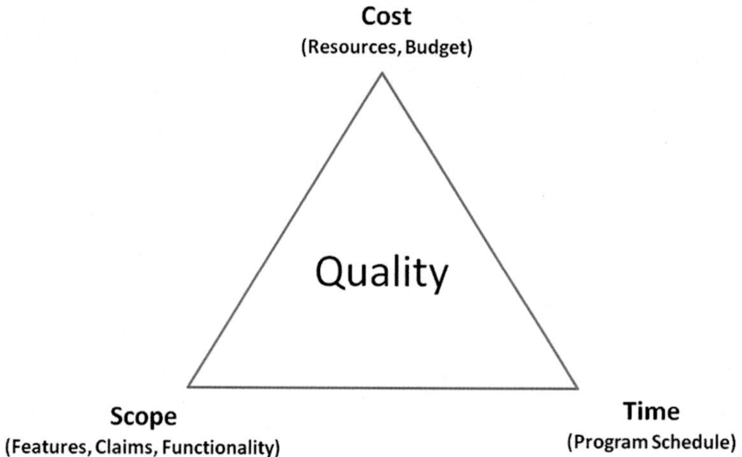

FIG. 28.9 The project management triangle, showing the relationship between cost scope and time. A change in one side of the triangle necessitates changes in one or more of the other sides.

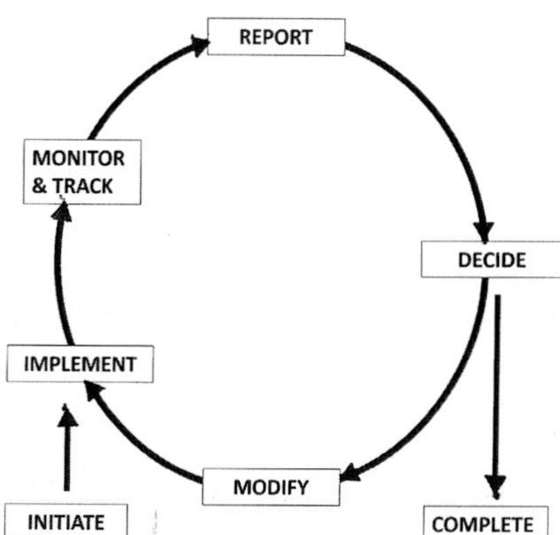

FIG. 28.10 The project cycle.

timeline and project resource components. It is the role of a PDT to optimize these three project dimensions and present a proposal for any necessary project modification to their R&D governance team.

As illustrated in Fig. 28.10, the project cycle consists of six stages [10]. The first stage, the *initiation stage*, encompasses the design and planning of the program, including the definition of the three project components (cost, scope, and time) which, even in a preliminary fashion, are documented in the TPP and the program charter. The initiation stage also includes creation of a PDT composed of individuals representing the many disciplines needed to complete the project. The second stage of the project cycle is called the *implementation stage*. During this stage, project planning, scheduling (timelines), and resource allocation actually start. For a drug development program, these first efforts will probably focus on projects that involve the preparation of drug substance for formulation screening and animal safety studies, and the start of these studies (e.g., see Chapter 30). The third stage of the project cycle is called the *monitoring and tracking stage*. The critically important point to be made regarding monitoring and tracking is to focus and limit attention on what is tracked so that linkage is established to the major milestones which will determine whether or not forward motion on the project is being made. The fourth stage of the project cycle is the *reporting stage*. The decision on what needs to be reported regarding project progress and variances, and to whom the information needs to be reported, should be based on what critical decisions will be made and by whom. Clearly, the level of detail reported to a PDT member is more than the level that senior management needs in order to make major decisions. Indeed, it is the role of the PDT to digest the current project information and to prepare Impact Reports and Actions Needed documents for those who make the resource allocation decisions necessary to keep the expected development program deliverables and timelines on track. The next stage is the *decision-*

making stage. A key point to remember regarding the decision-making stage is that a useful definition of a decision is "an allocation of resources." When a decision is made, resources must be added to a project, or taken away from a project, or maintained for that project. The final stage is the *completion/termination stage*. This stage is reached for each project cycle, and the outcome is determined by whether or not the project goals and objectives of that particular project cycle have been achieved.

A full development program can be thought of as a series of projects and project cycles that each contains these stages. From that perspective, the last stage for a project in early phase development will be "continue/terminate" rather than "complete/terminate." For example, a critical Phase 2 dose-exposure-response clinical study must be planned carefully, with alignment with and buy-in from key stakeholders in the organization, and then implemented, monitored, and reported. Based on the outcome of this Phase 2 study, a critical decision will be made as to whether or not to invest in a large, expensive, and lengthy Phase 3 confirmatory program.

Project planning and management tools

Several tools that are useful in the planning and management of biopharmaceutical programs are identified in Table 28.7 and are listed in the order in which they will be described. It is important to point out that these tools are useful only after the program objectives, goals, Go/No-Go decisions, decision criteria, and critical operating assumptions have been established. Each tool is intended for a specific purpose. Organizational context and culture are key considerations in selecting the tools to use and in deciding the level of rigor with which they will be applied. It is important *not* to force-fit the use of a tool into an organization that is not ready or willing to use it. Most if not all of these tools are implemented at the beginning of a program and continuously updated as additional information and knowledge are obtained, so as to reflect the new data that have been collected and changes in the external environment (competitive landscape, regulatory policy, healthcare policy).

Target product profile (TPP)

As mentioned earlier in this chapter, the TPP is a key document which captures critical product attributes that must be achieved by a development program. More details are provided in an earlier section of this chapter.

Business case

The business case is developed in tandem with the TPP. It sums up the development plan in terms of cost and timing to market and compares them to the revenue projections anticipated once product is commercially available. The business case document should clearly define assumptions and risks. The business case should outline the competitive landscape

TABLE 28.7 Project planning and management tools.
Target product profile
Business case
Target product claims
Program charter
Team charter
Milestone table/tracker
Communications plan
Product development plan
Detailed timeline with embedded work breakdown structure
Risk register
Action & decision log
Program goals/scorecard

and what risks and or opportunities are present. Where possible, scenario analysis should be incorporated to give a range of possible outcomes.

Target product claims

The target product claims document is generated from the TPP. It bridges the desired commercial messaging to the actual labeling that would go along with the product as it enters the marketplace. It should be an evergreen document that incorporates nonclinical, CMC, and clinical pharmacology data along with information regarding dose, regimen, and patient populations. It should be developed early in the program with confirmation provided by results of the Phase 3 program.

Target product label (TPL)

The TPL contains the language that will be submitted to regulatory authorities as part of the dossier submission. The information is a further refinement of the target product claims, stating the claims that are supported by adequate and sufficient evidence derived from the development program.

Program charter

The program charter can be thought of as a contract between the PDT and senior management. It states the goals of the development program, the time to achieve those goals, and the resources required to complete development of the asset. As previously described, the charter is typically developed by the PDT and approved by members of senior leadership.

Team charter

The team charter is used to establish team norms, operating principles, and mutual expectations. The charter also contains a list of the key members of the team. Their role and expected level of participation on the team is, as often specified in a RACI (Responsible, Accountable, Consulted, Informed) chart. Team charters are less formal than program charters, but are a valuable tool in establishing a healthy team that understands their role and the role of others.

Milestone table/tracker

Milestone tables consist of a tabulation of major drug development milestones. Whereas the Go/No-Go decisions are very project specific, development milestones are much more generic and can usually be applied to a wide variety of projects. Typical program milestones for pharmaceutical development are presented in Table 28.8. It is important that each organization decides on the milestones that it wishes to use and that it defines them very clearly. Some companies distinguish between milestones (progress point to be noted) and stage gates (decision points for future resource investment). Typically, subsets of milestones are considered to be the stage gates.

Communications plan

A communications plan is developed by the PDT and is meant to predefine how, who, when, and to whom critical communications will take place. It may contain general information on how the team will meet and capture meeting minutes and decisions. Depending on the sophistication of the organization, it may reference standard operating procedures and business practice documents that detail who will receive critical information (trial results) and how the information will be disseminated internally as well as externally.

Product development plan

The product development plan is a continuation of the TPP which lays out in a moderate level of detail all the major steps needed to develop a product to a regulatory approval. It should include all preclinical and clinical studies, formulation development work, any manufacturing or supply chain infrastructure enhancements, health economics research, and all regulatory agency interactions that are planned. The product development plan is the first step in developing a detailed timeline for product development. A key feature of the product development plan is the major assumptions that are associated with the development program (risk/benefit profile, efficacy signal, trial outcomes, etc.). When assumptions change,

TABLE 28.8 Typical program milestones.
Potential therapeutic target identified
Chemical lead identified
Clinical candidate selected
Pre-IND meeting with FDA and scientific advice meeting with EMA
First in human (FIH) clinical study initiated
End of Phase IIa meeting with FDA
Effective dose and dose regimen characterized for safety and for effectiveness
End of Phase II meeting with FDA and meetings with EMEA
Phase III clinical studies initiated
Phase III clinical studies completed
Pre-NDA meeting with FDA
NDA/BLA/MAA submitted
Risk evaluation and mediation studies (REMS) agreed to by FDA
NDA/BLA/MAA approved
Product launched
Postmarket surveillance program initiated

the PDT needs to revisit the product development plan to update it as necessary. There are many assumptions that can change during the development process. One example would be the need to modify later stage trials when a previously used validated end point tool gets changed or the standard of care in the specific disease state changes. The assumptions of using a certain tool and comparator early in the program are then no longer valid and the teams need to quickly adjust their strategy in the product development plan.

Detailed timeline with embedded work breakdown structure (WBS)

The WBS from the development plan should form the frame work for a *detailed timeline*. Whereas a development plan may have a WBS that contains 30–60 activities, the detailed timeline can contain upwards of 10,000 individual tasks. Each task should be linked to the tasks that need to be completed before it can be started. The benefit of linking tasks is many-fold, one of the most useful benefits being the ability to identify the *critical path* of the program. The critical path is all the activities that if delayed by even 1 day will delay the completion of the program. Each task should also have resources assigned to it. Assigning resources gives a twofold benefit. It helps the team identify who is accountable and it can also feed into a larger resource pool allowing managers to look at resource utilization across multiple programs.

The level of detail to track in plans and in WBSs varies greatly across organizations. Many companies have launched very elaborate, sophisticated tools to plan and track many detailed activities only to find that the resources required to maintain those plans exceed the value that is gained from trying to monitor detailed activities. For this reason, the senior management of each organization needs to clearly define and articulate their philosophy with regard to the level of detail to be tracked and the allocation of resources needed for the creation, maintenance, and updating of detailed product development plans, schedules, and resource requirements.

Gantt charts

The final execution plan for drug development should be captured in a Gantt chart of the detailed timeline. Gantt charts are horizontal bar charts (Fig. 28.11) that are used to view (1) the timeline (duration) of each task, activity, and objective; (2) the temporal relationship and possible interdependencies between various activities; and (3) the actual progress made on each

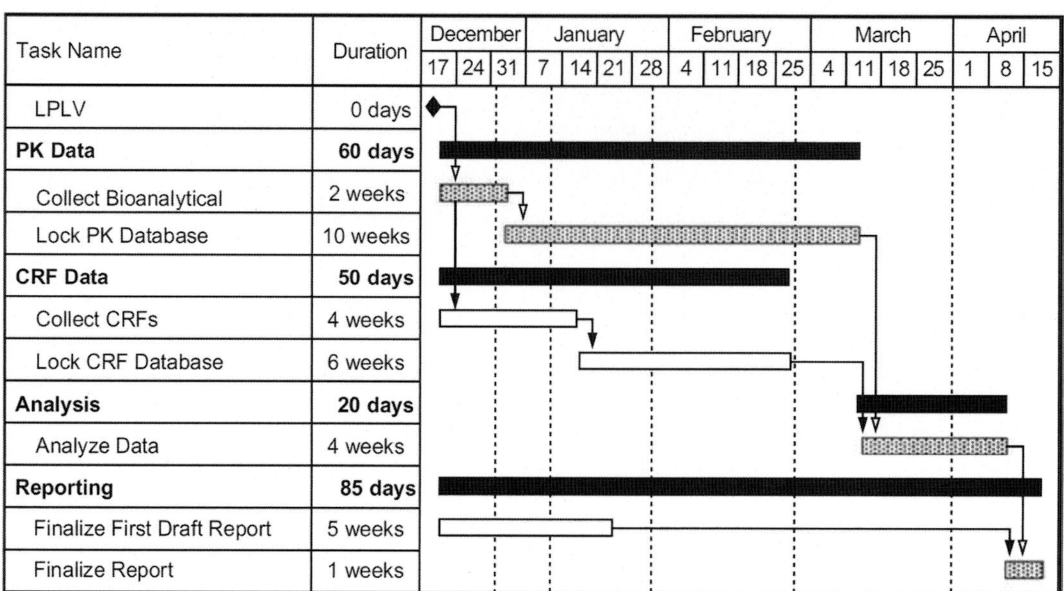

FIG. 28.11 A Gantt (bar) chart with the critical path activities indicated by the *stipples bars* and *arrows*. (*CRF*, case report form; *LPLV*, last patient, last visit; *PK*, pharmacokinetic.)

task, activity, and objective vs the original (baseline) project plan. The Gantt chart is the main project graphic used to track project progress and decision points, and usually a PowerPoint graphic of the key milestones and decision points from the Gantt chart is prepared and used for PDT meetings and R&D management team updates. A number of project-tracking software systems are available and provide the ability to view a chart of the whole project as well as just the high-level objectives (milestones and decision points).

Project progress is shown in a number of ways, for example, by shading a portion of the activity bar to indicate the proportion of the activity that has been completed (e.g., 75% shaded to represent that 75% of the subjects needed for a clinical study have been enrolled). A particularly effective way both to track project progress and to identify key activities that are lagging behind the agreed-upon schedule is to set up a comparison bar chart that includes the current bar chart schedule, the previous bar chart schedule, and the bar chart schedule that was originally planned. Project teams have found it very beneficial to view the project Gantt chart in a variety of presentations, such as a Gantt chart of all project activities that are scheduled to start within the next 90 days and a separate Gantt chart of all project activities that are scheduled to end within the next 90 days. To make the best use of PDT meeting time, it is advisable to have the project Gantt chart updated before each team meeting so that the team is fully informed of the current project timelines and any exceptions to the agreed-upon timelines. With a fully updated and informed project schedule, the project team can make the decisions and recommendations required to maintain the desired progress of the project.

As mentioned earlier, the project schedule is a consequence of the scope of the project objectives, availability of project resources, and timeline requirements. Projects can be scheduled to "complete no later than…," in which case objectives and resources have to be balanced appropriately. In other cases, the project objectives are established, the resources that are available for the project are allocated, and the product development team uses project management software to predict when the project is likely to be completed, given the limitations of the allocated resources. Clearly, allocation of more resources to a resource-limited project could accelerate the project significantly.

PERT/CPM charts

PERT (Performance Evaluation, Review, and Tracking) and CPM (Critical Path Method) charts (flow charts) are based on the flow, connectivity, and interdependency of project tasks, activities, and goals. A PERT chart (Fig. 28.12) depicts the activities in the order that they will need to be carried out, either in series or in parallel. These charts also identify which activities need to be completed (or initiated) before the next activity, which is dependent on it, can be initiated. It is important to point out that PERT and CPM charts are project planning and management tools that are used to ensure the integrity of the project design and planning process, but are rarely used as graphics to track and report on project progress.

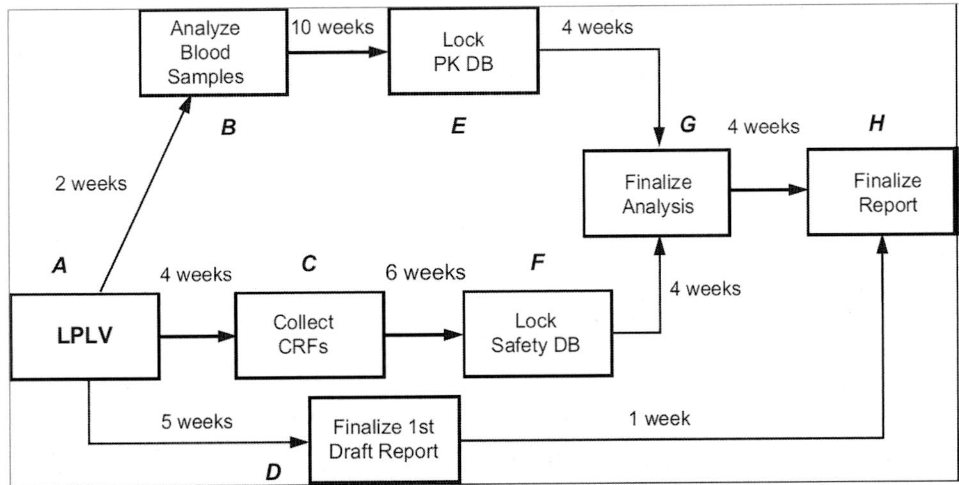

FIG. 28.12 A PERT chart showing three paths. Path 1 (A+D+H) will require 6 weeks. Path 2 (A+C+F+G+H) will require 18 weeks. Path 3 (A+B+E+G+H) is the longest, requiring 20 weeks, and is the critical path. (*CRF*, case report forms; *DB*, database; *LPLV*, last patient, last visit; *PK*, pharmacokinetic.)

CPM is the methodology used to identify the longest, or critical, path from project initiation to project completion. In Fig. 28.12, the critical path is Path 3 (A+B+E+G+H) since this path is the longest path from "A" to "H." The significance of the critical path is twofold. The first point is that if any activity on the critical path is delayed by 1 day, the whole project will be delayed by 1 day. The second point is that once the critical path activities have been identified, the PDT has four "critical path" jobs to focus on. The first job is to find a way to shorten the existing critical path. The second job is to track critical path activities very closely to ensure that there is no slippage. The third job is to track all of the activities that could possibly negatively impact the critical path to ensure that these "subcritical path" activities are initiated and completed as scheduled. The fourth job is to closely manage those activities that could create a new critical path if they were to be completed in a longer time frame than originally estimated.

Detailed budget and cost forecast model

The financial tracking of individual projects has become increasingly important for biopharmaceutical PDTs. In some organizations, a member of the R&D comptroller's office is a member of the team. In other cases, individuals from this office are available to support the team as requested. The PDT is asked on an annual basis to estimate the funding and human resources needed for the project over the next 36 months in order for the project to meet the goals that have been approved by the organization. The team is also asked to help track the project costs on a real-time basis and to make regular (e.g., quarterly or monthly) projections as to the "spend rate" over the next 12 months. Most financial models will contain a breakout of anticipated resources by month for a rolling 12–18-month period, and an annual projected resource requirement for the remainder of the project. It is also common to track and communicate the life of project spend. The life of project spend captures past, current, and future costs which can be used to understand the true cost of developing products over the entire development lifecycle.

Risk registers

A risk register is developed by a PDT as an inventory of critical activities, which if they were to have a negative outcome would significantly impede the project progress. By creating a project risk register, a PDT can use this valuable inventory of potential negative outcomes to proactively design well thought-out contingency project plans. Should adverse outcomes occur, these contingency plans could be rapidly deployed to maintain the forward motion of the project. This inventory of potentially negative impact outcomes also can be used proactively to modify the product development plan to minimize the risk posed by possible future negative outcomes. Thus the risk register inventory is a valuable resource for driving PDT goals, objectives, plans, and project team-meeting agendas.

Action/decision log

The action/decision log is a key document for maintaining the history of actions taken and decisions made by the PDT. As development programs are very lengthy and complex undertakings, team representatives will change over time and very few people will remain on the team from inception to completion. As new members transition onto the team, it is imperative that the team does not revisit previous decisions and actions. This will drastically slow down the development timeline. The action/decision log is also a good onboarding tool for new members. It gives a historical context to the issues that arose and how the team dealt with them.

Program goals dashboard/scorecard

Most organizations establish high-level goals to measure performance on a year-over-year basis. Attainment of the prespecified goals is often tied to variable compensation for those assigned to completing the milestones. It is important for the PDT to look at their development plan and, from the key milestones table, develop a scorecard that can be used to track performance against prespecified timelines. This scorecard should be maintained by the PDT and communicated to management on a regular interval (usually every month).

Project team management and decision-making

Industry project teams

In the pharmaceutical industry, the formal use of core product development teams (Core Team) to accelerate drug development began in the early 1980s. Rather than review the attributes and value of the team concept here, the reader is referred to the classic text on the subject by Katzenbach and Smith [11]. The current standard for biopharmaceutical product development team structure is the matrix team, which is composed of core-team members from the relevant functional organizations that are needed for the development of a new drug (i.e., discovery, toxicology, drug metabolism and pharmacokinetics, analytical, formulations, clinical, regulatory, manufacturing, and marketing), a PDT leader, and a program manager. Several alternatives for project leadership and project support are outlined in Table 28.9. Each alternative has its respective advantages and disadvantages, and each organization needs to choose the alternative that works best in its organizational culture.

It is the program manager's role to ensure that current program information has been incorporated into the various project planning and management tools that the organization is using. Using project management tools, the program manager develops various scenarios for review at decision-making meetings. Each core-team member represents the combined functions of his or her department and is supported by his or her own set of departmental team members and project

TABLE 28.9 Team leadership and project support alternatives.

Team leadership	Advantages	Disadvantages
Dual leadership: Technical process	Provides both strong technical AND process leadership	Two bosses, mixed signals
Technical (usually clinical)	Strong technical leadership	Limited management of process. Usually a part-time role in a full-time job
Full-time team leader	Team leader is dedicated to one or more projects	Might not have strong technical knowledge of the project. Might be leading multiple projects
Team support	**Advantages**	**Disadvantages**
Dedicated project manager	Provides both strong process and project planning and management support	None
None	None	Places excess burden on the project team leader to both lead and provide process and project planning and management support

planners and managers. Each core-team member is also a team leader of his or her respective project support functions, which may be called subteams (e.g., clinical subteam, regulatory subteam).

The term *matrix* refers to the fact that program team members have a dual reporting relationship and therefore are known as multiply supervised employees (MSEs). The traditional matrix team concept has performed adequately, but, as initially conceived, the performance evaluation of team members was conducted only by their departmental management, so that the focus of team members was usually centered on their functional department. However, this evaluation structure was modified in the early 1990s by having each team member's performance evaluated, at least in part, by his or her project team leader, and in some cases by other members of the project team. This change has greatly increased the effectiveness of the matrix team approach.

FDA review teams

The FDA is accountable to the American public to ensure the safety, efficacy, and quality of new drug and biological products. It is also accountable for a high-quality and efficient review process that produces timely and informed regulatory decisions. FDA utilizes Good Review Management Principles and Practices (GRMPPs) as a project management tool for review of PDUFA products [12]. GRMPPs is a tool that provides FDA consolidated review standard for new drug applications (NDAs), biologics license applications (BLAs), as well as review of IND submissions. GRMPPs creates a solid foundation for good review management that starts during product development. It ensures industry's responsibility for submission of a complete application to maximize review efficiency as well as ensures efficient management of an application by the FDA review team. It allows for better transparency to outside stakeholders on how FDA staff reviews an application. As discussed in Chapter 35, FDA review teams are involved in every step of the drug development process and provide scientific expertise and advice during Investigational New Drug Application (IND), marketing, and postmarketing application review. The FDA review team is responsible for reviewing the regulatory and scientific content of an applicant's IND submissions and providing advice on critical safety and efficacy issues. It is ideal for FDA to assemble a review team early and, if possible, to maintain the team throughout the lifecycle of the IND. Throughout the drug's development process, from pre-IND phase through marketing application submission, the review team gains expertise with the data submitted for that therapeutic drug and can foster scientific exchange and reach an accurate regulatory decision.

A *review* is the basis of FDA's decision to approve an application for marketing and is a comprehensive analysis of clinical trial data and other information prepared by FDA drug application reviewers. A review is divided into many sections that include regulatory, medical analysis, chemistry, clinical pharmacology, biopharmaceutics, pharmacology, statistics, microbiology, etc. The FDA review team generally consists of staff from multiple offices, representing different disciplines and areas of expertise. For example, review team from the Office of New Drugs (OND) provides clinical, nonclinical, and regulatory expertise on the full range of drugs and therapeutic biologics; staff from the Office of Pharmaceutical Quality (OPQ) provide expertise for drug product quality submissions; review staff from the Office of Clinical Pharmacology evaluate human pharmacokinetic/pharmacodynamic data; review staff from the Office of Safety and Epidemiology (OSE) evaluate the safety profile of the drugs; and the Office of Biostatistics evaluates statistical plans. Disciplines work together during the review process to contribute expertise to each component of the application. The primary reviewer from each discipline is responsible for conducting a scientific review on an assigned section of the application using his/her particular scientific discipline. The primary reviewer consults with their discipline team leader, peers, and others while developing the review and works collaboratively in a team environment. They are expected to raise review issues and provide potential solutions throughout the review. The primary reviewers work with their discipline team leaders for guidance and feedback as well as to resolve conflicts related to the discipline review area. The Cross-Discipline Team Leader (CDTL) is generally the medical team leader and provides day-to-day management of the review, performs secondary review of the overall application considering all discipline reviews, and ensures consistency of regulatory decisions and the overall direction of the review. The division director will consider all of the reviews and write a tertiary review, describing the basis for the regulatory decision that is binding for the sponsor/applicant. The Benefit-Risk (BR) Assessment is an important section of the primary review that weighs the demonstrated benefits against the risks posed by the drug and is the basis of FDA's regulatory decisions. Therefore this assessment draws on the conclusions reached in different sections of the review, such as efficacy and safety, therapeutic context, labeling recommendations, risk evaluation and mitigation strategies (REMS), and postmarketing requirements and commitments (PMRs/PMCs). The Benefit-Risk Framework (B-RF) summarizes the BR assessment and is an integral part of the review that is formatted to structure the reviewer team's thinking on the medical product's benefits and risks, in a way that effectively communicates the reasoning behind FDA's decisions to a broader audience (Fig. 28.13).

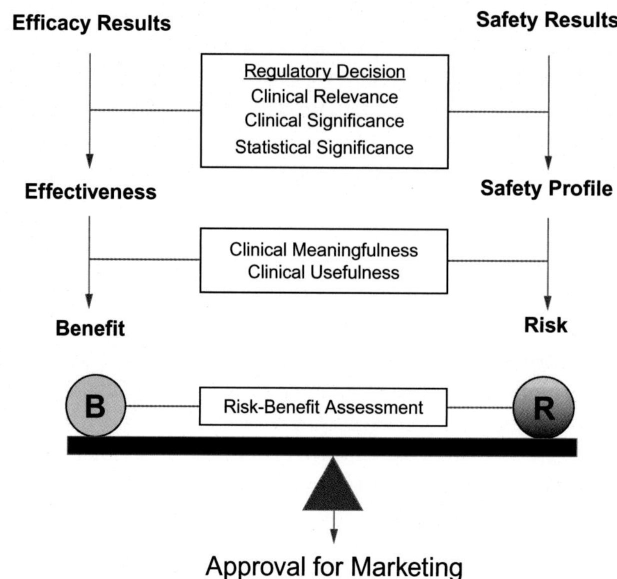

FIG. 28.13 Benefit vs Risk Framework that summarizes the benefit risk assessment.

Role of industry

For its part, industry is accountable for the quality and completeness of its regulatory applications and for the optimal use of drug development resources. The quality of applications submitted to the FDA is critical to achieving the timely and science-based regulatory decisions that are needed to achieve a shared public health goal of early availability of safe, effective, and high-quality drugs to the American Public. The CDTL works closely with the Regulatory Project Manager (RPM), who serves as the regulatory leader of the review team during the review of an application and they are the eyes and ears who communicate externally with sponsors and internally with review disciplines. The RPM is the primary point of the team's contact with regulated industry for all issues that arise over the course of a drug product's lifecycle and leads and facilitates all communications (oral and written) between the sponsor/applicant and review team members. The RPM facilitates and leads the coordination and tracking of all sponsor/applicant meeting requests. He or she works closely with the team leader and discipline reviewers in setting the agenda for sponsor/applicant meetings, facilitates discussion during the meeting, and issues comments and meeting minutes to the internal review team and the sponsor/applicant. The RPM manages the review process with the Cross-Discipline Team Leader for an application, coordinates all application review communications, maintains documentation of the review, conducts a regulatory review of the application and an initial labeling format review for prescribing information, and serves as the primary contact for review-related regulations and policies. The RPM oversees and ensures that the review team works within the new drug regulatory authority and all applicable regulatory precedence(s). They also manage the six-step NDA/BLA review process from presubmission activities through postaction activities using various project management models and tools (Fig. 28.14). The RPM identifies project management templates to utilize during the review of an NDA/BLA submission and establish templates to support the review of the application. They establish monitoring/controlling processes to support the scientific/regulatory review, take official regulatory action on the application, and close out processes to enhance postaction activities [13].

Effective PDT meetings

The ability to lead a meeting effectively is a skill that is most highly regarded in all types of organizations. Effective meetings rarely occur without good preparation and effective meeting management. A well-developed agenda is the most effective tool for holding a successful meeting. Indeed, in some organizations the mantra is "no agenda, no attenda." Having the right people attend the meeting is as important as having an effective agenda. This means that the team leader, the program manager, and all of the team members have a special responsibility to ensure that those who are needed at the meeting do indeed attend and are appropriately informed regarding the status of their function's activities and current

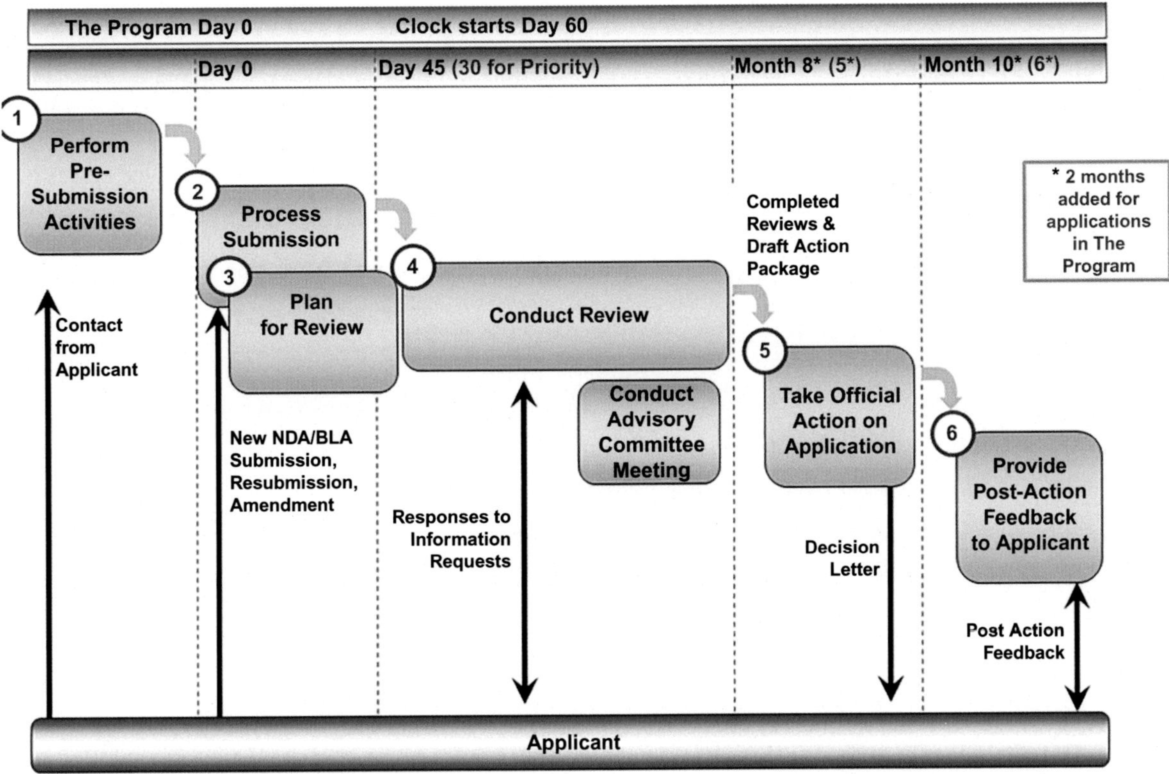

FIG. 28.14 The six-step NDA/BLA review process from presubmission activities through postaction activities.

results. With videoconferencing capabilities, many meetings can be very effective and productive even when not all the participants can be at the same physical site. It is important for one person to be responsible for ensuring that all of the remote-site participants receive meeting materials in advance of the meeting. It is not acceptable to delay a meeting while everyone is waiting for last minute distribution of critical documents to participants at another site. Most organizations have multimedia education tools in their libraries to help their staff develop effective meeting management skills.

Resource allocation

Resource allocation has become more important with the advent of prioritized portfolios. Once a portfolio is prioritized by the PMT, and the team has been informed of the program's priority, the core program team will allocate the resources made available for each constituent project in a manner that will provide for the most rapid progress to be made over a given budget period—usually 12 months. For those who manage a department, resource allocation takes on an added dimension, for although a department head may have adequate resources for all of the approved projects for the next 12 months, the need for the resources might not be evenly spaced over that time period. For example, the portfolio of projects might need 75% of the department's annual resources in the first 6 months and the remaining 25% in the second 6 months. Ideally, project team leaders, project managers, and department project management staff will resolve this mismatch by meeting and developing several alternative scenarios for senior management review and approval. For the decisions to be soundly based, management will ask each team to identify the impact of each alternative scenario on the overall program objectives, decisions, milestones, resources, and timelines.

Effective project decision-making

Decision trees

Decision trees began to be used in biopharmaceutical organizations during the mid-1990s as companies realized that a formalized decision-making process with prespecified criteria for success at each decision point could shorten the time needed for drug development program completion. Decision points for a specific biopharmaceutical program should focus on technical hurdles such as those in Table 28.10. An example of a high-level drug-development decision tree is provided in Fig. 28.15 (certain elements from the decision tree are included in Table 28.10). The key features of this decision tree are as follows: (1) the decision tree is driven by TPP criteria, (2) the decisions are "question-based," (3) the early clinical program is designed to determine the dose-exposure-response relationship for both safety and efficacy, and (4) the decision tree follows the "learn and confirm" paradigm [14].

Program teams are now being asked not only to construct decision trees, but also to develop contingency plans based on multiple "what-if" scenarios far in advance of the next decision points. The goal is to ensure that the program will not lose forward motion in the event of a "No" decision that requires rework or another loop through the program cycle, or a management decision that resources for a particular program are more urgently needed for another program.

TABLE 28.10 Examples of project-specific go/no-go decisions.[a]

Serious toxicity observed in dogs is NOT observed in primates, and therefore **tolerability meets TTP criteria**
A stable IV formulation has now been identified
PK & ADME profiles meet TPP criteria of adequate exposure
Dose-exposure-response (D-E-R) relationships for clinical safety and efficacy (S&E) established per TPP criteria
A process to reduce the high cost of goods has been achieved
The human safety profile observed is as predicted
Clinical activity is observed at 1/20th the highest no adverse effect (NAE) human blood levels
Synergy is demonstrated with the new combination product
Efficacy, safety, and value meet TPP goals
Highest survival ever observed is reported with this test medication

[a]*Bold indicates go decision criteria from Fig. 28.15.*

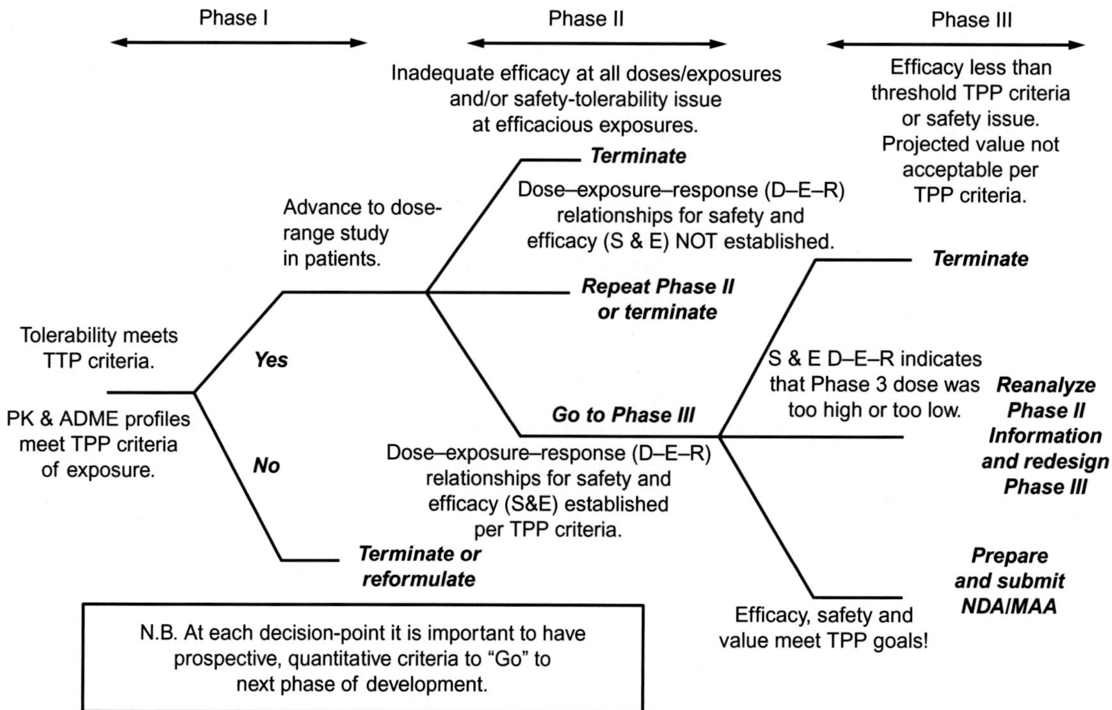

FIG. 28.15 Decision tree for a drug development project. The key features of the decision tree are summarized in the text.

Prespecified decision criteria

To facilitate the decision-making process, highly effective program teams should develop prespecified criteria for each decision point or contingency. These criteria provide the critical targets for the program and speed up the decision-making process. An example of clinical Go/No-Go decision criteria for a potential antihypertensive drug might be "lowers diastolic blood pressure by at least 10 mmHg for at least 6 months in at least 80% of the subjects treated with the middle of three doses, with a side-effect profile lower by 25% than that observed for the active control." One can imagine the debate that will occur if the blood pressure lowering observed at 6 months is only 8 mmHg. Finally, effective decision-making must include an assessment of resource allocation because, as previously emphasized, decision-making is in reality the selective allocation of resources.

Process leadership and benchmarking

It is appropriate to conclude this discussion of effective decision-making with some comments on process leadership and benchmarking. The ability to understand how all the complex pieces of drug development need to be integrated can only be learned through hands-on experience as a PDT team leader, project manager, or seasoned team member. Corporate management in the biopharmaceutical industry now counts on individuals with this experience to identify ways in which the drug development process can be improved to maximize the probability of commercial success and thereby add value to the organization.

Benchmarking has become an important tool for identifying ways in which an organization can quantify, and then exceed, industry standards (best practices) for the time, cost, and quality of the R&D activities that are needed to discover, evaluate, develop, and bring a new drug to market. Benchmarks can be as broad as "How long should it take from the FIH study to NDA submission?" to "How long should it take to design an approvable clinical protocol and case report form for a one-site clinical study?" The Centre for Medicines Research (CMR International) has been formally conducting benchmarking studies for the industry, and additional information can be found on their website [15].

The emphasis on both process leadership and benchmarking in the project planning and management domain of biopharmaceutical R&D truly illustrates the level of maturity and sophistication that this discipline has achieved.

Project management in nontraditional settings

This chapter has been written largely from the perspective of the for-profit biopharmaceutical industry. Product development also takes place in the nonprofit context, especially for global health. Many of the deadliest diseases are endemic in low- and middle-income countries (e.g., tuberculosis, malaria). Although there is little profit to be made treating or preventing these diseases, the world needs new products to treat or prevent them. Work in this area is done by nonprofit organization or public-private partnerships between nonprofits, governments, and industry. A full description of this environment is beyond the scope of this chapter. However, it should be appreciated that program and project management in this context is even more complex than it is in a more traditional industry context. The key stakeholders in these programs often have different, misaligned motivations and incentives. Frequently no one person or organization is clearly leading the efforts, further complicating the work. This leads to these development efforts being very inefficient when compared to product development in industry.

References

[1] NDA Partners LLC. Principles of optimal product development; 2019. Available from: https://ndapartners.com/news/show2.php?article=102.

[2] PMI Standards Committee. Guide to the project management body of knowledge (a PMBOK® guide). 5th ed. Newtown Square, PA: Project Management Institute; 2013.

[3] Baker SL. Perils of the internal rate of return; 2000. Available from: http://sambaker.com/econ/invest/invest.html.

[4] Kaitin KI, DiMasi JA. Pharmaceutical innovation in the 21st century: new drug approvals in the first decade, 2000–2009. Clin Pharmacol Ther 2011;89:183–8.

[5] DiMasi JA, Feldman L, Seckler A, Wilson A. Trends in risks associated with new drug development: success rates for investigational drugs. Clin Pharmacol Ther 2010;87:272–7.

[6] DiMasi JA, Reichert JM, Feldman L, Malins A. Clinical approval success rates for investigational cancer drugs. Clin Pharmacol Ther 2013;94:329–35.

[7] Tufts Center for the Study of Drug Development. Cardiovascular drug approval rate in the U.S. fell as development time rose. Impact report, vol. 19, no. 5; September/October 2017.

[8] Tufts Center for the Study of Drug Development. Diabetes drug development is riskier compared to all drug development. Impact report, vol. 18, no. 5; September/October 2016.
[9] CDER. Target product profile—a strategic development process tool. Draft guidance for industry. Rockville, MD: FDA; 2007. Available from: www.fda.gov/downloads/Drugs/GuidanceComplianceRegulatoryInformation/Guidances/ucm080593.pdf.
[10] Szakonyi R. How to successfully keep R & D projects on track. Mt Airy, MD: Lomond Publications Inc; 1988.
[11] Katzenbach C, Smith D. The wisdom of teams: creating the high-performance organization. New York, NY: HarperBusiness; 2003.
[12] CDER, CBER. Good review management principles and practices for new drug applications and biologics license applications. Guidance for industry and review staff. Silver Spring, MD: FDA; revised September 2018. Available from: https://www.fda.gov/media/72259/download.
[13] CDER. CDER 21st century review process desk reference guide (DRG); revised September 2014. Available from: https://www.fda.gov/media/78941/download.
[14] Sheiner LB. Learning versus confirming in clinical drug development. Clin Pharmacol Ther 1997;61:275–91.
[15] Clarivate. CMR international pharmaceutical R&D factbook. Available from: https://discover.clarivate.com/2019CMRFactbook; 2019.

Chapter 29

Drug discovery

Thomas J. Bateman
Merck & Co. Inc., Kenilworth, NJ, United States

Introduction

The discovery of new therapeutic agents to treat disease is a challenging, and continually evolving, responsibility of drug discovery scientists. A successful drug discovery strategy requires the navigation of a complex landscape of patient need (both in the number of patients and the burden of the disease), competition (current and future), and financial pressures. These financial pressures include regulatory pressures on new drug approvals as well as payor and political pressures on drug pricing [1]. The reward for successfully navigating this landscape is the opportunity to bring life-saving treatments to patients who need them. Given these challenges, detailed analyses of productivity are maintained to optimize discovery efforts and ensure organizational longevity. A key objective is to maintain sufficient innovation to replace the loss of exclusivity of key revenue generators, with the primary innovation being new drugs.

Following a lull in new drug discoveries in the early part of the 21st century, investigations were prevalent into the causes of waning productivity and into the ways in which it could be improved [2–4]. These investigations sparked new trends to enhance organizational efficiency and enable efficient decision making, including, the increased use of high-throughput screening and high-throughput synthesis approaches, enhanced use of in silico modeling to support compound selection, and selective and optimized experimentation to maximize data, minimize cycle times.

According to a recent analysis, the FDA's 5-year annual average new drug approval rate is now 43 drugs per year [5], nearly double the 5-year average output of 10 years ago, suggesting some success in the response of drug discovery scientists to this innovation challenge. In addition to an increase in productivity based on absolute number of approved molecules, an analysis by Wills and Lipkus [6], defining innovation based on new vs existing molecular shape, or new vs existing molecular scaffold, also showed that innovation has increased over the last several decades as assessed by these metrics. In addition to the continuous provision of new candidate drugs, the discovery effort must be achieved in a cost-effective manner, and organizational efficiency is critical to a company's survival. It was recently estimated that the average out-of-pocket cost per approved new compound was ~\$1.4 billion, which may exceed the revenue generated by the drug [7].

The core aspiration of any drug discovery effort is to identify a therapeutic that will modify disease in a manner that is beneficial to patients at a cost that is acceptable. Costs can be financial, in terms of out-of-pocket and societal costs, as well as the cost that side effects may levy on a patient's quality of life. This chapter discusses the drug discovery process, including the identification of a drug target and the assessment of the pharmacology, the selection of the appropriate modality, and the identification and optimization of chemical matter, leading to the selection of a clinical candidate (Fig. 29.1).

Due to the scope of the topic, the described optimization process focuses primarily on small-molecule therapeutics. However, alternative modalities (e.g., peptide, protein, antibody, siRNA, vaccine) are playing an increasingly important role in human disease intervention. Based on a recent assessment, antibody drugs currently make up 7 of the top 10 drugs based on sales [8, 9]. A thorough review of antibody drug discovery was recently published by Lu and colleagues [10].

Elements of drug discovery

Drug discovery teams

Drug discovery is a complex process that requires expertise in multiple disciplines, and, as such, discovery efforts are often carried out by a core team of specialists. Multidisciplinary teams typically include medicinal and computational chemists,

Atkinson's Principles of Clinical Pharmacology. https://doi.org/10.1016/B978-0-12-819869-8.00019-7

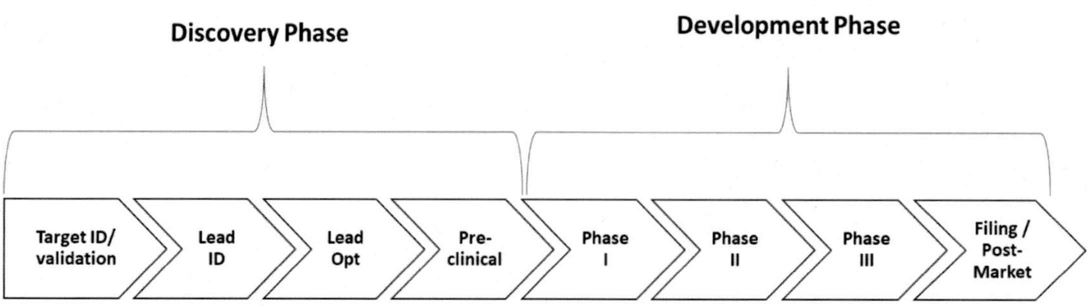

FIG. 29.1 Phases of drug discovery and development: target identification (ID) and validation, lead identification, lead optimization (Opt), preclinical, and clinical development.

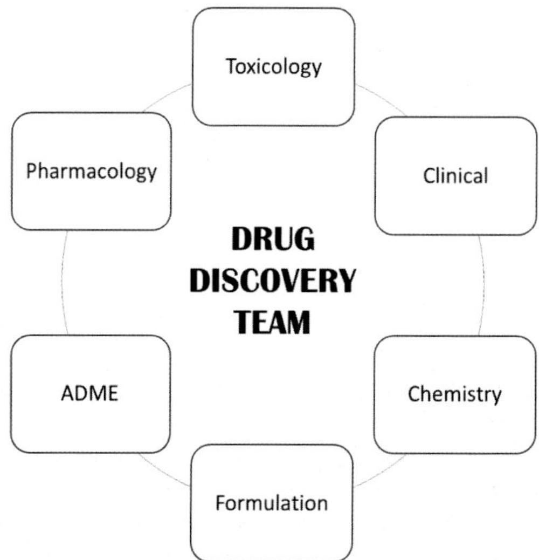

FIG. 29.2 Typical multidisciplinary representation on a drug discovery team.

molecular biologists, pharmacologists, ADME (absorption, distribution, metabolism, and excretion) specialists, formulation scientists, toxicologists, and clinical scientists [11] (Fig. 29.2).

The effective functioning of a team requires its members to supply both deep expertise in their designated scientific field, as well as a broader appreciation by the team of the overall drug discovery strategy. This is particularly pertinent when accepting a candidate molecule that, despite an overall profile that appears favorable, has a liability relevant to one team member's field of expertise. For example, while a formulation scientist may prefer a high solubility, high permeability molecule, many drugs do not meet these criteria, and as such, the team should be open to advance chemical matter outside this space provided adequate bioavailability is achievable. Given the necessity to balance the properties needed to make a successful drug, no single function drives the team, and team leadership is frequently situational, dependent on the issue at hand, and on the team member's disciplinary expertise [12].

Target selection

The selection of a therapeutic target requires an understanding of the underlying pathology of the disease being considered, as well as how the disease, or its progression, can be modulated through a drug's molecular interaction with the therapeutic target, or through the simultaneous modulation of multiple targets. If multiple targets are to be modulated simultaneously, an already complex optimization paradigm becomes more complex, in that it is difficult to design a molecule that appropriately balances modulation along multiple axes and to define the appropriate balance of modulation. As such, the modulation of a single target (sometimes termed a target-based approach) is often preferable when this is mechanistically feasible.

Heparin is an example of a molecule which modifies disease through the simultaneous modulation of multiple targets. Heparin enhances the inhibitory activity of the plasma protein antithrombin against several serine proteases of the coagulation system [13]. The resulting pharmacologic effect is the prevention of clot formation, which can be of therapeutic benefit in preventing thromboembolisms, including deep vein thrombosis, pulmonary embolism, or cerebral embolism. However, this inhibition of coagulation carries a risk of serious, potentially fatal, bleeding. Recognizing the limitations of heparin, drug discovery scientists set out in search of selective antithrombotic agents that targeted single nodes in the coagulation cascade. These newer anticoagulants included drugs that target FIIa (e.g., dabigatran), and drugs that target FXa (e.g., rivaroxaban and apixaban). The selective inhibitors were able to take advantage of an informed approach to target engagement and successfully optimized the balance between maximizing the desired antithrombotic effect, while minimizing the off-target risk of bleeding. The end result was an improved efficacy and safety profile of these selective inhibitors [14, 15], which has allowed these newer agents to dominate the marketplace, with both rivaroxaban and apixaban forecasted to be among the top 10 best-selling drugs for 2020 [16]. This example illustrates how, due to the relative ease of interpretation and optimization, it can be advantageous to modulate a single target.

The mapping of the human genome has provided a wealth of information on potential targets to modify disease processes [17] and currently genome-wide association studies are being utilized to identify genes encoding druggable human proteins and associated biomarkers [18], thus offering the potential for genetic validation of disease etiology. Our expanding knowledge base allows promising targets to be identified and enables informed interrogation of target modification. For some diseases, complex pathophysiological networks have been elucidated and quantitative systems pharmacology models have been built to simulate the impact of modifying nodes within these networks [19]. As our mechanistic understanding of disease improves, along with our ability to model and compute complex biological relationships, these systems pharmacology approaches hold great promise for informed disease intervention.

Further, the use of genetically modified animals has provided a preclinical tool to improve confidence that the target of interest can be beneficially modulated [20, 21]. These models are particularly useful for elucidating adverse effects that may be secondary to the desired pharmacology. By helping to elucidate on-target and off-target effects, mechanistic model-based understanding of the beneficial and adverse effects of a test agent is critical to an efficient drug discovery paradigm and enables a strategic response to experimental results [22]. As testing of candidate molecules progresses from in vitro studies, i.e., binding to isolated receptors or measuring a response in a cell-based system, to in vivo studies in nonclinical species, costs increase, and interpretation becomes more challenging [23] (Fig. 29.3).

In order to accelerate target validation, drug discovery teams are moving more quickly to advance toward more definitive in vivo proof-of-concept studies. In particular, genetic models can provide selective modulation of the target of interest in the absence of suitable chemical matter. A thorough collation of the molecular targets of approved drugs was recently compiled by Santos and colleagues [24]. They noted that, based on the nature of the target and its location, some modalities (e.g., small molecule, peptide, protein, antibody, siRNA, or vaccine) may be more or less amenable to effective therapeutic intervention.

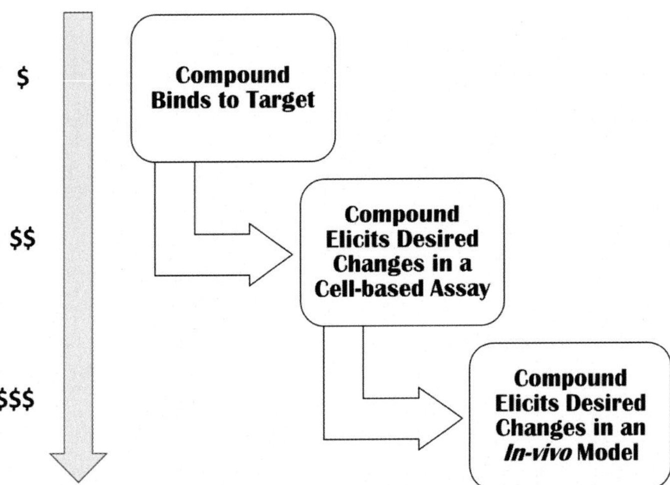

FIG. 29.3 Progression and relative costs associated with testing compound pharmacology.

Selection of a therapeutic modality

An appropriate therapeutic modality is best selected as early as possible after the target of interest is identified, as any investment in a suboptimal modality would be a fruitless effort. In selecting the appropriate modality to modify a disease process, key questions to consider include the following:

- Where is the target? Is the target location restricted? (e.g., the restriction of the blood–brain barrier to antibodies [25]).
- What are the pertinent aspects of patient convenience? (e.g., dosing route and frequency, patient comfort [26], fear of needles [27], lower incidence of side effects [28]).
- Is the target amenable to the desired modality? (Blocking protein–protein interaction surfaces may require inhibitors interacting over larger surface areas and small molecules may not be suitable).

Identification of leads

Library screening

Advances in automation and miniaturization, enabled by the development of new instrumentation, have dramatically changed the landscape of how chemical matter of interest is identified. Massive chemical libraries which are available from either internal inventory or from commercial sources can now be rapidly tested for their affinity against a target of interest [29] and significant investments are made to optimize the management of compound libraries [30]. Advances in molecular docking and computational power have expanded virtual screening paradigms in which the affinity of virtual compounds can be predicted and can be used to prioritize the selection of compounds for synthesis [31].

Identification and validation of hits

High-throughput screening may yield thousands of hits that need to be triaged. Following the screening of a compound library, the identified hits are confirmed and validated. Hits which appear to have adequate target affinity are either repurified or freshly synthesized in order to confirm the identity of the compound which elicited the desired response. Compounds of lower structural complexity may be prioritized as the ease with which analogs can be synthesized facilitates further lead optimization. High-throughput synthesis also allows additional experimentation that includes the combinatorial exploration of reaction variables such as solvents, catalysts, and reagents [32], and further enables the rapid and efficient identification of tool molecules and drug leads. When selecting chemical matter for further study, in addition to molecular properties, intellectual property must also be considered to ensure the selected development candidate is outside of the patent space of competitors.

High-throughput screening approaches, which rely on a rational selection of a target of interest, may not be ideally suited for the discovery of truly novel drugs. Phenotypic screening, in which collections of compounds are tested for their effects on cell-based systems or in animal models, provides an alternative approach. In fact, an analysis of FDA approvals between 1999 and 2008 determined that for drugs with new mechanisms of action, phenotypic screening exceeded target-based approaches in identifying first-in-class small-molecule drugs, with 28 and 17 of these drugs coming from phenotypic and target-based approaches, respectively [33]. However, phenotypic drug discovery is not without its challenges, as target deconvolution, the process of identifying the molecular targets responsible for the phenotypic response, is not trivial, and this is a key enabler to an informed drug discovery paradigm [34]. For this reason, organizations may apply both target-based high-throughput screening as well as phenotypic approaches in order to maximize the probability of finding promising leads.

Fragment-based screening

Fragment-based ligand discovery provides another avenue for generating advanced leads. A number of fragment-screening methods are now available that facilitate identification of low molecular weight ligands as a starting point for compound optimization [35]. These fragments often interact weakly with the target (typical equilibrium dissociation constant (KD) in the 100 s μM to low mM range) but provide a low molecular weight lead as a starting point that can be grown in size to increase binding affinity [36]. Once the crystal structure is obtained for the bound fragment ligand and target, medicinal chemists can use this powerful tool for informed structure modification to enhance binding efficiency.

Testing tool molecules in preclinical models

The term "tool molecule" describes early chemical matter that is adequate to robustly test the target in a relevant nonclinical in vivo model, but unlikely to be suitable for advancement into the clinic. In addition to demonstrating that a selected tool molecule is capable of binding to the target of interest, drug discovery teams seek further confirmation that this binding elicits the desired in vivo pharmacologic effect. Nonclinical in vivo pharmacology models extend the team's understanding of the effects of target modulation and can provide crucial evidence to support or refute further investment in the target. Extensive investment has been made into developing and validating in vivo models of disease in oncology [37], cardiovascular disease [38], analgesia [39], and metabolic disorders like diabetes [40] and obesity [41].

When these animal models of disease are used to interrogate a drug target, test compounds must meet basic prerequisites to allow for an effective and interpretable result. The compound must have acceptable potency and ADME properties to achieve exposures at the target site of action that are sufficient to achieve a level of target engagement that is expected to elicit a measured response. As described by Morgan and Van Der Graaf [42], the following "3 pillars" capture the key features required of a therapeutic agent, and these are applicable preclinically as they are for the clinic: (1) exposure at the target site of action, (2) binding to the pharmacological target, and (3) expression of pharmacology. It is highly desirable to have tool molecules early in the drug discovery process in order to validate the therapeutic potential and "druggability" of the target of interest. Unfortunately, nonclinical animal models, with a contrived reproduction of human disease states, cannot perfectly mimic the actual clinical condition and thus have inevitable limitations that need to be understood for correct interpretation of experimental results. The translation of exposure–response relationships from these preclinical models into the clinic is a field of extensive study for both efficacy [43] and safety [44] endpoints, the details of which will not be covered here.

Lead series

Around the time that the discovery team has identified optimized hits, capable of engaging the target in vivo, there typically are chemical compounds with a consistent pharmacophore structure that fall into a defined lead series. These lead series contain structurally similar compounds which are improved from hits and leads but are not fully optimized, and where data exists to understand and navigate remaining liabilities, such that there is a high degree of confidence that a clinical candidate can be identified from an analog within this series. Desirable lead series should be well positioned in terms of physicochemical properties and have clearly defined structure–activity relationships related to the modulation of potency, selectivity, and ADMET properties.

Approaches to lead optimization

It is now well appreciated that the identification of development candidates, projected to deliver clinical efficacy at a safe dose that is acceptable in size and frequency, requires a balance of suitable potency, selectivity, ADME, and toxicity properties (Fig. 29.4).

The balancing of these parameters creates a resourcing challenge for drug discovery organizations, as the desire to triage compounds as quickly and efficiently as possible. Experimental measurement of all properties for all chemical matter is not feasible, and this creates an incentive to perform screens to simply dismiss compounds that fall outside a designated cutoff. More comprehensive metrics which aim to define aggregate parameters of optimization also have been developed, some of which are described subsequently.

Ligand efficiency

Given current paradigms for identifying target hits, particularly the prevalence of high-throughput screening of in vitro target binding, the parameter of potency is often given a privileged position in the drug discovery process. However, potency alone is inadequate to make a drug, and the selection of only the most potent candidates for advancement would result in the dismissal of a significant fraction of potentially desirable candidates. There are various ligand efficiency metrics that can provide additional context to measured potency. One of the first such metrics was termed *ligand efficiency* (LE), in which binding affinity is normalized relative to the number of nonhydrogen atoms such that LE optimization indicates a greater potency expectation for higher MW molecules [45, 46]. LE is a relatively simple metric that can have utility in helping to control the molecular size of a series during optimization [47].

Another approach to evaluating ligand efficiency which has had a significant impact on compound optimization is lipophilic ligand efficiency termed LLE or LipE, which normalizes the potency of a molecule to its lipophilicity according to the equation:

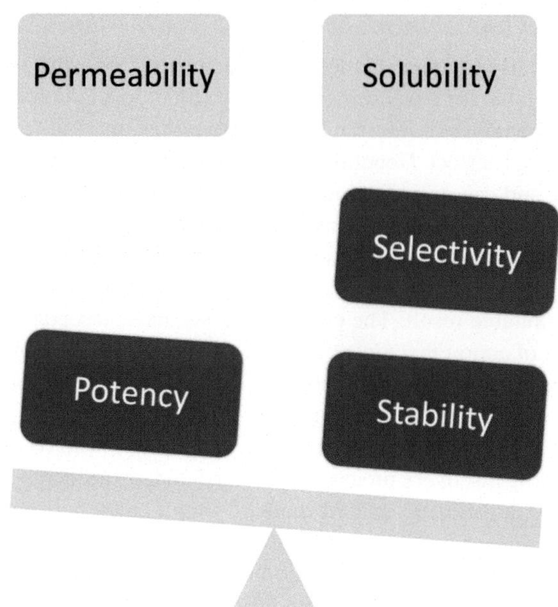

FIG. 29.4 Cartoon reflecting the challenge of finding a suitable balance of molecular properties.

$$LLE = LipE = pIC50 - logP \tag{29.1}$$

where pIC50 is the negative logarithm of the in vitro potency and log$P$ is the equilibrium of an unionized solute between water and an immiscible organic solvent [48].

Binding interactions include molecular interactions between the ligand and the receptor as well as the disruption of molecular interactions with the surrounding environment [49]. Underlying the utility of lipophilicity-normalized potency measurements is the concept that lipophilic molecules may have binding driven primarily by the favorable free energy of a hydrophobic molecule in a hydrophobic binding pocket vs the unfavorable free energy in a surrounding aqueous environment. These interactions tend to be promiscuous and not specific to the target of interest. Enthalpic interactions, on the other hand, including pi stacking, hydrogen bond formation, and ionic bond formation, can be designed to overcome the entropic penalty for the conformation constraint of the target and can be optimized for the intended target. Thermodynamic monitoring as optimization proceeds allows for an informed design of chemical modification that enhances enthalpic interactions and are more likely to produce molecules that are optimized across the multiple parameters that are required for successful drugs [50].

The influence of lipophilicity on potency, along with other parameters relevant to drug optimization, was recently described by Miller and colleagues [51]. However, the effects on individual parameters often counterbalance each other such that lipophilicity has no predictable effect on dose. For example, increasing lipophilicity tends to decrease unbound exposure through higher intrinsic clearance and unbound distribution, but also contributes to increased potency such that lower unbound concentrations are required for efficacy. This analysis reveals a potential pitfall in strategies that aim to optimize ligand design on single parameters in a sequential fashion, as molecules that are deemed to have "low potency" or "high intrinsic clearance" may be triaged, while the overall profile of some of these molecules may in fact be suitably druggable. This sequential approach further restricts the available chemical space, potentially excluding potentially druggable chemical matter and slowing (or preventing) the identification of a suitable candidate. Therefore, rather than a sequential screening paradigm, hypothesis-driven design cycles are increasingly favored [52] (Fig. 29.5).

Beyond relevance to the target of interest, physicochemical properties influence the molecular interactions that occur with the pool of macromolecules in the body, possibly leading to undesirable pharmacologic effects through engagement of off-targets [53]. This is further discussed subsequently under "mitigating the risk of toxicity."

Optimizing absorption

The "rule of 5," described by Lipinski and colleagues [54], is one of the most significant concepts that has influenced efforts to optimize the absorption of oral drugs. These authors described the common features of compounds that are likely to

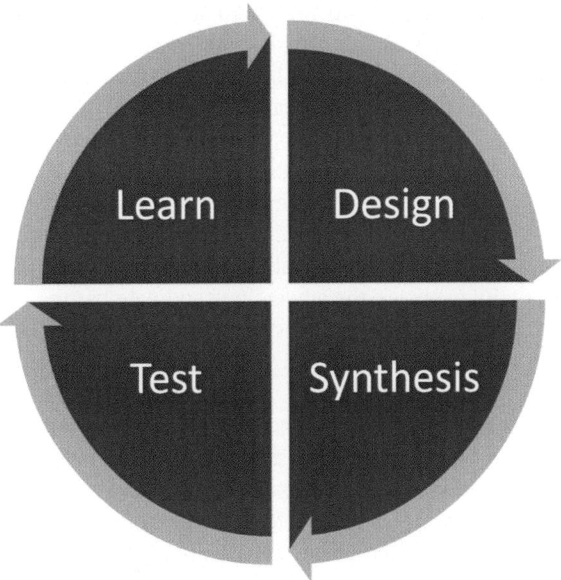

FIG. 29.5 Hypothesis-driven compound design cycle.

achieve adequate absorption through an appropriate balance of solubility and permeability. Features detrimental to absorption include (1) more than 5H-bond donors (expressed as the sum of OHs and NHs), (2) molecular weight greater than 500, (3) $\log P$ greater than 5, and (4) more than 10H-bond acceptors (expressed as the sum of Ns and Os). Despite the reliability of the rule of 5 to identify potential challenges to absorption, drug discovery efforts have often ventured beyond the chemical space defined by these rules and have done so with success. Approximately 6% of oral drugs fall outside of Lipinski space [55] and, considering that some targets require the disruption of protein–protein interactions with flat binding surfaces, deviation may be required. Perhaps the most extreme example of a successful drug operating outside the Lipinski space is Rybelsus, an oral formulation of semaglutide. Semaglutide is a modified peptide with a molecular weight over 4000, which was recently approved for control of blood sugar after demonstrating robust clinical efficacy [56]. Although the passive permeability of semaglutide is low as predicted, this restriction was circumvented by using the permeation enhancer sodium N-[8-(2-hydroxybenzoyl)aminocaprylate] (SNAC). The fact that semaglutide is efficacious at low systemic concentrations also allowed clinical efficacy to be obtained with an acceptably small oral dose [57].

Multiparameter optimization approaches

One way in which discovery teams aim to define lead optimization across all drug-like characteristics is through multiparameter optimization (MPO) of desirability characteristics. The approach involves assigning a desirability score to a range of parameters deemed relevant to optimization. An example of an MPO for central nervous system targeting drugs included scoring for physicochemical properties logP, logD, MW, TPSA (topological polar surface area), HBD (number of hydrogen bond donors), and pK_a with properties weighted equally or by a desirability score ranging from 0.0 to 1.0 for each property [9, 58]. It was noted in this example that if hard cutoffs had been applied at the design stage, some desirable compounds would have been eliminated from further consideration. Desirability weighting allows for an informed balance of optimization priorities and their relative importance for the safety and efficacy of a given candidate molecule [59]. It is also important to note that the utility of this approach will be determined by the parameters selected and the weights assigned, with MPO approaches that utilize multiple correlated parameters, or inappropriately balanced weighting, having the potential for bias.

Mitigating toxicity risk

Beyond understanding the projected pharmacology of a drug candidate, successful drug discovery requires a deep understanding of the adverse effects that might be anticipated. To begin with, it is crucial to distinguish if the adverse effect of the test compound is due to an on-target effect or an off-target effect [22]. Optimization of selectivity against the totality of potential off-target interactions represents one of the great challenges facing drug discovery scientists. When navigating off-target effects, compound design can be focused on improving the selectivity of the compound's affinity for the target of interest relative to the target of concern [60]. Commonly measured off-target potencies to inform selectivity in drug design include ion channels (e.g., hERG, Nav 1.5, Cav 1.2), which are implicated in potential cardiac toxicity [61], drug-metabolizing enzyme pathways (e.g., cytochrome P450s), nuclear receptors (e.g., pregnane X receptor (PXR), the aryl hydrocarbon receptor (AhR), and the constitutive androstane receptor (CAR)) which may precipitate drug–drug interactions through exaggeration of toxicity and reduction of efficacy, respectively [62]. As noted earlier, lipophilicity can correlate with higher affinity for any enzyme or receptor with a hydrophobic binding pocket, and as such, can lead to a correlation between potency for the target of interest and potency for undesirable off-targets with no change in the exposure multiples between these effects. A similar correlation is not expected for LLE optimization, unless the target of interest and the target of concern have a highly similar binding pocket. Targets with highly similar binding pockets to the target of interest are often tested experimentally to ensure the advancing candidate has the requisite selectivity against these off-targets [63]. Broad testing of off-target pharmacology against an array of receptors and ion channels has become common practice for advanced candidates. In addition, data analytics approaches are being explored to improve predictive capabilities in this space [64].

Navigation of on-target adverse effects hinges on an understanding of the exposure–response profile and an optimization of the exposure–time profile. In situations where a window exists between the desired pharmacologic effect and the undesirable adverse effect, the drug should be designed such that the exposure across time can remain above the level of effect and below the level of toxicity. This can be achieved through the design of molecules with a projected human half-life closely approximating the marketed dosing interval (e.g., a half-life of around 24 h for a once daily drug), with greater flexibility in the acceptable half-life for molecules with a greater therapeutic index. The projection of human pharmacokinetics and human dose is an underlying parameter that influences compound selection throughout the optimization process, and the tools and methodologies for the prediction of human dose are described in Chapter 31.

Clinical candidate selection

A lead compound that has been optimized to cross the considerable hurdles of target affinity, selectivity, solubility, permeability, and projected pharmacokinetic properties to achieve a desirable dose may be selected as a clinical candidate and advanced to preclinical development as described in Chapter 30.

Conflict of interest statement

Thomas Bateman is a full-time employee of Merck Sharp & Dohme Corp., a subsidiary of Merck & Co., Inc., Kenilworth, NJ, USA.

References

[1] Kang SY, Bai G, DiStefano M, Socal M, Yehia F, Anderson G. Comparative approaches to drug pricing. Annu Rev Public Health 2020;41:499–512.
[2] Pammolli F, Magazzini L, Riccaboni M. The productivity crisis in pharmaceutical R&D. Nat Rev Drug Discov 2011;10:428–438.
[3] Khanna I. Drug discovery in pharmaceutical industry: productivity challenges and trends. Drug Discov Today 2012;17:1088–1102.
[4] Paul S, Mytelka D, Dunwiddie C, Persinger C, Munos B, Linborg S, et al. How to improve R&D productivity: the pharmaceutical industry's grand challenge. Nat Rev Drug Discov 2010;9:203–214.
[5] Mullard A. 2018 FDA drug approvals. Nature Rev Drug Discov 2019;8:85–89.
[6] Wills T, Lipkus A. Structural approach to assessing the innovativeness of new drugs finds accelerating rate of innovation. ACS Med Chem Lett 2020;11:2114–2119.
[7] DiMasi J, Grabowski H, Hansen R. Innovation in the pharmaceutical industry: new estimates of R&D costs. J Health Econ 2016;47:20–33.
[8] Urquhart L. Top companies and drugs by sales in 2019. Nat Rev Drug Discov 2020;19:228.
[9] Wager TT, Hou X, Verhoest PR, Villalobos A. Central nervous system multiparameter optimization desirability: application in drug discovery. ACS Chem Nerosci 2016;7:767–775.
[10] Lu RM, Hwang YC, Lee CC, Tsai HZ, Li HJ, Wu HC. Development of therapeutic antibodies for the treatment of diseases. J Biomed Sci 2020;27:1–30.
[11] Stocks M. Chapter 3. The small molecule drug discovery process—from target selection to candidate selection. In: Ganellin CR, Jefferis R, Roberts SM, editors. Introduction to drug research and development. Waltham, MA: Academic Press; 2013. p. 81–126.
[12] Schneider A, Erden Z, Widmer H, Koch G, Billy C, Von Krogh G. Rethinking leadership in drug discovery projects. Drug Discov Today 2012;17:1258–1262.
[13] Gray E, Hogwood J, Mulloy B. The anticoagulant and antithrombotic mechanisms of heparin. In: Lever R, Mulloy B, Page CP, editors. Heparin—a century of progress. Handbook of Experimental Pharmacology, vol. 207. New York: Springer; 2012. p. 43–61.
[14] Jiang H, Meng J, Guo T, Zhou J-N, Wang Y-C, Wang J, et al. Comparison of apixaban and low molecular weight heparin in preventing deep venous thrombosis after total knee arthroplasty in older adults. Yonsei Med J 2019;60:626–632.

[15] Lazo-Langner A, Fleet JL, McArthur E, Garg AX. Rivaroxaban versus low molecular weight heparin for the prevention of venous thromboembolism after hip or knee arthroplasty: a cohort-based study. J Thromb Haemost 2014;1:1626–1635.

[16] Urquhart L. Top product forecasts for 2020. Nat Rev Drug Discov 2020;19:86.

[17] International Human Genome Sequencing Consortium. Initial sequencing and analysis of the human genome. Nature 2001;409:860–921.

[18] Finan C, Gaulton A, Kruger F, Lumbers RT, Shah T, Engmann J, et al. The druggable genome and support for target identification and validation in drug development. Sci Transl Med 2017;9:1–34.

[19] Helmlinger G, Sokolov V, Peskov K, Hallow K, Kosinsky Y, Voronova V, et al. Quantitative systems pharmacology: an exemplar model- building workflow with applications in cardiovascular, metabolic, and oncology drug development. CPT Pharmacometrics Syst Pharmacol 2019;8:380–395.

[20] Abuin A, Holt K, Platt K, Sands A, Zambrowicz B. Full-speed mammalian genetics: in vivo target validation in the drug discovery process. Trends Biotechnol 2002;20:36–42.

[21] Doyle A, McGarry M, Lee N, Lee J. The construction of transgenic and gene knockout/knockin mouse models of human disease. Transgenic Res 2012;21:327–349.

[22] Roberts R. Understanding drug targets: no such thing as bad news. Drug Discov Today 2018;23:1925–1928.

[23] Kenakin T. Chapter 11. The drug discovery process. In: A pharmacology primer: techniques for more effective and strategic drug discovery. 4th ed. San Diego: Academic Press; 2014. p. 281–320.

[24] Santos R, Ursu O, Gaulton A, Bento AP, Donadi R, Bologa C, et al. A comprehensive map of molecular drug targets. Nat Rev Drug Discov 2017;16:19–34.

[25] Freskgård PO, Urich E. Antibody therapies in CNS diseases. Neuropharmacology 2017;120:38–55.

[26] Blackwood C, Sanga P, Nuamah I, Keenan A, Singh A, Mathews M, et al. Patients' preference for long-acting injectable versus oral antipsychotics in schizophrenia: results from the patient-reported medication preference questionnaire. Patient Prefer Adherence 2020;14:1093–1102.

[27] Quante M, Thate-Waschke I, Schofer M. What are the reasons for patient preference? A comparison between oral and subcutaneous administration. Z Orthop Unfall 2012;150:397–403.

[28] Singh S, Tank N, Dwiwedi P, Charan J, Kaur R, Sidhu P, et al. Monoclonal antibodies: a review. Curr Clin Pharmacol 2018;13:85–99.

[29] Mayr L, Fuerst P. The future of high-throughput screening. J Biomol Screen 2008;13:443–448.

[30] Quintero C, Kariv I. Design and implementation of an automated compound management system in support of lead optimization. J Biomolec Screen 2009;14:499–508.

[31] Lyu J, Wang S, Balius T, Singh I, Levit A, Moroz Y, et al. Ultra-large library docking for discovering new chemotypes. Nat Res 2019;566:224–229.

[32] Buitrago Santanilla A, Regalado E, Pereira T, Shevlin M, Bateman K, Campeau LC, et al. Nanomole-scale high-throughput chemistry for the synthesis of complex molecules. Science 2015;347:49–53.

[33] Swinney D, Anthony J. How were new medicines discovered? Nat Rev Drug Discov 2011;10:507–519.

[34] Moffat J, Vincent F, Lee J, Eder J, Prunotto M. Opportunities and challenges in phenotypic drug discovery: an industry perspective. Nat Rev Drug Discov 2017;16:53543.

[35] Larsson A, Jansson A, Åberg A, Nordlund P. Efficiency of hit generation and structural characterization in fragment-based ligand discovery. Curr Opin Chem Biol 2011;15:482–488.

[36] Lamoree B, Hubbard R. Current perspectives in fragment-based lead discovery (FBLD). Essays Biochem 2017;61:453–464.

[37] Chen D, An X, Ouyang X, Cai J, Zhou D, Li QX. In vivo pharmacology models for cancer target research. In: Moll S, Carotta J, editors. Target identification and validation in drug discovery: Methods and protocols. 2nd ed Totowa, NJ: Humana Press; 2019. p. 183–211.

[38] Savoji H, Mohammadi M, Rafatian N, Toroghi MK, Wang EY, Zhao Y, et al. Cardiovascular disease models: a game changing paradigm in drug discovery and screening. Biomaterials 2019;198:3–26.

[39] Taneja A, Della Pasqua O, Danhof M. Challenges in translational drug research in neuropathic and inflammatory pain: the prerequisites for a new paradigm. Eur J Clin Pharmacol 2017;73:1219–1236.

[40] Shakya A, Chaudary SK, Garabadu D, Bhat HR, Kakoti BB, Ghosh SK. A comprehensive review on preclinical diabetic models. Curr Diabetes Rev 2020;16:104–116.

[41] Barrett P, Mercer J, Morgan P. Preclinical models for obesity research. Dis Model Mech 2016;9:1245–1255.

[42] Morgan P, Van Der Graaf P. Can the flow of medicines be improved? Fundamental pharmacokinetic and pharmacological principles toward improving phase II survival. Drug Discov Today 2012;17:419–424.

[43] Wong H, Bohnert T, Damian-Iordache V, Gibson C, Hsu C-P, et al. Translational pharmacokinetic-pharmacodynamic analysis in the pharmaceutical industry: an IQ consortium PK-PD discussion group perspective. Drug Discov Today 2017;22:1447–1459.

[44] Morissette P, Polak S, Chain A, Zhai J, Imredy J, Wildey MJ, et al. Combining an in silico proarrhythmic risk assay with a tPKPD model to predict QTc interval prolongation in the anesthetized Guinea pig assay. Toxicol Appl Pharmacol 2020;390:1–13.

[45] Abad-Zapatero CA, Metz J. Ligand efficiency indices as guideposts for drug discovery. Drug Discov Technol 2005;10:464–469.

[46] Kenny P. The nature of ligand efficiency. J Chem 2019;11:1–18.

[47] Murray C, Erlanson D, Hopkins A, Keseru G, Leeson P, Rees D, et al. Validity of ligand efficiency metrics. ACS Med Chem Lett 2014;5:616–618.

[48] Arnott J, Kumar R, Planey SL. Lipophilicity indices for drug development. J Appl Biopharm Pharmacokinet 2013;1:31–36.

[49] Lee LP, Tidor B. Optimization of binding electrostatics: charge complementarity in the barnase-barstar protein complex. Protein Sci 2001;10:362–377.

[50] Garbett N, Chaires J. Thermodynamic studies for drug design and screening. Expert Opin Drug Discov 2012;7:299–314.

[51] Miller RR, Madeira M, Wood HB, Geissler WM, Raab CE, Martin IJ. Integrating the impact of lipophilicity on potency and pharmacokinetic parameters enables the use of diverse chemical space during small molecule drug optimization. J Med Chem 2020;63:1256–1270.
[52] Andersson S, Armstrong A, Björe A, Bowker S, Chapman S, Davies R, et al. Making medicinal chemistry more effective application of lean sigma to improve processes, speed and quality. Drug Discov Today 2009;14:598–604.
[53] Leeson PD, Young RJ. Molecular property design: does everyone get it? ACS Med Chem Lett 2015;6:722–725.
[54] Lipinski C, Lombardo F, Dominy B, Feeney P. Experimental and computational approaches to estimate solubility and permeability in drug discovery and development settings. Adv Drug Del Rev 1997;23:3–25.
[55] DeGoey DA, Chen H-J, Cox PB, Wendt MD. Beyond the rule of 5: lessons learned from AbbVie's drugs and compound collection. J Med Chem 2018;61:2636–2651.
[56] Pratley R, Amod A, Tetens Hoff ST, Kadowaki T, Lingvay I, Nauck M, et al. Oral semaglutide versus subcutaneous liraglutide and placebo in type 2 diabetes (PIONEER 4): a randomised, double-blind, phase 3a trial. Lancet 2019;394:39–50.
[57] Sofogianni A, Tziomalos K. Oral semaglutide, a new option in the management of type 2 diabetes mellitus: a narrative review. Adv Ther 2020;37:4165–4174.
[58] Wager TT, Hou X, Verhoest PR, Villalobos A. Moving beyond rules: the development of a central nervous system multiparameter optimization (CNS MPO) approach to enable alignment of druglike properties. ACS Chem Nerosci 2010;1:435–449.
[59] Segall M. Multi-parameter optimization: identifying high quality compounds with a balance of properties. Curr Pharm Des 2012;18:1292–1310.
[60] Huggins D, Sherman W, Tidor S. Rational approaches to improving selectivity in drug design. J Med Chem 2012;55:1424–1444.
[61] Grant AO. Cardiac ion channels. Circ Arrhythm Electrophysiol 2009;2:185–194.
[62] Pelkonen O, Honkakoski P. Inhibition and induction of human cytochrome P450 enzymes: current status. Arch Toxicol 2008;82:667–715.
[63] Davis MI, Hunt JP, Herrgard S, Ciceri P, Wodicka LM, Pallares G, et al. Comprehensive analysis of kinase inhibitor selectivity. Nat Biotechnol 2011;29:1046–1051.
[64] Rao MS, Gupta R, Liguori MJ, Hu M, Huang X, Mantena SR, et al. Novel computational approach to predict off-target interactions for small molecules. Front Big Data 2019;2:1–17.

Chapter 30

Nonclinical drug development

Chris H. Takimoto[a], Michael J. Wick[b], Balaji Agoram[c], and Denise Jin[a]
[a]Gilead Sciences, Menlo Park, CA, United States, [b]Preclinical Research, XenoSTART, San Antonio, TX, United States, [c]Arcus Biosciences, Hayward, CA, United States

Introduction

Prior to entering clinical testing, a new molecular entity must first undergo a series of rigorous scientific assessments. These include pharmacologic evaluations of safety and efficacy, toxicology testing under carefully controlled conditions, and the thorough characterization of manufacturing processes. Nonclinical development, which spans the gap between drug discovery and clinical testing, encompasses all of these activities. The data resulting from these evaluations are subject to rigorous regulatory review prior to the initiation of first-in-human (FIH) trials.

Once a new molecular entity (NME) or drug candidate is selected for further development, the nonclinical testing process begins. In the United States, these nonclinical data form the basis for an Investigational New Drug (IND) application, which is a request for authorization from the Food and Drug Administration (FDA) to evaluate an investigational drug product in humans. The IND document includes detailed study results evaluating safety and efficacy pharmacology, toxicology profiles, manufacturing processes, and it also includes the proposed plan for the FIH clinical trial [1]. Specific IND-enabling tests are required both for small molecules and for biological agents, such as monoclonal antibodies; however, the manufacturing and optimization processes differ substantially for different types of therapeutics. This chapter describes the general process of nonclinical drug development, including the requirements for an FDA IND filing with specific examples taken from the field of oncology [2].

The IND document's organizational structure was established by the International Conference on Harmonization in their Common Technical Document (CTD) guidelines, which describe a mandatory standard format for regulatory agency submissions in the United States, European Union, and Japan [3]. The overall structure of the CTD is organized into five modules and it applies to a range of regulatory submission documents, including commercial INDs, New Drug Applications (NDAs), and Biological Licensing Applications (BLAs) (Fig. 30.1) [4]. Module 1 contains region-specific administrative information such as specific application forms; however, Modules 2, 3, 4, and 5 are common for all regions. Module 2 contains broad overview summaries starting with an introduction to the pharmaceutical product followed by a Quality Overall Summary covering Chemistry, Manufacturing, and Controls (CMC) topics [5]. It also includes Nonclinical [6] and Clinical [7] Overviews and Written and Tabulated Summaries. Module 3 contains CMC Quality information including the Body of Data relating to Drug Substance and Drug Product [5]. Module 4 is comprised of Nonclinical Study Reports [6] and Clinical Study Reports can be found in Module 5, which for an IND document includes the Phase 1 clinical protocol and informed consent documents [3, 7].

As outlined in the S9 FDA Guidance for the nonclinical evaluation of anticancer pharmaceuticals [2], the goals of testing are to (1) identify the pharmacological properties of the pharmaceutical agent, (2) establish a safe initial dose level for FIH exposure, and (3) understand the toxicological profile. For FIH studies in advanced cancer patients, nonclinical study specifics are defined in the ICH S9 guidance, while for most other indications, the ICH M3 guidance applies [8]. However, many additional components of nonclinical drug development are also required prior to clinical testing. For example, consistency in the chemical and physical properties of the active pharmaceutical ingredient (API) must be insured from the earliest small-scale syntheses for pharmacological studies to bulk API manufacturing for large clinical trials. These processes, broadly referred to as CMC, include the synthesis of the API under good manufacturing principles (GMP), bulk scale up of the manufacturing process, the selection and formulation of the dosage format, and the packaging of clinical trial materials. However, these important CMC activities are beyond the scope of this chapter [9], which will primarily focus on safety and efficacy pharmacology and toxicology studies.

In addition to the safety and toxicology testing required for an IND filing, the importance of characterizing the pharmacokinetic-pharmacodynamic (PKPD) properties of therapeutic candidates in nonclinical development has received

Atkinson's Principles of Clinical Pharmacology. https://doi.org/10.1016/B978-0-12-819869-8.00031-8

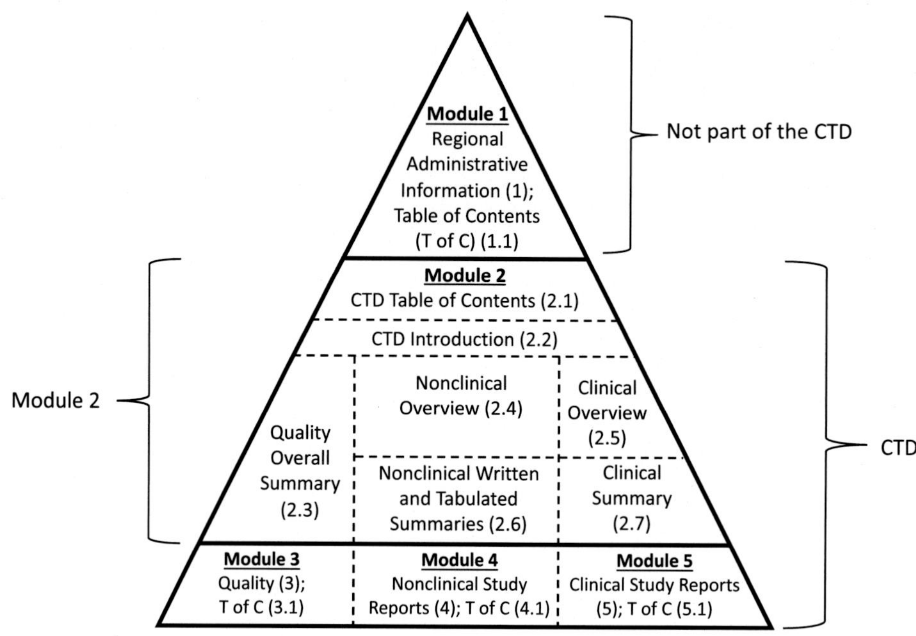

FIG. 30.1 Diagrammatic representation of the organization of the Common Technical Document used for Investigational New Drug Applications. *(Based on Food and Drug Administration. M4 organization of the common technical document for the registration of pharmaceuticals for human use: guidance for industry; 2017. Silver Spring. Available from: https://www.fda.gov/media/71551/download.)*

greater appreciation in recent years [10–12]. The early incorporation of PKPD principles into the analysis of preclinical data has multiple benefits, including accelerating lead optimization, streamlining early clinical development by identifying optimal clinical doses of therapeutics, and providing early warnings regarding possible clinical drug-drug interactions.

Components of nonclinical drug development

The nonclinical component of the IND document in Module 2 typically contains detailed information which is organized in three sections focused on the investigational agent's pharmacology, pharmacokinetics, and toxicology profiles [6] (Fig. 30.2). Pharmacology studies can be further subdivided into primary pharmacodynamic, secondary pharmacodynamic, and safety pharmacology studies [13]. The ICH S7A guidance defines primary pharmacodynamic studies as those being done to evaluate the drug's mode of action and/or effects related to the desired therapeutic target [13]. Secondary pharmacodynamic studies are those not related to the mode of action and/or the desired effects of a substance. For oncology therapeutics, primary pharmacodynamic evaluations on the mode of action are frequently conducted in vitro followed by antitumor efficacy evaluation done in vivo in relevant animal models. The in vivo evaluations should be conducted at doses that are tolerated in nonclinical species to inform clinical dose escalation plans, either as monotherapy and/or in combination with other agents [14]. Primary and secondary pharmacodynamic studies do not have to be conducted in compliance with formal good laboratory practice principles (GLP) [13]. Safety pharmacology studies are defined as those that investigate potentially undesirable drug effects on physiological functions occurring at drug exposures in the therapeutic dose range and above. Typically, these involve assessments of the drug's impact on a core battery of vital organs, including those in the cardiovascular [15], respiratory, and central nervous systems. Where feasible, they are generally done in compliance with GLP [13]. For anticancer agents, stand-alone safety pharmacology studies may not be necessary and, instead, these may be incorporated into later toxicologic evaluations [2]; however, standalone studies are more commonly required for agents in other indications [8]. Likewise, for biological agents, that are highly specific in their receptor targeting, it may also be sufficient to evaluate their safety pharmacology as part of the later toxicologic evaluation [13].

The nonclinical pharmacokinetics section for a small molecule therapeutic agent should include information on the absorption, distribution, metabolism, and excretion (ADME) of the product in relevant species, which most commonly are rodents, dogs, or primates. Information on plasma protein binding properties can also help with relative toxicity comparisons and with the extrapolation to humans. Understanding the pharmacology of potential metabolites and drug by-products is also important, especially when metabolites are present at exposures greater than 10% of the total drug-related exposure [8]. An early understanding of the exposure-response/safety relationships is critical at this stage of development [11].

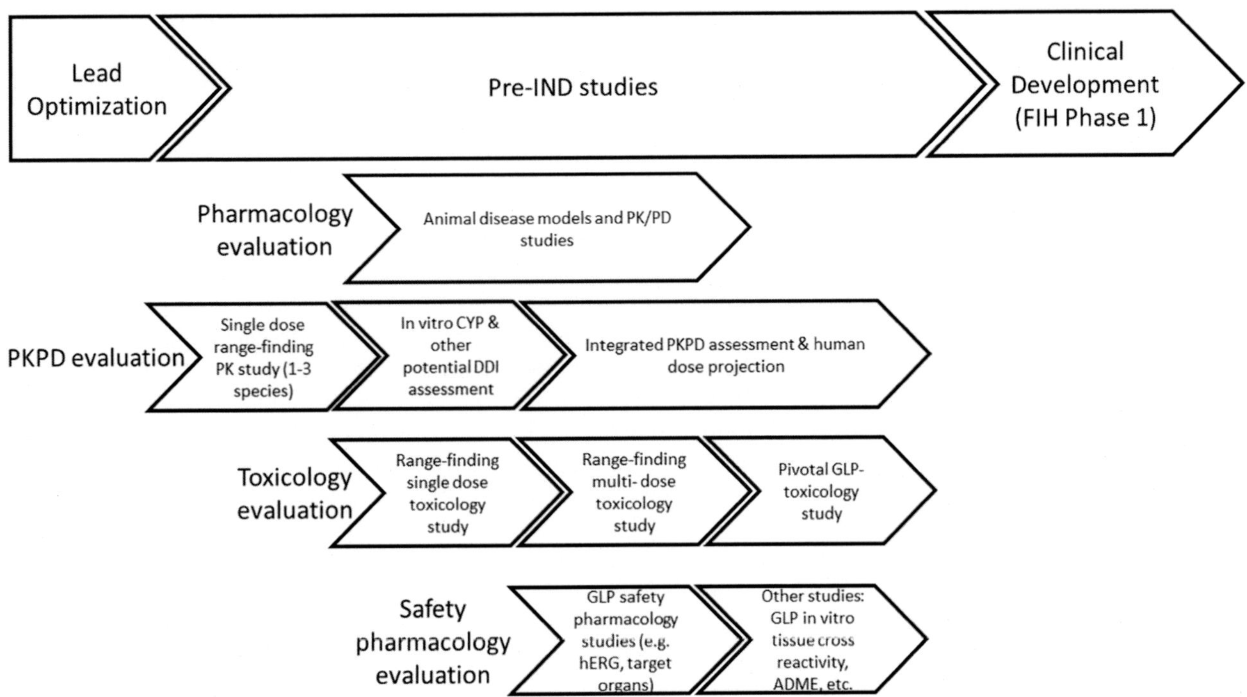

FIG. 30.2 Typical battery of studies conducted to enable an IND for a new chemical or biological entity in oncology. *ADME*, absorption, distribution, metabolism, and excretion; *CYP*, cytochrome P(450) enzyme; *FIH*, first in human; *GLP*, good laboratory practice; *PD*, pharmacodynamics; *PK*, pharmacokinetics.

For the toxicology sections, GLP conditions are generally not required for the initial studies, but this level of rigor is expected for pivotal nonclinical toxicology evaluations [14]. The toxicology studies that are submitted in the IND should utilize the expected clinical route of administration and include both clinical and histological tissue examinations. The histopathologic evaluation should be conducted over a range of doses, with an assessment of the reversibility of any findings. Careful attention should be paid to any irreversible or difficult to monitor toxicities, or to those that appear to be dose independent [14]. These studies will help identify potential target organs to be monitored in clinical testing and are critical for selecting the appropriate starting dose in the FIH trial. Other preclinical toxicity studies such as those analyzing local tolerance, embryofetal reproductive toxicology, genotoxicity, and phototoxicity should be considered for when the final marketing application is submitted, but these are not considered essential prior to initiating clinical trials in advanced cancer patients [2].

Nonclinical efficacy pharmacology

In vitro assessment of pharmacologic efficacy

The earliest in vitro studies of a new pharmaceutical agent are often integral to the drug discovery and screening process. Historically, anticancer screening strategies are used in vitro assays to identify agents with nonspecific growth inhibitory or cytotoxic activities. Modern approaches now screen for specific pharmacological properties utilizing well-characterized high-throughput technologies. Thus drug candidates are now selected on the basis of their pharmacological mechanism of action. In this process, molecular targets specific to cancer cells, but not present in normal tissues, are identified and used to screen drug libraries. As discussed in Chapter 29, modern discovery programs are designed to identify molecularly targeted drug candidates with inherent prespecified mechanisms of action. Likewise, biological agents are typically designed with a highly specific, well-characterized target in mind.

In oncology, in vitro assessments of pharmacologic efficacy are used to evaluate mechanisms of action and resistance, measure potency, provide early indications of selectivity of action, and identify potential predictive biomarkers. These studies are typically conducted in human tumor cell lines that represent a broad diversity of different cancer types [16]. Drug mechanisms can be further studied using cell lines which have been modified using gene editing tools such as CRISPR (clustered regularly interspaced short palindromic repeats)-based technologies [17]. Lead candidates can be further stratified through ex vivo studies using primary spheroid and stem-cell based organoid cultures derived from clinical or patient-derived xenograft tissues [18, 19]. These studies can enhance the extent to which drug mechanisms of action are understood and can identify potential tumor types to target in later clinical development. These early investigations can also elucidate potential molecular biomarkers of drug sensitivity or resistance that can serve as the basis for future patient enrichment strategies in clinical testing.

In vivo assessment of pharmacologic efficacy

Research in cancer biology has identified many properties that distinguish malignant cells from normal cells such as uncontrolled growth, metastasis, dedifferentiation, genetic plasticity, and drug resistance. Newer therapeutic strategies now under investigation include targets that interfere with the metastatic cascade, induce differentiation, interrupt autocrine or paracrine growth loops, block tumor angiogenesis, inhibit cell cycle and growth signal transduction, enhance tumor immunogenicity, and reverse drug resistance. Nonclinical evaluation of these strategies using in vitro systems is routine; however, many of these approaches can only be adequately assessed using in vivo animal model systems.

Tumor initiation, progression, and metastasis rely on select aspects of the heterogeneous primary tumor [20, 21]. Therefore successful evaluation of tumor biology and drug activity requires the appropriate selection of clinically relevant models. Mouse and rat models have several advantages over other animals for investigating mammalian biology. The release of a draft sequence of the mouse genome in 2002 [22] and the ongoing efforts to sequence the rat genetic code have enabled the identification of important mutations involved in the pathogenesis of human diseases, such as cancer, diabetes, arterial atherosclerosis, and hypertension. In addition, numerous genetically well-defined rodent lines with distinct phenotypic characteristics are readily available. Short generation times and relatively modest maintenance costs make these nonclinical models extremely attractive for examining the targeted activity of potential therapeutic agents.

A number of animal model systems have been developed that mimic the tumor microenvironments found in clinical situations. However, there are no perfect animal models for drug development. The adequacy of any specific animal model depends on its validity, selectivity, predictability, and reproducibility [23]. In cancer chemotherapy, animal models are selected to simultaneously demonstrate antitumor efficacy and acceptable systemic toxicity in an intact organism. Ideally, the tumor system under study should be genetically stable with homogeneous characteristics that mimic human tumor biology and do not vary over time. In oncology, a variety of diverse animal models for human tumors have been developed. These models can be broadly categorized into three groups: (1) spontaneous models, including those originating from natural or induced mutations; (2) genetically engineered models (GEMs), including transgenic and knockout animals; and (3) transplanted models, including implanted and orthotopic tumors.

Spontaneous in vivo models

Models resembling human disease states may arise spontaneously in animals that reach a certain age or period of development, or they may be induced by invasive interventions such as treatments with drugs, chemical toxins, or radiation. Cardiovascular drug development routinely utilizes a number of these models for research on hypertension, hypertrophic cardiomyopathies, and heart failure. One well-defined cardiac animal model is the Spontaneously Hypertensive Rat (SHR), originating from a colony of hypertensive Wistar rats developed in Kyoto, Japan [24, 25]. Another example is the obese Zucker rat, an animal model of noninsulin-dependent type 2 diabetes [26, 27]. In the Zucker rat, a single defect in the gene coding of the leptin receptor results in insulin resistance, hyperglycemia, and hypoinsulinemia.

In oncology, rodents with one or more naturally occurring genetic mutations comprise a majority of spontaneous animal tumor models. Examples include the spontaneous APC mutant Min mouse that develops adenomatous polyps that are precursors for invasive colon cancer [28], and the 7,12-dimethylbenz[α]anthracene (DMBA) or 1-methyl-1-nitrosourea (MNU) induced mammary carcinoma model for studying breast cancers [29]. Spontaneous models offer the advantages of orthotropic growth and clinically relevant metastatic spread via vascular and lymphatic vessels local to the primary tumor [30]. Although spontaneous tumors closely resemble the human clinical situation, a number of factors make these models poorly reproducible in controlled settings. For example, difficulties in experimental staging due to variability in the time and frequency of tumor induction can result in suboptimal animal numbers for comparative studies. Inconsistent tumor development due to local effects and extended experiment durations, ranging from several months to a year, also limit the utility of these specialized spontaneous models [21].

Genetically engineered in vivo models

An exciting area of ongoing research is the increasing use of genetically engineered models (GEMs) for preclinical drug testing. Transgenic and knockout mice are genetically altered to develop spontaneous endogenous tumors in a predictable fashion. Because of this, they can provide a versatile environment for testing novel experimental therapies. Advantages of these newer models include organ or site-specific targeting, natural growth rates and patterns of growth, and the use of immunocompetent animals [31, 32]. Use of GEMs has also improved the understanding of the role that individual and cooperative gene mutations play in tumorigenesis. However, the cost of these specialized models can be prohibitive, and in some cases, they may require a specific commercial license. Furthermore, the development of endogenous tumors often occurs later in the life span of these animals, which can delay experiment times. Finally, the diversity of available histological tumor types is low and the correlation between activity in GEM animal tumors and clinical anticancer activity has not been validated.

Transgenic mice provide a specialized tool and a model for a stepwise evolution of a particular disease state [33]. Transgenic mice arise from the introduction of a foreign gene into the pronucleus of a fertilized egg. This can be accomplished by microinjection [31, 32], retroviral infection [34], or embryonal stem cell transfer [35]. This latter technique involves the transfer of genetic material into embryonal stem cells that can then be transplanted into blastocysts to create a chimeric mouse. If the germ cells in the chimeric animal are derived from the embryonal stem cells, then the offspring of the animal will be transgenic and will express the inserted gene of interest. The capability of introducing and expressing a specific gene of interest in an intact organism provides a powerful means for manipulating the genetic milieu of an experimental animal.

Knockout mice are animals that have been genetically altered to remove both alleles of a specific gene [36]. This is accomplished by homologous recombination techniques that insert the defective gene into embryonic stem cells that are then isolated and injected into a blastocyst to generate heterozygous mice. Further inbreeding will generate homozygous "knockout" animals [36]. Knockout animals can be developed that are similar to transgenic animals in that they lack the function of a specific tumor suppressor gene, such as *p53*, and have a very high incidence of spontaneous tumor development [37]. If the tumor suppressor gene is required for viability of the animal during embryonic development, conditional knockout animals have been developed that selectively inactivate the gene of interest in specific tissues at defined periods in the animal's life span. Currently, these models are being extensively used in the study of carcinogenesis and chemoprevention, and their application in testing therapeutic agents is growing.

Transplanted in vivo models

Transplanted animal or human tumor xenograft models are some of the most widely used tools for studying experimental therapeutics in cancer. Established transplantable murine tumors have been extensively characterized and demonstrate excellent homogeneity and reproducibility [38]. Use of these syngeneic models, in which immortalized allografts from mouse cancer cell lines are transplanted into the same immunocompetent mouse strain, has increased dramatically since the explosion of immunotherapy use in cancer research. A major advantage of these models is that the host immune system remains intact allowing for analysis of immune effectors and downstream target analysis [39, 40]. However, their variable pathophysiology and growth patterns limit their usefulness in developing agents for human cancers [41]. In addition, results can be biased toward false positive results because selection has been based on ease of implementation, rapidity of growth, published drug sensitivities, and other attributes that facilitate experimental study design rather than clinical correlation.

An important advance in preclinical models for anticancer agents was the development of immunosuppressed mouse strains that allowed for the reproducible implantation and growth of human tumor cells in vivo. The first xenograft of a human colon cancer cell line into immunocompromised "nude" mice was reported in 1969 by Rygaard and Povlsen [42]. These mouse strains contained an autosomal recessive mutation in the *nu* (for nude) gene on chromosome 11. Homozygous mutations in the *nu* gene resulted in the absence of hair, poor growth, decreased fertility, an absent thymus gland, and a shortened life span [42, 43]. These animals exhibited a severe T-cell immunologic defect that impaired their ability to reject tissue transplants. Consequently, these animals tolerated the implantation and growth of human tumor cell xenografts because their suppressed immune system prevented the rejection of the human tumor cells. This discovery heralded a revolution in oncology experimental therapeutics [44]. Currently, xenograft tumors have been established for all common human solid tumors.

Mice lacking functional T- and B-cells referred to as severe combined immune deficiency (SCID) and those also lacking an intact natural killer (NK) cell system including nonobese diabetic (NOD-SCID) and NOD-SCID gamma (NSG) are routinely used for xenograft growth and studies in part due the increased ease of growth of some tumor types in these animals [45, 46]. The ability of SCID mice to support the growth of primary leukemia cell lines derived from patients with acute and chronic leukemia has led to the use of these animals as the primary models for testing agents with antileukemic activity [47]. However, the greater sensitivity of SCID mice to toxic drug effects and their greater expense has made them less popular than their nude counterparts as a platform for screening agents for activity against solid tumors. While use of syngeneic models is convenient in immune-oncology studies, recapitulating the human immune system in a mouse or "humanization" by injection of peripheral blood mononuclear cells (PBMCs) or CD34+ umbilical cord blood into NSG or similar mice provides an intact system that allows drug testing on growing human tumor models. This approach is not without limitations most notably of which are lack of reproducibility and graft versus host disease (GVHD) in animals from cell injection leading to a limited study duration that necessitates using only faster growing tumors [48–50].

For studies designed to screen drug candidates in vivo, subcutaneous implantation is the most common approach for growing human tumor xenografts in mice because of its simplicity and ease of access. After tumor cell suspensions are injected or tumor fragments implanted into the animal's flank, palpable subcutaneous tumors form over a period of days to weeks. Once a certain size is reached, screening studies are initiated, and tumor growth and drug treatment effects are easily followed by monitoring the dimensions of these tumors. The reliability and reproducibility of these models allows for rapid, high-throughput screening of many test agents in multiple tissue types. While subcutaneous implantation is most common, human xenografts can also be implanted in other sites. Implantation in the renal subcapsule has the advantage of requiring a relatively short inoculation time prior to drug treatment, making it particularly useful for short-term in vivo assays. However, technical requirements and inability to follow tumor growth limit the utility of this assay in broader drug screening.

Orthotopic xenograft models involve injecting cancer lines or implanting tumor fragments into anatomic sites corresponding to the cancer tissue type. The premise is to create a tumor environment that reflects the clinical situation, thereby allowing for antitumor activity testing that is more predictive of clinical efficacy. These models also are more likely to produce tumor metastases than subcutaneous tumor models, which lack the microenvironment and well-defined vessel system of organ systems. Orthotopic xenograft models have been developed for a number of different tumors, including renal cell carcinoma [51], central nervous system tumors [52], and pancreatic, prostate, colon, and lung cancers [53]. However, because of technical challenges, orthotopic xenografts are not as widely used as subcutaneously implanted tumors.

The utility and predictive value of xenograft models is critically dependent on the source of the cells or tissue that is used. Models derived from cell lines such as cell-derived xenografts (CDX) continuously grown in vitro produce mostly undifferentiated tumors that rarely resemble the histological architecture of the original human tumor. When injected subcutaneously, these models rapidly and reproducibly generate tumors for drug evaluation, but they rarely metastasize or become invasive and lack the components of the tumor microenvironment that are necessary to fully mimic the clinical condition. However, many of these models have well characterized genotypes and phenotypes and are useful for early characterization of targeted therapies. For example, cell-based xenograft models were used to identify drug leads targeting tumor cells with *BRAF* mutations, a useful target in melanoma [54].

Xenografts established by implanting clinical cancer samples directly into immunocompromised mice and serially passaging them for a limited number of times produce heterogeneous tumor models. These patient-derived xenograft (PDX) models often retain the histological architecture and molecular characteristics of the original sample [55, 56]. PDX models have become ubiquitous in oncology preclinical drug development and while CDX are still used in preliminary in vivo studies to assess drug activity, PDX models can be utilized to carry out "mouse clinical trials" (MCT) focused on specific indications, molecular targets, or both. These MCT trials can be initially designed to use large numbers of models with limited numbers of animals in the control and treatment groups, with the goal of identifying treatment-based efficacy patterns or sensitive models for follow-up studies that have adequate power to generate statistically sound results [57, 58]. Tumor samples collected from patients with progression following cancer treatment can be used to develop PDX which are valuable for understanding and overcoming drug resistance. Historically, models of drug resistance were developed by treating cells in vitro with *metronomic doses*, defined as continuous administration of low doses, of the target drug and injecting the resulting cells to create a resistant xenograft. Alternatively, the target drug was administered chronically to a tumor-bearing mouse until resistance developed. While these models had some success, resistance was often transient or required chronic drug administration to maintain [59, 60]. Development of longitudinal PDX models derived from the same patient at different points in the subject's clinical course, such as before and after treatment, may provide even greater value for researchers attempting to understand drug resistance [61].

Despite their popularity, xenograft models still have limitations [62]. The required use of immunocompromised animals limits the ability of these models to screen for investigational therapies such as immunomodulators that require an intact immune response. Infections are common in these animals and rigorous attention is required to maintain a sterile laboratory environment. In addition, subcutaneous xenograft implants may have higher growth rates, better organized tumor vasculature, and less overall necrosis than their clinical counterparts [63]. Retrospective reviews of the power of these models to predict the results of subsequent Phase 2 clinical trials revealed varying degrees of correlation based upon a number of factors, including tumor histology, drug class, and xenograft type. Breast tumor xenografts were generally not predictive of clinical activity; however, some lung adenocarcinoma xenografts did predict clinical activity in human trials [64–66]. In a retrospective study performed by the NCI of mostly cytotoxic chemotherapies, xenograft models predicted clinical activity about 33% of the time [65, 66]. It is unclear whether these models are as predictive for cytostatic and molecularly targeted therapies.

Nonclinical pharmacokinetics

A fully integrated pharmacokinetic (PK) and pharmacodynamic (PD) strategy is the hallmark of a well-designed drug development program. PKPD characterization of potential clinical drug candidates typically has the following objectives:

- Understand possible disposition mechanisms in humans, thereby providing insights into the safety profile of the molecule and anticipating potential interaction with concomitant drugs and/or organ dysfunction states
- Generate preclinical data to predict clinical PK behavior with sufficient confidence
- Understand the relationship between dose, exposure times, and PD effects to better predict human efficacious doses and schedules

Nonclinical pharmacokinetics aims to characterize the ADME profile of therapeutic candidates. Absorption of a molecular entity can be influenced by a number of factors, including the presence of transporters along the gastrointestinal tract, the presence of disease, and coadministered drugs and food [67]. As discussed in Chapter 4, oral permeability of small molecules can be predicted by measuring drug transport across a monolayer of Caco-2 human colon carcinoma cells [68]. Biologics, typically, are administered either intravenously, intramuscularly, or subcutaneously. After intravenous administration, biologics enter the blood stream directly but absorption is slow and occurs primarily through lymphatic drainage after subcutaneous and intramuscular administration. Typically, molecule-specific studies are not conducted to characterize the mechanism of subcutaneous or intramuscular absorption.

In addition to in vitro metabolic assessments, for small molecules there is a growing recognition of the importance of transporters in drug distribution and development of drug resistance. Drug distribution across tissues (e.g., blood-brain barrier) can be influenced by drug-specific transporters such as multidrug resistance-ATP binding cassette (MDR-ABC) transporters such as P-glycoprotein and multispecific solute carrier transporters such as organic anion/cation transporters [69]. Modified cell lines that differ from wild-type cells in their expression of specific drug resistance efflux transporters, such as the P-glycoprotein-mediated, multidrug resistance (MDR) gene, or the multidrug resistance protein (MRP), can be used to assess potential mechanisms of drug resistance [70]. Both MDR and MRP can confer drug resistance to a wide variety of natural product anticancer agents. These assessments can also provide early indications of the relative distribution of an agent, such as its likelihood of penetrating the blood-brain barrier. In addition, protein binding studies can help interpret the kinetics of free and bound drug concentrations, and absorption and distribution can be predicted by assessing the transport properties of novel agents in vitro [68]. In contrast to small molecules, biologics typically do not distribute intracellularly, and as described in Chapter 33, biologics such as monoclonal antibodies are typically confined to the vascular and interstitial space because of their large size. [71].

Metabolism testing of small molecules

The cytochrome P-450 (CYP) enzyme system plays a prominent role in drug metabolism, CYP enzyme-mediated drug interactions of clinical significance are common [72]. The risk of drug interactions due to metabolism by enzymes such as CYP3A4, 2D6, or 2C9 is now assessed in vitro using microsomes and cell lines that express these specific enzyme isoforms [73, 74]. It is now routine to conduct a battery of nonclinical in vitro tests of a drug candidate's potential to inhibit specific metabolic pathways, induce drug-metabolizing enzymes, or undergo metabolism by specific CYP isoforms [75]. Finally, if a drug is metabolized by an enzyme with a known pharmacogenetic polymorphism that may result in substantial pharmacokinetic variability in certain patient populations, this will need to be monitored during clinical testing [76]. While in vitro incubation studies with artificial cell systems can identify possible drug-drug interactions, they still do not quantify their magnitude, which determines their clinical significance. As discussed in Chapter 31, emerging technology using physiologically based PK modeling with commercially available software [e.g., GastroPlus (Simulations Plus, California) or SimCYP (Certara, United Kingdom)] can take into account the rate and extent of absorption at various doses, the extent of expression of various distribution transporters and metabolizing enzymes, and the impact of coadministered drugs on the expression of these enzymes so as to make quantitative predictions of the magnitude of clinical drug interactions. Thus these software tools provide the capability for the a priori identification of potential clinically significant interactions. In addition to hepatic CYP-450-mediated elimination, most small molecules also are subject to some level of renal elimination. Characterization of the extent of renal elimination during preclinical animal studies is useful to help assess the impact of renal insufficiency on drug disposition in patients.

Contrary to small molecules, biotherapeutics such as proteins and monoclonal antibodies are not cleared through CYP enzymes. They are typically converted to their constituent amino acids and recycled into the endogenous repertoire. So, drug interactions with other biotherapeutics and small molecules are typically not expected. But some antiinflammatory biologics have been shown to modulate expression of CYP450 enzymes, thus indirectly impacting exposure of substrate small molecules [77, 78]; however, no clinically significant interactions have been reported so far [79].

In vivo pharmacokinetic studies

Performing in vivo animal PK studies provides an opportunity to assess the combined impact of all ADME variables on the PK of the molecule. Rational scaling of the PK of the molecule to patients can be used to estimate whether the molecule is suitable for appropriate dosing in the clinic, for example whether sufficient exposure could be obtained after once a day oral dosing of the compound. Typically, in vivo PK information is gathered after single and multiple doses during preclinical testing of the molecule. While dedicated PK studies are typically done early during preclinical development, PK information can also be gathered from other studies, including pharmacological and toxicological testing studies. The first step requires the development of a sensitive and reliable analytical assay for the test compound and any associated metabolites. Currently, as described in Chapter 11, the most commonly employed analytical methods for small molecules utilize the liquid chromatography and mass spectrometry (LC/MS and LC/MS/MS). These technologies have largely supplanted standard high-performance liquid chromatography (HPLC) methods because of their greater specificity and sensitivity. For biologics, typically enzyme linked immunoassay (ELISA) methodologies are used to measure concentration of the candidate in serum. However, LCMS methodologies are also emerging as a more time-efficient alternative to immunoassays.

For most small molecules, formal PK studies are typically assessed in all toxicological species (e.g. mice, rat, and dogs). However, for many monoclonal antibodies, PK is typically only assessed in nonhuman primates (NHP) since these molecules do not interact with receptors in common toxicological species such as rats and mice. These nonclinical PK studies are typically conducted under non-GLP conditions [80]. An initial PK study in each toxicological species is usually conducted using administration of a single dose of the candidate through the intended route of administration. Data from this study is used to identify doses for the toxicological study and to better predict exposure after multiple dosing. PK after single and multiple dosing in the toxicological studies is also obtained to confirm exposure in the animals and to identify the thresholds at which various safety/toxicological events are observed. In addition, assessment of PK in pharmacology and efficacy studies is useful because it allows investigators to characterize the relationship between exposure and drug effects in a representative model of the target or disease pharmacology. This information is critical to predicting efficacious doses in humans. These studies can be done in healthy animals or in efficacy models such as xenograft models [81, 82] with the sole purpose of understanding drug mechanism of action [83]. The formation of antidrug antibodies (ADA) also needs to be measured in toxicology studies of biotherapeutics. Although ADA formation rates in NHP are not predictive of human ADA rates, their measurement in NHP studies is still very useful and may be helpful in interpreting anomalies in PK and PD and in identifying the cause of any toxicological events seen in these animals. Finally, radiolabeled drug distribution/mass balance studies in animals provide early indications of the tissue distribution and the ADME profile of a new agent.

Nonclinical safety pharmacology

Pharmacologic studies to assess drug safety are required to support the use of a new therapeutic in humans. The objectives of a safety pharmacology study are to identify undesirable or secondary/off-target pharmacodynamic effects of an agent that may be relevant to human safety and to evaluate the pathophysiologic effects of a substance observed in previous in vivo studies. The selection of safety pharmacologic endpoints can be made based upon the anticipated safety risks of the molecule. The tests could be in vitro and/or in vivo and are typically conducted after single doses using the expected route of administration. The core battery of tests involves the central nervous, cardiovascular, and respiratory systems. Other supplemental systems, such as gastrointestinal, genitourinary, could also be added to the core battery, depending on the initial risk assessment for the molecule and its therapeutic class [13].

Biotherapeutics such as monoclonal antibodies are typically more target specific and have fewer off-target side effects. So, in most cases, dedicated safety pharmacology studies are not required for these compounds. Safety endpoints are usually included in ongoing nonclinical toxicology or PK studies but dedicated safety pharmacology experiments may be required in some cases, depending on the drug's mechanism of action. For biotherapeutics such as monoclonal antibodies, a tissue cross reactivity study is recommended [84]. This study could identify possible off-target binding of these compounds. Extensive stand-alone safety pharmacology studies generally are not required for agents destined for use in late-stage cancer patients [13]. Formal safety pharmacology studies need to be conducted in compliance with GLP principles.

A common safety pharmacological concern is the potential for a new agent to cause serious ventricular arrhythmias. Drug-induced prolongation of the QTc interval can increase the risk of ventricular arrhythmias, especially Torsade de Pointes [15]. The duration of the QT interval reflects the late repolarization phase of the cardiac action potential, which is mediated by the efflux of potassium ions through the delayed rectifier potassium channels in the cardiac ventricles. Agents that inhibit potassium ion efflux prolong the QTc interval and increase the risk of serious cardiac arrhythmias. The human ether-a-go-go related gene (*hERG*) encodes the alpha subunit of the human potassium ion channel protein responsible for ion efflux. Nonclinical tests in cell lines expressing this protein can estimate the risk of QTc prolongation [15]. The US FDA recommends preclinical hERG channel testing coupled with in vivo QT assessments in a nonrodent species but may specify the need for additional follow-up studies on an individual basis. These data and all other relevant nonclinical information should be incorporated in a formal integrated risk assessment document that also considers the compound's chemical and pharmacological class. This assessment helps to define the necessary safeguards and precautions required for clinical testing and will determine the need to perform a thorough QTc study. Due to their large size, biotherapeutics typically do not interact with the hERG channel, so this test is typically not done. Similarly, genotoxicity testing is also not done due to the inability of these molecules to penetrate cell membranes.

Nonclinical toxicology

After a drug's primary pharmacological properties have been characterized and deemed optimal, the next key decision point is the candidate selection or NME designation. This step identifies the specific compound for further clinical evaluation and triggers a series of IND-enabling processes, the most extensive of which are the GLP toxicology studies. The IND-enabling toxicology studies should use the same drug formulation and route of administration that are planned for the clinical trial. The anticipated schedule and duration of treatment should also be approximated. While the IND-enabling GLP toxicology studies are pivotal for IND filing, they may be preceded by single or multiple dose-range finding studies to determine the doses to administer and specific safety measurements to monitor in the GLP study. These non-GLP toxicology studies are typically progressively longer ranging from single to a few doses at the anticipated clinical dosing frequency. For small molecules, toxicology testing usually includes a rodent and nonrodent species, most often dogs. Biological agents often do not bind to the analogous rodent receptors and ligands; therefore, toxicological testing is typically conducted in NHP. These experiments should be designed to assess both the severity of acute toxicities and the time needed for recovery. Toxicokinetic evaluations are included in most GLP-toxicology studies [2] to provide an indication of the exposures which are potentially safe and nontoxic. One of the important goals of the GLP toxicology study is to identify a no-adverse event dose level (NOAEL) and measures of exposure associated with the NOAEL dose. For biotherapeutics, ADA formation is also monitored to help identify possible causes of loss of exposure and immune-mediated toxicities in animals.

For oncology agents, reproductive toxicology, including embryonic and fetal toxicology studies, may be deferred until the marketing application is submitted [2]. In rare cases, these studies may not be needed at all, especially for known genotoxic agents that target rapidly dividing cells, or for known developmental toxins. Reproductive toxicology is typically performed in two different species, although biologicals may use only one relevant species when other options are not available. Fertility and early embryonic development studies are not required for agents used to treat patients with advanced cancer; likewise, pre- and postnatal toxicology studies are also not warranted for most oncology indications.

Starting dose selection for FIH studies

An important goal of nonclinical development is to select a safe starting dose to be used in FIH trials. While FIH trials have been historically safe, two recent incidents have highlighted risks associated with FIH testing of novel therapeutic compounds. The first is the Tegenero/Northwick Park incident, in which six healthy volunteer subjects were severely injured in a FIH study of a super agonist anti-CD28 antibody that unexpectedly induced a cytokine storm after a single dose [85, 86].

The second incident is the Rennes incident in which a fatal severe adverse event occurred in a healthy volunteer during testing of BIA-102474-101, a fatty acid amide hydroxylase inhibitor [87]. These incidents have focused attention on nonclinical testing, nonclinical to clinical PKPD translation, and the design of FIH trials, especially as regards dose selection.

Traditionally, identification of the starting and top doses in the FIH trial has been based mainly on the NOAEL dose by calculating human equivalent doses and applying a further safety factor to account for animal-to-human translation uncertainties [88]. However, in light of the recent incidents and acknowledgment of the complex pharmacology of emerging modalities that renders animal testing more uncertain, a more holistic approach that analyzes all preclinical data within a PKPD framework is warranted [89]. Since for many targeted therapies, toxicity typically is dose related and results from an extension of the drug's underlying pharmacology, these guidelines have recommended the use of pharmacology-based metrics such as minimum anticipated biological effect level (MABEL) for FIH dose selection [90].

The general practice in FIH oncology studies is to minimize exposing patients to suboptimal doses, so starting doses are typically pharmacologically active. For small molecules, the FIH dose has traditionally been based on 1/10 the dose that causes severe toxicity in 10% of animals (STD_{10}) in rodent studies. However, if nonrodents are more appropriate, then 1/6 the highest nonseverely toxic dose (HNSTD) is used. The HNSTD is the highest dose level that does not produce evidence of life-threatening or irreversible toxicity. However, in recent years, FIH dose selection in oncology studies has also tended to follow the integrated PKPD-based approach referred to previously. Furthermore, in FIH oncology studies, the highest anticipated dose is *not* limited by the doses or exposures tested in nonclinical studies, but the planned dose escalation increments should reflect the steepness of the dose-toxicity curve. In Phase 1 trials in advanced stage cancer patients, the duration of treatment may continue according to patient response and toleration of the experimental therapy and additional toxicology studies are not required for extended clinical use. Phase 2 studies may be supported by existing nonclinical data and the accumulated clinical Phase 1 experience. However, additional nonclinical repeat-dose GLP toxicology studies of at least 3 months duration may be required to support large Phase 3 trials, and these can also be used to support the marketing application. New drug combination regimens do not require special toxicology studies; instead, in vivo efficacy pharmacology studies of the combination may suffice [2]. The recommended nonclinical toxicology treatment schedules required to support initiation of oncology clinical trials are presented in Table 30.1.

Model based development bridging nonclinical to clinical

The traditional approach to guide FIH dose selection is to utilize human equivalent dose (HED) of the NOAEL or HNSTD obtained from preclinical toxicology testing [88]. In this approach, the toxicological dose—either NOAEL or HNSTD obtained from the most appropriate animal species—is converted to a HED using allometry principles, by either scaling based on body weight or body surface area. While this approach is simple and easy to follow, it also has a number of limitations. It does not take into account factors such as species-specific differences in expression of CYP isoforms and other transporter proteins, genomic impact on PK and PD across different human populations, effect of coadministered drugs on

TABLE 30.1 Nonclinical toxicology treatment schedules of anticancer pharmaceuticals to support initial clinical trials.

Clinical schedule	Nonclinical treatment schedule[a]
Once every 3–4 weeks	Single dose
Daily for 5 days every 3 weeks	Daily for 5 days
Daily for 5–7 days, alternating weeks	Daily for 5–7 days, alternating weeks (2-dose cycles)
Once a week for 3 weeks, 1 week off	Once a week for 3 weeks
Two or three times a week	Two or three times a week for 4 weeks
Daily	Daily for 4 weeks
Weekly	Once a week for 4–5 doses

[a]*The timing of the toxicity assessment(s) in the nonclinical studies should be scientifically justified based on the anticipated toxicity profile and the clinical schedule. For example, a sacrifice shortly after the dosing phase to examine early toxicity and a later sacrifice to examine late onset of toxicity should be considered. The treatment schedules described in the table do not specify recovery periods. The treatment schedules described in this table should be modified as appropriate for molecules with extended pharmacodynamic effects, long half-lives, or potential for anaphylactic reactions. In addition, the potential effects of immunogenicity should be considered.*

Modified from Food and Drug Administration. Guidance for industry: S9 nonclinical evaluation for anticancer pharmaceuticals; 2010. Rockville. Available from: https://www.fda.gov/media/73161/download.

PKPD, and differences in pharmacology between animal and human species for target-specific toxicology. In recent years, an integrated PKPD modeling approach has been proposed to characterize time course of exposure and PD effect of therapeutic candidates during preclinical development and rationally extrapolate these results to humans to guide FIH dose selection. This approach has been described in a guideline that also recommends identifying alternative pharmacology or toxicology parameters, such as MABEL, that can be used to identify starting and maximum doses and exposures in FIH and subsequent human clinical trials [89].

The general modeling principle based on the MABEL approach is to predict pharmacological response in humans by integrating in vitro and in vivo preclinical data, utilizing translational modeling from preclinical PK/PD to clinical PK/PD to inform FIH dose selection. This approach includes mechanistic/quantitative modeling to: (1) translate animal PK to human PK; (2) relate predicted human PK and pharmacological activity by integrating all nonclinical pharmacological data, including in vitro (e.g., receptor binding and activation), in vivo (animal models exploring drug effect on PD markers and/or disease models), and clinical data (e.g., information on prior compounds targeting similar pathways) into a unified prediction of human dose-exposure-PD and efficacy endpoints. A few examples that illustrate this rational process of translating nonclinical data into valuable human predictions are illustrated as follows.

(1) Human PK projection:
   a. Therapeutic candidates exhibit linear PK: predict human PK from preclinical PK in relevant species using allometric scaling or species-invariant time methods [91, 92]
   b. Therapeutic candidates with nonlinear PK: can utilize nonlinear Michaelis-Menten models with adjustment to account for species-specific differences.
   c. Monoclonal antibodies (mAb) exhibit nonlinear PK due to target-mediated drug disposition (TMDD):
      i. PK models described by the Michaelis-Menten equation for the nonlinear elimination can be used with adjustment to account for target expression levels and binding affinities across species [92]
      ii. Full TMDD models can be developed when data are sufficient to describe synthesis/turnover of the target, nonspecific drug clearance, drug-receptor binding, and internalization of the drug-receptor complex [93, 94]
   d. Physiologically based pharmacokinetic (PBPK) approach: parameter sensitivity analysis should be performed to consider the key ADME properties of the therapeutic candidates and evaluate the uncertainty [95]

(2) FIH dose selection and human PKPD extrapolation:
   a. MABEL approach for FIH dose selection to consider biological drug-receptor interaction and multiple factors that affect the dose-receptor occupancy relationship [96, 97]
   b. Translational PKPD modeling: the use of biomarker or receptor occupancy (RO) as a surrogate to extrapolate exposure-target modulation in preclinical models to identify target efficacious concentration/dose for clinical antitumor efficacy in oncology drug development [81, 82]

Other approaches such as those utilizing predicted human PK with EC_{50}/IC_{50} based on in vitro activity data and in vitro binding affinity, K_D to estimate human pharmacological activity, and RO, respectively [98], have been discussed when preclinical in vivo pharmacological activity data are not available. In summary, mechanistic-based translational PKPD modeling provides critical insights to better guide FIH dose selection and study design.

Nonclinical development of immuno-oncology therapeutics

The development of powerful new therapeutics that augment the antitumor activity of the body's own immune system has heralded the dawn of a new era of immuno-oncology (IO) therapeutics. The clinical activity of antibodies such as ipilimumab targeting CTLA-4 [99], and nivolumab [100] and pembrolizumab [101] that target PD-1 has validated inhibitory checkpoint molecules as important therapeutic targets. These agents block inhibitory signals in the adaptive immune system unleashing a T-cell-mediated antitumor response even in patients with highly advanced tumors. However, despite the impressive durability of some of these IO responses, only a minority of patients respond to these treatments. Thus there is a substantial need for improved IO therapies and novel new combinations that can extend these seminal advances.

Despite this progress, the nonclinical development of IO therapies presents a number of daunting challenges to the drug development scientist. First, the specificity and complexity of the immune system renders the use of traditional animal models such as human tumor xenografts in immunocompromised animals largely irrelevant for preclinical testing. Instead, the safety and efficacy pharmacology of IO therapeutics must be tested in alternative models, such as genetically engineered spontaneous tumors or syngeneic models in animals with intact immune systems. Often surrogate agents must be employed to circumvent the inability of some IO therapeutics to target the same molecule across different species [102]. But such approaches are complicated by differences between human and murine immune systems, and the absence of some human IO targets in mice. A better alternative may be the use of animals genetically engineered to express a humanized immune system; however, these tools are still in relatively early stages of development [103].

These complexities also impact the nonclinical safety evaluation of IO agents. For IO agents with established cross species activity, toxicological studies are generally conducted in nonhuman primates, most often cynomolgus monkeys. However, cynomolgus monkeys and murine models have underpredicted toxicity in humans [104]. This risk is compounded by the development of newer agonist IO therapies, such as those that target CD40, OX40, and 4-1BB [105] and these have the potential to generate amplified immune responses. The severe morbidity induced in healthy volunteers in the FIH study of Tegenero's CD28 super agonist, TGN-1412, is a cogent reminder of the potential risks of uncontrolled immune responses [85].

The heightened expectation of clinical activity has changed the nature of early phase IO trials. In FIH Phase 1 IO trials, it is not unusual to observe rapid dose escalation followed by increasingly large expansion cohorts [106, 107]. The FIH KEYNOTE study of pembrolizumab had over 1200 patients and led to its initial approval less than 4 years after initiating clinical testing [108]. This places an even higher premium on the robustness of nonclinical data packages because of the scale of these early phase studies and the condensed timeframe available for studying a drug's clinical behavior in these accelerated trials. In addition, traditional FIH Phase 1 study designs may not be well designed for evaluating newer IO therapies. For example, immune-related adverse events can have a late onset, occurring outside of the typically short dose limiting toxicity (DLT) monitoring period used for classic anticancer agents [104]. Furthermore, IO agents such as nivolumab, pembrolizumab, and durvalumab may not demonstrate linear exposure-response/toxicity curves [109] and may demonstrate time-varying kinetics [110] further complicating the determination of the maximum tolerated dose (MTD). Flat fixed dosing of IO agents independent of body weight or surface areas is increasingly common because monoclonal antibody distribution does not strongly relate to body size [111]. One solution is to base IO dose selection for future studies on formal PKPD modeling that can be implemented in earlier stages of drug development [11]. The groundwork for this quantitative understanding of pharmacological behavior must first be established in nonclinical testing and carried through seamlessly into early phase clinical trials.

Despite these multiple challenges, the promise of newer, more efficacious IO therapies has never been greater. Cellular immunotherapies, such as chimeric antigen receptor T cells, are generating impressive durable responses in diseases such as acute lymphocytic leukemia [112] and diffuse large cell non-Hodgkin's lymphoma [113]. Also, new negative checkpoint inhibitors of the innate immune system are enhancing the antitumor effects mediated by first responder cells such as macrophages [114, 115]. Prior to entering into FIH clinical trials, the nonclinical development of these newer IO therapeutics will still require well-designed safety and efficacy pharmacology studies including a thorough understanding of an agent's pharmacokinetics and pharmacodynamics, and detailed toxicologic evaluations. These studies are needed to generate scientifically robust and carefully analyzed nonclinical data packages that will serve as the foundation for the clinical evaluation of the next generation of transformational IO therapeutics.

References

[1] CDER. Guideline on the preparation of investigational new drug products (human and animal). Guidance for industry. Rockville: FDA; 1991. Available from: https://www.fda.gov/media/71017/download.

[2] Food and Drug Administration. Guidance for industry: S9 nonclinical evaluation for anticancer pharmaceuticals. Rockville. Available from: https://www.fda.gov/media/73161/download; 2010.

[3] Molzon J. The common technical document: the changing face of the new drug application. Nat Rev Drug Discov 2003;2:71–4.

[4] Food and Drug Administration. M4 organization of the common technical document for the registration of pharmaceuticals for human use: guidance for industry. Silver Spring. Available from: https://www.fda.gov/media/71551/download; 2017.

[5] Food and Drug Administration. M4Q: the CTD—quality: guidance for industry. Silver Spring. Available from: https://www.fda.gov/media/71581/download; 2017.

[6] Food and Drug Administration. M4S: the CTD—safety: guidance for industry. Silver Spring. Available from: https://www.fda.gov/media/71628/download; 2017.

[7] Food and Drug Administration. M4E(R2): the CTD—efficacy: guidance for Industry. Silver Spring. Available from: https://www.fda.gov/media/93569/download; 2017.

[8] Food and Drug Administration. Guidance for industry: M3(R2) nonclinical safety studies for the conduct of human clinical trials and marketing authorization for pharmaceuticals. Silver Spring. Available from: https://www.fda.gov/media/71542/download; 2010.

[9] Cauchon NS, Oghamian S, Hassanpour S, Abernathy M. Innovation in chemistry, manufacturing, and controls-a regulatory perspective from industry. J Pharm Sci 2019;108:2207–37.

[10] Mager DE, Woo S, Jusko WJ. Scaling pharmacodynamics from in vitro and preclinical animal studies to humans. Drug Metab Pharmacokinet 2009;24:16–24.

[11] Agoram BM, Martin SW, van der Graaf PH. The role of mechanism-based pharmacokinetic-pharmacodynamic (PK-PD) modelling in translational research of biologics. Drug Discov Today 2007;121018–24.

[12] Jamei M. Recent advances in development and application of physiologically-based pharmacokinetic (PBPK) models: a transition from academic curiosity to regulatory acceptance. Curr Pharmacol Rep 2016;2:161–9.

[13] Food and Drug Administration. Guidance for industry: S7A safety pharmacology studies for human pharmaceuticals. Rockville. Available from: https://www.fda.gov/media/72033/download; 2001.

[14] Senderowicz AM. Information needed to conduct first-in-human oncology trials in the United States: a view from a former FDA medical reviewer. Clin Cancer Res 2010;16:1719–25.

[15] Food and Drug Administration. Guidance for industry: S7B the non-clinical evaluation of the potential for delayed ventricular repolarization (QT inteval prolongation) by human pharmaceuticals. Rockville. Available from: https://www.fda.gov/media/72043/download; 2005.

[16] Monks A, Scudiero D, Skehan P, Shoemaker R, Paull K, Vistica D, et al. Feasibility of a high-flux anticancer drug screen using a diverse panel of cultured human tumor cell lines. J Natl Cancer Inst 1991;83:757–66.

[17] Bahreini A, Li Z, Wang P, Levine KM, Tasdemir N, Cao L, et al. Mutation site and context dependent effects of ESR1 mutation in genome-edited breast cancer cell models. Breast Cancer Res 2017;19:60.

[18] Clevers H. Modeling development and disease with organoids. Cell 2016;165:1586–97.

[19] Shuford S, Wilhelm C, Rayner M, Elrod A, Millard M, Mattingly C, et al. Prospective validation of an ex vivo, patient-derived 3D spheroid model for response predictions in newly diagnosed ovarian cancer. Sci Rep 2019;9:11153.

[20] Talmadge JE, Fidler IJ. Cancer metastasis is selective or random depending on the parent tumour population. Nature 1982;297:593–4.

[21] Talmadge JE, Wolman SR, Fidler IJ. Evidence for the clonal origin of spontaneous metastases. Science 1982;217:361–3.

[22] Waterston RH, Lindblad-Toh K, Birney E, Rogers J, Abril JF, Agarwal P, et al. Initial sequencing and comparative analysis of the mouse genome. Nature 2002;420:520–62.

[23] Khleif SN, Curt GA. Animal models in drug development. In: Holland JF, Bast BR, Morton DL, Frei E, Kufe DW, Weischelbaum RR, editors. Cancer medicine. Baltimore, MD: Williams & Wilkins; 1997. p. 855–68.

[24] Bing OH, Conrad CH, Boluyt MO, Robinson KG, Brooks WW. Studies of prevention, treatment and mechanisms of heart failure in the aging spontaneously hypertensive rat. Heart Fail Rev 2002;7:71–88.

[25] Tsotetsi OJ, Woodiwiss AJ, Netjhardt M, Qubu D, Brooksbank R, Norton GR. Attenuation of cardiac failure, dilatation, damage, and detrimental interstitial remodeling without regression of hypertrophy in hypertensive rats. Hypertension 2001;38:846–51.

[26] Kasiske BL, O'Donnell MP, Keane WF. The Zucker rat model of obesity, insulin resistance, hyperlipidemia, and renal injury. Hypertension 1992;19 (1 Suppl):I110–5.

[27] Van Zwieten PA, Kam KL, Pijl AJ, Hendriks MG, Beenen OH, Pfaffendorf M. Hypertensive diabetic rats in pharmacological studies. Pharmacol Res 1996;33:95–105.

[28] Thompson MB. The Min mouse: a genetic model for intestinal carcinogenesis. Toxicol Pathol 1997;25:329–32.

[29] Tsubura A, Lai YC, Miki H, Sasaki T, Uehara N, Yuri T, et al. Review: animal models of N-methyl-N-nitrosourea-induced mammary cancer and retinal degeneration with special emphasis on therapeutic trials. In Vivo 2011;25:11–22.

[30] Berger M. Is there a relevance of anticancer drug development. In: Fiebig H, Burger B, editors. Relevance of tumor models for anticancer drug development. Basel: Karger; 1999. p. 15–27.

[31] Rosenberg MP, Bortner D. Why transgenic and knockout animal models should be used (for drug efficacy studies in cancer). Cancer Metastasis Rev 1998;17:295–9.

[32] Thomas H, Balkwill F. Assessing new anti-tumour agents and strategies in oncogene transgenic mice. Cancer Metastasis Rev 1995;14:91–5.

[33] Burger A, Fiebig H. Screening using animal systems. In: Baguley B, Ker D, editors. Anticancer drug development. San Diego: Academic Press; 2001. p. 285–97.

[34] Jaenisch R. Retroviruses and embryogenesis: microinjection of Moloney leukemia virus into midgestation mouse embryos. Cell 1980;19:181–8.

[35] Hooper M, Hardy K, Handyside A, Hunter S, Monk M. HPRT-deficient (Lesch-Nyhan) mouse embryos derived from germline colonization by cultured cells. Nature 1987;326:292–5.

[36] Majzoub JA, Muglia LJ. Knockout mice. N Engl J Med 1996;334904–7.

[37] Donehower LA. The p53-deficient mouse: a model for basic and applied cancer studies. Semin Cancer Biol 1996;7:269–78.

[38] Rockwell S. In vivo-in vitro tumour cell lines: characteristics and limitations as models for human cancer. Br J Cancer Suppl 1980;41(Suppl. 4): 118–22.

[39] Sanmamed MF, Chester C, Melero I, Kohrt H. Defining the optimal murine models to investigate immune checkpoint blockers and their combination with other immunotherapies. Ann Oncol 2016;27:1190–8.

[40] Buque A, Galluzz L. Modeling tumor immunology and immunotherapy in mice. Trends Cancer 2018;4:599–601.

[41] Staquet MJ, Byar DP, Green SB, Rozencweig M. Clinical predictivity of transplantable tumor systems in the selection of new drugs for solid tumors: rationale for a three-stage strategy. Cancer Treat Rep 1983;67:753–65.

[42] Rygaard J, Povlsen CO. Heterotransplantation of a human malignant tumour to "Nude" mice. Acta Pathol Microbiol Scand 1969;77:758–60.

[43] Flanagan SP. 'Nude', a new hairless gene with pleiotropic effects in the mouse. Genet Res 1966;8:295–309.

[44] Neely JE, Ballard ET, Britt AL, Workman L. Characteristics of 85 pediatric tumors heterotransplanted into nude mice. Exp Cell Biol 1983;51:217–27.

[45] Okada S, Vaeteewoottacharn K, Kariya R. Application of highly immunocompromised mice for the establishment of patient-derived xenograft (PDX) models. Cell 2019;8:889.

[46] Shultz LD, Goodwin N, Ishikawa F, Hosur V, Lyons B, Greiner DL. Human cancer growth and therapy in immunodeficient mouse models. Cold Spring Harb Protoc 2014;2014:694–708.
[47] Uckun FM. Severe combined immunodeficient mouse models of human leukemia. Blood 1996;88:1135–46.
[48] Ali N, Flutter B, Sanchez Rodriguez R, Sharif-Paghaleh E, Barber LD, Lombardi G, et al. Xenogeneic graft-versus-host-disease in NOD-scid IL-2Rgammanull mice display a T-effector memory phenotype. PLoS One 2012;7, e44219.
[49] Covassin L, Laning J, Abdi R, Langevin DL, Phillips NE, Shultz LD, et al. Human peripheral blood CD4 T cell-engrafted non-obese diabetic-scid IL2rgamma(null) H2-Ab1 (tm1Gru) Tg (human leucocyte antigen D-related 4) mice: a mouse model of human allogeneic graft-versus-host disease. Clin Exp Immunol 2011;66:269–80.
[50] Yaguchi T, Kobayash A, Inozume T, Morii K, Nagumo H, Nishio H, et al. Human PBMC-transferred murine MHC class I/II-deficient NOG mice enable long-term evaluation of human immune responses. Cell Mol Immunol 2018;15:953–62.
[51] Fidler IJ. Rationale and methods for the use of nude mice to study the biology and therapy of human cancer metastasis. Cancer Metastasis Rev 1986;5:29–49.
[52] Shapiro WR, Basler GA, Chernik NL, Posner JB. Human brain tumor transplantation into nude mice. J Natl Cancer Inst 1979;62:447–53.
[53] Hoffman RM. Fertile seed and rich soil: the development of clinically relevant models of human cancer by surgical orthotopic implantation of intact tissue. In: Teicher BA, editor. Anticancer drug development guide: preclinical screening, clinical trials and approval. Totowa, NJ: Humana Press; 1997. p. 127–44.
[54] Solit DB, Garraway LA, Pratilas CA, Sawai A, Getz G, Basso A, et al. BRAF mutation predicts sensitivity to MEK inhibition. Nature 2006;439:358–62.
[55] Annibali D, Leucci E, Hermans E, Amant F. Development of patient-derived tumor xenograft models. Methods Mol Biol 1862;2019:217–25.
[56] Hidalgo M, Amant F, Biankin AV, Budinska E, Byrne AT, Caldas C, et al. Patient-derived xenograft models: an emerging platform for translational cancer research. Cancer Discov 2014;4:998–1013.
[57] Gao H, Korn JM, Ferretti S, Monahan JE, Wang Y, Singh M, et al. High-throughput screening using patient-derived tumor xenografts to predict clinical trial drug response. Nat Med 2015;21:1318–25.
[58] Guo S, Jiang X, Mao B, Li QX. The design, analysis and application of mouse clinical trials in oncology drug development. BMC Cancer 2019;19:718.
[59] Herrera-Abreu MT, Palafox M, Asghar U, Rivas MA, Cutts RJ, Garcia-Murillas I, et al. Early adaptation and acquired resistance to CDK4/6 inhibition in estrogen receptor-positive breast cancer. Cancer Res 2016;76:2301–13.
[60] Kita K, Fukuda K, Takahashi H, Tanimoto A, Nishiyama A, Arai S, et al. Patient-derived xenograft models of non-small cell lung cancer for evaluating targeted drug sensitivity and resistance. Cancer Sci 2019;110:215–24.
[61] Germann UA, Furey BF, Markland W, Hoover RR, Aronov AM, Roix JJ, et al. Targeting the MAPK signaling pathway in cancer: promising preclinical activity with the novel selective ERK1/2 inhibitor BVD-523 (Ulixertinib). Mol Cancer Ther 2017;16:2351–63.
[62] Gura T. Systems for identifying new drugs are often faulty. Science 1997;278:1041–2.
[63] Steel GG, Courtenay VD, Peckham MJ. The response to chemotherapy of a variety of human tumour xenografts. Br J Cancer 1983;47:1–13.
[64] Fiebig HH, Maier A, Burger AM. Clonogenic assay with established human tumour xenografts: correlation of in vitro to in vivo activity as a basis for anticancer drug discovery. Eur J Cancer 2004;40:802–20.
[65] Johnson JI, Decker S, Zaharevitz D, Rubinstein LV, Venditti JM, Schepartz S, et al. Relationships between drug activity in NCI preclinical in vitro and in vivo models and early clinical trials. Br J Cancer 2001;84:1424–31.
[66] Voskoglou-Nomikos T, Pater JL, Seymour L. Clinical predictive value of the in vitro cell line, human xenograft, and mouse allograft preclinical cancer models. Clin Cancer Res 2003;9:4227–39.
[67] Agoram B, Woltosz WS, Bolger MB. Predicting the impact of physiological and biochemical processes on oral drug bioavailability. Adv Drug Deliv Rev 2001;50(Suppl. 1):S41–67.
[68] Wilson G. Cell culture techniques for the study of drug transport. Eur J Drug Metab Pharmacokinet 1990;15:159–63.
[69] Szakacs G, Varadi A, Ozvegy-Laczka C, Sarkadi B. The role of ABC transporters in drug absorption, distribution, metabolism, excretion and toxicity (ADME-Tox). Drug Discov Today 2008;13:379–93.
[70] Jansen WJ, Hulscher TM, van Ark-Otte J, Giaccone G, Pinedo HM, Boven E. CPT-11 sensitivity in relation to the expression of P170-glycoprotein and multidrug resistance-associated protein. Br J Cancer 1998;77:359–65.
[71] Wang W, Wang EQ, Balthasar JP. Monoclonal antibody pharmacokinetics and pharmacodynamics. Clin Pharmacol Ther 2008;84:548–58.
[72] Flockhart DA, Oesterheld JR. Cytochrome P450-mediated drug interactions. Child Adolesc Psychiatr Clin N Am 2000;9:43–76.
[73] Iwatsubo T, Hirota N, Ooie T, Suzuki H, Shimada N, Chiba K, et al. Prediction of in vivo drug metabolism in the human liver from in vitro metabolism data. Pharmacol Ther 1997;73:147–71.
[74] Thummel KE, Wilkinson GR. In vitro and in vivo drug interactions involving human CYP3A. Annu Rev Pharmacol Toxicol 1998;38:389–430.
[75] Food and Drug Administration. In vitro drug interaction studies—cytochrome P450 enzyme- and transporter-mediated drug interactions guidance for industry. Silver Spring. Available from: https://www.fda.gov/media/134582/download; 2020.
[76] Food and Drug Administration. Clinical drug interaction studies—cytochrome P450 enzyme- and transporter-mediated drug interactions guidance for industry. Silver Spring. Available from: https://www.fda.gov/media/134581/download; 2020.
[77] Lee JI, Zhang L, Men AY, Kenna LA, Huang SM. CYP-mediated therapeutic protein-drug interactions: clinical findings, proposed mechanisms and regulatory implications. Clin Pharmacokinet 2010;49:295–310.
[78] Girish S, Martin SW, Peterson MC, Zhang LK, Zhao H, Balthasar J, et al. AAPS workshop report: strategies to address therapeutic protein-drug interactions during clinical development. AAPS J 2011;13:405–16.

[79] Harvey RD, Morgan ET. Cancer, inflammation, and therapy: effects on cytochrome p450-mediated drug metabolism and implications for novel immunotherapeutic agents. Clin Pharmacol Ther 2014;96:449–57.
[80] Bjornsson TD, Callaghan JT, Einolf HJ, Fischer V, Gan L, Grimm S, et al. The conduct of in vitro and in vivo drug-drug interaction studies: a PhRMA perspective. J Clin Pharmacol 2003;43:443–69.
[81] Yamazaki S, Lam JL, Zou HY, Wang H, Smeal T, Vicini P. Mechanistic understanding of translational pharmacokinetic-pharmacodynamic relationships in nonclinical tumor models: a case study of orally available novel inhibitors of anaplastic lymphoma kinase. Drug Metab Dispos 2015;43:54–62.
[82] Lindauer A, Valiathan CR, Mehta K, Sriram V, de Greef R, Elassaiss-Schaap J, et al. Translational pharmacokinetic/pharmacodynamic modeling of tumor growth inhibition supports dose-range selection of the anti-PD-1 antibody pembrolizumab. CPT Pharmacometrics Syst Pharmacol 2017;6:11–20.
[83] Hooker AC, Dunn-Sims E, Fairman D, Mead A, Van Der Graaf P, Karlsson MO. Modeling exposure-response relationships in the rat self-administration model. In: Population Approach Group Europe; 2010. p. 19. Abstr 1884 www.page-meeting.org/?abstract=1884.
[84] Food and Drug Administration. Guidance for industry: guidance for submission of immunohistochemistry applications to the FDA. Rockville. Available from: https://www.fda.gov/media/73622/download; 1998.
[85] Suntharalingam G, Perry MR, Ward S, Brett SJ, Castello-Cortes A, Brunner MD, et al. Cytokine storm in a phase 1 trial of the anti-CD28 monoclonal antibody TGN1412. N Engl J Med 2006;355:1018–28.
[86] Walker M, Makropoulos D, Achuthanandam R, Bugelski PJ. Recent advances in the understanding of drug-mediated infusion reactions and cytokine release syndrome. Curr Opin Drug Discov Devel 2010;13:124–35.
[87] Eddleston M, Cohen AF, Webb DJ. Implications of the BIA-102474-101 study for review of first-into-human clinical trials. Br J Clin Pharmacol 2016;81:582–6.
[88] Food and Drug Administration. Guidance for industry estimating the maximum safe starting dose in initial clinical trials for therapeutics in adult healthy volunteers. Rockville. Available from: https://www.fda.gov/media/72309/download; 2005.
[89] European Medicines Agency. Guideline on strategies to identify and mitigate risks for first-in-human and early clinical trials with investigational medicinal products. London. Available from: https://www.ema.europa.eu/en/documents/scientific-guideline/guideline-strategies-identify-mitigate-risks-first-human-early-clinical-trials-investigational_en.pdf; 2017.
[90] Muller PY, Milton M, Lloyd P, Sims J, Brennan FR. The minimum anticipated biological effect level (MABEL) for selection of first human dose in clinical trials with monoclonal antibodies. Curr Opin Biotechnol 2009;20:722–9.
[91] Nnane IP, Xu Z, Zhou H, Davis HM. Non-clinical pharmacokinetics, prediction of human pharmacokinetics and first-in-human dose selection for CNTO 5825, an anti-interleukin-13 monoclonal antibody. Basic Clin Pharmacol Toxicol 2015;117:219–25.
[92] Dong JQ, Salinger DH, Endre CJ, Gibbs JP, Hsu CP, Stouch BJ, et al. Quantitative prediction of human pharmacokinetics for monoclonal antibodies: retrospective analysis of monkey as a single species for first-in-human prediction. Clin Pharmacokinet 2011;50:131–42.
[93] Luu KT, Bergqvist S, Chen E, Hu-Lowe D, Kraynov E. A model-based approach to predicting the human pharmacokinetics of a monoclonal antibody exhibiting target-mediated drug disposition. J Pharmacol Exp Ther 2012;341:702–8.
[94] Vugmeyster Y, Rohde C, Perreault M, Gimeno RE, Singh P. Agonistic TAM-163 antibody targeting tyrosine kinase receptor-B: applying mechanistic modeling to enable preclinical to clinical translation and guide clinical trial design. MAbs 2013;5:373–83.
[95] Miller NA, Reddy MB, Heikkinen AT, Lukacova V, Parrott N. Physiologically based pharmacokinetic modelling for first-in-human predictions: an updated model building strategy illustrated with challenging industry case studies. Clin Pharmacokinet 2019;58:727–46.
[96] Agoram BM. Use of pharmacokinetic/ pharmacodynamic modelling for starting dose selection in first-in-human trials of high-risk biologics. Br J Clin Pharmacol 2009;67:153–60.
[97] Betts AM, Clark TH, Yang J, Treadway JL, Li M, Giovanelli MA, et al. The application of target information and preclinical pharmacokinetic/ pharmacodynamic modeling in predicting clinical doses of a Dickkopf-1 antibody for osteoporosis. J Pharmacol Exp Ther 2010;333:2–13.
[98] Saber H, Gudi R, Manning M, Wearne E, Leighton JK. An FDA oncology analysis of immune activating products and first-in-human dose selection. Regul Toxicol Pharmacol 2016;81:448–56.
[99] Hodi FS, O'Day SJ, McDermott DF, Weber RW, Sosman JA, Haanen JB, et al. Improved survival with ipilimumab in patients with metastatic melanoma. N Engl J Med 2010;363:711–23.
[100] Brahmer JR, Tykodi SS, Chow LQ, Hwu WJ, Topalian SL, Hwu P, et al. Safety and activity of anti-PD-L1 antibody in patients with advanced cancer. N Engl J Med 2012;366:2455–65.
[101] Hamid O, Robert C, Daud A, Hodi FS, Hwu WJ, Kefford R, et al. Safety and tumor responses with lambrolizumab (anti-PD-1) in melanoma. N Engl J Med 2013;369:134–44.
[102] Bornstein GG, Klakamp SL, Andrews L, Boyle WJ, Tabrizi M. Surrogate approaches in development of monoclonal antibodies. Drug Discov Today 2009;14:1159–65.
[103] Rongvaux A, Takizawa H, Strowig T, Willinger T, Eynon EE, Flavell RA, et al. Human hemato-lymphoid system mice: current use and future potential for medicine. Annu Rev Immunol 2013;31:635–74.
[104] Ochoa de Olza M, Oliva M, Hierro C, Matos I, Martin-Liberal J, Garrald E. Early-drug development in the era of immuno-oncology: are we ready to face the challenges? Ann Oncol 2018;29:1727–40.
[105] Mayes PA, Hance KW, Hoos A. The promise and challenges of immune agonist antibody development in cancer. Nat Rev Drug Discov 2018;17:509–27.
[106] Food and Drug Administration. Expansion cohorts: use in first-in-human clinical trials to expedite development of oncology drugs and biologics guidance for industry. Silver Spring. Available from: https://www.fda.gov/media/115172/download; 2018.

[107] Iasonos A, O'Quigley J. Adaptive dose-finding studies: a review of model-guided phase I clinical trials. J Clin Oncol 2014;32:2505–11.

[108] Kang SP, Gergich K, Lubiniecki GM, de Alwis DP, Chen C, Tice MAB, et al. Pembrolizumab KEYNOTE-001: an adaptive study leading to accelerated approval for two indications and a companion diagnostic. Ann Oncol 2017;28:1388–98.

[109] Tabrizi M, Zhang D, Ganti V, Azad G. Integrative pharmacology: advancing development of effective immunotherapies. AAPS J 2018;20:66. https://doi.org/10.1208/s12248-018-0229-2.

[110] Liu C, Yu J, Li H, Liu J, Xu Y, Song P, et al. Association of time-varying clearance of nivolumab with disease dynamics and its implications on exposure response analysis. Clin Pharmacol Ther 2017;101:657–66.

[111] Hendrikx J, Haanen J, Voest EE, Schellens JHM, Huitema ADR, Beijnen JH. Fixed dosing of monoclonal antibodies in oncology. Oncologist 2017;22:1212–21.

[112] Maude SL, Laetsch TW, Buechner J, Rives S, Boyer M, Bittencourt H, et al. Tisagenlecleucel in children and young adults with B-cell lymphoblastic leukemia. N Engl J Med 2018;378:439–48.

[113] Schuster SJ, Bishop MR, Tam CS, Waller EK, Borchmann P, McGuirk JP, et al. Tisagenlecleucel in adult relapsed or refractory diffuse large B-cell lymphoma. N Engl J Med 2019;380:45–56.

[114] Advani R, Flinn I, Popplewell L, Forero A, Bartlett NL, Ghosh N, et al. CD47 blockade by Hu5F9-G4 and rituximab in non-hodgkin's lymphoma. N Engl J Med 2018;379:1711–21.

[115] Takimoto CH, Chao MP, Gibbs C, McCamish MA, Liu J, Chen JY, et al. The macrophage 'do not eat me' signal, CD47, is a clinically validated cancer immunotherapy target. Ann Oncol 2019;30:486–9.

Chapter 31

Preclinical prediction of human pharmacokinetics

Malcolm Rowland[a,b]

[a]Centre for Applied Pharmacokinetic Research, Manchester School of Pharmacy, University of Manchester, Manchester, United Kingdom, [b]Department of Bioengineering and Therapeutic Sciences, Schools of Pharmacy and Medicine, University of California San Francisco, CA, United States

Introduction

Pharmacokinetics is an important property of a drug. It determines the temporal profiles of drugs and their metabolites in blood and tissues, which in turn drive the magnitude and temporal pattern of response following drug administration. Poor pharmacokinetic properties of a drug limit its clinical utility. Too rapid elimination normally necessitates frequent administration causing inconvenience for the patient and may raise the dose of drug needed to ensure that the exposure of drug in the body remains at a sufficiently high level and for long enough during a dosing interval to maintain an adequate therapeutic response; too slow elimination creates potential problems when trying to remove drug in the event of intoxication, and may take too long to reach adequate levels of exposure during accumulation following normal repetitive dosing associated with chronic therapy. Poor oral absorption may also limit the use of this common and convenient route of administration. For these and other reasons, such as reducing the wasted time, effort, and resources bringing poor compounds into clinical development, it is important to try to ensure that new drugs under development are likely to have desirable pharmacokinetic features at potential therapeutic doses, prior to actual administration to humans. In addition, accurate prediction of human pharmacokinetics gained from preclinical information, often coupled with in vitro human receptor occupation data or in vivo animal efficacy data, helps to design Phase 1 studies and to calculate the appropriate drug doses and hence the total amount of drug needed to be produced to meet early clinical evaluation. If calculations show that the anticipated therapeutic maintenance dose of a drug is particularly high, this together with other adverse features, may be grounds to stop its development.

This chapter contains a brief discussion of the three preclinical approaches to this prediction of pharmacokinetics in humans: allometry, physiologic modeling, incorporating in vitro and physiologic data, and microdosing. All three approaches involve extrapolation of one form or another; allometry involves extrapolating across animal species, physiologic modeling involves extrapolation of in vitro data to in vivo, while microdosing involves extrapolating data by dose.

Most applications have been with small molecular weight compounds (MW < 1000) that can distribute extensively into tissues and are predominantly eliminated via hepatic metabolism/biliary excretion and renal excretion. Prediction of human pharmacokinetics of biologics, such as monoclonal antibodies, which because of their large molecular size have restrictive tissue distribution, and often are eliminated outside of the liver and kidney by intracellular endosomal degradation, currently rely almost exclusively on allometry.

Allometry

Allometry, which is the oldest of the approaches and still widely applied in biology, is concerned with the study of the relationship between the size and function of components of the body, and growth or size of the whole body. Adolph [1] observed that many physiologic processes and organ sizes show a relatively simple power–law relationship with body weight when these are compared among mammals. The allometric equation proposed by Adolph is as follows:

$$P = a(BW)^m \tag{31.1}$$

where P = physiologic property or anatomic size, a = empirical coefficient, BW = body weight, and m = allometric exponent.

Atkinson's Principles of Clinical Pharmacology. https://doi.org/10.1016/B978-0-12-819869-8.00007-0

Note that a is not dimensionless; its value depends on the units in which P and BW are measured, while the exponent, m, is dimensionless and independent of the system of units. Note further that if $m=1$, then P is directly proportional to BW, a common approximation when considering tissue or organ mass, such as heart weight (Fig. 31.1A) and skeletal muscle mass. If $m<1$, P increases less rapidly than BW, or expressed per unit of body weight, *P decreases* as body weight *increases*. This is frequently found with physiologic functions, such as glomerular filtration rate (Fig. 31.1B), cardiac output, tissue blood flow rate, and daily heat production, with a value of m centered on 0.75 in all these cases [1, 2]. Note also that the data in Fig. 31.1 are displayed as log–log plots. This transformation not only allows data for mammals of widely differing body weights, ranging between 20 g for a mouse and about 200,000 kg for a blue whale (Fig. 31.1A), to be displayed on one graph, but also linearizes (Eq. 31.1)

$$\log P = \log a + m \log BW \tag{31.2}$$

with the slope of the line providing the value of m.

While useful, general allometric correlations, such as $m=1$ for organ weight, can obscure some interesting and important interspecies differences. Brain size in humans and nonhuman primates, for example, is considerably larger than would be expected from scaling brain data of other mammals. Some implications of this have been discussed with reference to regional drug delivery to the brain [3].

Use of allometry to predict human pharmacokinetic parameters

Given that pharmacokinetic data are invariably gathered in safety assessment species (such as mouse, rat, dog, or monkey) and those used in preclinical efficacy assessment, to gain exposure–response information, which better extrapolates across species than does dose, allometry remains a common approach to prediction of human pharmacokinetics [4, 5]. Also, noting that body composition tends to vary relatively little among mammalian species it is expected that, as with skeletal muscle mass, the volume of distribution of a drug should vary in direct proportion to body weight (i.e., $m=1$). This reflects the fact that a drug's distribution volume is simply a function of the affinity tissues have for the drug and the size of the various tissues. On the other hand, the value of m for drug clearance, being a measure of functional activity, like glomerular filtration rate, is expected, and often found, to be close to 0.75. As shown in Fig. 31.2, the chemotherapeutic agent, cyclophosphamide, is a drug that meets these expectations [4].

Although the difference in m between 0.75 and 1 appears small, as shown in Fig. 31.3 [6], the predicted value of a physiologic property varies substantially across this range of the exponential coefficient in moving from mouse to man, given the 3500-fold difference in body weight (20 g vs 70,000 g). In more concrete terms, if $m=0.75$ for clearance of a particular drug, the clearance per unit body weight in a 20-g mouse [$20^{(0.75-1)}$ or $1/20^{0.25}$] would expected to be $[(70{,}000)/(20)]^{0.25}$, or almost 8 times that in a 70-kg human. Furthermore, if the distribution volume is similar on a L/kg basis between the two species (e.g., cyclophosphamide) then, as a rough approximation, the elimination half-life ($0.693(V/BW)/(CL/BW)$) would be 8 times shorter in the mouse than human. For example, 8 h in a human would be pharmacokinetically equivalent on a time scale to 1 h in a mouse. This chronologic difference should be kept in mind when undertaking safety assessment studies in small animals in which, for example, twice daily dosing may appear to be frequent but could be associated with substantial "drug holiday" periods, during which the drug has been largely eliminated well before the end of each 12-h dosing interval.

Dedrick et al. [7] used similar reasoning to demonstrate that methotrexate plasma concentration *vs.* time data for several species were virtually superimposable, when plasma concentrations were normalized for dose/BW and chronological time was converted to an "equivalent time" by dividing it by species body weight raised to the 0.25 power (Fig. 31.4). The form of the correlation should, in principle, be useful for interspecies prediction of plasma concentration–time data for other drugs. This is true for drugs that are primarily renally eliminated unchanged, because renal clearance is generally highly correlated with glomerular filtration rate [8] and also for hepatic clearance of drugs for which elimination is so efficient that clearance is limited by delivery of compound to the liver, and therefore controlled by blood flow. However, it does not apply nearly so well for many other more stable compounds, as discussed later.

Another property for which m is approximately 0.75 is body surface area, which is the reason why physiologic functions are often said to vary in direct proportion to body surface area, both across and within species. For example, clinical dose calculations based on drug clearance are often expressed per 1.73 m^2, which is the average body surface area of a 70-kg adult. Actually, the value of m for surface area is closer to 0.67 (2/3) than 0.75 (¾), but in practice the difference in prediction on scaling between 0.67 and 0.75 is acceptably small. Dosing on a m^2 basis, which involves calculation usually from height and weight, can be prone to administration errors, and is only warranted if body size is an important determinant of clearance within the target patient population. This is invariably the case when scaling PK data from adults to children, but may be less so within an adult population, when other factors such as genetics, disease, and coadministered drugs may dominate.

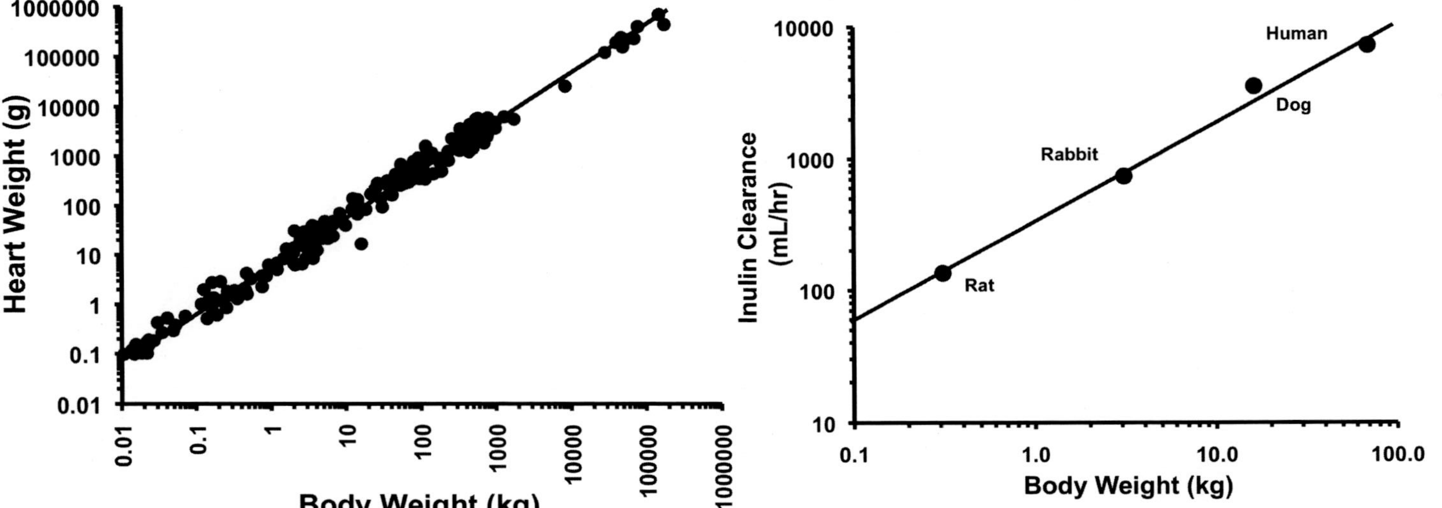

FIG. 31.1 Allometric relationships between body weight of mammals and (A) Heart weight, for 104 species spanning the weight range from mouse to blue whale; (B) Inulin clearance, a measure of glomerular filtration rate. Note that the data are displayed as log–log plots, and that the slope of the line (m) is approximately 1 for heart weight and 0.75 for glomerular filtration rate. *(Data abstracted from Prothero J. Heart weight as a function of body weight in mammals. Growth 1979;43;139–150 (heart weight) and Adolph EF. Quantitative relations in the physiological constitutions of mammals. Science 1949;109:579–585 (inulin clearance)).*

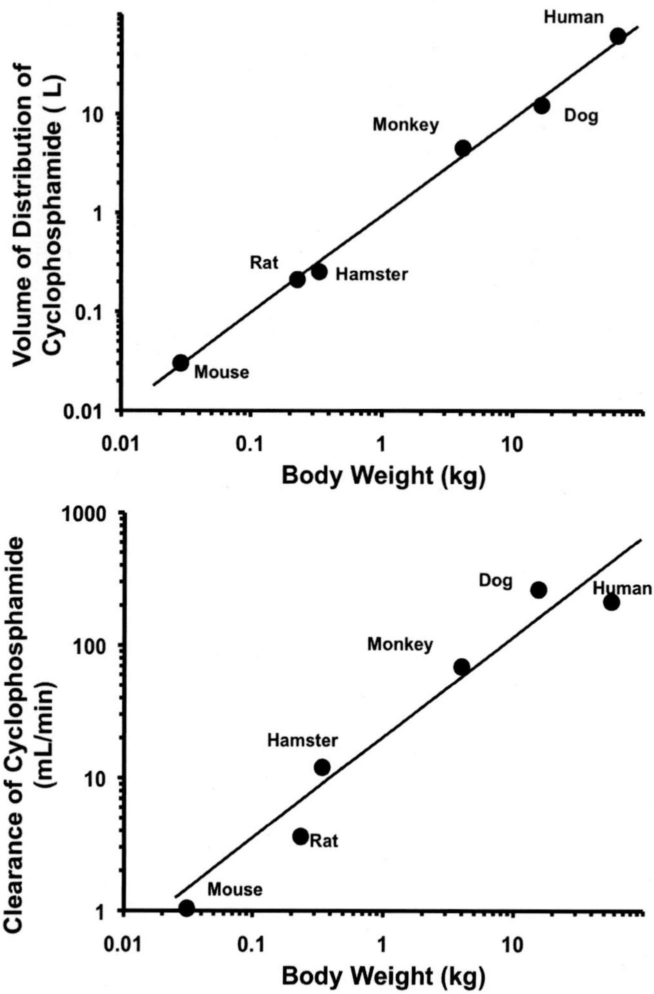

FIG. 31.2 Allometric relationship between (A) volume of distribution and (B) clearance of cyclophosphamide and body weight among mammals. The exponents are 1.0 and 0.75, respectively. Note the differences in the scales of the y-axes of the two graphs. *(Redrawn from Boxenbaum H. Interspecies scaling, allometry, physiological time, and the ground plan of pharmacokinetics. J Pharmacokinet Pharmacodyn 1982;10:201–227.)*

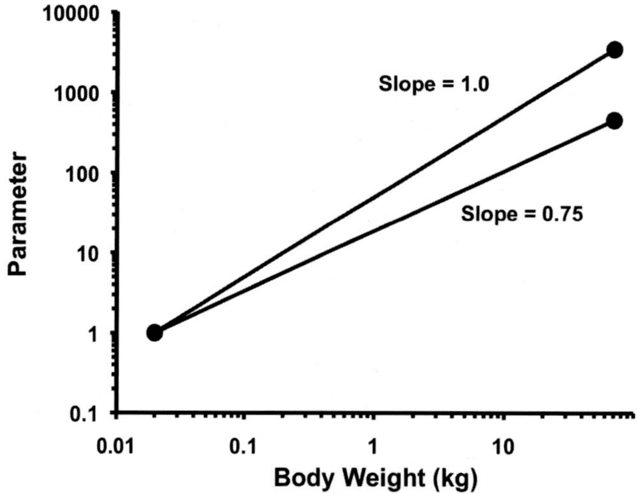

FIG. 31.3 Although exponents of 0.75 and 1 on relating a physiologic parameter to body weight do not appear to differ greatly, when applied across animal species that differ greatly in body weight, in this case from 0.02 kg (mouse) to 70 kg (human), the differences in the projected parameter values become large, eightfold in this case. The value of the parameter is arbitrarily set at 1 for mouse. *(Reproduced with permission from Rowland M, Tozer TN. Clinical pharmacokinetics and pharmacodynamics: concepts and application. Baltimore: Lippincott Williams & Wilkins; 5th ed, 2020; pp 665.)*

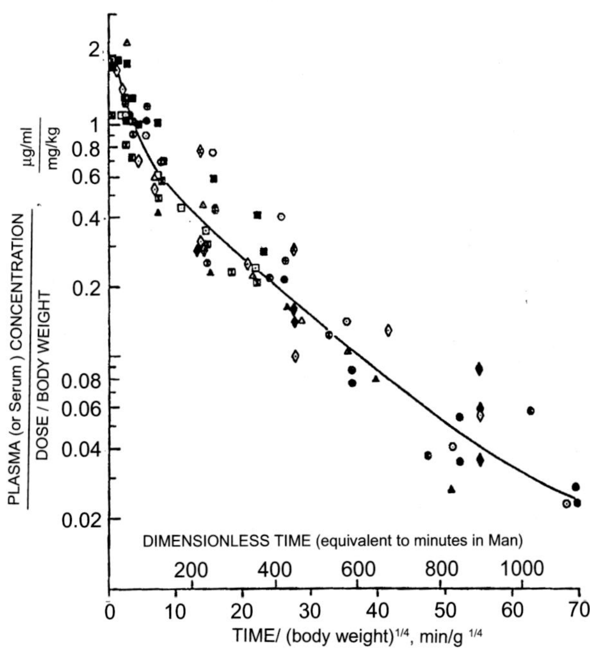

FIG. 31.4 Plot of plasma concentrations of methotrexate after intravenous (IV) or intraperitoneal (IP) injection normalized for each species to dose per kg body weight versus time divided by kg body weight raised to the 0.25 power. Observations: mice, *diamonds* (IV 0.3 mg/kg; IP 4.5, 45, 450 mg/kg), rats (IP 0.5, 6, 13.5, 25 mg/kg), rhesus monkey *solid triangles* (IV 0.3 mg/kg), beagle dog, *open triangle* (IV 0.2 mg/kg), adult patients, *squares* (IV 0.1, 1, 10 mg/kg). *(Reproduced with permission from Dedrick R, Bischof KB, Zaharko, DS. Interspecies correlation of plasma concentration history of methotrexate (NSC-740). Cancer Chemother Rep 1970;54:95–101.)*

Deviation from expectation

It is perhaps not surprising that allometric scaling frequently fails, given the simplistic assumptions set against the known complexity of biological systems. Various modifications of this scaling have been proposed to overcome discrepancies. One reason that predictions of human distribution volume fail is that there sometimes are large interspecies differences in plasma protein binding. With greater plasma binding more drug within the body resides in plasma and the volume of distribution is correspondingly smaller. Consequently, distribution volume predictions often are substantially improved when corrections for these differences in plasma binding are made, indicating that interspecies differences in the composition and binding of compounds to individual tissues, such as skeletal muscle and heart, may be small. Occasionally, distribution of a drug to tissues in an animal differs even after correcting for differences in plasma binding signifying differences in tissue composition across species.

Many proposals have been made for correcting clearance when the exponential coefficient m deviates substantially from 0.75 [4]. However, these proposals have invariably been based on retrospective analysis of the body of combined animal *and* human data. Unfortunately, these proposals may be of little value to those engaged in prospectively predicting human pharmacokinetics of a new chemical entity during preclinical drug development. Indeed, in an analysis of all the recommended correction strategies adopting the prospective approach, none systemically improved the allometric predictability of clearance over that with $m = 0.75$ after correcting for differences in plasma protein binding [9]. Failure to predict human clearance allometrically is particularly noticeable with relatively stable compounds, that is, ones with low clearance. This is because for such compounds clearance is more heavily dependent on the activity of either metabolic enzymes or transporters, rather than organ blood flow rate, which often show large interspecies differences in both specificity and activity, whereas allometry assumes that the only variable is body size. Today, these low clearance compounds are the most prevalent ones emerging from early in vitro screens of biologic stability (before in vivo studies), as these tend to have longer half-lives, facilitating such favorable features as once daily or even less frequent administration coupled with lower doses needed to maintain therapeutic concentrations.

Beyond clearance, another common reason that allometric predictions fail is that most drugs are developed for oral administration and gastrointestinal absorption is another major source of uncertainty. Unlike clearance and volume of distribution, the extent of oral absorption, bioavailability, is not dependent on body weight per se and so does not scale allometrically. In addition, the formulations of compounds used in preclinical development are often very different from those given to humans. For example, it is not uncommon to administer to animals a suspension or a solution of the compound in a powerful water miscible solvent, such as polyethylene glycol 400, to maximize the likelihood of good absorption whereas humans often receive solid dosage forms, such as capsules or tablets, from which drug must disintegrate, disperse, and dissolve to be absorbed. This difference in formulation frequently becomes an important problem when dealing with sparingly soluble compounds, as formulation then has a profound effect on the absorption characteristics of the compound. Moreover, while the monkey might be thought to behave more similarly to humans than rat or dog, this has not proved always to be the case with respect to oral absorption; dog is generally the default species when evaluating solid dosage forms. As a result of such discrepancies, considerable caution is warranted if only allometric scaling of pharmacokinetics is relied on to guide initial dose selection in Phase I clinical trials.

Physiologic pharmacokinetics

Conceptually, the second approach, widely known as *physiologically based pharmacokinetics* (PBPK), is not new. As described in Chapter 3, the physiologic approach can be traced back to the 1930s but languished for many years, viewed by many in drug development as too complex and demanding, although it has been more widely employed in predicting human exposure to environmental chemicals, where often human data are lacking. However, more recently, the approach has gained substantial momentum and wide application in drug development, including prediction of human PK, with the increasing knowledge of the processes controlling ADME (absorption, distribution, metabolism and excretion) processes, the increasingly ability of in vitro methods to accurately predict quantitatively events in vivo, coupled with the availability of user-friendly commercially supported software platforms that provide not only the models but also a vast amount of relevant physiological, anatomic, and biochemical data [10]. In particular, in contrast to allometry (and microdosing) which cease to have utility once Phase 1 data become available, PBPK, which is highly mechanistic, can predict the impact of genetics, disease, drug–drug interaction, and age encountered during clinical drug development and beyond.

PBPK is predicated on the realization that absorption, distribution, and elimination processes of a drug involve a complex set of interactions between drug and all tissues of the body which, together with recirculation of body fluids, particularly blood, result in the observed concentration–time profile in tissues and systemic circulation. In principle, it is possible to describe these events in mathematical terms and, if sufficient data are available, to predict the time course of drug and metabolite(s) in different species and at specific anatomic sites [10]. Such physiologic models have been developed to predict the pharmacokinetics of numerous compounds in humans, using a combination of anatomic, physiologic, and biochemical data, *systems properties* that are independent of the drug, coupled with drug-specific data, comprising a mixture of physicochemical information, such as solubility and lipophilicity, and in vitro metabolic and transporter experimental data gained using human tissue components, such as microsomes, hepatocytes, and enterocytes (intestinal epithelial cells). Emphasis in the following section is on prediction of human pharmacokinetics, but much of the initial validation of the methods has been made in animals, and it is not uncommon to establish the appropriateness of a physiologic model for a particular drug in an animal, often the rat, prior to its application to predict events in humans. As confidence in this approach has increased the need for preclinical validation has diminished.

Because PBPK involves the building up and integration of the component processes to predict whole body pharmacokinetics it is often referred to as a *bottom-up approach*, in contrast to the modeling of in vivo data to obtain global estimates of the parameters controlling the ADME processes of a drug, which is designated as a *top-down approach*. In practice, once Phase 1 data and beyond become available these are used to update and refine the preclinical PBPK model in a *middling-out approach*.

The use of in vitro methods to predict clearance in vivo is well established [11]. Fig. 31.5 [12] illustrates this application using human hepatic expression systems containing minute amounts of the common CYP isoforms, which are primarily responsible for eliminating approximately 50% of all marketed small MW drugs [13]. More commonly microsomes and hepatocytes are employed. In this method, the in vitro metabolic activity data of the compound, after correcting for any nonspecific binding, is scaled proportionately to the corresponding amount of enzyme in the liver and integrated into a mathematical model, such as the well-stirred model of hepatic elimination (Chapter 7), with other information, including binding of compound within blood, hepatic blood flow, and in some cases hepatocyte membrane permeability and transporters [14]. Despite continual improvement in the in vitro methods, there is still a degree of uncertainty and also a tendency for underprediction of hepatic clearance in vivo, which are not fully understood and require the introduction of correction factors [11]. One reason for the underprediction may be associated with how differences in protein binding between in vitro systems and in vivo are taken into account, predicated on the assumption that reactions are driven by the unbound concentration [15]. A reason for uncertainty is that in vitro systems are inherently unstable,

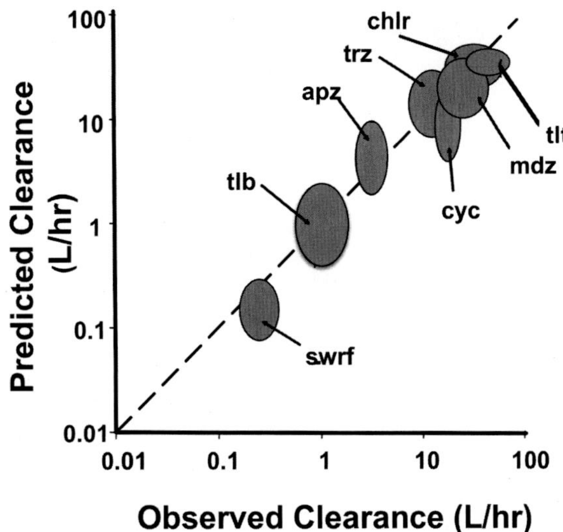

FIG. 31.5 Log–log plot showing a generally good accord between predicted and observed clearance in humans, including interindividual variability, for eight drugs predominantly eliminated by CYP enzymes. Prediction using a model of hepatic elimination is based on a combination of physiologic, biochemical, and demographic data together with drug-specific human data, including in vitro metabolic microsomal activity, and plasma and microsomal binding. The *ellipses* delineate the 90% confidence intervals for both predictions and observations; the *dotted line* is the line of identity. Apz, alprazolam; chlor, chlorzoxazone; cyc, cyclosporine; mdz, midazolam; swarf, S-warfarin; tlb, tolbutamide; tlt, tolterodine; trz, triazolam. *(Abstracted from Howgate EM, Rowland Yeo K, Proctor NJ, Tucker GT, Rostami-Hodjegan A. Prediction of in vivo drug clearance from in vitro data. I: impact of inter-individual variability. Xenobiotica 2006;36:473–497.)*

and for some compounds metabolism is so slow that within the period of viability there is insufficient turnover of the compound to allow a reliable estimate of clearance. To overcome this last deficiency more stable hepatocyte systems have appeared in recent years, with some promising results [16]. More widely, microfluidically linked organ-on-a-chip technology is emerging as a powerful approach to in vitro–in vivo extrapolation in PBPK [17].

An estimate of the distribution of compound to individual tissues and organs forms an essential component of the PBPK model and would be a major limitation if, as in the past, this required the need to obtain experimental human (or animal) drug tissue data. However, this limitation has been largely overcome for many compounds by taking advantage of the fact that tissue affinity is a function of the physicochemical properties of the compound, such as lipophilicity and degree of ionization in tissues, and the binding components within tissues, which are predominantly neutral lipids and phospholipids for neutral compounds and acidic phospholipids for bases, through ion pairing of the cationic form of the base, particularly for bases $pK_a > 7$, which are predominantly ionized at physiologic pHs [18]. Another factor for ionized bases is trapping in the acidic environment of lysozymes [19]. The concentrations of these constituents vary among tissues but are relatively fixed and known for a particular tissue. This knowledge has allowed the successful in silico prediction of tissue distribution in many cases, as shown for example in Fig. 31.6 [18]. Exceptions are generally those in which the drug has a high affinity for a specific tissue binding constituent that accounts for much of the drug in the body. Examples are some sulfonamide drugs, such as chlorthalidone, highly, and almost exclusively, bound to carbonic anhydrase, which resides predominantly within erythrocytes; doxorubicin, which interacts extensively with DNA; and digoxin, which binds to tissue Na^+-K^+ ATPase. If animal in vivo data or human microdose data (see later) are available the parameters of the PBPK model can be updated prior to Phase 1 studies.

Physiologic models of absorption, particularly oral absorption, are often more complex than those of elimination and tissue distribution, as can readily be seen in Fig. 31.7 [20], where the gastrointestinal tract is divided into a series of sequentially connected compartments to accommodate the known heterogeneity of luminal dimension, content, structure, motility, and enzyme and transporter activity along the gastrointestinal tract. Again, much of this drug independent information is now known. The net rate of intestinal absorption of a compound from the gastrointestinal tract is the sum of its rates of entry from each segment into the associated mesenteric blood, which then collectively drains into the hepatic portal vein and passes through the liver before entering the general circulation. Hence, the overall systemic bioavailability of an oral dose is a function of three components operating in sequence: the fraction of the ingested dose that enters the apical membrane of the enterocyte (which is dependent on dissolution of the solid, stability in gut lumen, and permeation of the membrane); the fraction entering the enterocyte that avoids gut wall metabolism and intestinal efflux

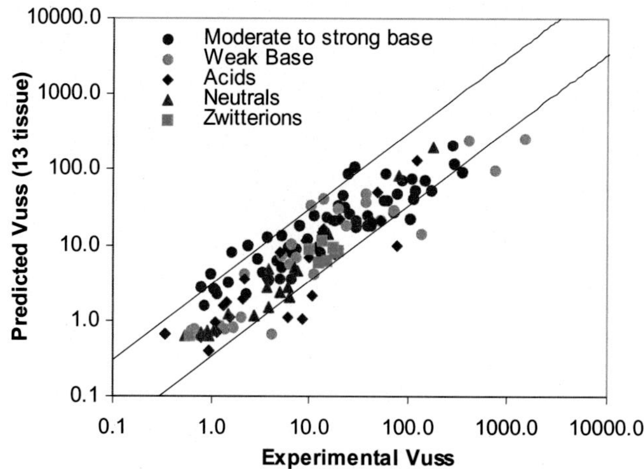

FIG. 31.6 Correlation between observed unbound volume of distribution at steady state ($V_{u,ss}$) and predicted values using a physiologic model of drug tissue distribution for a set of 140 diverse compounds in humans. The predicted values were based on a combination of the physicochemical properties of the compounds together with knowledge of the composition of the important binding constituents within tissues. The lines are threefold on either side of the line of identity. *(Reproduced with permission from Rodgers T, Rowland M. Mechanistic approaches to volume of distribution predictions: understanding the processes. Pharm Res 2007;24:918–933.)*

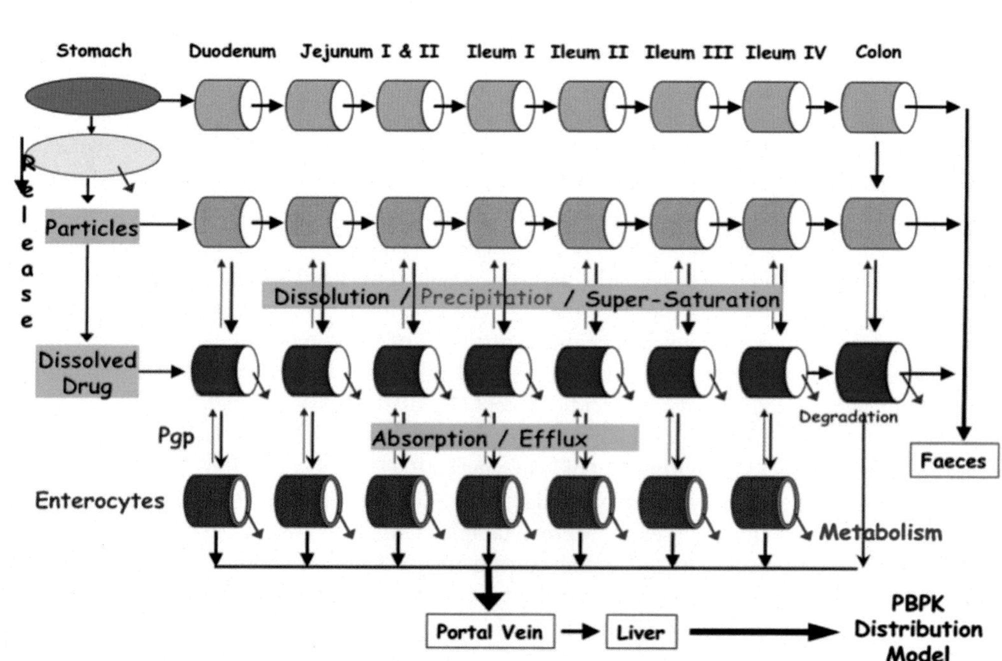

FIG. 31.7 An Advanced Dissolution Absorption and Metabolism (ADAM) model of events in the gastrointestinal tract. The intestine is divided into segments each comprising four compartments to account for luminal solid, particulate and dissolved drug and drug passing through the enterocytes subject to metabolism and transport. Absorbed drug enters the physiologically based pharmacokinetic (PBPK) model characterizing systemic events via the hepatic portal vein. *(Modified from Jamei M, Turner D, Yang J, Neuhoff S, Polak S, Rostami-Hodjegan A, et al. Population-based mechanistic prediction of oral drug absorption. AAPS J 2009;11:225–237.)*

to enter the portal blood; and finally the fraction entering the portal blood that escapes loss on passage through the liver to enter the general circulation. Not surprisingly, developing drugs that are fully orally bioavailable is challenging. Progress has also been profitably made toward development of physiologic models to accommodate other routes of drug administration, such as transdermal [21] and inhalation [22], and to represent events within specific target tissues such as brain [23] and solid tumors [24].

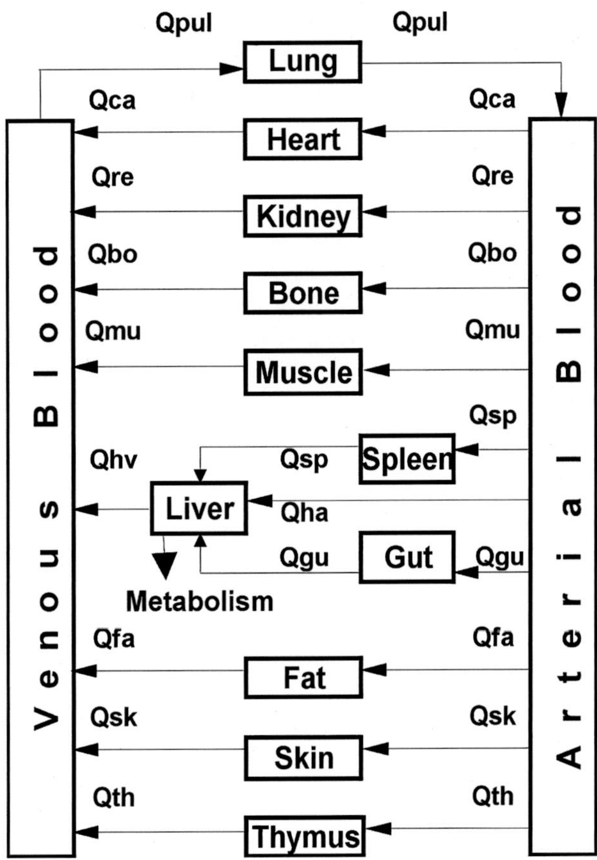

FIG. 31.8 A whole body physiologically based pharmacokinetic model. Q refers to blood flow, subsequent initials refers to specific tissues or organs. Input can be into any site of the body. Elimination is depicted as occurring from only liver and kidneys, whereas it can occur also at other sites for some drugs. Some drugs undergo enterohepatic cycling, which involves biliary secretion into the small intestine followed by subsequent intestinal reabsorption. The model can be extended to include a similar model for formed metabolites.

More generally, although there are still issues with the methodology, PBPK modeling for first in human prediction has advanced substantially during the past decade [25, 26]. These models can be depicted with flow diagrams indicating the anatomic relationships among various organs and tissues, as shown in Fig. 31.8. The degree of complexity of the model, in terms of the number of tissue compartments and events within them, varies with the application. In some cases, tissues such as those that are well perfused, which include the liver, kidneys, lungs, and heart, and which have comparable kinetics of drug distribution, may be lumped together as a single compartment. Previously this was often done to reduce the complexity of the model to facilitate faster numerical integration of the rate equations, but with the computing power and speed now available this is not a serious limitation.

The accumulation of a drug within a compartment is described by an appropriate mass balance equation, such as eq. (7.2), the equation for the well-stirred model of hepatic drug elimination that was derived in Chapter 7. As a further illustration, consider the accumulation with time of a drug in the kidney, which is assumed to eliminate the drug by a combination of glomerular filtration and saturable secretion, without tubular reabsorption. It is further assumed that the drug is unbound in plasma, evenly distributed between plasma and blood cells, and that the concentration within the compartment is uniform and equal to that in the emergent venous blood.

$$V_K \frac{dC_K}{dt} = Q_K C_A - Q_K C_{V,K} - GFR \cdot C_A - \left[\frac{T_{\max,K} C_{V,K}}{K_{m,K} + C_{V,K}}\right] \tag{31.3}$$

where V = volume of kidney compartment, C = drug concentration, t = time, Q = blood flow rate, $T_{max,K}$ = maximum rate of renal secretion, K_m = Michaelis–Menten constant, GFR = glomerular filtration rate, and the subscripts K, A, and V refer to kidney, arterial, and venous blood, respectively.

Similar equations can be written for all relevant compartments. Once parameters are determined or chosen, the resulting set of equations can be solved numerically to yield predictions of the concentration of the drug in each of the compartments as a function of time. Of course, the simplifying assumptions earlier can be, and often are, refined to include much more detail concerning plasma and tissue binding, transport at the level of the blood capillary and cell membrane, and spatial nonuniformity, especially when dealing with gastrointestinal drug absorption. Similar equations can be written for all relevant compartments and for metabolites.

Fig. 31.9 [27] compares a prediction of the expected blood concentration–time profile of cyclosporine with the observed concentrations measured in patients following oral administration of this immunosuppressive drug which is used to suppress rejection of an organ transplant. Cyclosporine is a neutral, lipophilic, sparingly soluble compound that is almost exclusively metabolized by CYP3A4. In this example, the prediction was based on a combination of tissue distribution information gained from animal studies, metabolism from human hepatic tissue in vitro, and absorption from prior data for a microemulsion formulation of the drug. The compartment sizes and blood flow rates were taken from published data. In this case, the prediction provides a good approximation to the observed data. But had it been necessary or desired, the parameters of the model could be updated to better fit the observed in vivo data, after first exploring the sensitivity of the blood profile to changes in each of the parameters to identity the important components of the model.

Examination of Eq. (31.3), or its counterpart for any eliminating organ, shows that blood flow and organ elimination interact. In general, clearance is taken to relate rate of elimination to systemic concentration. However, the driving force for elimination occurs within the cells of the eliminating organ, and the rate of the reaction related to the unbound concentration there is referred to as the *intrinsic clearance*, CL_{int} as it is intrinsic to the cell and independent of external factors, such as blood flow and binding within blood. Because the organ cannot eliminate more drug than reaches it by blood flow, the absolute upper limit on the organ's contribution to rate of elimination is $Q \bullet C_{V,K}$. This is known as a *blood flow or perfusion rate limitation*. This occurs when the drug is an excellent substrate for the elimination processes, in which case its intrinsic clearance is much greater than blood flow. Under these circumstances organ clearance approaches blood flow, and as organ blood flow scales allometrically so too does the clearance of such drugs. Also, for such drugs, because clearance is not limited by cellular eliminating activity, even if clearly seen in vitro the effects of enzyme induction or inhibition on clearance are expected to be attenuated in vivo. More often, however, the intrinsic clearances of modern drugs are relatively low, in which case the rate-controlling step is no longer blood flow but intrinsic clearance itself or, for more polar compounds, cell membrane permeability. Then, the impact of inhibitors and inducers of enzymes or transporters should be readily apparent in vivo. In practice, these expectations are borne out experimentally.

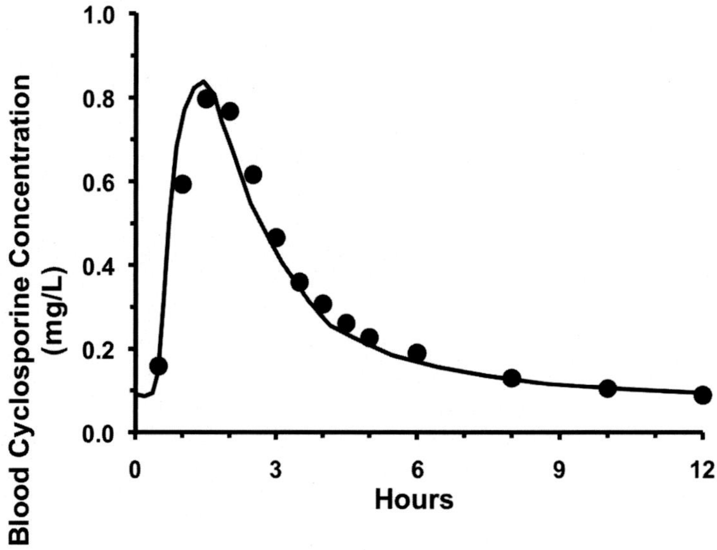

FIG. 31.9 Observed (•) and predicted (*solid line*) blood cyclosporine concentration–time profile within a dosing interval at steady state in renal transplant patients receiving 1.5 mg/kg orally twice daily. Measured data are the mean observations in 18 patients. The predictions were generated with the whole body physiologic model depicted in Fig. 31.8, together with drug-specific information, including in vitro drug metabolism, intestinal permeability, binding within blood, and dissolution data together with animal tissue distribution data. *(Redrawn from Kawai R, Matthew D, Tanaka C, Rowland M. - Physiologically-based pharmacokinetics of cyclosporine A: extension to tissue distribution kinetics in rats and scale-up to human. J Pharmacol Exp Ther 1998;287:457–468.)*

As mentioned allometry is the default method for predicting human PK of monoclonal antibodies. However, it ignores the known differences in the activity and distribution of FcRn (neonatal Fc receptor) that controls the trafficking of antibodies, reducing their otherwise relatively rapid elimination, and thereby extending their half-lives often from days to weeks, making them more convenient and economical to administer. PBPK modeling, which allows for the inclusion of human in vitro data, shows promise [28] and may well be the way forward in prediction of human PK of the multitude of emerging bioengineered manipulations of monoclonal antibodies and fragments. The third option is microdosing.

Microdosing

Microdosing is also relatively recent but unlike PBPK, which is highly mechanistic, it is an empirical approach to human pharmacokinetic prediction made possible by the development of the ultrasensitive analytical techniques discussed in Chapter 11 [10]. It involves administering to humans a minute, safe, subtherapeutic dose (a microdose) of the test compound (not greater than 0.1 mg/adult) and proportionally scaling the observed pharmacokinetic profile, and hence dose, to the desired concentration–time profile intended to be evaluated in the Phase 1 study. It has regulatory support as a component for example of the exploratory IND (e-IND, [29]). The attractiveness of a microdose, in addition to needing very little compound, is its high safety profile (generally requiring only testing over a range of single doses in one species, usually rat) so therefore can be administered to humans very much earlier than normal. Microdosing has tended to be used when there is little confidence in allometry, because for example the allometric exponent is very different than the usually accepted default values mentioned previously, an accepted warning signal, and there are problems in in vitro:in vivo extrapolation as part of PBPK, due to either involvement of poorly understood enzymes or transporters [30] or because enzymatic turnover of compound is too slow to gain a reliable estimate of metabolic activity (intrinsic clearance) in microsomes or hepatocytes. However, because of its relatively high predictive success coupled with it helping at a very early stage to optimize the PBPK model (see later), particularly if the compound is administered intravenously (to characterize disposition parameters, clearance, and volume of distribution, which tend to be linear over a wide dose range due to the dilution linked to often extensive tissue distribution), there is an argument to be made that microdosing should always be considered, even if ultimately it is not pursued. Because microdosing is strictly not a preclinical activity nor part of the normal Phase 1 program, it has been termed a Phase 0 approach [31].

The microdose approach is based on two simple ideas. First, there is no better pharmacokinetic predictor of humans than humans, and second, the assumption that the pharmacokinetics of the compound is dose proportional, that is, parameters, such as clearance, volume of distribution, and bioavailability, do not change with dose between a microdose and a therapeutic dose. Although essentially all processes within the body are eventually saturable if the dose is large enough, which clearly would violate the assumption of dose proportionality, and needs to be accommodated to avoid serious errors in prediction of human pharmacokinetics at therapeutic doses, it turns out that this assumption of linearity holds reasonably well for many compounds over the dose range of interest, especially when the therapeutic dose is below 50 mg, as shown in Fig. 31.10 [32] for midazolam. Exceptions to this assumption of linearity occasionally are encountered and often can be anticipated from in vitro studies [33].

One particular form of nonlinearity is *target-mediated drug disposition* (TMDD) seen at very low rather than high doses, which arises when at low doses most of the drug in the body is bound to the pharmacologic target, a situation due to a combination of two factors. One is an extremely avid affinity of the drug for its target, that is very high potency, and the other is restrictive tissue distribution. A class of compounds that characteristically display TMDD are monoclonal antibodies. As dose is increased the target is readily saturated being only a very small body constituent, although it may be highly localized. There are also many highly potent small molecules but most, especially basic and neutral lipophilic compounds, bind so extensively and nonspecifically to many tissue components so as to dominate distribution, thereby obscuring target binding, and linear PK behavior prevails. However, there are exceptions [34,35] such as the highly potent compounds warfarin [36] and bosentan [37] that have a relatively low affinity for tissue constituents. And, there are likely to be more examples in the future with the desire for ever greater potency, linked to the drive for low dose compounds as these are not only drug sparing but also have less chance of evoking drug–drug interactions and nonspecific toxicity. In both cases of high and low dose saturation, attempts are being made to improve prediction of human PK by coupling microdose results with in vitro characterization of the saturable process(es) incorporated into a PBPK model, which is not restricted to assuming linearity.

Another limitation of microdosing arises because at the minute doses administered test compounds are invariably sufficiently soluble to dissolve in the dosing solution. Accordingly, microdosing cannot be used to assess the performance of solid formulations, including tablets and capsules, a particular issue for poorly soluble compounds when dissolution of the

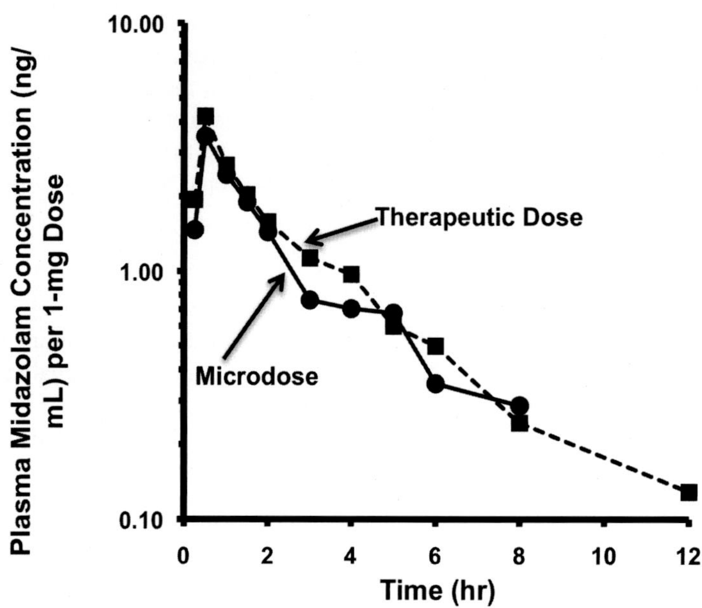

FIG. 31.10 An oral microdose (100-µg) (*circles*) successfully predicts the pharmacokinetics following a therapeutic oral dose of midazolam (7.5 mg) (*squares*), as evidenced by the virtual superposition of the plasma concentration–time profiles when normalized to a common 1-mg dose. Data are geometric means of observations in six subjects receiving the two 75-fold different doses on separate occasions. *(Redrawn from Lappin GKW, Kuhnz W, Jochemsen R, Kneer J, Chaudhary A, Oosterhuis B, et al. Use of microdosing to predict pharmacokinetics at the therapeutic dose: experience with 5 drugs. Clin Pharmacol Ther 2006;80:203–215.)*

drug critically determines its absorption. Nevertheless, early warning of a poor pharmacokinetic profile when compound is given in solution is useful as it generally portends to serious problems that are unlikely to be readily overcome by formulation efforts.

Direct comparison of the predictive performance between the three methods is limited. An analysis comparing allometry with PBPK of 107 orally administered compounds (none of which were administered as a microdose), representing typical drugs under current development, was equivocal [25]. There were failures with both methods, especially in the prediction of oral bioavailability, indicating that there is still need for improvement. However, further improvement is not possible with either allometry or microdosing, as these involve simple scaling, whereas it is possible with PBPK. Indeed, the performance of this last method is continuing to improve as we learn more about the qualitative and quantitative factors controlling various physiologic processes and continue to develop in vitro methods with improved in vivo predictability. Accordingly, because of its many advantages, including extension to all phases and situations encountered in preclinical and clinical drug development, and is resource and animal sparing features, PBPK is predicted to become the standard approach for the preclinical prediction of human pharmacokinetics. In the meanwhile, given current limitations all three methods, allometry, PBPK, and microdosing are needed.

References

[1] Prothero J. Heart weight as a function of body weight in mammals. Growth 1979;43:139–150.

[2] Adolph EF. Quantitative relations in the physiological constitutions of mammals. Science 1949;109:579–585.

[3] Dedrick RL, Oldfield EH, Collins JM. Arterial drug infusion with extracorporeal removal. I. Theoretic basis with particular reference to the brain. Cancer Treat Rep 1984;68:373–380.

[4] Boxenbaum H. Interspecies scaling, allometry, physiological time, and the ground plan of pharmacokinetics. J Pharmacokinet Pharmacodyn 1982;10:201–227.

[5] Mahmood I. Interspecies pharmacokinetic scaling: Principles and applications of allometric scaling. Rockville, MD: Pine House Publishers; 2005. 374 p.

[6] Rowland M, Tozer TN. Clinical pharmacokinetics and pharmacodynamics: concepts and application. 5th ed Baltimore: Lippincott Williams & Wilkins; 2020. pp 665.

[7] Dedrick R, Bischof KB, Zaharko DS. Interspecies correlation of plasma concentration history of methotrexate (NSC-740). Cancer Chemother Rep 1970;54:95–101.

[8] Mahmood I. Interspecies scaling of renally secreted drugs. Life Sci 1998;63:2365–2371.

[9] Ring BJ, Chien JY, Adkison KK, Jones HM, Rowland M, Jones RDO, et al. PhRMA CPCDC initiative on predictive models of human pharmacokinetics, part 3: comparative assessment of prediction methods of human clearance. J Pharm Sci 2011;100:4090–4110.

[10] Rowland M, Peck C, Tucker GT. Physiologically-based pharmacokinetics in drug development and regulatory science. Ann Rev Pharmacol Toxicol 2011;51:45–73.

[11] Howgate EM, Rowland Yeo K, Proctor NJ, Tucker GT, Rostami-Hodjegan A. Prediction of *in vivo* drug clearance from *in vitro* data. I: impact of inter-individual variability. Xenobiotica 2006;36:473–497.

[12] Wood FL, Houston JB, Hallifax D. Clearance prediction methodology needs fundamental improvement: trends common to rat and human hepatocytes/microsomes and implications for experimental methodology. Drug Metal Dispos 2017;45:1178–1188.

[13] Clarke SE, Jones BC. Hepatic cytochromes P450 and their role in metabolism-based drug–drug interactions. In: Rodriguez AD, editor. Drug–drug interactions. New York: Marcel Dekker; 2002. p. 55–88.

[14] El-Kattan AF, Varma MVS. Navigating transporter sciences in pharmacokinetics characterization using the extended clearance classification system. Drug Metab Dispos 2018;46:729–739.

[15] Bowman CM, Benet LZ. An examination of protein binding and protein facilitated uptake relating to *in vitro-in vivo* extrapolation. Eur J Pharm Sc 2018;123:502–514.

[16] Da-Silva F, Boulenc X, Vermet V, Compigne P, Gerbal-Chaloin S, Daujat-Chavanieu S, et al. Improving prediction of metabolic clearance using quantitative extrapolation of results obtained from human hepatic micropatterned cocultures model and by considering the impact of albumin binding. J Pharm Sci 2018;107:1957–1972.

[17] Prantil-Baun R, Novak R, Das D, Somayaji MR, Przekwas A, Ingber DE. Physiologically based pharmacokinetic and pharmacodynamic analysis enabled by microfluidically linked organs-on-chips. Ann Rev Pharmacol Toxicol 2018;58:37–64.

[18] Rodgers T, Rowland M. Mechanistic approaches to volume of distribution predictions: understanding the processes. Pharm Res 2007;24:918–933.

[19] Schmitt MV, Lienau P, Fricker G, Reichel A. Quantitation of lysosomal trapping of basic lipophilic compounds using in vitro assays and in silico predictions based on the determination of the full pH profile of the endo-/lysosomal system in rat hepatocytes. Drug Metab Dispos 2019;47:49–57.

[20] Jamei M, Turner D, Yang J, Neuhoff S, Polak S, Rostami-Hodjegan A, et al. Population-based mechanistic prediction of oral drug absorption. AAPS J 2009;11:225–237.

[21] Polak S, Tylutki Z, Holbrook M, Wisniowska B. Better prediction of the local concentration–effect relationship: the role of physiologically based pharmacokinetics and quantitative systems pharmacology and toxicology in the evolution of model-informed drug discovery and development. Drug Discov Today 2019;24:1344–1354.

[22] Kolli AR, Kuczac AK, Martin F, Hayes AW. Bridging inhaled aerosol dosimetry to physiologically based pharmacokinetic modeling for toxicological assessment: nicotine delivery systems and beyond. Crit Rev Toxicol 2019;49:725–741.

[23] Liu X, Smith BJ, Chen C, Callegari E, Becker SL, Chen X, Cianfrogna J, Doran AC, Doran SD, Gibbs JP, Hosea N, Liu J, Nelson FR, Szewc MA, Van Deusen J. Use of a physiologically based pharmacokinetic model to study the time to reach brain equilibrium: an experimental analysis of the role of blood-brain barrier permeability, plasma protein binding, and brain tissue binding. J Pharmacol Exp Ther 2005;313:1254–1262.

[24] He H, Liu C, Wu Y, Zhang X, Fan J, Cao Y. A multiscale physiologically-based pharmacokinetic model for doxorubicin to explore its mechanisms of cytotoxicity and cardiotoxicity in human physiological context. Pharm Res 2018;35:174–184.

[25] Poulin P, Jones RDO, Jones HM, Gibson CR, Rowland M, Chien JY, et al. PHRMA CPCDC initiative on predictive models of human pharmacokinetics, part 5: prediction of plasma concentration–time profiles in human by using the physiologically-based pharmacokinetic modeling approach. J Pharm Sci 2011;100:4127–4157.

[26] Miller NA, Reddy MB, Heikkinen AT, Lukacova V, Parrott N. Physiologically based pharmacokinetic modelling for first-in-humanpredictions: an updated model building strategy illustrated with challenging industry case studies. Clin Pharmacokin 2019;58:727–746.

[27] Kawai R, Matthew D, Tanaka C, Rowland M. Physiologically-based pharmacokinetics of cyclosporine A: extension to tissue distribution kinetics in rats and scale-up to human. J Pharmacol Exp Ther 1998;287:457–468.

[28] Jones HM, Zhang Z, Jasper P, Luo H, Avery LB, King LE, et al. A physiologically-based pharmacokinetic model for the prediction of monoclonal antibody pharmacokinetics from *in vitro* data. CPT Pharmacometrics Syst Pharmacol 2019;8:738–747.

[29] Burt T, Yoshida K, Lappin G, Vuong L, John C, de Wildt SN, Sugiyama Y, Rowland M. Microdosing and other phase 0 clinical trials: facilitating translation in drug development. Clin Transl Sci 2016;9:74–88.

[30] CDER. Exploratory IND studies. Guidance for industry. Rockville: FDA; 2006. Internet at https://www.fda.gov/media/72325/download.

[31] Burt T, Young G, Lee Y, Kusuhara H, Langer O, Rowland M, et al. Phase-0 including microdosing approaches: time for mainstream application in drug development? Nat Rev Drug Discov 2020;19:801–818.

[32] Lappin GKW, Kuhnz W, Jochemsen R, Kneer J, Chaudhary A, Oosterhuis B, et al. Use of microdosing to predict pharmacokinetics at the therapeutic dose: experience with 5 drugs. Clin Pharmacol Ther 2006;80:203–215.

[33] Bosgra S, Vlaming ML, Vaes WH. To apply microdosing or not? Recommendations to single out compounds with non-linear pharmacokinetics. Clin Pharmacokinet 2016;55:1–15.

[34] van Waterschoot RAB, Parrott NJ, Olivares-Morales A, Lavé T, Rowland M, Smith DA. Impact of target interactions on small-molecule drug disposition: an overlooked area. Nat Rev Drug Discov 2018;17:299.

[35] Levy G, Mager DE, Cheung WK, Jusko WJ. Comparative pharmacokinetics of coumarin anticoagulants L: physiologic modeling of S-warfarin in rats and pharmacologic target-mediated warfarin disposition in man. J Pharm Sci 2003;92:985–994.

[36] Li R, Kimoto E, Niosi M, Tess DA, Lin J, Tremaine LM, et al. A study on pharmacokinetics of bosentan with systems modeling, part 2: prospectively predicting systemic and liver exposure in healthy subjects. Drug Metab Dispos 2018;46:357–366.

[37] Jones HM, Butt RP, Webster RW, Gurrell I, Dzygiel P, Neil Flanagan N, et al. Clinical micro-dose studies to explore the human pharmacokinetics of four selective inhibitors of human Nav1. 7 voltage-dependent sodium channels. Clin Pharmacokinet 2016;55:875–887.

Chapter 32

Phase 1 clinical studies

Robert Joseph Noveck[a] **and Martina Dagmar Sahre**[b]
[a]*Noveck Consultancy, Durham, NC, United States,* [b]*Office of Clinical Pharmacology, Food and Drug Administration, Silver Spring, MD, United States*

Introduction

The entry of a novel molecular entity into human beings for the first time is unquestionably a very exciting event for clinical pharmacologists and other practitioners involved in drug development. This chapter will concentrate on considerations for first-in-human (FIH) studies which are the beginning of testing a drug in humans (Chapter 1, Fig. 1.1).

Safety in humans is always the primary concern for FIH studies and with the use of novel adaptive approaches in study designs and recent innovations in the fields of prediction, using physiologically based models (Chapter 31) and in vitro experiments, our understanding and capacity to better anticipate drug exposure and resulting safety issues in FIH trials are now widely used to support the IND filings that are required before initiating these studies [1]. Hence, FIH studies provide an extraordinary opportunity to apply and integrate the principles of clinical pharmacology, using preclinical pharmacokinetic, pharmacodynamic, and toxicologic information while launching a new molecule on a rational path for clinical development [2, 3].

Healthy volunteers and patients in phase 1 studies

Phase 1 studies, especially FIH studies, are often conducted in healthy participants due to the interest in observing safety and tolerability, and pharmacokinetic data in a setting that is free from the influence of disease or other confounding variables. Those FIH studies that are conducted in patients are often conducted with compounds that may have toxicity that would be unacceptable in healthy participants, for example in oncology. However, with the changing landscape of oncology targets and mechanisms of action, it is becoming more common for potential (noncytotoxic) therapeutics to be studied in healthy participants. In this case, no medical benefit from participating in the trial is expected. However, these volunteers usually receive compensation for the inconveniences of participating in the study. One limitation of conducting FIH studies in healthy participants is that it limits the ability to observe the desired therapeutic effect. For example, if an agent is intended to correct metabolic deficiencies, or to lower elevated blood pressure, there may be no detectable changes in healthy participants.

Starting dose and dose escalation

Starting dose considerations for FIH studies are predicated on a need to protect trial participants from unnecessary risk while achieving the objectives of the study, which are to assess the safety and tolerability of a drug at doses that may later be studied in Phase 2 and 3 studies, as well as to gain important pharmacokinetic and, at times, pharmacodynamic information.

Starting doses can be based on several considerations. A commonly used metric is to base the starting dose on a "no observed adverse event level" (NOAEL), determined from preclinical animal testing. The NOAEL from the most sensitive and relevant animal species is then used to determine a starting dose (see also Chapter 30) [4]. However, the starting dose determined in this way can be too high in some cases. While it is rare, the combination of the NOAEL approach and results from animal species that were not appropriate to assess risk has led to problems with grave consequences for study participants [5]. Newer approaches suggest taking the totality of data into account, including potency, species differences, and in vitro models of exposure-response relationships and receptor occupancy. Important markers are the minimal anticipated biological effect level (MABEL), as well as the anticipated pharmacologically active dose (PAD). In addition, as clinical data becomes available, models that aid predictions from animals to man are refined and provide further guidance to a better understanding of the preclinical to clinical relationships [6, 7].

Atkinson's Principles of Clinical Pharmacology. https://doi.org/10.1016/B978-0-12-819869-8.00040-9

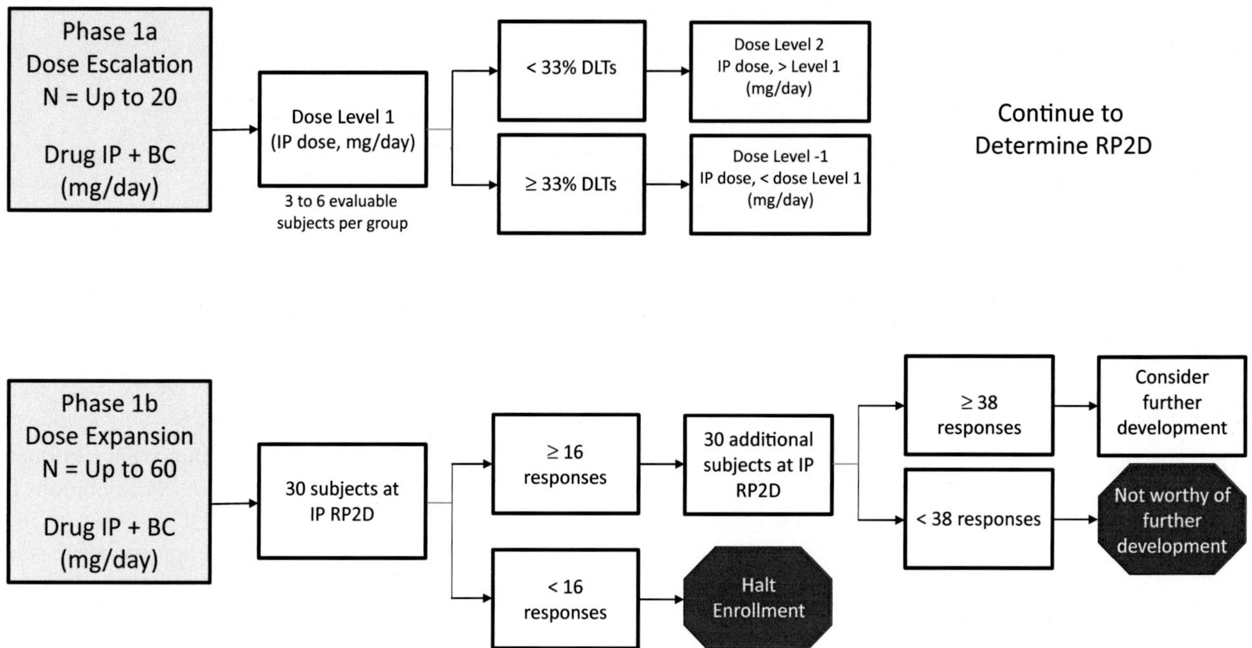

FIG. 32.1 Early cancer trial design. *(Figure developed from Simon R, Freidlin B, Rubinstein L, Arbuck SG, Collins J, Christian MC. Accelerated titration designs for phase I clinical trials in oncology. J Natl Cancer Inst 1997;89:1138–1147; Tourneau CJ, Lee J, Siu LL. Dose escalation methods in phase I cancer clinical trials, J Natl Cancer Inst 2009;101:708–720; Hansen AR, Graham DM, Pond GR, Siu LL. Phase 1 trial design: is 3 + 3 the best? Cancer Control 2014;21:200–208.)*

In determining human safety there has been an emphasis upon defining the *maximum tolerated dose* (MTD) as a study endpoint. Whereas determination of the MTD is important from the standpoint of clinical toxicology, in the past, the MTD has been selected in many cases as the dose for subsequent clinical trials, resulting in the registration and initial marketing of drug doses that are inappropriately high for some clinical conditions [8]. More recently, in FIH oncology trials where the nomenclature is not fully standardized, adaptive designs are frequently used to gain efficiency while maintaining safety. Phase 1 trials have been described as Phase 1a and 1b, simply to indicate first and second parts within a protocol (Fig. 32.1). This approach has been used to identify the *maximum tolerated dose* (MTD) in one part (Phase 1a), and then through *dose expansion*, identify the *Recommended Phase 2 Dose* (RP2D) in the other part (Phase 1b) [9–11]. Other exploratory FIH studies, described as "Phase 0," are described in Chapter 31 and have goals that are somewhat different from classic Phase 1 trials [12].

Dose escalation is based on evaluation of safety and pharmacokinetic data that becomes available throughout the trial. Every protocol defines stopping rules and criteria for the escalation of doses, which are based on adverse event rates and severity but can include exposure assessments as well. More recently, for added safety, the use of *sentinel participants* has been advocated as a way of increasing the safety of FIH studies (i.e., a single participant receives a dose of the experimental agent, and another participant receives placebo, and both are evaluated before other participants are enrolled into the cohort) [3]. This procedure is sometimes also used for subsequent cohort dose levels as well.

A modified Fibonacci scheme has traditionally been one of the more widely used methods for dose step increases. There are variations, but a common step increase is shown in Fig. 32.2. In this approach, step increases are preplanned and continue until stopping rules are triggered.

Pharmacologically guided dose escalation is a method in which data is assessed while it is accrued as the trial is ongoing. In this method, dose escalation steps are based on a combination of observed toxicity and the expectation that the toxicity at a given exposure in animals is predictive of the toxicity at the same exposure in humans [13, 14]. Dose escalation steps are then adapted based on target AUC or other pharmacokinetic markers. There are other designs that use data as it becomes available in the trial. For example, the *continuous reassessment method* is based on observed toxicity rates and prediction of likelihood of a participant experiencing toxicity. These methods have been replacing standard Fibonacci schemes in many oncology studies [9].

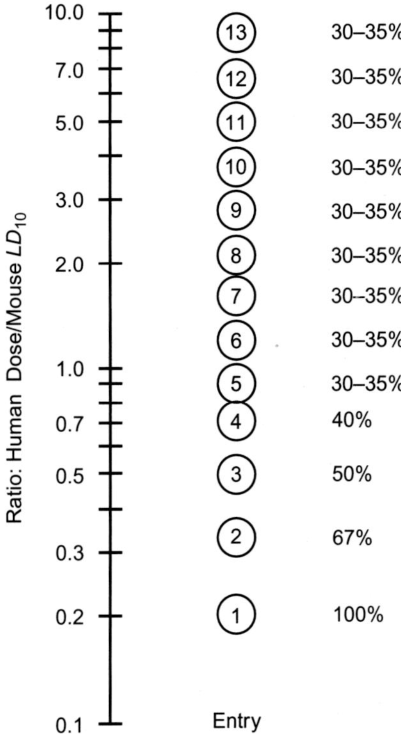

FIG. 32.2 Modified Fibonacci dose escalation procedure, expressed as a ratio of the human dose to a reference dose in mice (e.g., the 10% lethal dose (LD10)). Human studies typically start at one-tenth the murine dose, expressed on the basis of body surface area. If tolerated, the next dose is initially doubled, then the percentage change at each escalation step decreases. *(Reproduced from Collins JM, Zaharko DS, Dedrick RL, Chabner BA. Potential roles for preclinical pharmacology in phase I trials. Cancer Treat Rep 1986;70:73–80.)*

Many trials use expansion cohorts to increase efficiency in drug development, especially in oncology. Expansion cohorts are patient cohorts that are added after the dose escalation phase to obtain either more safety data, data in specific patient populations, assessment of a biomarker, or even preliminary efficacy data [15].

Limitations of the use of preclinical species data to predict human exposure and toxicity

Interspecies differences in drug metabolism

The data in Table 32.1 for iododeoxydoxorubicin (I-Dox) were obtained during FIH studies conducted by Gianni et al. [16]. There was greater exposure to the parent drug in mice and to the hydroxylated metabolite (I-Dox-ol) in humans. Overall, there was a 50-fold difference in the relative AUC metabolite/parent drug exposure ratios for humans and mice. Because I-Dox and I-Dox-ol are approximately equieffective and equitoxic, these exposure comparisons are also indicative of pharmacologic response. This extreme example of an interspecies difference in drug metabolism was comparable to studying

TABLE 32.1 AUC values in plasma for iododeoxydoxorubicin (I-Dox) and its metabolite (I-Dox-ol) in mouse and human equitoxic doses.

Compound	Mouse (mM·h)	Human (mM·h)
I-Dox	5.0	0.3
I-Dox-ol	1.2	4.0

Data from Gianni L, Vigano L, Surbone A, et al. Pharmacology and clinical toxicity of 40-iodo-40-deoxydoxorubicin: an example of successful application of pharmacokinetics to dose escalation in phase I trials. J Natl Cancer Inst 1990;82:469–477.

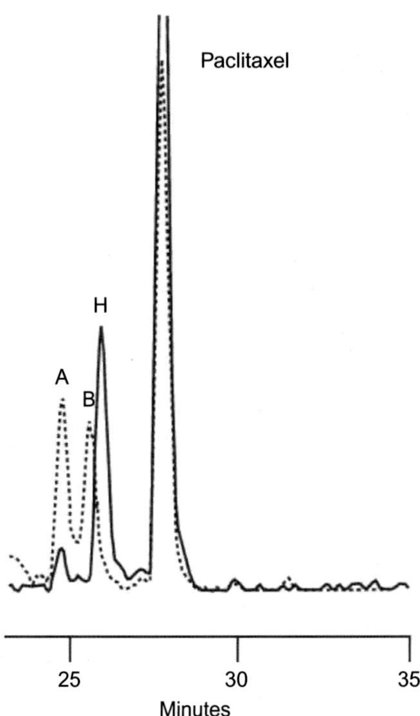

FIG. 32.3 High-performance liquid chromatograms comparing in vitro paclitaxel metabolism by hepatic microsomes from rats *(dotted line)* and humans *(solid line)*. The major human metabolite, designated peak "H," was not formed by rats. *(Adapted from Jamis-Dow CA, Klecker RW, Katki AG, Collins JM. Metabolism of taxol by human and rat liver in vitro: a screen for drug interactions and interspecies differences. Cancer Chemother Pharmacol 1995;6:107–114.)*

one molecule (the parent) in mice and then (unintentionally) studying a different molecule (the metabolite) in humans. The similarity in potency of the parent molecule and metabolite was fortuitous and ordinarily not expected, especially for both desirable and adverse effects.

Fig. 32.3 illustrates an interspecies difference in paclitaxel metabolism [17]. The principal metabolite formed in humans was not produced by rat microsomes. This example illustrates the potential of in vitro studies to discover interspecies differences in metabolism. In most cases it is no longer necessary, and certainly not advisable, to wait for in vivo Phase 1 studies to discover such differences. For that reason, regulatory authorities around the world have encouraged early consideration of interspecies metabolic comparisons.

Active metabolites

During FIH studies with the investigational anticancer drug penclomedine, it was discovered that exposure to parent drug concentrations was less than 1% of the exposure to its metabolite, demethylpenclomedine [18]. As shown in Fig. 32.4, exposure to the parent drug was very brief, while the metabolite accumulated during the course of a 5-day treatment cycle. Because the toxicity of the parent molecule limits the amount of tolerable exposure to the metabolite, which provides the antitumor effect, the penclomedine example clearly demonstrates the danger of not knowing which molecules are circulating in the body. If this type of information is determined early enough in drug development, the metabolite can be selected to replace the parent molecule as the lead development candidate.

There is stunning similarity of the penclomedine story to the history of terfenadine (Seldane), a highly successful antihistamine product that was withdrawn from marketing. In early clinical studies, it was not appreciated that the major source of clinical benefit was derived from its metabolite, fexofenadine (Allegra; see structures in Chapter 1, Fig. 1.2). It became obvious that the metabolite should have been the lead compound only after cardiotoxicity was subsequently discovered for the parent drug but not the metabolite.

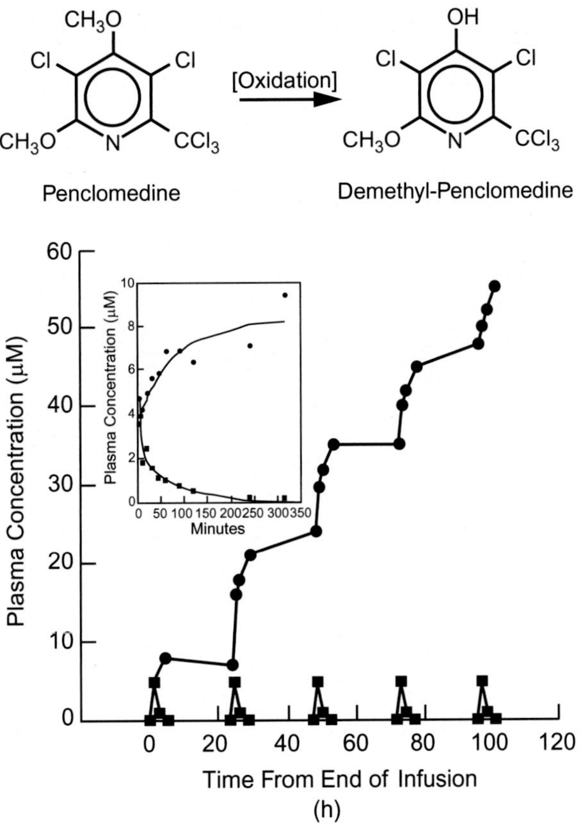

FIG. 32.4 The investigational anticancer drug, penclomedine, was administered to patients once a day for 5 consecutive days. The parent drug disappeared rapidly from plasma, whereas the demethyl metabolite accumulated over the course of therapy. *(Adapted from Hartman NR, O'Reilly S, Rowinsky EK, et al. Murine and human in vivo penclomedine metabolism. Clin Cancer Res 996;2:953–962.)*

Beyond toxicity

The study of toxicity without consideration of efficacy is inherently unsatisfying. Indeed, when patients participate in Phase 1 trials, there is usually therapeutic intent. Although there is only a low probability of success in many settings, the obligation is to maximize that chance. As it becomes more common to seek "proof-of-concept" or mechanistic evaluations during Phase 1, an increased emphasis on demonstrating therapeutic activity—the usual domain for Phase 2 studies—looms on the horizon. By monitoring a target biomarker, both proof-of-concept and dose determination might be achieved simultaneously. Further, by enrolling in the trial, patients who have favorable expression profiles of the target, an "enriched" population is obtained with a higher likelihood of response if the therapeutic concept has merit. For "accessible" targets such as blood pressure or heart rate, these concepts are not new. The techniques of external, noninvasive imaging described in Chapter 18 now permit real-time monitoring of targets such as in situ regions of the human brain that were previously considered inaccessible. Fowler et al. [19] reported a study of the inhibition of monoamine oxidase, type B (MAO-B) by lazabemide (Fig. 32.5). A dose of 25 mg twice a day inhibited most MAO-B activity in subjects and doubling the dose to 50 mg abolished all detectable activity. Also, brain activity for MAO-B had returned to baseline values within 36 hours of the last dose of lazabemide. This example of MAO-B inhibition demonstrates the successful investigation in early human studies of three areas of fundamental interest in developing drug therapy (Table 32.2): monitoring impact at the desired target, evaluating the dose-response relationship (dose ranging), and determining an appropriate dose interval from recovery of enzyme activity.

The expansion of Phase 1 studies to include goals formerly reserved for Phase 2 evaluation is only one direction of change. Simultaneously, the toxicity goals of Phase 1 studies are being decoupled from evaluations of drug absorption, distribution, metabolism, and excretion (ADME) to include additional objectives early in development [20]. As described in Chapter 31, both the United States and the European regulators now permit microdose studies that include both metabolism and excretion components as well as tracer doses for imaging [12]. In both regulatory sectors, the preclinical requirements for FIH studies are substantially reduced for situations in which doses are kept low to minimize risk to study participants. This structural change facilitates the type of translational research that has been described as Phase 0 or pre-Phase 1.

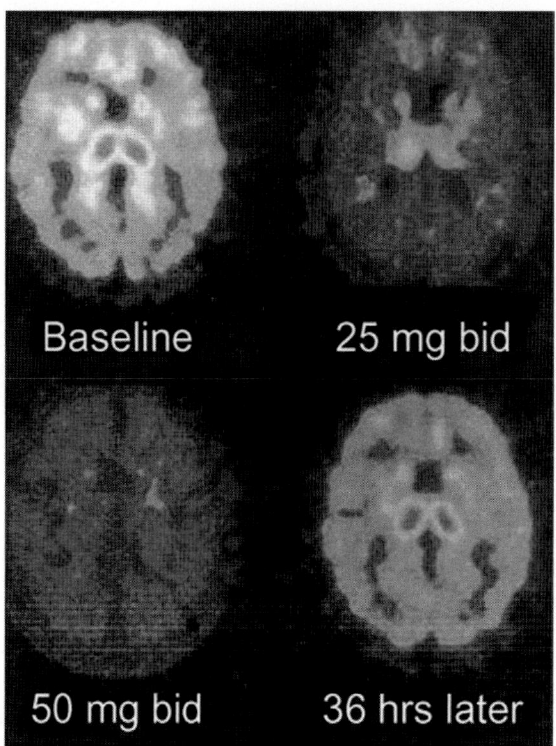

FIG. 32.5 PET scans showing dose dependency and time dependency of lazabemide inhibition of monoamine oxidase, type B in human brain. *(From Fowler JS, Volkow ND, Logan J, Schlyer DJ, MacGregor RR, Wang G-J, et al. Monoamine oxidase B (MAO B) inhibitor therapy in Parkinson's disease: the degree and reversibility of human brain MAO B inhibition by Ro 19 6327. Neurology 1993;43(10):1984. https://doi.org/10.1212/WNL.43.10.1984.)*

TABLE 32.2 Therapeutic issues for drug development.
• Does treatment impact the desired target?
• What is the minimum/maximum acceptable dose?
• What dose (therapeutic course) interval is appropriate?

These developments provide an opportunity to change the traditional goals of early drug development and to reengineer the entire drug development pipeline. However, this blurring of the traditional lines of demarcation between clinical phases of drug development has its pitfalls and disorienting aspects, and not all development organizations will adopt such changes. Indeed, there should always be a place for diversity in approaches to drug development. Nonetheless, the early harvesting of benefits from investments in biomarkers presents exciting new opportunities for clinical pharmacologists and other stakeholders in drug development. Recently, an international consortium of pharmaceutical stakeholders addressed the critical topic of FIH starting dose and published recommendations using data-driven and a risk-based approach [21].

Acknowledgment

The authors wish to acknowledge Dr. Jerry M. Collins for his previous contributions in writing this chapter.

References

[1] Food and Drug Administration, Center for Drug Evaluation and Research. Physiologically based pharmacokinetic analyses—Format and content guidance for industry, https://www.fda.gov/regulatory-information/search-fda-guidance-documents/physiologically-based-pharmacokinetic-analyses-format-and-content-guidance-industry; 2018. [Accessed 15 November 2020].

[2] Peck CC, Barr WH, Benet LZ, Collins J, Desjardins RE, Furst DE, et al. Opportunities for integration of pharmacokinetics, pharmacodynamics, and toxicokinetics in rational drug development. Clin Pharmacol Ther 1992;51:465–73.

[3] Shen J, Swift B, Mamelok R, Pine S, Sinclair J, Attar M. Design and conduct considerations for first-in-human trials. Clin Transl Sci 2019;12:6–19.

[4] Food and Drug Administration, Center for Drug Evaluation and Research. Estimating the maximum safe starting dose in initial clinical trials for therapeutics in adult healthy volunteers guidance for industry, https://www.fda.gov/regulatory-information/search-fda-guidance-documents/estimating-maximum-safe-starting-dose-initial-clinical-trials-therapeutics-adult-healthy-volunteers; 2005. [Accessed 15 November 2020].

[5] Dowsing T, Kendall MJ. The Northwick Park tragedy—protecting healthy volunteers in future first-in-man trials. J Clin Pharm Ther 2007;32:203–7.

[6] Miller NA, Reddy MB, Heikkinen AT, Lukacova V, Parrott N. Physiologically based pharmacokinetic modelling for first-in-human predictions: an updated model building strategy illustrated with challenging industry case studies. Clin Pharmacokinet 2019;58:727–46.

[7] Liu D, Song H, Song L, Liu Y, Cao Y, Jiang J, et al. A unified strategy in selection of the best allometric scaling methods to predict human clearance based on drug disposition pathway. Xenobiotica 2016;46:1105–11.

[8] Rolan P. The contribution of clinical pharmacology surrogates and models to drug development—a critical appraisal. Br J Clin Pharmacol 1997;44:219–25.

[9] Simon R, Freidlin B, Rubinstein L, Arbuck SG, Collins J, Christian MC. Accelerated titration designs for phase I clinical trials in oncology. J Natl Cancer Inst 1997;89:1138–47.

[10] Tourneau CJ, Lee J, Siu LL. Dose escalation methods in phase I cancer clinical trials. J Natl Cancer Inst 2009;101:708–20.

[11] Hansen AR, Graham DM, Pond GR, Siu LL. Phase 1 trial design: is 3 + 3 the best? Cancer Control 2014;21:200–8.

[12] Food and Drug Administration, Center for Drug Evaluation and Research. Guidance for industry, investigators, and reviewers: Exploratory IND studies guidance for industry, https://www.fda.gov/regulatory-information/search-fda-guidance-documents/exploratory-ind-studies; 2006. [Accessed 15 November 2020].

[13] Collins JM, Grieshaber CK, Chabner BA. Pharmacologically-guided phase I trials based upon pre-clinical development. J Natl Cancer Inst 1990;82:1321–6.

[14] Collins JM, Zaharko DS, Dedrick RL, Chabner BA. Potential roles for preclinical pharmacology in phase I trials. Cancer Treat Rep 1986;70:73–80.

[15] Food and Drug Administration, Center for Drug Evaluation and Research. Expansion cohorts: Use in first-in-human clinical trials to expedite development of oncology drugs and biologics guidance for industry, https://www.fda.gov/regulatory-information/search-fda-guidance-documents/expansion-cohorts-use-first-human-clinical-trials-expedite-development-oncology-drugs-and-biologics; 2018. [Accessed 15 November 2020].

[16] Gianni L, Vigano L, Surbone A, Ballinari D, Casali P, Tarella C, et al. Pharmacology and clinical toxicity of 40-iodo-40-deoxydoxorubicin: an example of successful application of pharmacokinetics to dose escalation in phase I trials. J Natl Cancer Inst 1990;82:469–77.

[17] Jamis-Dow CA, Klecker RW, Katki AG, Collins JM. Metabolism of taxol by human and rat liver in vitro: a screen for drug interactions and interspecies differences. Cancer Chemother Pharmacol 1995;6:107–14.

[18] Hartman NR, O'Reilly S, Rowinsky EK, Collins JM, Strong JM. Murine and human in vivo penclomedine metabolism. Clin Cancer Res 1996;2:953–62.

[19] Fowler JS, Volkow ND, Wang G-J, Dewey SL. PET and drug research and development. J Nucl Med 1999;40:1154–63.

[20] Food and Drug Administration, Center for Drug Evaluation and Research. Clinical drug interaction studies—Cytochrome P450 enzyme- and transporter-mediated drug interactions guidance for industry, https://www.fda.gov/regulatory-information/search-fda-guidance-documents/clinical-drug-interaction-studies-cytochrome-p450-enzyme-and-transporter-mediated-drug-interactions; 2020. [Accessed 15 November 2020].

[21] Leach MW, Clarke DO, Dudal S, Han C, Li C, Yang Z, Brennan FR, et al. Strategies and recommendations for using a data-driven and risk-based approach in the selection of first-in-human starting dose: an international consortium for innovation and quality in pharmaceutical development (IQ) assessment. Clin Pharmacol Ther 2021;109(6):1395–416. https://doi.org/10.1002/cpt.2009. 32757299.

Chapter 33

Pharmacokinetic and pharmacodynamic considerations in the development of biotechnology products and large molecules

Pamela D. Garzone[a] and Yow-Ming C. Wang[b]

[a]*Anixa Biosciences, San Jose, CA, United States,* [b]*Office of Clinical Pharmacology, Office of Translational Sciences, Center for Drug Evaluation and Research, Food and Drug Administration, Silver Spring, MD, United States*

Introduction

Biologics currently account for more than 25% of FDA approved entities, and this percentage is expected to increase. The number of FDA approvals reached an all-time high in 2018 and included novel biologics such as antibody drug conjugates, cytotoxic fusion proteins, and bi-specific antibodies [1]. In 2010, the FDA approved 15 new molecular entities and 6 new biologics. Biologics accounted for slightly more than 25% of the approved entities and this percentage has remained steady until 2018, which as noted, reached an all-time high [2] (Fig. 33.1). Since 2014, cancer therapeutics have been the top disease category for which biologics have been developed, and the oncology segment is also the top segment of the growing rare disease market.

For the purpose of this chapter, a macromolecule is defined as a large molecule, with a molecular mass in kilodaltons (kDa), such as a protein or glycoprotein, or a monoclonal antibody, consisting of either an intact immunoglobulin or its fragments. Well-known macromolecules that have been approved and are currently marketed are listed in Table 33.1. This chapter presents information on proteins and mAbs currently marketed or under investigation and discusses methodology used to assay macromolecules, interspecies scaling of macromolecules, pharmacokinetic (PK) characteristics of macromolecules, and pharmacodynamics (PD) of macromolecules.

Monoclonal antibodies

Monoclonal antibodies (mAbs) were initially considered "magic bullets" offering, for the first time, targeted therapy against specific tumor surface antigens. The development of mAbs as diagnostic aids and as therapy was made possible by advances in hybridoma technology [3]. The first murine monoclonal antibody trial was published in 1982 [4]. However, in the 1980s and early 1990s most of the murine mAbs failed in clinical trials. The major drawback was the inefficient interaction of the Fc component of the mouse antibody with human effector functions [5]. The repeated administration of mouse antibodies to humans also resulted in the production of a human antimouse antibody (HAMA) response that reduced the effectiveness of the murine antibody or resulted in allergic reactions in humans.

The first murine mAb was approved for marketing in 1986, when Orthoclone (a cluster of differentiation [CD]3-specific antibody) or OKT3 was approved for treating patients with graft versus host disease. Presently, CD3 is an important target of bi-specific antibodies that are designed to engage and redirect T-cells to tumors. Now, humanized and fully human antibodies, engineered so that HAMA response is negligible, have become mainstream therapy (Table 33.1). The following sections describe how engineered antibodies can be produced to meet these requirements.

Monoclonal antibody structure and production

A successful antibody needs to be potent and specific [6]. The basic structure of an immunoglobulin (Ig) antibody, IgG, is shown in Fig. 33.2. The IgG molecule consists of an Fc region and one Fab region which provide multivalency, high avidity,

Atkinson's Principles of Clinical Pharmacology. https://doi.org/10.1016/B978-0-12-819869-8.00011-2

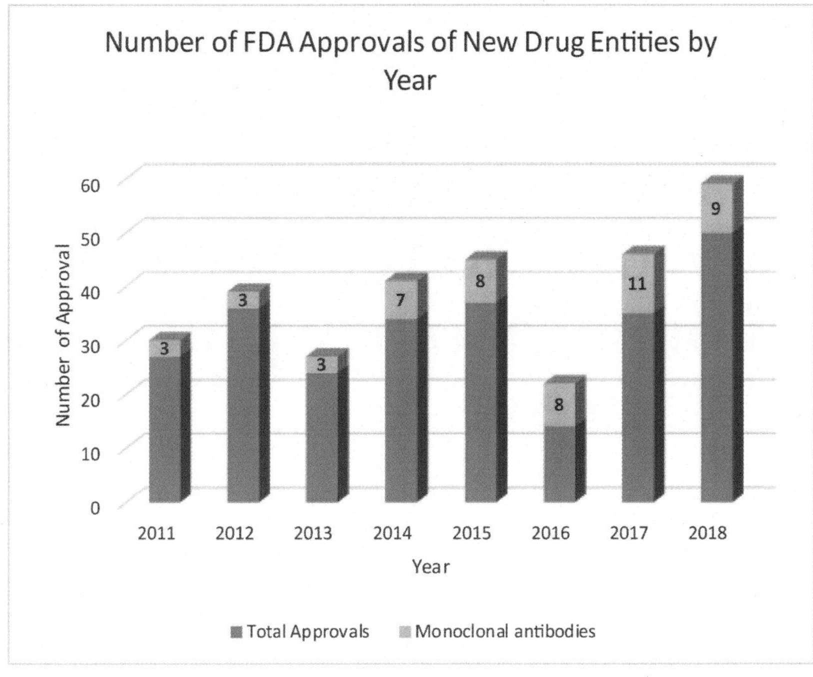

FIG. 33.1 Graph of number of approved drugs and percentage that were biologics. *Created with data from FDA (CDER) 2018 Advancing health through innovation 2018 new drug therapy approvals report. Internet at: https://www.fda.gov/files/drugs/published/New-Drug-Therapy-Approvals-2018_3.pdf.*

TABLE 33.1 Summary of currently marketed macromolecules.

Name	International nonproprietary name (INN)	Company	Target	Type	Year of first FDA approval	Therapeutic indication(s)
Ajovy	Fremanezumab	Teva	GCRPαβ	Humanized IgG_1	2018	Prevention of migraines
Ultomiris	Ravulizumab	Alexion Pharmaceuticals	Complement component 5	Humanized $IgG_{2/4}$	2018	Treatment of paroxysmal nocturnal hemoglobinuria
Lumoxiti	Moxetumomab pasudotox	Astra Zeneca	Anti-CD22 immunotoxin	Fv fragment fused to Pseudomonas exotoxin	2018	Treatment of adult patients with relapsed or refractory hairy cell leukemia (HCL) who have received at least two prior systemic therapies
Takhzyro	Lanadelumab	Shire	Kallikrein	Human IgG_1	2018	Hereditary angioedema
Poteligeo	Mogamulizumab	Kyowa Hallo Kirin	CCR4	Humanized, glyco-engineered IgG_1, κ-chain	2018	Adult T-cell leukemia or lymphoma
Aimovig	Erenumab	Amgen and Novartis	Calcitonin gene related peptide (CGRP)	Human IgG_1	2018	Prevention of migraines in adults
Bavencio	Avelumab	Merck Sharp & Dohme Limited	PD-L1	Human IgG_1	2017	Metastatic Merkel cell carcinoma
Dupixent	Dupilumab	Regeneron Pharmaceuticals Inc	IL-4Rα	Human IgG_4	2017	Asthma; dermatitis
Imfinzi	Durvalumab	Astrazeneca UK	PD-L1	Human $IgG_{1/\kappa}$	2017	Metastatic urothelial carcinoma

TABLE 33.1 Summary of currently marketed macromolecules—cont'd

Name	International nonproprietary name (INN)	Company	Target	Type	Year of first FDA approval	Therapeutic indication(s)
Ocrevus	Ocrelizumab	Genentech (Roche)	CD20	Humanized $IgG_{1\kappa}$	2017	Multiple sclerosis
Siliq	Brodalumab	Valeant Pharmaceuticals international	IL-17RA	Human $IgG_{2/\kappa}$	2017	Psoriasis
Amjevita	Adalimumab	Amgen Europe	TNFα	Human IgG_1	2016	Arthritis; juvenile rheumatoid arthritis; psoriatic arthritis; rheumatoid colitis; ulcerative Crohn's disease; psoriasis; spondylitis; ankylosing
Zinplava	Bezlotoxumab	Merck Sharp & Dohme Limited	*C. difficile* toxin B	Human monoclonal antitoxin antibody	2016	Enterocolitis; pseudomembranous
Cinqair	Reslizumab	Teva Pharmaceuticals Limited	IL-5	Human $IgG_{4/\kappa}$	2016	Asthma
Lartruvo	Olaratumab	Eli Lilly	PDGFR-α	Human IgG_1	2016	Sarcoma
Inflectra	Infliximab	Hospira UK Limited	TNFα	Chimeric human-murine IgG_1	2016	Spondylitis; ankylosing; arthritis; rheumatoid colitis; ulcerative arthritis; psoriatic Crohn's Disease; psoriasis
Darzalex	Daratumumab	Janssen-Cilag	CD38	Human $IgG_{1/\kappa}$	2015	Multiple myeloma
Empliciti	Elotuzumab	Bristol-Myers Squibb	SLAMF7	Human IgG_1	2015	Multiple myeloma
Portrazza	Necitumumab	Eli Lilly	EGFR	Human IgG_1	2015	Carcinoma, nonsmall cell lung
Anthim	Obiltoxaximab	Elusys Therapeutics INC	PA component of B. anthracis toxin	Chimeric (mouse/ human) $IgG_{1/\kappa}$	2016	Anthrax infection
Tecentriq	Atezolizumab	Genentech (Roche)	PD-L1	Human IgG_1	2016	Metastatic nonsmall cell lung cancer
Cosentyx	Secukinumab	Novartis Europharm	interleukin-17A	Human $IgG_{1/\kappa}$	2015	Arthritis; psoriatic psoriasis; spondylitis; ankylosing
Nucala	Mepolizumab	GlaxoSmithKline	IL-5	Human $IgG_{1/\kappa}$	2015	Asthma
Opdivo	Nivolumab	Bristol-Myers Squibb Pharma	PD-1	Human IgG_4	2015	Carcinoma; nonsmall cell lung carcinoma; renal cell Hodgkin disease melanoma
Praluent	Alirocumab	sanofi-aventis groupe	PCSK9	Human IgG_1	2015	Dyslipidemias
Praxbind	Idarucizumab	Boehringer Ingelheim International GmbH	dabigatran etexilate	Human FaB	2015	Hemorrhage
Repatha	Evolocumab	Amgen	LDL-C/ PCSK9	Human IgG_2	2015	Dyslipidemias; hypercholesterolemia

Continued

TABLE 33.1 Summary of currently marketed macromolecules—cont'd

Name	International nonproprietary name (INN)	Company	Target	Type	Year of first FDA approval	Therapeutic indication(s)
Unituxin	Dinutuximab	United Therapeutics Europe	GD2	Human $IgG_{1/\kappa}$	2015	Neuroblastoma
Blincyto	Bevacizumab	Amgen Europe	CD19	BiTEs	2014	Precursor cell lymphoblastic leukemia-lymphoma
Keytruda	Pembrolizumab	Merck Sharp & Dohme Limited	PD-1	Human IgG_4	2014	Melanoma
Cyramza	Ramucirumab	Eli Lilly	VEGF	Human IgG_1	2014	Stomach neoplasms
Entyvio	Vedolizumab	Takeda Pharma	Integrin-$\alpha 4\beta 7$	Humanized IgG_1	2014	Colitis; ulcerative Crohn's disease
Sylvant	Siltuximab	Janssen-Cilag International	cCLB8	Chimeric $IgG_{1\kappa}$	2014	Giant lymph node hyperplasia
Lemtrada	Alemtuzumab	Sanofi	CD52	Humanized IgG_1	2014	Multiple sclerosis
Kadcyla	Trastuzumab emtansine	Roche	HER2	Humanized IgG_1 as ADC	2013	Breast cancer
Gazyvaro	Obinutuzumab	Roche	CD20	Humanized IgG_1	2013	CLL
Perjeta	Pertuzumab	Roche	HER2	Humanized IgG_1	2012	Breast cancer
Adcetris	Brentuximab	Seattle Genetics	CD30 (conjugate of Mab and MMAE)	Chimeric IgG_1 as ADC (antibody drug conjugate)	2011	Hodgkin lymphoma (HL), systemic anaplastic large cell lymphoma (ALCL)
ABthrax	Raxibacumab	HGS (Human Genome Sciences Inc.)	Bacillus anthracis protective antigen	Human IgG_1	2012	Prevention and treatment of inhalation anthrax

and specificity. It should be noted that IgG sequences are conserved across species such that considerable homology between mouse and human variable regions exists [7]. Mouse antibodies can be further engineered by molecular cloning and expression of the variable region of IgG to be more human, or they can be fully human. Fully human mAbs, derived from transgenic mice or human antibody libraries, are the current state-of-the-art of mAb bioengineering [8].

Monoclonal antibodies, by definition, are produced by a single clone of hybridoma cells, i.e., a single species of antibody molecule (Fig. 33.3) [8]. However, engineered monoclonal antibodies can be chimeras, in which the Fv region from mouse IgG is fused with the variable region of the human IgG. Monoclonal antibodies can be humanized so that only the complementary determining regions of the murine variable region are combined into the human variable region. In addition to being full length, mAbs can be single-chain IgG, the simplest fragment being the scFv (single-chain variable fragment). The scFv can be a monomer, dimer, or tetramer; this multivalency results in a significant increase in functional affinity [9]. Further, in addition to the diversity of engineered antibodies, other molecules can be attached to the antibody, such as toxins, radionuclides, and biosensors for targeting, imaging, or diagnosing. These are commonly referred to as antibody drug conjugates, or ADC.

The production of antibodies appears to be simple (Fig. 33.3). However, their commercialization is challenging. The need for specificity makes the market small; thus the costs of doing clinical trials for small markets are unattractive to most

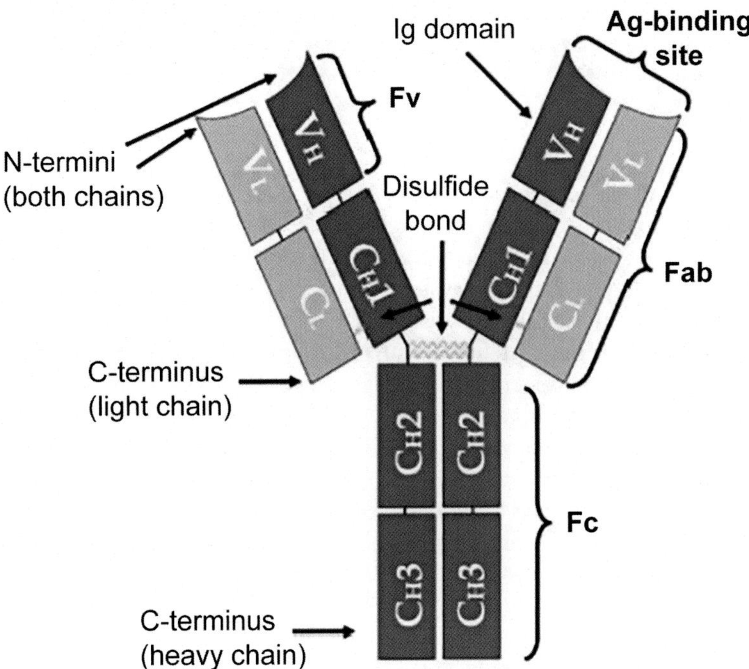

FIG. 33.2 Structure of prototypical IgG and single-chain Fv (scFv) antibody molecules. The large solid-line box encloses the divalent Fab′ molecules; the small dotted line box, the Fab′ fragment; the large dashed-line box, the Fc components; and the small dashed-line box, the Fv components which are the antigen-binding sites. The variable light-chain region is designated V_L and variable heavy-chain region is designated V_H. Other definitions: constant region domains, C_{H1}, C_{H2}, C_{H3}; hinge, Hi; constant light region, C_L; linker region, Lkr. Conserved N-linked (–N–N–) carbohydrates are located in the Fc domain; cysteine bond (–S–S–) join heavy and light chains. *Reprinted by permission of Edizioni Minerva Medica from Q J Nucl Med 1999;43(2):132–139.*

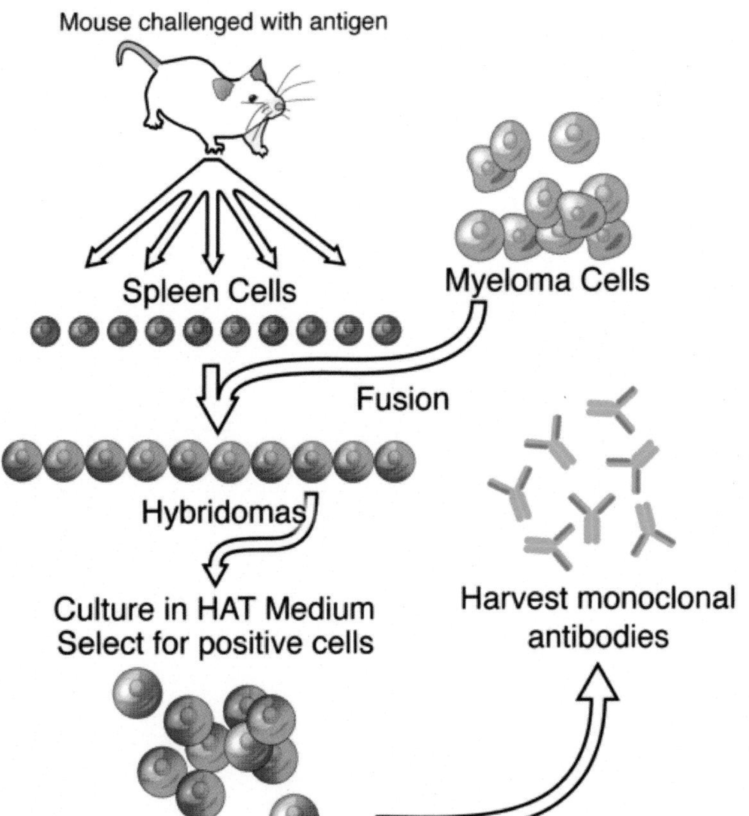

FIG. 33.3 Cartoon depicting monoclonal antibody production. A mouse is immunized by injection of an antigen to stimulate the production of antibodies targeted against it. The antibody-forming cells are isolated from the mouse's spleen. Monoclonal antibodies are produced by fusing single antibody-forming cells to tumor cells grown in culture. The resulting cell is called a *hybridoma*. Each hybridoma produces relatively large quantities of identical antibody molecules. By allowing the hybridoma to multiply in culture it is possible to produce a population of cells, each of which produces identical antibody molecules. These antibodies are called *monoclonal antibodies* because they are produced by the identical offspring of a single, cloned antibody-producing cell. *Abbreviation:* HAT is a culture medium that contains hypoxanthine, aminopterin, and thymidine. http://en.wikipedia.org/wiki/Monoclonal_antibodies. *Reproduced from Internet at: https://en.wikipedia.org/wiki/Monoclonal_antibody#/media/File:Monoclonals.png) (licensed under Creative Commons Attribution-Share Alike 3.0 Unported license).*

companies. Quality control of the production and manufacture of monoclonal antibodies is another issue, since a high degree of purification and low degree of contamination is necessary before approval. Finally, a major limitation is the stability of the mammalian cells expressing the immunoglobulin [10].

Pharmacokinetic properties of monoclonal antibodies

Many of the factors affecting the PK of mAbs are similar to those affecting other macromolecules, and these principles are explored in the following sections. However, the optimal mAb dose and schedule also are determined by several additional factors, such as the avidity of the antibody and the specific antibody-antigen system, the species used in nonclinical studies to inform human dosing, and the mAb itself. Dose selection influences mAb distribution into organs and tissues and liver uptake. At lower doses target-mediated clearance may be observed, particularly with mAbs directed at cell surface targets. With increasing dose, saturation of binding sites, including nonspecific binding, is expected to occur and results in decreased clearance and greater availability of the antibody to the target.

The most characteristic features of mAbs are their low blood clearance and prolonged elimination half-life. It has been demonstrated for both intact mAbs and fragments that clearance is inversely related to molecular size (Table 33.2) [11, 12]. Detailed investigations have been undertaken to explore the specific IgG structures that may affect clearance and half-life. In particular, the Fc receptor, FcRn (neonatal MHC class I-related receptor), has been shown to play a central role in determining IgG half-life, and specific sequences in the C_{H2} and C_{H3} regions of IgG regulate clearance rate through their interaction with FcRn [13].

While the prolonged half-life of a mAb is usually advantageous, allowing for infrequent administration, it also has some disadvantages. For example, mAbs with the longest half-lives and lowest clearance rates diffuse poorly across tumor membranes. This feature can result in significant exposure to normal tissues and organs when effective antitumor doses are administered. In contrast, scFv fragments, one of the smallest functional amino acid sequences of antibodies, have more rapid clearance and better penetration of tumor mass than intact mAbs, yet retain high-affinity binding (Table 33.3) [13]. Also, tumor-to-blood concentration ratios appear to be higher and less heterogeneous with multivalent scFvs than with intact antibody. $F(ab)_2$ elimination clearance appears to be similar to intact IgG, but with a faster distribution to tissues from blood and a higher uptake in kidneys. Other fragments, such as Fab′, $sc(Fv)_2$, $(scFv)_2$, and scFv, have lower uptake in tissues due to their rapid elimination. For example, approximately 90% of scFvs are cleared from the body in 24 hours. Lastly, the charge of a mAb has been shown to affect PK and tissue distribution due to electrostatic and hydrophobic interactions between mammalian cell membrane lipid bilayers and negatively charged proteins [14]. Factors that may influence the effects of charge on mAb PK and tissue distribution include the magnitude of the change in isoelectric point (pI), the IgG isotype (i.e., IgG_1, IgG_2, IgG_4), the location of the charge (e.g., variable region vs the constant region of the IgG molecule), and the binding avidity. Cationization, the chemical conversion of surface carboxyl groups on aspartate or glutamate to primary amino groups, can raise the pI of macromolecules [15]. Raising the pI of mAbs has been shown to increase the rate of clearance of an IgG_{2a} cationized mAb from the blood, resulting in higher tissue concentrations relative to a native

TABLE 33.2 Proposed human plasma clearance of different antibody molecules

Antibody molecule	Molecular weight (kD)	Relative plasma clearance (*CL*)
Native intact human IgG	150	≈21 days
Fully human/humanized	150	↓
Chimeric human-mouse IgG	150	
Whole mouse IgG	150	
$F(ab)_2$	110	
Fab′	50	
Single chain Fv (scFv)	25	≈1 day

Adapted from Iznaga-Escobar N, Mishra Ak, Perez-Rodriguez R. Methods Find Exp Clin Pharmacol 2004; 26:123–127.

TABLE 33.3 Tumor, kidney and blood distribution, as percentage of dose per gram of iodinated antibody fragments of CC49.

Antibody fragment	Tissue	Time (h)				
		0.5	4.0	24.0	48.0	72.0
scFv	Tumor/Blood/ Kidneys	4.74/4.66/41.24	2.93/1.32/2.65	1.06/0.06/0.15	0.72/0.04/0.07	0.27/0.05/0.06
$(scFv)_2$	Tumor/Blood/ Kidneys	5.94/19.27/32.83	6.91/2.56/2.93	4.29/0.10/0.42	2.56/0.07/0.13	1.92/0.07/0.08
$Sc(Fv)_2$	Tumor/Blood/ Kidneys	6.12/18.30/27.85	6.78/2.17/2.32	4.29/0.07/0.36	2.62/0.06/0.12	1.94/0.07/0.07
Fab′	Tumor/Blood/ Kidneys	4.87/9.63/138.34	5.91/2.38/21.50	2.96/0.1/0.37	2.15/0.06/0.16	ND[a]/ND/ND
$F(ab')_2$	Tumor/Blood/ Kidneys	14.63/30.15/11.48	25.82/16.32/9.78	28.06/1.68/2.10	19.42/0.36/0.52	13.11/0.16/0.25
IgG	Tumor/Blood/ Kidneys	8.95/28.32/7.0	30.66/24.20/5.29	37.83/11.01/2.19	42.42/5.34/1.18	ND/ND/ND

[a]*ND, not determined.*
Adapted from Colcher D, Pavlinkova G, Beresford G, et al. Ann NY Acad Sci 1999;880:263–280.

IgG_{2a} mAb in mice [15, 16]. In contrast, in mice given IgG_4 antibodies with pIs ranging from 7.2 to 9.2, the elimination half-life increased with increasing pI [17].

As noted earlier, the earliest mAbs were derived entirely from mouse proteins and caused highly immunogenic reactions in patients. This reaction, the HAMA response, was against both the constant and the variable regions of the proteins. In addition to the signs and symptoms of the HAMA response that included the classic allergic hallmarks of urticaria, anaphylaxis, and fever, this response resulted in attenuated mAb activity due to the formation of neutralizing antibodies and rapid clearance of the resulting immune complex. Although the HAMA response has been mitigated by the development of humanized or fully human antibodies, these antibodies still can elicit antiallotypic or antiidiotypic antibody responses [12].

Bi-specific antibodies

Bi-specific antibodies (BsAbs) are antibodies in various configurations (Fig. 33.4). The commonality of all of the constructs is the utilization of the variable domains, e.g., two pairs of V_L and V_H, one for one target and the other for another target, producing a hybrid. The constructs are not limited to engaging just 2 binding targets. The constructs can bind to more than 2, such as the tri-specifics which can bind to 3 sites. Specific advantages of bi-specific antibodies are as follows: (1) specificity is good even though engaging more than one target; (2) the many constructs from scFv fragments to full IgG antibodies have different PK properties which can be tailored for use; and (3) instead of 2 separate antibodies being produced, there is efficient production of the hybrid.

As previously noted, hybridoma technology enabled the production of murine antibodies, such as the murine antibody, OKT3 (Orthoclone), the first mAb directed toward the cluster of differentiation-3 (CD3) on the surface of T-cells. Hybridoma technology proved to be cumbersome and inefficient. Since the first attempt of combining antibody fragments of differing specificities [18], advances in technology have resulted in the production of monoclonal antibodies of any configuration, specificity, and stability.

First generation bi-specifics were products of protein digestion [18], reducing the IgG antibody to individual components such as a Fab' and then, with crosslinking reagents, creating heterodimers. Unfortunately, these constructs were very unstable, hard to purify, and had reduced activity.

Quadroma technology—the somatic fusion of two different hybridoma cells producing monoclonal antibodies with the desired specificity—was another approach to the production of bi-specific antibodies. Molecules produced by quadroma technology retained immune effector functions of antibody-dependent cellular cytotoxicity (ADCC) and complement-dependent cytotoxicity (CDC) and unlike crosslinked antibodies, these bi-specifics were pure and stable. The main

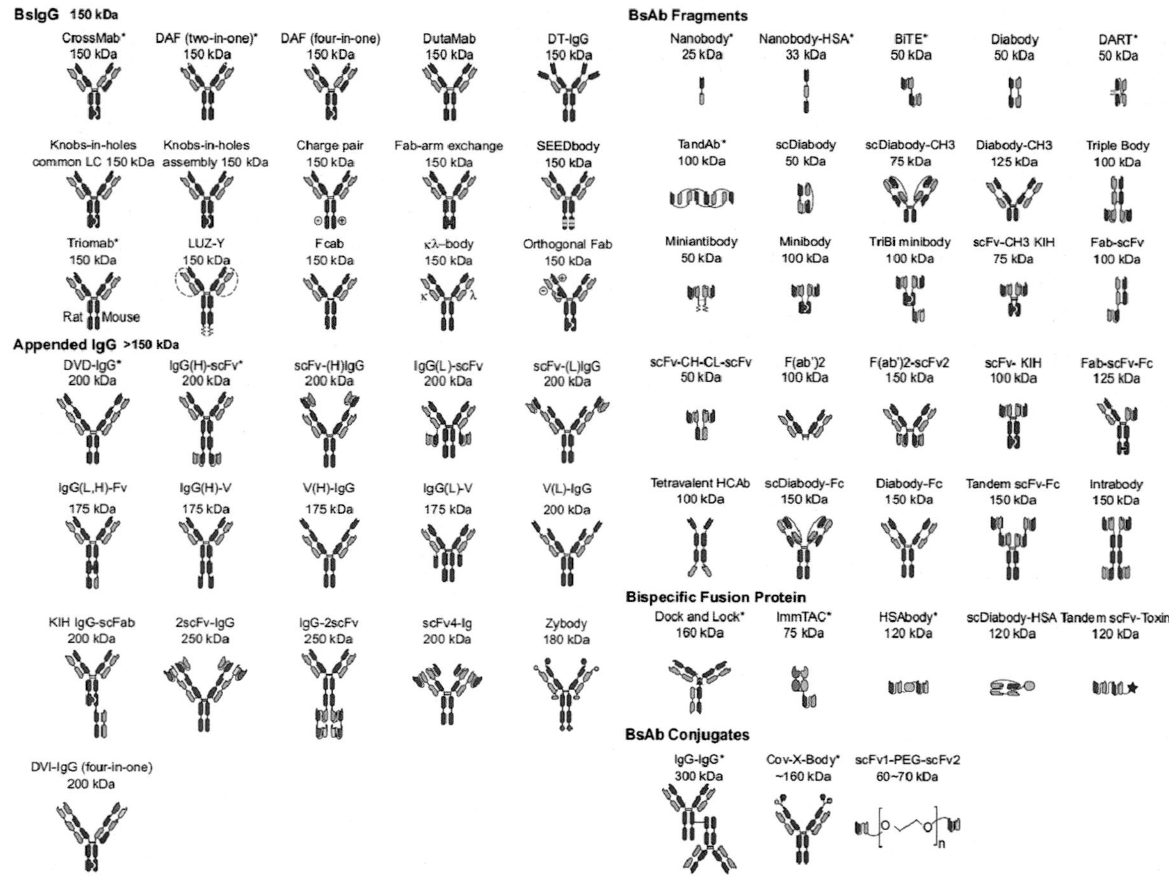

FIG. 33.4 Bi-Specific Formats and Combinations. *Reproduced with permission from Spies C, Zhai Q, Carter PJ. Alternative molecular formats and therapeutic applications for bispecific antibodies. Mol Immunol 2015;67:95–106 (open access article under the CC BY-NC-ND license: http://creativecommons.org/licenses/by-nc-nd/4.0/).*

limitation was that each component was assembled randomly, producing unwanted and nonfunctional paired antibodies, such as the pairing of two heavy chains instead of pairing of one light and one heavy chain.

To overcome the problem of unwanted pairing, a technology referred to as "Knob into hole (KiH)" was developed. This technology, originally used in *E. coli* as an expression host but can also be used in mammalian hosts [19], allows for heterodimerization by making complementary mutations in the CH3 domain of each heavy chain that is coupled with disulfide bridges in the hinge region. Even with this technology, homodimerization can still occur and production yields can be unsatisfactory [20].

Efficient approaches to produce mono- and multivalent bi-specific antibodies are the subject of intense evaluation. Notwithstanding, with molecular cloning technology, BsAbs are now constructed with some or all of the constant domains of an antibody. Formats include IgG and non-IgG formats. Multiple names are emerging that describe bi-specific fragments such as dimers, diabodies, tri-body, tetrabody, di-diabodies (Fig. 33.4). Different formats differ in molecular size, stability, flexibility, compactness, ease of production, valency of antigen binding, and mode of interaction with target and effector cells. There is probably no one format suitable for all applications [21].

The choice of IgG isoforms to be used in bi-specifics is typically optimized for particular properties such as increased potency. This was the case of changing from an IgG_1 to an IgG_4 with hinge stabilization to enhance agonist properties of the FIXa/FX bi-specific antibody [22]. It is also possible that an IgG_4 format may be optimal for immune synapse connections due to its compactness compared with an IgG_1 isoform [23]. Also, Kapelski et al. demonstrated IgG isotypes have different avidities for a particular target as was the case for a CD3 bi-specific that had 10X weaker binding to CD3 compared with CD19 with an IgG_2 isoform.

The various domain combinations constituting a platform have been trademarked and are briefly described. CrossMab (Roche) is based on the crossover of the antibody domain within one Fab-arm of a bi-specific IgG antibody to enable the specific binding of the light antibody chains to its heavy counterparts to prevent unwanted side products. In addition, it was desired to keep the natural IgG architecture with minimal mutations to maintain favorable properties of pharmacokinetics, stability, production, and low immunogenicity. This technology has been used to develop additional bi-, tri-, and tetravalent bi-specific constructs as well as non-Fc tandem antigen-binding fragment (Fab)-based antibodies [24].

The BiTE (Amgen) format recombinantly links the four minimal variable domains of heavy and light chains required for two antigen-binding specificities via polypeptide linkers: one variable region targets CD3 on T-cells and the other binds to tumor surface antigen. The resulting 55-kDa, nonglycosylated molecule is a single polypeptide with 1 N- and 1 C-terminus. BiTEs combine tumor cell targeting with selective T-cell activation at low picomolar concentrations, leading to tumor lysis. Because of their relatively small size, <50 kD, they have volumes of distribution similar to plasma volume, are easily excreted by the kidneys following the rapid catabolism into amino acids, and thus require prolonged continuous intravenous administration [25]. In spite of this disadvantage, the low molecule weight enables significant tumor uptake that was shown to be sustained over several days despite the short elimination half-life, as was demonstrated with the CD3/EpCam BiTE in tumor models [26].

Blinatumomab

T-cells recruited by blinatumomab do not require ex vivo prestimulation or in vivo costimulation, but are strictly dependent on the presence of $CD19^+$ normal or malignant B-cells for activation. Its small size brings target and effector cells in close proximity, enabling the formation of cytolytic synapses [27]. In addition, blinatumomab's monovalent engagement of the tumor cell receptor (TCR) complex prevents systemic activation of effector cells in the absence of target cells.

Blinatumomab was approved in 2014 for the treatment of B-cell acute lymphoblastic leukemia (ALL). An open label single-arm trial of 185 patients with ALL [28] formed the basis for its approval. In this study, the complete response (CR) rate was 32% with a median relapse-free survival of 6.7 months (range <0.1–16.5 months). Minimal residual disease response (MRD; $<10^{-4}$) was achieved. Subsequently, blinatumomab has been studied in relapsed/refractory diffuse large B-cell lymphoma [29]. Blinatumomab monotherapy induced responses in 43% of evaluable patients, the CR rate was 19%, and the longest progression-free survival (PFS) recorded was 20.1 months. More importantly, treatment with stepwise dose escalation over 14 days (blinatumomab at 9 μg/day in the first week, 28 μg/day in the second week, and 112 μg/day thereafter) accompanied by primary prophylaxis with dexamethasone administration before the start and before every step improved tolerability.

Linear drug disposition, and not target-mediated drug disposition (TMDD), has been observed for blinatumomab within the range of doses studied. PK/PD relationships for tumor response, cytokine release, and B-cell aplasia were explored in patients with non-Hodgkin's lymphomas [30]. The relationship between blinatumomab concentrations and reduction in tumor size was highly variable due to baseline tumor burden, different dosing regimens that included flat and stepped dosing, and duration of treatment. Nonetheless, there was an exposure-dependent reduction in tumor size and the inhibitory sigmoid E_{max} model predicted that a dose of 47 $\mu g/m^2$/day for 28 days would result in at least a 50% reduction in tumor size in most patients. Since B-cell depletion was rapid, with B-cell levels dropping to zero within 48 hours in almost all patients receiving doses of $\geq 5\ \mu g/m^2$/day, regardless of B-cell levels at baseline, the evaluation with an E_{max} model was precluded. Lastly, cytokine serum C_{max} generally increased with blinatumomab dose, particularly above 15 $\mu g/m^2$/day. Stepwise dosing (5–15–60 $\mu g/m^2$/day) showed less pronounced cytokine elevation after first dose and subsequent dose steps, compared with a flat dose of 60 $\mu g/m^2$/day.

Dual affinity retargeting

Dual affinity retargeting, DART (Macrogen), is another format that separates variable domains of heavy and light chains of the 2 antigen binding specificities on 2 separate polypeptide chains [31]. DART molecules are stable, are effective in T-cell cytotoxicity, and can be modified to incorporate an Fc function to extend the elimination half-life for convenient dosing [32].

Duobody technology

Duobody (Genmab) technology is a platform for creating full length IgG_1 antibodies that retain Fc effector function of antibody-dependent cellular cytotoxicity (ADCC) and complement-dependent cytotoxicity (CDC). As expected, the elimination half-life of Duobodies is similar to native IgG_1, approximately 10–15 days.

The most common indication for bi-specifics is cancer and the most common component of these bi-specifics, whether it's an scFv, Fab, or full IgG molecule, is a CD3 arm that is humanized or fully human (Table 33.4). In this way, the CD3 simultaneously engages $CD8^+$ and $CD4^+$ T-cells (expressing CD3) and redirects them to the tumor, resulting in lysis of cancer cells (expressing the targeted tumor antigen).

Multiple factors can affect T-cell redirection activity, such as differential affinities of the targeting arms, as shown by the example of a CLL1/CD3 knob-in-hole IgG_1 BsAb [47]. Structural characteristics of the target, such as accessibility and distance of the epitope from the membrane and BsAb flexibility, can contribute to efficient T-cell redirection. T-cell

TABLE 33.4 T-cell redirecting Bi-specifics for the treatment of cancer.

Construct	Fc	Molecules	Route of Administration	Half-Life	Ref.
BiTE 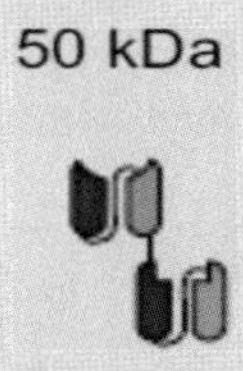 50 kDa	No Fc	CD3/CD19 *Blinatumomab*	CI	Mouse 1.2–2.5 h Chimpanzee 1.2–2.6 h Human 2.1 h	[33]
		CD3/EGFR$_{VIII}$	CI	Mouse 2.5 h	[34]
		CD3/EpCAM *solitomab*	CI	Human 4.5 h	[35]
		CD3/PSMA *pasotuxizumab*	IV SC	Mouse 8 h Mouse 11 h	[36]
DART 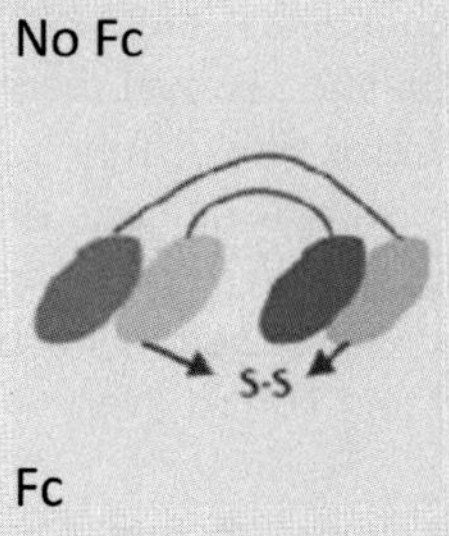 No Fc S-S Fc	No Fc; two chains one variable region light (VL) and one heavy (VH) chain arranged in the order VL (1)-VH(2) and VL (2)-VH (1)	CD3/CD123	IV	Cynomolgus Monkey 3.5 h	[37]
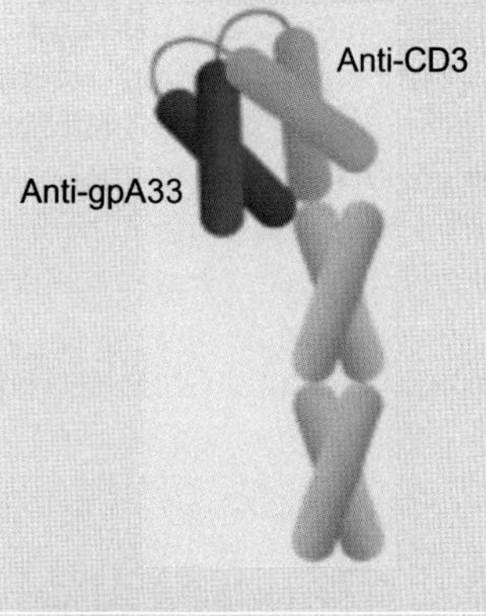 Anti-CD3 Anti-gpA33	Fc domain introduced at C-termini of heterodimer, modified to avoid binding to FcγR receptors, binds to FcRn	CD3/GPA33	IV	Cynomolgus Monkey 7 days	[38]
		CD3/B7H3	IV	Cynomolgus monkey: 114–135 h	[39]
		CD3/P-cadherin	IV	Mouse 105.7 h	[40]
ADAPTIR (modular protein technology) 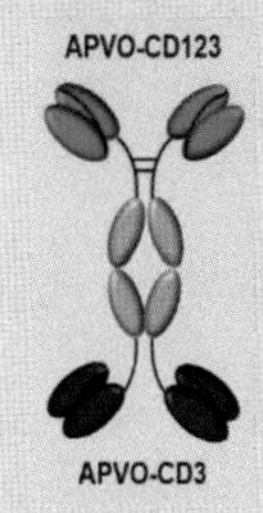 APVO-CD123 APVO-CD3	Two sets of binding domains linked to an immunoglobulin Fc domain to extend the half-life of the molecule in vivo	CD3/PSMA	IV	Mouse 96.5 h Cynomolgus monkey 108 h	[41] [42]
TRiTac 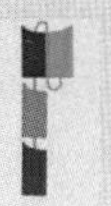	No Fc but has albumin binding site to extend half-life	CD3/PSMA	IV	Cynomolgus Monkey 3.3 days	[43]

TABLE 33.4 T-cell redirecting Bi-specifics for the treatment of cancer—cont'd

Construct	Fc	Molecules	Route of Administration	Half-Life	Ref.
ATTACK 110kD	No Fc	CD3/EGFRVIII			[44]
EM801	Heterodimeric Fc region with intact FcRn binding (bi-valent)	CD3/BCMA	IV SC	Cynomolgus Monkey 110h (mean across 3 dose levels 125h (CL reported as 2 mL/hr/kg)	[45]
	IgG_4 Fc and bivalent (VH) BCMA	CD3_F2B/ BCMA	IV	Mouse 8.5 days Cynomolgus Monkey 12.8 days	[46]
	Full-length bi-specific humanized IgG_1 in a knob-and-hole format Mutations introduced in the Fc domain to reduce interactions with Fcγ receptors	CD3/CLL-1	IV	Mouse: approx. 3 days Cynomolgus Monkey: approx. 5 days	[47]

engagement requires mimicry of the immune synapse (IS) which is achieved by bridging the T-cell receptor complex (via CD3 binding) to the target cell (via binding to a target cell surface antigen). The IS intercellular distance of ~15 nm is approximately the same distance as the Fab arm span of an IgG_1 [24]. Lastly, modulating the size and amino acid composition of the linker in a CD19/CD3 tandem diabody indicated that an optimal length and flexibility is required for efficient cytotoxic activity [48]. IgG_2 isoforms are less suitable for T-cell redirection than their IgG_1- or IgG_4 counterparts; the degree of saturation in binding of CD3 on T-cells was ~25% lower for the IgG_2 subclass [23].

Equally attractive molecules to target in a bi-specific format include tyrosine kinases, antiangiogenics, T-cell costimulatory and checkpoint inhibitory molecules because they are associated with cellular proliferation, migration, differentiation, and death. The optimal size of a bi-specific is a size that persists in the circulation without administration by continuous infusion and good tumor penetration is not known but may reside in the range of 75–85 kD, such as scFv-Fab combinations [49].

While most attention and publications of bi-specifics are cancer therapies, bi-specifics are also being evaluated in autoimmune diseases and in hemophilia (Table 33.5). The first bi-specific for an indication other than cancer, emicizumab, was approved in 2018 for patients with Hemophilia A.

Emicizumab

Emicizumab (ACE910), a recombinant humanized bi-specific monoclonal antibody of factor IX (FIXa) and factor X (FX) to restore hemostasis in people with hemophilia A, acts as a factor VIII (FVIII) mimetic by binding simultaneously to activated FIXa and FX [63]. This particular asymmetric native IgG structure was the only format recognizing FIXa and FX with each arm.

TABLE 33.5 Bi-specific antibodies lacking CD3 arm and used in the treatment of cancer and other indications.

Construct	Fc	Molecule	Route of administration	Half-life	Ref.
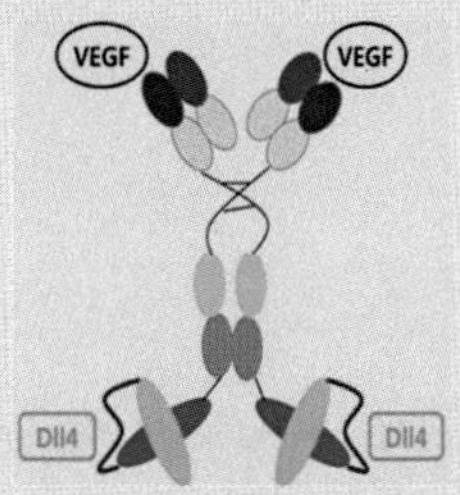	IgG_2 bi-valent with Fc	DLL4/VEGF Cancer Navicixizumab	IV	Human 11.4 days	[50]
TandAb Tetravalent di-diabody 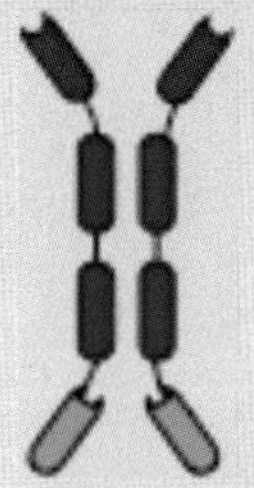	No Fc	CD30/CD16A Cancer	IV	Human 19 h	[51] [52]
ADAPTIR 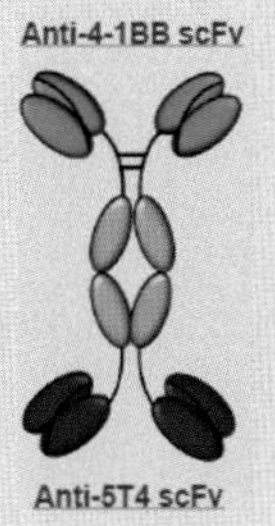	Two sets of binding domains linked to an immunoglobulin Fc domain	4-1BB/5T4 Cancer	IV	Cynomolgus monkey 5.1–5.9 days	[53]
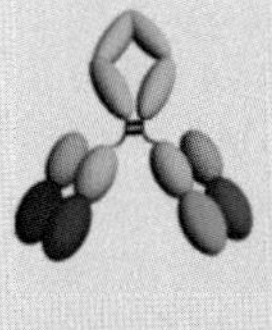	Humanized native IgG_4 with Fc	FIXa/Fx Hemophilia A *Emicizumab*	SC	Cynomolgus monkey 23–27 days Cynomolgus monkey hemophilia A model 19.4 days Human 27.8±8.1 days	[54] [55] [56]
Dual Variable domain DVD 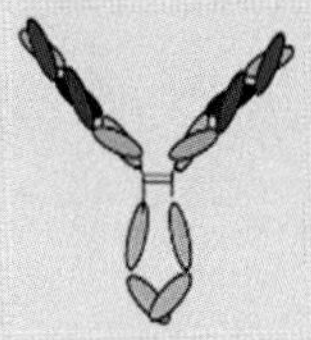	Humanized IgG with Fc region joined to 2 complementary determining regions	IL-1α/IL-1β Osteoarthritis *Lutikizumab (ABT-981)*	IV SC SC	Mouse 10.5 days Rat 10.0 days Monkey 10.4 days Mouse 20.3 Rat 12.0 Monkey 8.0 Human 10–14 days	[57] [58]
		DLL4/VEGF Cancer ABT-165	IV	Cynomolgus monkeys >5 days	[59]

TABLE 33.5 Bi-specific antibodies lacking CD3 arm and used in the treatment of cancer and other indications—cont'd

Construct	Fc	Molecule	Route of administration	Half-life	Ref.
ABT-122	Heterodimer IgG-electrostatic Fc pairing and light chain crossover	TNFα/IL-17A Psoriatic arthritis, rheumatoid arthritis Plaque psoriasis	IV SC	Human 4.3–9.7 days Human 5.3 days	[60]
Crossmab CrossMab$^{CH1\text{-}CL}$	IgG_1 with heavy chain dimerization	ANG2/VEGFA Renal Cell Carcinoma *Vanucizumab*	IP IV	Mouse 177 h Human 6–9 days	[61] [62]

CI, continuous infusion; *IV*, intravenous; *Sc*, subcutaneous; *IP*, intraperitoneal.

TABLE 33.6 Examples of immunoassays used to quantitate macromolecules.

Assay acronym	Assay description
ECLIA	Electrochemiluminescence immunoassay
ELISA	Enzyme-linked immunosorbent assay
RIA	Radioimmunoassay
IRMA	Immunoradiometric assay
RRA	Radioreceptor assay

Subcutaneously administered emicizumab showed high bioavailability in cynomolgus monkeys [54] and once-weekly administration significantly reduced spontaneous bleeding symptoms in a primate model of acquired hemophilia A [64]. In its first-in-human phase 1 study, emicizumab demonstrated linear PK profile with a mean elimination half-life ranging 28-34 days in Japanese and Caucasian subjects, and single subcutaneous doses of 1 mg/kg had favorable safety and tolerability in healthy subjects [65]. Subsequently, in the first-in-patient 12-week, phase 1 study, once-weekly subcutaneous emicizumab at 0.3, 1, or 3 mg/kg was well tolerated and substantially reduced annualized bleeding rates (ABRs) in patients with severe hemophilia A, both with and without inhibitors [56]. A population PK/PD model was developed to refine the relationship between the pharmacokinetics of emicizumab and reduction in bleeding frequency [66]. A one-compartment model with first-order absorption and elimination was employed as the structural model for SC dosing and Repeated Time-To-Event modeling was used to characterize the exposure-response relationship of emicizumab in patients. Results of the modeling identified a maintenance dose of 1.5 mg/kg as the minimal dose to provide a median steady-state trough concentration of 45 μg/mL with every week dosing; large interindividual variability in the exposure-response was observed such that the target efficacious exposure prediction would need to be prospectively confirmed with a larger sample size of patients in a late stage clinical trial.

Assay of macromolecules

The most common types of assays employed to quantitate protein and mAb concentrations in biologic matrices are listed in Table 33.6. Radioimmunoassays (RIA), radioreceptor assays (RRA), and immunoradiometric assays (IRMA) require radioactivity and have been largely replaced by enzyme-linked immunosorbent assays (ELISAs), which are based on antibody recognition of an antigenic epitope (i.e., a molecular region on the surface of a molecule capable of binding to the specific antibody). More recently, electrochemiluminescence (ECL) immunoassays have been developed and utilized in drug development because they provide a modest improvement in sensitivity and extended dynamic assay range.

The bioanalysis of macromolecules is far more complex than the assays of small molecules that are described in Chapter 11. Unlike small molecules, which can be extracted from matrices and subsequently analyzed, macromolecules are analyzed in a matrix containing other proteins that may cause interference, or soluble ligands that can be upregulated and prevent binding of the assay reagents to protein's or mAb's epitope. An example of an interfering substance is rheumatoid factor (RF), a heterophilic antibody that is a normal secondary immune response to many antigens. RF interferes with many assays of IgG mAbs by binding to the Fc portion of IgG, but this interference can be circumvented by using antiidiotype (anti-ID) antibodies in the assay construct. Antiidiotype antibodies are antigenic determinants created by the combining site of an antibody, called *idiotypes,* and the antibodies elicited to the idiotypes, called anti-ID antibodies. Anti-idiotypic antibodies are those directed against the hypervariable regions of an antibody.

Macromolecules that have a particularly complex structure—such as trastuzumab-DM1, a humanized IgG_1 specific for human HER2 receptor that is conjugated to the cytotoxic maytansine derivative DM1 which binds to microtubules—require orthogonal assay methods to fully characterize their PK/PD and to further our understanding of the biology of these molecules. Such orthogonal methods include multiple ELISAs, to measure total, bound, and free antibody; liquid chromatography and tandem mass spectrometry (LC-MS/MS) for free cytotoxin; bioactivity assays; and affinity capture-mass spectrometry (AC-MS). For further detail, the reader is referred to a review of the bioanalysis of macromolecules [67] and to a report on the consensus of the AAPS Ligand-binding Assay Bioanalytical Focus Group on strategies for determining total and free concentrations of mAbs [68].

The bioanalysis of bi-specific antibodies is even more challenging than monoclonal antibodies. The challenges encountered for bi-specifics include biotransformation or in vivo instability of the molecule, avoidance of steric hindrance effect due to binding to two targets, and decision of what to measure, i.e., the intact form of bi-specific with two functional domains vs. the moiety with one particular target binding domain. Assay formats typically used include (1) measurement of the intact form of the bi-specific with two reagents (capture and detection), each binding to a different functional domain; (2) measurement of forms with one selected functional domain which binds to the capture reagent and uses anti-Fc reagents for detection; and (3) measurement of all soluble forms (a total assay) by employing two anti-Fc antibodies, one for capture and one for detection. The decision of which assay and/or format to use in a drug development program is dependent on the engagement of the targets, the mechanism of action, and an understanding of the biology and the specific goals the drug developer wants to accomplish. For instance, the functional assay may be used to evaluate loss of activity due to ADA. As with all assays used in nonclinical and clinical studies, following the FDA guidance on assay validation [69] is paramount for consistent and robust results.

Interspecies scaling of macromolecules: predictions in humans

As discussed in Chapter 31 and elsewhere [70], interspecies scaling is based upon allometry or physiology. Protein PK parameters such as volume of distribution (V_d), elimination half-life ($t_{1/2}$), and elimination clearance (CL) have been scaled across species using the standard allometric equation [71]:

$$Y = aW^b \tag{33.1}$$

In this equation, Y is the parameter of interest, the coefficient a is the value of the parameter at one unit of body weight, W is body weight, and b is the allometric exponent. For convenience, this equation is linearized to:

$$\log Y = \log a + b \log W \tag{33.2}$$

In this form, $\log a$ is the y-intercept and b is the slope of the line. In Fig. 33.5, representative linearized plots of CL and initial volume of distribution (V_1) are shown for recombinant growth hormone (GH) across four species.

Allometric equations for V_1 and CL for some representative macromolecules are presented in Table 33.7 [71–76]. The theoretical exponent approximations for V_1 (mL) and CL (mL/min) are $aW^{0.8}$–$aW^{1.0}$ and $aW^{0.6}$–$aW^{0.8}$, respectively. Parameter estimates can be normalized for body weight simply by subtracting 1.0 from the exponent. In Table 33.8 the predicted parameter estimates derived from the allometric equations in Table 33.7 are compared with the corresponding parameter estimates reported in humans [77, 78]. The observed values of V_1 for the macromolecules listed fall within the expected range of observed results. However, the observed clearances of FIX and IL-12 were not predicted from allometry. Factors such as species specificity in the endothelial binding of FIX [79] or saturation of clearance mechanisms may account for the inability to predict these parameters in humans.

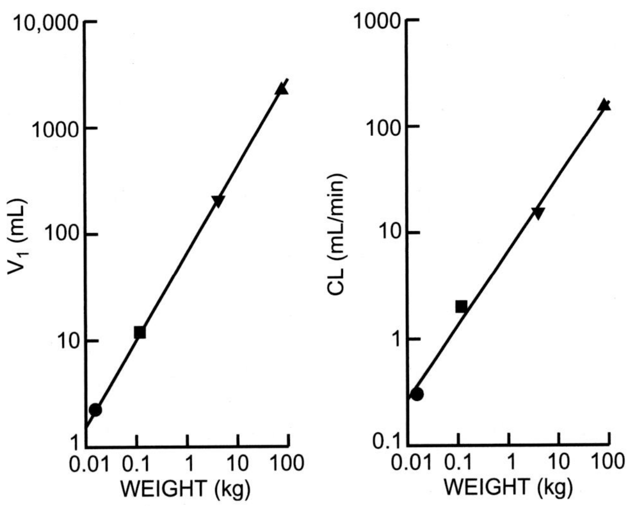

FIG. 33.5 Log-log plots of V_1 and CL vs body weight for recombinant human growth hormone: mouse (●), rat (▪), cynomolgous monkey (▼), human (▲). *Reproduced with permission from Mordenti J, Chen SA, Moore JA, et al. Pharm Res 1991;8:1351–1359.*

TABLE 33.7 Allometric equations for representative macromolecules.

Macromolecule	Allometric equations V_1 (mL)	Allometric equations CL (mL/h)	Ref(s)
Factor IX[a]	$87W^{1.26}$	$14W^{0.68}$	[72, 73][b]
Factor VIII[a]	$44W^{1.04}$	$10W^{0.69}$	[74]
Interleukin-12[a]	$65W^{0.85}$	$8W^{0.62}$	[75, 76][b]
Growth hormone[c]	$68W^{0.83}$	$7W^{0.71}$	[71]
Tissue plasminogen activator[c]	$91W^{0.93}$	$17W^{0.84}$	[71]

[a]Based on parameter estimates in at least two species.
[b]Allometric equations determined from PK parameter estimates reported in published literature.
[c]Based on parameter estimates in at least four species.

TABLE 33.8 Prediction of human pharmacokinetic parameters based on allometric scaling.

Macromolecule	V_1 Predicted (mL)	V_1 Observed (mL)	V_1 Expected range[a] (mL/kg)	CL Predicted (mL/h)	CL Observed (mL/h)	CL Expected range[a] (mL/h)	Ref (s).
Factor IX	18,380	10,150	9190–27,570	248	434[b]	124–372	[77]
Factor VIII	3617	3030	1809–5426	195	174	98–293	[74]
Interleukin-12	2406	3360	1203–3609	113	406	57–170	[78]
Growth hormone	2243	2432	1122–3365	148	175	74–222	[71]
Recombinant tissue plasminogen activator	5814	4450	2907–8721	646	620	323–969	[71]

[a]For comparison with observed results, an expected range is chosen that is 0.5 to 1.5 times the predicted value.
[b]Calculated from Fig. 1 of White G, Shapiro A, Ragni M, et al. Semin Hematol 1998;35(Suppl 2):33–38 [77].

TABLE 33.9 Allometric equations for EGF mAb PK parameters.

Parameter (Y)	Coefficient (a)	Exponent (b)	r
V_d (mL)	219	0.84	0.92
CL (mL/h)	4.07	0.85	0.94

Adapted from Duconge J, Fernandez-Sanchez E, Alvarez D. Biopharm Drug Dispos 2004;25:177–186.

TABLE 33.10 Comparison of EGF PK parameters predicted from allometric equations and estimated in cancer patients.

Parameter (Y)	Predicted PK parameter estimate[a]	Estimated PK parameter in cancer patients
V_d (L/kg)	0.01	0.04
CL (mL/h/kg)	0.22	0.98

[a]*Calculated from the allometric equations in Table 7, Duconge J, Fernandez-Sanchez E, Alvarez D, et al. Biopharm Drug Dispos 2004;25:177–186.*

Allometric scaling also has been applied to mAbs [80, 81]. Duconge and coworkers conducted PK studies in mice, rats, rabbits, and dogs after a single administration of 16 mg/kg, 8 mg/kg, 1.5 mg/kg, and 0.2 mg/kg, respectively, of a murine mAb ior EGF/r^3 [80]. Three female patients with nonsmall cell lung cancer were also studied. They were participating in a Phase I trial and received a single IV infusion of 400 mg. EGF concentrations were analyzed either by a radioreceptor assay (mice and rats) or a sandwich ELISA method (rabbits, dogs, and humans). The allometric equations for V_d and CL were calculated according to the standard methods and with incorporation of a complex Dedrick plot, similar to that used in Fig. 32.4. The results of the allometric analysis are presented in Table 33.9. A comparison between the predicted and calculated PK parameters in cancer patients is presented in Table 33.10. The actual clearance in patients with cancer was four-fold greater than the predicted value. The authors proposed that the observed variance suggests that patients with cancer possess additional clearance processes that are not present in healthy subjects or predictable from studies in normal animals. However, even with this disparate result the authors used their 0.85 allometric scaling factor for CL to assist in designing dose regimens for a clinical trial [82].

Mahmood et al. [81] further demonstrated that simple allometry using PK parameter estimates from at least three species, resulting in an exponent for CL in the range of 0.5–0.9, predicted human clearance reasonably well. Others have proposed that allometry based on single-species studies of macromolecules in monkeys, and using the theoretical exponent of 0.8 for CL, accurately predicts human CL [83, 84]. In both cases, the authors determined PK parameters within a dosage range that was assumed to be linear. Recently, it has been shown that classifying mAbs based on whether or not the mAb antigen target was either soluble or membrane bound enables human CL to be reasonably predicted with an exponent of either 0.85 for solid or 0.90 for membrane-bound targets [85]. Other factors to be considered in deciding whether or not interspecies scaling would be predictive of human PK parameter estimates include: (1) binding characteristics, (2) receptor density, (3) size and charge of molecule, (4) end-terminal carbohydrate characteristics, (5) degree of sialylation, and (6) saturation of elimination pathways. These factors are known to influence clearance and distribution volumes, as will be discussed in subsequent sections. For example, clearance may involve several mechanisms, including immune-mediated clearance that results in nonconstant clearance rates. The interspecies predictability of clearance in this situation would be questionable.

In spite of the limitations, interspecies scaling can be used to relate dosages across species in toxicology studies, to predict human PK parameter estimates for macromolecules, and, as discussed in Chapters 31 and 32, to guide dose selection in Phase I clinical trials. However, an understanding of the characteristics of the macromolecule is important for the interpretation and application of these results.

Safe starting doses of monoclonal and Bi-specific antibodies in first-in-human (FIH) studies

In a 2006 Phase I study, TGN1412, an agonist mAb targeting CD28, was administered to healthy volunteers and resulted in cytokine storm, an adverse event that is often fatal [86]. As this event had not been predicted by preclinical studies, the

TABLE 33.11 Steps in determining MABEL.

1. Assess relevant in vitro binding characteristics (e.g., via Biacore)
2. Determine receptor occupancy either by in vitro or in vivo methods, or by both (i.e., confirm in vivo, the in vitro findings)
3. Obtain concentration-effect data from in vivo studies
4. Establish the mechanism-based PK/PD model and integrate the pharmacology data
5. Account for species differences in binding affinity, potency, target expression and rate of turnover, target-mediated clearance, duration of effects
6. Use allometry to scale PK parameters to humans and refine PK/PD model to predict human dosages
7. Identify maximum recommended starting dose (MRSD)

Adapted from Muller PY, Milton M, Lloyd P, et al. Curr Opin Biotech 2009; 20:722–729.

selection of safe starting doses for mAbs has subsequently received considerable attention and discussion in the pharmaceutical and regulatory communities. In response to this case, the Committee for Medicinal Product (CHMP) of the European Medicines Agency (EMA) issued guidelines highlighting considerations that should be taken to mitigate safety risks, such as those seen with TGN1412 [87]. In particular, the guidelines emphasize application of the concept of "minimum anticipated biological effect," or MABEL. The steps for determining MABEL are outlined in Table 33.11. The integration of all information, including toxicology, mAb pharmacology, PK/PD modeling, and interspecies scaling, will result in improved decisions regarding safe starting doses and dose-escalation intervals in both healthy volunteers and subjects with discasc [88].

An even more sophisticated mechanism-based PK/PD model has been proposed for FIH dose selection that incorporates factors such as receptor occupancy and target cell (blood) depletion [89]. The purpose of the model is to predict a mAb's pharmacology at the proposed dosages in order to guide both initial and subsequent dose selection. The model incorporates in vitro measures of affinity binding of the mAb to blood cells and in vivo monkey PK and target cell depletion data. These data were fit to the PK/PD model and the resulting PK parameters were allometrically scaled to humans. The human model used the same structure as that for the monkey, but the mAb binding affinity was adjusted to that of humans in order to simulate PK, receptor occupancy, and target cell depletion profiles (Fig. 33.6). Prior to building models of this type, it is important to establish that the humanized or fully human mAb being studied cross-reacts with monkey, in order to reliably extrapolate in vivo PK and PD, and that its binding affinity to the target cell is similar in the two species.

T-cell redirecting bi-specific antibodies have different binding affinities to the CD3 arm relative to the target antigen arm and are very potent such that utilizing receptor occupancy (RO) data in establishing the FIH dose for T-cell redirecting bi-specifics may result in toxicity at the initial dosages. In support of this, a retrospective analysis of IND submissions of bi-specific antibodies [90] concluded that the FIH doses were at, too close to, or above human maximum tolerated dose (MTD) or highest human dose (HDD) for 67% of those INDs when RO was used. Methods to determine the MABEL to support FIH dose, other than receptor occupancy, have been employed and include determining the pharmacologic activity based on the most sensitive in vitro assay [91] or a more sophisticated approach employing an in vitro MABEL/in vivo PK/PD mechanistic model [92].

Pharmacokinetic characteristics of macromolecules

Endogenous concentrations

Unlike chemically synthesized molecules, many of the macromolecules, e.g., non-mAb form of proteins, currently marketed are naturally occurring substances in the body. This presents some unique challenges for estimating PK parameters. Most commercially available ELISAs were developed to quantitate exogenously administered proteins and do not distinguish between the native protein in the body and the exogenously administered protein. Clearly, concentrations of endogenous proteins, which can fluctuate because of stimulation or feedback control (such as insulin growth factor, IGF-1), can result in erroneous parameter estimates. There are several approaches to deal with the problem posed by detectable endogenous protein concentrations.

In a study by Cheung et al. [93], the investigators administered erythropoietin subcutaneously to 30 healthy volunteers. Blood sampling times included a predose sample and samples collected multiple times postadministration. In the predose sample, erythropoietin was detected in all subjects at concentrations in the physiological range (<7 to 30 IU/mL) with the exception of a subject whose baseline concentration of 48 IU/mL exceeded the normal physiologic range. Prior to estimating PK parameters, the investigators subtracted each predose concentration from all concentrations detected

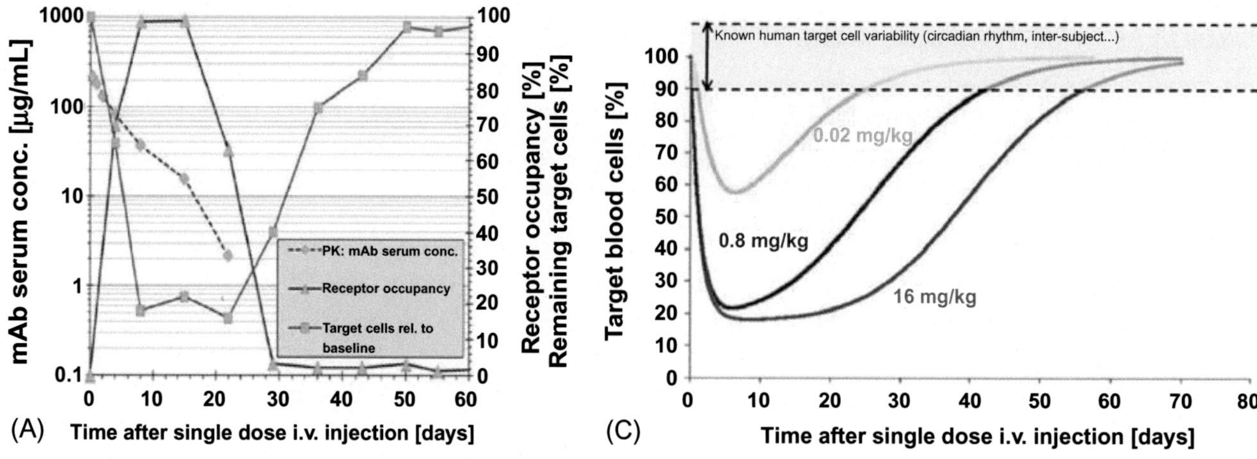

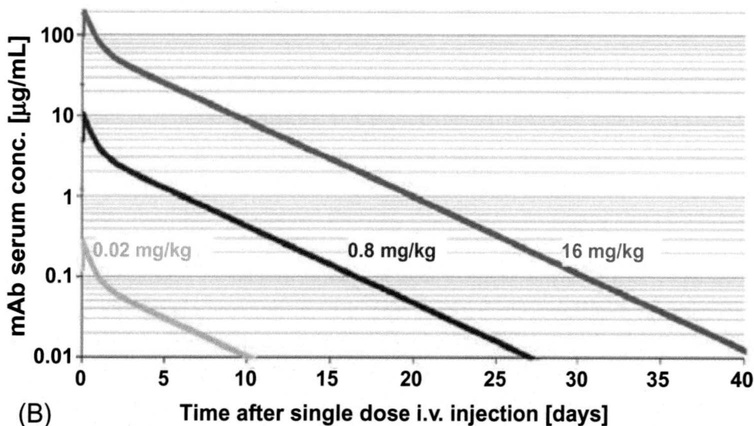

FIG. 33.6 MABEL determination for a mAb binding to blood-based cell surface receptors. (A) Data from one monkey used to build the PK/PD monkey model. Depletion of target cells as percentage of remaining target cells in circulation, relative to baseline (on right axis) is modulated by receptor occupancy (RO), expressed as % occupied receptors from all available receptors at a specific time point. When mAb serum concentration (on left axis, logarithmic scale) falls below ≈ 10 µg/mL for this mAb, a decrease in RO is observed followed by recovery of target cell counts. (B) Simulation of human PK following three single IV doses with a half-life hypothesized to be ≈ 3.5 days. (C) Simulation of human target cell depletion dose-response for the three IV doses. On this figure, MABEL corresponds to a dose <0.02 mg/kg, where suppression of target cells is minimal and transient. *Reproduced with permission from Yu J, Karcher H, Feire AL, Lowe PJ. AAPS J 2011;13:169–178.*

postadministration. The underlying assumption for this approach was that the low endogenous concentrations remained relatively stable over the postadministration sampling period. However, data were not presented to confirm or refute this assumption.

Another approach for dealing with this problem has been proposed for GH by Veldhuis and colleagues [94]. These investigators used a deconvolution method to minimize the influence of circulating endogenous GH on PK parameter estimates derived from exogenously administered growth hormone. In this method, diurnal variation in the 24-h secretory rate of GH is estimated by approximating endogenous plasma GH concentration data with cubic spline smoothing controlled by setting a maximum limit for the weighted residual square sum [95]. Patient-specific parameters can be estimated from individual endogenous hormone concentrations or from group means.

Another option is to estimate PK parameters from the sum of exogenous and endogenous protein concentrations detected after the exogenous administration of the protein. The basic assumption is that the PK parameter estimates are not significantly altered by the presence of endogenous protein concentrations. This generally is true in the very early part of the concentration vs time profile when the endogenous concentration may represent less than 10% of the total concentration. However, in the example depicted in Fig. 33.7, endogenous concentrations are oscillating and pulsatile, reaching peaks during the sampling period that are greater than 100-fold the initial basal values [96]. This illustrates how changes in endogenous protein concentrations over the sampling period can influence model fitting and confound PK parameter estimation.

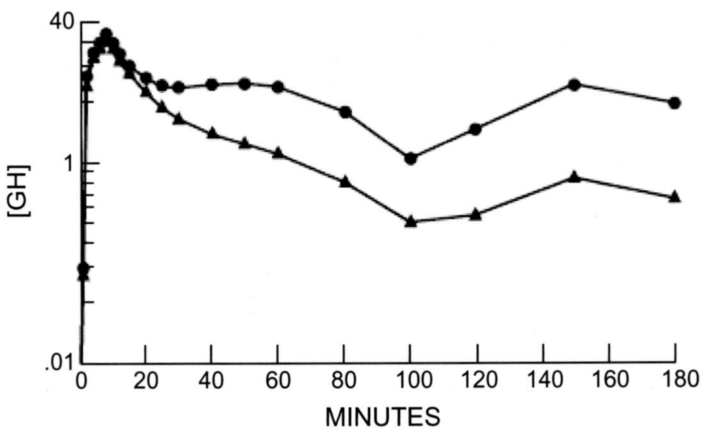

FIG. 33.7 Simulated effects of increasing basal growth hormone (GH) concentrations on measured total GH concentrations at various times during and after an 8-min infusion of recombinant human growth hormone (rhGH) using basal concentrations 10 times (▲) and 100 times (●) the observed preinfusion value of 0.042 ng/mL. *Reproduced with permission from Bright GM, Veldhuis JD, Iranmanesh A, et al. J Clin Endocrinol Metab 1999;84:3301–3308.*

TABLE 33.12 Bioavailability of macromolecules after extravascular routes of administration.

	Route of administration			
Macromolecule	SC[a]	IP[a]	Other	Ref(s)
Erythropoietin	22.0%	2.9%	–	[97]
Granulocyte-macrophage colony-stimulating factor	83.0%	–	–	[98]
GH	49.5%	–	7.8%–9.9%[b]	[99]
Interferon α_{2b}	>100%	42.0%	>100 %[c]	[100, 101]
Interleukin-11	65%	–	–	[102]
Alemtuzumab[d]	53%	–	–	[103]
Golimumab	51%	–	–	[104]

[a]*SC, subcutaneous; IP, intraperitoneal.*
[b]*Nasal administration.*
[c]*Intramuscular administration.*
[d]*Calculated from AUC after IV administration (Summary Basis of Approval; Drugs@FDA), and after SC administration (Montagna M, Montillo M, Avanzini MA, et al., Haematologia 2011; 96:932–936) [103].*

Finally, a crossover study design can be employed such that subjects are randomized to placebo or treatment on one occasion and to the alternate regimen on a second occasion, assuring an adequate washout period between the two occasions. The endogenous concentrations determined in the same subjects after placebo administration can be subtracted from the matching sample collected after treatment administration. This design accommodates intrasubject variability and variations in endogenous concentrations due to pulsatile secretion but assumes that the endogenous concentrations on two separate study days are similar.

Thus it is important to recognize that current analytical methods cannot distinguish endogenous protein concentrations from exogenous concentrations. Administering radiolabeled proteins would allow for exogenous and endogenous proteins to be distinguished, but there are experimental limitations to the use of radiolabeled proteins. Although the accuracy of PK parameter estimation may be impacted by the presence of endogenous concentrations, study designs and data analysis methods can be employed that take endogenous concentration into consideration.

Absorption

The absolute bioavailability of representative macromolecules following extravascular administration is presented in Table 33.12 [97–104]. It is apparent that bioavailability is variable with different molecules and with different routes of administration, reflecting individual molecule characteristics. However, the bioavailability of mAbs generally has been found to be in the 50%–60% range after subcutaneous (SC) administration [105, 106]. In one report, the bioavailability of interferon α after SC or intramuscular (IM) administration was actually greater than 100% relative to an intravenous (IV) bolus injection [100]. This implausible result may reflect the inability of the immunoradiometric assay to distinguish proteolytic fragments of interferon α from the intact molecule, the slow absorption phase of either the SC or IM routes, or a saturable elimination process. The authors did not elucidate which of these factors might have contributed to their observation.

Flip-flop pharmacokinetics of macromolecules

When the absorption rate constant (k_a) is greater than the elimination rate constant (k_e), elimination of the molecule from the body is the rate-limiting step and the terminal portion of the concentration-time curve is primarily determined by the elimination rate. However, as discussed in Chapter 4, if k_a is less than k_e, absorption is rate limiting and the terminal phase of the curve reflects the absorption rate. This phenomenon is illustrated for several molecules in Table 33.13 [96, 100, 107–109]

In the absence of concentration-time profiles after IV administration, it is impossible to estimate the actual elimination rate constant, and the interpretation of absorption and elimination rates after SC administration of macromolecules must be performed cautiously. It is for this reason surprisingly that so few published pharmacokinetic studies include IV administration to assess whether or not the macromolecule follows flip-flop pharmacokinetics.

Factors affecting absorption from subcutaneous sites

Two very important principles on the absorption of macromolecules after SC administration were elucidated by Supersaxo et al. [110]. First, in the range of the molecular weight of the various molecules tested (246–19,000 Da), there was a linear relationship between molecular weight and absorption by the lymphatic system (Fig. 33.8). Second, the authors concluded that molecules with a molecular weight greater than 16,000 Da are absorbed mainly by the lymphatic system that drains the SC injection site, whereas molecules with a molecular weight of less than 1000 Da are absorbed almost entirely by blood

TABLE 33.13 Absorption and apparent elimination rates of macromolecules after SC and IV administration.

Macromolecule	Route of administration	k_a (h^{-1})	Apparent k_e (h^{-1})	Ref(s)
GH	SC	0.23±0.04	0.43±0.05	[96, 107]
	IV		2.58	
IFN-α_{2b}	SC	0.24	0.13	[100]
	IV		0.42	
Erythropoietin	SC	0.0403±0.002	0.206±0.004	[108, 109]
	IV		0.077	

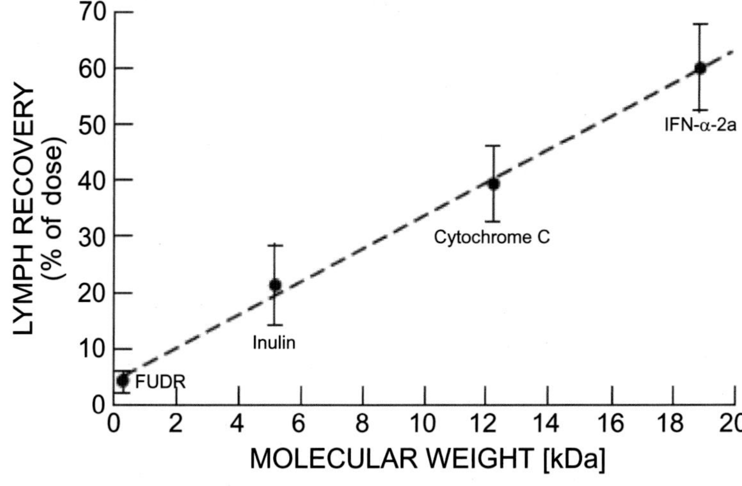

FIG. 33.8 Correlation between molecular weight (MW) and cumulative recovery of IFN-α-2a (MW 19,000), cytochrome c (MW 12,300), inulin (MW 5200), and 5-fluoro-2′-deoxyuridine (FUDR, MW 246.2) in the efferent lymph from the right popliteal lymph node following SC administration into the lower part of the right hind leg of sheep. Each point and bar shows the mean and standard deviation of three experiments performed in three separate sheep. The line drawn represents a least-squares fit of the data (r=0.988, P<0.01). *Reproduced with permission from Supersaxo A, Hein WR, Steffen H. Pharm Res 1990;7: 167–169.*

capillaries. The authors hypothesized that macromolecules are absorbed preferentially by lymphatic rather than blood capillaries because lymphatic capillaries lack the subendothelial basement membrane present in continuous blood capillaries, and may also have 20- to 100-nm gaps between adjacent endothelial cells.

Others have proposed that absorption from the lymphatics cannot be the only factor contributing to the observed bioavailability of macromolecules after SC administration, and that other factors such as an increase in blood flow, proteolysis at the site of injection, or the physical and electrostatic interaction of macromolecules with other components of the interstitium, such as the fibrous collagen network and glycosaminoglycans, also play a role [104, 111, 112]. In the case of mAbs, there is no evidence to suggest the proteolysis occurs at the injection site since the binding of IgG isotypes to the FcRn may protect mAbs from degradation or contribute to transport across the interstitium to blood capillaries.

Although molecular weight is a key factor affecting the absorption of SC administered macromolecules, injection site may also influence the absorption. For example, the absorption half-life was significantly longer, 14.9 vs 12.3 h, after injection of recombinant human erythropoietin (RhEPO) into the thigh than after injection into the abdomen [113]. Also, the concentration vs time profile displayed a double peak after injection into the thigh that was more pronounced than after the abdominal injection (Fig. 33.9). However, these differences are clinically irrelevant, and no statistically significant differences were observed in the area under the curve (*AUC* 5684 vs. 6185 U·h/L), in the maximum concentration (C_{max} 175 vs. 212 U/L), or in the time of maximum concentration (t_{max} = 10 h) for thigh vs. abdomen, respectively.

In another study, recombinant human GH was absorbed faster after SC injection into the abdomen compared with the absorption after SC injection into the thigh [114]. C_{max} was higher (29.7 ± 4.8 mU/L) and t_{max} was faster (4.3 ± 0.5 h) after injection into the abdomen than after injection into the thigh (23.2 ± 3.9 mU/L and 5.9 ± 0.4 h, respectively). It is possible that thcsc absorption differences may be dependent on lymphatic drainage at the two injection sites and may reflect differences in lymph flow. However, mean IGF-1 and insulin growth factor-binding protein 1 (IGFBP-1) concentrations, a PD marker of GH effect, were unaffected by the site of injection. Other effects independent of injection site were blood glucose, and serum insulin and glucagon levels. Thus site of injection is clinically irrelevant for GH, as well as for recombinant erythropoietin.

The influence of injection site on mAb absorption also has been studied [104]. In an open-label, randomized, and parallel designed PK study, 100 mg doses of golimumab were administered either SC to the upper arm, abdomen, or thigh, or IV to healthy adult men. Similar to the results with protein macromolecules, the bioavailability of golimumab was not significantly different, suggesting that injection site had little effect on bioavailability. The mean absolute bioavailability of golimumab was 52% following SC injection in the upper arm, 47% following SC injection into the abdomen, and 54% following SC injection into the thigh, and no significant differences in C_{max}, t_{max}, or $AUC_{0-\infty}$ were observed. Further, the coefficient of variation (CV) in $AUC_{0-\infty}$ following SC injection was approximately 30% and was only slightly greater than

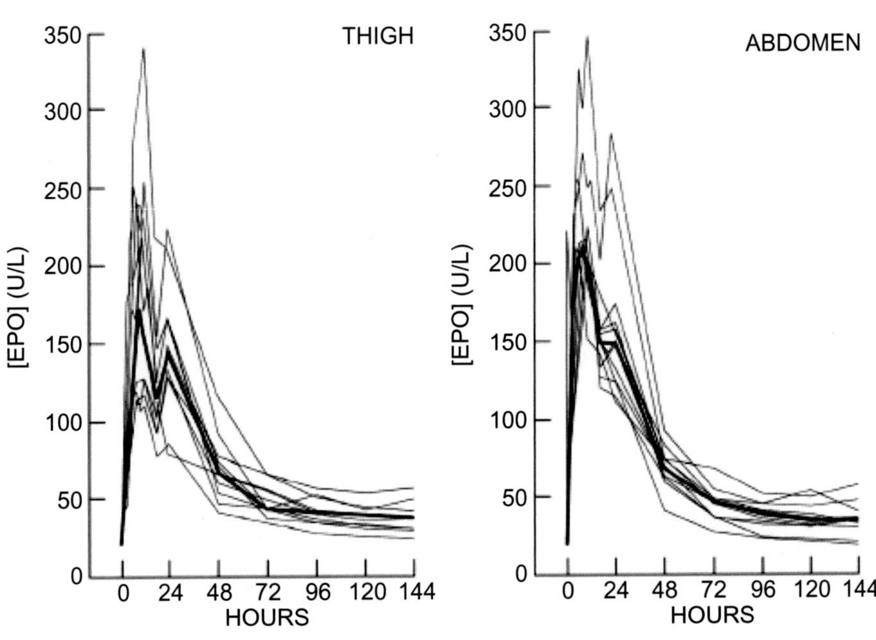

FIG. 33.9 Serum erythropoietin (EPO) concentrations as a function of time after SC injection of 100 U/kg of recombinant human erythropoietin into the thigh and abdomen of 11 healthy volunteers. The *bold curve* represents the median. *Reproduced with permission from Jensen JD, Jensen LW, Madsen JK, et al. Eur J Clin Pharmacol 1994;46:333–337.*

that associated with IV administration (approximately 25% CV), suggesting the SC administration does not result in increased observed variability in estimates of these PK parameters.

In summary, there is no single factor that can account for the finding that macromolecules have reduced bioavailability after SC administration. However, molecular weight, injection site, proteolysis of proteins at injection site, or interactions of exogenously administered macromolecules with constituents within the interstitium may affect their absorption characteristics and should be considered both in designing clinical trials and in treating patients.

Distribution

As discussed in Chapter 3, proteins and mAbs distribute initially into the plasma volume and then more slowly into the interstitial fluid space. It can be seen from Table 33.14 that the initial distribution volume of interleukin-2 (IL-2), IL-12, granulocyte colony-stimulating factor (G-CSF), and recombinant tissue plasminogen activator (rt-PA) approximates that of plasma volume. In contrast, the initial distribution volume of FIX is approximately twice that of plasma volume. On the other hand, the volume of distribution at steady state ($V_{d(ss)}$) for IL-12, G-CSF), and rt-PA is considerably smaller than the $V_{d(ss)}$ of inulin, a marker for extracellular fluid space (ECF) [72, 73, 115–120]. When distribution volume estimates are much less than expected values for ECF, they could reflect the slow transport of large molecules across membranes and the fact that either assay sensitivity or sampling time has been inadequate to characterize the true elimination phase of the compound.

The issue of inadequate sampling time is exemplified by the PK results for mAbs that are presented in Table 33.15 [121]. The reported values of V_1 and $V_{d(ss)}$ are not that different, and both are similar to intravascular space estimates that usually range from 2 to 3 L/m^2. These low V_{ss} estimates for macromolecules suggest not only that equilibrium between the

TABLE 33.14 Distribution volume of representative macromolecules.

Macromolecule	MW (kDa)	V_1 (mL/kg)	$V_{d(ss)}$ (mL/kg)	Ref(s)
Inulin[a]	5.2	55	164	[115]
Factor IX	57	136[b]	271[b]	[72]
Interleukin-2	15.5	60	112	[116, 117]
Interleukin-12	53	52	59	[75]
Granulocyte colony-stimulating factor	20	44	60	[118, 119]
Recombinant tissue plasminogen activator	65	59	106	[120]

[a]*Inulin values used as a reference for plasma volume (V_1) and extracellular fluid space ($V_{d(ss)}$).*
[b]*Calculated from Fig. 1 of White G, Shapiro A, Ragni M. Semin Hematol 1998;35(Suppl 2):33–38 [77].*

TABLE 33.15 Pharmacokinetics of marketed monoclonal antibodies.

mAbs	Molecular weight (kD)	$t_{1/2}$[a] (Days)	V_1[a] (L)	$V_{d(ss)}$[a]
Avastin	149	13–15	3	3.5–4.5 L
Erbitux	152	ND[b]	2.7–3.4	2–3 L/m^2
Raptiva	150	6–7.5[c]	NR[d]	9 L[e]
Humira	148	12–18	3	5 L
Campath	150	1–14[f]	NR[d]	7–28 L

[a]*All values extracted from the Summary Basis for Approval review posted on www.accessdata.fda.gov/scripts/cder/drugsatfda/.*
[b]*Used clearance instead of $T_{1/2}$ since it has nonlinear PK at dosages greater than 200 mg/m^2.*
[c]*Average $t_{1/2}$ based on noncompartmental methods and after subcutaneous administration (see Ref. [121]).*
[d]*NR, not reported.*
[e]*Calculated as V/F.*
[f]*Campath has nonlinear PK in the range of 3–30 mg three times weekly.*

intravascular and extravascular compartments is slow but also that measured plasma concentrations at steady state may not be a good guide to the actual, active concentrations at the site of action. On the other hand, binding of macromolecules and mAbs to receptors or other binding sites could significantly increase apparent distribution volumes that would otherwise be much smaller (e.g., Factor IX in Table 33.14) [122].

Finally, it is important to note that the PK studies submitted to support approval of a Biological License Application (BLA) for the most part are based on noncompartmental methods that assume linear, first-order kinetics, even though this clearly is not the case for the majority of the monoclonal antibodies currently marketed, such as cetuximab (Erbitux). Unfortunately, little attention has been paid to the fact that the use of noncompartmental methods to describe the PK of mAbs greatly oversimplifies their complex properties and, as pointed out in Chapter 8, is inappropriate.

Binding to α_2-macroglobulin

α_2-Macroglobulin, one of the major proteins in the serum, is highly conserved across species and can bind many molecules, such as cytokines, enzymes, lipopolysaccharide (LPS), and ions such as zinc and nickel [123]. α_2-Macroglobulin is found in extravascular secretions, such as lymph. It exists in two forms: an electrophoretically slow native form, and a fast form, an α_2-macroglobulin-protease complex that results in a conformational change that increases electrophoretic mobility. This conformational change results in exposure of a hydrophobic region that can bind to cell surface receptors such as those on hepatocytes.

There is evidence suggesting that α_2-macroglobulin plays an important role in human immune function. Specifically, studies have shown that the fast form can inhibit antibody-dependent cellular toxicity and natural killer (NK) cell-mediated cytolysis [124], as well as superoxide production by activated macrophages [125].

As presented in Table 33.16, α_2-macroglobulin can bind to a number of exogenously administered proteins. Three different mechanisms for this binding have been identified [126]. The binding can be noncovalent and reversible. An example of this type of binding is seen with growth factors such as tissue growth factor-β (TGF-β). Second, the binding to α_2-macroglobulin can be covalent [127] and the third mechanism involves covalent linkages with proteinase reactions [128]. Subsequent to the binding, the PK and PD properties of the macromolecule may be altered. The binding of α_2-macroglobulin is associated with variable results: the α_2-macroglobulin-cytokine complex may interfere with bioassay results (e.g., nerve growth factor) [126], serve as a carrier (e.g., TGF-β) [126], prevent proteolytic degradation (e.g., IL-2) [129], or enhance removal of the protein from the circulation (e.g., tissue necrosis factor-α) [123].

Binding to other proteins

Insulin-like growth factor-1 (IGF-1) is produced by many tissues in the body and has approximately 50% structural homology with insulin. In plasma, IGF-1 exists as "free" IGF-1 and "bound" IGF-1, and its physiology, as depicted in Fig. 33.10, is very complex [130]. To date, eight binding proteins (designated IGFBP-1 through 8) have been identified, with IGFBP-3 being the most abundant. The binding proteins vary in molecular weight, distribution, concentration in biological fluids, and binding affinity [131]. It is important to note that the interactions between the binding proteins and their physiologic role are poorly understood, but probably serve to modulate the clearance and/or biological effects of IGF-1.

Metabolism

Monoclonal antibodies undergo catalytic degradation, unlike small molecules. However, there are effects of these mAbs on metabolic pathways, in particular the P450 cytochrome system that is discussed here. Table 33.17 summarizes the effects of various cytokines on the cytochrome P450 (CYP) mixed function oxidase system [132]. With the exception of IL-2, these cytokines depress the activity of CYP enzymes. Data on cytokine-mediated depression of drug-metabolizing ability has

TABLE 33.16 Binding of macromolecules to Alpha$_2$-macroglobulin.

Macromolecule	Physiological effect	Relevance of binding
Nerve growth factor	Stimulates nerve growth	Interferes with assay
Interleukin-1	Regulates proliferation of thymocytes	Regulates cell activity
Interleukin-2	Impairs proliferation of T-cells	Inactivates cytokine
Tissue growth factor β	Stimulates growth of kidney fibroblasts	Functions as carrier; accelerates clearance

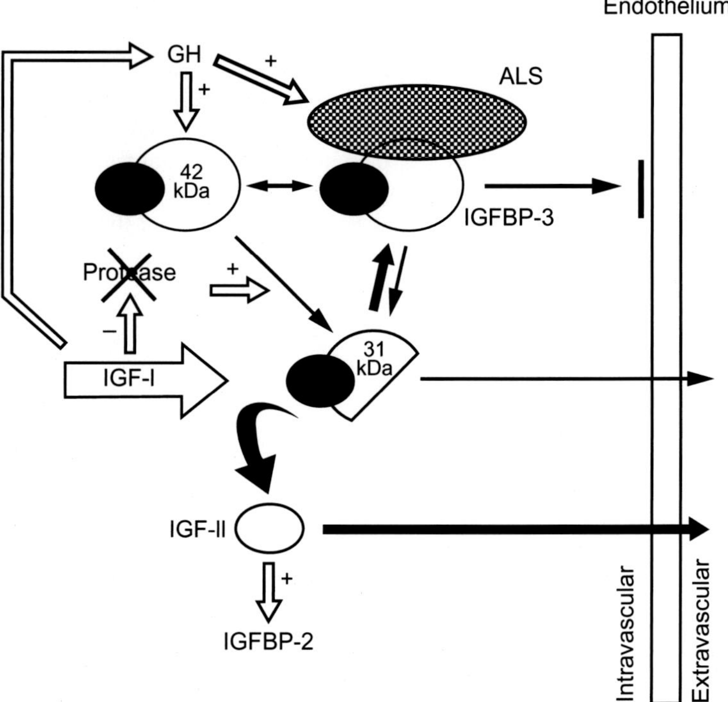

FIG. 33.10 Hypothetical model of the effects of insulin-like growth factor (IGF-1). Open arrows show regulating influences. Plasma IGF-1 consists of free and bound IGF-1. Insulin-like growth factor-binding protein-3 (IFGBP-3) exists in two forms, a 42-kDa complete form or a 31-kDa fragment. IGF-1 drives the reaction toward binding with the acid-labile subunit (ALS) to form a ternary complex, which is retained in the intravascular space. IFG-1 also suppresses growth hormone (GH) secretion, decreasing the synthesis of IGFBP-3. *Reproduced with permission from Blum WF, Jensen LW, Madsen JK. Acta Paediatr Suppl 1993;82 (Suppl 391):15–19.*

TABLE 33.17 Effect of various macromolecules on P450 isoenzymes.

Macromolecule	Isoenzyme	Effects
Interferon-α	CYP2C11	Decreased mRNA and enzyme levels
Interleukin-1	CYP2C11	Decreased mRNA and enzyme levels
	CYP2D	Decreased mRNA and enzyme levels
Interleukin-2	CYP2D1	Increased mRNA and enzyme levels
Interleukin-6	CYP2C11	Decreased mRNA and enzyme levels
Tumor necrosis factor	CYP2C11	Decreased enzyme levels

been obtained primarily in rodents under conditions of inflammation or infection [133]. The reduction in drug biotransformation capacity parallels a decrease in total CYP content and enzyme activity and is due primarily to a downregulation of CYP gene transcription, but modulation of RNA and enzyme inhibition may also be involved [133, 134].

As presented in Table 33.17, the expression of CYP2C11 and CYP2D isoenzymes is frequently suppressed by cytokines. These two CYP gene families are constitutively expressed in male and female rats. In the rat, CYP2C is under developmental and pituitary hormone regulation. Although there is approximately 70% cDNA-deduced amino acid sequence homology with the human CYP2C, caution is needed in extrapolating these observations on CYP2C regulation from rats to humans [135]. In both rats and humans, there is polymorphic expression of the CYP2D and CYP2D1 isoenzymes which exhibit debrisoquine 4-hydroxylase activity. However, this gene family has evolved differently in rats than in humans. Specifically, the rat has four genes that are approximately 73%–80% similar while the human has three genes that are 89–95% similar. Thus results in rat studies may not be predictive of results in humans because of the difference in number of genes, their regulation, and their complexity [136].

In vitro study results have been consistent with those obtained in vivo. For example, in primary rat hepatocyte cultures, IL-1, tumor necrosis factor (TNF), and interleukin-6 (IL-6) concentrations ranging from 0.5 to 10.0 ng/mL suppressed the expression of CYP2C11 mRNA [135]. It is interesting to note that in rat liver microsomes, IL-2 increased both the amount of immunoreactive CYP2D protein and its mRNA [136]. In human primary hepatocytes, IL-1β, IL-6, and TNF-α caused a decrease in all mRNAs and CYP isoenzyme activities. Moreover, interferon γ (IFN-γ) was shown to decrease CYP1D2 and CYP2E1 mRNA but had no effect on CYP2C or CYP3A mRNAs [132].

The in vitro effects of IL-6 on the CYP 450 isoenzymes were confirmed by Dickmann et al. [137], who found that IL-6 increased acute phase reactants (e.g., C-reactive protein), downregulated all CYP P450 isoform mRNA expression and, at concentrations greater than 500 pg/mL, suppressed induction of CYP1A2 by omeprazole and of CYP3A4 by rifampicin. In addition, in the presence of an anti-IL-6 mAb in the human primary hepatocyte culture, IL-6 suppression of CYP1A2 activity was completely abolished but the suppression of CYP3A4 was not, although there was a shift in the EC_{50} to the right by approximately 19-fold and 13-fold, respectively, in two different donors.

The clinical significance of the aforementioned findings is unknown. A report by Khakoo et al. [138] did not demonstrate a PK interaction between IFN-α_{2b} and ribavirin, or an additive effect of the combination therapy on safety assessments. In another study, administration of IFN-α prior to cyclophosphamide administration significantly impaired the metabolism of cyclophosphamide and 4-hydroxycyclophosphamide. In contrast, the administration of IFN-α after cyclophosphamide resulted in higher 4-hydroxycyclophosphamide concentrations and produced a significant decrease in leukocyte count [139].

The interaction between IL-2 and doxorubicin was explored in patients with advanced solid tumors [140]. Doxorubicin was given alone, and 3 weeks later patients received the combination of rhIL-2 (18 mIU/m^2 given SC on days 1–5) and doxorubicin. Doxorubicin PK was assessed for 48 hours after each administration period. SC injections of rhIL-2 did not affect doxorubicin PK, but doxorubicin given before IL-2 prevented IL-2-induced lymphocyte rebounds, although it did not qualitatively alter nonmajor histocompatibility complex-restricted cytotoxicity.

Schmitt et al. [141] evaluated the effects of an IL-6 receptor antagonist monoclonal antibody, tocilizumab, in patients with rheumatoid arthritis (RA), a disease characterized by elevated concentrations of IL-6. In this study of 12 patients with RA, the effects of tocilizumab on simvastatin, a CYP3A4 substrate, were used as an indirect measure of CYP3A4 activity. Simvastatin was administered on days 1, 13, and 43, and tocilizumab was given IV on Day 8. Tocilizumab reduced simvastatin *AUC* by one-half, corresponding to a doubling of simvastatin clearance over baseline values. In addition, C-reactive protein (CRP) levels that were markedly elevated at baseline were observed to be maximally reduced 1 week after tocilizumab administration, and this nadir occurred at the same time that the effects of tocilizumab on simvastatin were maximal. Taken together, these results constitute one of the first reports of a concurrent drug-disease and drug-drug interaction.

Tocilizumab has been used in the management of cytokine release syndrome observed after the administration of CD3 bi-specifics and chimeric antigen receptor T-cell therapies (CAR-T) [142]. In this setting, the acute treatment of patients with severe CRS is critical; the impact of potential interactions is more of a concern with the chronic treatment of a disease such as RA.

Finally, as mAbs persist in the body for a long time, patients should be monitored for a prolonged period of time, even after stopping the mAb, since the effects on CYP activity may also persist.

Although these examples illustrate that various cytokines administered exogenously can affect CYP protein content, mRNA, and enzyme activities, and reports that evaluate the extent and clinical significance of corresponding PK or PD changes are emerging in the literature with increasing frequency [143], little is known regarding the catabolism of proteins that are either currently marketed or under investigation. The absence of suitable biological assays or other analytical methods for identifying and quantitating protein degradation products obviously limits evaluation of this catabolism. Similarly, the catabolism of mAbs, in particular the catabolism of the IgG molecule, is complex and not well understood [144]. Monoclonal antibody catabolism reflects the basal metabolic rate of the body, as well as the function of phagocytic cells [monocytes, macrophages of the reticuloendothelial system (RES)]. There is also a relationship between IgG concentration and catabolism that is specific for each IgG molecule—the higher the IgG concentration, the shorter the survival time. To explain this characteristic of immunoglobulins, Brambell et al. [145] hypothesized, and Junghans and Anderson [146] have confirmed, that there is a specific, saturable receptor (FcRn) for each immunoglobulin that, when bound, protects the IgG from degradation. The IgG isotypes differ from one another in their amino acid sequence and Fc-fragment with survival half-lives of approximately 20 days for IgG_1, IgG_2, and IgG_4, but 7 days for IgG_3 [7]. The location and mechanism of IgG metabolism is not known but is believed to involve uptake by pinocytic vacuoles, release of proteolytic enzymes, and subsequent degradation of unbound IgG.

Elimination

Renal excretion

The renal excretion of proteins is size dependent and glomerular filtration is rate limiting. It has been suggested that the renal clearance rate of macromolecules, relative to the glomerular filtration rate of inulin, decreases with increasing molecular radius [147]. The following general conclusions are based on studies using indirect methods to estimate glomerular sieving coefficients. Small proteins (< 25 kDa) cross the glomerular barrier, and filtration accounts for most of their plasma clearance; the degree of sieving is independent of biologic activity, and the filtered load of protein is directly related to plasma concentration. The effect of molecular charge is negligible for these small proteins, whereas charge retards glomerular filtration of anionic proteins as large as albumin (approximately 70 kDa). Subsequent to glomerular filtration, macromolecules may undergo hydrolysis and tubular reabsorption, mainly in endocytotic vesicles located in the apical regions of renal tubular cells [148].

Consistent with these concepts, bi-specifics with molecular weights ≤50 kD without an Fc region result in rapid clearance and short elimination half-life. The half-life of bi-specifics can be extended by maintaining the Fc region or other means to extend the half-life such as pegylation and conjugation with albumin or full-length antibodies. All the variables affecting the PK of monoclonal antibodies, in addition to size, such as glycosylation and charge, may have more of an impact on the PK of bi-specifics.

Hepatic clearance

In addition to physical characteristics, the clearance of glycoproteins, structural components of macromolecules, is mediated by cell surface receptors for specific terminal carbohydrates and monosaccharides (Table 33.18). There are at least eight such receptors, the most well known of these being the Ashwell or asialoglycoprotein receptor [149]. Once the glycoprotein ligand binds to its receptor, it is internalized by endocytosis and degraded. The degrees of glycosylation, sialylation, or fucosylation are all factors that determine the clearance of these glycoproteins.

Clearance of rt-PA appears to be mediated by the mannose/*N*-acetylglucosamine specific receptor on hepatic reticuloendothelial cells. To confirm that the mannose receptor is involved, Lucore et al. [150] evaluated the clearance of rt-PA from the blood circulation of rabbits. Analysis of sequential blood samples by fibrin autography indicated that circulating free tissue plasminogen activator (t-PA, approximately 55 kDa) was predominant, but that minimal amounts of high molecular weight complexes of approximately 110 and 170 kDa also were present. Competition experiments were conducted to determine the effect of glycosylation on rt-PA clearance. As shown in Fig. 33.11, coadministration of rt-PA with *p*-aminophenyl-α-D-mannopyranoside-bovine serum albumin [BSA (BSA-Man)] prolonged both the α-phase and β-phase half-lives of rt-PA. The fact that BSA-Man inhibits the clearance of rt-PA suggests that the MAN-GlcNAc-specific glycoprotein receptor contributes to its clearance. In contrast, coadministration of rt-PA with asialofetuin did not alter the α-phase and β-phase half-lives of rt-P, suggesting that the galactose receptor does not mediate clearance. This study demonstrates that the nature and extent of the glycosylation have a direct effect on the clearance of rt-PA and its interaction with the mannose receptors in the liver.

Production of recombinant proteins using Chinese hamster ovary (CHO) cells, or other mammalian cells, results in a glycosylation pattern that differs from that of recombinant proteins produced by bacteria such as *Escherichia coli* in that CHO-produced proteins are heavily glycosylated whereas those produced by bacteria are not glycosylated. Fig. 33.12 depicts the results of an experiment comparing the plasma concentration vs time profile of granulocyte-macrophage colony-stimulating factor (GM-CSF) produced by CHO cells with that produced by *E. coli* [151]. After IV administration, the *E. coli*-produced GM-CSF had a significantly shorter α-phase half-life than did CHO-produced GM-CSF, but there was

TABLE 33.18 Cell surface receptors for the clearance of carbohydrates and monosaccharides.

Specificity[a]	Cell type
Gal/Gal/NAc	Liver parenchymal cells (asialoglycoprotein receptor)
Gal/GalNAc	Liver Kupffer and endothelial cells, peritoneal macrophages
Man/GlcNAc	Liver Kupffer and endothelial cells, peritoneal macrophages
Fuc	Liver Kupffer cells

[a]*Abbreviations:* Gal, *D-galactose;* NAc, N-*Acetylglucosamine;* Glc, *D-glucose;* Man, *D-mannose;* Fuc, *Fucose.*

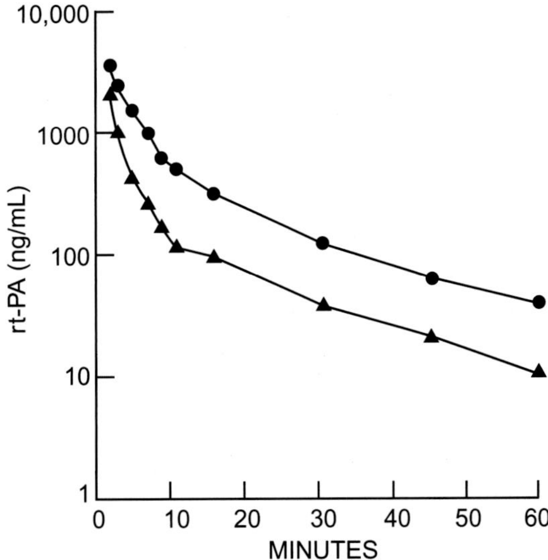

FIG. 33.11 Clearance of different forms of recombinant tissue plasmin activator (rt-PA) in rabbits after administration of rt-PA alone (▲) or in combination with *p*-aminophenyl-α-D-mannoside bovine serum albumin (●). *Reproduced with permission from Lucore CL, Fry ETA, Nachowiak DA, Sobel BE, et al. Circulation 1988;77:906–914.*

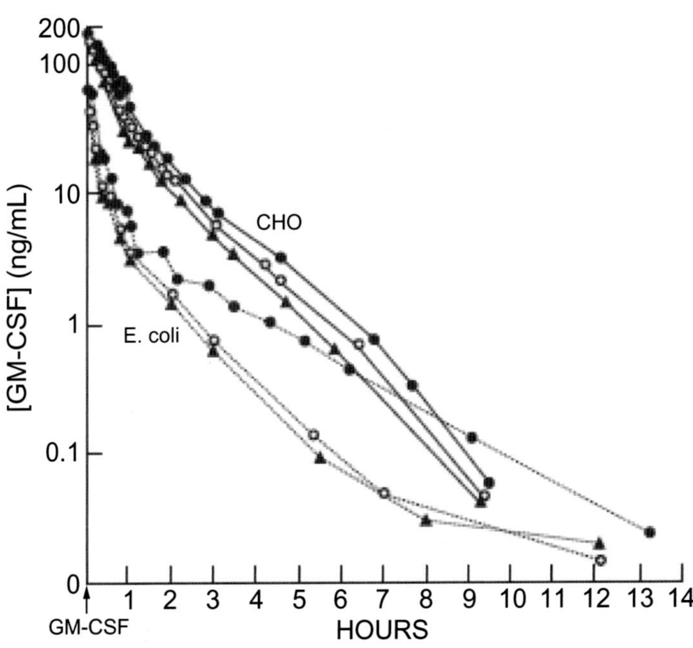

FIG. 33.12 Granulocyte-macrophage colony-stimulating factor (GM-CSF) serum concentration vs time profiles for three patients after IV bolus injection of 8 μg/kg Chinese hamster ovary (CHO)-produced GM-CSF *(solid lines)*, and for three patients who received *E. coli*-produced GM-CSF *(dotted lines)* (one patient received 5.5 μg/kg and two patients received 3 μg/kg). *Reproduced with permission from Hovgaard D, Mortensen BT, Schifter S, Nissen NI. Eur J Haematol 1993;50:32–36.*

no significant difference in the terminal half-life. The *AUC* of the glycosylated GM-CSF was approximately four to five times higher (6.3 μg min/mL) than the *AUC* of the nonglycosylated product (1.27 μg min/mL). However, since no difference in neutrophil counts was observed, the choice of one product over the other may only be a theoretical concern.

Similar to GM-CSF, granulocyte colony-stimulating factor (G-CSF) is available as either the glycosylated or nonglycosylated form of the protein. In vitro studies suggest that the glycosylated form is more stable and of a higher potency than the nonglycosylated form [152, 153]. The PK of these two forms of G-CSF were evaluated in 20 healthy volunteers [154]. As shown in Fig. 33.13, the nonglycosylated form was more rapidly absorbed after SC administration and produced a higher C_{max} (14.23 vs. 11.85 pg/mL), but there was little difference in the elimination-phase half-life (2.75 vs. 2.95 h, respectively).

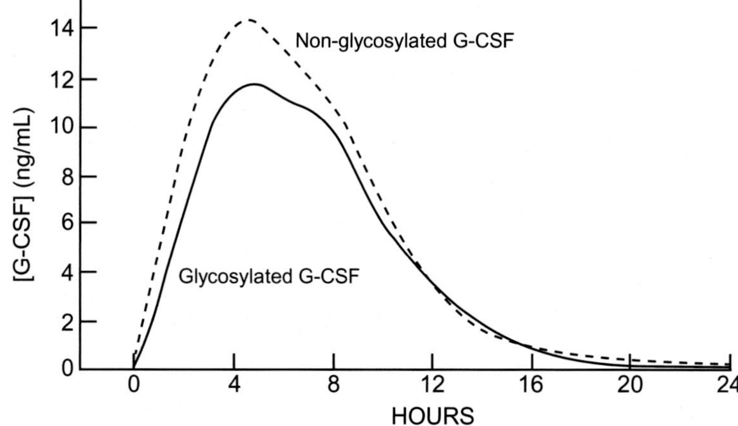

FIG. 33.13 Comparison of serum concentration vs time profiles in healthy subjects after SC administration of glycosylated G-CSF (—) and nonglycosylated G-CSF (- - -). *Reproduced with permission from Watts MJ, Addison L, Long SG, et al. Eur J Haematol 1997;98:474–479.*

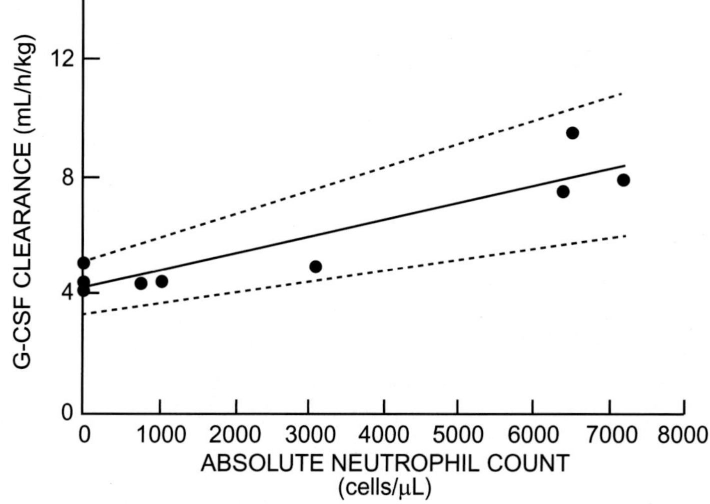

FIG. 33.14 Relationship between G-CSF clearance and absolute neutrophil count (r=0.85, P=0.00025). The dotted lines represent the 95% confidence intervals of the regression. *Reproduced with permission from Ericson SG, Gao H, Gericke GH, Lewis LD. Exp Hematol 1997;25:1313–1325.*

The AUC for the nonglycosylated form was approximately 1.2 times higher than that of the glycosylated form. However, despite these PK differences, the progenitor cell count was significantly higher with the glycosylated product, confirming the in vitro potency results.

The results with G-CSF are dissimilar from those produced after IV administration of GM-CSF, where it was found that the C_{max} was higher and the α-half-life was longer for the glycosylated than for the nonglycosylated form. The reason for these differences is unknown, but it is apparent that the comparison and subsequent interpretation of study results is dependent on knowing the production source of the protein and the structural features that may influence the potency, PK, and/or PD of individual proteins.

Monoclonal antibody structural features, such as carbohydrate side chains, influence tissue uptake and clearance [12]. For example, Morell and colleagues [155] demonstrated that removal of sialic acid residue from the carbohydrate side chain of mouse IgG_1 increased its clearance and shortened its half-life. They also demonstrated increased clearance and liver uptake of asialo-α_2 macroglobulin and asialohaptoglobin. Elimination of intact mAbs by the kidney is restricted so clearance is mainly due to catabolism, even though catabolites may be renally eliminated.

Finally, clearance may change over time for macromolecules whose clearance is mediated by cell surface receptors and, in the case of mAbs, antigens. This is illustrated by an experiment in three patients with metastatic breast cancer who received a continuous infusion of G-CSF for 2 consecutive days [119]. Absolute neutrophil counts were obtained every morning, and there was a very strong positive correlation between neutrophil count and G-CSF clearance (Fig. 33.14). Clearance on day 2 was 4.6 mL/h/kg, increasing to 8.3 mL/h/kg on day 9. Thus neutrophil production may mediate the clearance of G-CSF.

The role of target-mediated disposition and binding affinities to the targets may also affect the PK of bi-specifics; however, there is a paucity of information regarding these factors in the pharmacokinetics of bi-specific antibodies. A search of PubMed did not result in any publications identifying target mediated clearance other than publications on simulations that incorporate TMDD to include sequential binding to two targets [156, 157]. It is highly probable that TMDD also occurs with bi-specific antibodies and should be considered in modeling of concentration vs. time and response data.

In summary, there are multiple characteristics of proteins that influence their PK; some of these are listed in Table 33.19.

Application of sparse sampling and population kinetic methods

There have been attempts to study the PK of macromolecules by applying the sparse sampling strategy and population kinetic methods described in Chapter 9 [108, 158, 159]. In one study, erythropoietin was administered SC to 48 healthy adult male Japanese volunteers [108]. The population mean values estimated for k_a, k_e, V_d and the endogenous erythropoietin production rate were $0.043\,h^{-1}$, $0.206\,h^{-1}$, 3.14 L, and $15.7\,IU\,h^{-1}$, respectively. The good correlation between predicted and observed concentration values shown in Fig. 33.15 supports the choice of model, as does the fact that the values for k_e and V_d determined by this analysis were similar to those reported for IV erythropoietin with the standard two-stage method of determining population PK parameters described in Chapter 9. However, given the flip-flop PK characteristics of erythropoietin (Table 33.13), the comparison to the IV parameter estimates may be misleading. In fact, the population PK estimates for k_e are dissimilar to those obtained by other authors after SC administration of erythropoietin [93].

TABLE 33.19 Characteristics that affect the pharmacokinetics of macromolecules.

Physical characteristics	Size, structure, net charge
Posttranslational modifications	Degree of glycosylation, sialylation, fucosylation
Protein binding	Plasma proteins, induced proteins
Route of administration	Transient peaks and trough, sustained concentrations
Duration of administration	Time-dependent changes in elimination clearance
Frequency of administration	Up- or downregulation of receptors

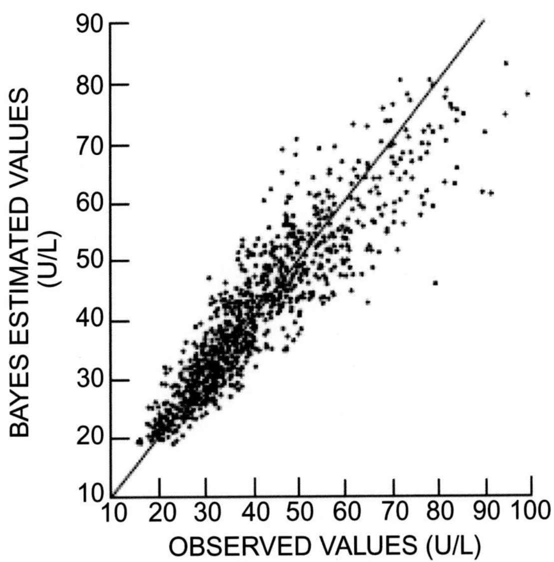

FIG. 33.15 Correlation between observed and predicted erythropoietin concentration values analyzing sparse sampling data with a population pharmacokinetic model (no *r* value given). *Reproduced with permission from Hayashi W, Kinoshita H, Yukawa E, Higuchi S. Br J Clin Pharmacol 1998;46:11–19.*

Population PK methods also were used to analyze the concentration vs time profiles of IFN-α in 27 patients with chronic hepatitis C virus infection who received an SC injection of this macromolecule [158]. The investigators reported that the absorption rate was best described by two processes: an initial zero-order process, accounting for 24% of net absorption, followed by a first-order process that had a rate constant of $0.18\,h^{-1}$. The authors noted that this value for k_a is consistent with the $0.13\,h^{-1}$ reported by Radwanski et al. [100], and both results confirm that IFN-α is slowly absorbed after SC administration.

Population PK of sibrotuzumab, a humanized mAb directed against fibroblast activation protein (FAP), which is expressed in the stromal fibroblasts in >90% of malignant epithelial tumors, was analyzed in patients with advanced or metastatic carcinoma after multiple IV infusions of doses ranging from $5\,mg/m^2$ to a maximum of 100 mg [159]. The PK model consisted of two distribution compartments with parallel first-order and Michaelis-Menten elimination pathways from the central compartment. Body weight was significantly correlated with both central and peripheral distribution volumes, the first-order elimination clearance, and V_{max} of the Michaelis-Menten pathway. Of interest was the observation that body surface area (BSA) was inferior to body weight as a covariate in explaining interpatient variability.

It is well known that for IV mAbs in general, and mAbs used in oncology in particular, dosing is based on weight or BSA. In recent years, the concept of BSA-based dosing for small molecules in oncology has been questioned [160]. The purpose of adjusting dosages based on BSA is the observation that clearance of many anticancer agents was related to glomerular filtration rate. However, the correlation of nonrenal clearance with BSA has not been demonstrated and the clearance of many anticancer agents is a function of hepatic enzyme activity. Although the objective of adjusting dosages based on weight or BSA is to reduce the pharmacokinetic variability, this has been disputed by Baker et al. [161], who found that only 5 of 33 drugs evaluated demonstrated a reduction in interpatient variability with BSA-adjusted dosages. Currently, oncologic IgG_1 mAbs such as trastuzumab, bevacizumab, and rituximab are dosed based on body weight, but it has been proposed by several authors [162, 163] that fixed dosing of mAbs performs as well as weight-based dosing and may offer advantages over weight-based dosing. This illustrates that it is important to assess during early development the contribution of differences in weight, BMI, or BSA to the observed intersubject variability in PK parameter estimates in order to make better decisions regarding the optimal basis for dose selection in late-stage clinical trials and in subsequent clinical practice.

Pharmacodynamics of macromolecules

The relationship between circulating protein concentrations following exogenous administration and PD endpoints, either for efficacy or for safety, has been explored for a number of proteins, such as IGF-1, recombinant Factor IX and Factor VIII, interleukins (IL-2), and mAbs, such as rituximab, golimumab, and omalizumab. Several conclusions emerge from the currently published data: these relationships are complex and not easily explained by a simple E_{max} model, the endpoints are not clear cut (except for those macromolecules intended to substitute for endogenous proteins that are deficient), effects of disease on PD must be evaluated, and there is a high likelihood of regimen dependency.

Models

The principles of receptor occupancy discussed in Chapter 19 and several of the PK/PD models described in Chapter 20 have been employed to explore the relationship between circulating protein or mAb concentrations and pharmacodynamic endpoints. For example, a dog model of hemophilia was used to study the activity of recombinant FIX [164]. Activity was determined in a bioassay, a modified one-stage partial thromboplastin time assay with pooled human plasma as the internal standard. As shown in Fig. 33.16, the relationship between activity and recombinant FIX concentration was linear ($r^2 = 0.86$), suggesting that for every 34.5 ng/mL of FIX there is a corresponding 1% increase in FIX activity. In 11 males with hemophilia B, it was necessary to use a sigmoid E_{max} model to describe the relationship between FIX activity and concentration (unpublished observations) and FIX serum concentrations of approximately 46 ng/mL were necessary to obtain a 1% increase in FIX activity. This translates into a 20% increase in the dosage of recombinant FIX necessary to achieve the same efficacy as plasma-derived FIX.

The indirect response model shown in Fig. 33.17 was used to describe the relationship between the administration of GH and IGF-1 in nonhuman primates [165]. The realistic assumption was made that the production of IGF-1 varied over time and, as shown in Fig. 33.18, the model provided a reasonable characterization of the induction of IGF-1 after both single and multiple GH doses. However, one limitation to this simple model is its inability to account for the role of the IGFBPs in the

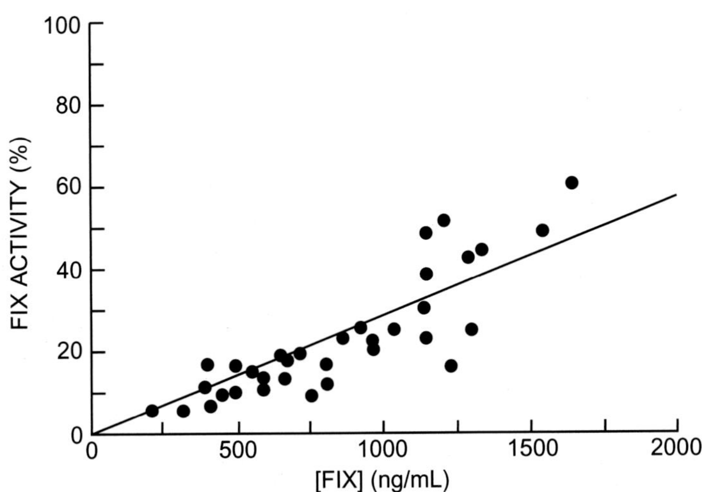

FIG. 33.16 The relationship between Factor IX (FIX) activity (determined by a modified one-stage partial thromboplastin assay) and FIX concentration in hemophilia B dogs after an infusion of 50 μg/kg FIX over 10 min. *Reproduced with permission from Schaub R, Garzone P, Bouchard P, et al. Semin Hematol 1998;35(Suppl. 2):28–32.*

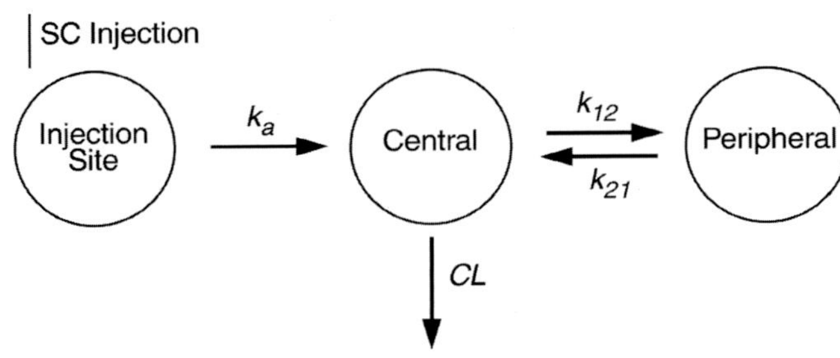

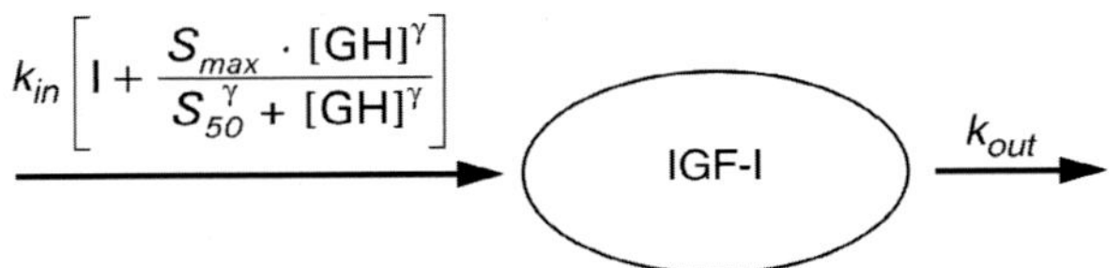

FIG. 33.17 Pharmacokinetic model for recombinant human growth hormone (rhGH) coupled with an indirect response model for IGF-1 induction by rhGH. The Hill equation was used to model IGF-1 induction by rhGH. Abbreviations: k_a, absorption rate of rhGH after SC injection; *CL*, elimination clearance of rhGH; k_{12} and k_{21}, intercompartmental transfer rates of rhGH; IGF-1, total IGF concentration; and k_{in}, basal formation rate of IGF-1. Stimulation of IGF-1 production is modeled by the Hill function shown in brackets, where S_{max} = maximum IGF stimulation of k_{in} by rhGH, S_{50} = rhGH concentration for 50% maximal stimulation of k_{in}, [GH] = rhGH concentration, n = the Hill coefficient, and k_{out} = elimination rate of IGF-1. *Modified from Sun YN, Lee JH, Almon RR, Jusko WJ. J Pharmacol Exp Ther 1999;289:1523–1532.*

responses to both GH and IGF-1. Thus others have proposed more complex models that account for the induction of IGFBPs [166–168] that can have an impact on IGF-1 and GH dosage regimens [167–169] and, more recently, for mAbs targeting the IGF-1 receptor [169].

Table 33.20 presents the PK/PD models used to predict dosage regimens for different mAbs with different IgG isotypes [170–176]. The models use population PK methods to describe the mAb concentration time course and include parameters describing receptor occupancy and binding, biomarker expression, downstream cell-signaling events, and disease severity indexes. These publications establish PK/PD paradigms that can be the basis for more sophisticated, complex models capable of describing complex dynamic interactions between administered macromolecules, cells, and disease states.

Regimen dependency

Regimen dependency was first shown for the antitumor efficacy of IL-2. Mice given 12 injections of a 1500-unit dose of this cytokine showed greater tumor inhibition than those mice that received 2 doses of 9000 units [177]. Similar results were

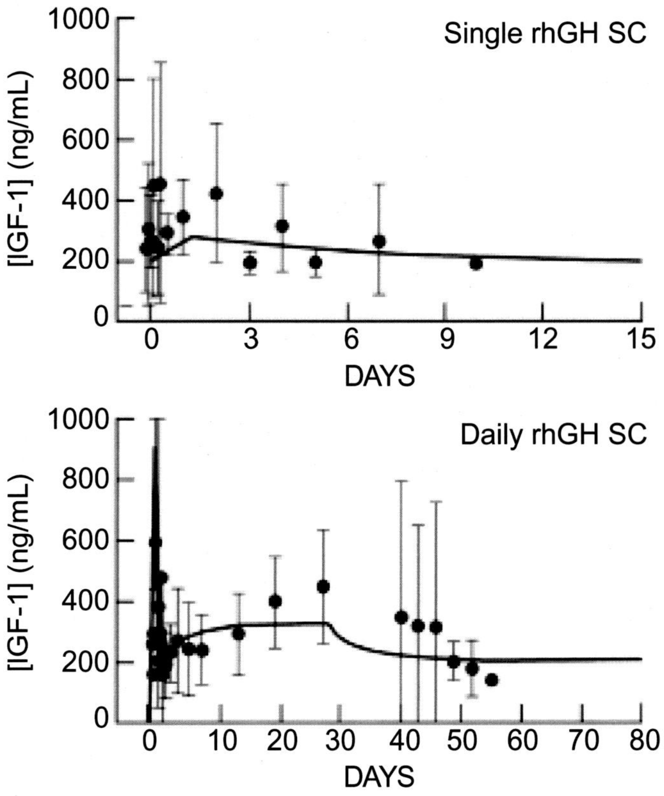

FIG. 33.18 Total IGF-1 concentrations resulting from single *(upper panel)* and daily *(lower panel)* SC injections of rhGH. Data points and bars represent the mean and standard deviation of results from four monkeys. Solid lines are the values that were simulated from the model shown in Fig. 32.15. *Reproduced with permission from Sun YN, Lee JH, Almon RR, Jusko WJ. J Pharmacol Exp Ther 1999;289:1523–1532.*

TABLE 33.20 Pharmacokinetic and pharmacodynamic models used to predict dosing regimens of mAbs.

mAb/IgG Isotype	Target	Disease	PD endpoint	PK/PD model	Ref.
Abciximab/Fab fragment	GP 11b/111a (CD41)	Coronary artery disease (angioplasty)	Ex vivo platelet aggregation	Mechanism-based model with target mediated disposition	[170]
Efalizumab[a]/IgG_1	CD11a	Psoriasis	CD11a	Mechanism based receptor mediated Pop PK	[171]
Golimumab/IgG_1	TNF-α	RA	ACRN	Inhibitory indirect response modelPop PK	[172]
Omalizumab/IgG_1	IgE	Asthma	Total and free IgE	Feedback modelPop PK	[173]
Otelixizumab/IgG_1 (aglycosylated)	CD3	PsoriasisType 1 Diabetes	$CD4^+$ & $CD8^+$ T-cell countsCD3 T-cell receptors	Direct response PDPop MM PK	[174]
Rituximab/IgG_1	CD20	FollicularNHL	Progression-free survival	Drug-disease time to event modelPop PKTPP model	[175]
Volociximab /IgG_4	$\alpha_5\beta_1$ integrin	Cancer	Free $\alpha_5\beta_1$ (on monocytes)	Mechanism-based receptor binding Pop PK	[176]

[a]*Withdrawn from the market in 2009.*

obtained in a Phase I clinical trial in which patients with renal cell carcinoma were given one of three schedules of IL-2 at an IV dosage of 1.0 or 3.0×10^6 U/m^2/day given either as a 24-h continuous infusion, as a single daily bolus injection, or as a combination of one-half of the dose by bolus injection and the remaining one-half by 24-hour infusion [178]. At least three patients received each schedule. Two of the 23 patients with renal cell carcinoma had a partial response and acceptable toxicity with the combined bolus and continuous infusion regimen. On the other hand, disease progressed in the patients that received the same dose as a daily bolus injection.

Other investigators have also described regimen dependency for IL-12 given IV [78, 179] and SC [180]. For example, Motzer and colleagues [180] treated patients with renal cell carcinoma with IL-12, administered on days 1, 8, and 15 either as a fixed dose of 1.0 μg/kg or as a series of escalating doses, where the dose was escalated for each patient from week 1 to week 2 to a target dose level of 0.5, 0.75, 1.0, 1.25, or 1.5 μg/mL. Mean peak concentrations of IL-12 and IFN-γ were greater after patients received their initial 1.0-μg/kg dose on the fixed-dose regimen (peak concentrations of 1092 ± 275 pg/mL and 250 pg/mL, respectively) than after they received the same dose on day 15 as part of the dose-escalation scheme (353 ± 79 pg/mL and 126 pg/mL, respectively). More severe toxicity was encountered with the single, fixed-dose regimen, and the maximum tolerated dose was lower (1.0 μg/kg) than that achievable with the escalation scheme (1.5 μg/kg). As a result, Phase II trials with this cytokine were begun with a regimen in which doses were escalated to 1.25 μg/kg.

This observation of tolerance has been utilized for the T-cell redirecting bi-specific antibodies' toxicity of cytokine release syndrome (CRS) as previously discussed with the stepped dosing of blinatumomab. The event of cytokine release has been shown to be related to monocyte activation (and not T-cell activation per se), which results in systemic production of toxic cytokines [181]. One therapeutic approach is to administer antibodies that inhibit the IL-6 ligand binding to the receptor such as tocilizumab or sarilumab that directly blocks the IL-6 receptor. The other approach employed has been intrasubject dose escalation. Intrasubject dose escalation results in better tolerance of doses by introducing lower doses of the product before higher doses are administered [90]. In this setting, the maximum tolerated dose (MTD) may be higher than the MTD obtained when naïve subjects receive the higher dose.

Pharmacokinetics and pharmacodynamics in biosimilar drug development

The Public Health Services (PHS) Act section 351(k) stipulates that drug developers must submit biological license applications (BLAs) to obtain marketing authorization for biosimilar and interchangeable products in the United States. The 351 (k) BLAs must contain data demonstrating biosimilarity, or interchangeability, of the proposed biosimilar/interchangeable product to a biological product already licensed (US-licensed reference product). As described before, characterizing PK and PD properties of novel biological products plays a key role in advancing novel biological products through stages of drug development and supporting a 351(a) BLA. In biosimilar drug development, PK and PD data are a critical component of regulatory submissions to establish biosimilarity to the reference product and to demonstrate that there are no clinically meaningful differences between the proposed biosimilar product and the reference product [182].

Biosimilars are approved under an abbreviated pathway by demonstrating biosimilarity, compared with demonstrating safety and efficacy for novel biological products that follow the regular approval pathway, per section 351(a) of PHS Act. Comparative analytical assessments are the foundation of a biosimilar program. The comparative clinical PK, PD, and immunogenicity data contribute to the totality of evidence in establishing biosimilarity, whereas comparative clinical efficacy data may or may not be necessary depending on the identified residual uncertainty in overall data supporting biosimilarity. As an example, the clinical program for 5 of 23 approved biosimilars in the United States, as of July 23, 2019 [183], did not contain a comparative study with clinical efficacy endpoints. These five programs included biosimilar filgrastim [184], pegfilgrastim (NCT02650973, [185]), and epoetin alfa [186, 187] which relied on PK and PD data to support the demonstration of biosimilarity. The remaining 18 approved biosimilars (adalimumab, bevacizumab, etanercept, infliximab, rituximab, and trastuzumab) obtained approval based on data from PK studies and comparative assessments of immunogenicity and efficacy endpoints.

PK similarity

The purpose of PK similarity studies is to detect clinically meaningful differences, should they exist, in systemic exposure. Achieving similar systemic exposure of the biosimilar and reference product(s) in the PK similarity study is important because the systemic exposure is generally a driver of treatment effects. Prior knowledge of the PK properties of the reference product(s) as well as the extent of analytical similarity of the proposed biosimilar to the reference product are essential for designing a successful and efficient PK similarity study. The design considerations of PK similarity studies which must meet prespecified acceptance criteria for similarity assessments include crossover vs parallel-arm, the study population (healthy subjects vs patients), the dose and the route of administration, the study duration, and the PK sampling schedule. For instance, sources of PK variability such as intersubject variability of PK parameter estimates influence the sample size of the study and the selection of the study population. For products that are approved for more than one route of administration, a study with extravascular dosing would provide more comprehensive comparative data, including the characteristics of absorption and systemic elimination. A good understanding of the PK properties facilitates the selection of study duration and sampling schedule to capture an adequate profile for evaluating the PK similarity between two products.

PD similarity

Achieving similar PD responses between the biosimilar and reference product(s) can further streamline biosimilar development programs when the selected PD biomarkers are relevant to the mechanism(s) of action and are adequately sensitive for the evaluation of clinically meaningful differences between products. So far, PK, PD, and immunogenicity similarity data supported the FDA's approval of five biosimilar products, two filgrastim biosimilars, two pegfilgrastim biosimilars, and one biosimilar epoetin alfa. The biomarkers used to assess PD similarity were absolute neutrophil count (ANC) and $CD34^+$ cells for filgrastim, ANC for pegfilgrastim, and reticulocyte counts and hemoglobin for epoetin alfa. The PD similarity evaluation was based on a comparison of temporal PD profiles following either a single-dose (ANC, reticulocyte) or multiple-dose administration ($CD34^+$, hemoglobin). Issues such as the lack of clarity in the mechanism(s) of action or the limited availability of well-characterized or suitable PD biomarkers for many biologics may limit broad application of this approach. Nonetheless, there is great potential for using PD biomarkers to support biosimilar programs, because the biomarkers do not need to be established surrogate biomarkers for efficacy. In this respect, the use of PD biomarkers for biosimilar development represents a new area for innovation and is likely to have a big impact by repurposing existing PD biomarkers, traditionally secondary or exploratory endpoints in a clinical trial to now become primary endpoints [188]. Importantly, the FDA's guidance [182] lays out five characteristics to consider which will serve to shape the roadmap for evidentiary standards of biomarkers in biosimilar development. This will require reviewing literature to identify potential biomarkers relevant to the mechanism(s) of action, conducting pilot studies to collect clinical data evaluating the suitability of the biomarker sensitivity to detect meaningful differences, and confirming the validity of bioanalytical methods used in monitoring the biomarkers' temporal profiles [189].

Bioanalytical technologies

The bioanalytical methodologies used to measure concentrations of drugs and biomarkers need to have adequate precision and accuracy for detecting clinically meaningful differences between the biosimilar product and the reference product, should they exist. The draft ICH M10 guidance [190] provides regulatory expectations regarding validation of the bioanalytical methods used to measure PK and PD analytes. Although PK assay methodologies are generally well established during the development of reference products, biosimilar development also requires thoughtful selection of critical reagents for the ligand binding assays (LBA) and careful evaluation of the performance of the bioanalytical methods. Due to the diversity of PD biomarkers, methods for PD biomarker measurements can encompass a wide range of technologies, including, but not limited to, liquid chromatography-tandem mass spectroscopy (LC/MS-MS) for smaller analytes, LBA for proteins, and flow cytometry for cell counts. While the ICH M10 guidance does not address all assay methodologies, the best practices for validation of various method types are available in published scientific literature.

Modeling and simulation

Use of in silico technologies such as population modeling of PK and/or PD data can enhance the probability of success in demonstrating a lack of clinically meaningful differences in PK and PD between two products [191, 192]. For example, estimating the source of variability contributing to observed data can inform the selection of the study population and reduce its sample size. Temporal PK and PD profiles generated from model-based simulations provide greater details regarding dose-response and dose-exposure relationships that can guide the selection of study dose(s), study duration, and sampling schedule. Biosimilar development programs can leverage many publicly available in silico tools from novel drug development programs and from published literature.

References

[1] Kaplona H, Reichert JM. Antibodies to watch in 2019. MAbs 2019;11:219–238.

[2] FDA (CDER). Advancing health through innovation 2018 new drug therapy approvals report. Internet at: https://www.fda.gov/files/drugs/published/New-Drug-Therapy-Approvals-2018_3.pdf; 2018.

[3] Coté RJ, Morrissey DM, Houghtone AN, Beattie EJ, Oettgen HF, Old LJ. Generation of human monoclonal antibodies reactive with cellular antigens. Proc Natl Acad Sci U S A 1983;80:2026–2030.

[4] Sears HF, Atkinson B, Mattis J, Ernst C, Herlyn D, Steplewski A, et al. Phase-1 clinical trial of monoclonal antibody in treatment of gastrointestinal tumours. Lancet 1982;1:762–765.

[5] Mellstedt H. Monoclonal antibodies in human cancer. Drugs Today (Barc) 2003;39(Suppl. C):1–16.

[6] Hoet RM, Cohen EH, Kent RB, Rookey K, Schoonbroodt S, Hogan S, et al. Generation of high-affinity human antibodies by combining donor-derived and synthetic complementarity-determining-region diversity. Nat Biotechnol 2005;23:344–348.

[7] Roguska MA, Pedersen JT, Keddy CA, Henry AH, Searle SJ, Lambert JM, et al. Humanization of murine monoclonal antibodies through a variable domain resurfacing. Proc Natl Acad Sci 1994;91:969–973.

[8] Anon. Monoclonal antibody production. (Internet at https://en.wikipedia.org/wiki/Monoclonal_antibody#/media/File:Monoclonals.png.).

[9] Batra SK, Jain M, Wittel UA, Chauhan SC, Colcher D. Pharmacokinetics and biodistribution of genetically engineered antibodies. Curr Opin Biotechnol 2002;13:603–608.

[10] Colcher D, Goel A, Pavlinkova G, Beresford G, Booth B, Batra SK. Effects of genetic engineering on the pharmacokinetics of antibodies. Q J Nucl Med 1999;43:132–139.

[11] Miller K, Meng G, Liu J, Hurst A, Hsei V, Wong WL, et al. Design, construction, and *in vitro* analysis of multivalent antibodies. J Immunol 2003;170:4854–4861.

[12] Iznaga-Escobar N, Ak M, Perez-Rodriguez R. Factors affecting the pharmacokinetics of monoclonal antibodies: a review article. Methods Find Exp Clin Pharmacol 2004;26:123–127.

[13] Colcher D, Pavlinkova G, Beresford G, Booth BJ, Batra SK. Single-chain antibodies in pancreatic cancer. Ann N Y Acad Sci 1999;880:263–280.

[14] Putnam WS, Prabhu S, Zheng Y, Subramanyam M, Wang YMC. Pharmacokinetic, pharmacodynamic and immunogenicity comparability assessment strategies for monoclonal antibodies. Trends Biotechnol 2010;28:509–516.

[15] Pardridge WM, Kang YS, Yang J, Buciak JL. Enhanced cellular uptake and in vivo biodistribution of a monoclonal antibody following cationization. J Pharm Sci 1995;84:943–948.

[16] Lee HJ, Pardridge WM. Monoclonal antibody radiopharmaceuticals: cationization, pegylation, radiometal chelation, pharmacokinetics, and tumor imaging. Bioconjug Chem 2003;14:546–553.

[17] Igawa T, Tsunoda H, Tachibana MA, Mimoto F, Moriyama C, et al. Reduced elimination of IgG antibodies by engineering the variable region. Protein Eng Des Sel 2010;23:385–392.

[18] Nisonoff A, Rivers MM. Recombination of a mixture of univalent antibody fragments of different specificity. Arch Biochem Biophys 1961;93:460–462.

[19] Shatz W, Chung S, Bing L, Marshall B, Tejada M, Phung W, Sandoval W, Kelley RF, Scheer JM. Knobs-into-holes antibody production in mammalian cell lines reveals that asymmetric afucosylation is sufficient for full antibody-dependent cellular cytotoxicity. MAbs 2013;5:872–881.

[20] Wei H, Cai H, Jin Y, Wang P, Zhang Q, Lin Y, Wang W, Cheng J, Zeng XT, Zhour A. Structural basis of a novel heterodimeric Fc for bispecific antibody production. Oncotarget 2017;8:51037–51049.

[21] Spies C, Zhai Q, Carter PJ. Alternative molecular formats and therapeutic applications for bispecific antibodies. Mol Immunol 2015;67:95–106.

[22] Kai M, Motoki K, Yoshida H, Emuta C, Chisaka Y, Tsuruhata K, Endo C, Muto M, Shimabe M, Nishiyama U, et al. Switching constant domains enhances agonist activities of antibodies to a thrombopoietin receptor. Nat Biotechnol 2008;26:209–211.

[23] Kapelski S, Cleiren E, Attar RM, Philippar U, Häsler J, Chiu ML. Influence of the bispecific antibody IgG subclass on T cell redirection. MAbs 2019;11:1012–1024.

[24] Klein C, Schaefer W, Regula JT. The use of CrossMAb technology for the generation of bi- and multispecific antibodies. MAbs 2016;8:1010–1020.

[25] Stieglmaier J, Benjamin J, Nagorsen D. Utlizing the BiTE (bispecific T-cell engager) platform for immunotherapy of cancer. Expert Opin Biol Ther 2015;15:1093–1099.

[26] Warnders FJ, Waaijer SJ, Pool M, Lub-de Hooge MN, Friedrich M, Terwisscha van Scheltinga AG, et al. Biodistribution and PET imaging of labeled bispecific T cell-engaging antibody targeting EpCAM. J Nucl Med 2016;57:812–817.

[27] Radar C. DARTS take aim at BiTEs. Blood 2011;117:4043–4044.

[28] von Stackelberg A, Locatelli F, Zugmaier G, Handgretinger R, Trippett TM, Rizzari C, et al. Phase 1/Phase2 study in pediatric patients with relapsed/refractory B-cell precursor acute lymphoblastic leukemia (BCP-ALL) receiving blinatumomab treatment. Blood 2016;34:4381–4389.

[29] Viardot A, Goebeler M, Hess G, Neumann S, Pfreundschuh M, Adrian N, et al. Phase 2 study of the bispecific T-cell engager (BiTE) antibody blinatumomab in relapsed/refractory diffuse large B-Cell lymphoma. Blood 2016;127:1410–1416.

[30] Hijazi Y, Klinger M, Kratzer A, Wu B, Baeuerle PA, Kufer P, et al. Pharmacokinetic and pharmacodynamic relationship of blinatumomab in patients with non-Hodgkin lymphoma. Curr Clin Pharmacol 2018;13:55–64.

[31] Johnson S, Burke S, Huang L, Gorlatov S, Li H, Wang W, et al. Effector cell recruitment with novel Fv-based dual-affinity re-targeting protein leads to potent tumor cytolysis and in vivo B-cell depletion. J Mol Biol 2010;399:436–449.

[32] Fisher TS, Hooper AT, Lucas J, Clark TH, Rohner AK, Peano B, et al. A CD3-bispecifc molecule targeting P-cadherin demonstrates T cell-mediated regression of established solid tumors in mice. Cancer Immunol Immunother 2018;67:247–259.

[33] Blinatumomab Summary Basis of Approval. (Internet at, https://www.accessdata.fda.gov/drugsatfda_docs/nda/2014/125557Orig1s000TOC.cfm).

[34] Schaller TH, Foster MW, Thompson JW, Spasojevic I, Normantaite D, Moseley MA, et al. Pharmacokinetic analysis of a novel human EGFRvIII: CD3 bispecific antibody in plasma and whole blood using a high-resolution targeted mass spectrometry approach. J Proteome Res 2019;18:3032–3041.

[35] Kebenko M, Goebeler ME, Wolf M, Hasenburg A, Seggewiss-Bernhardt R, Ritter B, et al. A multicenter phase 1 study of solitomab (MT110, AMG 110), a bispecific EpCAM/CD3 T-cell engager (BiTE) antibody construct, in patients with refractory solid tumors. J Oncol Immunol 2018;7:1–10.

[36] Friedrich M, Raum T, Lutterbuese R, Voelkel M, Deegen P, Rau D, et al. Regression of human prostate cancer xenografts in mice by AMG 212/ BAY2010112, a novel PSMA/CD3-bispecific BiTE antibody cross-reactive with non-humanprimate antigens. Mol Cancer Ther 2012;11:2664–2673.

[37] Campagne O, Delmas A, Fouliard S, Chenel M, Chichili GR, Li H, et al. Integrated pharmacokinetic/pharmacodynamic model of a bispecific CD3xCD123 DART molecule in nonhuman primates: evaluation of activity and impact of immunogenicity. Clin Cancer Res 2018;24:2631–2641.

[38] Moore PA, Shah K, Yang Y, Alderson R, Roberts P, Long V, et al. Development of MGD007, a gpA33 x CD3- bispecific DART protein for T-cell immunotherapy of metastatic colorectal. cancer. Mol Cancer Ther 2018;17:1761–1772.

[39] Moore PA, Chichili GR, Alderson R, Li H, Brown J, Huang L, et al. MGD009, a B7-H3 x CD3 bispecific dual-affinity re-targeting (DART) molecule directing T cells to solid tumors. In: Keystone symposia conference, March 6–10, 2016, Whistler, British Columbia, Canada; 2016.

[40] Root AR, Cao W, Li B, LaPan P, Meade C, Sanford J, et al. Development of PF-06671008, a highly potent anti-P-cadherin/anti-CD3 bispecific DART molecule with extended half-life for the treatment of cancer. Antibodies (Basel) 2016;5:6. https://doi.org/10.3390/antib5010006.

[41] Hernandez-Hoyos G, Seell T, Bader R, Bannink J, Chenault RA, Daugherty M, et al. Mor209/ES414, a novel bispecific antibody targeting PSMA for the treatment of metastatic castration-resistant prostate cancer. Mol Cancer Ther 2016;15:2155–2165.

[42] Comeau MR, Gottschalk R, Daugherty M, Sewell T, Misher L, Jeannette B, et al. APVO436, a bispecific anti-CD123 x anti-CD3 ADAPTIR molecule for redirected T-cell cytotoxicity with limited cytokine release, is well tolerated in repeat dose toxicology studies in cynomolgus macaques. Cancer Res 2019;79(13 Suppl). https://doi.org/10.1158/1538-7445.AM2019-LB-199. Abstract LB-199.

[43] Lemon B, Aaron W, Austin R, Baeuerle PA, Jones A, Jones SD, et al. HPN424, a half-life extended, PSMA/CD3-specific TriTAC for the treatment of metastatic prostate cancer. In: AACR Poster 2018; 2018. Internet at: https://www.harpoontx.com/file.cfm/43/docs/AACR_2018_Poster_HPN424.pdf.

[44] Harwood SL, Alvarez-Cienfuegos A, Nunez-Prado N, Compteb M, Hernandez-Perezc S, Merinod N, et al. ATTACK, a novel bispecific T cell-recruiting antibody with trivalent EGFR binding and monovalent CD3 binding for cancer immunotherapy. Oncoimmunology 2018;7:e1377874.

[45] Seckinger A, Delgado JA, Moser S, Hose D, Paiva B, Vu MD. Target expression, generation, preclinical activity and pharmacokinetics of the BCMA- T cell bi-specific antibody EM801 for multiple myeloma treatment. Cancer Cell 2017;31:396–410.

[46] Trinklein ND, Pham D, Schellenberger U, Buelowa B, Boudreau A, Choudhry P, et al. Efficient tumor killing and minimal cytokine release with novel T-cell agonist bi-specific antibodies. MAbs 2019;11:639–652.

[47] Leong SR, Sukumaran S, Hristopoulos M, Totpal K, Stainton S, Lu E, et al. An anti-CD3/anti–CLL-1 bispecific antibody for the treatment of acute myeloid leukemia. Blood 2017;129:609–618.

[48] Le Gall F, Reusch U, Little M, Kipriyanov SM. Effect of linker sequences between the antibody variable domains on the formation, stability and biological activity of a bispecific tandem diabody. Protein Eng Des Sel 2004;17:357–366.

[49] Du J, Cao Y, Liu Y, Wang Y, Zhang Y, Fu G, et al. Engineering bifunctional antibodies with constant regime fusion architectures. J Am Chem Soc 2017;139:18607–18615.

[50] Jimeno A, Moore KN, Gordon M, Chugh R, Diamond JR, Aljumaily R, et al. A first-in-human phase 1a study of the bispecific anti-DLL4/anti-VEGF antibody navicixizumab (OMP-305B83) in patients with previously treated solid tumors. Investig New Drugs 2019;37:461–472.

[51] Rothe A, Sasse S, Topp MS, Eichenauer DA, Hummel H, Reiners KS, et al. A phase 1 study of the bispecific anti-CD30/CD16A antibody construct AFM13 in patients with relapsed or refractory Hodgkin lymphoma. Blood 2015;125:4024–4031.

[52] Reusch U, Burkhardt C, Fucek I, Le Gall F, Le Gall M, Hoffmann K, et al. A novel tetravalent bispecific TandAb (CD30/CD16A) efficiently recruits NK cells for the lysis of CD30+ tumor cells. MAbs 2014;6:727–738.

[53] Nelson M, Mille R, Bader R, Werchau D, Nilsson A, Ljung L, et al. Potent tumor-directed T-cell activation and tumor inhibition induced by ALG. APV-527,4-1BB x 5T4 ADAPTIR bispecific antibody. In: Abstract (P642) presented at SITC, Washington DC, Nov; 2019. p. 642. https://sitc.sitcancer.org/2019/abstracts/titles/index.php?filter=Immune-stimulants+and+immune+modulators.

[54] Muto A, Yoshihashi K, Takeda M, Kitazawa T, Soeda T, Igawa T, et al. Anti-factor IXa/X bispecific antibody (ACE910): hemostatic potency against ongoing bleeds in a hemophilia A model and the possibility of routine supplementation. J Thromb Haemost 2014;12:206–213.

[55] Kitazawa T, Igawa T, Sampei Z, Muto A, Kojima T, Soeda T, et al. A bispecific antibody to factors IXa and X restores factor VIII hemostatic activity in a hemophilia A model. Nat Med 2012;18:1570–1576.

[56] Shima M, Hanabusa H, Taki M, Matsushita T, Sato T, Fukutake K, et al. Factor VIII-mimetic function of humanized bispecific antibody in hemophilia A. N Engl J Med 2016;374:2044–2053.

[57] Lacy SE, Wu C, Ambrosi DJ, Hsieh CM, Bose S, Miller R, et al. Generation and characterization of ABT-981, a dual variable domain immunoglobulin (DVD-IgTM) molecule that specifically and potently neutralizes both IL-1a and IL-1b. MAbs 2015;7:605–619.

[58] Kosloski MP, Goss S, Wang SX, Liu J, Loebbert R, Medema JK, et al. Pharmacokinetics and tolerability of a dual variable domain immunoglobulin ABT-981against IL-1α and IL-1β in healthy subjects and patients with osteoarthritis of the knee. J Clin Pharmacol 2016;56:1582–1590.

[59] Li Y, Hickson JA, Ambrosi DJ, Haasch DL, Foster-Duke KD, Eaton LJ, et al. ABT-165, a dual variable domain immunoglobulin(DVD-Ig) targeting DLL4 and VEGF demonstrates superior efficacy and favorable safety profiles in preclinical models. Mol Cancer Ther 2018;17:1039–1050.

[60] Akpalu DE, Frederick B, Nnane IP, Yao Z, Shen F, Ort T, et al. Pharmacokinetics, pharmacodynamics, immunogenicity, safety, and tolerability of JNJ-61178104, a novel tumor necrosis factor-alpha and interleukin-17A bispecific antibody, in healthy subjects. J Clin Pharmacol 2019;59:968–978.

[61] Schaefer W, Regula JT, Bähner M, Schanzer J, Croasdale R, Dürr H, et al. Immunoglobulin domain crossover as a generic approach for the production of bi-specific IgG antibodies. MAbs 2011;108:11187–11192.

[62] Hidalgo M, Martinez-Garcia M, Le Tourneau C, Massard C, Garralda E, Boni V, et al. First-in-human Phase I study of single-agent vanucizumab, a first-in-classbispecific anti-angiopoietin-2/anti-VEGF-A antibody, in adult patients with advanced solid tumors. Clin Cancer Res 2017;24:1536–1545.

[63] Sampei Z, Igawa T, Soeda T, Okuyama-Nishida Y, Moriyama C, Wakabayashi T, et al. Identification and multidimensional optimization of an asymmetric bispecific IgG antibody mimicking the function of factor VIII cofactor activity. PLoS One 2013;8(2)e57479.

[64] Muto A, Yoshihashi K, Takeda M, Kitazawa T, Soeda T, Igawa T, et al. Anti-factor IXa/X bispecific antibody ACE910 prevents joint bleeds in a long-term primate model of acquired hemophilia A. Blood 2014;124(20):3165–3171.

[65] Uchida N, Sambe T, Yoneyama K, Fukazawa N, Kawanishi T, Kobayashi S, et al. A first-in-human phase 1 study of ACE910, a novel factor VIII-mimetic bispecific antibody, in healthy subjects. Blood 2016;127:1633–1641.

[66] Yoneyama K, Schmitt C, Kotani N, Levy GG, Kasai R, Iida S, et al. A pharmacometric approach to substitute for a conventional dose-finding study in rare diseases: example of Phase III dose selection for emicizumab in hemophilia A. Clin Pharmacokinet 2018;57:1123–1134.

[67] Myler HA, Given A, Kolz K, Mora JR, Hristopoulos G. Biotherapeutic bioanalysis: a multi-indication case study review. Bioanalysis 2011;3:623–643.

[68] Lee JW, Kelley M, King LE, Yang J, Salimi-Moosavi H, Tang MT, et al. Bioanalytical approaches to quantify "total" and "free" therapeutic antibodies and their targets: technical challenges and PK/PD applications over the course of drug development. AAPS J 2011;13:99–110.

[69] FDA Guidance. Bioanalytical method validation guidance for industry, Internet at: https://www.fda.gov/media/70858/download; 2018.

[70] Chappell WR, Mordenti J. Extrapolation of toxicological and pharmacological data from animals to humans. Adv Drug Res 1991;20:1–116.

[71] Mordenti J, Chen SA, Moore JA, Ferraiolo BL, Green JD. Interspecies scaling of clearance and volume of distribution data for five therapeutic proteins. Pharm Res 1991;8:1351–1359.

[72] Schaub R, Garzone P, Bouchard P, Rup B, Keith J, Brinkhous K, et al. Preclinical studies of recombinant factor IX. Semin Hematol 1998;35(Suppl. 2):28–32.

[73] Brinkhouse KM, Sigman JL, Read MS, Stewart PF, McCarthy KP, Timony GA, et al. Recombinant human Factor IX: replacement therapy, prophylaxis, and pharmacokinetics in canine hemophilia B. Blood 1996;88:2603–2610.

[74] Mordenti J, Osaka G, Garcia K, Thomsen K, Licko V, Meng G. Pharmacokinetics and interspecies scaling of recombinant human factor VIII. Toxicol Appl Pharmacol 1996;136:75–78.

[75] Nadeau RR, Ostrowski C, Ni-Wu G, Liberator DJ. Pharmacokinetics and pharmacodynamics of recombinant human interleukin-12 in male rhesus monkeys. J Pharmacol Exp Ther 1995;274:78–83.

[76] Rakhit A, Yeon MM, Ferrante J, Fettner S, Nadeau R, Motzer R, et al. Down-regulation of the pharmacokinetic–pharmacodynamic response to interleukin-12 during long-term administration to patients with renal cell carcinoma and evaluation of the mechanism of this "adaptive response" in mice. Clin Pharmacol Ther 1999;65:615–629.

[77] White G, Shapiro A, Ragni M, Garzone P, Goodfellow J, Tubridy K, et al. Clinical evaluation of recombinant factor IX. Semin Hematol 1998;35 (Suppl. 2):33–38.

[78] Atkins MB, Robertson MJ, Gordon M, Lotze MT, DeCoste M, DuBois JS, et al. Phase 1 evaluation of intravenous recombinant human interleukin 12 (rhIL-12) in patients with advanced malignancies. Clin Cancer Res 1997;3:409–417.

[79] Wolberg AS, Stafford DW, Erie DA. Human factor IX binds to specific sites on the collagenous domain of collagen IV. J Biol Chem 1997;272:16717–16720.

[80] Duconge J, Fernandez-Sanchez E, Alvarez D. Interspecies scaling of the monoclonal anti-EGF receptor ior EGF/r^3 antibody disposition using allometric paradigm: is it really suitable? Biopharm Drug Dispos 2004;25:177–186.

[81] Mahmood I. Interspecies scaling of protein drugs: prediction of clearance from animals to humans. J Pharm Sci 2004;93:177–185.

[82] Duconge J, Castillo R, Crombet T, Alvarez D, Matheu J, Vecino G, et al. Integrated pharmacokinetic–pharmacodynamic modeling and allometric scaling for optimizing the dosage regimen of the monoclonal ior EGF/r^3 antibody. Eur J Pharm Sci 2004;21:261–270.

[83] Wang W, Prueksaritanont T. Prediction of human clearance of therapeutic proteins: simple allometric scaling method revisited. Biopharm Drug Dispos 2010;31:253–263.

[84] Oitate M, Masubuchi N, Ito T, Yabe Y, Karibe T, Aoki T, et al. Prediction of human pharmacokinetics of therapeutic monoclonal antibodies from simple allometry of monkey data. Drug Metab Pharmacokinet 2011;26:423–430.

[85] Ling J, Zhou H, Jiao Q, Davis HM. Interspecies scaling of therapeutic monoclonal antibodies: initial look. J Clin Pharmacol 2009;49:1382–1402.

[86] Suntharalingam G, Perry MR, Ward S, Brett SJ, Castello-Cortes A, Brunner MD, et al. Cytokine Storm in a Phase 1 trial of the anti-CD28 monoclonal antibody TGN1412. New Engl J Med 2006;355:1018–1028.

[87] Committee for Medicinal Products for Human Use. Guideline on strategies to identify and mitigate risks for first-in-human clinical trials with investigational medicinal products, London: EMEA/CHMP; 2007. Internet at: http://www.emea.europa.eu/docs/en_GB/document_library/Scientific_guideline/2009/09/WC500002988.pdf.

[88] Muller PY, Milton M, Lloyd P, Sims J, Brennan FR. The minimum anticipated biological effect level (MABEL) for selection of first human dose in clinical trials with monoclonal antibodies. Curr Opin Biotechnol 2009;20:722–729.

[89] Yu J, Karcher H, Feire AL, Lowe PJ. From target selection to minimum acceptable biological effect level for human study: use of mechanism-based PK/PD modeling to design safe and efficacious biologics. AAPS J 2011;13:169–178.

[90] Saber H, Del Valle P, Ricks TK, Leighton JK. An FDA oncology analysis of CD3 bispecific constructs and first-in human dose selection. Regul Toxicol Pharmacol 2017;90:448–456.
[91] Dudal S, Hinton H, Giust AM, Bacac M, Muller M, Fauti T, et al. Application of a MABEL approach for a T-cell-bispecific monoclonal antibody: CEA TCB. J Immunother 2016;39:279–289.
[92] Chen X, Haddish-Berhane N, Moore P, Clark T, Yang Y, Li H, et al. Mechanistic projection of first-in-human dose for bispecific immunomodulatory P-cadherin LPDART: an integrated PK/PD modeling approach. Clin Pharmacol Ther 2016;100:232–241.
[93] Cheung WK, Goon BL, Guilfoyle MC, Wacholtz MC. Pharmacokinetics and pharmacodynamics of recombinant human erythropoietin after single and multiple subcutaneous doses to healthy subjects. Clin Pharmacol Ther 1998;64:412–423.
[94] Veldhuis JD, Evans WS, Johnson ML. Complicating effects of highly correlated model variables on nonlinear least-squares estimates of unique parameter values and their statistical confidence intervals: estimating basal secretion and neurohormone half-life by deconvolution analysis. In: Johnson ML, Veldhuis JD, editors. Methods in neurosciences. vol. 28. Academic Press; 1995. p. 130–138.
[95] Albertsson-Wikland K, Rosberg S, Libre E, Lundberg LO, Groth T. Growth hormone secretory rates in children as estimated by deconvolution analysis of 24-h plasma concentration profiles. Am J Phys 1989;257:E809–E814.
[96] Bright GM, Veldhuis JD, Iranmanesh A, Baumann G, Maheshwari H, Lima J. Appraisal of growth hormone (GH) secretion: evaluation of a composite pharmacokinetic model that discriminates multiple components of GH input. J Clin Endocrinol Metab 1999;84:3301–3308.
[97] Macdougall IC, Roberts DE, Neubert P, Dharmasena AD, Coles GA, Williams JD. Pharmacokinetics of intravenous, intraperitoneal, and subcutaneous recombinant erythropoietin in patients on CAPD. A rationale for treatment. Contrib Nephrol 1989;76:112–121.
[98] Cetron JS, Bury RW, Lieschke GJ, Morstyn G. The effects of dose and route of administration on the pharmacokinetics of granulocyte-macrophage colony stimulating factor. Eur J Cancer 1990;26:1064–1069.
[99] Lauresen T, Grardjean B, Jørgensen JOL, Christiansen JS. Bioavailability and bioactivity of three different doses of nasal growth hormone (GH) administered to GH-deficient patients: comparison with intravenous and subcutaneous administration. Eur J Endocrinol 1996;135:309–315.
[100] Radwanski E, Perentisis G, Jacobs S, Oden E, Affrime M, Symchowicz S, et al. Pharmacokinetics of interferon alpha-2b in healthy volunteers. J Clin Pharmacol 1987;27:432–435.
[101] Schuller J, Czejka MJ, Schernthaner G, Wirth M, Bosse C, Jager W, et al. Pharmacokinetics of interferon-alfa-2b after intrahepatic or intraperitoneal administration. Semin Oncol 1992;19(Suppl. 3):98–104.
[102] Aoyama K, Uchida T, Takanuki F, Usui T, Watanabe T, Higuchi S, et al. Pharmacokinetics of recombinant human interleukin-11 (rhIL-11) in healthy male subjects. Br J Clin Pharmacol 1997;43:571–578.
[103] Montagna M, Montillo M, Avanzini MA, Tinelli C, Tedeschi A, Visai L, et al. Relationship between pharmacokinetic profile of subcutaneously administered alemtuzumab and clinical response in patients with chronic lymphocytic leukemia. Haematologia 2011;96:932–936.
[104] Xu Z, Wang Q, Zhuang Y, Frederick B, Yan H, Bouman-Thio E, et al. Subcutaneous bioavailability of golimumab at 3 different injection sites in healthy subjects. J Clin Pharmacol 2010;50:276–284.
[105] Plosker GL, Keam SJ. OmalizuMab: a review of its use in the treatment of allergic asthma. BioDrugs 2008;22:189–204.
[106] Smith DA, Minthorn EA, Beerahee M. Pharmacokinetics and pharmacodynamics of mepolizumab, an anti-interleukin-5 monoclonal antibody. Clin Pharmacokinet 2011;50:215–227.
[107] Kearns GL, Kemp SF, Frindik JP. Single and multiple dose pharmacokinetics of methionyl growth hormone in children with idiopathic growth hormone deficiency. J Clin Endocrin Metabol 1991;72:1148–1156.
[108] Hayashi W, Kinoshita H, Yukawa E, Higuchi S. Pharmacokinetic analysis of subcutaneous erythropoietin administration with non-linear mixed effect model including endogenous production. Br J Clin Pharmacol 1998;46:11–19.
[109] Kindler J, Eckardt KU, Ehmer B, Jandeleit K, Kurtz A, Schreiber A, et al. Single-dose pharmacokinetics of recombinant human erythropoietin in patients with various degrees of renal failure. Nephrol Dial Transplant 1989;4:345–349.
[110] Supersaxo A, Hein WR, Steffen H. Effect of molecular weight on the lymphatic absorption of water-soluble compounds following subcutaneous administration. Pharm Res 1990;7:167–169.
[111] Kagan L, Turner MR, Balu-Iyer SV, Mager DE. Subcutaneous absorption of monoclonal antibodies: role of dose, site of injection, and injection volume on rituximab pharmacokinetics in rats. Pharm Res 2012;29:490–499.
[112] Porter CJ, Charman SA. Lymphatic transport of proteins after subcutaneous administration. J Pharm Sci 2000;89:297–310.
[113] Jensen JD, Jensen LW, Madsen JK. The pharmacokinetics of recombinant human erythropoietin after subcutaneous injection at different sites. Eur J Clin Pharmacol 1994;46:333–337.
[114] Laursen T, Jørgensen JOL, Christiansen JS. Pharmacokinetics and metabolic effects of growth hormone injected subcutaneously in growth hormone deficient patients: thigh versus abdomen. Clin Endocrinol 1994;40:373–378.
[115] Odeh YK, Wang Z, Ruo TI, Wang T, Frederiksen MC, Pospisil PA, et al. Simultaneous analysis of inulin and $^{15}N_2$-urea kinetics in humans. Clin Pharmacol Ther 1993;53:419–425.
[116] Sculier JP, Body JJ, Donnadieu N, Nejai S, Glibert F, Raymakers N, et al. Pharmacokinetics of repeated i.v. bolus administration of high doses of r-met-Hu interleukin-2 in advanced cancer patients. Cancer Chemother Pharmacol 1990;26:355–358.
[117] Konrad MW, Hemstreet G, Hersch EM, Mansell PW, Mertelsmann R, Kolitz JE, et al. Pharmacokinetics of recombinant interleukin-2 in humans. Cancer Res 1990;50:2009–2017.
[118] Watari K, Ozawa K, Takahashi S, Tojo A, Tani K, Kamachi S, et al. Pharmacokinetic studies of intravenous glycosylated recombinant human granulocyte colony-stimulating factor in various hematological disorders: inverse correlation between the half-life and bone marrow myeloid cell pool. Int J Hematol 1997;66:57–67.

[119] Ericson SG, Gao H, Gericke GH, Lewis LD. The role of PMNs in clearance of granulocyte colony-stimulating factor (G-CSF) *in vivo* and *in vitro*. Exp Hematol 1997;25:1313–1325.

[120] Tanswell P, Seifried E, Su PCAF, Feuerer W, Rijken DC. Pharmacokinetics and systemic effects of tissue-type plasminogen activator in normal subjects. Clin Pharmacol Ther 1989;46:155–162.

[121] Mortensen DL, Walicke PA, Wang X, Kwan P, Kuebler P, Gottlieb AB, et al. Pharmacokinetics and pharmacodynamics of multiple weekly subcutaneous efalizumab doses in patients with plaque psoriasis. J Clin Pharmacol 2005;45:286–288.

[122] Huang JD. What can the volume of distribution of macromolecular drugs indicate? Drug Metab Pharmacokinet 2010;25:510–520.

[123] James K. Interactions between cytokines and alpha-2 macroglobulin. Immunol Today 1990;11:163–166.

[124] Dickinson AM, Shenton BK, Alomran AH, Donnelly PK, Proctor SJ. Inhibition of natural killing and antibody-dependent cell-mediated cytotoxicity by the plasma protease inhibitor alpha 2-macroglobulin (alpha 2M) and alpha 2M protease complexes. Clin Immunol Immunopathol 1985;36:259–265.

[125] Hoffman M, Feldman SR, Pizzo SV. α_2-macroglobulin "fast" forms inhibit superoxide production by activated macrophages. Biochim Biophys Acta 1983;760:421–423.

[126] Feige JJ, Negoescu A, Keramidas M, Souchelnitskiy S, Chambaz EM. Alpha 2-macroglobulin: a binding protein for transforming growth factor-beta and various cytokines. Horm Res 1996;45:227–232.

[127] Huang JS, Huang SS, Deuel TF. Specific covalent binding of platelet-derived growth factor to human plasma alpha 2-macroglobulin. Proc Natl Acad Sci U S A 1984;81:342–346.

[128] LaMarre J, Wollenberg GK, Gonias SL, Hayes MA. Cytokine binding and clearance properties of proteinase-activated alpha 2-macroglobulin. Lab Investig 1991;65:3–14.

[129] Legrès LG, Pochon F, Barray M, Gay F, Chouaib S, Delain E. Evidence for the binding of a biologically active interleukin-2 to human alpha 2-macroglobulin. J Biol Chem 1995;83:81–84.

[130] Blum WF, Jensen LW, Madsen JK. Growth hormone insensitivity syndromes: a preliminary report on changes in insulin-like growth factors and their binding proteins during treatment with recombinant insulin-like growth factor I. Kabi Pharmacia Study Group on Insulin-like Growth Factor I Treatment in Growth Hormone Insensitivity Syndromes. Acta Paediatr Suppl 1993;82(Suppl. 391):15–19.

[131] Kostecka Y, Blahovec J. Insulin-like growth factor binding proteins and their functions. Endocr Regul 1999;33:90–94.

[132] Abdel-Razzak ZA, Loyer P, Fautrel A, Gautier JC, Corcos L, Turlin B, et al. Cytokines down-regulate expression of major cytochrome P-450 enzymes in adult human hepatocytes in primary culture. Mol Pharmacol 1993;44:707–715.

[133] Morgan ET. Regulation of cytochrome P450 during inflammation and infection. Drug Metab Rev 1997;9:1129–1188.

[134] Chen JQ, Ström A, Gustafsson JA, Morgan ET. Suppression of the constitutive expression of cytochrome P-450 2C11 by cytokines and interferons in primary cultures of rat hepatocytes: comparison with induction of acute-phase genes and demonstration that CYP2C11 promoter sequences are involved in the suppressive response to interleukins 1 and 6. Mol Pharmacol 1995;47:940–947.

[135] Gonzalez FJ. Molecular biology of cytochrome P450s. Pharmacol Rev 1989;40:243–287.

[136] Kurokohchi K, Matsuo Y, Yoneyama H, Nishioka M, Ichikawa Y. Interleukin-2 induction of cytochrome P450-linked monooxygenase systems of rat liver microsomes. Biochem Pharmacol 1993;45:585–592.

[137] Dickmann LJ, Patel SK, Dan RA, Wienkers LC, Slatter JG. Effects of interleukin-6 (IL-6) and an anti-IL-6 monoclonal antibody on drug-metabolizing enzymes in human hepatocyte culture. Drug Metab Dispos 2011;39:1415–1422.

[138] Khakoo S, Glue P, Grellier L, Wells B, Bell A, Dash C, et al. Ribavarin and interferon alfa-2b in chronic hepatitis C: assessment of possible pharmacokinetic and pharmacodynamic interactions. Br J Clin Pharmacol 1998;46:563–570.

[139] Hassan M, Nilsson C, Olsson H, Lundin J, Osterborg A. The influence of interferon-alpha on the pharmacokinetics of cyclophosphamide and its 4-hydroxy metabolite in patients with multiple myeloma. Eur J Haematol 1999;63:163–170.

[140] Le Cesne A, Vassal G, Farace F, Spielmann M, Le Chevalier T, Angevin E, et al. Combination interleukin-2 and doxorubicin in advanced adult solid tumors: circumvention of doxorubicin resistance in soft-tissue sarcoma? J Immunother 1999;22:268–277.

[141] Schmitt C, Kuhn B, Zhang X, Kivitz AJ, Grange S. Disease–drug–drug interaction involving tocilizumab and simvastatin in patients with rheumatoid arthritis. Clin Pharmacol Ther 2011;89:735–740.

[142] Shimabukuro-Vornhagen A, Gödel P, Subklewe M, Stemmler HJ, Schlößer HA, Schlaak M, et al. Cytokine release syndrome. J Immunother Cancer 2018;6:56. https://doi.org/10.1186/s40425-018-0343-9.

[143] Huang SM, Zhao H, Lee JI, Reynolds K, Zhang L, Temple R, et al. Therapeutic protein–drug interactions and implications for drug development. Clin Pharmacol Ther 2010;87:497–503.

[144] Morell A, Terry WD, Waldmann TA. Metabolic properties of IgG subclasses in man. J Clin Invest 1970;49:673–680.

[145] Brambell FWR, Hemmings WA, Morris LG. A theoretical model of γ-globulin catabolism. Nature 1964;203:1352–1355.

[146] Junghans RP, Anderson CL. The protection receptor for IgG catabolism is the β_2 microglobulin-containing neonatal intestinal transport receptor. Proc Natl Acad Sci U S A 1996;93:5512–5516.

[147] Venkatachalam MA, Rennke HG. The structural and molecular basis of glomerular filtration. Circ Res 1978;43:337–347.

[148] Maack T, Johnson V, Kau ST, Figueiredo J, Sigulem D. Renal filtration, transport, and metabolism of low-molecular-weight proteins: a review. Kidney Int 1979;16:251–270.

[149] Ashwell G, Harford J. Carbohydrate-specific receptors of the liver. Annu Rev Biochem 1982;51:531–554.

[150] Lucore CL, Fry ETA, Nachowiak DA, Sobel BE. Biochemical determinants of clearance of tissue-type plasminogen activator from the circulation. Circulation 1988;77:906–914.

[151] Hovgaard D, Mortensen BT, Schifter S, Nissen NI. Comparative pharmacokinetics of single dose administration of mammalian and bacterially-derived recombinant human granulocyte-macrophage colony stimulating factor. Eur J Haematol 1993;50:32–36.

[152] Moonen P, Mermod JJ, Ernst JF, Hirschi M, DeLamarter JF. Increased biological activity of deglycosylated recombinant human granulocyte-macrophage colony stimulating factor produced by yeast or animal cells. Proc Natl Acad Sci U S A 1987;84:4428–4431.

[153] Kauskansky K. Role of carbohydrate in the function of human granulocyte-macrophage colony stimulating factor. Biochemistry 1987;26:4861–4867.

[154] Watts MJ, Addison L, Long SG, Hartley S, Warrington S, Boyce M, et al. Crossover study of the haematological effects and pharmacokinetics of glycosylated and non-glycosylated G-CSF in healthy volunteers. Br J Haematol 1997;98:474–479.

[155] Morell AG, Gregoriadis G, Scheinberg HI, Hickman J, Ashwell G. The role of sialic acid in determining the survival of glycoproteins in the circulation. J Biol Chem 1971;246:1461–1467.

[156] Gibiansky L, Gibiansky E. Target mediated drug disposition model for drugs that bind to more than one targert. J Pharmacokinet Pharmacodyn 2010;37:323–346.

[157] Chudasama VL, Zutshi A, Singh AAK, Mager DE, Harrold JM. Simulations of site-specific target mediated pharmacokinetic models for guiding the development of bispecific antibodies. J Pharmacokinet Pharmacodyn 2015;42:1–18.

[158] Chatelut E, Rostaing L, Grégoire N, Payen JL, Pujol A, Izopet J, et al. A pharmacokinetic model for alpha interferon administered subcutaneously. Br J Clin Pharmacol 1999;47:365–367.

[159] Kloft C, Graefe E-U, Tanswell P, Scott AM, Hofheinz R, Amelsberg A, et al. Population pharmacokinetics of sibrotuzumab, a novel therapeutic monoclonal antibody, in cancer patients. Investig New Drugs 2004;22:39–52.

[160] Felici A, Verweij J, Sparreboom A. Dosing strategies for anticancer drugs: the good, the bad and body-surface area. Eur J Cancer 2002;38:1677–1684.

[161] Baker SD, Verweij J, Rowinsky EK, Donehower RC, Schellens JHM, Grochow LB, et al. Role of body surface area in dosing of investigational anticancer agents in adults 1991–2001. J Natl Cancer Inst 2002;94:1883–1887.

[162] Ng CM, Lum BI, Gimenez V, Kelsey S, Allison D. Rationale for fixed dosing of pertuzumab in cancer patients based on population pharmacokinetic analysis. Pharm Res 2006;23:1275–1284.

[163] Wang DD, Zhang S, Zhao H, Men AY, Parivar K. Fixed dosing versus body size-based dosing of monoclonal antibodies in adult clinical trials. J Clin Pharmacol 2009;49:1012–1024.

[164] Evans JP, Brinkhouse KM, Brayer GD, Reisner HM, High KA. Canine hemophilia B resulting from a point mutation with unusual consequences. Proc Natl Acad Sci U S A 1989;86:10095–10099.

[165] Sun YN, Lee JH, Almon RR, Jusko WJ. A pharmacokinetic/pharmacodynamic model for recombinant human growth hormone. Effects on induction of insulin-like growth factor 1 in monkeys. J Pharmacol Exp Ther 1999;89:1523–1532.

[166] Baxter RC. Insulin-like growth factor (IGF) binding proteins: the role of serum IGFBPs in regulating IGF availability. Acta Paediatr Scand Suppl 1991;372:107–114.

[167] Carroll PV, Umpleby M, Alexander EL, Egel VA, Callison KV, Sonksen PH, et al. Recombinant human insulin-like growth factor-I (rhIGF-I) therapy in adults with type 1 diabetes mellitus: effects on IGFs, IGF-binding proteins, glucose levels and insulin treatment. Clin Endocrinol 1998;49:739–746.

[168] Mandel SH, Moreland E, Rosenfeld RG, Gargosky SE. The effect of GH therapy on the immunoreactive forms and distribution of IGFBP-3, IGF-I, the acid-labile subunit, and growth rate in GH-deficient children. Endocrine 1997;7:351–360.

[169] Gualberto A. Figitumumab (CP-751,871) for cancer therapy. Expert Opin Biol Ther 2010;10:575–585.

[170] Mager DE, Mascelli MA, Kleiman NS, Fitzgerald JF. Simultaneous modeling of abciximab plasma concentration and ex vivo pharmacodynamics in patients undergoing coronary angioplasty. J Pharmacol Exp Ther 2003;307:969–976.

[171] Ng CM, Joshi A, Dedrick RL, Garovoy MR, Bauer RJ. Pharmacokinetic–pharmacodynamic–efficacy analysis of efalizumab in patients with moderate to severe psoriasis. Pharm Res 2005;22:1088–1100.

[172] Hu C, Xu A, Zhang Y, Rahman MU, Davis HM, Zhou H. Population approach for exposure–response modeling of golimumab in patients with rheumatoid arthritis. J Clin Pharmacol 2011;51:639–648.

[173] Lowe PJ, Renard D. Omalizumab decreases IgE production in patients with allergic (IgE-mediated) asthma; PK/PD analysis of a biomarker, total IgE. Br J Clin Pharmacol 2011;72:306–320.

[174] Wiczling P, Rosenweig M, Vaickus L, Jusko WJ. Pharmacokinetics and pharmacodynamics of a chimeric/humanized anti-CD3 monoclonal antibody, Otelixizumab (TRX4), in subjects with psoriasis and with type 1 diabetes mellitus. J Clin Pharmacol 2010;50:494–506.

[175] Ternant D, Hénin E, Cartron G, Tod M, Paintaud G, Girard P. Development of a drug–disease simulation model for rituximab in follicular non-Hodgkin's lymphoma. Br J Clin Pharmacol 2009;68:561–573.

[176] Ng CM, Bai S, Takimoto CH, Tang MT, Tolcher AW. Mechanism-based receptor-binding model to describe the pharmacokinetic and pharmacodynamic of an anti-α5β1 integrin monoclonal antibody (volociximab) in cancer patients. Cancer Chemother Pharmacol 2010;65:207–217.

[177] Vaage J, Pauly JL, Harlos JP. Influence of the administration schedule on the therapeutic effect of interleukin-2. Int J Cancer 1987;39:530–533.

[178] Sosman JA, Kohler PC, Hank J, Moore KH, Bechhofer R, Storer B, et al. Repetitive weekly cycles of recombinant human interleukin-2: responses of renal carcinoma with acceptable toxicity. J Natl Cancer Inst 1988;80:60–63.

[179] Leonard JP, Sherman ML, Fisher GL, Buchanan LJ, Larsen G, Atkins MB, et al. Effects of single dose interleukin-12 exposure on interleukin-12-associated toxicity and interferon-gamma production. Blood 1997;90:2541–2548.

[180] Motzer RJ, Rakhit A, Schwartz LH, Olencki T, Malone TM, Sandstrom K, et al. Phase 1 trial of subcutaneous human interleukin-12 in patients with advanced renal cell carcinoma. Clin Cancer Res 1998;4:1183–1191.

[181] Li J, Piskol R, Ybarra R, Chen YJJ, Li J, Slaga D, et al. CD3 bispecific antibody–induced cytokine release is dispensable for cytotoxic T cell activity. Sci Transl Med 2019;11:eaax8861. https://doi.org/10.1126/scitranslmed.aax8861.

[182] CDER, CBER. Clinical pharmacology data to support a demonstration of biosimilarity to a reference product. Guidance for industry, Silver Spring, MD: FDA; 2016. Internet at: https://www.fda.gov/media/88622/download.

[183] CDER, CBER. Purple book lists of licensed biological products with reference product exclusivity and biosimilarity or interchangeabiltiy evaluations. Internet at: https://www.fda.gov/drugs/therapeutic-biologics-applications-bla/purple-book-lists-licensed-biological-products-reference-product-exclusivity-and-biosimilarity-or; 2020.

[184] Yao HM, Ottery FD, Borema T, Harris S, Levy J, May TB, et al. PF-06881893 (Nivestym), a filgrastim biosimilar, versus US-licensed filgrastim reference product (US-Neupogen((R))): pharmacokinetics, pharmacodynamics, immunogenicity, and safety of single or multiple subcutaneous doses in healthy volunteers. BioDrugs 2019;33:207–220.

[185] Waller CF, Tiessen RG, Lawrence TE, Shaw A, Liu MS, Sharma R, et al. A pharmacokinetics and pharmacodynamics equivalence trial of the proposed pegfilgrastim biosimilar, MYL-1401H, versus reference pegfilgrastim. J Cancer Res Clin Oncol 2018;144:1087–1095.

[186] Stalker D, Ramaiya A, Kumbhat S, Zhang J, Reid S, Martin N. Pharmacodynamic and pharmacokinetic equivalences of epoetin hospira and epogen ((R)) after multiple subcutaneous doses to healthy male subjects. Clin Ther 2016;38:1090–1101.

[187] Stalker D, Reid S, Ramaiya A, Wisemandle WA, Martin NE. Pharmacokinetic and pharmacodynamic equivalence of epoetin hospira and epogen after single subcutaneous doses to healthy male subjects. Clin Ther 2016;38:1778–1788.

[188] Wang Y, Strauss DG, Huang SM. Use of pharmacodynamic/response biomarkers for therapeutic biologics regulatory submissions. Biomark Med 2019;13:805–809.

[189] Li J, Florian J, Campbell E, Schrieber SJ, Bai JPF, Weaver JL, et al. Advancing biosimilar development using pharmacodynamic biomarkers in clinical pharmacology studies. Clin Pharmacol Ther 2020;107:40–42.

[190] ICH. Harmonized guideline—bioanalytical method validation, M10. Draft version, Internet at: https://database.ich.org/sites/default/files/M10_EWG_Draft_Guideline.pdf; 2019.

[191] Dodds M, Chow V, Markus R, Perez-Ruixo JJ, Shen D, Gibbs M. The use of pharmacometrics to optimize biosimilar development. J Pharm Sci 2013;102:3908–3914.

[192] Zhu P, Sy SKB, Skerjanec A. Application of pharmacometric analysis in the design of clinical pharmacology studies for biosimilar development. AAPS J 2018;20:40. https://doi.org/10.1208/s12248-018-0196-7.

Chapter 34

Design of clinical development programs

Megan A. Gibbs[a,b,c], Bengt Hamren[a,b,c], David W. Boulton[a,b,c], Helen Tomkinson[a,b,c], and Renee Iacona[d]

[a]*Astra Zeneca Global Clinical Pharmacology and Quantitative Pharmacology, Gaithersburg, MD, United States,* [b]*Astra Zeneca Global Clinical Pharmacology and Quantitative Pharmacology, Gothenburg, Sweden,* [c]*Astra Zeneca Global Clinical Pharmacology and Quantitative Pharmacology, Cambridge, United Kingdom,* [d]*Astra Zeneca Oncology Biometrics, Gaithersburg, MD, United States*

Clinical development is the scientific process of exploring and confirming the product attributes and therapeutic role of potential new medical treatments. This chapter provides an overview of the clinical development of a pharmaceutical product for medical use, introducing and discussing the principles of clinical development and application of those principles on both a programmatic and a study level. While the development process is continuous, beginning during the discovery of an innovative potential pharmaceutical product and ending with the replacement of the innovative pharmaceutical by a more effective or safer alternative treatment, the process follows an orderly path of evidence-based, goal-directed development. This chapter focuses on the clinical development and registration of an innovative pharmaceutical product in the treatment of patients or of an additional indication for an existing pharmaceutical product.

Introduction

Clinical development is the scientific process of exploring and confirming the product attributes and therapeutic role of potential new medical treatments. This chapter provides an overview of the clinical development of a pharmaceutical product for medical use, introducing and discussing the principles of clinical development and application of those principles on both a programmatic and a study level. While the development process is continuous, beginning during the discovery of an innovative potential pharmaceutical product and ending with the replacement of the innovative pharmaceutical by a more effective or safer alternative treatment, the process follows an orderly path of evidence-based, goal-directed development.

This chapter focuses on the clinical development and registration of an innovative pharmaceutical product in the treatment of patients or of an additional indication for an existing pharmaceutical product. The chapter covers clinical development spanning the traditional phases that are diagrammed in Fig. 1.1 (Chapter 1). Coverage includes the conduct of first in human, proof of mechanism (PoM), proof of concept (PoC), and confirmatory clinical trials, registration and postapproval, including new indications and new formulations, risk management plans, postmarket studies, and clinical trials conducted as part of risk evaluation and mitigation strategies authorized by the Food and Drug Administration Amendments Act (FDAAA) of 2007 [1]. The chapter also covers the development of both biological agents and small molecules, noting some areas that distinctly apply to each of these two therapeutic classes, but does not cover the development of nonpharmaceutical treatments, medical procedures, or medical devices, and does not discuss nonhuman development, although some development principles involving medical device and veterinary use products may be similar.

The clinical development process has allowed the introduction of many important new medical treatments that have improved public health and offered relief to countless patients. An example of the substantial public health impact of clinical development is the progress made in the treatment of patients with multiple sclerosis. Multiple sclerosis is the most common autoimmune disorder of the nervous system, has the potential to cause significant disability, and contributes significant public health morbidity [2]. Prior to the 1990s, therapy was nonspecific and supportive. As noted in a 1951 medical textbook [3]:

> *As yet there is no satisfactory treatment for the syndrome of multiple sclerosis, despite the large amount of published material concerning this subject.*

Atkinson's Principles of Clinical Pharmacology. https://doi.org/10.1016/B978-0-12-819869-8.00034-3

Following a prescribed clinical development pathway, a number of agents including the injectable medications (Interferon beta 1a and 1 b and Glatiramer), oral medications (Teriflunomide, Fingolimod, Cladribine, Siponimod, Dimethyl fumarate, diroximel fumarate, and ozanimod), and infused medications (Alemtuzumab, mitoxantrone, ocrelizumab, and natalizumab) have now been introduced to modify the course of multiple sclerosis [2–6]. While not able to repair already existing damage, the agents reduce the frequency and intensity of relapse. However, in the case of natalizumab, it was withdrawn from the market because of multifocal leukoencephalopathy only to be reintroduced later to the market clearly highlighting the complexity to treatment in this area. The medical introduction of these agents was the result of comprehensive and systematic clinical development programs [7, 8].

Importantly, the clinical development process is not stagnant. Rather, it is dynamic and evolves as science and medicine advance and as the information needs required by regulators, prescribers, patients, and payers continue to expand. It is the dynamic and improving capability of the clinical development process that assures its ability to continue to support significant medical and public health advancements.

Principles of clinical development

Clinical development is a scientific process that adheres to the principles of proper scientific conduct, to ethical principles applying to human research, to legal and regulatory requirements, and to the numerous technical guidances provided by governments and professional societies. Companies develop disease area strategies coupled with business and commercial drivers to design and develop medications in areas of unmet medical need. Further, as the costs of drugs increase, trial efficiency and informed development decisions have escalated the need for new technologies such as digital health, data and Artificial Intelligence, and the expansion of real-world data to inform drug development decisions.

Proper scientific conduct

Proper scientific conduct requires adherence to the principles of scientific excellence and integrity. All research should be soundly based on well-grounded prior evidence and, in accordance with this, clinical development requires a solid scientific foundation for the intervention being tested. The pathology and pathophysiology of the disorder under study should be examined and the actions of the studied intervention appropriately understood. Occasionally, empiric observations arise in clinical or preclinical studies that are unexpected and poorly understood on the basis of known pathophysiology and pharmacology. In these cases, attempts should be made to further understand the pharmacology and physiology underlying the observation. If this is not possible, or if studies fail to advance understanding, clinical development should proceed cautiously and with full consideration of the benefit–risk of the intervention.

Scientific misconduct, violation of integrity, and the occurrence of fraud have been reported in both preclinical and clinical investigations throughout the world. There is appropriate and particularly intense scrutiny of clinical development, since it involves human subjects and is closely linked with clinical therapeutics. This has caused an increasing emphasis on ensuring integrity through training, guidance, oversight, regulation, and law. It is the obligation of all scientists engaged in clinical development to assure that the highest standards of scientific conduct and integrity are always maintained.

Ethical principles

Ethical issues and concerns are prominent in the conduct of clinical development. Numerous agencies have issued reviews of the ethical principles of clinical research. These include ethical guidance issued by the US Department of Health, Education, and Welfare (now the Department of Health and Human Services) in the Belmont Report [9], by the World Medical Association in the Declaration of Helsinki [10], and by the Council for International Organizations of Medical Sciences in its International Ethical Guidelines for Health-Related Research Involving Humans [11]. It is a fundamental requirement that clinical development respects the rights and well-being of all participating human subjects. External, objective review of the proposed clinical study by an independent review body (e.g., institutional review boards, regulatory agencies) is always required along with ongoing assessment of risks and benefits as substantial new information becomes available. This requires proper clinical study monitoring, data integration and review, and, for larger trials, may require an external, independent data safety monitoring board. A final rule on the Investigational New Drug Safety Reporting Requirements for Human Drug and Biological Products recently issued by the US Food and Drug

Administration (FDA) [12] notes that, among other criteria, sponsors of clinical development must report an adverse event as a suspected adverse reaction if:

> *an aggregate analysis of specific events observed in a clinical trial (such as known consequences of the underlying disease or condition under investigation or other events that commonly occur in the study population independent of drug therapy) indicates those events occur more frequently in the drug treatment group than in a concurrent or historical control group.*

Adherence to this final rule requires diligent and regular study monitoring, data review, and analysis.

Legal and regulatory requirements

Clinical development occurs within a framework of increasing international, national, and local laws and regulation. The legal framework surrounding clinical development is substantially focused on preapproval investigational activities, regulatory submission for approval, approval process, and postapproval commitments and requirements. Although laws and regulations affecting these areas have been most notably increased in the EU, United States, Japan, and affiliated regions such as Australia, New Zealand, and Canada, laws and regulations also are becoming increasingly stringent in emerging market areas such as China, India, Latin America, and Russia.

In the United States, the FDA is the agency primarily charged with overseeing the regulation of clinical development activities, regulatory submissions, drug approval, and postapproval activities. The evolution of the legal framework impacting FDA-regulated clinical development in the United States is discussed in Chapter 35 and has been summarized elsewhere [13]. A substantial recent addition to this legislation is the Food and Drug Administration Amendments Act (FDAAA) that in 2007 greatly increased the responsibilities of the FDA, provided it with new authorities, and reauthorized several FDA critical programs such as PDUFA, BPCA, and PREA. The Act [1]:

- Extensively expands the authority of the FDA to require sponsors to conduct and report on postmarketing studies and clinical trials. It defines a postmarketing requirement (PMR) as a study or trial that a sponsor is required by statute or regulation to conduct postapproval, and a postmarketing commitment (PMC) as a study or trial that a sponsor agrees to in writing, but is not required by law, to conduct postapproval;
- Introduces Risk Evaluation and Mitigation Strategies (REMS) as a tool to be used when "necessary to ensure that the benefits of the drug outweigh the risks of the drug";
- Requires the FDA to develop and maintain a website with comprehensive safety information about approved drug products. Among other things, the FDA must prepare a summary analysis of adverse reaction reports received for each drug 18 months after approval or after use of the drug by 10,000 individuals, whichever is later;
- Requires the FDA to conduct a regular biweekly screening of the Adverse Event Reporting System database and post a quarterly report on its website of "any new safety information or potential signal of a serious risk" identified within the last quarter;
- Requires the NIH (through the National Library of Medicine) to issue regulations that markedly expand the clinical trial registry and results databank;
- Establishes the Reagan-Udall Foundation to advance regulatory science and product safety; and
- Creates templates to immediately implement provisions regarding conflicts of interest waivers and disclosure of financial information for Advisory Committee members.

The body of Congressional Acts authorizes the FDA to issue regulations that have the strength of law and are codified in the Code of Federal Regulations (CFR) [14]. Particularly pertinent to clinical development are CFR Title 21, Part 50: Protection of Human Subjects; Part 56: Institutional Review Boards; Part 312: Investigational New Drug Application; Part 314: Applications for FDA Approval to Market a New Drug; and Part 316: Orphan Drugs.

In addition to these acts and amendments, the Patient Protection and Affordable Care Act (PPACA) [15] and the Health Care and Education Reconciliation Act of 2010 [16] include numerous health-related provisions to take effect over a 4-year period, including expanding Medicaid eligibility, subsidizing insurance premiums, providing incentives for businesses to provide health care benefits, prohibiting denial of coverage/claims based on preexisting conditions, establishing health insurance exchanges, and support for medical research including a specific focus on comparative treatment clinical research.

In 2016, 21st Century Cures Act (Cures Act) was signed into law. This Act is designed to help accelerate medical product development and bring new innovations and advances to patients faster and more efficiently and incorporates the perspectives of patients into the development of drugs, biological products, and devices. The Cures Act is intended to enable modernization of clinical trial designs, including the use of real-world evidence, and clinical outcome assessments. It also established new expedited product development programs, including the Regenerative Medicine Advanced

Therapy (RMAT) that offers a new expedited option for certain eligible biologics products and the Breakthrough Devices program, designed to speed the review of certain innovative medical devices and established intercenter institutes to help coordinate activities in major disease areas between the drug, biologics, and device centers such as the Oncology Center of Excellence.

These substantive changes will have an impact on clinical development that is uncertain but will almost assuredly increase the emphasis on rigorously demonstrating the additional and comparative benefit of proposed new pharmaceutical treatments.

Regulatory guidance

In addition to regulation, the FDA issues guidance documents and other notes, representing the Agency's current thinking on a particular subject. Several guidances are issuances of the International Conference on Harmonization (ICH) approved guidelines. These documents cover both brad and focused areas and are discussed in Chapter 35.

Directives, guidelines, and position papers pertinent to clinical development are also regularly issued by the European Medicines Agency (EMA), established by the European Union (EU) and beginning operations in 1995. The EMA guides, evaluates, and oversees pharmaceutical development, approval, and postapproval activities in EU member states. The directives, guidelines, and position papers of the EMA assume legal and regulatory status as they are approved by the EU Parliament and as they are adopted by EU member states. Although independent national regulatory agencies continue to exist, the EMA brings a comprehensive EU viewpoint on issues of clinical development and regulatory applications. The EMA also provides the opportunity for scientific advice meetings with clinical development sponsors. In addition, meetings with national regulatory agencies can also assist clinical development in the EU. The EMA website presents a complete listing of directives, guidelines, and position papers [17].

Since its establishment in April 2004, the Japanese Pharmaceuticals and Medical Devices Agency (PMDA) has become increasingly transparent and informative on the clinical development of new pharmaceutical products [18]. The PMDA is the Japanese regulatory agency which works together with the Japanese Ministry of Health, Labour and Welfare to protect the public health by assuring the safety, efficacy, and quality of pharmaceuticals and medical devices. The PMDA conducts scientific reviews of pharmaceutical and medical device regulatory applications and oversees and assists in their clinical development in Japan. Scheduled meetings between sponsors and the PMDA also are important in facilitating clinical development of pharmaceutical products in Japan.

China's regulatory complexity and timelines historically have excluded or delayed China's inclusion in "Global" clinical development programs. For multinational pharmaceutical companies, the historical approach to register a drug in China was to execute an imported drug registration path whereby the drug is already approved in a major market (e.g., EU, United States, or Japan) and the "Global" registration package is bridged to the Chinese population by conducting at least one Phase 3 study and Clinical Pharmacology study in first-generation Chinese subjects resident in China. The advantage of this approach is a high probability of success, since the drug has been approved by another major health authority. However, the main disadvantage of this approach is the China approval timelines delay the availability of the new drug to Chinese patients who may benefit from it by 5 years or more. Multinational companies can also have a faster route to approval by implementing an independent China development program if the manufacturing of the drug and drug product is conducted in China, often with Chinese partner firms [19]. However, the need for early planning, significant early investment to establish the manufacturing when it may not be clear what the chances of success for the drug candidate might be, are practical barriers to this approach.

China's National Medical Products Administration (NMPA) began to overhaul the country's regulatory framework in 2018 in acknowledgment of the aforementioned challenges. Major changes have been implemented to address the Chinese lag to market, including an improved and shortened drug review process for both Investigational New Drug (IND) and New Drug Authorization (NDA) reviews, acceptance of clinical data from outside China and alignment and integration of International Council on Harmonisation (ICH) guidelines whereby Chinese regulatory guidances generally mirror those of other major health authorities. The goals of these changes are to have new drug approval and launch timelines in China more proximal to the approvals in other major markets by facilitating China to participate in the global clinical trial programs. A minimum number of patients from China (e.g., 100 patients per arm in a Phase 3 study and a local Clinical Pharmacology study) would be needed along with a separate China clinical study report and a Clinical Pharmacology ethic sensitivity evaluation. This approach substantially closes the approval gap between China and other major markets. It is important to be aware of any potential for ethnic sensitivity from the PK, PD, safety/tolerability, and/or efficacy perspectives and if such characteristics exist that suggest, for example, a different dose may be appropriate for Chinese patients, then a parallel China clinical program may be considered. It is also important to plan early for China participation in the clinical development program. For global clinical development programs, regulatory advice and guidance should routinely be obtained from the EU, United States, Japanese, and Chinese pharmaceutical regulatory authorities prior to the initiation of clinical development and periodically throughout the development process.

International Conference on Harmonisation of Technical Requirements for Registration of Pharmaceuticals for Human Use (ICH)

In the early 1990s, the International Conference on Harmonisation of Technical Requirements for Registration of Pharmaceuticals for Human Use (ICH) was initiated to harmonize the drug development regulatory guidances in the EU, United States, and Japan. ICH membership includes academic, regulatory, and pharmaceutical industry experts from the EU, United States, and Japan [20]. Six ICH conferences have been held since 1991 along with many meetings of the Steering Committee and Expert Working Groups. ICH guidelines have been issued on quality, safety, efficacy, and multidisciplinary topics, with the five-step process for implementation outlined by ICH for each of the three corresponding regions [21]. Formal implementation in the United States occurs with the issuance of an approved FDA guidance such as Structure and Content of Clinical Study Reports (ICH E3), Good Clinical Practice: Consolidated Guideline (ICH E6), General Considerations for Clinical Trials (ICH E8), Statistical Principles for Clinical Trials (ICH E9), and Organization of the Common Technical Document (ICH M4).

Good clinical practice

Clinical research is the core activity of clinical development, and it is essential that clinical development scientists adhere to the principles of good clinical research design, conduct, analysis, and reporting. The ICH Guideline for Good Clinical Practice (GCP) (ICH E6) [22] presents many of these principles and has been adopted by regulatory authorities in the EU, United States, Japan, and many other nations as the guideline for clinical research. Among the topics and functions covered in the guideline are the following:

- Institutional Review Board/Independent Ethics Committee (responsibilities, composition, functions, operations, procedures, and records);
- Investigator (qualifications, resources, compliance, handling of investigational product(s), informed consent of trial subjects, records, and reports);
- Sponsor (trial management, data handling, record keeping, quality control/assurance, financing, monitoring, handling of safety information, and reporting obligations);
- Clinical Trial Protocol (trial design and objective, selection and treatment of subjects, assessment of efficacy and safety, statistics, data handling, and clinical trial reporting);
- Investigator's Brochure (general considerations and contents for this document, which contains a summary of preclinical and clinical data known up to that point for use by investigators in clinical trials);
- Essential Documents (essential documents and their handling before, during, and after clinical trial conduct); and
- Standards for data quality and integrity.

GCP areas of particular focus for clinical development include:

- Ethics committee/IRB approval of protocols and updates during study conduct;
- Subject's informed consent and privacy protection; protocol violations;
- Sponsor monitoring of investigative sites as required by standard procedures;
- Source data verification, including the verification of patients, matching of case report form data to source documents (e.g., medical records), record retention, and the audit trail for all case report form changes (i.e., who made them, why, and when);
- Timely reporting of serious adverse events to sponsors, ethics committees, and regulatory authorities; and
- The conduct of audits to assure GCP compliance by both sponsor and regulatory authorities.

International (outside EU, United States, Japan, China) and US state regulation

The laws and regulations guiding and impacting clinical development are rapidly increasing as clinical research expands to more commonly involve areas outside of the EU, United States, Japan, and China to regions or countries such as Australasia, South America (Brazil in particular), Switzerland, South Africa, Russia, and India [23]. These laws and regulations should be reviewed and considered before planning a global clinical development program. In addition, state regulations may impact clinical development in the United States, and most often address investigator financial disclosure [24] or agreements requiring health plans to pay for the routine medical care a patient receives while participating in a clinical trial [25].

Business regulation

For clinical development sponsors that are for-profit pharmaceutical firms, not-for-profit business organizations, or academic or governmental institutions, numerous laws and regulations addressing intellectual property, business conduct, or conflict of interest may also impact clinical development. Intellectual property concerns are increasingly important and are becoming increasingly complex with the global expansion of clinical research operations. They are important to consider as clinical development is planned, reviewed, and analyzed.

A number of laws and regulations govern the interactions of sponsors with investigators and with governmental officials. The US Federal Corrupt Practices Act specifically addresses relationships with foreign government officials. The US antitrust regulations are particularly important because of the increasing importance of cross-sponsor cooperation in the advancement of numerous precompetitive scientific areas, such as the validation of biomarkers for use in clinical development. Several groups have directly addressed this issue through the creation of innovative, carefully defined structures. One example is the Biomarkers Consortium, a public-private partnership created to identify and qualify new biological markers. Members include the Foundation for the National Institutes of Health (FNIH), the National Institutes of Health (NIH), the FDA, the US Centers for Medicare & Medicaid Services (CMS), the Pharmaceutical Research and Manufacturers of America (PhRMA), the Biotechnology Industry Organization (BIO), and patient advocacy organizations [26, 27]. Other examples of across-Pharmaceutical Industry collaborative groups are the European Federation of Pharmaceutical Industries and Associations (EFPIA) and the International Consortium for Innovation and Quality in Pharmaceutical Development (IQ Consortium, or IQ) who work on topics pertinent to the industry and provide input to regulatory bodies on a wide variety of topics [28, 29]. Continued support for broad-based, cross-sponsor precompetitive collaboration is essential to advancing biomarkers, and proteomic and pharmacogenomic markers.

Sponsors of clinical development that are publicly held firms must also consider securities regulations that govern the release and sharing of information. Compliance with these regulations is mandatory and is determined by the materiality of the information. For a small biotechnology organization with few projects, the results of a single study or the occurrence of a single adverse reaction may be material, while the same information may not be material to a larger pharmaceutical organization with multiple projects.

Data privacy

Clinical development must also consider the impact of laws and regulations concerning data privacy, including the European Commission's Directive on Data Protection [30] and the US Privacy Rule enacted under the Health Insurance Portability and Accountability Act of 1996 (HIPAA) [31]. The increasingly multinational conduct of clinical development programs enhances the importance of adhering to privacy regulations. Clinical development design, conduct, analysis, and reporting must consider data privacy, while maintaining auditable data verification, allowing the composite pooling of appropriate data, and supporting the clinical trial data usage in all global areas. Informed consent is essential with full disclosure of the extent of necessary data collection, the need for verification, and the use of the data to support appropriate monitoring and regulatory requirements. Knowledge of and adherence to the scientific, ethical, legal, and regulatory principles of clinical development not only is essential but also assures full support for the clinical research enterprise and allows for continuous improvements of the clinical development process within this framework.

Evidence-based, goal-directed clinical development

Clinical development of a drug or biologic candidate is traditionally divided into the four phases shown in Fig. 1.1: Phase 1, in which the pharmacokinetic, pharmacodynamic, and early safety properties of the drug are determined, generally in healthy volunteers; Phase 2, in which proof of efficacy along with safety and toleration is demonstrated in the targeted disease state and a dose response is determined; Phase 3, in which selected doses are tested in larger numbers of subjects in order to confirm safety and efficacy; and postapproval Phase 4, in which new indications or use of the drug in special situations is examined. Over the years, it has been recognized that this paradigm is overly simplistic and gives the incorrect impression that these activities are chronologically separated and that drug development is a linear process. In fact, many

"Phase 1" studies, such as drug-drug interaction studies or bioequivalence studies, are often done later in development, and many Phase 1 studies, even first-in-human studies, are done in patients, not healthy volunteers.

Modern drug development programs therefore have come to be characterized as having different somewhat overlapping stages, focused first on "learning" and then on "confirming," as outlined as follows [32]:

- Nomination for development by discovery—after it has been demonstrated that the molecule in question has adequately characterized in vitro and in vivo pharmacology and has the appropriate pharmaceutical properties. This includes suitable potency and specificity for the desired target and effectiveness in animal models of the intended disease states to be treated, if such models exist. It also often includes demonstration of an acceptable genetic and short-term toxicology profile.
- Proof of mechanism (PoM)—demonstrating that the drug or biologic candidate in man gets to its target tissues at levels sufficient to engage the target and to have an effect on pharmacodynamic markers or biomarkers, showing that the agent exerts its intended mechanism (i.e., blocks or stimulates the appropriate receptors, inhibits the relevant enzymes, or has an effect on a closely related downstream activity). Typically, tens of study subjects are treated short term (days to weeks) to establish PoM.
- Proof of concept (PoC)—demonstrating that the candidate has a desirable effect on the appropriate endpoints in the relevant disease state(s) at a dose that is adequately tolerated with an acceptable level of serious adverse events. Generally, hundreds of study subjects are treated for weeks to months in order to establish PoC.
- Confirmatory clinical trials—demonstrating with a high degree of rigor, often with replicate studies, that the candidate has desirable effects on efficacy endpoints suitable for registration and has an acceptable safety profile, with risks that are outweighed by the benefit conferred. Such programs typically involve thousands of study subjects, many of which may be treated for one to several years if chronic diseases are being targeted.

As emphasized in Chapter 17, the appropriate choice of biomarkers or clinical endpoints suitable for PoM, PoC, or confirmation trials is integral to the candidate development program. However, the demonstration of an "acceptable safety profile" or "tolerability" is also a critical factor in designing a development program.

Two major issues impact the design of all development programs: the resource requirements for each development phase, and candidate drug attrition.

Exponential growth of resource requirements as a clinical development program progresses

The cost of a complete development program adequate to meet regulatory requirements for registration costs was estimated to be \$800 million in 2003 [33, 34]. Clinical trials account for the largest proportion of this cost, and this is a function of the number of study subjects enrolled, the duration of the trial, and the complexity of the endpoints being measured. The clinical activities required for PoC trials generally take 2–3 years and have direct costs in the range of \$10–\$50 million. Confirmatory clinical trials generally require 2 to >5 years to complete at a direct cost of \$100–\$500 million or more (Fig. 34.1).

High attrition at all phases of clinical development

Of every 100 molecules nominated for development, about 15 will become marketed pharmaceuticals. Failures occur in all phases of development, and candidate drug "survival" rate is roughly 50%–65% in Phase 1, 25%–40% in Phase 2, and 50%–66% in Phase 3, Fig. 34.2 [33]. Furthermore, about 15%–20% of candidates submitted for regulatory approval never become marketed. These percentages have not shown improvement over the past one to two decades, and if anything have recently become somewhat worse. Candidate survival rates vary somewhat by therapeutic area and are somewhat higher for biologics (overall survival about 30%) vs small molecules (overall survival about 15%) [34, 35].

The primary reasons for attrition at the PoM phase are failure to achieve suitable tissue penetration or failure to affect desired pharmacodynamic endpoints or biomarkers, followed by adverse preclinical toxicology findings that emerge during long-term toxicology studies. Lack of tolerability or other safety issues are additional causes of early failure in early clinical trials. The predominant reasons for failure at the PoC phase are lack of effectiveness in the disease being tested followed by issues of clinical safety. Even in the confirmatory phase, failure to demonstrate benefit remains a primary cause for failure, as do safety issues which arise as larger populations are examined [36].

With all the advances over the past two decades in understanding the underlying basic science of disease pathways, one would have expected attrition rates to improve rather than to stagnate or worsen. The continuing high attrition rate is partly due to more stringent evidentiary requirements for evaluating drug candidates because of an intensified focus on the safety

Core content

Finding the optimum balance between efficacy and safety

The impact of Clinical and Quantitative Pharmacology on the drug development process

Candidate Selection

Shaping the clinical pharmacology plan

CPQP work with DMPK to develop the right clinical pharmacology plan needed to ensure a robust and informed decision is made on the approval of a candidate drug.

Key questions

- What will be the best way to test the efficacy and safety of the drug in the clinic?
- What options are there for formulation?

Phase 1

Defining the dose and understanding exposure

Modelling, simulation and bio-analytics from CPQP provide the clinical team with a recommended FTIM starting dose; a plan for dose escalation and a deeper understanding of how the drug interacts with the human body

Key questions

- What is the correct starting dose for the drug and how do we escalate the dose during the trial?
- What is the correlation between the dose and the probability of an adverse event?
- How will the change in dose impact the biomarkers needed?
- What is the overall exposure of the drug in the human body?

Answering these questions help CPQP define the right doses to take into phase 2

Phase 2

Modelling the right dose for the right patient

CPQP create models that provide the clinical team with a deeper understanding how the balance of efficacy and safety are impacted by real world variables and commercial teams with insight on how the drug performs against standard of care

Key questions

- What difference do factors such as age or impairments have on the efficacy and safety of the drug?
- How does food intake or use of other drugs impact the ADME in patients?
- What potential Phase 3 restrictions would still provide an advantage over SOC?

Collaborating with commercial team to provide answers to these questions shapes the Phase 3 clinical trial

Phase 3

Informing the regulatory submission

To support the regulatory submission CPQP creates models for deeper dives into patient profiles designed to broaden the protocol and develops the clinical pharmacology package that describes the pharmacokinetics and outlines all ADME evidence

Key questions

- Which patient populations need further ADME evidence?
- What evidence is required to broaden the protocol?
- What intrinsic and extrinsic factors do we need to demonstrate?
- How do you define the right end point and how do you correlate this to the biomarker?

Answering these questions will help ensure the regulatory submission provides the evidence needed for the optimum commercial label

On market

Enhancing the label to broaden the reach

From delivering the post marketing studies required by regulators to new indication studies, CPQP continues to support the development of label enhancements that help to broaden the long-term reach of the drug.

Key questions

- What post marketing studies will be required?
- What models or simulation will help understand other drug combinations that should be considered?
- What real world evidence do we need to support label enhancements?
- How does the safety and efficacy compare with potential new entrants?
- Which additional patient populations should be considered?

By working with commercial teams to answer these questions CPQP can enhance the lifetime value of the drug

FIG. 34.1 Role of clinical pharmacology throughout the drug development continuum.

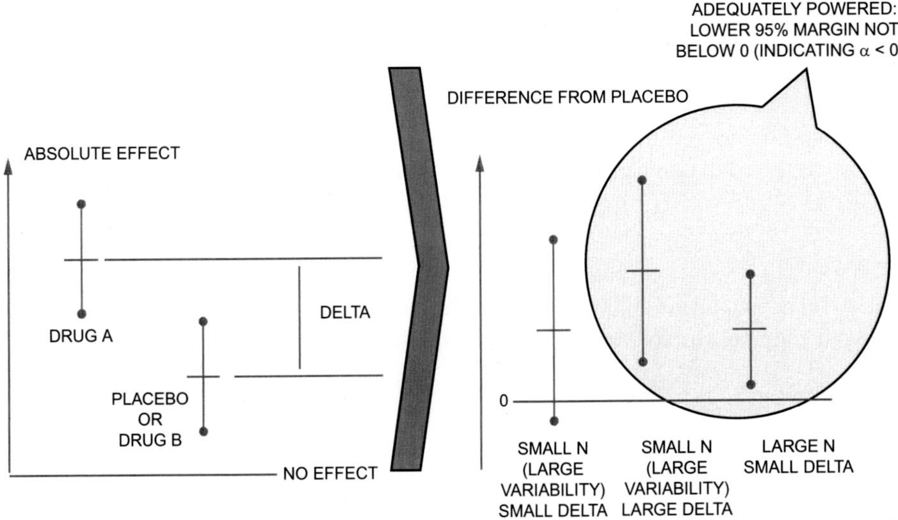

FIG. 34.2 Project and success rates and reasons for failure. *(Reproduced with permission from Nat Rev Drug Discov).*

of drug candidates in development, and partly due to the fact that most candidates currently are developed for diseases for which treatments already exist. Hence market acceptance, if not regulatory acceptance, requires most new agents to have either a better safety profile or more pronounced efficacy than existing drugs. This presents an ever higher hurdle as our therapeutic armamentarium improves.

The high failure rates are also partly due to the massive proliferation of previously unexplored targets that basic science has produced over the past two decades as hundreds of new cytokine, kinase, and other enzymatic and signal transduction pathways have been elucidated. For example, agents to inhibit the effect of IL-1, TNF-α, and P-38 MAP kinase all showed good efficacy in preclinical models of rheumatoid arthritis. However, in clinical trials, only anti-TNF-α showed a high degree of effectiveness and revolutionized therapy for the disease [37, 38], whereas anti-IL-1 showed modest efficacy [39], and P-38 MAP kinase inhibitors failed to have any lasting positive impact on the disease and are no longer being developed for rheumatoid arthritis [40, 41]. Over the past decades, significant efforts have been made to reduce attrition and optimize the large investments required for both drug discovery and development. It is now more common to use genomics, proteomics, and other data such as phenotyping coupled with artificial intelligence (AI) and machine learning (ML) to improve target identification and to identify patients most likely to benefit from treatment. Companies are also adopting more rigor when evaluating new targets and compounds and in making go/no go decisions. One such approach is the 5R concept where every project is rated with respect to right target, right patient, right tissue/exposure, right safety, and right commercial potential. This approach has enabled more consistent and scientific-driven decision making and has been shown to increase productivity and efficiency [36, 42]. There are also advances in the types of drug modalities that are being tested, far beyond small molecules, peptides, and monoclonal antibodies. Novel modalities, such as antisense oligonucleotides, silencing/modified RNA, and gene and cell therapy, are being evaluated to engage targets that traditionally were not reachable by small molecules. These efforts, coupled with a precision medicine approach to identify the patient groups most appropriate to have a beneficial clinical response, are thought to decrease attrition. Although attrition will likely remain high also over time, these new approaches provide hope that novel treatments will be made available to patients with unmet medical needs.

Key milestones: Proof of mechanism, proof of concept, and confirmation

Since failure is the norm and resource requirements rise exponentially as programs progress, clinical development programs are designed to fail as early as possible, but are also designed so that failure at each step yields critical information for follow-on programs. Programs that make it through stringent early hurdles are then run to succeed. Therefore a well-designed program should focus on establishing or failing to establish PoM and PoC, and then on building the basis for success during confirmatory clinical trials. PoC is the inflection point after which a well-designed program which has not failed should be designed for success in the confirmatory phase. A well-designed program which does fail at the PoM or PoC stage also should provide key feedback for the drug discovery scientists. In particular, it should provide answers as to whether the agent failed because it did not reach the target tissue in adequate levels or because of unanticipated toxicity, both of which can possibly be designed out of a follow-on candidate, or whether it failed to impact the disease in question because the pharmacologic rationale underlying target selection was flawed. With this information in hand, drug discovery scientists can either produce new candidates that have the same mechanism of action but which correct the particular defect that caused the prior molecule to fail, or abandon the target and move on to new ones. The promise of new approaches to expedite knowledge obtained from failed trials such as digital technologies and artificial intelligence to evaluate enormous datasets has not yet been fully realized. However, model-informed approaches such as model-based meta-analysis are now employed to compare drug effects to comparators in the POC stage [43].

Proof of mechanism trials

These trials provide critical information for designing the clinical trials that make up the subsequent development program. Studies to assess PoM are designed with endpoints to answer the following questions:

- Does the candidate at a tolerated dose achieve suitable tissue levels at the target tissues, and does it bind to or inhibit its target?
- Does the agent have its desired pharmacologic activity at the site of action?
- Is there evidence that the mechanism targeted has a clinically relevant effect on the disease?
- Are safety and tolerability acceptable?

A well-designed POM trial should either confirm that the candidate meets all of the earlier mentioned requirements, or, if not, which hurdle failed and why. It should do so by exposing the fewest study subjects to the candidate for the shortest possible time, both to minimize human exposure to an unknown new agent and to minimize resource usage since at this stage failure is the likely outcome. As discussed in Chapter 17, endpoints for early trials are generally biomarkers but there generally is progression to more clinically established trial endpoints in later phases of development. Several examples of how endpoints evolve from pharmacodynamic markers or biomarkers to more established clinical endpoints as development progresses are presented in Table 34.1 [44–47].

TABLE 34.1 Endpoint selection in a development program.[a]

Disease to be treated	Possible PoM endpoints	Possible PoC endpoints	Regulatory approval endpoints
Rheumatoid arthritis	CRP, cytokine levels in blood or joint	DAS, ACR-20	DAS, ACR-20, radiographic change, functional outcomes
Alzheimer's disease	Hippocampal imaging	ADAS-cog	ADAS-cog, clinician global change score
Multiple sclerosis	CNS and systemic markers of inflammation	MRI lesions	Number of relapses, neurological status
Osteoarthritis disease modification	Cartilage degradation products, anabolic markers (none yet validated)	Possibly signs and symptoms (e.g., WOMAC), possibly imaging modalities (e.g., MRI)	Radiographic change (joint space narrowing), functional status
Type 2 diabetes mellitus	Fasting plasma glucose, oral glucose tolerance test	HbA1c after 1 month	HbA1c at 6 months
Chronic kidney disease	Biomarkers of target engagement	Improvement in proteinuria	eGFR slope and/or a composite of renal outcomes
Rapidly acting treatments for asthma or chronic obstructive airways disease	FEV_1, methacholine challenge test	Serial FEV1 (e.g., maximum FEV_1 response and duration of response, or the FEV_1 area under the curve above baseline)	Exacerbation rates

[a]*Abbreviations: CRP, C-reactive protein; DAS, disease activity score for RA [43]; ACR-20, American College of Rheumatology 20% improvement score for an individual study subject which shows a 20% improvement over their baseline score in terms of the number of affected joints and other related factors [44]; ADAS-cog, Alzheimer's Disease Assessment Scale, Cognitive Subscale [45]; eGFR, estimated glomerular filtration rate; HbA1c, glycated hemoglobin A1c; MRI, magnetic resonance imaging; WOMAC, Western Ontario and McMaster University osteoarthritis index [46].*

Proof of concept trials

Should the candidate achieve PoM, studies to assess PoC should focus on answering related questions:

- Is the pharmacologic activity of relevance to treating the symptoms of the disease, and, for chronic diseases, is it likely to be of relevance to the natural history or progression of the disease?
- Is the drug adequately tolerated at a dose that achieves the desired pharmacologic effects, taking into account the inherent limitations of relatively small trial size (hundreds of subjects) and short duration (weeks to months)?

Since these studies should be of the shortest possible duration to answer these questions, endpoints are focused on factors which can respond fairly quickly to an intervention, but which are also predictive of longer-term benefit. Sometimes these endpoints will be "hard clinical endpoints" that measure symptom improvement; sometimes they will be biomarkers or imaging tests that predict longer-term improvement. Examples for various chronic diseases are provided in Table 34.1, along with possible endpoints that would be examined in a PoC trial.

There are other considerations which also enter into deciding whether a drug candidate has achieved PoC, such as whether the agent is sufficiently well behaved from a pharmaceutic and pharmacokinetic perspective, whether it shows signs of differentiation from existing agents, and whether there is a clear set of endpoints and study designs accepted by regulatory authorities for the claims being sought [48].

Should the candidate fail in this phase, information again is passed back to drug discovery regarding whether this was a failure of the target to impact the disease, despite prior PoM showing that the pharmaceutical affected the target (as was the case with the P-38 MAP kinase inhibitors), or whether this was a failure due to toxicity. If the latter, the data generated by a well-designed program should also be able to address whether the toxicity was related to the target itself or to the particular agent being used.

Should a candidate pass the PoC phase, subsequent trials enroll more subjects who are treated for longer durations. However, before moving to confirmatory Phase 3 trials, additional trials, sometimes called "Phase 2b" trials, are often conducted. The major purpose of such trials is to refine selection of the dose that optimally balances efficacy and safety, to "derisk" the confirmation phase by conducting larger, longer-duration trials to ascertain whether beneficial effects observed in PoC trials can be replicated, and to acquire a larger safety database. Dose selection is sometimes folded into pre-PoC trials, especially if adaptive designs are used, as discussed later.

Confirmatory trials to support registration

Phase 3 confirmatory trials are often designed after consulting with regulatory authorities at an "end of Phase 2 meeting" with the appropriate review division at the US FDA, at a scientific advice session with the Committee on Human Medicinal Products of the EMA, or at meetings with national regulatory agencies in Europe and the Japanese PMDA. By this point, there should be sufficient knowledge of how the drug candidate behaves so that agreement can be reached with regulatory authorities regarding the a priori specification of clinically relevant endpoints that will be included in designing the confirmatory trials. There must also be agreement on many of the study design aspects reviewed later in this chapter.

Examples of possible endpoints for confirmatory trials are included in Table 34.1. These endpoints are usually widely accepted scales of clinical benefit in a given disease state, such as the ACR-20 for rheumatoid arthritis [45] or the Alzheimer's Disease Assessment Scale cognitive subscale (ADAS-cog) for Alzheimer's disease [49]. Often it is required that the candidate shows benefit in more than one endpoint in order to establish claims, such as improvement in ADAS-cog plus improvement in the physician's global assessment for Alzheimer's disease [49]. Specific recommended endpoints for selected disease states are outlined in both FDA [50] and EMA [17] development guidances. Because confirmatory trials provide the vast majority of patient exposure to the pharmaceutical candidate, they also are instrumental in meeting registration requirements for an adequate safety database.

Subsequent clinical trials

At the time the candidate is under review for marketing approval, and even after the drug is marketed, there are new questions which are raised:

- *Will very rare adverse effects occur that were not seen in the preregistration database?* This question is often best answered by pharmacovigilance and epidemiologic surveillance, rather than by clinical trials, and such activities form an integral part of the risk management plan for the drug.

- *Will the agent be safe and effective in a more broadly defined population than was studied in the preregistration development program?* For instance, can it be given to patients with concomitant morbidity, such as congestive heart failure? Clinical trials to address this question often make up part of what traditionally was called "Phase 4."
- *Will adverse events with an initially low background rate in the population being treated increase with prolonged drug treatment?* Such effects, for example a 30% increase in the incidence of stroke, MI, or cardiac death, are very hard to detect in a preregistration program. Large event-based outcomes trials often will be needed after registration to answer this question.
- *Will the agent be effective in conditions similar to those studied in the initial development program?* For example, will a drug developed for rheumatoid arthritis be useful in ankylosing spondylitis or psoriatic arthritis? Such separate development programs with both PoC and confirmatory phases often are conducted after an agent is initially marketed for a related condition. Because such programs take advantage of the vast knowledge developed in the initial dossier, such as safety data, dose response for the parent disease, and PK/PD data, these programs can be smaller and faster than the original program.

Clinical development of a drug candidate spans the gamut from the time the candidate is first introduced into man through its life cycle as a marketed agent. Throughout the process, the questions being asked by clinical trials, and the trial design and endpoints being measured, evolve with the specific needs of the program at that time. Initially the program is designed around likely failure, so early clinical trials seek to assess the relevance of the underlying pharmacology. During the next development phase, clinical trials are designed to learn the optimum dose and regimen for drug administration. Subsequently, the program seeks to establish efficacy, based on specific endpoints that have been agreed upon in meetings with regulatory authorities as representing effectiveness in the relevant disease state, while establishing an adequate safety database. Finally, the same process is used to conduct additional trials to look at related indications or broader populations and enhance knowledge of the agent's safety.

Specific design issues in clinical development programs

Individual clinical trials are the building blocks of the development program, and, in addition to those mentioned earlier, there are many other design factors that must be considered for each clinical trial if it is to play its role effectively in the development program.

Ethical design considerations

Ethical principles are embodied in the Declaration of Helsinki as well as in GCP guidelines, and designers of a clinical program must consider the ethical implications of study design as each clinical protocol is written. Every study is required to have a valid, testable hypothesis. For example, does treatment with the drug candidate have a specified impact on a given endpoint? Generally, studies testing therapeutic efficacy are done in patients with the disease who stand to benefit from the treatment. Often, however, early trials in humans to assess pharmacokinetic and pharmacodynamic parameters are done in healthy volunteers, since this provides a more standardized, more predictable population with less comorbidity. However, if the drug candidate has high potential risks, ethical considerations dictate doing even these early trials in patients. In some areas, such as oncology, even first-in-human trials are designed to be of sufficient length to provide potential benefit to cancer patients.

There has been much controversy over the ethical use of placebos. The Declaration of Helsinki justifies the use of a placebo only if no other treatment exists, or if compelling scientific reasons dictate its use. In general, placebo-controlled trials are performed in nonprogressive, nonlife-threatening conditions, or if performed in progressive chronic disease, such trials are of short duration (often 12 weeks or less) and are usually followed by an extension phase in which every study subject receives an active treatment. Placebo-controlled trials are often necessary to provide a clear assessment of drug effect, and in many circumstances are required by regulatory agencies for proof of effectiveness. The alternative to a placebo-controlled trial is a noninferiority trial, which compares an active drug with a known alternative. Such trials present both design and interpretation issues, as discussed later in this chapter. The ideal study design has been stated to be a design that includes both placebo and active control: the placebo arm to provide the reference for the population, and the active control to confirm that the trial is capable of demonstrating efficacy. Temple and Ellenberg [51, 52] summarize the issues with the use of placebos and conclude that placebos generally remain necessary to establish the efficacy of a new pharmaceutical candidate, and that placebo use also generally remains ethically acceptable when used for a limited duration of time not associated with significant morbidity mostly in therapy areas exclusive of oncology. In the oncology space, placebo-controlled trials are not as common due to the grievous illness and limited life span of patients in this therapy area, and are acceptable to regulatory agencies which require hard endpoints such as mortality in the absence of placebo control.

Study populations

Considerations in selecting a study population with a given disease include the choice of including either a patient population with little comorbidity and limited complications of the disease, or a population with more comorbidity or more disease complications. The former population oftentimes provides a clearer assessment of drug effect, since there are fewer confounders in the assessment of both safety and efficacy. However, it leaves open the question of whether the observed therapeutic benefits and safety profile can be generalized to more "real-world" disease populations who often have complications and comorbidities. Studying the latter population introduces more confounders but provides a more realistic assessment. In general, early phase development programs focus on a restricted population (i.e., before PoC), but during the confirmatory phase include a broader population, so that by the time of dossier submission a population has been treated that is more representative of the patients who will use the agent in medical practice. In addition, there are regulatory expectations that the elderly, the young, and other special populations will be included in adequate numbers by the time a development program is completed.

Study design paradigms

There are several fundamental trial designs that are reviewed from a regulatory and statistical perspective in the ICH E9 guidelines [53]. Each trial design has its advantages and disadvantages. However, in general, trials are randomized, so that subjects are assigned to different treatment regimens by an algorithm rather than by the investigator's choice, and double-blind, so that neither the investigator treating the study subjects nor the subjects themselves know which treatment regimen they are allocated to. Where trials are not double-blind (investigator and/or patient know the treatment regimen), regulators will expect the study to have endpoints that are not subjective, for example, mortality rate. Additionally, if the trial is not double-blind, sponsors may choose to create a "sponsor blind" set up (sponsor does not know treatment arm assigned even if the investigator/patient have this information) in order to protect trial integrity.

Cross-over studies

Early development-phase studies frequently use a cross-over design in which subjects receive each of several different treatments for several days, often with a several-day washout period between treatments, and then are assigned to another of the treatment regimens. The different arms of the study to which subjects are randomized receive the treatments in different order. Such studies allow each subject to serve as his or her own control, eliminating confounding patient selection factors due to imbalances in age, gender, genetic makeup, disease duration and severity, and other individual factors. However, interpretation of cross-over studies can be confounded because key measurements may change over the time of the study or the effects of the prior treatment may linger beyond the washout period. As a result, cross-over designs are generally feasible only for small numbers of study subjects and are mainly used in early phase development studies such as drug interaction studies and relative bioavailability studies.

Cohort studies

Another design predominantly used in early development is the cohort study, in which small groups of subjects (often 10–12) are randomized either to the active agent or to placebo, often with more subjects receiving drug than placebo. Subsequent cohorts often are treated with higher doses of the study drug or different combinations of study drug and other agents. These studies afford the assessment of safety and PK in one cohort before the next cohort is treated and lend themselves to early evaluation of agents about which little safety data exist. By incorporating different dosing regimens, cohort studies allow rapid ascertainment of the maximum tolerated dose and rapidly add key PK and PD insights. It also is common to pool the placebo groups from the various cohorts and compare that entire placebo group to the various cohorts receiving the candidate drug. As with cross-over designs, these studies are generally limited to short treatment durations and small numbers of subjects, and can be confounded by temporal shifts between cohorts. In addition, a large amount of variability is introduced if the different cohorts are evaluated by different investigators at different study sites, often making results difficult or impossible to interpret. Hence, as with cross-over studies, cohort studies best lend themselves to early development and are best suited to single-investigator settings and are most commonly employed as first-in-human studies.

Parallel group studies

Most safety and efficacy data in a development program are acquired by means of parallel group studies in which subjects are randomly allocated to two or more treatment arms. Patients in each arm usually receive one treatment regimen for the duration of the study, but there are variations in which the regimens are modified for each treatment arm at a prespecified study time point. Parallel group studies are amenable to any treatment duration and can be scaled up over multiple sites, since any confounding introduced by time or by study site differences will be more or less equally applied to each arm of the study. Since regulatory agencies often require studies of 1 year or longer to show evidence of durable efficacy and acceptable toxicity in many chronic diseases, such studies, almost by definition, must be parallel group studies. The major drawback of these studies is that the treatment arms can be imbalanced by factors that can affect the outcome, such as significant comorbidity that can affect safety assessments or the fact that patients with the most severe disease at baseline tend to show the greatest improvement during the study as they "regress to the mean." Enrolling larger numbers of study subjects and stratifying them by prognostic factors known to affect the study outcome (i.e., putting equal numbers from each stratification factor into each treatment group) are two common ways to mitigate these confounders.

Adaptive study designs

Increasing use is being made of adaptive study designs in which the study data are sampled and the study modified under controlled circumstances that are specified in the study protocol. Examples include early termination of a study for futility (statistical demonstration based on partial results that there is a very low probability of showing a drug effect), modification of study size based on observed variability in results (more variability than planned will require a larger study size, less variability a smaller study size), or reallocation of study subjects to various treatment arms or cohorts based on prior results in order to maximize the number of patients allocated to treatment-dose groups or regimens with the highest therapeutic index [54]. These techniques can be very powerful in increasing the efficiency of clinical development. At the same time, they can become quite challenging from an operational perspective, as the repeated interim analyses called for by some of the more complex adaptive designs require extraordinary steps to protect data integrity while data are being rapidly acquired and analyzed [55]. Some adaptive design features, such as futility analysis and modification of study size based on a blinded assessment of variability, are well accepted by regulatory authorities even in pivotal confirmatory trials. However, other adaptive designs, especially those that seek to combine the learning (pre-PoC) and confirming phases into one study, are generally still considered only suitable for exploratory trials both by the FDA [56] and by regulators elsewhere [57]. Despite these caveats, elements of adaptive design, while rarely used just a decade ago, are now finding their way into most clinical development programs because of the increased efficiency that they can add to these programs.

Confirmatory studies may also be designed with dual primary endpoints such that a positive outcome could be seen with either or both endpoints and such designs will require prespecification of how type 1 error will be controlled for the trial. Use of dual primary endpoints may also support earlier interim analysis readouts from one endpoint while the trial continues for the other dual primary endpoint. Regulatory acceptance of such designs centers around prespecification of type 1 error control, sufficient information for both safety and efficacy from the interim analysis, and level of effect observed at the interim but such interim analyses have led to accelerated drug development mainly in the Oncology therapy area.

Additional adaptive designs in the POM/POC space include umbrella, basket, and platform trial designs. In umbrella trials, patients are enrolled with a common indication but may have different biomarker/genetic drivers and consists of many tests of various drugs in this population in one trial so the drug arms vary dependent on the biomarker/genetic drivers. Basket trials help evaluate if a drug would work well in patients with a certain genetic/biomarker driver. For example, a basket trial involving patients with BRAF genetic mutations helped lead to the FDA approval of vemurafenib in patients with rare heme malignancy Erdheim-Chester Disease (ECD) [58]. Platform trials, sometimes called multiarm, multistage trials, evaluate several treatments against a patient population and interim analyses for either safety or efficacy may lead to stopping arms and arms being added to the trial and various other scenarios [59].

In the confirmatory space, the seamless Phase 2 and 3 trial design in which a Phase 2 has an analysis and upon reaching a prespecified criteria is expanded in sample size to now seek confirmation of safety and efficacy. Such Phase 2/3 trials have operational and logistical complexities to be considered including endpoint for the Phase 2 trial to determine if Phase 3 expansion will occur, timing of the analysis, and whether the Phase 2 trial continues to enroll while the interim occurs, just to name a few example parameters that would need to be planned up front.

Statistical considerations underlying the number of study subjects

As noted previously, every clinical trial should have a hypothesis to be tested. Generally, such a hypothesis for a superiority study is that the active treatment will have a specified difference, or *effect size*, compared to placebo or the comparator drug.

For example, for a rheumatoid arthritis study it could be postulated that the active agent in the trial will produce an ACR-20 response (see Table 34.1) in at least 25% more of the study subjects given the experimental therapy than those receiving placebo [45]. Generally, the study is designed to validate the hypothesis that the observed difference has a 95% chance of being more than 25 units if any similar population is studied, and that the likelihood of the observed difference in the study being due to chance or confounders alone is less than 5% ($\alpha = 0.05$), the level most commonly required to conclude that a result is "statistically significant." The larger the number of study subjects enrolled, the more likely the findings will achieve this level of certainty, because increasing the number of subjects reduces the impact of variability due to random "noise." Likewise, the larger the effect size is for a given number of study subjects, the more likely the effect will achieve this degree of certainty because the "signal-to-noise ratio" is larger. The likelihood that a study will achieve the desired goal based on a given effect size is termed the study *power*. The number of study subjects per treatment arm required to achieve a given power is a function of the inherent variability of the study population, the study endpoint, and the effect size. Generally, studies are powered to 80%–90%, meaning that the designers expect 80%–90% certainty that if the agent they are testing truly has the desired effect size designed into the study, it will manifest itself with statistical significance when the study is completed.

These concepts are illustrated in Fig. 34.2. While it is impossible to generalize over the vast array of study designs, diseases, endpoints, and pharmaceuticals, generally tens to hundreds of subjects per arm are required. If one intends to impact an infrequent outcome, the number of study patients can be in the thousands or tens of thousands. Small increases in variability, small decreases in anticipated effect size, or small changes in desired power (e.g., going from 80% to 90%) have very large impacts on the number of patients required for each treatment group—often many-fold the size of the change in the input parameter. Additionally, trials designed with dual primary endpoints may also find that the sample size is driven more for one of the endpoints that requires a larger sample size and therefore the alternative dual primary endpoint may be overpowered and therefore detect a result that is smaller than the effect size intended; the consequence could be that the regulatory acceptability of the result will be subject to whether it's clinically relevant for the disease setting.

Noninferiority studies

Noninferiority studies, in which one active agent is compared to another to show that their effect is similar, add additional complexities. The approach is outlined in Fig. 34.3. These studies are powered to demonstrate that the lower 95% confidence bound of the difference between the experimental agent and the established agent is no worse than a specified amount. For instance, if two antibiotics are being compared for community-acquired pneumonia, the study might be powered to show that the lower 95% confidence bound of the cure rate for the experimental agent stays above the −5% noninferiority margin. That way we can say with 95% confidence that the experimental agent at worst cures 5% fewer pneumonias than the established antibiotic. At best, it may cure the same amount or more, but it is the worst-case scenario that the study must be powered for. How much worse the experimental agent can be and still be considered "noninferior" can become a major issue, involving clinical judgment, health policy, and statistics. A large noninferiority margin is of little use because it allows for the experimental agent to be sufficiently worse than the established agent that the clinical relevance of the findings is called into question. Conversely, very small noninferiority margins, requiring very tight confidence

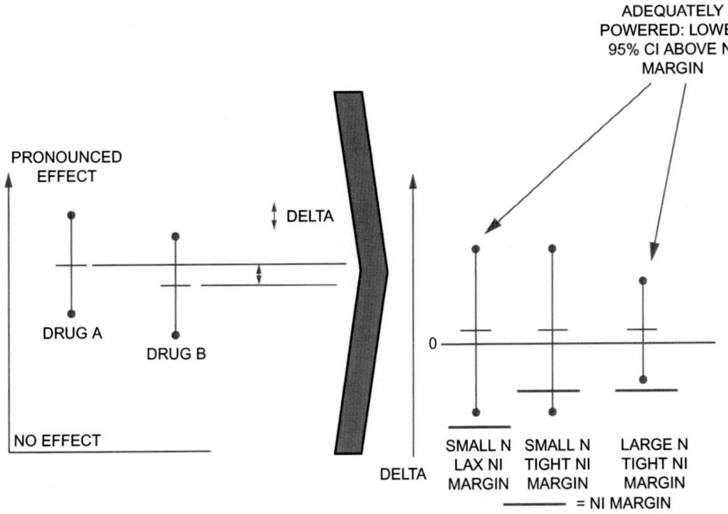

FIG. 34.3 Statistical considerations for superiority trials (N = number of subjects per treatment group that is used in the power calculations, Delta = expected effect size).

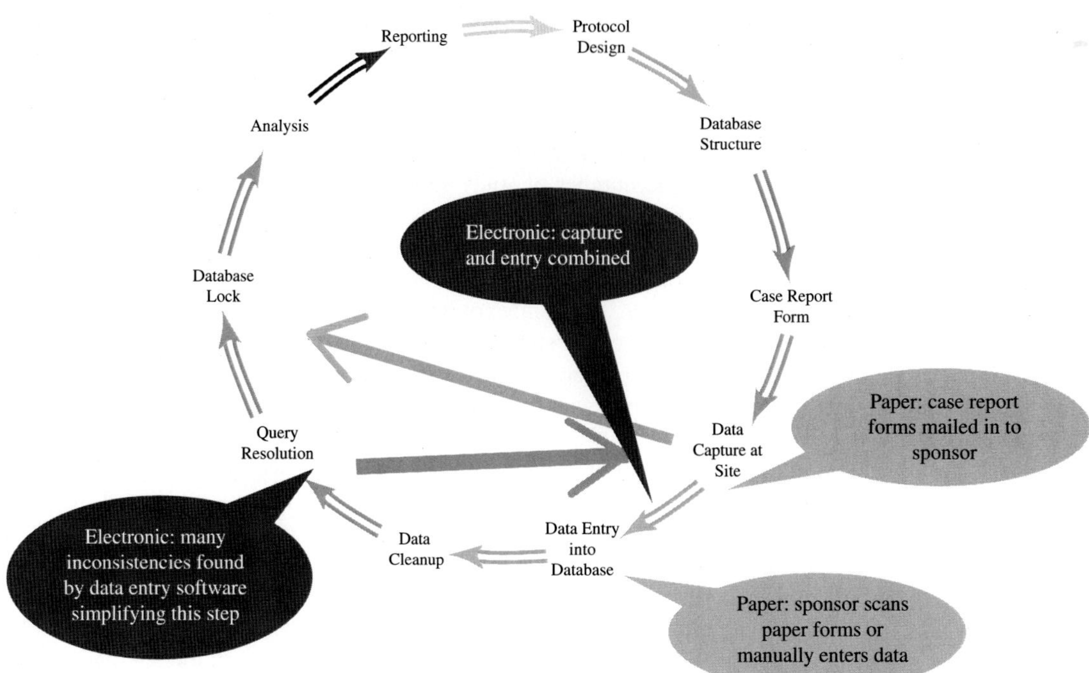

FIG. 34.4 Statistical considerations for noninferiority trials (delta = between treatment difference in effect, CI = confidence interval, NI = noninferiority).

bounds, require inordinately large numbers of patients per treatment arm. The right balance is often difficult to ascertain, and sometimes may not exist. The FDA, for instance, in its influenza guidance does not consider noninferiority studies to be valid evidence of effectiveness partly because there is no consensus on what a meaningful noninferiority margin might be [60]. In other areas, such as community-acquired pneumonia [61], where sufficient data on effectiveness of active agents exist and placebo studies would be unethical, regulatory agencies accept noninferiority studies, but in this and other conditions caution the sponsor that extensive justification of the noninferiority margin used is required [62]. Despite the issues associated with these trials, many recent new drug applications, particularly for antibacterial agents, have relied on noninferiority designs in the key pivotal trials that support the registration dossier [63]. These study designs will also be heavily relied upon in any comparative effectiveness program (Fig. 34.4).

The impact of safety assessment on development programs

Whereas efficacy is measured with specific endpoints and prespecified differences between treatments that are incorporated into the hypothesis testing of a clinical trial, safety is holistic, oftentimes unpredictable, and its evaluation must be comprehensive. While many unsafe potential drug candidates are weeded out in preclinical assessment, this does not assure safety in the clinic and many types of adverse events are difficult to predict from in vitro or in vivo preclinical data. While studies can be designed to test specific safety-related hypotheses using a formal statistical powering method (e.g., there will be x% fewer cases of renal failure on an experimental transplant drug vs standard of care), most preregistration [64] knowledge of candidate drug safety is accrued by treating as many patients as possible for as long as possible. Modern drug development programs typically vastly exceed the minimum requirements set by ICH for the amount of required patient exposure to an experimental agent by the time the dossier is filed for approval, as presented in Table 34.2 [65], which compares a typical development program for a chronic disease to the ICH guidelines. However, the typical drug development programs typically vastly exceed the minimum requirements set by ICH for the required duration of patient exposure to an experimental agent by the time the dossier is filed for approval.

Large databases are required not only to characterize more common adverse events but also to detect rare but severe events such as agranulocytosis, toxic epidermal necrolysis, or fulminant hepatic necrosis. These life-threatening conditions often occur at rates of 1 in 10,000 to 1 in 100,000 for drugs known to cause them. For instance, a database with 6000 patients exposed to an experimental agent would have about a 50% chance of detecting an adverse event that occurs at a rate of 1 in 10,000, and a single event could be dismissed as chance alone. The likelihood of such a database containing two such

TABLE 34.2 Size of a preregistration safety database.

Study subjects' exposure to investigational drug	ICH guideline (# of subjects)	Size of a contemporary chronic use drug database (# of subjects)[a]
Total exposure to new drug	1500	2498
Duration >3 months		2237
Duration >6 months		1979
Duration >1 year	100	1698
Duration >2 years		821
Duration >3 years		153

[a]*Data from Pfizer, Inc. Advisory Committee Briefing Document EXUBERA—Endocrinologic and Metabolic Drugs Advisory Committee 2005. Internet at, www.fda.gov/ohrms/dockets/ac/05/briefing/2005-4169B1_01_01-Pfizer-Exubera.pdf [60].*

events, which would begin to raise serious concerns about the candidate, is only about 12%. Therefore drug development programs must be constructed to be of adequate size to characterize safety with a reasonable degree of certainty.

Power calculations based on efficacy hypotheses generally dictate the size of the component studies in a drug development program. Often the aggregate drug exposure provided by these studies is inadequate either in number of subjects treated or duration of treatment, or in both, to fully characterize safety to a degree suitable for registration. Hence, the development program must incorporate other types of studies to accrue adequate exposure data. For example, additional efficacy studies can be performed that test alternate hypotheses while adding to the size of the safety database. Such studies also have the advantage of providing exposure to placebo and/or additional comparative agents, helping to place safety data observed with the experimental candidate in a broader context. Alternatively, it is common practice to allow subjects completing double-blind studies to enter extension studies. Such studies provide long-term exposure and offer study subjects the opportunity to remain on treatment should they have a good response. This not only enhances patient recruitment into the studies but also places the entire program on a solid ethical foundation.

Many development programs must be designed to meet an even more difficult safety challenge than detecting very rare events by demonstrating that a drug candidate does not increase the amount of low-level background morbid events. Certain drug classes such as oral antidiabetic agents or cyclooxygenase inhibitors have the potential to increase the rate of major adverse cardiovascular events (MACE) (i.e., strokes, nonfatal myocardial infarctions, and cardiac deaths). These events occur at a background rate of several occurrences per 100 patient-years in many of the populations being treated for chronic diseases such as arthritis or diabetes. For example, design of an outcome trial to demonstrate that a drug candidate does not cause an increase in the rate of MACE events can take an approach similar to that of a noninferiority study by being powered to show that the occurrence of MACE events in a population treated with the new agent (often for 1–2 years) at worst (upper confidence bound) does not exceed by more than a given percentage the rate observed with a comparator treatment. Thus if the outcomes trial were powered for 20% and the background rate of MACE events was 5% per year, the trial would need to show with 95% confidence that MACE events for the experimental treatment were less than 6% (i.e., 20% more than 5%). These safety studies are major undertakings, and their size grows exponentially as the background rate of events of interest falls or the noninferiority margin is reduced. As seen in Table 34.3, if the rate of MACE events is 4% per year for both the experimental drug and background therapy, it would take 743 study subjects per arm to show that the experimental drug did not increase MACE events by more than 80% with a 95% confidence level, and 5076 subjects per arm to show that the same agent with a true rate identical to background therapy did not increase the rate of MACE events by more than 30%.

Current FDA guidelines for antidiabetic drug development require at the time of registration that the safety database is large enough, or that an outcomes trial exists, to demonstrate a no more than 80% increase in MACE events over background or comparator treatments, and that a postapproval commitment be made to study sufficient subjects to establish this at the 30% level [66]. As concerns for the cardiovascular safety of commonly used drugs increase, such requirements are likely to become more common features of other clinical development programs. This methodology can also be applied to address concerns that a pharmaceutical agent could potentially increase other major health events, such as infection or cancer, over an existing background rate. Finally, as in the earlier mentioned example of antidiabetic drugs, the clinical

TABLE 34.3 Size of event-based outcomes trials.

Percent of subjects with event	Upper 95% CI = 1.1	Upper 95% CI = 1.3	Upper 95% CI = 1.8	Upper 95% CI = 2.0
1%	173,354	19,339	2747	1765
4%	44,961	5076	743	483
10%	19,414	2244	347	231
15%	13,840	1630	264	178

development program for drug safety does not end at the time of dossier submission but postapproval clinical trials, coupled with epidemiology and pharmacovigilance, continue as long as the agent remains in medical use.

Conduct of clinical development

Number and location of study sites for global clinical development programs

Small trials conducted early in development are often conducted at one or only a few study sites. As programs progress into large parallel group trials, tens or hundreds of study sites become the norm. Modern large multicenter trials are often global in scope. Advantages of global trials include access to large numbers of qualified study subjects that would be difficult to recruit solely in North America or Western Europe. This also expands the diversity of the study population, making it more representative of the ultimate users of the drug. It may also enhance the validity of the development program to foreign regulatory authorities, provided that sufficient numbers of study subjects from their respective country or region are enrolled to give them confidence that the study results can be generalized to their jurisdiction [67].

Historically, data quality was suspect from trials conducted in regions outside of North America and Western Europe. However, with the adoption of electronic data capture and global standards such as GCP this is no longer a significant issue. Likewise, statistical methodologies have been developed for dealing with regional variability [68]. Despite these advances, cultural, regulatory, and operational barriers continue to impede the conduct of global trials [69]. However, large global trials that are coordinated with global development programs and use the same pivotal studies for simultaneous filing in major regions of the world are rapidly becoming the norm in clinical development programs.

Data flow and data quality

A significant part of GCP is concerned with data quality and integrity. Sponsors of clinical trials must assure themselves and regulatory authorities through comprehensive and consistent monitoring of activities at every study site that GCP standards were maintained and that the data were collected as specified by the study protocol. These monitoring activities must also assure that every study subject's data is valid and can be verified by examination of source documents such as medical records and office notes. Data, whether entered on paper case report forms or electronically, must have an audit trail indicating when the data were entered, why and when any changes were made, and the persons who entered and changed the data. Before study data can be analyzed, the data must have been verified, inconsistencies checked with the study site and resolved, and the database "locked" for analysis.

The advent of electronic data capture has streamlined this process by enabling study sites to enter data directly through an internet portal into the study database and has been one of the key enablers of global clinical trials. Data entry software has even provided automated recognition of some data inconsistencies. It also has facilitated the adoption of adaptive designs for which electronic data capture provides the rapid data turnaround that is required to make the protocol-specified changes in study design that are based on the acquired data.

Use of Independent Data Monitoring Committees (IDMCs) and adjudication committees

For the past several decades, large clinical trials with outcomes related to survival, mortality, or major events such as myocardial infarction have used IDMCs to monitor unblinded data as these were acquired during a study and, under appropriate circumstances, advise the sponsor to modify or terminate the study. Although generally not required under regulatory law,

IDMCs have become more widespread and are now used in the majority of large confirmatory trials, and even smaller PoC trials for some indications. Generally, an IDMC should be used for any trial in which a clinically important difference in significant morbidity is possible between treatment arms. An IDMC is equally appropriate to safeguard against the risk of increased adverse events or mortality in the experimental treatment arm or against worse outcomes, such as more disease progression, in the nonexperimental or placebo arms of a study.

The composition of IDMCs includes clinicians, preferably with experience in drug safety and expertise in the disease under study, and statisticians who operate independently of the sponsor. Their roles and responsibilities are defined by a charter that generally specifies committee membership and rules of operation, the milestones at which the board will review data, the specific data that the board will review, and what the board is allowed to communicate back to the sponsor without compromising the integrity of the study. It is critical that communication back to the sponsor be limited to what is absolutely necessary in order to avoid revealing information about how the respective study arms are performing, which could influence further conduct of the study outside of the specific IDMC remit and thus unblind the study. Often the board is restricted to making recommendations to the sponsor including the following examples: continue the study unchanged, eliminate one or more arms in the study, modify the dose of one of the treatments in the study, or terminate the study entirely. Occasionally boards are provided with specific "stopping rules," so that the board will recommend termination or modification of the study if a prespecified difference is observed between treatment groups. The FDA [70] and EMA [71] each have guidance documents for IDMCs that elaborate the benefits (independent oversight of study conduct, protection of patient safety) and risks (particularly the potential of interim analyses to bias future study conduct) and provide practical guidance regarding the composition, operation, and remit of these committees.

Somewhat related in function to IDMCs are adjudication committees, which are groups of independent experts who review study data, often in a blinded fashion unlike the case with IDMCs, in order to assess whether specific criteria are met for important study events. Most cardiovascular outcomes trials, for instance, have a committee to adjudicate data acquired about every suspected MACE event and use prespecified criteria to determine whether the incident under review truly represents a MACE event, to be counted as an endpoint for the trial, or some other type of adverse event. Similarly, a blinded adjudication committee might be used in an oncology study to provide an unbiased assessment of tumor progression.

Special topics

Personalized medicine

The optimal therapy of individual patients has been a long-standing goal of clinical pharmacologists and has been enhanced by the incorporation of therapeutic drug monitoring and pharmacokinetics into clinical care. Recent advances in pharmacogenetics and pharmacogenomics represent an extension of this effort to "personalize" medicine. As discussed in previous chapters, genomic and biological markers have played key roles in the clinical development of a number of drugs, and the evolving process and evidentiary standards of diagnostic validation and "fit-for-purpose" utilization are important considerations for clinical development scientists [72]. Recent examples include the HER2 assay for trastuzumab in the treatment of breast and gastric cancer, the KRAS mutation assay for cetuximab and panitumumab in the treatment of colon cancer, the EGFR mutational assay for erlotinib in the treatment of lung cancer, the HIV CCR5 tropism assay for maraviroc in the treatment of HIV, and the HLA-B 5701 assay for abacavir in the treatment of HIV.

Incorporation of a genomic or biomarker diagnostic should be considered during exploratory development (pre-PoC) along with the development of a diagnostic assay that is validated, standardized, practical, scalable, and affordable at the time of regulatory registration. The pace and clinical development relevance of personalized medicine is anticipated to increase, so clinical development scientists must be aware of personalized medicine advances in the therapeutic and pharmacologic areas relevant to their research.

Model-informed drug (discovery and) development (MIDD)

During the past two decades, new approaches to improve efficiency and confidence throughout the drug development stages have emerged and become more commonly applied. One of these approaches is called model-informed drug (discovery and) development (MIDD) which is based on the concept presented by Lewis Sheiner [32] to think of early development (up to Phase 3 pivotal testing) as a learning platform where one should design informative Phase 1 and 2 trials, coupled with use of PKPD and other modeling techniques to inform decisions. The consistent application of MIDD can help reduce attrition and improve cycle times, as exemplified in higher confidence in selecting the right dose at start of Phase 3, or when assessing whether the candidate drug has a favorable differentiation profile vs standard of care of competitors [73]. Regulatory authorities are also promoting the concept of MIDD and workshops and positions papers have been produced. In 2015 and 2016 both EFPIA (European Federation of Pharmaceutical Industries and Associations) and EMA have published papers describing the role and value of MIDD to both enhance efficiency and also to facilitate the regulatory review process [73–76]. FDA has expanded the application of MIDD and as part of their PDUVA VI commitment, have set-up a MIDD pilot program where the sponsor is invited to engage FDA to discuss and align the MIDD strategy for a given project [73, 74, 77, 78].

Artificial Intelligence and digital and Mobile medicine in drug development

Interest in the application of Artificial Intelligence (AI) to drug discovery and development has exponentially increased in recent times. An obvious use of AI would be its application to translating Informed Consent forms into various languages. However, more significant approaches to the application of AI vary by function and the questions or problems to be considered. Actually, almost every aspect of drug development may have a potential application due to the ability of the technique to "learn" from vast datasets and to provide insights that may have been missed by manual analysis of the huge amount of data that drug discovery generates.

In particular, drug discovery generates a huge amount of data on potential chemical, in vitro and in vivo characteristics for a drug candidate's potential toxicity, efficacy, and PK. Furthermore, manually integrating data from other sources (e.g., databases, literature, abstracts, etc.) is an enormous task. Particularly time consuming is the manual analysis of large datasets to identify potential new drug candidate. Artificial intelligence, using machine learning and deep learning algorithms, can accelerate the process of optimizing chemical structures which may maximize the benefit-risk ratio of drug candidates during drug discovery and also may be useful in clinical pharmacology and later stages of drug development [79]. The potential application of AI in other areas of drug development is almost limitless: including real-world data, image recognition—analyzing pathology slide or clinical images for identifying and measuring tumors or other lesions; analyzing clinical databases for unexpected safety or efficacy signals; outcomes predictions by analyzing clinical trajectories; identifying responders and nonresponders; and many, many more applications.

As digital technology has become more portable, easy to use, and affordable, it has begun to find more common usage in clinical trials. This technology may take the form of new imaging tools, the use of mobile devices, swallowable and implantable sensors, and other applications that collect data on patients many times a day. These approaches combined with at-home sampling are allowing for much more data to be collected outside of the clinic and for a much more detailed picture of a drug candidate's profile. In many instances this influx of data is married to AI technology to more fully interrogate the increased amount of data.

Elderly and pediatric populations

Clinical development programs should gather sufficient information to assess benefit and risk and provide adequate treatment guidance for the population of patients likely to receive the new treatment following approval. Since most disease states occur more frequently in elderly patients, there has been special emphasis on assuring adequate participation of elderly subjects in clinical development programs. Advanced age alone should generally not exclude clinical trial participation, especially in confirmatory clinical trials. Rather, exclusion criteria should be medically appropriate and based on the pharmacology of the new treatment and the characteristics of the disease under study. The clinical development program should recognize that age-related physiological changes, as described in Chapter 25, may impact the PK or PD response to a new treatment. In addition, elderly clinical trial participants generally use more concomitant medications and have more concurrent medical illnesses. For these reasons, clinical development programs should: (1) in early development, specifically investigate the comparative PK of a new pharmaceutical treatment in elderly and young patients; (2) include adequate numbers of elderly participants in clinical trials; and (3) specifically review the aggregate efficacy and safety results in elderly and young clinical trial participants. There is specific ICH guidance on the inclusion of elderly subjects in clinical development programs [80, 81].

It is important that infants and children have access to new pharmaceutical treatments and that adequate information be available on their use in the pediatric population. There is increasing focus on assuring these goals and on the pediatric clinical development of new pharmaceutical products. In the United States, the Pediatric Research Equity Act (PREA) of 2003 requires the FDA and sponsor to agree on the conduct and timing of the pediatric studies, with their possible deferral pending the acquisition of appropriate preliminary information. If the new pharmaceutical treatment is not anticipated to have pediatric application, a specific FDA waiver of pediatric development must be obtained [82]. In addition, the Best

Pharmaceuticals for Children Act (BPCA) of 2002 incentivizes pediatric clinical development by providing an additional 6 months of marketing exclusivity for products that have a pediatric data package which is accepted by the FDA [83]. In the EU, regulatory approval applications must include the results of pediatric studies conducted in compliance with a Pediatric Investigation Plan (PIP), unless a deferral has been granted, or unless pediatric development is inappropriate or not necessary [84]. The PIP is binding and must be agreed to in advance by the sponsor and the Pediatric Committee of the EMA. If changes are required during clinical development of the new pharmaceutical product, modification of the plan must be requested from the Pediatric Committee. Compliance with the PIP is checked at the time of application for marketing authorization but also provides the pharmaceutical product with eligibility for a 6-month extension of market exclusivity in the EU.

There are a number of ethical concerns particular to the conduct of pediatric clinical development. These include the process of obtaining informed consent, which raises issues of even subtle coercion or influence. In general, written informed consent must be obtained from both parents or a legal guardian, as well as assent from children able to understand, and consent from older children and adolescents. In each instance a full disclosure of risks and benefits must be made using appropriate and understandable language [85, 86].

Orphan drugs

Specific legislative and regulatory actions have been taken in the EU, United States, and Japan to support the development of new pharmaceutical treatments for patients with rare diseases [87–90]. These actions are intended to address and incentivize the clinical development of designated candidates and a request for orphan drug designation may be made at any time during the drug development process. Table 34.4 presents the specific orphan drug definitions, actions, and incentives for each of the three regions. In addition to the disease prevalence restriction, legislation enabling orphan product development in the United States requires that applications for orphan product designation demonstrate that the candidate drug has "promise" for efficacy in treating the rare disease; however, the designation may occur at any time during the drug

TABLE 34.4 Orphan drug definitions, regulatory actions, and incentives in the EU, United States, and Japan.

Legislation (year)	Definition	Regulatory actions	Incentives
EU Orphan Medicinal Product Regulation (2000)	Disorder that affects <5/10,000 people in the EU, or the treatment is intended for a life-threatening, seriously debilitating, or serious and chronic condition in the EU, and that without incentives it is unlikely that the marketing of the medicinal product would generate sufficient return to justify the necessary investment	• EMA Scientific Advice and protocol assistance • Reduction of fees or fee waivers will be considered for all types of pre- and post-authorization activities	• 10-year period of market exclusivity for the orphan drug indication • Tax incentives • Incentives made available by EU and Member States
US Orphan Drug Act (1982)	Disorder that affects <200,000 people in the United States, or that affects >200,000 persons but is not expected to recover the costs of developing and marketing the treatment drug	• Creation of Office of Orphan Products Development (OOPD) • FDA written recommendations concerning required clinical studies • Possible fast-track regulatory review of marketing application	• 7-year period of market exclusivity for the orphan drug indication • Tax incentives • Orphan Drug Product Grants Program
Japan Orphan Drug Pharmaceutical Affairs Law Revisions (1993)	Disorder that affects <50,000 people in Japan (corresponding to <4/10,000 people) and is incurable and without alternative treatment, or the efficacy and expected safety of the drug must be excellent in comparison with other available drugs	• Fast-track Marketing Authorization procedure • Regulatory consultation • Specific mention of global clinical trial acceptability	• Up to a 10-year period of market exclusivity for the orphan drug indication • Tax incentives • Possible financial support for development costs

development continuum. As reported by the FDA, the Orphan Drug Act has been successful in promoting the development of more than 300 new pharmaceutical treatments for rare diseases since 1983, compared to fewer than 10 such treatments in the prior decade [91]. In the single area of rare neurological diseases, over 27 new treatments have been introduced in the United States between 1983 and 2009, covering the areas of movement disorders (14 treatments), seizures (7 treatments), sleep (3 treatments), pain (2 treatments), and spinal cord spasticity (1 treatment) [92].

Clinical development programs for orphan drug indications should adhere to the same principles, guidance, and good practice that apply to all clinical development. In order to address the rarity of the diseases under study, combined and collaborative efforts are being proposed to accelerate biomarker validation, improve patient access, and accelerate research and development in rare diseases [93]. Clinical development scientists involved with orphan drug development should consider these and other available resources.

Comparative effectiveness

Increasing importance is being placed on comparing the efficacy and safety profiles of new pharmaceutical products with those of existing treatments, and there is particular emphasis on the need for direct comparative studies. In these studies, the active comparator serves as the reference for the proposed new pharmaceutical candidate, oftentimes instead of placebo. The importance of comparative effectiveness has been highlighted in the evaluations of many regulatory and reimbursement agencies, including the UK National Institute for Health and Clinical Excellence (NICE) [94] and the US Department of Health and Human Services Agency for Healthcare Research and Quality (AHRQ) [95]. Both NICE and AHRQ sponsor reviews in which the efficacy and safety data of newly approved treatments are compared to already existing therapies. The importance of comparative effectiveness is further emphasized by the fact that specific funding has been allocated by the US government for comparative effectiveness research in both the Patient Protection and Affordable Care Act (PPACA) of 2009 [15] and the American Recovery and Reinvestment Act of 2009, which includes the establishment of a US Federal Coordinating Council for Comparative Effectiveness Research [96].

There are significant challenges in the acquisition of the comparative effectiveness data that should be considered when planning a clinical development program. These include:

- Selection of the most appropriate comparator agent, which may depend on the medical practice environment in which the trials take place;
- Dose and administration regimen of the comparator and experimental agents;
- Specific endpoints for comparison;
- Specific population to be studied (e.g., allowed concurrent illness and concomitant medications, disease severity at baseline, demographic entry criteria); and
- Specific conditions under which the study is conducted. This is particularly important since the relatively strict conditions required for randomized, controlled clinical trials oftentimes cannot replicate the less controlled environment of medical practice. The most relevant comparative effectiveness data obviously are those data collected in an environment that most closely reflects medical practice.

In addition, there are a number of substantial issues in designing trials that are intended to show noninferiority or therapeutic equivalence rather than superiority. One particular concern is in selecting a noninferiority margin that is clinically meaningful and is supported by prior clinical investigation, yet also allows for a feasible clinical trial design. Because of these substantial challenges, while most drug development programs include comparative data, they also continue to depend on the use of placebo to establish the effectiveness of the pharmaceutical candidate and to provide a reference point for determining the treatment-emergent safety and toleration profile. For many indications in the United States, this is a required evidentiary standard for efficacy.

Combination treatments

It is becoming apparent that there often is value in using two or more pharmaceutical agents together to treat numerous diseases, including hypertension, diabetes, infectious disease, and cancer. While we will only discuss the combined use of two or more pharmaceutical agents administered as a single entity, there are other examples in which two different regulated entities are combined, such as a drug and device (e.g., a drug-eluting coronary stent) or a drug and diagnostic (e.g., the use of trastuzumab and the HER-2 diagnostic). As stated by the US FDA Office of Combination Products [97]:

Combination products have the potential to provide enhanced therapeutic advantages compared to single entity devices, drugs, and biologics. More and more combination products are incorporating cutting-edge, novel technologies that hold great promise for advancing patient care. Combination products may include drug-delivery systems, gene therapy systems, personalized medicine drug–device combinations, biological–device combinations, nanotechnology, and other innovative products for diagnostic and therapeutic treatments of cardiovascular, metabolic, oncologic, and other disorders.

Traditionally, combination pharmaceuticals were single entities that contained an investigational new drug and an already approved drug that was commonly used in the population for which the combination was targeted. The combination product generally would have the following characteristics:

- The constituents act on the same disease or symptom via different mechanisms and in doing so may act to produce a greater therapeutic effect than either one could individually, or may produce similar efficacy with improved safety/toleration than either one could individually (e.g., combined angiotensin-converting enzyme or angiotensin receptor blocker and calcium channel blocker agents);
- The constituents act on distinct diseases or symptoms that commonly occur together where the combination product may offer improved convenience and compliance (e.g., combined hypolipidemic and antihypertensive agents);
- One constituent is used to markedly improve the PK or PD profile of the investigational new drug. Examples include:
  - Ritonavir/lopinavir where lopinavir is an inhibitor of the HIV-1 protease and ritonavir inhibits the CYP3A-mediated metabolism of lopinavir, thereby providing increased plasma levels of lopinavir; and
  - Nivolumab/Ipilimumab where Nivolumab blocks the action of the checkpoint inhibitor PD-1 and Ipilimumab blocks the action of the checkpoint inhibitor CTLA-4 thus taking the brakes off the immune system and allowing T-cell proliferation and activation; and
  - Venclexta/azacitidine where Venclexta blocks the antiapoptotic protein Bcl2 and azacitidine a hypomethylation agent becomes incorporated into DNA preventing methylation; and
  - Amoxicillin/clavulanate potassium which is an oral antibacterial combination consisting of the semisynthetic antibiotic, amoxicillin and the β-lactamase inhibitor, clavulanate potassium.

Initiation of combination product global development should begin after regulatory consultation with EU [98], United States [97], and Japanese regulatory agencies [57]. Historically this has occurred after the efficacy, safety, and toleration of the investigational drug has been established as a single agent for treating the disease or symptom under study. This would usually require completion of a PoC trial and substantial confirmatory trial. The efficacy, safety, and toleration data of the already approved drug component would be summarized and available for review in the approval authorization submission. After completing some preclinical animal safety studies with the combination product, clinical development traditionally beg with a study of the PK/PD response of the investigational and approved drugs given alone and in combination. Based on these results, a broad, dose-ranging clinical study then would be conducted to examine the efficacy, safety, and toleration of the investigational and approved agents given alone and in combination. One example of such a broad dose-ranging study is one that was conducted to examine the combined use of the calcium channel blocker amlodipine and the angiotensin receptor blocker valsartan [99]. Using a two-study paradigm, the dose ranging covered a fourfold range of amlodipine doses (2.5–10 mg once daily) and an eightfold range of valsartan doses (40–320 mg once daily) administered alone and in combination. Depending on the required efficacy, safety, and toleration database, and the required combination product labeling, further confirmatory trials might be needed based on the results of the broad dose-ranging studies.

It is now increasingly recognized that new pharmaceutical treatments for certain diseases or conditions require drug combinations in order to show meaningful efficacy that cannot be obtained when either agent is used alone. For example, combination therapy may be needed because an infectious agent or oncology treatment develops resistance to single-agent therapy, because redundant pathophysiological mechanisms reduce the effectiveness of single-agent antihypertensive therapy, or because the body's own immune system must be switched on before an oncology agent can be effective. To respond to this need, the FDA has issued guidance for the combined development of two or more investigational pharmaceutical agents [100]. The guidance notes that this approach generally should be used: (1) for agents to treat a serious disease, (2) where there is a strong pathophysiological rationale, (3) where there are favorable preclinical data supporting the combination use, and (4) where there are data supporting the inappropriateness of single-agent use. The guidance mentions the need to establish the safety and PK of both new investigational new drugs as single entities, if feasible, and in the combination to support dose selection for Phase 2. It also refers to the design of a clinical development plan that allows the contribution of each component to be established. Once again, this may require dosing the agents as single entities or otherwise to demonstrate that the combination is superior to one of the drugs alone Xavier and Sander [101] note that while combination drug therapy may be more effective, it may also be antagonistic or suppressive, and emphasize that the thorough understanding of the pathophysiology of the disease to be treated and the selection of drugs with appropriate mechanisms of action form the foundation for the clinical development of rational combination therapy.

Transparency

There is increasing emphasis on the transparency of clinical development, including clinical trial conduct, clinical trial reporting, and regulatory review and oversight. There not only is general support for more timely reporting of all clinical trial results but greater transparency is also advocated to address concerns regarding key issues such as the selective reporting of clinical trial results and patient access to clinical development programs. As a result of the 1997 FDA Modernization Act, the National Institutes of Health (NIH), through its National Library of Medicine (NLM), collaborated with the FDA to develop a clinical trials registry (www.ClinicalTrials.gov). The basic registry contains information about a trial's purpose, participant entry criteria, investigative site location, and contact information for obtaining more details. The 2007 FDA Amendments Act [102] required the NLM to markedly expand the clinical trial registry and results databank, which now presents information on the following:

- Clinical studies of all diseases and studies of devices (previously, only trials of drugs and biologics for serious or life-threatening diseases or conditions were required to be registered);
- An increased amount of clinical trial information and summary data tables including the following:
- Baseline participant characteristics taken at the beginning of a trial that may include demographic and physiologic characteristics,
- Participant flow to indicate the number of participants at each stage of the trial,
- Outcomes data, including prespecified primary and secondary outcomes and relevant statistical analyses,
- Tables for reporting serious adverse events and other frequent adverse events observed during the trial.

Trial results posting is now required for Phase 2 through Phase 4 interventional studies involving drugs, biological products, and medical devices approved by the FDA that have at least one trial site in the United States or are conducted under a US IND [103].

In addition to the NLM website and publication, additional clinical trial result registries include web sites sponsored by the US National Cancer Institute at NIH (www.cancer.gov/clinicaltrials) as well as a number of individual pharmaceutical organizations. In the EU, EudraCT (https://eudract.ema.europa.eu/index.html) is a database of all clinical trials in the European Community that was established in accordance with Directive 2001/20/EC.

References

[1] H.R. 3580. Food and Drug Administration Amendments Act of 2007. Public Law 110-85. Available from: https://www.congress.gov/bill/110th-congress/house-bill/3580; 2007.

[2] Greenberg BM, Ratchford JN, Calabresi PA. Multiple sclerosis. In: Waldman SA, Terzic A, editors. Pharmacology and therapeutics: Principles to practice. Philadelphia, PA: Saunders; 2009. p. 685–702 [chapter 46].

[3] Cecil RL, Loeb RF. A textbook of medicine. 8th ed. Philadelphia, PA: W. B. Saunders; 1951.

[4] Kappos L, Radue E-W, O'Connor P, Polman C, Hohlfeld R, Calabresi P, et al. A placebo-controlled trial of oral fingolimod in relapsing multiple sclerosis. N Engl J Med 2010;362(5):387–401.

[5] Paolicelli D, Direnzo V, Trojano M. Review of interferon beta-1b in the treatment of early and relapsing multiple sclerosis. Biol Theory 2009; 3:369–76.

[6] The IFNB Multiple Sclerosis Study Group. Interferon beta-1b is effective in relapsing-remitting multiple sclerosis. I. Clinical results of a multi-center, randomized, double-blind, placebo-controlled trial. Neurology 1993;43(4):655–61.

[7] Francis G, Collins W, Burtin P. Fingolimod (NDA 22–527) briefing document. Available from: https://pdfs.semanticscholar.org/f98c/a444894e2df16cb9ac253d2193144cf88e25.pdf; 2010.

[8] U.S. Food and Drug Administration. FDA approves new oral drug to treat multiple sclerosis. Available from: https://www.fda.gov/news-events/press-announcements/fda-approves-new-oral-drug-treat-multiple-sclerosis.

[9] U.S. Department of Health and Human Services. The Belmont report: Ethical principles and guidelines for the protection of human subjects of research. Available from: https://www.hhs.gov/ohrp/sites/default/files/the-belmont-report-508c_FINAL.pdf; 1979.

[10] World Medical Association. Declaration of Helsinki: Ethical principles for medical research involving human subjects. Helsinki. Available from: https://www.wma.net/policies-post/wma-declaration-of-helsinki-ethical-principles-for-medical-research-involving-human-subjects; 1964.

[11] Council for International Organizations of Medical Sciences. International ethical guidelines for health-related research involving humans. Geneva. Available from: https://cioms.ch/wp-content/uploads/2017/01/WEB-CIOMS-EthicalGuidelines.pdf; 2016.

[12] U.S. Food and Drug Administration. Investigational new drug safety reporting requirements for human drug and biological products and safety reporting requirements for bioavailability and bioequivalence studies in humans. Available from: https://www.fda.gov/drugs/investigational-new-drug-ind-application/final-rule-investigational-new-drug-safety-reporting-requirements-human-drug-and-biological-products; 2015.

[13] U.S. Food and Drug Administration. FDA 101: An overview of FDA's regulatory review and research activities. Available from: https://www.fda.gov/about-fda/what-we-do/fda-101-overview-fdas-regulatory-review-and-research-activities#framework; 2020.

[14] CFR. Title 21: Food and drugs. Available from: https://www.fda.gov/medical-devices/medical-device-databases/code-federal-regulations-title-21-food-and-drugs; 2018.

[15] U.S. Department of Health and Human Services. Patient Protection and Affordable Care Act. Available from: https://www.congress.gov/111/plaws/publ148/PLAW-111publ148.pdf; 2010.

[16] Health Care and Education Reconciliation Act of 2010. Pub. L. No. 111-152 Stat. 124 Stat. 1029; March 30, 2010.

[17] European Medicines Agency. Human medicines: Regulatory information. Available from: https://www.ema.europa.eu/en/human-medicines-regulatory-information.

[18] Pharmaceutical and Medical Devices Agency (Japan). Home page. Available from: https://www.pmda.go.jp/english/index.html.

[19] Su L. Drug development models in China and the impact on multinational pharmaceutical companies. FDLI update [Internet]. (September/October). Available from: https://www.sidley.com/~/media/files/publications/2013/09/drug-development-models-in-china-and-the-impact-__/files/view-article/fileattachment/fdli-article- -ling-su- -2013.pdf; 2013.

[20] International Council on Harmonisation. ICH home page. Available from: https://www.ich.org.

[21] International Council on Harmonisation. ICH guidelines. Available from: https://www.ich.org/page/ich-guidelines.

[22] International Council on Harmonisation. Guideline for good clinical practice (ICH E6[R2]). Available from: https://www.ema.europa.eu/en/documents/scientific-guideline/ich-e-6-r2-guideline-good-clinical-practice-step-5_en.pdf; 2016.

[23] McAuslane N, Cone M, Collins J, Walker S. Emerging markets and emerging agencies: a comparative study of how key regulatory agencies in Asia, Latin America, the Middle East, and Africa are developing regulatory processes and review models for new medicinal products. Drug Inf J 2009;43(3):349–59.

[24] Ramesh VC. State legislation relating to transparency and disclosure of health and hospital charges. Available from: https://sites.google.com/a/healthbillmap.com/www/home/articles/statelegislationrelatingtotransparencyanddisclosureofhealthandhospitalcharges.

[25] National Conference of State Legislatures. Clinical trials: What are states doing? Available from: https://www.ncsl.org/research/health/clinical-trials-what-are-states-doing-2010.aspx; 2010.

[26] Altar CA. The Biomarkers Consortium: on the critical path of drug discovery. Clin Pharmacol Ther 2008;83(2):361–4.

[27] Zerhouni EA, Sanders CA, von Eschenbach AC. The Biomarkers Consortium: public and private sectors working in partnership to improve the public health. Oncologist 2007;12(3):250–2.

[28] Wagner JA, Prince M, Wright EC, Ennis MM, Kochan J, Nunez DJ, et al. The Biomarkers Consortium: practice and pitfalls of open-source precompetitive collaboration. Clin Pharmacol Ther 2010;87(5):539–42.

[29] Wagner JA, Wright EC, Ennis MM, Prince M, Kochan J, Nunez DJ, et al. Utility of adiponectin as a biomarker predictive of glycemic efficacy is demonstrated by collaborative pooling of data from clinical trials conducted by multiple sponsors. Clin Pharmacol Ther 2009;86(6):619–25.

[30] European Commission. Data protection: Rules for the protection of personal data inside and outside the EU. Available from: https://ec.europa.eu/info/law/law-topic/data-protection_en.

[31] Anon. Health Insurance Portability and Accountability Act of 1996. Available from: https://aspe.hhs.gov/report/health-insurance-portability-and-accountability-act-1996; 1996.

[32] Sheiner LB. Learning versus confirming in clinical drug development. Clin Pharmacol Ther 1997;61(3):275–91.

[33] DiMasi JA, Hansen RW, Grabowski HG. The price of innovation: new estimates of drug development costs. J Health Econ 2003;22(2):151–85.

[34] Ledley FD, McCoy SS, Vaughan G, Cleary EG. Profitability of large pharmaceutical companies compared with other large public companies. JAMA 2020;323(9):834–43.

[35] DiMasi JA, Feldman L, Seckler A, Wilson A. Trends in risks associated with new drug development: success rates for investigational drugs. Clin Pharmacol Ther 2010;87(3):272–7.

[36] Morgan P, Brown DG, Lennard S, Anderton MJ, Barrett JC, Eriksson U, et al. Impact of a five-dimensional framework on R&D productivity at AstraZeneca. Nat Rev Drug Discov 2018;17(3):167–81.

[37] Saag KG, Teng GG, Patkar NM, Anuntiyo J, Finney C, Curtis JR, et al. American College of Rheumatology 2008 recommendations for the use of nonbiologic and biologic disease-modifying antirheumatic drugs in rheumatoid arthritis. Arthritis Rheum 2008;59(6):762–84.

[38] Smolen JS, Landewé R, Breedveld FC, Dougados M, Emery P, Gaujoux-Viala C, et al. EULAR recommendations for the management of rheumatoid arthritis with synthetic and biological disease-modifying antirheumatic drugs. Ann Rheum Dis 2010;69(6):964–75.

[39] Gartlehner G, Hansen RA, Jonas BL, Thieda P, Lohr KN. The comparative efficacy and safety of biologics for the treatment of rheumatoid arthritis: a systematic review and metaanalysis. J Rheumatol 2006;33(12):2398–408.

[40] Cohen SB, Cheng T-T, Chindalore V, Damjanov N, Burgos-Vargas R, Delora P, et al. Evaluation of the efficacy and safety of pamapimod, a p38 MAP kinase inhibitor, in a double-blind, methotrexate-controlled study of patients with active rheumatoid arthritis. Arthritis Rheum 2009;60(2):335–44.

[41] Damjanov N, Kauffman RS, Spencer-Green GT. Efficacy, pharmacodynamics, and safety of VX-702, a novel p38 MAPK inhibitor, in rheumatoid arthritis: results of two randomized, double-blind, placebo-controlled clinical studies. Arthritis Rheum 2009;60(5):1232–41.

[42] Cook D, Brown D, Alexander R, March R, Morgan P, Satterthwaite G, et al. Lessons learned from the fate of AstraZeneca's drug pipeline: a five-dimensional framework. Nat Rev Drug Discov 2014;13(6):419–31.

[43] Mandema JW, Gibbs M, Boyd RA, Wada DR, Pfister M. Model-based meta-analysis for comparative efficacy and safety: application in drug development and beyond. Clin Pharmacol Ther 2011;90(6):766–9.

[44] Bellamy N, Buchanan WW, Goldsmith CH, Campbell J, Stitt LW. Validation study of WOMAC: a health status instrument for measuring clinically important patient relevant outcomes to antirheumatic drug therapy in patients with osteoarthritis of the hip or knee. J Rheumatol 1988;15(12): 1833–40.

[45] Felson DT, Anderson JJ, Boers M, Bombardier C, Furst D, Goldsmith C, et al. American College of Rheumatology. Preliminary definition of improvement in rheumatoid arthritis. Arthritis Rheum 1995;38(6):727–35.

[46] Fransen J, van Riel PLCM. The disease activity score and the EULAR response criteria. Rheum Dis Clin North Am 2009;35(4):745–57. vii–viii.

[47] Rosen WG, Mohs RC, Davis KL. A new rating scale for Alzheimer's disease. Am J Psychiatry 1984;141(11):1356–64.

[48] Cartwright ME, Cohen S, Fleishaker JC, Madani S, McLeod JF, Musser B, et al. Proof of concept: a PhRMA position paper with recommendations for best practice. Clin Pharmacol Ther 2010;87(3):278–85.

[49] Reisberg B, Schneider L, Doody R, Anand R, Feldman H, Haraguchi H, et al. Clinical global measures of dementia. Position paper from the International Working Group on Harmonization of Dementia Drug Guidelines. Alzheimer Dis Assoc Disord 1997;11(Suppl. 3):8–18.

[50] U.S. Food and Drug Administration. Guidance, compliance, and regulatory information. Available from: https://www.fda.gov/drugs/guidance-compliance-regulatory-information; 2020.

[51] Ellenberg SS, Temple R. Placebo-controlled trials and active-control trials in the evaluation of new treatments. Part 2: practical issues and specific cases. Ann Intern Med 2000;133(6):464–70.

[52] Temple R, Ellenberg SS. Placebo-controlled trials and active-control trials in the evaluation of new treatments. Part 1: ethical and scientific issues. Ann Intern Med 2000;133(6):455–63.

[53] International Council on Harmonisation. ICH harmonised tripartite guideline: Statistical principles for clinical trials (ICH E9). Geneva. Available from: https://database.ich.org/sites/default/files/E9_Guideline.pdf; 1988.

[54] Dragalin V. An introduction to adaptive designs and adaptation in CNS trials. Eur Neuropsychopharmacol 2011;21(2):153–8.

[55] Wang S-J, Hung HMJ, O'Neill R. Adaptive design clinical trials and trial logistics models in CNS drug development. Eur Neuropsychopharmacol 2011;21(2):159–66.

[56] U.S. Food and Drug Administration. Adaptive designs for clinical trials of drugs and biologics. Guidance for industry. Rockville, MD: U.S. Department of Health and Human Services; 2019. Available from: https://www.fda.gov/media/78495/download.

[57] Ando Y, Hirakawa A, Uyama Y. Adaptive clinical trials for new drug applications in Japan. Eur Neuropsychopharmacol 2011;21(2):175–9.

[58] Diamond EL, Subbiah V, Lockhart AC, Blay J-Y, Puzanov I, Chau I, et al. Vemurafenib for BRAF V600-mutant Erdheim-Chester disease and Langerhans cell histiocytosis: analysis of data from the histology-independent, phase 2, open-label VE-BASKET study. JAMA Oncol 2018;4(3):384–8.

[59] Saville BR, Berry SM. Efficiencies of platform clinical trials: a vision of the future. Clin Trials 2016;13(3):358–66.

[60] U.S. Food and Drug Administration. Influenza: Developing drugs for treatment and/or prophylaxis. Guidance for industry. Rockville, MD: U.S. Department of Health and Human Services; 2011. Available from: https://www.fda.gov/media/73339/download.

[61] U.S. Food and Drug Administration. Community-acquired bacterial pneumonia: Developing drugs for treatment. Guidance for industry. Rockville, MD: U.S. Department of Health and Human Services; 2020. Available from: https://www.fda.gov/media/75149/download.

[62] U.S. Food and Drug Administration. Antibacterial drug products: Use of noninferiority trials to support approval. Guidance for industry. Rockville, MD: U.S. Department of Health and Human Services; 2010. Available from: https://www.fda.gov/media/71215/download.

[63] U.S. Government Accountability Office. New Drug Approval: FDA's consideration of evidence from certain clinical trials. Available from: https://www.gao.gov/assets/310/308301.pdf; 2010.

[64] U.S. Food and Drug Administration. The extent of population exposure to assess clinical safety: For drugs intended for long-term treatment of non-life-threatening conditions. Guideline for industry. Rockville, MD: U.S. Department of Health and Human Services; 1995. Available from: https://www.fda.gov/media/71180/download.

[65] Pfizer Endocrinologic and Metabolic Drugs Advisory Committee. Advisory Committee briefing document: Exubera. Pfizer; 2005. Available from: https://wayback.archive-it.org/7993/20170405084235/https:/www.fda.gov/ohrms/dockets/ac/05/briefing/2005-4169B1_01_01-Pfizer-Exubera.pdf.

[66] U.S. Food and Drug Administration. Diabetes mellitus: Evaluating cardiovascular risk in new antidiabetic therapies to treat type 2 diabetes. Guidance for industry. Rockville, MD: U.S. Department of Health and Human Services; 2008. Available from: https://www.fda.gov/media/71297/download.

[67] Uyama Y, Shibata T, Nagai N, Hanaoka H, Toyoshima S, Mori K. Successful bridging strategy based on ICH E5 guideline for drugs approved in Japan. Clin Pharmacol Ther 2005;78(2):102–13.

[68] Quan H, Li M, Chen J, Gallo P, Binkowitz B, Ibia E, et al. Assessment of consistency of treatment effects in multiregional clinical trials. Ther Innov Regul Sci 2010;44(5):617–32.

[69] Saillot J-L, Paxton M. Industry efforts on simultaneous global development. Drug Inf J 2009;43(3):339–47.

[70] U.S. Food and Drug Administration. Establishment and operation of clinical trial data monitoring committees. Guidance for clinical trial sponsors. Rockville, MD: U.S. Department of Health and Human Services; 2006. Available from: https://www.fda.gov/media/75398/download.

[71] European Medicines Agency. Guideline on data monitoring committees. Available from: https://www.ema.europa.eu/en/documents/scientific-guideline/guideline-data-monitoring-committees_en.pdf; 2006.

[72] Woodcock J. Assessing the clinical utility of diagnostics used in drug therapy. Clin Pharmacol Ther 2010;88(6):765–73.

[73] Lalonde RL, Kowalski KG, Hutmacher MM, Ewy W, Nichols DJ, Milligan PA, et al. Model-based drug development. Clin Pharmacol Ther 2007;82 (1):21–32.
[74] EFPIA MID Workgroup, Marshall SF, Burghaus R, Cosson V, Cheung SY, Chenel M, et al. Good practices in model-informed drug discovery and development: practice, application, and documentation. CPT Pharmacometrics Syst Pharmacol 2016;5(3):93–122.
[75] European Medicines Agency. EFPIA-EMA modelling and simulation workshop report. In: EMA-EFPIA Modelling and Simulation Workshop; 30 Nov–1 Dec 2011; London, UK; 2011.
[76] Wang Y, Zhu H, Madabushi R, Liu Q, Huang SM, Zineh I. Model-informed drug development: current US regulatory practice and future considerations. Clin Pharmacol Ther 2019;105(4):899–911.
[77] Jain L, Mehrotra N, Wenning L, Sinha V. PDUFA VI: it is time to unleash the full potential of model-informed drug development. CPT Pharmacometrics Syst Pharmacol 2019;8(1):5–8.
[78] Zhu H, Huang SM, Madabushi R, Strauss DG, Wang Y, Zineh I. Model-informed drug development: a regulatory perspective on progress. Clin Pharmacol Ther 2019;106(1):91–3.
[79] Zhavoronkov A, Vanhaelen Q, Oprea TI. Will artificial intelligence for drug discovery impact clinical pharmacology? Clin Pharmacol Ther 2020;107(4):780–5.
[80] International Council on Harmonisation. ICH harmonised tripartite guideline: Studies in support of special populations: Geriatrics. Geneva: ICH E7; 1993. Available from: https://database.ich.org/sites/default/files/E7_Guideline.pdf.
[81] International Council on Harmonisation. ICH topic E7. Studies in support of special populations: Geriatrics. Questions and answers. Available from: https://www.ema.europa.eu/en/documents/scientific-guideline/ich-e-7-studies-support-special-populations-geriatrics-questions-answers-step-5_en.pdf; 2010.
[82] U.S. Food and Drug Administration. How to comply with the Pediatric Research Equity Act. Guidance for industry. Rockville, MD: U.S. Department of Health and Human Services; 2005. Available from: https://www.fda.gov/media/72274/download.
[83] U.S. Food and Drug Administration. Qualifying for pediatric exclusivity under section 505A of the Federal Food, Drug, and Cosmetic Act. Guidance for industry. Rockville, MD: U.S. Department of Health and Human Services; 1999. Available from: https://www.fda.gov/media/72029/download.
[84] European Medicines Agency. Paediatric medicines: An overview. Available from: https://www.ema.europa.eu/en/human-regulatory/overview/paediatric-medicines-overview. [Accessed 3 February 2021].
[85] Gill D, Kurz R. Practical and ethical issues in pediatric clinical trials. Appl Clin Trials 2003;121(9):41–4.
[86] International Council on Harmonisation. Guideline on clinical investigation of medicinal products in the pediatric population. Geneva: ICH E11; 2017. Available from: https://www.ema.europa.eu/en/documents/scientific-guideline/ich-e11r1-guideline-clinical-investigation-medicinal-products-pediatric-population-revision-1_en.pdf.
[87] Orphan Drug Act. Stat. HR 5238; 1981.
[88] European Medicines Agency. Orphan designation: Overview. Available from: https://www.ema.europa.eu/en/human-regulatory/overview/orphan-designation-overview. [Accessed 1 February 2021].
[89] Mehta A, Beck M, Sunder-Plassmann G. Fabry disease: Perspectives from 5 years of FOS. Oxford: Oxford PharmaGenesis; 2006.
[90] Shirigami M, Nakai K. Development of orphan drugs in Japan: effects of a support system for development of orphan drugs in Japan. Drug Inf J 2000;34:829–37.
[91] U.S. Food and Drug Administration. Office of Orphan Products Development. Available from: https://www.fda.gov/about-fda/office-clinical-policy-and-programs/office-orphan-products-development; 2019.
[92] Burke KA, Freeman SN, Imoisili MA, Coté TR. The impact of the Orphan Drug Act on the development and advancement of neurological products for rare diseases: a descriptive review. Clin Pharmacol Ther 2010;88(4):449–53.
[93] Institute of Medicine. Rare diseases and orphan products: Accelerating research and development. Washington, DC: National Academies Press; 2010. Available from: https://www.nap.edu/catalog/12953/rare-diseases-and-orphan-products-accelerating-research-and-development.
[94] National Institute for Health and Care Excellence. Improving health and social care through evidence-based guidance (home page). Available from: https://www.nice.org.uk.
[95] Agency for Healthcare Research and Quality. Home page. Available from: https://www.ahrq.gov.
[96] Anon. American Recovery and Reinvestment Act of 2009; January 6, 2009.
[97] U.S. Food and Drug Administration Combination products: Therapeutic and diagnostic products that combine drugs, devices, and/or biological products. Available from: https://www.fda.gov/combination-products.
[98] European Medicines Agency. Guideline on clinical development of fixed combination medicinal products. Available from: https://www.ema.europa.eu/en/documents/scientific-guideline/guideline-clinical-development-fixed-combination-medicinal-products-revision-2_en.pdf.
[99] Philipp T, Smith TR, Glazer R, Wernsing M, Yen J, Jin J, et al. Two multicenter, 8-week, randomized, double-blind, placebo-controlled, parallel-group studies evaluating the efficacy and tolerability of amlodipine and valsartan in combination and as monotherapy in adult patients with mild to moderate essential hypertension. Clin Ther 2007;29(4):563–80.
[100] U.S. Food and Drug Administration. Codevelopment of two or more new investigational drugs for use in combination. Guidance for industry. Rockville, MD: U.S. Department of Health and Human Services; 2013. Available from: https://www.fda.gov/media/80100/download.
[101] Xavier JB, Sander C. Principle of system balance for drug interactions. N Engl J Med 2010;362(14):1339–40.
[102] Food and Drug Administration Amendments Act (FDAAA) of 2007. Stat. H.R. 3580; September 27, 2007.
[103] Tse T, Williams RJ, Zarin DA. Reporting "basic results" in ClinicalTrials.gov. Chest 2009;136(1):295–303.

Chapter 35

The role of the FDA in guiding drug development

Elimika Pfuma Fletcher[a], Rajanikanth Madabushi[a], Chandrahas G. Sahajwalla[a], Lawrence J. Lesko[b], and Shiew-Mei Huang[a]

[a]*Office of Clinical Pharmacology, Office of Translational Sciences, Center for Drug Evaluation and Research, U.S. Food and Drug Administration, Silver Spring, MD, United States,* [b]*Center for Pharmacometrics and Systems Pharmacology, College of Pharmacy, University of Florida, Lake Nona in Orlando, FL, United States*

Introduction

The US Food and Drug Administration (FDA) plays a central role in guiding drug development. This chapter provides a brief overview of the FDA and discusses the various ways that the FDA gets involved in guiding drug development. It is written with a focus on drugs submitted in Investigational New Drug (IND) applications, New Drug Applications (NDAs), and Biologics License Applications (BLAs) that are the responsibility of the Center for Drug Evaluation and Research (CDER) in FDA.

The drug development process is defined here as one that includes the preclinical and clinical phases of drug development following the selection of a lead molecule by the sponsor and includes the regulatory review phase that is intended to lead to marketing authorization. This process is complex, time consuming, and costly and components of drug development generally continue beyond an initial approval. A typical new molecular entity (NME), if approved for marketing, has gone through extensive preclinical pharmacology/toxicology evaluation followed by a clinical evaluation stage that lasts, on average, 5–7 years [1]. With an average of 6–10 months required for regulatory review, the entire process, from preclinical evaluation to market approval, may take up to 15 years. Published cost estimates range from $314 million to $2.8 billion dollars in direct and lost-opportunity costs for a new drug. The current attrition rate of drugs is high and can vary across products and therapeutic area. A 2016 publication reported that only 12% of drugs that entered Phase 1 received regulatory approval, highlighting the need for more predictive and informative drug development [1–3].

One of the goals of the drug development process is to provide effective drugs to patients as quickly as possible, and to manage the risks associated with these drugs in the best way possible. That is, the benefit/risk ratio should be appropriate for the indication. In addition, it is critical to obtain data during drug development to achieve therapeutic individualization for specific patient populations (e.g., pediatric patients or patients with a relevant pharmacogenomic marker). To help achieve these goals, the FDA has an accountable role in providing transparent scientific review, regulations, and communication. The FDA not only reviews the designs and results of studies submitted by the drug developer but also plays a critical role in guiding drug development decisions by providing drug developers with advice and insights to guide drug development. The regulatory authority of the FDA is stipulated in 21 USC 393, which confers on the FDA the dual mission of (1) promoting the public health by promptly and efficiently reviewing clinical research, and by taking appropriate and timely action on the marketing of regulated products and (2) protect public health by ensuring the regulated products are safe and effective (for drugs and devices).

Evolution of the FDA's role in drug regulation

The history of legislature relevant to drug regulation is summarized in Table 35.1 [4].

Strength, purity, and labeling: The FDA's mission began with a focus on strength, purity, and labeling. The 1906 Food and Drugs Act prohibited interstate commerce in misbranded and adulterated foods, drinks, and drugs. In 1912 Congress enacted the Sherley Amendment to the Food and Drug Act to prohibit labeling medicines with false therapeutic claims intended to defraud the purchaser.

Atkinson's Principles of Clinical Pharmacology. https://doi.org/10.1016/B978-0-12-819869-8.00024-0

TABLE 35.1 Chronology and key components of selected pharmaceutical legislation.

Date	Legislation	Key components
1906	Food and Drugs Act	Drugs meet standards of strength and purity
1938	Food, Drug and Cosmetic Act (FD&C Act)	Manufacturers need to show safety of a drug before marketing
1945	Penicillin Amendment	FDA testing and certification of safety and effectiveness of all penicillin products
1962	Kefauver-Harris Amendments	Drugs need to be safe and effective
1983	Orphan Drug Act	Incentives (tax deduction and market exclusivity) for developing drugs for rare diseases
1992	Prescription Drug User Fee Act (PDUFA)	Provides FDA resources and defines review timelines
1997	FDA Modernization Act (FDAMA)	Significant amendments to the FD&C Act.[a] Reauthorized PDUFA (PDUFA 2)
2002	PDUFA 3	BPCA, Bioterrorism and response Act
2007	FDA Amendments Act (FDAAA)	Reauthorization of PDUFA, MDUFA, FDAMA, BPCA, PREA and amendments related to FDA to assess/manage drug risks and to create a foundation (Reagan-Udall)[b]
2009	Biologics Price Competition and Innovation (BPCI) Act	Establishes an abbreviated approval pathway for "biosimilars"
2012	Food and Drug Administration Safety and Innovation Act (FDASIA)	Reauthorization of PDUFA (PDUFA V). Promotes innovation, increases stakeholder involvement in FDA processes, and enhances the safety of the drug supply chain
2017	Food and Drug Administration Reauthorization Act (FDARA)—21st Century Cures	Reauthorization of PDUFA (PDUFA V1). Includes enhanced transparency and communication and enhanced regulatory science and decision tools

[a]Details of the amendments can be found in the following website: https://www.fda.gov/about-fda/fdas-evolving-regulatory-powers/milestones-us-food-and-drug-law-history and https://www.fda.gov/industry/prescription-drug-user-fee-amendments/pdufa-vi-fiscal-years-2018-2022.
[b]MDUFA/MA, Medical device User Fee and Modernization Act; BPCA, Best Pharmaceuticals for Children Act; PREA: Pediatric Research Equity Act.

Focus on safety: Over the years, a number of public health safety disasters have contributed to the evolution of drug regulations that currently impact drug development. For example, 107 deaths in 1937 were linked to sulfanilamide elixir, which was dissolved in the poisonous solvent diethylene glycol. The legal basis the FDA used for involvement in this case was related to misbranding because the product did not contain alcohol as the name elixir would suggest [5]. This case increased the cries for action and prompted Congress to enact the Federal Food, Drug and Cosmetic Act (FDCA) of 1938 that required sponsors to demonstrate that new drugs are safe before they can be marketed.

A Mission beyond safety—Considering benefit/risk: Some amendments to the FDCA expanded the regulatory role of the FDA to include considering effectiveness. The 1945 Penicillin Amendment required FDA testing and certification of safety and effectiveness of all penicillin products, and this was extended to other antibiotics in later amendments (these specific provisions were abolished in 1980 as subsequent amendments rendered them redundant). It was the thalidomide tragedy that ushered in the 1962 Kefauver-Harris Drug Amendment. Thalidomide was a sleeping pill, used off-label by pregnant women for morning sickness, that caused birth defects in thousands of babies in Western Europe (see Chapter 24 for detailed discussion). The drug was kept off the US market by efforts of an FDA medical officer named Dr. Frances Kelsey. The 1962 amendment that was prompted by this tragedy required sponsors to prove the effectiveness, in addition to safety, of their products to the FDA before marketing. In addition, the FDA contracted with the National Academy of Sciences/National Research Council to evaluate the effectiveness of 4000 drugs approved between 1938 and 1962 on the basis of safety alone, and the recommendations were implemented in 1968, referred to as drug efficacy study implementation (DESI).

Regulation increasing access: Several laws were enacted to increase market access or to address the needs of understudied populations. In 1984 the Drug Price Competition and Patent Term Restoration Act (Hatch-Waxman Amendment) allowed for approval of generic products, while giving some patent protection for brand name products. This 1984 amendment also introduced a pathway known as 505(b)(2) that permitted the FDA to rely on information not developed by the applicant, such as literature data or agency's findings of efficacy and safety for a reference approved product by another applicant [6]. These efforts were intended to increase market competition and prescribing options.

In addition, several legislative efforts have aimed to increase drug development in understudied populations such as for patients with rare diseases, and specific populations, such as pediatric patients. For example, the Orphan Drug Act was passed in 1983 with changes and incentives targeted at promoting development of drugs for treating rare diseases. In addition, legislature to encourage drug development in pediatric patients includes the 1997 FDA Modernization Act (FDAMA) that included marketing exclusivity incentives for pediatric evaluation. In addition, the Pediatric Research Equity Act (PREA) was introduced in 2013 to require pediatric studies for a new active ingredient, indication, dosage form, dosing regimen, or route of administration, unless waivers and deferrals were obtained. These and other laws have encouraged drug development in understudied populations.

Beyond premarket safety and effectiveness: Several postmarketing safety issues, such as the cardiovascular safety concerns associated with the postmarketing use of Vioxx® and Avandia®, led to calls for strengthening premarketing safety assessments and postmarketing surveillance [7, 8]. The 2007 FDA Amendments Act (FDAAA) mandated the FDA to establish an active postmarket risk identification and analysis system that analyzed safety data from multiple sources. The FDA, in collaboration with various stakeholders, established the Sentinel System for this purpose [9, 10]. FDAAA additionally provided the FDA with authority to require postmarket safety evaluations to assess possible serious risks associated with the drugs.

As described before, the FDA authority has evolved from the early focus on purity and labeling to a focus on benefit/risk analyses considering both pre- and postmarketing information. The FDA's charge in promoting public health has required the agency to develop and continue to evolve its evidence-based approach to drug regulation.

FDA's role in guiding drug development—A science-driven agency

Part of the FDA mission is to take appropriate and timely action on the marketing of regulated products. This has meant that the agency has developed and maintained a science-driven regulatory approach to help foster innovation while serving to protect the American public.

An example is related to the bioavailability problems with digoxin that led to a greater awareness of the need for better manufacturing regulatory standards to ensure high-quality drug products for the American public. As reported in 1971 by Lindenbaum et al. [11], digoxin tablets marketed by different manufacturers, and even different lots produced by the same manufacturer, showed substantial variation in the rate and extent of oral absorption. This was particularly alarming since, as emphasized in Chapter 2, digoxin has a narrow therapeutic window. Consequently, dissolution-rate testing requirements for digoxin tablets were initiated by the FDA in 1974 and that effectively improved the uniformity of performance of digoxin tablets and oral formulations of other NMEs and generic drugs.

The agency has come a long way in its drive toward implementing a science-based application of regulations. A great example is the evolution of the FDA's Office of Clinical pharmacology (OCP) from strictly a biopharmaceutics focus to a broader focus on therapeutic individualization (*the role of OCP is further discussed at the end of this chapter*) [12]. Therapeutic individualization has been an important aspect of drug development with information increasingly available about the causes of variability in pharmacokinetics, pharmacodynamics, and response because of technology advancements (e.g., modeling and genomic sequencing). As a result, current drug labeling includes sections that provide information for the use of drugs in specific populations, such as those with renal and hepatic impairment, and for specific contexts related to concomitant administration of drugs. In addition, as described in Chapter 12, there are many examples of approved product labels with therapeutic individualization based on pharmacogenomic markers that have an impact on drug exposure and/or response [13].

The 2004 FDA Critical Path White Paper ("Innovation/Stagnation: Challenge and Opportunity on the Critical Path to New Medical Products") addressed a slowdown in innovative medical therapies submitted to the FDA for approval [14]. The report described the urgent need to modernize the medical product development process to make product development more predictable and less costly. This report initiated the FDA Critical Path Initiative (CPI), which is a national strategy to utilize modern scientific and technical tools to evaluate and predict the safety, effectiveness, and manufacturability of medical products. This initiative sought to enhance collaborations with other government agencies, global organizations, academia, industry, patient advocacy groups, and other stakeholders. In addition, it aimed to foster the development of new tools, methods, and approaches to enhance innovation and efficiency in drug development [15, 16].

Because of its regulatory perspective, the FDA is uniquely positioned to work with a variety of stakeholders to coordinate, develop, and/or disseminate solutions to scientific hurdles in product development [17, 18]. In 2011 the FDA developed a strategic plan aimed at advancing regulatory science. This initiative emphasizes the critical need for regulatory scientists to be equipped with innovative approaches to make science-based regulatory decisions and expedite drug development. Drug regulatory paradigms that incorporate novel regulatory science will need to continue to evolve if they are to reduce the uncertainties currently inherent in evaluating drug response. The key to the future successful development of regulatory science will be an understanding of the drivers and challenges underlying drug development, and this will require intense collaboration among all stakeholders [19]. The ultimate value of these efforts will be reflected in the quality of the data and regulatory submissions provided by drug developers and the resulting products that reach patients.

The 2017 21st Century Cures Act highlights FDA's continuous focus on science-based regulation and describes efforts to advance a new era of medicine. It includes provisions for using real-world evidence (RWE), patient-focused drug development, innovative clinical trial designs, and model-informed drug development (MIDD). MIDD is defined as the use of exposure-based, biological, and statistical models derived from preclinical and clinical data to facilitate decision-making. These examples highlight some of the ways in which the FDA continues as a partner in advancing innovation in drug development while protecting public health (see Chapter 36).

FDA approval processes and special designations designed to accelerate drug development

The FDA mission mandated by Congress includes the prompt and efficient review of clinical research relevant to the regulatory process and the taking of appropriate and timely action. The FDA not only reviews the designs and results of studies submitted by the sponsor, but also plays a critical role in guiding drug development decisions by providing sponsors with advice and insights during drug development.

Legislation that introduced user fees (i.e., PDUFA) included some mandated performance goals and timelines for FDA review in order to increase the transparency and accountability of the review process. PDUFA IV (FDAAA) defined an efficient "twenty-first century review" process and PDUFA V addressed issues related to increased communications with sponsors [20]. In addition to mandating general review timelines for most drugs, additional approaches were introduced to enhance the drug development process for drugs that treat serious diseases. These include fast-track designation, accelerated approval (Subpart H, 21 CFR 314.500–560), priority reviews, and breakthrough therapy designations (Table 35.2). These specific programs offer benefits to aid sponsors both during the development and review process and serve as an important component of the transparent and efficient review process that is desired [21].

TABLE 35.2 FDA expedited programs for serious conditions.

Program	Qualification	Benefit
Accelerated approval pathway	For drugs to treat a serious condition for an unmet medical need	An approval pathway that allows approval based on a surrogate endpoint. This surrogate marker has to be a measure reasonably likely to predict clinical benefit and the clinical benefit will need to be established postmarketing
Breakthrough therapy designation	For a drug that treats a serious condition and preliminary clinical evidence indicates the drug may demonstrate substantial improvement over available therapy	• Benefits of fast track • Intensive guidance on efficient drug development beginning as early as phase 1 • Organizational commitment involving senior managers
Fast-track designation	For drugs that treat serious conditions and fill an unmet medical need	Benefits of the designation include: • more frequent meetings and communications with the FDA • ability to submit a rolling review (submit completed sections of NDA/BLA for FDA review before the entire application is complete) • eligible for accelerated approval or priority review if criteria are met
Priority Review Designation	Drug that treats a serious condition and, if approved, would provide a significant improvement in safety or effectiveness	Shorter review clock (6 months vs standard 10 months)

In addition to the programs designed to increase efficiency in general, the FDA has authorities under the FDCA to help cope with emergency situations. Under the Emergency Use Authorization (EUA) authority, the FDA can allow use of unapproved medical products or unapproved uses of approved medical products in the absence of adequate, approved, and available alternatives. This authority specifically applies to emergencies related to serious or life-threatening conditions caused by chemical, biological, radiological, and nuclear (CBRN) threat agents. This authority has been used to allow for access to therapeutic drugs, diagnostic products, personal protective equipment, and other medical devices during a pandemic such as COVID-19 [22].

The role of FDA in facilitating drug development through communication

Effective communication and mutual trust between the FDA, sponsors, and the public is essential to achieving the goals of the drug development process in an efficient, successful, and informative manner. Well-constructed meetings held face to face or by teleconference between sponsor representatives and FDA staff are a key part of direct communication. However, less direct but critical communications can also occur through domestic and international guidances, FDA presentations at advisory committee, professional and public meetings, and scientific publications. In addition, developers can learn about the FDA's current thinking, including its precedent-setting decisions, through FDA reviews of applications for marketing authorization that are publicly available [23]. These sources of information combine to provide transparency and accountability that should facilitate drug development and help to reduce uncertainty about the regulatory review process.

Formal sponsor meetings

The FDA has a formal process for holding meetings with sponsors to discuss scientific and clinical issues related to specific drug development programs. These formal meetings are consistent with the FDA's goal of facilitating drug development by providing advice and assuring a transparent review process. Policies and procedures for requesting, scheduling, and conducting formal meetings between CDER and a sponsor are described in the FDA Guidance for Industry entitled "Formal Meetings Between the FDA and Sponsors or Applicants" [24].

Although these meetings are voluntary, they are quite common and generally helpful. The meetings can be held based on the time frame during the drug development process or by focus area. Examples are meetings held before the submission of an Investigational New Drug Application (pre-IND), at the end of Phase 1 (EOP1), the end of Phase 2 (EOP2), and before NDA/BLA submission (Pre-NDA or Pre-BLA). In addition, certain meetings can focus on specific disciplines or topics (e.g., chemistry) including the meetings introduced with PDUFA 6—model-informed drug development (MIDD) and complex innovative trial designs (CID) meetings [25]. Important interactions between a pharmaceutical company and the FDA can also occur during review of a submitted NDA or BLA to discuss any outstanding issues in an application. In addition, following market authorization, the FDA continues to be involved with the development and approval of new uses or new dosage forms for an approved product.

Each of these meetings can have a major impact on decisions made during the drug development process. The questions that are raised and discussed at each of these meetings need to be appropriate for the drug's stage of development. For example, pre-IND meetings that are held early in the drug development process are extremely valuable to both the FDA and the sponsor because they routinely focus on critical issues (e.g., drug safety) related to the initial trial for the IND and plans for the drug development program and are held before the sponsor has expended substantial resources in the conduct of clinical trials. These meetings may help sponsors minimize the risk of a *clinical hold*, which the FDA may impose on a study or study site during any phase of clinical development if it finds that human subjects are or would be exposed to unreasonable and significant risk of illness or injury.

Later meetings such as EOP2 meetings can have a primary objective of discussing the design of pivotal trials and the studies that would be needed for a regulatory submission in a target indication. Topics can range from patient population, dose selection, endpoints, and statistical plans. The sponsor could seek advice on the utility of clinical pharmacology approaches and tools such as modeling and simulation and pharmacogenomics to guide study design and address therapeutic individualization [26].

Pre-NDA/Pre-BLA meetings are intended to focus on the content and format of the sponsor's marketing application, and to familiarize the reviewers from various disciplines with the application that will be submitted. Any issues that remain to be resolved [e.g., problems or questions related to CMC (chemistry, manufacturing, and control)] may also be discussed at this meeting. Pre-NDA meetings serve to identify any other pending issues which may otherwise result in a *refuse-to-file* (RTF) action when an NDA is submitted to the Agency for review.

Given the relatively short time that can be allotted for each meeting (1–2h), the agenda, topics, and quality of these meetings are important determinants of their utility. Both the sponsor and the FDA share the responsibility for planning and conducting these meetings in an optimally productive way. To ensure a high-quality meeting with substantive agreements or understanding about issues, the meetings should be focused on the most important questions or issues, designed with a specific purpose in mind, and have the necessary background information available that are appropriate for the agenda. Proper timing of the meeting is important if the meeting involves a discussion of drug development plans. For example, in planning a meeting to discuss a clinical trial protocol, the sponsor should allow sufficient time so that the meeting is held before the clinical study has begun; otherwise the sponsor's and the FDA's resources may be wasted. The meetings are sometimes held in-person or via teleconference. In some cases, the FDA may respond to the questions and content of the written materials submitted by a sponsor instead of granting a meeting, referred to as a Written Response Only (WRO) [24].

Besides meetings that are specific to a drug development program, the FDA offers meetings focused on topics and initiatives of interest to sponsors or various stakeholders. An example would be a meeting related to the qualification of drug development tools (DDT). DDTs may include biomarkers, clinical outcome assessments, and animal models for medical countermeasures (products that can have potential use for public health emergencies stemming from CBRN or a naturally occurring disease) meant to facilitate drug development. As discussed for biomarkers in Chapter 17, the qualification would be for a specific context of use that could be applied to various drug development programs. Of note, the fit-for purpose (FFP) initiative includes discussion of DDTs that are considered evolving in nature and cannot be given formal qualification. Another relevant type of meeting is the Critical Path Innovation Meeting (CPIM) in which investigators from industry, academia, scientific consortia, patient advocacy groups, and other government agencies can apply to the FDA for a meeting to discuss a proposed methodology or technology that might enhance drug development. It is a nonregulatory, nonbinding, drug product-independent meeting [27, 28].

Public meetings

In addition, to closed meetings that may be between FDA and a sponsor or relevant stakeholder, the FDA also holds public meetings to discuss a specific product with an advisory committee (AC) or to review a general therapeutic topic. In specific circumstances, some AC meetings may have both closed door (e.g., discussion of proprietary data with AC members) and public components. A calendar of public meetings is always available on the FDA website with options for in-person or remote participation. In many cases, there is an open public hearing period that will allow any member of the public to speak on the topic if preregistered as a speaker [29].

Advisory Committee meetings facilitate the regulatory review and FDA approval process by bringing together external experts to address specific questions to help resolve scientific or clinical issues that are related to the drug development process or to approval of a specific product. Slides and handouts presented at public meetings, including AC meetings, are generally placed on the public FDA website [29]. Public workshops could be hosted solely by the FDA or with partners, such as Centers of Excellence in Regulatory Science and Innovation (CERSI), Duke Margolis, scientific professional societies, or various consortia. These meetings can serve to enhance scientific discourse on specific topics relevant to drug development. An example is the FDA CERSI workshop on pediatric ontogeny held in May 2019 [30, 31]. Another example is the FDA-American Society for Clinical Pharmacology and Therapeutics (ASCPT) workshop on transporters in March 2017 [30].

The role of FDA in developing guidance and policy to inform drug development

In addition to meetings, the FDA advises sponsors by communicating their current thinking and policy in guidance and policy documents, and by interpreting laws, rules, and regulation [32]. This helps reduce concerns around regulatory uncertainty and allows sponsors to better plan their development programs. Guidance documents authored by the FDA or by the International Conference on Harmonization (ICH) are a widespread, effective, and transparent way that the FDA communicates with sponsors.

The development of guidances proceeds by a process known as Good Guidance Practices (21 CFR 10.115) and includes an appropriate level of meaningful public input [33]. The FDA recognizes the value to sponsors of transparency, consistency, and predictability in regulatory decision-making, and guidances for industry are developed as good-faith efforts to share with sponsors the current FDA thinking on a given topic. Guidances are intended to provide sponsors with assurances that FDA staff intends to interpret statutes and regulations in a consistent manner across its various clinical divisions.

However, if inconsistent interpretations of guidances occur among CDER's therapeutic review divisions, which is possible, the sponsors can communicate with the FDA about the inconsistencies and try to understand or resolve them [34].

In addition, to facilitate more consistency the FDA has implemented various measures, including good review management practices [35], 21st century performance standards [36, 37], and organizational changes [38] to improve the review process. This includes the CDER initiative to modernize the New Drugs Regulatory Program that began in 2017 and started implementation in 2020. The initiative is based on problem-focused, interdisciplinary, team-based approaches focused on six pillars: scientific leadership, interdisciplinary integrated assessments, systematic benefit/risk monitoring, talent management, operational excellence, and knowledge management [38].

Guidances cover a wide range of topics that focus on standards of quality, preclinical animal toxicology requirements, ethical standards for the conduct of clinical trials, and documentation requirements for submissions. Other guidances with a clinical focus include topics related to biopharmaceutics, clinical pharmacology, clinical trial design, and therapeutic area specific topics. These are publicly available on the FDA website [32].

One of the most important guidances was issued by the FDA in 1998 and is entitled "Providing Clinical Evidence of Effectiveness for Human Drug and Biological Products" [39], with a companion guidance later issued in 2019 [40]. This guidance provides advice and describes experience in drawing evidence of effectiveness from all clinical phases of drug development. In particular, it provides context on situations in which exposure–response information may provide primary evidence of effectiveness in drug development. Among these examples are approval of new formulations and new doses or dosing regimens of approved drug products. Other noteworthy guidances related to clinical pharmacology include those that pertain to exposure–response, drug–drug interaction, renal impairment, pediatrics, bioavailability, and food effect [32].

Through its guidances, the FDA also facilitates and encourages the use of emerging scientific technology and knowledge. For example, to enable scientific progress in the field of pharmacogenomics and to facilitate the use of pharmacogenomic data in informing regulatory decisions, the FDA has issued several guidance documents related to pharmacogenomics and maintains on the public FDA site a list of resources relevant to pharmacogenomics [13]. Another example is a guidance published on format and content for the growing field of Physiologically Based Pharmacokinetic (PBPK) Analyses [41]. Thus through guidance, the FDA can articulate its current thinking on acceptability, limitations, and opportunities in specific areas.

Guidance documents also focus on new legislative requirements and explain the FDA's current thinking in order to help prepare industry to implement the relevant requirements. An example is the introduction of an "abbreviated pathway" for approval of biologics that are "biosimilar" to marketed US reference products, as provided in the 2009 Biologics Price Competition and Innovation (BPCI) Act. Under the authority of this act, the FDA has approved 26 biosimilar products as of May 2020. Over the last decade, the FDA published several guidance documents that are available online and describe the "totality of evidence" approach used in evaluating biosimilars. In addition, resources for drug developers, healthcare providers, and patients related to biosimilars and biosimilar development programs are publicly available [42].

Another example is the 2017 amendment to the Pediatric Research Equity Act, referred to as the Research to Accelerate Cures and Equity (RACE) Act, with an effect date of August 2020. This act allows the FDA to require pediatric evaluation within an original application for an NME intended for treating adult cancers that is directed at a molecular target that is substantially relevant to the growth or progression of a pediatric cancer. The FDA published two guidance documents in 2019 and 2020 to address the current thinking of the agency ahead of implementation of this act [43, 44]. In addition, the FDA held public meetings and provided resources on its external facing website [45].

In the current globalized world, drug development is also global, and companies have to interact with several regulatory agencies that may have different standards and requirements. The International Council for Harmonization (ICH) provides opportunities for harmonization of guidance/guidelines on a chosen topic [46]. The ICH consists of 16 Members that are agencies or organizations, and 32 Observers. The ICH guidelines are harmonized guidelines that apply to all the regions that adopt the specific guideline [47]. A recent example of this is the M9 guideline on Biopharmaceutics Classification System-based Biowaivers. BCS-based waivers were not recognized across regulatory agencies or applied in a consistent manner. The guideline aimed at harmonizing and streamlining global drug development [48]. As sponsors continue to seek regulatory certainty and regulatory agencies depend on data and products from various parts of the world, communication and collaboration among regulatory agencies is important. The initiative of achieving harmonized guidelines is one such area of collaboration.

Although various staff within the FDA contribute to the issuance of guidances, the FDA organizational structure reflects the integral part of policy development to its work. The agency has policy staff, groups, and offices throughout its organizational structure. For example, the Office of Clinical Pharmacology (OCP) has a dedicated Guidance and Policy Team [49]. The policy staff along with other staff in the FDA work to ensure a transparent communication of current thinking of the agency.

The role of the FDA office of clinical pharmacology

The role of clinical pharmacology at the FDA has expanded over the past 20 years. The Division of Biopharmaceutics, which reviewed basic pharmacokinetic and bioavailability/bioequivalence studies, has evolved to become the current Office of Clinical Pharmacology (OCP), which is focused on ensuring that the right dose is given to the right patient [12]. OCP grew from about 30 scientific staff and now has over 200 staff with diverse knowledge and skill sets. OCP's core functions are regulatory review, policy development, and research, which are enhanced by its work in communication and stakeholder engagement. The 2019 OCP annual report highlights some of the important work the staff of this office did in that year, including conducting ~2400 reviews, engaging with sponsors in >2100 meetings, and responding to >250 consults. Consults include OCP's Chemical Informatics Program that conducts structure-based safety assessments (e.g., genetic toxicity, carcinogenicity, hepatotoxicity, and cardiotoxicity) to inform regulatory decision-making [50].

MIDD is an important component of the work done in OCP. The MIDD pilot program established as part of PDUFA VI highlighted the importance of MIDD in drug development. OCP is the lead office for this multidisciplinary program that provides sponsors an opportunity to engage with regulators on MIDD strategy issues during drug development [25, 51]. A specific example of an MIDD application is the use of drug concentration-QTc modeling as a primary analytical approach for assessing the QTc interval prolongation risk of new drugs [52].

OCP has played a central role in guidance and policy development. The office has instituted a lifecycle process for guidances and policies that is focused on modernizing existing guidances and developing policies on contemporary topics. These documents are written either entirely within OCP or in collaboration with other offices to provide a clinical pharmacology perspective.

As described before, regulatory research is an important component of our science-driven agency. OCP conducts regulatory research related to various clinical pharmacology topics that contribute to both regulatory review and the wider the scientific field. The office has a dedicated research group, the Division of Applied Regulatory Science (DARS), that has various translational research capabilities including in vitro and in vivo lab work and in silico computational modeling and informatics. Regulatory research plays an important role in informing regulatory policy and review work. For example, OCP conducted regulatory research on concentration-QTc modeling that resulted in updates to the ICH E14 guideline to reflect the acceptance of the approach [51]. In 2019 alone, OCP staff authored over 150 manuscripts.

OCP reflects the science-driven nature of the Agency whose mission is focused on protecting public health. Along with the Agency, OCP continues to evolve to meet the challenge of protecting public health in the ever-advancing world.

Disclaimer

The views expressed in this chapter do not necessarily represent the FDA's official view.

References

[1] Wouters OJ, McKee M, Luyten J. Estimated research and development investment needed to bring a new medicine to market, 2009-2018. JAMA 2020;323:844–853.

[2] DiMasi JA, Grabowski HG, Hansen RW. Innovation in the pharmaceutical industry: new estimates of R&D costs. J Health Econ 2016;47:20–33.

[3] US Food and Drug Administration n.d. CDER NDA and BLA Approval Times (Internet at, https://www.fda.gov/drugs/nda-and-bla-approvals/nda-and-bla-approval-times).

[4] US Food and Drug Administration. n.d. Milestones in U.S. Food and Drug Law History; Silver Spring, MD: FDA (Internet at https://www.fda.gov/about-fda/fdas-evolving-regulatory-powers/milestones-us-food-and-drug-law-history).

[5] US Food and Drug Administration. Sulfanilamide disaster. June 1981 FDA Consumer Magazine; Silver Spring, MD: FDA June 1981 Issue; (Internet at https://www.fda.gov/files/about%20fda/published/The-Sulfanilamide-Disaster.pdf).

[6] Guidance for Industry for Applications Covered by Section 505(b)(2) (Internet at, https://www.fda.gov/media/72419/download).

[7] US Food and Drug Administration. COX-2 selective (includes Bextra, Celebrex, and Vioxx) and non-selective non-steroidal anti-inflammatory drugs (NSAIDS). In: Postmarket drug safety information for patients and providers. Silver Spring, MD: FDA; April 7, 2005 (Internet at, www.fda.gov/drugs/drugsafety/postmarketdrugsafetyinformationforpatientsandproviders/ucm103420.htm).

[8] US Food and Drug Administration. Updated risk evaluation and mitigation strategy (REMS) to restrict access to rosiglitazone-containing medicines including Avandia, Avandamet, and Avandaryl. In: FDA drug safety communication. Silver Spring, MD: FDA; May 18, 2011 (Internet at, www.fda.gov/Drugs/DrugSafety/ucm255005.htm).

[9] Staffa JA, Dal Pan GJ. Regulatory innovation in postmarketing risk assessment and management. Clin Pharmacol Ther 2012;91:555–557.

[10] US Food and Drug Administration. FDA's sentinel initiative. Silver Spring, MD: FDA; March 9, 2020 (Internet at https://www.fda.gov/safety/fdas-sentinel-initiative/fdas-sentinel-initiative-background).

[11] Lindenbaum J, Mellow MH, Blackstone MO, Butler VP Jr. Variation in biologic availability of digoxin from four preparations. N Engl J Med 1971;285:1344–1347.

[12] US Food and Drug Administration. Office of clinical pharmacology. Silver Spring, MD: FDA; January 23, 2020 (Internet at, https://www.fda.gov/about-fda/center-drug-evaluation-and-research-cder/office-clinical-pharmacology).

[13] US Food and Drug Administration. Pharmacogenomics: overview of the genomics and targeted therapy group; March 30, 2018 (Internet at, https://www.fda.gov/drugs/science-and-research-drugs/pharmacogenomics-overview-genomics-and-targeted-therapy-group).

[14] US Food and Drug Administration. Critical path initiative. Silver Spring, MD: FDA; April 23, 2018 (Internet at https://www.fda.gov/science-research/science-and-research-special-topics/critical-path-initiative).

[15] Buckman S, Huang S-M, Murphy S. Medical product development and regulatory science for the 21st century: the critical path vision and its impact on health care. Clin Pharmacol Ther 2007;81:141–144.

[16] Barratt RA, Bowens SL, McCune SK, Johannessen JN, Buckman SY. The critical path initiative: leveraging collaborations to enhance regulatory science. Clin Pharmacol Ther 2012;91:380–383.

[17] US Food and Drug Administration. A Strategic Plan: Advancing Regulatory Science at FDA; August 2011 (Internet at, https://www.fda.gov/media/81109/download).

[18] US Food and Drug Administration. Advancing regulatory science. Silver Spring, MD: FDA; April 10, 2019 (Internet at, https://www.fda.gov/science-research/science-and-research-special-topics/advancing-regulatory-science).

[19] Honig PK, Huang S-M. Regulatory science and the role of the regulator in biomedical innovation. Clin Pharmacol Ther 2012;91:347–352.

[20] PDUFA V. n.d. (Internet at, www.fda.gov/NewsEvents/Testimony/ucm261396.htm; www.thepinksheet.com/nr/FDC/SupportingDocs/Pink/2011/PDUFA_V_draft_commitment_letter.pdf).

[21] US FDA Guidance for Industry. Expedited programs for serious conditions—drugs and biologics; May 2014. (Internet at, https://www.fda.gov/files/drugs/published/Expedited-Programs-for-Serious-Conditions-Drugs-and-Biologics.pdf).

[22] US Food and Drug Administration. Emergency use authorization; May 2020. (Internet at, https://www.fda.gov/emergency-preparedness-and-response/mcm-legal-regulatory-and-policy-framework/emergency-use-authorization).

[23] US Food and Drug Administration. Drugs@FDA: FDA-approved drugs; June 2020. (Internet at, https://www.accessdata.fda.gov/scripts/cder/daf/index.cfm).

[24] US FDA Guidance for Industry. Formal meetings between the FDA and sponsors or applicants of PDUFA products; December 2017. (Internet at, https://www.fda.gov/media/109951/download).

[25] Madabushi R, Benjamin JM, Grewal R, et al. The US Food and Drug Administration's model-informed drug development paired meeting pilot program: early experience and impact. Clin Pharmacol Ther 2019;106:74–78.

[26] US FDA Guidance for Industry. End-of-phase 2A meetings; September 2009. (Internet at, https://www.fda.gov/regulatory-information/search-fda-guidance-documents/end-phase-2a-meetings).

[27] US Food and Drug Administration. Drug development tool (DDT) qualification programs. Silver Spring, MD: FDA; February 20, 2020 (Internet at https://www.fda.gov/drugs/development-approval-process-drugs/drug-development-tool-ddt-qualification-programs).

[28] US Food and Drug Administration. Critical path innovation meetings (CPIM). Silver Spring, MD: FDA; June 26, 2019 (Internet at, https://www.fda.gov/drugs/new-drugs-fda-cders-new-molecular-entities-and-new-therapeutic-biological-products/critical-path-innovation-meetings-cpim).

[29] US Food and Drug Administration. Advisory committees. Silver Spring, MD: FDA; March 31, 2020 (Internet at, https://www.fda.gov/advisory-committees).

[30] US Food and Drug Administration. FDA meetings, conferences and workshops. Silver Spring, MD: FDA; March 31, 2020 (Internet at, https://www.fda.gov/news-events/fda-meetings-conferences-and-workshops).

[31] Burckart GJ, van den Anker JN. Pediatric ontogeny: moving from translational science to drug development. J Clin Pharmacol 2019;59(Suppl 1):S7–S8.

[32] US Food and Drug Administration. Guidances (Drugs). Silver Spring, MD: FDA; March 31, 2020 (Internet at, https://www.fda.gov/drugs/guidance-compliance-regulatory-information/guidances-drugs).

[33] Good guidance practices (Final Rule). Federal Register 65FR182; September 29, 2000.

[34] Milne CP, Kaitin KI. FDA review divisions: performance levels, and the impact on drug sponsors. Clin Pharmacol Ther 2012;91:393–404.

[35] US FDA Guidance for Review Staff and Industry. Good review management: principles and practices for PDUFA products. Rockville, MD: FDA; April 2000 (Internet at, www.fda.gov/downloads/Drugs/GuidanceComplianceRegulatoryInformation/Guidances/UCM079748.pdf).

[36] CDER. Manual of policies and procedures. Using the 21st century review process desk reference guide. Silver Spring, MD: FDA; November 8, 2010 (Internet at, www.fda.gov/downloads/AboutFDA/CentersOffices/OfficeofMedicalProductsandTobacco/CDER/ManualofPoliciesProcedures/UCM233003.pdf).

[37] US Food and Drug Administration. CDER 21st century review process desk reference guide. Silver Spring, MD: FDA; 1 April 2020. April 1st 2020; (Internet at, https://www.fda.gov/media/78941/download).

[38] US Food and Drug Administration. Modernizing FDA's new drugs regulatory program. Silver Spring, MD; FDA; January 17, 2020 (Internet at https://www.fda.gov/drugs/regulatory-science-research-and-education/modernizing-fdas-new-drugs-regulatory-program).

[39] US FDA Guidance for Industry. Providing clinical evidence of effectiveness for human drug and biological products; 1998. (Internet at https://www.fda.gov/regulatory-information/search-fda-guidance-documents/providing-clinical-evidence-effectiveness-human-drug-and-biological-products).

[40] US FDA Guidance for Industry. Demonstrating substantial evidence of effectiveness for human drug and biological products; 2019. (Internet at, https://www.fda.gov/media/133660/download).

[41] US FDA Guidance for Industry. Physiologically based pharmacokinetic analyses—format and content. (Internet at, https://www.fda.gov/media/101469/download).

[42] US Food and Drug Administration. Biosimilars; February 2020. (Internet at https://www.fda.gov/drugs/therapeutic-biologics-applications-bla/biosimilars).

[43] US FDA Guidance for Industry. FDARA implementation guidance for pediatric studies of molecularly targeted oncology drugs: amendments to Sec. 505B of the FD&C Act; December 2019. (Internet at https://www.fda.gov/media/133440/download).

[44] US FDA Guidance for Industry. Pediatric study plans for oncology drugs: transitional information until full implementation of FDARA Section 504 Questions and Answers; January 2020. (Internet at, https://www.fda.gov/media/134155/download).

[45] US Food and Drug Administration. Pediatric oncology; August 2018. (Internet at, https://www.fda.gov/about-fda/oncology-center-excellence/pediatric-oncology).

[46] Lindström-Gommers L, Mullin T. International conference on harmonization: recent reforms as a driver of global regulatory harmonization and innovation in medical products. Clin Pharmacol Ther 2019;105:926–931.

[47] The International Council for Harmonisation (ICH). ICH official website; April 2020 (Internet at, https://www.ich.org/).

[48] International Council for Harmonisation Guideline. M9 biopharmaceutics classification system-based biowaivers; October 2018. (Internet at, https://www.fda.gov/media/117974/download).

[49] Madabushi R, Pfuma Fletcher E, Florian J, Milligan L, Ramamoorthy A, Yang X, et al. Role of guidance and policy in enhancing the impact of clinical pharmacology in drug development, regulation, and use [published online ahead of print, 2020 May 19]. Clin Pharmacol Ther 2020. https://doi.org/10.1002/cpt.1849.

[50] US Food and Drug Administration. 2019 Office of clinical pharmacology annual report. April 2020 (Internet at, https://www.fda.gov/media/134935/download).

[51] US Food and Drug Administration. Model-informed drug development pilot program; February 2020. (Internet at, https://www.fda.gov/drugs/development-resources/model-informed-drug-development-pilot-program).

[52] Garnett C, Bonate PL, Dang Q, et al. Scientific white paper on concentration-QTc modeling. J Pharmacokinet Pharmacodyn 2018;45:383–397 [correction published in J Pharmacokinet Pharmacodyn. 2018;45:399].

Chapter 36

Emerging clinical pharmacology topics in drug development and precision medicine

Qi Liu[a], Jack A Gilbert[b,c], Hao Zhu[a], Shiew-Mei Huang[a], Elizabeth Kunkoski[d], Promi Das[b,c], Kimberly Bergman[a], Mary Buschmann[b,c], and M. Khair ElZarrad[d]

[a]*Office of Clinical Pharmacology, Office of Translational Sciences, Center for Drug Evaluation and Research, U.S. Food and Drug Administration, Silver Spring, MD, United States,* [b]*Department of Pediatrics, University of California San Diego School of Medicine, La Jolla, CA, United States,* [c]*Scripps Institution of Oceanography, UCSD, La Jolla, CA, United States,* [d]*Office of Medical Policy, Center for Drug Evaluation and Research, U.S. Food and Drug Administration, Silver Spring, MD, United States*

Introduction

Science is constantly evolving. As a result, novel tools as well as new issues are arising for clinical pharmacologists. In this chapter, we will discuss some emerging topics in clinical pharmacology, including model-informed drug development, real-world data and real-world evidence, and digital health technologies, as well as the microbiome and its impact on drug effect and treatment outcome.

Model-informed drug development

Model-informed drug development (MIDD) refers to the application of a wide variety of quantitative models to inform drug development and to assist regulatory decision making [1]. Empirical (e.g., statistical models or machine learning models) or mechanistic models (e.g., physiologically based pharmacokinetic (PBPK) models and quantitative systems pharmacology (QSP) models), which serve as a quantitative platform, integrate current understanding about diseases, patients, and pharmacological effect. As an evolving concept, MIDD reflects an accumulation of knowledge and experience through decades of practice. Historically, different terms, such as model-based drug development, have been applied to describe the effort to apply quantitative models to streamline clinical development programs. Given the high cost and high attrition rate in new drug development, MIDD recently has become more appealing and commonly adopted in drug development programs [2, 3]. This section provides an overview of MIDD-related applications, and outlines current and future trends in MIDD (Fig. 36.1).

MIDD applications

Drug development can be considered as learn-and-confirm or learn-and-apply process [4]. For many years, modeling has been successfully applied in various phases of drug development. Broadly considered, MIDD is an essential tool for dosage optimization/selection, clinical program/trial design, identification of supportive evidence of efficacy, and new policy development [1].

Dosage optimization/selection

Identification of the optimal dose for patients may be a challenging task in some drug development programs. MIDD approaches have the potential to fill in knowledge gaps and to determine optimal dosing. Following are some examples in which MIDD has been of value in dose optimization and selection.

Modeling and simulation can be applied to evaluate doses or dosing regimens that are not studied in clinical trials. Paliperidone palmitate is a long-acting injectable antipsychotic indicated for the treatment of schizophrenia. A gradual release of the active moiety from the formulation ensures that plasma concentrations can be maintained within a desirable

Atkinson's Principles of Clinical Pharmacology. https://doi.org/10.1016/B978-0-12-819869-8.00028-8

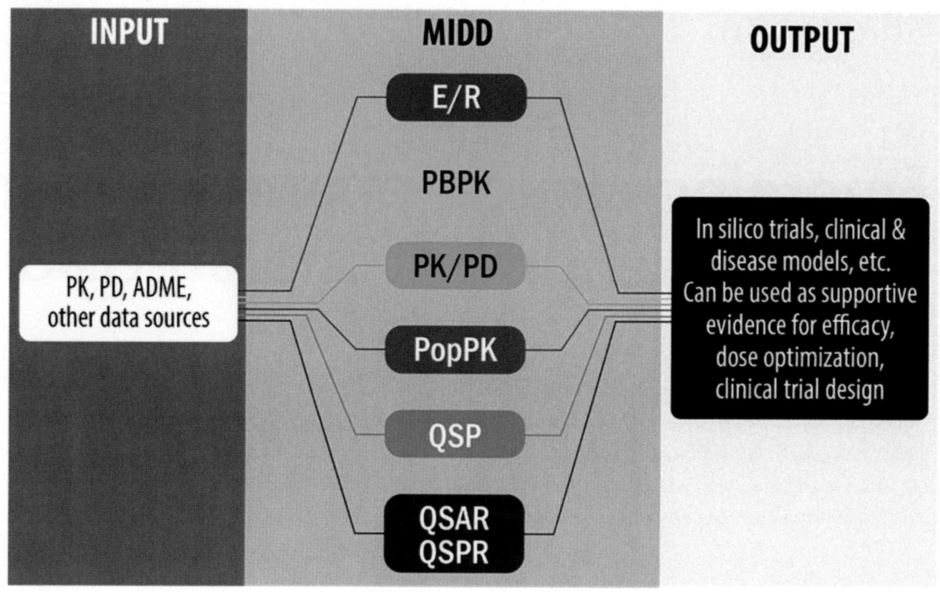

FIG. 36.1 MIDD overview. *ADME*, absorption, distribution, metabolism, excretion; *PK/PD*, pharmacokinetic/pharmacodynamic; *QSAR*, quantitative structure-activity relationship; *QSP*, quantitative systems pharmacology; *QSPR*, quantitative structure-property relationship. *Figure kindly prepared by Giang Ho.*

range over a dosing interval of 4 weeks at steady state. However, steady-state concentration cannot be reached even after 3 to 4 months of repeated dosing because the slow rate of drug release results in a very long apparent half-life of the drug due to flip-flop pharmacokinetics (see Chapter 4) [5]. Modeling and simulation were successfully applied to evaluate alternative loading dose regimens so that drug concentrations could reach the desirable range shortly after treatment was initiated. So, in combination with the understanding of the safety profile of paliperidone palmitate, a loading dose regimen with two repeated injections in the first week was approved in the U.S, even though it had never been directly studied in clinical trials [6, 7].

A MIDD approach also has been used to facilitate dose optimization after the initial approval of a drug. Vilazodone is indicated for treating patients with major depressive disorder. In the initial development program, only a 40-mg dose was evaluated and it demonstrated significant superiority over placebo in three randomized, double-blind clinical trials. However, the clinical trial data showed a flat exposure-efficacy relationship, whereas the exposure-safety relationship was steep. The modeling results suggested that a lower dose of 20mg might have similar efficacy but a better safety profile. A postmarketing, fixed-dose clinical trial was performed using placebo, 20mg, and 40mg vilazodone in major depressive disorder patients. As predicted, compared to the 40-mg dose, 20-mg vilazodone demonstrated almost identical efficacy with reduced safety risks. Accordingly, the product label was amended so that 20mg was added as one of the recommended doses for vilazodone [8].

Clinical trial design

Different trial design components (e.g., trial duration, dosing regimens, patient selection, endpoint identification, and sampling schedule) can be optimized through modeling and simulation to enhance the efficiency of clinical trials.

The following example demonstrates that an alternative endpoint may be considered in schizophrenia trials based on an MIDD approach. The Positive and Negative Syndrome Scale (PANSS) at week 6–8 is typically used as the primary efficacy endpoint for trials conducted in schizophrenia patients with an acute exacerbation. U.S. FDA has applied a modeling approach to systematically evaluate clinical data submitted in new drug applications (NDAs) over the past 15 years. Analyses using item-response theory [9] suggest that not all of the 30 items in PANSS are necessary to characterize syndrome severity in schizophrenia patients enrolled in the efficacy trials. Instead, a modified PANSS reflecting the most relevant 19 items may be adequate, and good concordance has been demonstrated on conclusions regarding drug efficacy between observations at Week 6 and Week 4 using the 19-item modified PANSS. These modeling results suggest that trial efficiency can be improved by using a modified PANSS with a shortened trial duration (i.e., 4 weeks) as an alternative primary endpoint [10].

Identification of evidence for efficacy

Supportive evidence of efficacy can be identified through MIDD approaches. A significant exposure/dose-response relationship implying that higher dose/exposure leads to improved treatment effect may provide critical evidence to support approval of a new product. In drug development programs for rare diseases, or diseases suitable for the FDA Animal Rule pathway, modeling and simulation may allow efficacy findings to be extended to a new patient population.

The approval of boceprevir provides a good example. Boceprevir is indicated for the treatment of Hepatitis C. Previously treated patients were excluded from the initial clinical trials in treatment-naïve patients. However, the resulting clinical data were analyzed by using a novel MIDD approach which predicted a similar treatment response in previously treated patients. After product approval, this prediction was confirmed by clinical trials in previously treated patients [11].

New policy development

The accumulation of experience in MIDD has led to the implementation of new policies and guidance to facilitate drug development. An illustrative example is the pediatric development program for antiepileptic drugs. Traditionally, dedicated pediatric efficacy and safety clinical trials were required to support the approval of antiepileptic drugs in pediatric patients. This has generally resulted in a significant delay (~ 7 years) between the adult approval of these drugs and the addition of pediatric-related labeling [12]. To shorten the lag time for the approval of pediatric indications for antiepileptic drugs, a policy has been developed to allow full extrapolation of efficacy findings from adults to pediatric patients 2 years and older. A collaborative effort from U.S. Food and Drug Administration (FDA), academia, and industry generated a policy employing an MIDD approach to demonstrate similar exposure-response relationships between adults and pediatric patients 2 years of age and older. This draft guidance was published in 2018 [13]. Several products are listed in Table 36.1 that have been approved using the expedited MIDD-informed approach outlined in this guidance.

Active research using MIDD approaches is being conducted in different disease areas, such as schizophrenia, bipolar disorder, Parkinson's disease, lung cancer, and rheumatoid arthritis. As a result, new policy has been developed to streamline clinical programs that incorporates these approaches. For instance, a new draft guidance was published in 2019 that allows efficacy findings to be extrapolated from children 6-12 years of age to adolescents and adults for several central nervous system stimulant products used for treating attention deficit and hyperactivity disorder [14]. New guidance documents also have been developed or updated in recent years to promote the utility of MIDD approaches in drug development programs for the treatment of infectious diseases (e.g., bacterial skin infection [15], HIV-1 infection [16], HCV infection [17], respiratory syncytial virus infection [18], pulmonary tuberculosis [19]), hypertension [20], and ulcerative colitis [21], etc.

Current and future trends in MIDD

Built upon decades of practice and technical refinement, MIDD is being widely applied in drug development and recent regulatory and organizational developments have been designed to enhance communication among all stakeholders who seek to apply this approach. Several emerging techniques have demonstrated the capability to further expand the scope of MIDD, so it is anticipated to play an increasingly critical role in efficient drug development and crucial regulatory decision making in the future.

TABLE 36.1 An overview of new drugs approved for the treatment of partial onset seizure in pediatric patients 4 years and older following the full extrapolation approach.

Drug name	Indication[a]	Approval basis	Dosing determination
Eslicarbazepine	Partial onset seizure in pediatric patients	Extrapolation	Matching exposure level in adults
Lacosamide			
Pregabalin			
Brivaracetam			

[a]*Note: The products were approved based on an early guidance published in 2018. Pediatric indication was extrapolated to patients 4 years and older.*

FDA's current MIDD initiatives

Currently, the FDA is embarked on several initiatives to enhance MIDD under the Prescription Drug User Fee Act (PDUFA) VI. These new MIDD initiatives reflect an extension of the Agency's continuous effort in past decades to promote innovation in drug development. The core of the initiatives is the MIDD Paired Meeting Pilot Program, which was started in 2018. The Agency has committed to accept 2-4 submissions under the program each quarter. Paired sponsor meetings are designed to facilitate in-depth discussion between drug developers and FDA's multidisciplinary review team members with the objective to best apply MIDD methodologies in a specific development program. Thus far, the program has accepted submissions for oncology, cardiovascular, dermatology, antiviral, and neurology products. A wide range of development issues, including dose determination for first-in-human studies, postmarketing dosing changes, and Phase 2/3 clinical trial design has been discussed. This program is expected to enhance early and detailed discussion between regulators and developers on the application of MIDD with the objective of streamlining and facilitating clinical development [22].

Additionally, the FDA has agreed to update MIDD-related guidance and host public workshops to engage the scientific community in a broad discussion on MIDD best practices and technical detail. In line with this effort, the FDA published the format and content guidance on PBPK modeling in 2018 [23] and the revised draft population pharmacokinetic guidance in 2019 [24]. To facilitate scientific exchange and experience sharing, FDA has hosted workshops on dose selection for oncology products [25] and PBPK modeling [26], and plans to host additional workshops on disease progression modeling, and modeling for immunogenicity.

Future trends in MIDD

Continued evolution of state-of-the-art technologies, some of which will be discussed further in the subsequent sections of this chapter, can be expected to expand the scope of MIDD and reshape future drug development. For instance, current inclusion and exclusion criteria in most pivotal efficacy and safety trials tend to exclude patients with potentially confounding variables or diseases. The real-world data, such as electronic health record information that is collected through daily medical practice, may serve as a complementary data source for understanding heterogenous patient response [27]. This information could, if complete and reliable, be used to characterize risk and benefit profiles in subgroups of patients, and to optimize selection of drug treatment and dose. Artificial intelligence (AI) and machine learning (ML) techniques can be employed to provide an empirical tool to manage medical information that is not routinely handled by MIDD approaches. For example, active efforts are being undertaken to link medical images (e.g., CT or MRI scan) with treatment response by using deep learning techniques [28]. Novel modeling techniques are under development to process digital biomarker data collected through software applications (apps) installed on portable or wearable devices [29]. There is also the potential for conducting trials that are integrated into healthcare systems and for using data generated during clinical care or decentralized clinical trials in which data is collected outside of traditional healthcare settings, as in the home. These developments obviously will require more complicated MIDD approaches for trial design. In the meantime, mechanistic models, including PBPK and QSP models, can be used to link results from early research to clinical findings. With accumulated experience, mechanistic models may provide valuable insights on drug disposition, safety, efficacy, and potential drug-drug interactions. So, it is apparent that emerging MIDD approaches, most of which are already under development, will provide opportunities to transform new drug development.

Real-world data and real-world evidence

Real-world data (RWD) are data relating to patient health status and/or the delivery of healthcare routinely collected from a variety of sources other than controlled clinical trials. RWD includes many different types of data, including electronic health records (EHRs), claims and billing data, product and disease registries, and data gathered through personal devices and health applications (Fig. 36.2) [30–32]. The term *real world evidence* (RWE) is defined as clinical evidence regarding the usage, or the potential benefits or risks of a drug, derived from RWD. Drug development and treatment optimization are expensive processes in terms of both the time and money invested. The use of real-world evidence (RWE) derived from real-world data (RWD) has been identified as a potential opportunity for augmenting the evidence derived from controlled clinical trials and for lowering drug development cost and improving its efficiency. Accordingly, the 21st Century Cures Act requires FDA to establish a program to evaluate the potential use of RWE [30, 33].

The use of RWD and RWE in healthcare research is not new. For example, pharmacoepidemiologists and health economists have been using such data routinely to monitor postmarket adverse events, to support coverage decisions, and to

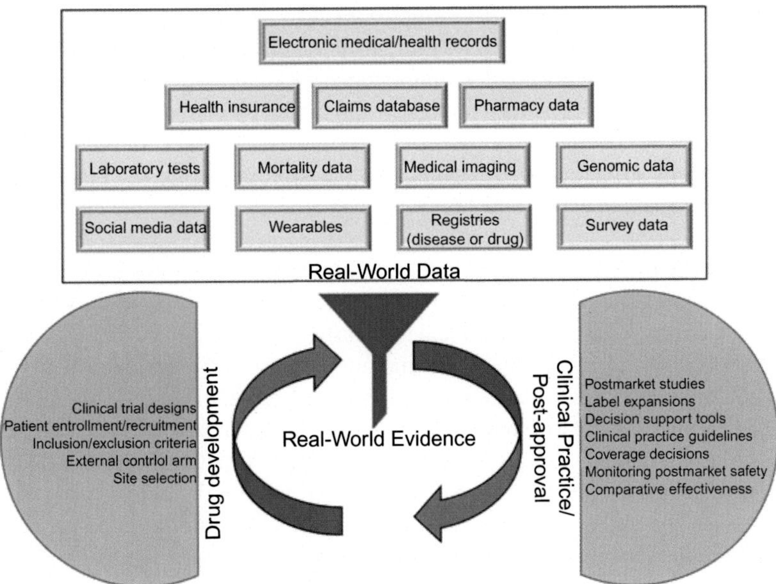

FIG. 36.2 Transformation of real-world data into real-world evidence. *Reproduced with permission from Ramamoorthy A, Huang SM. Clin Pharmacol Ther 2019;106:10–18.*

develop treatment guidelines. A mandate in the 2010 Patient Protection and Affordable Care Act (PPACA) requires all medical practitioners to use electronic medical records (EMRs) for their patients. As of 2015, 96% of nonfederal, acute-care hospitals utilize an EHR that is certified by Health and Human Services (HHS), and 87% of office-based physicians had adopted an EHR [34]. In addition, the use of digital health technologies (DHTs), such as wearable sensors and smart phone applications, makes it possible for patients to generate a large amount of their own health data on a continuous basis. So in the healthcare field, we have a vast wealth of RWD in this digital age.

The utility of RWD in advancing clinical pharmacology

As can be gleaned from previous chapters, clinical pharmacology is concerned with the impact of various intrinsic factors (e.g., age, gender, body weight, and organ dysfunction) and extrinsic factors (e.g., concomitant medications, smoking, and food) on interpatient and intrasubject variability in drug exposure and response, and with how consideration of these factors contributes to precision medicine. Thus the primary mission of the clinical pharmacologist is to find the right drug at the right dose (including dosing regimen and administration route) at the right time (for example, the sequence of therapies) for each patient. Clinical pharmacology also contributes to an understanding of the benefit/risk ratio in different patients and the development of relevant therapeutic monitoring and management strategies. In addition, clinical pharmacology, as a translational science, often contributes to the establishment of drug development tools, such as biomarkers and disease modeling. It is becoming apparent that RWD can be used to augment traditional clinical trial data across these areas.

Filling the knowledge gap between clinical trials and real-world clinical practice

Patients enrolled in clinical trials are somewhat homogeneous in that they must meet certain eligibility criteria, while in real-world practice drugs are likely prescribed to a more heterogeneous patient population. However, it is most informative if trials are designed to reflect as much as possible, the real-world heterogeneity of the expected patient population. RWD may help characterize and identify real-world patients to include in clinical trials. In a retrospective cohort study, O'Connor et al. [35] used EHR data to evaluate how quickly immune checkpoint inhibitors of programmed cell death 1 protein (PD-1 inhibitors) were adopted in clinical practice and to ascertain whether the patients who were enrolled in the clinical trials that lead to the FDA approval differed from patients treated subsequently in clinical practice. The study was of interest because anticancer therapies for an unmet medical need may sometimes be approved based on relatively small studies, and it is important to understand their use in the real-world general population. In this study, most eligible real-world patients were being treated with PD-1 inhibitors within 4 months of FDA approval, with more patients older than 65 years in clinical practice (approximately 60%) than in the pivotal clinical trials (approximately 40%) [36]. In two follow-up studies using the data from the same EHR system, the proportion of patients aged 75 years or older receiving these immunotherapies was found to also increase with time. For example, in the second quarter of 2017 (approximately 2 years after nivolumab was approved for nonsmall cell lung cancer), approximately 1/3 of the patients with nonsmall cell lung cancer who received these treatments were 75 years or older when they started treatment with these immunotherapies. Reassuringly, both studies suggested that older patients did not have worse treatment outcomes than younger patients [36, 37]. It is important to note that the utility of current RWD sources can help evaluate the safety of therapeutic products; however, further study is needed to ascertain their role in establishing therapeutic efficacy. Also needing further exploration are the potential of RWD to augment the data collected in randomized trials and to expand the knowledge on how therapeutics are used across healthcare systems and patient populations.

The eligibility criteria for some clinical trials can be overly restrictive, thereby limiting the representation of the population that will take the drug in clinical practice. This can pose a challenge for patient access to these trials and may impact the subsequent generalizability of clinical trial conclusions. Currently the clinical trial participation rate in the United States is low [38, 39]. Attempts are underway to make eligibility criteria more inclusive and representative of the patients who will use the medication in practice. RWD can be used to guide eligibility criteria development. Lichtman et al. [40] reviewed patient data from Kaiser Permanente Northern California (KPNC) to explore whether changes in standard eligibility criteria would enable greater numbers of cancer patients to participate in clinical trials. Data for all KPNC patients diagnosed with breast, colon, lung, and bladder cancer between 2013 and 2014 ($n = 12,881$) were compared with the cutoff parameters commonly found in clinical trial eligibility criteria. The authors found that inclusion/exclusion criteria based on renal function had a significantly negative impact on patient eligibility and recommended that, if renal toxicity and clearance are not of concern, then CL_{Cr} values of >30 mL/min should be satisfactory for inclusion of patients in cancer trials [40].

In addition to cautious patient selection based on restrictive eligibility criteria, rigorous efforts are made throughout a trial's duration to ensure patient adherence to the protocol. While these approaches may be useful in controlling variability, they can also lead to significant discrepancies between the clinical trial setting/outcome and clinical practice setting/outcome. RWD can be of particular help in understanding the use pattern and effectiveness of the drug in the clinical practice after it is approved. This may be especially relevant to payors as the lack of adherence that is often seen in clinical practice not surprisingly will affect the assessment of effectiveness outcome.

Supporting benefit/risk assessment and management strategy in subpopulations

There is a need to understand drug usage and clinical outcome in certain patients who may be underrepresented or absent in the clinical trials conducted in drug development programs, such as patients with organ dysfunction, patients on certain concomitant medications, ultra/poor drug metabolizers, elderly patients, or pregnant women. Based on RWD and RWE, we may be able to better understand the benefit/risk ratio of the drug in these patient subgroups and develop relevant treatment monitoring and management strategies. At the time of initial approval, the impact of hepatic or renal dysfunction on the pharmacokinetics of many immune checkpoint inhibitors is known, but the associated clinical outcomes are not well characterized. Liu et al. [41] used longitudinal, deidentified patient-level EHR data to evaluate the real-world clinical outcomes of immune checkpoint inhibitors in patients with baseline liver or renal impairment. They found that patients with poor baseline liver function had progressively worse treatment outcomes, including shorter overall survival, while baseline renal dysfunction did not appear to be a correlate of treatment outcomes. Using data from a longitudinal, observational study of patients with chronic hepatitis C from a consortium of academic and community centers, Saxena et al. [42] evaluated safety and efficacy of sofosbuvir-containing regimens in hepatitis C-infected patients with impaired renal function (estimated glomerular filtration rate, eGFR $\leq$ 45 mL/min/1.73 m [2]). The authors found that sofosbuvir-containing treatments remain highly efficacious in patients with renal dysfunction; however, these patients had higher rates of serious adverse events regardless of ribavirin concomitant therapy, which necessitated careful monitoring and aggressive management of adverse events during treatment. Using RWD from the same system, Terrault et al. [43] found that the concomitant therapy with proton pump inhibitors (PPI) in regimens containing ledipasvir and sofosbuvir was associated with an approximately twofold lower chance of achieving sustained virologic response compared to regimens in which PPI were not used. This is consistent with the fact that PPI can decrease ledipasvir absorption and systemic exposure because ledipasvir's solubility decreases as pH increases. Oshikoya et al. [44] analyzed data from a deidentified DNA biobank linked to the EHR and demonstrated that children with CYP2D6 poor or intermediate metabolizer phenotypes were at greater risk for risperidone adverse events. The authors concluded that preprescription genotyping could identify this high-risk subset so that an alternate therapy, risperidone dose reduction, and/or increased safety monitoring could be implemented.

RWD can also be used to support indication expansion in populations that are hard to study. One example is the use of palbociclib in combination with endocrine therapy to treat male patients with breast cancer. Although Palbociclib had been approved for treating women with breast cancer, the rarity of breast cancer in men made randomized trials infeasible in this population. The real-world use pattern, safety, and response of this treatment regimen in men, generated from an insurance database, the EHR system, and the drug developer's global safety database, played a role to support this indication expansion [45].

Optimizing treatment selection and dose

RWD and RWE can be used to help select the optimal treatment and dosing regimen for different patient populations. Although this may not lead to definitive conclusions, it can generate interesting hypothesis for further testing. Wei et al. [46] characterized the dose-response of simvastatin and atorvastatin using EMRs and concluded that atorvastatin was more efficacious, more potent, and demonstrated less interindividual variability than simvastatin. Although this finding is interesting, it may need to be confirmed in a randomized comparative study. Graham et al. [47] performed a retrospective cohort study of patients with nonvalvular atrial fibrillation enrolled in US Medicare who initiated anticoagulant therapy with warfarin, or a standard dose of the nonvitamin K antagonist new oral anticoagulants (NOACs): dabigatran, rivaroxaban, or apixaban. Among patients with similar baseline characteristic, those treated with standard-dose NOAC for nonvalvular atrial fibrillation and warfarin had a more favorable benefit-harm profile than those treated with warfarin. The RWD also suggested that dabigatran and apixaban were associated with a more favorable benefit-harm profile than rivaroxaban. Using RWD from two United Kingdom primary care databases, Vinogradova et al. [48] evaluated the risks and benefits of dabigatran, rivaroxaban, apixaban versus warfarin in a real-world setting. The authors compared risks for bleeding, stroke, venous thromboembolism, and mortality among nearly 200,000 patients (about half with atrial fibrillation) who received initial prescriptions for dabigatran, rivaroxaban, apixaban, and warfarin. The authors concluded from their RWD that apixaban was the safest of the drugs studied, with a decreased risk of major bleeding events in both patients with atrial fibrillation and patients without atrial fibrillation. However, the authors also found that low-dose (less than 10 mg daily) apixaban was associated with increased risks of all-cause mortality compared with warfarin. Mueller [49] subsequently reviewed this publication and commented that it was possible that low-dose apixaban was given preferentially to complex patients with the highest underlying risk for both bleeding and mortality. Thus, due to lack of randomization, these real-world findings could have been subject to confounding and bias. This example highlights an important limitation of RWD and RWE: when there is no randomization the data can be hard to interpret and causal inferences are of limited value. On the other hand, it is possible to conduct a randomized pragmatic study in the real-world setting. For example, a pragmatic study by Patient-Centered Outcomes Research Institute, called Aspirin Dosing: A Patient-centric Trial Assessing Benefits and Long-term Effectiveness (ADAPTABLE), will randomly assign 20,000 patients with established coronary heart disease to either low-dose (81 mg) or high-dose (325 mg) aspirin therapy [50]. It is anticipated that this pragmatic, point-of-care study will determine which aspirin dose is better for patients with established cardiovascular disease.

Opportunistic real-world blood sampling can facilitate pragmatic pharmacokinetic (PK) research that is needed to optimize dosing for subpopulations, such as pediatric patients in whom serial blood sampling is challenging. Van Driest et al. [51] determined fentanyl PK in children after cardiac surgery using leftover blood specimens and EMR data generated during clinical care. Using a population PK approach, the authors estimated PK parameters for this population and established that the relationship between PK parameters and weight was nonlinear. They used simulations to show that allometric model-adjusted per kg fentanyl dosing led to more consistent therapeutic fentanyl concentrations than fixed per kg dosing. This case demonstrates that population PK modeling using opportunistic real-world samples can be used for PK assessment and dose optimization.

RWD can also be used to help understand whether dosing in the real-world setting is similar to that used in pivotal clinical trials and recommended in subsequent labeling [52, 53]. Using EMR data linked to administrative claims, White et al. [54] analyzed the real-world dosing patterns of three drugs approved by the FDA for fibromyalgia—pregabalin, duloxetine, and milnacipran and found that only approximately 1/3 of patients with fibromyalgia were prescribed these drugs at the recommended starting dose. Patients using pregabalin were the most likely cohort to receive lower than label-recommended starting doses and the least likely to receive the recommended maintenance doses. The authors concluded that that factors other than label recommendations, such as an individual's tolerability and opioid use, may be influencing the real-world dosing pattern.

Assisting in drug development

RWD can also be used to improve the efficiency of drug development. As discussed earlier, RWD can be used to guide the eligibility criteria of the clinical trials. In addition, other aspects of clinical trial design/planning (e.g., selection of clinical sites, estimation of enrollment speed/trial duration) can also be guided by RWD. Other areas of interest include the use of RWD for disease modeling and the development of biomarkers and endpoints. For example, the combined data from patient registries and longitudinal cohort studies supported the qualification of total kidney volume measured at baseline as a prognostic enrichment biomarker to be used in combination with patient age and baseline eGFR, to help identify those autosomal dominant polycystic kidney disease patients who are at greater risk for a substantial decline in renal function [55].

Limitations of RWD

An inherent limitation of RWD is that the data sources are not designed for a research purpose so the quality of the data is often suboptimal. In general, data elements captured in RWD may differ from those needed to provide regulatory evidence. RWD data also have variable structures. Missing data and coding errors are more common in RWD than in datasets from clinical trials. Best practices are needed to ensure the quality of RWD when they are used to support important clinical and regulatory decisions [56]. Much RWD currently exists as unstructured data. Technology needs to be developed to facilitate the appropriate utilization of unstructured data and to improve the future collection of RWD. RWD data sources can also be fragmented in that various sources of information for a patient may exist in different electronic systems that lack cross-communication. In addition, there are many different data platforms and diverse data standards, which can hinder the use of RWD. Adopting common data standards and making different electronic systems interoperable will be critical if RWD and RWE are to be used optimally.

Confounding and bias are challenges that could limit the potential to make useful inferences from RWD. Randomization is the best way to overcome these issues and could be used in the real-world setting of pragmatic trials. Sometimes, propensity score, the probability of treatment assignment conditional on observed baseline characteristics, or instrumental variables might be used to address potential confounding factors. In some cases, inferences based on RWE can be supported by combining RWD with other information, such as knowledge of mechanism of action and clinical trial data.

Future trends

Multiple challenges must be addressed before the full potential of RWD is realized. Technological advances in informatics, statistical methodologies, and machine learning (ML) tools, among other areas, are all important developments needed to further the utility of RWD in producing relevant evidence capable of supporting regulatory and healthcare-related decision making and policy development. The following sections highlight a few areas in which technological innovations are proving to be key to exploiting the full potential of RWD.

Making sense of the data

Among the challenges that hinder the full utilization of RWD are variable data quality, structure, standards, and formats, and the lack of communication between data sources. To use EHR as an example, there are multiple systems that represent different standards with variable specifications that prevent linkages and interoperability with other data sources. The standards used and data quality may also differ between organizations that utilize the same EHR system. In addition to these challenges, the likelihood of capturing certain data elements may also be variable and inconsistent. Clearly, the complexity of this scenario represents a substantial obstacle to the optimal use of RWE. As a result, multiple organizations are working on addressing these challenges by exploring an array of technological and analytical tools. Artificial intelligence (AI) tools, such as ML and natural language processing (NLP), are increasingly being developed and explored to aid in analyzing, organizing, and scanning through RWD datasets in order to identify signals of interest. Such tools are also being developed to bridge gaps in data by linking different sources of data. For example, automated tools are being explored to scan massive amounts of drug safety data to identify potential red flags [57]. Also, NLP and ML techniques are being developed to identify specific trends and natural experiments that are not typically detectable using current approaches [58–60]. Multiple AI techniques are also being utilized and explored to help organize, link, and identify gaps in RWD sources, such as insurance claims and EHR.

A cloud-based analytical ecosystem

The volume and diversity of RWD requires robust hosting and analytics infrastructures to support the use and processing of these data to produce relevant evidence. These infrastructures can also facilitate near real-time data capture and robust analytics to augment randomized clinical trials and can also enable implementation of innovative clinical trial designs, such as clinical trials that are conducted in healthcare settings (clinical trials with pragmatic elements), adaptive clinical trials, and decentralized clinical trials. Because cloud-based data platforms can provide the needed flexibility and the capacity to handle RWD in a responsive manner, they will allow for a near real-time flow of data and for an analysis of the data that is sufficiently rapid to provide relevant information to support timely healthcare or research decisions [61, 62].

The mosaic of evidence

As the scientific community continues to explore the use of RWD to augment data from traditional, randomized clinical trials, and as we gain knowledge and experience in managing and analyzing data from these sources, there will be a trend for evidence to be shaped as a composite from multiple data sources. Technological tools will continue to be developed, not only to help us organize and analyze RWD, but also to provide additional pieces of the puzzle that identify data reflecting important outcomes [29, 63, 64]. Digital health technologies (DHTs) are being developed at a rapid pace. Tools for passive sensing, to capture patient-reported outcomes (PROs), and to identify outcomes generated using digital tools and trackers, are also being increasingly explored and introduced. The development of these advances must be accompanied by a shared understanding on how to validate them and how to effectively organize and analyze the generated data.

Digital health technologies

Medical practice has traditionally relied on periodic in-person visits between patients and physicians. Patient evaluations and medical tests are performed during these visits, and physicians rely on patient recollection to report their experiences between visits. Although important, these periodic encounters may not provide a complete understanding of patient experience or overall health. For example, everyday fluctuations in glucose levels, heart rate, blood pressure, mental state, strength, and fatigue are likely to be missed. Because of a rapidly evolving digital ecosystem, continuous patient-generated data are increasingly becoming a reality through the integration of DHTs into our daily lives. DHTs use computing platforms, connectivity, software, and/or sensors to collect data from patients on a day-to-day basis. DHTs may include wearable, implantable, or ingestible sensors (e.g., accelerometers, continuous glucose monitors, heart rate monitors, digital ingestion tracking system), or environmental sensors placed in a patient's home or immediate environment (e.g., video recorders or motion sensors). DHTs may also include software applications that run on general-purpose computing platforms (e.g., mobile telephones, tablets), associated general-purpose hardware (e.g., camera, microphone, accelerometer), and specialized hardware (e.g., handheld spirometers).

DHTs permit measurement of a growing range of clinical events or characteristics and can acquire data remotely from anyone. The increasing trend of individuals to monitor their own health as part of day-to-day activities allows for the continuous recording and analysis of physiological or pathological data (e.g., ambulatory blood pressure, temperature, cardiac rhythm, blood glucose level, oxygen saturation) and allows the frequency and/or intensity of physiological or pathological events to be measured (e.g., coughs, breaths, steps, sleep, eye movement, falls, seizures, arrhythmias). The overwhelming quantity of RWD available via DHTs opens a plethora of monitoring opportunities. The ubiquity of mobile telephones that include cameras means that most individuals have the ability to photograph lesions or record movement disorders or patient behavior. Sensors provide opportunities to acquire data directly from infants or cognitively impaired individuals who are unable to report their experiences. They may also be used to measure the mental or physical ability of patients to perform defined tasks, such as tests of visual acuity, auditory acuity, fine motor coordination, muscle strength, forced expiratory volume (FEV1), and memory [29, 64].

The utility of DHTs to advance clinical pharmacology and medical research

The ability to frequently, or even continuously, capture data remotely from patients and/or healthy people may improve the understanding of the pharmacodynamic activity and clinical effects of medical products (Fig. 36.3). Such data can also provide valuable information on the effects of medical products on routine daily living activities directly from the patient's environment. The high-density data of collection offered by DHTs provides a more complete dynamic profile of patient data than traditional discrete measurements and may improve the sensitivity of detecting important changes. For example, in a Phase 1 trial, the transient heart rate increase after amphetamine challenge was captured by a continuous monitoring approach using a wearable device, but could not be detected in the conventional data that was collected at discrete time points [65]. DHTs can also be used to monitor patient adherence, when a patient takes their medicine and the number of doses taken. This information can be used to improve patient adherence by providing a convenient and automated way to

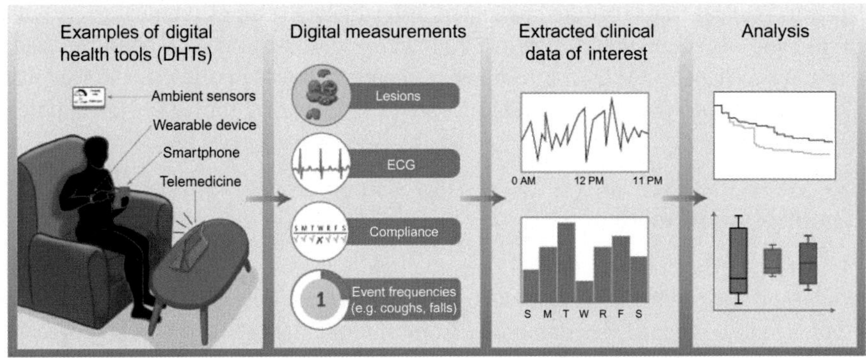

FIG. 36.3 Clinical trial utilization of digital health tools (DHTs). *Figure kindly prepared by Giang Ho.*

send reminders to subjects to take medication, complete an electronic diary (e-diary), or attend a follow-up appointment. If DHT measurements of pharmacodynamic activity and clinical effects can be analyzed together with the drug concentrations or the treatment timing and dosing information, it can improve understanding of the exposure-response relationship of the drug and can help guide better treatment selection and dosing recommendations. The information collected by DHTs may also facilitate interpretation of adverse events. DHTs may also be used to support Clinical Outcome Assessments (COAs) by providing more convenient way to capture patient-reported outcomes (PRO), clinician-reported outcomes (CRO), and other observer-reported outcomes (ObsRO).

Remote data collection via DHTs has great potential to facilitate clinical investigations. DHTs utilized in decentralized clinical trials (DCTs) will enable data capture from participants directly without the additional cost and effort incurred when patients need to travel to the investigator [66]. Thus DCTs may result in greater convenience for study participants by saving time and overcoming geographic restrictions and socioeconomic and demographic barriers. This promise is being increasingly realized with the increasing utilization of telemedicine and DHTs in decentralized settings. In DCTs, some or all study-related procedures and data acquisition can take place at locations remote from the investigator, with no or minimal disruption to the daily life of study participants.

The design of DCTs allows for elements of decentralization, augmented by DHTs, to be applied selectively. In a fully decentralized model, all clinical investigation-related activities are implemented remotely (i.e., subject data acquisition and interaction is done through telemedicine, DHTs, and/or local healthcare providers). In a partially decentralized model (a hybrid model), some of the clinical investigation-related activities are implemented remotely while others are centralized. For example, some study subjects may be seen at centralized sites, while others may be followed remotely. Nevertheless, a number of hurdles exist in the implementation of a DCT. Jurisdictional laws governing telemedicine are still evolving. Physicians engaging in telemedicine may need to be licensed in the state in which the subject is located or may require a separate telemedicine license or certificate. Coverage from private payers, Medicaid, or Medicare may not cover telemedicine services or may not provide the same coverage for in-person services. Shipping restrictions may limit pharmacist participation. Variability in local healthcare practice may introduce variability in outcomes measured, making it difficult to assess a medical product's effect. However, these challenges can be addressed with appropriate planning and foresight, and DCTs can be expected to bring clinical research more conveniently to the patient.

Key considerations for the use of DHTs

DHTs may pose data privacy and security risks and concerns. End-user licensing agreements and terms of service for DHTs often release data to DHT vendors and other third parties who are not directly participating in clinical research. With appropriate planning and foresight, patient privacy can be protected. Security can be enhanced through the use of advanced encryption or distributed ledger technology. Integration of DHTs also requires other logistical and ethical considerations. Sim et al. [67] discussed the challenges of integrating mobile health data into clinical care. Such challenges include how the inclusion and presentation of data will fit into an already complicated and overstretched workflow. There are also multiple technical considerations regarding the validation of both the technology and associated software that are used. The authors highlighted the need for additional resources to perform critical functions, such as technical support and training patients on how to use technology. There are ethical implications relating to equity and patient autonomy. There is a need to consider economic factors in technology adoption among lower-income, disabled, elderly, and rural populations, which are also linked to digital literacy skills. The considerations compel invested parties to proactively ensure that the mobile health frontier is safe, fair, and just for all patients.

One of the most crucial steps in implementing DHT in a successful clinical investigation will be selecting the most appropriate DHT. A variety of factors should be evaluated in selecting a particular DHT, including the clinical event or characteristic being measured and the purpose and design of the clinical investigation. Other selection criteria include the technical aptitude; ability and willingness of the study population; and the type, method, and duration of data collection. Subject environment should also be considered, whether there is the availability of a network and electronic systems that can manage frequent or continuous data streams. Some studies may accommodate a "bring-your-own" approach in which study subjects use their own personal DHTs to collect data during the investigation. Manufacturers will need to consider whether the benefits and risks of this approach can ensure appropriate data collection and privacy.

Another key to successful implementation of DHTs in a clinical investigation will be feasibility studies to ensure that the DHT is appropriate for the proposed clinical investigation. Findings from such studies may improve the design and functionality of the DHT, improve user satisfaction, inform the instructions for use and training for study subjects and personnel, and demonstrate if the DHT achieves its intended goal. Izmailova et al. [68] assessed the performance of two wearable DHTs and the operational feasibility of deploying them to augment data collection in a residential Phase 1 clinical trial. The authors identified one DHT as "not fit-for-purpose" because of artifacts that necessitated time-consuming manual review. The other wearable DHT was identified as suitable for monitoring mobility, collecting derived sleep data, and facilitating interpretation of vital sign data. The authors emphasize the importance of a fit-for-purpose evaluation of wearable DHTs prior to deployment in drug development studies. Bakker et al. [69] reviewed feasibility studies that advocated using DHTs in clinical research and developed a searchable, living database to promote standardization of feasibility methods and to support the efficient and effective adoption of DHTs in clinical research. This database is maintained by the Clinical Trials Transformation Initiative (CTTI).

The future convergence of innovative technologies

Advances in DHT, the adoption of cloud-based infrastructure, and the increased availability of multiple streams of large health datasets, coupled with advances in analytics and informatics, are shaping the future of medical research, therapeutic development, and healthcare. Infrastructures, training programs, and collaborations need to be established that can maximize the benefits of this transformation. Although technology provides the necessary tools to answer key questions in a fast and efficient manner, much more work is needed to shed light on key areas, such as developing novel endpoints that take advantage of advances in DHTs. Technology can also help refine benchmarks of clinical efficacy (e.g., clinical scales, patient-reported outcomes, hospitalization, mortality) and provide meaningful indicators of clinical outcome. Technology is facilitating an evolution in clinical trials designs and enabling innovative designs, such as decentralized clinical trials, adaptive clinical trials, and trials in a healthcare setting.

The continued development of increasingly sophisticated analytical and predictive tools is needed to further advance the parallel development of DHT. AI approaches, such as ML and NLP, are being increasingly explored to facilitate therapeutic development. Recently, AI utilizing deep learning to facilitate early drug discovery was shown to be ground breaking in developing a compound to target a kinase involved in fibrosis and other diseases [70]. Although the potential for AI to accelerate and facilitate the development of therapeutics is significant, we are only at the early stages of understanding the full promise of such tools and methods. Through the convergence of the innovations discussed previously, drug discovery and clinical trials are poised to become more robust and efficient. Collectively, these trends will facilitate drug development, regulatory decision making, clinical care, and ultimately improve public health.

The microbiome and its impact on therapy response

Given the importance of the microbiome in various human diseases, it is unsurprising that microbial organisms, their metabolism, and their interaction with the immune system may also play a role in patient response to therapy (Fig. 36.4). A combination of human observational studies, as well as studies in germ-free and conventional animal models, have adequately demonstrated that the microbiome is involved in the maturation and regulation of the host immune system. Recent evidence has shown that modulating the human gut microbiome can influence response to drug-based therapies, for example cancer immunotherapy. In the age of precision medicine, several studies have demonstrated that microbial composition in mice can be optimized to result in improved therapeutic response. Therefore it is essential to understand the factors influencing the gut microbiome and therapeutic response as the microbiome plays an important role in anticancer immunosurveillance, immunotherapy, and immune system modulation.

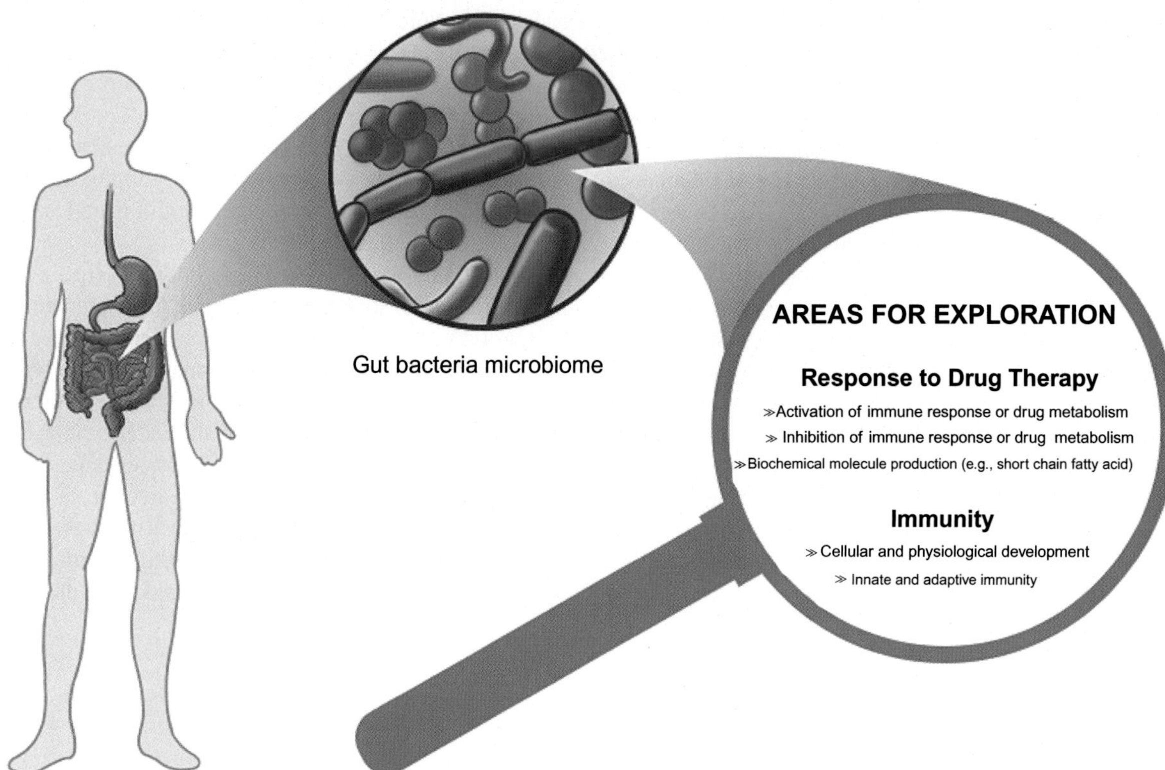

FIG. 36.4 Gut microbiome and its impact on immunity and drug response. *Figure kindly prepared by Giang Ho.*

The influence of the gut microbiome on immunity

Defective control of the immune system has been recognized as the primary factor leading to cancer initiation and progression. Tumor-specific markers and their differential metabolic factors have been identified as indicators of the success or failure of cancer therapy [71]. However, as these specific markers continue to evolve in response to selection pressure, a multitude of factors that contribute to the overall immune status have been established in a new holistic model [72]. Recent findings have also demonstrated that the gut microbiome can affect response to cancer therapy [73].

Trillions of microbes exist in the body where they are as abundant as human cells and regularly interact throughout the body and throughout development. Therefore it is not surprising that the microbiome plays an operational role in numerous human physiological systems, including immunity [74, 75]. The immune system is not only able to differentiate between self and non-self-antigens, which is the basis for immune tolerance, but also permits and even encourages the establishment of commensal microbes while restricting opportunistic bacterial invasion and infection. The microbiome influences both innate and adaptive immunity across many different levels. Evidence for this comes from observing physiological development in germ-free (GF) mice, which tend to have numerous defects in immune system development. These defects include reduced size and functionality of Peyer's patches and draining mesenteric lymph nodes (mLNs), absence of an intestinal mucous layer and gut-associated lymphoid tissue, and altered immunoglobulin A (IgA) secretion [76–79].

A link between gut microbial composition and anticancer therapeutic efficacy

Commensal microbial metabolism has a fundamental influence on host cellular physiology and development, but commensal microbial antigens can also influence local and systemic inflammation, which can have far-reaching consequences for host health. In 2013 Iida et al. [80] proposed in a groundbreaking study that commensal bacteria could alter inflammation in the tumor microenvironment and showed that disruption of the gut microbiota by antibiotic therapy impaired response to different chemotherapeutic agents, such as CpG-oligonucleotide immunotherapy and platinum chemotherapy. In addition, GF mice with implanted subcutaneous tumors showed an inadequate response to CpG-oligonucleotide treatment, which was attributed to the lack of microbiota and a consequent reduction in cytokine and tumor necrosis factor production. The similar poor tumor response in GF mice treated with platinum was thought to result from a reduced concentration of reactive oxygen species (ROSs) and cytotoxicity. As these therapeutic interventions lacked efficacy in the absence of microbiota, these authors proposed using microbial intervention to influence therapeutic outcome and also hypothesized that treatments or lifestyle choices that affect the microbiome may influence therapeutic efficacy. Therefore maintenance of an intact, functional microbiota appears to be essential for optimal response to cancer therapy.

Cyclophosphamide (CTX) is an alkylating agent that is widely used in chemotherapy. Viaud et al. [81] demonstrated that nonmyeloablative doses of CTX disrupt the intestinal barrier and alter the microbiota of tumor-bearing mice. This results in translocation of certain commensal Gram-positive bacteria from the intestine to mesenteric lymph nodes and the spleen where they stimulate generation of "pathogenic" T helper 17 (pTh17) cells which inhibit cancer growth. This pTh17 response was reduced in tumor-bearing GF or antibiotic-pretreated mice that received CTX and their tumors were resistant to CTX therapy. However, the antitumor efficacy of CTX was partially restored following adoptive transfer of pTh17 cells into vancomycin-treated mice.

As intestinal bacteria are potent modulators of systemic immune responses, the microbiota was investigated in patients with acute graft-versus-host disease (GVHD) after allogeneic blood/marrow transplantation (allo-BMT) or allogeneic hematopoietic-cell transplantation (allo-HCT). Following allo-HCT, patients with a greater proportion of a bacterial group composed mostly of *Eubacterium limosum* had a decreased risk of relapse or progression of GVHD [82]. Similarly, subjects with a greater proportion of genus *Blautia* generally had reduced GVHD mortality after allo-BMT [83].

Additional research studies suggest that specific bacterial species could be used not only as biomarkers but might have potential as actual biotherapeutic agents. In one study, oral administration of a *Bifidobacterium*-probiotic to melanoma-implanted mice was found to have antitumor effects that were comparable to and synergistic with checkpoint blockade following treatment with programmed cell death protein 1 ligand 1 (PD-L1). These effects were mediated by an augmentation in dendritic cell function that increased CD8+ T cell priming and accumulation in the tumor microenvironment [84]. Similarly, Vétizou et al. [85] investigated the response of sarcoma-implanted mice to a CTLA-4 blocking antibody. Tumors implanted in GF and antibiotic pretreated mice did not respond but responsiveness was restored in these mice following gavage with *Bacteroides fragilis*. The authors then treated GF mice with microbial transplants of feces from melanoma patients who were being treated with the CTLA-4 blocker, ipilimumab. They found that good tumor responses to CTLA-4 blocking antibody were only found in mice whose fecal transplants facilitated colonization of *Bacteroides fragilis* and *Bacteroides thetaiotaomicron*. These findings both suggest that it may be helpful to manipulate the microbiota in order to optimize immunotherapy.

Mechanistic link between microbial function and immunotherapy

The microbiota influences immunotherapy in a number of ways: first, as an effector to reach out from the GI tract via circulation to the tumor microenvironment, and second, as an activator or inhibitor of an immune response. In support of the first function, bacteria capable of converting gemcitabine to an inactive metabolite were hypothesized to have migrated from the duodenum to the tumor microenvironment of human pancreatic ductal adenocarcinomas, thereby conferring tumor resistance to this drug [86]. In support of the second function, studies have suggested that shared similarity for T-cell epitopes between tumor and bacterial antigens could cause sensitized cross-reactive T cells to further augment tumor antigenicity [87, 88]. In this way, the bacterial antigens of the microbiota could exert important antitumor effects. Furthermore, commensal genomic DNA could act as a natural adjuvant and modulate regulatory and effector T cell (Treg/Teff) equilibrium [89]. Notably, the unmethylated cytosine phosphate guanosine dinucleotides that are found abundant in the prokaryotic DNA of gut microbiota are potent activators of the Toll-like receptor 9 (TLR9) signaling system that is needed to stimulate the inflammatory cytokine production by Teff that is needed to provide an immune response. Thus another way in which gut commensals could strengthen antitumor immunity is by enhancing antigenicity and adjuvanticity.

In addition, gut microbiota can produce bioactive molecules as a result of their metabolism of dietary enteric contents. Short-chain fatty acids (SCFA) are examples of microbial metabolic products that have immunomodulatory effects [90, 91]. SCFAs such as lactate, acetate, butyrate, and propionate are formed from the fermentation of complex carbohydrates in the anaerobic environment of the gut. Intestinal epithelial cells consume these metabolites as their primary energy source and regulate production of pro-inflammatory cytokines by TL4 and TL5 in a dose-dependent manner [92], as well as the generation and function of extrathymic Treg [93], and dendritic cells [94]. They inhibit histone deacetylases, thereby blunting both T-cell dependent and independent antibody responses that play a role in autoimmune diseases [95]. Gut microbiota can also form N-acylamides that mimic eukaryotic signaling molecules and can act as ligands for G-protein coupled receptors to further modulate immune response outside of the gastrointestinal tract [96]. These N-acylamides regulate immunological functions by communicating as signaling molecules, epigenetic regulators, and inflammation switchers which in turn could affect antitumor immunity.

Impact of microbial metabolism on drug therapy

Early pharmacogenomic research proposed polymorphism analysis of the bacterial repertoire of metabolic enzymes and the human genome to explore a possible source of variability in drug efficacy and toxicity. As an example, members of the UDP-glucuronosyltransferase (UGT) enzyme family, which inactivates some drugs, were genotyped to determine the distribution of polymorphisms across different bacterial species and hosts. Similar genotyping of other drug-metabolizing hepatic enzymes, such as members of the cytochrome (CYP) P450 superfamily, has also been performed. However, these approaches characterized drug metabolism in the human liver and intestinal mucosa, and as such could not be broadly translated to microbiota. However, recent advances in high-throughput sequencing methodologies for microbial organisms, analytical molecular separation techniques, and GF mouse models have provided a new dimension to our understanding of gut microbiota-mediated biotransformation of exogenous compounds and have led to a new field of pharmacomicrobiomics that is based on pharmacogenomics and pharmacometabolomics [97].

The most important microbial enzymatic reactions involved in metabolizing drugs are hydrolysis and reduction. As discussed in Chapter 4, the interactions of such reactions between the gut microbiome's enzymatic pool and drugs can either lead to drug activation or inactivation, or even transformation to a toxic compound. To gain systematic understanding of the determinants of microbiome drug metabolism and interactions, their microbial gene products need to be identified and measured [98]. Additional experiments with gnotobiotic animals need to be conducted to further establish the role of enteric bacteria in drug metabolism. However, it already appears that there is a mechanistic link between gut metagenome and genomics, and interindividual microbial variation in drug metabolism.

Future therapeutic applications of microbiome science

Validation of correlative associations across multiple cohorts in a prospective clinical trial would be essential if microbiome science is to be applied to patient care. Existing preclinical research suggests several strategies for using microbiome knowledge to improve clinical cancer therapy. For example, administration of antibiotics to cancer patients undergoing immunotherapy should be treated with caution due to its potential to disrupt immune-regulatory bacteria. Additionally, microbiome profiling before and after therapy could be used to guide treatment decisions, by determining the proportion of potential effector taxa and biomarkers that could predict therapeutic outcome.

There is a range of specific and nonspecific intervention strategies that could be used to manipulate the microbiota in order to achieve an overall health benefit or a specific clinical outcome. For example, for a particular treatment, a fecal microbiota transplant (FMT) from therapeutic responders could be used to deliver a specific beneficial effect by conveying favorable response status to potential nonresponders. However, FMT is associated with many uncertainties that warrant further investigation, such as standardization of product, complications associated with introduction of foreign bacteria, and other adverse health consequences. Alternatively, modulating the existing commensal community with diet, probiotics, or prebiotics produces variable and only temporary effects based on the initial state of an individual's microbiome. Therefore it is important to identify the consequences of specific (e.g., FMT) versus general (e.g., dietary) therapies to determine the most effective strategy. Importantly, probiotics or microbially derived small molecule therapies could be considered specific effectors. However, to date the FDA has not approved a probiotic therapeutic as a drug product.

One of the most important considerations is the inherent complexity of the microbiome, especially considering its high interindividual and intrastrain level variability, which likely results in a correspondingly highly variable response outcome within a typical human population. This makes it challenging to identify the critical elements from the various modalities that contribute to the impact of microbes on therapeutic efficacy. Functional metabolic variation between microbe strains or subspecies could cause different drug interactions, as well as different interactions with the host and disease condition, even if two individuals have a shared microbiome at the species level. Also, an identical strain could contribute very different functional outcomes in two discrete microbiomes, due to the influence of the entire microbiota on a single microorganism's metabolism. In the future, microbiome-enabled therapeutic interventions could potentially become standard of care for many drug-based therapeutic strategies, and serve as both biomarkers of response and agents for augmenting efficacy. The full potential of personalized treatment will only be realized by understanding the biological mechanisms that link specific bacterial strains to host immunity and physiological response.

References

[1] Wang Y, Zhu H, Madabushi R, Liu Q, Huang SM, Zineh I. Model-informed drug development: current US regulatory practice and future considerations. Clin Pharmacol Ther 2019;105(4):899–911.
[2] Madabushi R, Wang Y, Zineh I. A holistic and integrative approach for advancing model-informed drug development. CPT Pharmacometrics Syst Pharmacol 2019;8(1):9–11.
[3] Zhu H, Huang SM, Madabushi R, Strauss DG, Wang Y, Zineh I. Model-informed drug development: a regulatory perspective on progress. Clin Pharmacol Ther 2019;106(1):91–93.
[4] Sheiner LB. Learning versus confirming in clinical drug development. Clin Pharmacol Ther 1997;61(3):275–291.
[5] Zhou RQ, Ji HC, Liu Q, Zhu CY, Liu R. Leveraging machine learning techniques for predicting pancreatic neuroendocrine tumor grades using biochemical and tumor markers. World J Clin Cases 2019;7(13):1611–1622.
[6] Wang S, Liu Q, Zhu E, Yin J, Zhao W. MST-GEN: an efficient parameter selection method for one-class extreme learning machine. IEEE Trans Cybern 2017;47(10):3266–3279.
[7] Samtani MN, Vermeulen A, Stuyckens K. Population pharmacokinetics of intramuscular paliperidone palmitate in patients with schizophrenia: a novel once-monthly, long-acting formulation of an atypical antipsychotic. Clin Pharmacokinet 2009;48(9):585–600.
[8] U.S. Package Insert of Vibryd® (vilazodone). https://www.accessdata.fda.gov/drugsatfda_docs/label/2020/022567s021lbl.pdf; 2020. Accessed 19 March 2020.
[9] Yang FM, Kao ST. Item response theory for measurement validity. Shanghai Arch Psychiatry 2014;26(3):171–177.
[10] Younis IR. Clinical trial database analyses to inform regulatory guidances: improving the efficiency of schizophrenia clinical trials, https://isctm.org/public_access/Feb2018/Presentations/S2-Younis.pdf; 2018. Accessed.
[11] FDA. Artificial intelligence and machine learning in software as a medical device, https://www.fda.gov/medical-devices/software-medical-device-samd/artificial-intelligence-and-machine-learning-software-medical-device#news; 2020. Accessed 17 July 2020.
[12] Mulugeta YL, Zajicek A, Barrett J, et al. Development of drug therapies for newborns and children: the scientific and regulatory imperatives. Pediatr Clin N Am 2017;64(6):1185–1196.
[13] FDA. Guidance for industry: drugs for treatment of partial onset seizures: full extrapolation of efficacy from adults to pediatric patients 2 years of age and older, https://www.fda.gov/media/130449/download; 2020. Accessed 19 March 2020.
[14] FDA. Guidance for industry: attention deficit hyperactivity disorder: developing stimulant drugs for treatment, https://www.fda.gov/media/124334/download; 2020. Accessed 19 March 2020.
[15] FDA. Guidance for industry: acute bacterial skin and skin structure infections: developing drugs for treatment, https://www.fda.gov/media/71052/download; 2020. Accessed 19 March 2020.
[16] FDA. Guidance for industry: human immunodeficiency virus-1 infection: developing antiretroviral drugs for treatment, https://www.fda.gov/media/86284/download; 2020. Accessed 19 March 2020.
[17] FDA. Guidance for industry: chronic hepatitis C virus infection: developing direct-acting antiviral drugs for treatment; 2016.
[18] FDA. Guidance for industry: respiratory syncytial virus infection: developing antiviral drugs for prophylaxis and treatment, https://www.fda.gov/media/79486/download; 2020. Accessed 19 March 2020.
[19] FDA. Proposed regulatory framework for modifications to artificial intelligence/machine learning (AI/ML)-based software as a medical device (SaMD)—discussion paper and request for feedback, https://www.fda.gov/files/medical%20devices/published/US-FDA-Artificial-Intelligence-and-Machine-Learning-Discussion-Paper.pdf; 2019. Accessed 17 July 2019.
[20] FDA. Guidance for industry: hypertension indication: drug labeling for cardiovascular outcome claims, https://www.fda.gov/media/134777/download; 2020. Accessed 19 March 2020.
[21] FDA. Guidance for industry: ulcerative colitis: clinical trail endpoint, https://www.fda.gov/files/drugs/published/Ulcerative-Colitis--Clinical-Trial-Endpoints-Guidance-for-Industry.pdf; 2020. Accessed 19 March 2020.
[22] Madabushi R, Benjamin JM, Grewal R, et al. The US Food and Drug Administration's model-informed drug development paired meeting pilot program: early experience and impact. Clin Pharmacol Ther 2019;106(1):74–78.
[23] FDA. Guidance for industry: physiologically based pharmacokinetic analyses—format and content guidance for industry, https://www.fda.gov/media/101469/download; 2020. Accessed 19 March 2020.
[24] FDA. Guidance for industry: population pharmacokinetics, https://www.fda.gov/media/128793/download. Accessed 19 March 2020.
[25] FDA-ISoP Public Workshop. Model informed drug development (MIDD) for oncology products, https://www.fda.gov/drugs/news-events-human-drugs/fda-isop-public-workshop-model-informed-drug-development-midd-oncology-products; 2020. Accessed 19 March 2020.
[26] FDA Public Workshop. Development of best practices in physiologically based pharmacokinetic modeling to support clinical pharmacology regulatory decision-making, https://www.fda.gov/drugs/news-events-human-drugs/development-best-practices-physiologically-based-pharmacokinetic-modeling-support-clinical; 2020. Accessed 19 March 2020.
[27] Sherman RE, Anderson SA, Dal Pan GJ, et al. Real-world evidence—what is it and what can it tell us? N Engl J Med 2016;375(23):2293–2297.
[28] Liu Q, Zhu H, Liu C, et al. Application of machine learning in drug development and regulation: current status and future potential. Clin Pharmacol Ther 2020;107(4):726–729.
[29] Mehta NWJ, Wang Y, Zhu H, Liu Q. The use of mobile technology in drug development. Clin Pharmcol Ther 2020.
[30] Public Law: 114–255. https://www.govinfo.gov/content/pkg/PLAW-114publ255/pdf/PLAW-114publ255.pdf; 2020. Accessed 19 March 2020.
[31] FDA. Use of real-world evidence to support regulatory decision-making for medical devices. Guidance for Industry and Food and Drug Administrative Staff, https://www.fda.gov/media/99447/download; 2020. Accessed 19 March 2020.

[32] FDA. Use of electronic health record data in clinical investigations. Guidance for Industry, https://www.fda.gov/media/97567/download; 2020. Accessed 19 March 2020.

[33] FDA. Real-world evidence, https://www.fda.gov/science-research/science-and-research-special-topics/real-world-evidence; 2020. Accessed 19 March 2020.

[34] Technology TOotNCfHI. Health IT Dash board, https://dashboard.healthit.gov/quickstats/quickstats.php; 2020. Accessed 19 March 2020.

[35] O'Connor JM, Fessele KL, Steiner J, et al. Speed of adoption of immune checkpoint inhibitors of programmed cell death 1 protein and comparison of patient ages in clinical practice vs pivotal clinical trials. JAMA Oncol 2018;4(8), e180798.

[36] Khozin S, Carson KR, Zhi J, et al. Real-world outcomes of patients with metastatic non-small cell lung cancer treated with programmed cell death protein 1 inhibitors in the year following U.S. regulatory approval. Oncologist 2019;24(5):648–656.

[37] Khozin S, Miksad RA, Adami J, et al. Real-world progression, treatment, and survival outcomes during rapid adoption of immunotherapy for advanced non-small cell lung cancer. Cancer 2019;125(22):4019–4032.

[38] Institute of Medicine (US) Forum on Drug Discovery, Development, and Translation. Transforming clinical research in the United States: challenges and opportunities: workshop summary, Washington (DC): National Academies Press (US); 2010. 2, The state of clinical research in the United States: an overview https://www.ncbi.nlm.nih.gov/books/NBK50886. Accessed 19 March 2020.

[39] Unger JM, Vaidya R, Hershman DL, Minasian LM, Fleury ME. Systematic review and meta-analysis of the magnitude of structural, clinical, and physician and patient barriers to cancer clinical trial participation. J Natl Cancer Inst 2019;111(3):245–255.

[40] Lichtman SM, Harvey RD, Damiette Smit MA, et al. Modernizing clinical trial eligibility criteria: recommendations of the American Society of Clinical Oncology-Friends of Cancer Research Organ Dysfunction, Prior or Concurrent Malignancy, and Comorbidities Working Group. J Clin Oncol 2017;35(33):3753–3759.

[41] Liu Q, Sharon E, Zineh I, et al. Organ dysfunction (dys) and clinical outcomes in patients (pts) treated with immune checkpoint inhibitors (ICIs). J Clin Oncol 2019;37(15_suppl):2569.

[42] Saxena V, Koraishy FM, Sise ME, et al. Safety and efficacy of sofosbuvir-containing regimens in hepatitis C-infected patients with impaired renal function. Liver Int 2016;36(6):807–816.

[43] Terrault NA, Zeuzem S, Di Bisceglie AM, et al. Effectiveness of ledipasvir-sofosbuvir combination in patients with hepatitis C virus infection and factors associated with sustained virologic response. Gastroenterology 2016;151(6):1131–1140.e1135.

[44] Oshikoya KA, Neely KM, Carroll RJ, et al. CYP2D6 genotype and adverse events to risperidone in children and adolescents. Pediatr Res 2019;85 (5):602–606.

[45] Bartlett CH, Mardekian J, Yu-Kite M, et al. Real-world evidence of male breast cancer (BC) patients treated with palbociclib (PAL) in combination with endocrine therapy (ET). J Clin Oncol 2019;37(15_suppl):1055.

[46] Wei WQ, Feng Q, Jiang L, et al. Characterization of statin dose response in electronic medical records. Clin Pharmacol Ther 2014;95(3):331–338.

[47] Graham DJ, Baro E, Zhang R, et al. Comparative stroke, bleeding, and mortality risks in older medicare patients treated with oral anticoagulants for nonvalvular atrial fibrillation. Am J Med 2019;132(5):596–604.e511.

[48] Vinogradova Y, Coupland C, Hill T, Hippisley-Cox J. Risks and benefits of direct oral anticoagulants versus warfarin in a real world setting: cohort study in primary care. BMJ 2018;362:k2505.

[49] Mueller P. Direct-Acting Oral Anticoagulants vs. Warfarin in "Real-World" Patients, NEJM Journal Watch Web site; 2018. https://www.jwatch.org/na47096/2018/08/23/direct-acting-oral-anticoagulants-vs-warfarin-real-world. Accessed 19 March 2020.

[50] Johnston A, Jones WS, Hernandez AF. The ADAPTABLE trial and aspirin dosing in secondary prevention for patients with coronary artery disease. Curr Cardiol Rep 2016;18(8):81.

[51] Van Driest S, Marshall M, Hachey B, et al. Pragmatic pharmacology: population pharmacokinetic analysis of fentanyl using remnant samples from children after cardiac surgery. Br J Clin Pharmacol 2016;81(6):1165–1174.

[52] Kish JK, Ward MA, Garofalo D, et al. Real-world evidence analysis of palbociclib prescribing patterns for patients with advanced/metastatic breast cancer treated in community oncology practice in the USA one year post approval. Breast Cancer Res 2018;20(1):37.

[53] MacLean E, Cisar L, Mehle K, Eremina D, Quigley JM. Real-world axitinib use in the united states: a retrospective study using linked datasets. J Manag Care Spec Pharm 2016;22(6):723–732u.

[54] White C, Kwong WJ, Armstrong H, Behling M, Niemira J, Lang K. Analysis of real-world dosing patterns for the 3 FDA-approved medications in the treatment of fibromyalgia. Am Health Drug Benefits 2018;11(6):293–301.

[55] FDA. Biomarker qualification review for total kidney volume, https://www.fda.gov/media/93143/download; 2020. Accessed 19 March 2020.

[56] Miksad RA, Abernethy AP. Harnessing the power of real-world evidence (RWE): a checklist to ensure regulatory-grade data quality. Clin Pharmacol Ther 2018;103(2):202–205.

[57] Ball R, Toh S, Nolan J, Haynes K, Forshee R, Botsis T. Evaluating automated approaches to anaphylaxis case classification using unstructured data from the FDA Sentinel System. Pharmacoepidemiol Drug Saf 2018;27(10):1077–1084.

[58] Herlands W, McFowland E, Wilson AG, Neill DB. Automated local regression discontinuity design discovery. In: Proceedings of the 24th ACM SIGKDD international conference on knowledge discovery & data mining, London, United Kingdom; 2018.

[59] Hernandez-Boussard T, Monda KL, Crespo BC, Riskin D. Real world evidence in cardiovascular medicine: ensuring data validity in electronic health record-based studies. J Am Med Inform Assoc 2019;26(11):1189–1194.

[60] Dabic S, Azarbaijani Y, Karapetyan T, et al. Development of an integrated platform using multidisciplinary real-world data to facilitate biomarker discovery for medical products. Clin Transl Sci 2020;13(1):98–109.

[61] National Academies of Sciences, Engineering, and Medicine, Health and Medicine Division; Board on Health Sciences Policy, Forum on Drug Discovery, Development, and Translation. Real-world evidence generation and evaluation of therapeutics: proceedings of a workshop, Washington (DC): National Academies Press (US); 2017. https://pubmed.ncbi.nlm.nih.gov/28211655/. Accessed 19 March 2020.
[62] Ellis CA, Gu P, Sendi MSE, Huddleston D, Sharma A, Mahmoudi B. A cloud-based framework for implementing portable machine learning pipelines for neural data analysis. Conf Proc IEEE Eng Med Biol Soc 2019;2019:4466–4469.
[63] FDA's MyStudies Application (App). https://www.fda.gov/drugs/science-and-research-drugs/fdas-mystudies-application-app; 2020. Accessed 19 March 2020.
[64] Coran P, Goldsack JC, Grandinetti CA, et al. Advancing the use of mobile technologies in clinical trials: recommendations from the clinical trials transformation initiative. Digit Biomark 2019;3(3):145–154.
[65] Izmailova ES, McLean IL, Hather G, et al. Continuous monitoring using a wearable device detects activity-induced heart rate changes after administration of amphetamine. Clin Transl Sci 2019;12(6):677–686.
[66] Clinical Trials Transformation Initiative. Project: decentralized clinical trials, https://www.ctti-clinicaltrials.org/projects/decentralized-clinical-trials; 2020. Accessed 19 March 2020.
[67] Sim I. Mobile devices and health. N Engl J Med 2019;381(10):956–968.
[68] Izmailova ES, McLean IL, Bhatia G, et al. Evaluation of wearable digital devices in a phase I clinical trial. Clin Transl Sci 2019;12(3):247–256.
[69] Bakker JP, Goldsack JC, Clarke M, et al. A systematic review of feasibility studies promoting the use of mobile technologies in clinical research. NPJ Digit Med 2019;2:47.
[70] Zhavoronkov A, Ivanenkov YA, Aliper A, et al. Deep learning enables rapid identification of potent DDR1 kinase inhibitors. Nat Biotechnol 2019;37(9):1038–1040.
[71] Snyder A, Makarov V, Merghoub T, et al. Genetic basis for clinical response to CTLA-4 blockade in melanoma. N Engl J Med 2014;371(23):2189–2199.
[72] Blank CU, Haanen JB, Ribas A, Schumacher TN. The "cancer immunogram". Science 2016;352(6286):658–660.
[73] Kroemer G, Zitvogel L. Cancer immunotherapy in 2017: the breakthrough of the microbiota. Nat Rev Immunol 2018;18(2):87–88.
[74] Morgan XC, Huttenhower C. Chapter 12: human microbiome analysis. PLoS Comput Biol 2012;8(12)e1002808.
[75] Sender R, Fuchs S, Milo R. Revised estimates for the number of human and bacteria cells in the body. PLoS Biol 2016;14(8)e1002533.
[76] Weinstein PD, Cebra JJ. The preference for switching to IgA expression by Peyer's patch germinal center B cells is likely due to the intrinsic influence of their microenvironment. J Immunol 1991;147(12):4126–4135.
[77] Deplancke B, Gaskins HR. Microbial modulation of innate defense: goblet cells and the intestinal mucus layer. Am J Clin Nutr 2001;73(6):1131S–1141S.
[78] Macpherson AJ, Hunziker L, McCoy K, Lamarre A. IgA responses in the intestinal mucosa against pathogenic and non-pathogenic microorganisms. Microbes Infect 2001;3(12):1021–1035.
[79] Smith K, McCoy KD, Macpherson AJ. Use of axenic animals in studying the adaptation of mammals to their commensal intestinal microbiota. Semin Immunol 2007;19(2):59–69.
[80] Iida N, Dzutsev A, Stewart CA, et al. Commensal bacteria control cancer response to therapy by modulating the tumor microenvironment. Science 2013;342(6161):967–970.
[81] Viaud S, Saccheri F, Mignot G, et al. The intestinal microbiota modulates the anticancer immune effects of cyclophosphamide. Science 2013;342(6161):971–976.
[82] Peled JU, Devlin SM, Staffas A, et al. Intestinal microbiota and relapse after hematopoietic-cell transplantation. J Clin Oncol 2017;35(15):1650–1659.
[83] Jenq RR, Taur Y, Devlin SM, et al. Intestinal blautia is associated with reduced death from graft-versus-host disease. Biol Blood Marrow Transplant 2015;21(8):1373–1383.
[84] Sivan A, Corrales L, Hubert N, et al. Commensal Bifidobacterium promotes antitumor immunity and facilitates anti-PD-L1 efficacy. Science 2015;350(6264):1084–1089.
[85] Vetizou M, Pitt JM, Daillere R, et al. Anticancer immunotherapy by CTLA-4 blockade relies on the gut microbiota. Science 2015;350(6264):1079–1084.
[86] Geller LT, Barzily-Rokni M, Danino T, et al. Potential role of intratumor bacteria in mediating tumor resistance to the chemotherapeutic drug gemcitabine. Science 2017;357(6356):1156–1160.
[87] Balachandran VP, Luksza M, Zhao JN, et al. Identification of unique neoantigen qualities in long-term survivors of pancreatic cancer. Nature 2017;551(7681):512–516.
[88] Routy B, Le Chatelier E, Derosa L, et al. Gut microbiome influences efficacy of PD-1-based immunotherapy against epithelial tumors. Science 2018;359(6371):91–97.
[89] Hall JA, Bouladoux N, Sun CM, et al. Commensal DNA limits regulatory T cell conversion and is a natural adjuvant of intestinal immune responses. Immunity 2008;29(4):637–649.
[90] den Besten G, van Eunen K, Groen AK, Venema K, Reijngoud DJ, Bakker BM. The role of short-chain fatty acids in the interplay between diet, gut microbiota, and host energy metabolism. J Lipid Res 2013;54(9):2325–2340.
[91] Rooks MG, Garrett WS. Gut microbiota, metabolites and host immunity. Nat Rev Immunol 2016;16(6):341–352.
[92] Iraporda C, Errea A, Romanin DE, et al. Lactate and short chain fatty acids produced by microbial fermentation downregulate proinflammatory responses in intestinal epithelial cells and myeloid cells. Immunobiology 2015;220(10):1161–1169.

[93] Arpaia N, Campbell C, Fan X, et al. Metabolites produced by commensal bacteria promote peripheral regulatory T-cell generation. Nature 2013;504 (7480):451–455.

[94] Gurav A, Sivaprakasam S, Bhutia YD, Boettger T, Singh N, Ganapathy V. Slc5a8, a Na+-coupled high-affinity transporter for short-chain fatty acids, is a conditional tumour suppressor in colon that protects against colitis and colon cancer under low-fibre dietary conditions. Biochem J 2015;469 (2):267–278.

[95] White CA, Pone EJ, Lam T, et al. Histone deacetylase inhibitors upregulate B cell microRNAs that silence AID and Blimp-1 expression for epigenetic modulation of antibody and autoantibody responses. J Immunol 2014;193(12):5933–5950.

[96] Cohen LJ, Esterhazy D, Kim SH, et al. Commensal bacteria make GPCR ligands that mimic human signalling molecules. Nature 2017;549(7670):48–53.

[97] Mariam Reyad R, Rama S, Ramy KA. The human microbiome project, personalized medicine and the birth of pharmacomicrobiomics. Curr Pharmacogenomics Person Med 2010;8(3):182–193.

[98] Gilbert JA, Quinn RA, Debelius J, et al. Microbiome-wide association studies link dynamic microbial consortia to disease. Nature 2016;535(7610):94–103.

Appendix I

Abbreviated table of Laplace transforms

TABLE I.1 Table of operations ($\mathscr{L}$).

Time domain	Laplace domain
$F(t)$	$f(s)=\int_0^\infty F(t)e^{-st}dt$
1	$^1/_s$
A	$^A/_s$
$F'(t)$	$sf(s)-F(0)$
$F''(t)$	$s^2f(s)-sF(0)-F'(0)$

TABLE I.2 Table of inverse operations ($\mathscr{L}^{-1}$).

Laplace domain	Time domain
$\frac{1}{s}$	1
$\frac{1}{s-a}$	e^{at}
$\frac{1}{(s-a)^2}$	te^{at}
$\frac{1}{s(s-a)}$	$\frac{1}{a}(e^{at}-1)$
$\frac{1}{(s-a)(s-b)}\quad a\neq b$	$\frac{1}{a-b}(e^{at}-e^{bt})$

Appendix II

Answers to study problems—Chapters 2–5

Arthur J. Atkinson, Jr.

Department of Pharmacology, Feinberg School of Medicine, Northwestern University, Chicago, IL, United States

Answers to study problems—Chapter 2

Note how dimensional analysis has been performed by including units in the calculations.

Problem 1: Answer—E

$$V_d = \frac{Dose}{C_0} = \frac{80\text{mg}}{4\text{mg/L}} = 20\text{L}$$

Problem 2: Answer—A

$$V_d = 2.0\text{L/kg} \cdot 80\text{kg} = 160\text{L}; \ \ t_{1/2} = 3\text{h}$$

Therefore

$$CL_E = \frac{\ln 2 \cdot V_d}{t_{1/2}} = \frac{\ln 2 \cdot 160\text{L}}{3\text{h}} = 37\text{L/h}$$

and the infusion rate should be

$$I = C_{ss} \cdot CL = 4\text{mg/L} \cdot 37\text{L/h} = 148\text{mg/h} = 2.5\text{mg/min}$$

Problem 3: Answer—C

The gentamicin plasma level fell to half of its previous value in the 5-h interval between blood draws. Therefore $t_{1/2} = 5\text{h}$ and $\text{k} = \ln 2/t_{1/2} = 0.139\ \text{h}^{-1}$

$$CF = \frac{1}{(1 - e^{-k\tau})}$$

Since $\tau = 8\text{h}$,

$$CF = \frac{1}{(1 - e^{-1.11})} = \frac{1}{0.67} = 1.49$$

Therefore the expected steady-state peak level is: 1.49 • 10 μg/mL = 15 μg/mL.

Problem 4: Answer—C

The target level of 12 μg/mL is one-half the toxic level of 24 μg/mL. Therefore one should wait one half-life before restarting the aminophylline infusion.

$$t_{1/2} = \frac{0.693V_d}{CL} \quad V_d = 60\text{kg} \cdot 0.45\text{L/kg} = 27\text{L}$$

$$CL = \frac{I}{C_{ss}} = \frac{(0.5\text{mg/kg} \cdot \text{h}) \cdot (60\text{kg})}{24\text{mg/L}} = 1.25\text{L/h}$$

Therefore

$$t_{1/2} = \frac{0.693 \cdot 27\text{L}}{1.25\text{L/h}} = 15\text{h}$$

Problem 5: Answer—D

Given that once-daily doses are administered, it requires 3.3 half-lives to reach 90% of the eventual steady-state level:

$$3.3 \cdot 7\text{days} = 23\text{days}$$

Problem 6: Answer—D

On admission the digoxin plasma level was 2.4 ng/mL and it fell to 1.9 ng/mL 24 h later. Hence, the daily excretion fraction is 0.5/2.4 = 0.208 (the excretion fraction with normal renal function = 1/3). Therefore levels can be expected to fall by 0.208 every 24 h as follows:

Hospital Day:	0	1	2	3	4	5	6
Digoxin Level:	2.4 ng/mL	1.9 ng/mL	1.50 ng/mL	1.19 ng/mL	0.94 ng/mL	0.74 ng/mL	0.59 ng/mL
"More Days":	–	–	1	2	3	4	5

We can see that levels can be expected to reach the 0.6 ng/mL target on the sixth day after stopping digoxin, or *five more days after the level of 1.9 ng/mL was measured.*

Problem 7: Answer—E

Three half-lives are needed for plasma levels to fall from 8 to 1 μg/mL:

Level:	8 μg/mL	→	4 μg/mL	→	2 μg/mL	→	1 μg/mL
Half-lives:	0		1		2		3

Since the elimination-phase half-life is given as 2 h, three half-lives would require 6 h. However, the question asks for a dosing interval that would allow peak levels *to exceed 8 μg/mL and fall below 1 μg/mL.* The only dosing interval offered that is longer than 6 h is 8 h. Currently, most patients would be treated with gentamicin by administering this drug in larger doses at a 24-h interval (see Chapter 3).

Problem 8: Answer—D

Since phenytoin is eliminated by Michaelis-Menten kinetics, Eq. (2.6) applies:

$$Dose/\tau = \frac{V_{\max}}{K_m + \overline{C}_{ss}} \cdot \overline{C}_{ss} \tag{II.1}$$

Rearranging:

$$(Dose/\tau)K_m + (Dose/\tau)\overline{C}_{ss} = V_{\max}\overline{C}_{ss}$$

Two simultaneous equations can be set up, one for the concentration measured at each previously administered dose.

$$300\text{mg/day} \cdot K_m + 300\text{mg/day} \cdot 5\mu g/\text{mL} = 5\mu g/\text{mL} \cdot V_{\max} \tag{II.2}$$

$$600\text{mg/day} \cdot K_m + 600\text{mg/day} \cdot 30\mu g/\text{mL} = 30\mu g/\text{mL} \cdot V_{\max} \tag{II.3}$$

These can be simplified to:

$$300\text{mg/day} \cdot K_m + 1500\text{mg}^2/\text{L} \cdot \text{day} = 5\text{mg/L} \cdot V_{\max} \tag{II.4}$$

$$600\text{mg/day} \cdot K_m + 18{,}000\text{mg}^2/\text{L} \cdot \text{day} = 30\text{mg/L} \cdot V_{\max} \tag{II.5}$$

By multiplying Eq. (II.4) by 2 and subtracting it from Eq. (II.5) we obtain:

$$15{,}000\text{mg}^2/\text{L} \cdot \text{day} = 20\text{mg/L} \cdot V_{\max}$$

Therefore

$$V_{\max} = 750\text{mg/day}$$

Substituting this value for $V_{\max}$ into Eq. (II.4) yields:

$$300\text{mg/day} \cdot K_m + 1500\text{mg}^2/\text{L} \cdot \text{day} = 5\text{mg/L} \cdot 750\text{mg/day}$$

$$300\text{mg/day} \cdot K_m = 2250\text{mg}^2/\text{L} \cdot \text{day}$$

$$K_m = 7.5\text{mg/L}$$

We can now substitute these parameters into Eq. (II.1) to estimate the dose that will provide a phenytoin level of 15 μg/mL.

$$Dose/\tau = \frac{750\text{mg/day}}{7.5\text{mg/L} + 15.0\text{mg/L}} \cdot 15\text{mg/L}$$

$$Dose/\tau = 500\,\text{mg/day}$$

Answers to study problems—Chapter 3

Problem 1

We are given that $CF_{obs} = 1.29$ and $\tau = 12\text{h}$.

Since

$$k_{eff} = \frac{1}{\tau}\ln\left[\frac{CF_{obs}}{CF_{obs} - 1}\right]$$

$$k_{eff} = \frac{1}{12}\ln\left[\frac{1.29}{0.29}\right] = 0.124$$

Therefore

$$t_{1/2eff} = \frac{\ln 2}{0.124} = 5.6\text{h}$$

Problem 2

Part a

Although a number of software packages are available to facilitate analysis of this type of data, most of them require the kineticist to provide initial estimates of the parameter values. The technique of "curve peeling" is classically used for this purpose and also provides an initial evaluation of data quality.

The first step is to graph the experimental data (●) in a semilogarithmic plot of drug concentration-vs-time as shown in Fig. II.1. Then draw a line (beta line) through the terminal exponential phase and back-extrapolate it to the y-axis. Read the y-intercept (B') and half-life of this line ($\beta_{t1/2}$) from the graph. Next, as presented in Table II.1, obtain the difference (alpha values in the table) between the experimental data points lying above the back-extrapolated line and the corresponding values on the back-extrapolated beta line (beta values in the table) at each data time point.

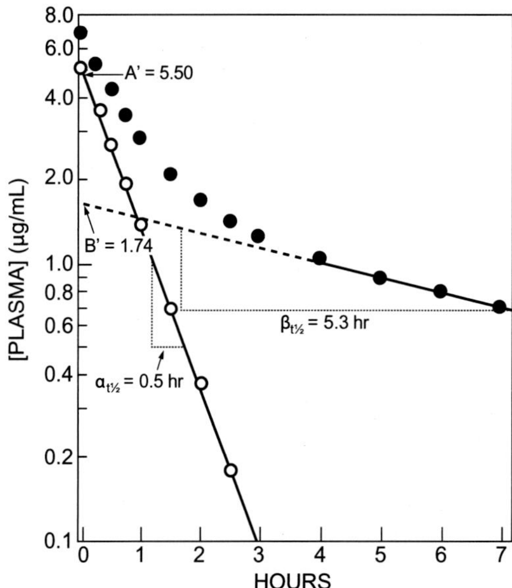

FIG. II.1 Curve peel of the data (●) that are plotted on semilogarithmic coordinates. The points for the α-curve (○) are obtained by subtracting back-extrapolated β-curve values from the experimental data, as presented in Table II.1.

TABLE II.1 Results of curve peel.

Time (h)	[Plasma] (μg/mL)	Beta value (μg/mL)	Alpha value (μg/mL)
0.10	6.3	1.7	4.6
0.25	5.4	1.7	3.7
0.50	4.3	1.6	2.7
0.75	3.5	1.6	1.9
1.0	2.9	1.5	1.4
1.5	2.1	1.43	0.67
2.0	1.7	1.34	0.36
2.5	1.4	1.25	0.15

The alpha values (○) are then plotted on the graph (Fig. II.1) and are used to draw a second line (alpha line) from which the y-intercept (A') and $\alpha_{t1/2}$ are obtained. Criteria that can be used to assess data quality at this point are: (1) the number of points that lie on each of the exponential lines, and (2) the scatter of the points about the alpha and beta lines.

The values for α and β are obtained from their half-life estimates as follows:

$$\alpha = \frac{\ln 2}{\alpha_{t1/2}} = \frac{\ln 2}{0.5\text{h}} = 1.39\text{h}^{-1}$$

$$\beta = \frac{\ln 2}{\beta_{t1/2}} = \frac{\ln 2}{5.3\text{h}} = 0.131\text{h}^{-1}$$

Please Note: Although it might seem easier to calculate α and β directly from the graph as slopes, this is complicated by the fact that most semilogarithmic graph paper uses a $\log_{10}$ scale rather than a natural log scale on the *y*-axis. The best way to circumvent this difficulty is to calculate the values of α and β from their respective half-lives.

The intercept values of $A' = 5.50\,\mu\text{g/mL}$ and $B' = 1.74\,\mu\text{g/mL}$ are normalized as follows:

$$A = \frac{A'}{A' + B'} = \frac{5.50}{5.50 + 1.74} = 0.76$$

$$B = \frac{B'}{A' + B'} = \frac{1.74}{5.50 + 1.74} = 0.24$$

As shown here, normalization is a technique for converting the sum of A and B to 1 and is required because we have stipulated that the administered dose is 1 in our derivation of the equations for calculating the model parameters.

Part b

The parameters of the two compartment model shown in Fig. II.2 can be calculated as follows.

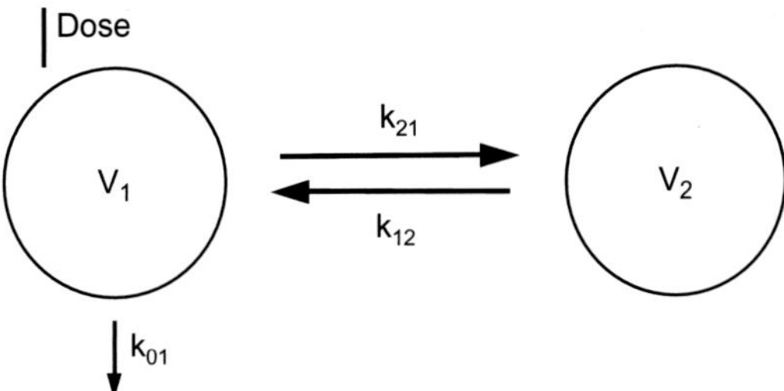

FIG. II.2 Diagram of the two-compartment model used to analyze the experimental data.

From Eq. (3.11):

$$k_{01} = \frac{1}{A/\alpha + B/\beta} = \frac{1}{\frac{0.76}{1.39} + \frac{0.24}{0.131}} = 0.42\text{h}^{-1}$$

From Eq. (3.14):

$$k_{12} = \beta A + \alpha\beta = (0.131)(0.76) + (1.39)(0.24) = 0.43\text{h}^{-1}$$

From Eq. (3.16):

$$k_{21} = \frac{AB(\alpha - \beta)^2}{k_{12}} = \frac{(0.76)(0.24)(1.39 - 0.13)^2}{0.43} = 0.67\text{h}^{-1}$$

Part c

$$V_1 = \frac{Dose}{A' + B'} = \frac{100\text{mg}}{(5.50 + 1.74)\text{mg/L}} = 13.8\text{L}$$

The elimination clearance is:

$$CL_E = k_{01} \cdot V_1 = (0.42\text{h}^{-1})(13.8\text{L}) = 5.8\text{L/h}$$

Similarly,

$$CL_I = k_{21} \cdot V_1 = (0.67\text{h}^{-1})(13.8\text{L}) = 9.25\text{L/h}$$

Part d

$$V_2 = \frac{CL_I}{k_{12}} = \frac{9.25\text{L/h}}{0.43\text{h}^{-1}} = 21.5\text{L}$$

$$V_{d(ss)} = V_1 + V_2 = 13.8\text{L} + 21.5\text{L} = 35.3\text{L}$$

Compare this value with

$$V_{d(area)} = \frac{CL_E \cdot t_{1/2\beta}}{\ln 2} = \frac{5.8\text{L/h} \cdot 5.3\text{h}}{\ln 2} = 44\text{L}$$

and

$$V_{d(extrap)} = \frac{Dose}{B'} = \frac{100\text{mg}}{1.74\text{mg/L}} = 57.5\text{L}$$

The reason that $V_{d(ss)}$ is smaller than either of these two estimates is that neither the half-life equation used to calculate $V_{d(area)}$ nor the single compartment model implied in calculating $V_{d(extrap)}$ makes any provision for the contribution of intercompartmental clearance to the prolongation of the elimination-phase half-life. Therefore these estimates must compensate for this by increasing the estimate of distribution volume, which in these approaches is the only way that half-life can be prolonged without affecting elimination clearance.

Answers to study problems—Chapter 4

Problem 1

AUC *after a single intravenous drug dose*

We have shown that after a single drug dose,

$$F \cdot D = CL \cdot AUC$$

When the dose is administered intravenously it is completely absorbed, so $F = 1$, and

$$AUC_{IV} = \frac{D_{IV}}{CL}$$

$\text{AUC}_{0\rightarrow\tau}$ *after an oral dose at steady state*

The mean steady-state concentration ($\overline{C}_{ss}$) with oral dosing is

$$\overline{C}_{ss} = \frac{F \cdot D_{oral}/\tau}{CL}$$

where the dose (D_{oral}) divided by the dosing interval (τ) is the dosing rate. As shown in Fig. II.3, the area under the plasma-level-vs-time curve during a steady-state dosing interval is equivalent to the area of a rectangle whose height equals $\overline{C}_{ss}$ and whose base equals τ. In other words,

$$AUC_{0\rightarrow\tau(oral)} = \overline{C}_{ss} \cdot \tau$$

Substituting for $\overline{C}_{ss}$,

$$AUC_{0\rightarrow\tau(oral)} = \frac{F \cdot D_{oral}/\tau}{CL} \cdot \tau = \frac{F \cdot D_{oral}}{CL}$$

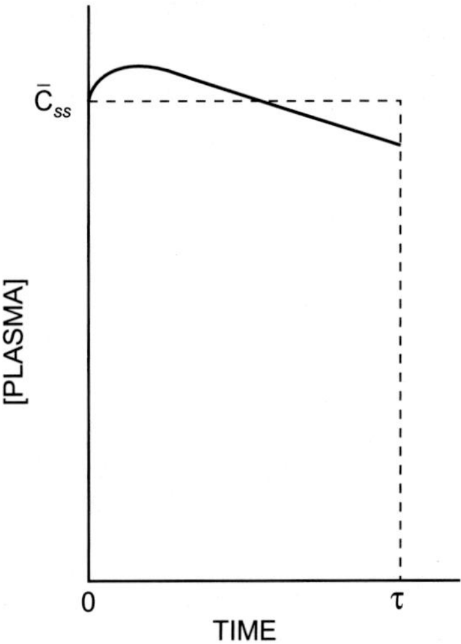

FIG. II.3 Diagram of a plasma level-vs-time curve during a dosing interval at steady state. $\overline{C}_{ss}$ is the average plasma concentration during the dosing interval τ. $AUC_{0\text{-}\tau}$ is equal to the area given by the product $\overline{C}_{ss} \cdot \tau$.

Therefore it can be seen by inspection that

$$\frac{AUC_{0\to\tau(oral)}}{D_{oral}} = F \cdot \frac{AUC_{IV}}{D_{IV}}$$

and that the extent of absorption of the oral dose formulation is

$$\%Absorption = \frac{D_{IV} \cdot AUC_{0\to\tau(oral)}}{D_{oral} \cdot AUC_{IV}} \times 100$$

Problem 2

We are asked to obtain $X(t)$ from the convolution of $G(t)$ and the disposition function $H(t)$, where the input function $G(t)$ is a constant intravenous drug infusion:

$$X(t) = G(t)*H(t)$$

Since the operation of convolution in the time domain corresponds to multiplication in the domain of the subsidiary algebraic equation given by Laplace transformation, we can write the subsidiary equation as

$$x(s) = g(s) \cdot h(s)$$

The intravenous infusion provides a constant rate of drug appearance in plasma (I), so

$$G(t) = I$$

Since $\mathscr{L}\ 1 = 1/s$,

$$g(s) = \frac{I}{s}$$

We have shown previously (see derivation of Eq. 4.3) that the Laplace transform of the disposition function is

$$h(s) = \frac{1}{s+k}$$

Therefore the subsidiary equation for the output function is

$$x(s) = \frac{I}{s} \cdot \frac{1}{s+k}$$

and $\mathscr{L}^{-1}\ x(s)$ is

$$X(t) = \frac{I}{k}\left(1 - e^{-kt}\right)$$

Problem 3

Part a

From the equation derived earlier for $X(t)$, we see that steady state is only reached when $t=\infty$. At infinite time

$$X_\infty = \frac{I}{k}$$

Since $C_{ss}=X_\infty/V_d$ and $k=CL_E/V_d$,

$$C_{ss} = \frac{I}{CL_E}$$

Note that this is Eq. (2.2) that we presented in Chapter 2. In the problem that we are given, $I=2$ mg/min, and $V_{d(area)}=1.9$ L/kg • 70 kg = 133 L.

Therefore

$$CL_E = \frac{\ln 2 \cdot V_{d(area)}}{t_{1/2}} = \frac{0.693 \cdot 133\text{L}}{90\,\text{min}} = 1.02\text{L/min}$$

and

$$C_{ss} = \frac{2\text{mg/min}}{1.02\text{L/min}} = 2.0\mu\text{g/mL}$$

Note: Many nurses who work in cardiac intensive care units know that the expected steady-state lidocaine level in µg/mL simply equals the infusion rate in mg/min (usual therapeutic range: 2–5 µg/mL). Somewhat higher levels occur in patients with congestive heart failure or severe hepatic dysfunction.

Part b

Since

$$X(t) = \frac{I}{k}\left(1 - e^{-kt}\right)$$

When $t=\infty$,

$$X_\infty = \frac{I}{k}$$

Therefore for any fraction of the eventual steady state,

$$X(t)/X_\infty = \left(1 - e^{-kt}\right)$$

When 90% of the eventual steady-state level is reached,

$$0.90 = \left(1 - e^{-kt_{0.90}}\right)$$

$$e^{-kt_{0.90}} = 0.10$$

$$kt_{0.90} = \ln 10 = 2.30$$

Since

$$k = \frac{\ln 2}{90\,\text{min}} = 0.0077\,\text{min}^{-1}$$

It follows that

$$t_{0.90} = \frac{2.30}{0.0077\,\text{min}^{-1}} = 299\,\text{min}$$

Note: Because it takes so long for an infusion to provide stable therapeutic drug concentrations, lidocaine therapy of life-threatening cardiac arrhythmias is usually begun by administering an intravenous loading dose together with an infusion.

Part c

Since $t_{1/2} = 90\,\text{min}$, this corresponds to 3.3 half-lives. *Note:* This result for a continuous intravenous infusion was previously presented in Chapter 2.

Answer to study problem—Chapter 5

Part a

$t_{1/2} = 6.2\,\text{h}$; $CL_E = 233\,\text{mL/min} = 14.0\,\text{L/h}$; % Renal excretion = 85.5%

$$CL_R = 0.855\,CL_E = 12.0\,\text{L/h}$$

$$CL_{NR} = 0.145\,CL_E = 2.03\,\text{L/h}$$

$$V_{d(area)} = \frac{CL_E \cdot t_{1/2}}{\ln 2} = \frac{(14.0\text{L/h})(6.2\text{h})}{\ln 2} = 125\text{L}$$

Therefore if CL_{NR} for *N*-acetylprocainamide (NAPA) is unchanged in functionally anephric patients, the expected elimination-phase half-life would be

$$t_{1/2} = \frac{(\ln 2)V_{d(area)}}{CL_{NR}} = \frac{(\ln 2)(125\text{L})}{2.03\text{L/h}} = 42.7\text{h}$$

Note: The mean NAPA elimination half-life actually measured in six functionally anephric patients was 41.9h (Stec GP, Atkinson AJ Jr, Nevin MJ, Thenot J-P, Ruo TI, Gibson TP, Ivanovich P, del Greco F. *N*-Acetylprocainamide pharmacokinetics in functionally anephric patients before and after perturbation by hemodialysis. Clin Pharmacol Ther 1979;26:618–28).

Part b

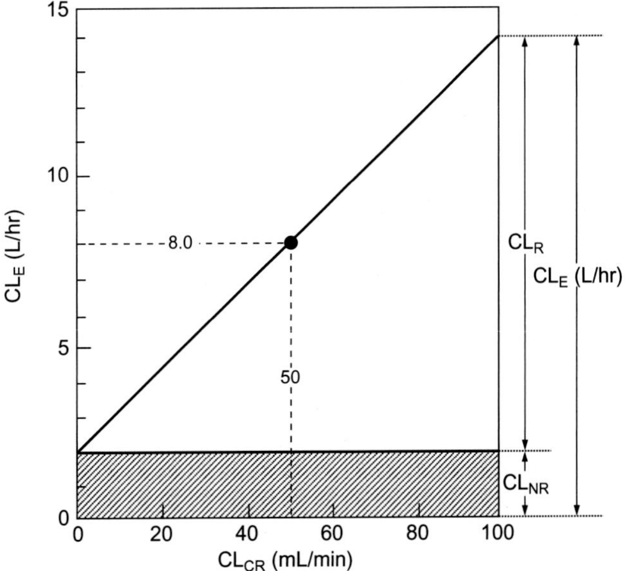

FIG. II.4 Nomogram for estimating *N*-acetylprocainamide (NAPA) elimination clearance in patients with impaired renal function. The hypothetical patient described in Part b of the problem has a creatinine clearance of 50mL/min and would be expected to have a NAPA elimination clearance of 8.0L/h.

From Fig. II.4:

When $CL_{CR} = 50\,\text{mL/min}$, expected $CL_E = 8.0\,\text{L/h}$

By direct calculation:

When $CL_{CR} = 50\,\text{mL/min}$, $CL_R = (50/100)(12\,\text{L/h}) = 6.0\,\text{L/h}$

Since $CL_{NR} = 2.0\,\text{L/h}$: $CL_E = CL_R + CL_{NR} = 8.0\,\text{L/h}$

Part c

The 8-h dosing interval is maintained.

$$\text{Adjusted dose} = (8/14)(1\,\text{g}) = 0.57\,\text{g}$$

This would reduce fluctuation between peak and trough levels but would be awkward if only 0.5 g tablets were available.

Part d

The 1-g dose is maintained and the interval is adjusted. The usual 8-h interval corresponds to: 8 h/6.2 h = 1.3 half-lives when renal function is normal.

Expected half-life when $CL_{CR} = 50\,\text{mL/min}$:

$$t_{1/2} = \frac{(\ln 2)V_{d(area)}}{CL_E} = \frac{(\ln 2)(125\text{L})}{8.0\text{L/h}} = 10.8\text{h}$$

$$\text{Adjusted dose interval} = (1.3)(10.8\,\text{h}) = 14\,\text{h}$$

In practice, a 12-h dose interval would be selected to increase patient convenience.

Index

Note: Page numbers followed by *f* indicate figures, *t* indicate tables, *b* indicate boxes, and *s* indicate schemes.

B

C

D

G

H

P

Q

S

T

X

Y

Z